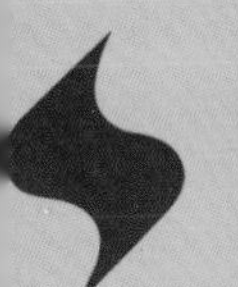

STEDMAN'S

Medical Terminology

SECOND EDITION

STEDMAN'S
Medical Terminology

SECOND EDITION

Judi L. Nath, Ph.D.

Professor

Biology & Health Sciences

Lourdes University

Sylvania, Ohio

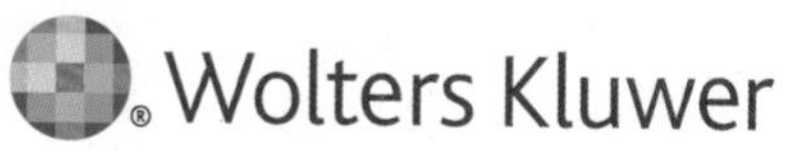

Philadelphia • Baltimore • New York • London
Buenos Aires • Hong Kong • Sydney • Tokyo

Senior Acquisitions Editor: Jonathan Joyce
Product Development Editor: Staci Wolfson
Editorial Assistant: Tish Rogers
Marketing Manager: Leah Thomson
Production Project Manager: David Orzechowski
Design Coordinator: Stephen Druding
Art Director: Jennifer Clements
Manufacturing Coordinator: Margie Orzech
Prepress Vendor: Aptara, Inc.

2nd edition

9 8 7 6 5 4 3 2 1

Printed in China

978-1-4963-1711-7
Library of Congress Cataloging-in-Publication Data
available upon request

LWW.com

■ PREFACE

Welcome to the second edition of *Stedman's Medical Terminology*! Written by a professional with decades of teaching, education, and authoring experience, this text-workbook uses effective strategies to learn medical terminology. This text and its ancillary materials introduce beginning medical terminology students to a variety of word parts and medical terms necessary to succeed in today's health care settings. It is a perfect match for a medical terminology course that seeks to provide students with a thorough understanding of medical terminology through the use of term tables and an abundance of exercises. It is also appropriate for the independent learner who wants to learn medical language through repetition and application. *Stedman's Medical Terminology* uses a hands-on "text-workbook" approach in which sections of related terms and visuals are immediately followed by a series of exercises. This method allows you to immediately recall and apply what you have learned. To gain the most from this approach, you should study the text and accompanying visuals in tandem, and then move to the term tables, and finally work through the exercises until each word part or medical term is set in your memory.

Organization of the Book

Learning medical terminology is the key to successful communication in the health care environment, and each of the book's 16 chapters are geared toward preparing you for fluency in medical language. Chapters 1 and 2 introduce medical terminology by explaining word structure and how medical terms are formed, and Chapter 3 presents common terms related to the whole body. Chapters 4 through 15 cover each body system and include moderate coverage of anatomy and physiology and the terms needed to understand the content later in the chapter. These chapters cover the material in the order you would find in a typical anatomy and physiology textbook. The book finishes with a chapter devoted to oncology and cancer terms that draws on the terminology presented in each of the preceding chapters. Appendices serve as quick references for word parts and their meanings, abbreviations, and other essential medical information.

Features

Purposeful attention has been put into incorporating the elements that will effectively help you gain a solid understanding of the language of health care. Seeking to move beyond simple rote memorization, *Stedman's Medical Terminology* steps up the text-workbook approach with the following features:

- **Logical Grouping of Terms.** Throughout the text, terms are grouped in clearly defined categorical tables to promote ease of use and understanding. These distinct categories include anatomy and physiology, word parts (combining forms, prefixes, and suffixes), adjectives and other related terms, medical conditions, laboratory tests and procedures, surgical interventions and therapeutic procedures, medications, and drug therapies, specialties and specialists, and abbreviations.

- **Meaningful Progression of Exercises.** Each chapter contains a variety of engaging and effective exercises to appeal to all learners. As you move through each new set of terms, the exercises progress in a meaningful way through five steps of learning:

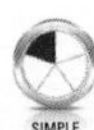

Simple Recall: promotes commitment to memory through simple term-and-definition type exercises

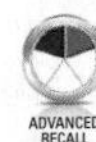

Advanced Recall: builds upon the Simple Recall exercises by presenting similar content in a different way

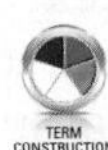

Term Construction and Deconstruction: draws on the core method of learning medical terminology and allows you to practice building and understanding terms based on the meaning of the word parts

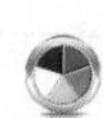

Comprehension: requires you to make connections and demonstrate a deeper understanding of the terminology in the chapter

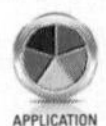

Application and Analysis: prepares you for life beyond the classroom by demonstrating how terms are used in the "real world" while also building critical thinking skills

Each chapter culminates in a Chapter Review that encompasses terms from throughout the chapter. Illustration activities, pronunciation reviews, and spelling exercises round out the available exercises.

- **Real-world Application.** Case-based exercises, case studies, and authentic medical records allow you to associate what you are learning with its application in the real world. Medical record scenarios place you in an allied health profession for a "real-life" connection.
- **Robust Art Program.** Vibrant photos, figures, and illustrations bring key concepts to life, allow you to link the art with the text, and further your understanding of difficult concepts. A stunning 16-page Stedman's Anatomy Atlas serves as a comprehensive reference for the structures of each body system.
- **Coverage of Key Content.** In response to feedback from instructors and former students, Stedman's Medical Terminology includes pharmacology terms within each of the body systems chapters. In addition, blood and immunity are covered in their own chapter (Chapter 9) to ensure comprehensive coverage of these two important topics, and an entire chapter is devoted to Oncology (Chapter 16).
- **Additional Features.** Study Tips and Extra! Extra! boxes scattered throughout the text include additional information to aid in learning and to make the subject more relevant.

Electronic Student Resources at www.thepoint.lww.com/StedmansMedTerm2e

Use of the student ancillaries is highly encouraged and can be fun! They have been carefully thought out and provide you with different ways of learning this vast amount of medical terms. The electronic student resources are referenced directly in the textbook and include a variety of exercises, games, and additional information for each chapter. Engage with:

- Electronic flash cards
- Interactive activities such as Concentration, Roboterms (Hangman), Word Anatomy, Quiz Show, Complete the Case, Medical Records Review, Look and Label, Image Matching, Spelling Bee, and more!

- Chapter quizzes and a final exam
- Animations and videos that build upon the content in the text
- Flash card anatomy that allows you to create and print your own cards
- Audio glossary/dictionary
- Descriptions of various health professions careers

Premium Online Course

Also available for adoption, the *Stedman's Medical Terminology* Premium Online Course is a complete, ready-to-go course designed to be used in conjunction with the textbook. The course is customized to the text by chapter, and features content and activities that are unique to the online course. Contact your Lippincott Williams & Wilkins Sales Representative for more information.

Instructor Resources

Visit thePoint at www.thepoint.lww.com/StedmansMedTerm2e to access resources designed specifically to help instructors teach more effectively and to save time. There you will find:

- *Instructor's test generator*, encompassing individual chapter tests and a comprehensive exam
- *PowerPoint slides* with lecture notes for each chapter
- *Lesson plans* for each chapter that are easy to follow
- *Classroom handouts* for each chapter
- *Image bank* of figures and photos from each chapter
- *Animations and videos* to enhance learning
- *Medical record library* for additional practice
- And more!

A solid understanding of medical terminology provides an essential foundation for any career in health care. The *Stedman's Medical Terminology* product suite makes learning and teaching medical terminology a rewarding and exciting process.

Steps to Success:
How to Use *Stedman's Medical Terminology*

Stedman's Medical Terminology offers an engaging and hands-on way to learn the language of health care. Using a text-workbook approach and a meaningful progression of exercises, it will provide you with the knowledge you need to communicate successfully in the health care world. Along the way, you'll encounter special features and tools that will help you navigate and understand the material presented. This section explains how to get the most out of each chapter so you can take your new language with you into your chosen health care profession!

Chapter Outline presents a concise overview of the chapter content. Read it to understand what is covered in the chapter, and then use it as roadmap to help you easily navigate the material.

Learning Outcomes list fundamental learning goals for the chapter and indicate what you should be able to do after completing the chapter. Review these before beginning the chapter to identify the learning tasks you will need to complete so that you know what to study. When you have finished the chapter exercises and the activities with the Student Resources, review the Learning Outcomes to assess your level of mastery.

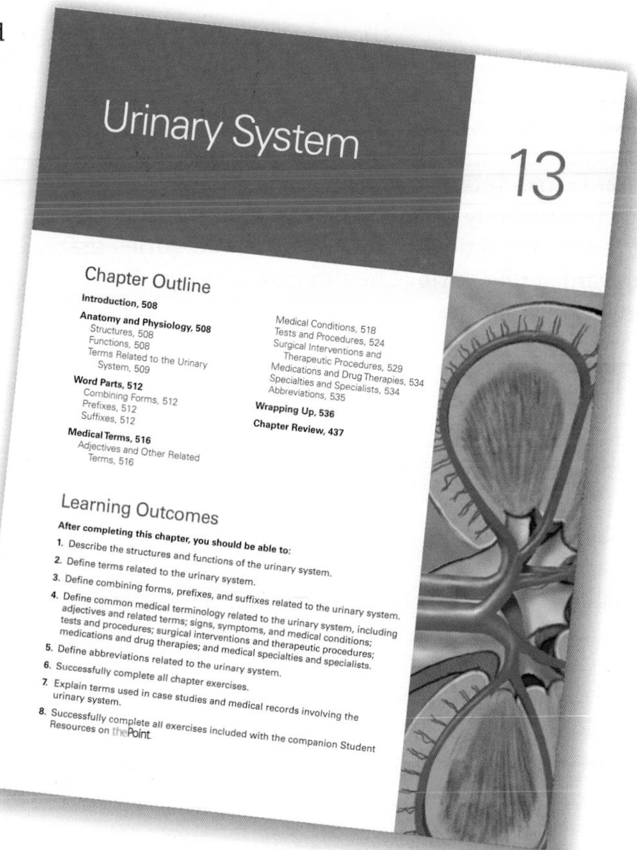

Urinary System

13

Chapter Outline

Introduction, 508

Anatomy and Physiology, 508
Structures, 508
Functions, 508
Terms Related to the Urinary System, 509

Word Parts, 512
Combining Forms, 512
Prefixes, 512
Suffixes, 512

Medical Terms, 516
Adjectives and Other Related Terms, 516
Medical Conditions, 518
Tests and Procedures, 524
Surgical Interventions and Therapeutic Procedures, 529
Medications and Drug Therapies, 534
Specialties and Specialists, 534
Abbreviations, 535

Wrapping Up, 536

Chapter Review, 437

Learning Outcomes

After completing this chapter, you should be able to:

1. Describe the structures and functions of the urinary system.
2. Define terms related to the urinary system.
3. Define combining forms, prefixes, and suffixes related to the urinary system.
4. Define common medical terminology related to the urinary system, including adjectives and related terms; signs, symptoms, and medical conditions; tests and procedures; surgical interventions and therapeutic procedures; medications and drug therapies; and medical specialties and specialists.
5. Define abbreviations related to the urinary system.
6. Successfully complete all chapter exercises.
7. Explain terms used in case studies and medical records involving the urinary system.
8. Successfully complete all exercises included with the companion Student Resources on thePoint.

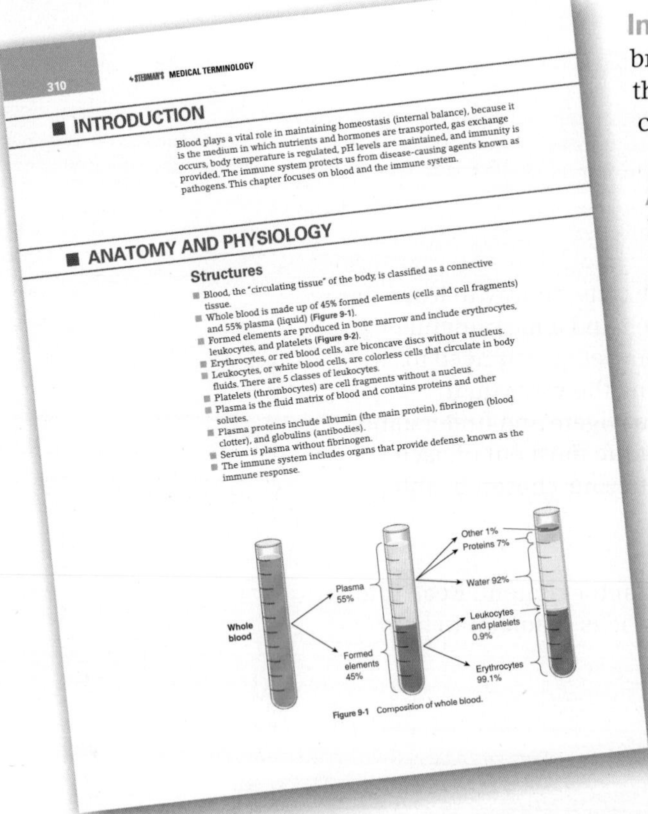

310 STEDMAN'S MEDICAL TERMINOLOGY

INTRODUCTION

Blood plays a vital role in maintaining homeostasis (internal balance), because it is the medium in which nutrients and hormones are transported, gas exchange occurs, body temperature is regulated, pH levels are maintained, and immunity is provided. The immune system protects us from disease-causing agents known as pathogens. This chapter focuses on blood and the immune system.

ANATOMY AND PHYSIOLOGY

Structures

- Blood, the "circulating tissue" of the body, is classified as a connective tissue.
- Whole blood is made up of 45% formed elements (cells and cell fragments) and 55% plasma (liquid) (Figure 9-1).
- Formed elements are produced in bone marrow and include erythrocytes, leukocytes, and platelets (Figure 9-2).
- Erythrocytes, or red blood cells, are biconcave discs without a nucleus.
- Leukocytes, or white blood cells, are colorless cells that circulate in body fluids. There are 5 classes of leukocytes.
- Platelets (thrombocytes) are cell fragments without a nucleus.
- Plasma is the fluid matrix of blood and contains proteins and other solutes.
- Plasma proteins include albumin (the main protein), fibrinogen (blood clotter), and globulins (antibodies).
- Serum is plasma without fibrinogen.
- The immune system includes organs that provide defense, known as the immune response.

Figure 9-1 Composition of whole blood.

Introduction sets the stage for the chapter and gives a brief overview of what is to come. In essence, it signals that you are about to begin the main content of the chapter.

Anatomy and Physiology, the first section of each body system chapter, provides the context for learning the chapter's medical terms. Essential facts and detailed, full-color illustrations showing the body system's key structures and functions are included. If you have not previously studied Anatomy and Physiology, use this information to familiarize yourself with the specific body system. If you have already studied Anatomy and Physiology, this section can serve as a refresher on key concepts.

Word Parts Tables list the combining forms, prefixes, and suffixes for terms related to the chapter's topic or the chapter's body system. Study the meanings of these word parts to help you build medical terms and develop your vocabulary. Use your understanding of word parts to help break down unfamiliar terms to figure out their meanings.

Medical Terms Tables present need-to-know terms for the specific body system covered. The terms are organized into practical, clearly defined categories that are relevant across various health care settings. As you review each of the tables, read the terms, practice the pronunciations, and study the meanings. Learn the synonyms listed to expand your vocabulary and understanding. Note that related terms are grouped together, so that you can more easily recognize their connection to specific body structures.

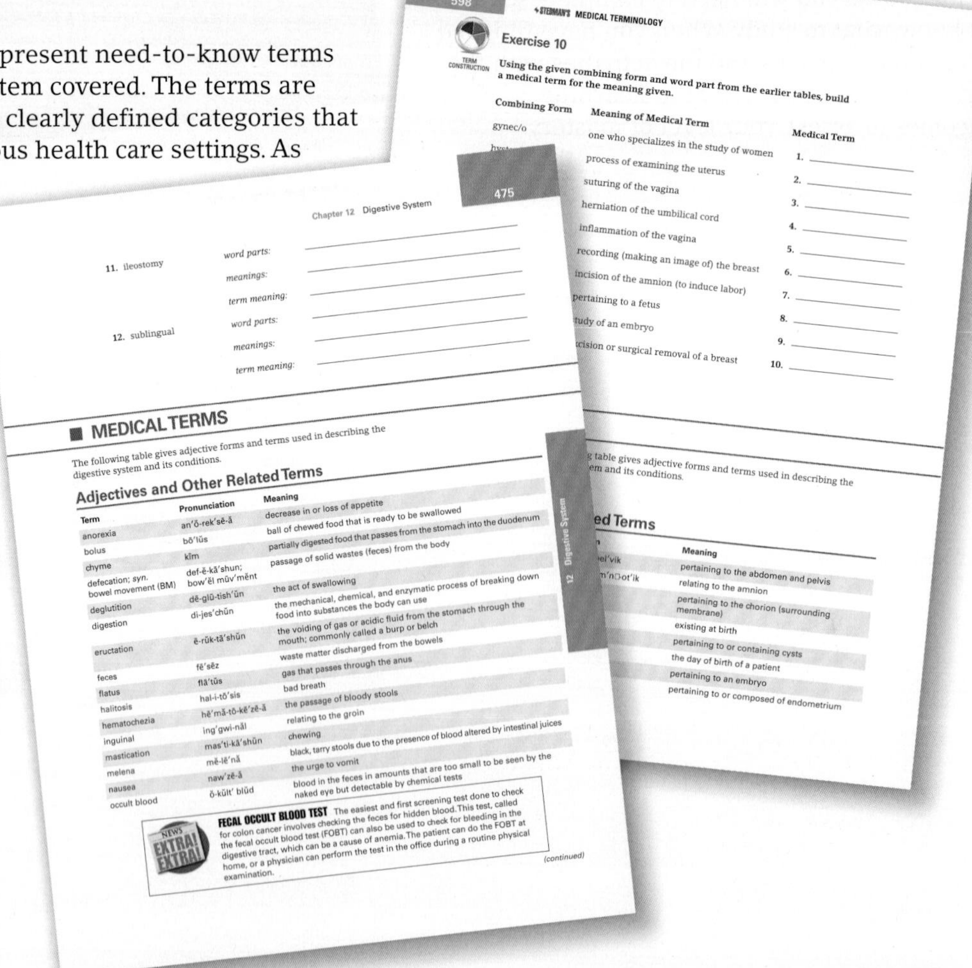

598 STEDMAN'S MEDICAL TERMINOLOGY

Exercise 10

TERM CONSTRUCTION

Using the given combining form and word part from the earlier tables, build a medical term for the meaning given.

Combining Form	Meaning of Medical Term	Medical Term
gynec/o	one who specializes in the study of women	1.
	process of examining the uterus	2.
	suturing of the vagina	3.
	herniation of the umbilical cord	4.
	inflammation of the vagina	5.
	recording (making an image of) the breast	6.
	incision of the amnion (to induce labor)	7.
	pertaining to a fetus	8.
	study of an embryo	9.
	excision or surgical removal of a breast	10.

Chapter 12 Digestive System 475

11. ileostomy	word parts:	
	meanings:	
	term meaning:	
12. sublingual	word parts:	
	meanings:	
	term meaning:	

MEDICAL TERMS

The following table gives adjective forms and terms used in describing the digestive system and its conditions.

Adjectives and Other Related Terms

Term	Pronunciation	Meaning
anorexia	an'ō-rek'sē-ă	decrease in or loss of appetite
bolus	bō'lŭs	ball of chewed food that is ready to be swallowed
chyme	kīm	partially digested food that passes from the stomach into the duodenum
defecation; syn. bowel movement (BM)	def-ĕ-kā'shun; bow'ĕl mūv'mĕnt	passage of solid wastes (feces) from the body
deglutition	dē-glū-tish'ŭn	the act of swallowing
digestion	di-jes'chŭn	the mechanical, chemical, and enzymatic process of breaking down food into substances the body can use
eructation	ē-rŭk-tā'shŭn	the voiding of gas or acidic fluid from the stomach through the mouth; commonly called a burp or belch
feces	fē'sēz	waste matter discharged from the bowels
flatus	flā'tŭs	gas that passes through the anus
halitosis	hal-i-tō'sis	bad breath
hematochezia	hē'mă-tō-kē'zē-ă	the passage of bloody stools
inguinal	ing'gwi-năl	relating to the groin
mastication	mas'ti-kā'shŭn	chewing
melena	mĕ-lē'nă	black, tarry stools due to the presence of blood altered by intestinal juices
nausea	naw'zē-ă	the urge to vomit
occult blood	ŏ-kŭlt' blŭd	blood in the feces in amounts that are too small to be seen by the naked eye but detectable by chemical tests

NEWS EXTRA! EXTRA! **FECAL OCCULT BLOOD TEST** The easiest and first screening test done to check for colon cancer involves checking the feces for hidden blood. This test, called the fecal occult blood test (FOBT) can also be used to check for bleeding in the digestive tract, which can be a cause of anemia. The patient can do the FOBT at home, or a physician can perform the test in the office during a routine physical examination.

(continued)

12 Digestive System

Medications and Drug Therapies are integrated into the chapters and reflect common pharmacologic interventions for disorders related to the chapter's topic or body system. Learning these in context will help you link medical conditions with the drugs used to treat them.

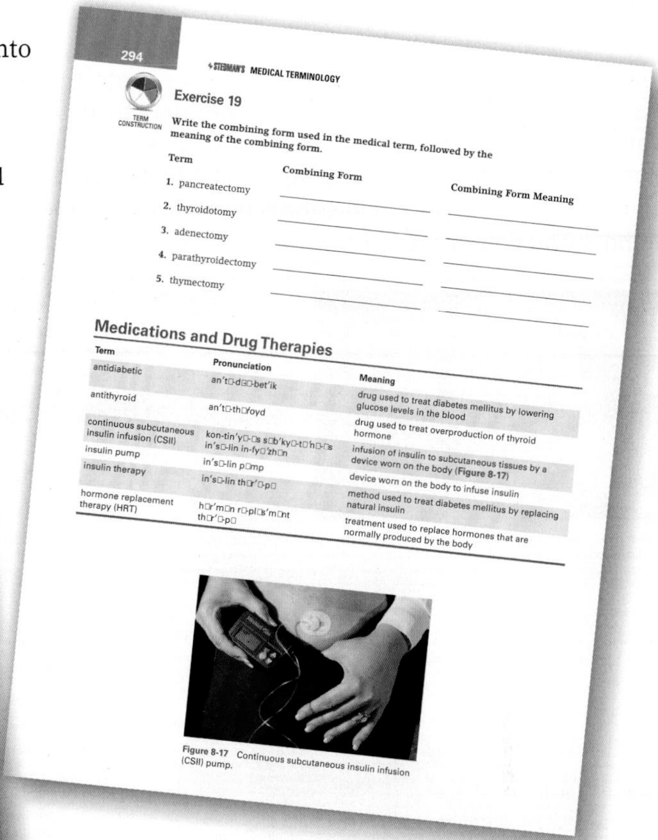

294 STEDMAN'S MEDICAL TERMINOLOGY

TERM CONSTRUCTION

Exercise 19

Write the combining form used in the medical term, followed by the meaning of the combining form.

Term	Combining Form	Combining Form Meaning
1. pancreatectomy		
2. thyroidotomy		
3. adenectomy		
4. parathyroidectomy		
5. thymectomy		

Medications and Drug Therapies

Term	Pronunciation	Meaning
antidiabetic	an'tē-dī-ă-bet'ik	drug used to treat diabetes mellitus by lowering glucose levels in the blood
antithyroid	an'tē-thī'royd	drug used to treat overproduction of thyroid hormone
continuous subcutaneous insulin infusion (CSII)	kon-tin'yū-ŭs sŭb'kyū-tā'nē-ŭs in'sŭ-lin in-fyū'zhŭn	infusion of insulin to subcutaneous tissues by a device worn on the body (Figure 8-17)
insulin pump	in'sŭ-lin pŭmp	device worn on the body to infuse insulin
insulin therapy	in'sŭ-lin thār'ă-pē	method used to treat diabetes mellitus by replacing natural insulin
hormone replacement therapy (HRT)	hōr'mōn rē-plās'mĕnt thār'ă-pē	treatment used to replace hormones that are normally produced by the body

Figure 8-17 Continuous subcutaneous insulin infusion (CSII) pump.

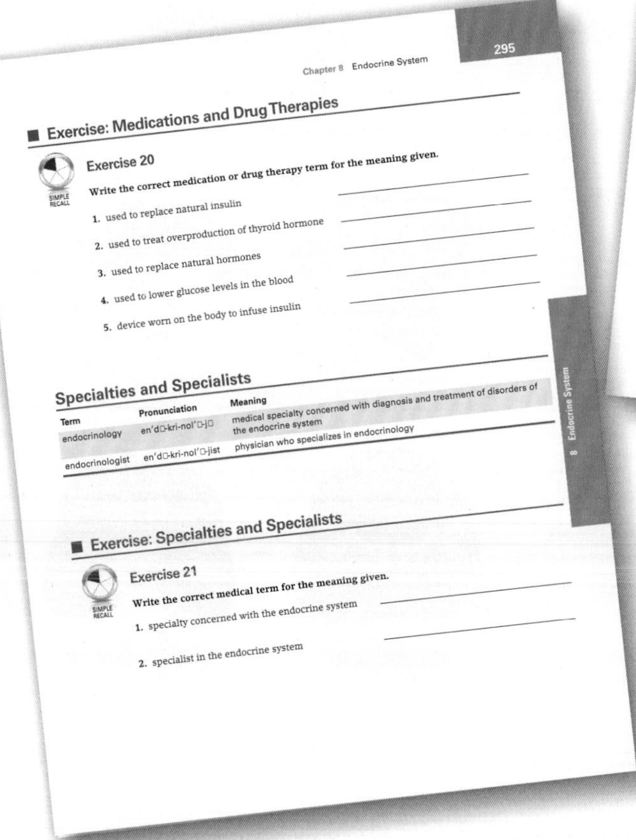

Chapter 8 Endocrine System 295

Exercise: Medications and Drug Therapies

SIMPLE RECALL

Exercise 20

Write the correct medication or drug therapy term for the meaning given.

1. used to replace natural insulin ________
2. used to treat overproduction of thyroid hormone ________
3. used to replace natural hormones ________
4. used to lower glucose levels in the blood ________
5. device worn on the body to infuse insulin ________

Specialties and Specialists

Term	Pronunciation	Meaning
endocrinology	en'dō-kri-nol'ŏ-jē	medical specialty concerned with diagnosis and treatment of disorders of the endocrine system
endocrinologist	en'dō-kri-nol'ŏ-jist	physician who specializes in endocrinology

8 Endocrine System

Exercise: Specialties and Specialists

SIMPLE RECALL

Exercise 21

Write the correct medical term for the meaning given.

1. specialty concerned with the endocrine system ________
2. specialist in the endocrine system ________

Exercises using varied formats and styles appear throughout this text-workbook after each chapter section. Questions progress from basic recall to activities involving higher-level critical thinking. Complete each exercise as it is presented, to gain practice and to steadily build your knowledge and reinforce learning. Check your understanding before continuing on to the next section.

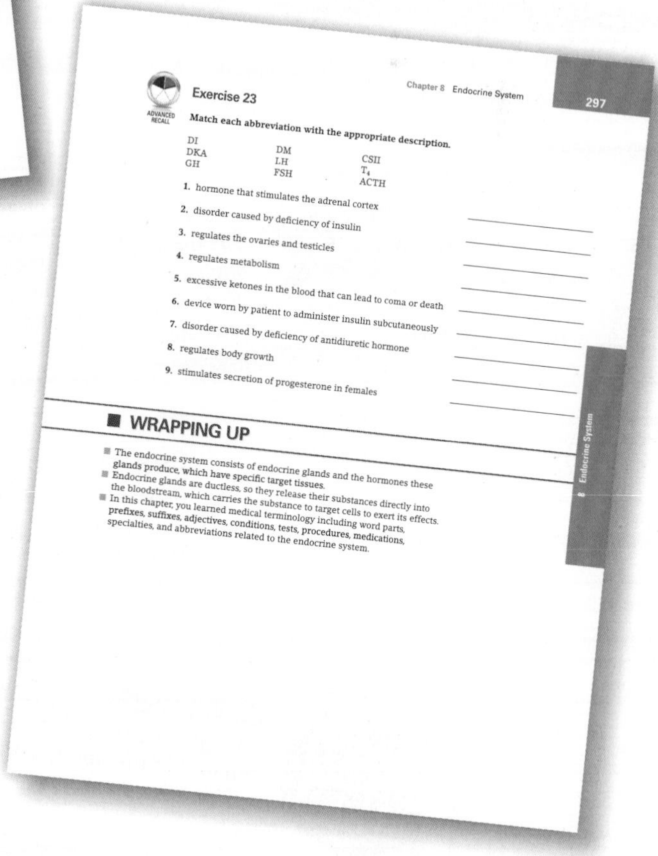

Chapter 8 Endocrine System 297

ADVANCED RECALL

Exercise 23

Match each abbreviation with the appropriate description.

DI	DM	CSII
DKA	LH	T_4
GH	FSH	ACTH

1. hormone that stimulates the adrenal cortex ________
2. disorder caused by deficiency of insulin ________
3. regulates the ovaries and testicles ________
4. regulates metabolism ________
5. excessive ketones in the blood that can lead to coma or death ________
6. device worn by patient to administer insulin subcutaneously ________
7. disorder caused by deficiency of antidiuretic hormone ________
8. regulates body growth ________
9. stimulates secretion of progesterone in females ________

WRAPPING UP

- The endocrine system consists of endocrine glands and the hormones these glands produce, which have specific target tissues.
- Endocrine glands are ductless, so they release their substances directly into the bloodstream, which carries the substance to target cells to exert its effects.
- In this chapter, you learned medical terminology including word parts, prefixes, suffixes, adjectives, conditions, tests, procedures, medications, specialties, and abbreviations related to the endocrine system.

8 Endocrine System

Wrapping Up lists some important concepts and signals that you are at the end of the chapter. It is a signpost that lets you know you have completed the chapter's content and now you should be ready for the end-of-chapter review questions and real-world exercises.

Full-Color Illustrations and Photographs offer detailed views of selected medical terms and key concepts. Images of x-rays, CT scans, MRI scans, and other diagnostic tests provide additional real-life examples. Review each of the anatomic drawings and photographs together with the related terms to make visual connections, which aid memory and comprehension.

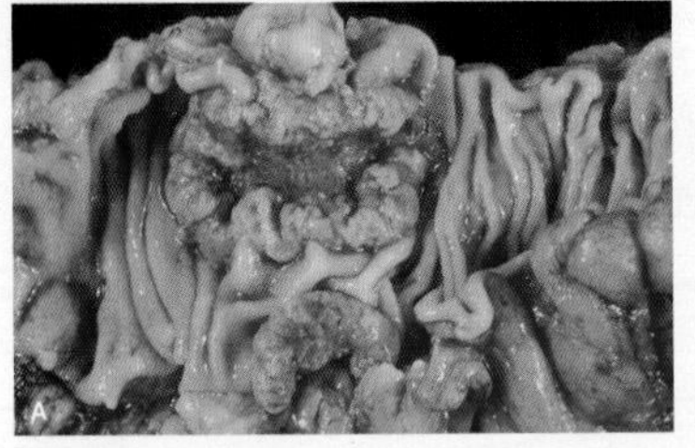

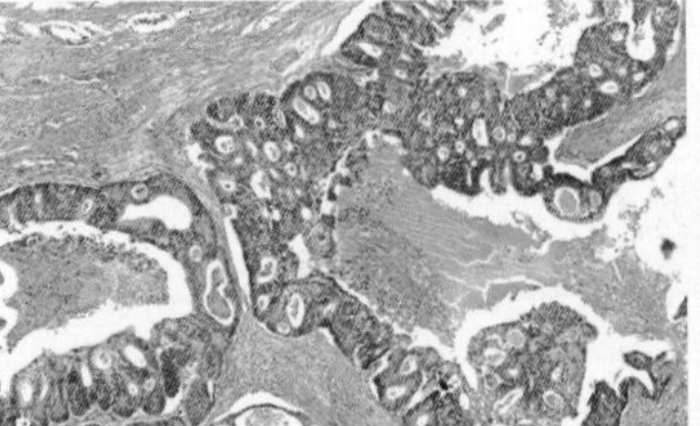

Figure 16-4 Adenocarcinoma of the colon. **A.** A resected colon shows an ulcerated mass with enlarged, firm, rolled borders. **B.** Microscopically, this adenocarcinoma consists of moderately differentiated glands.

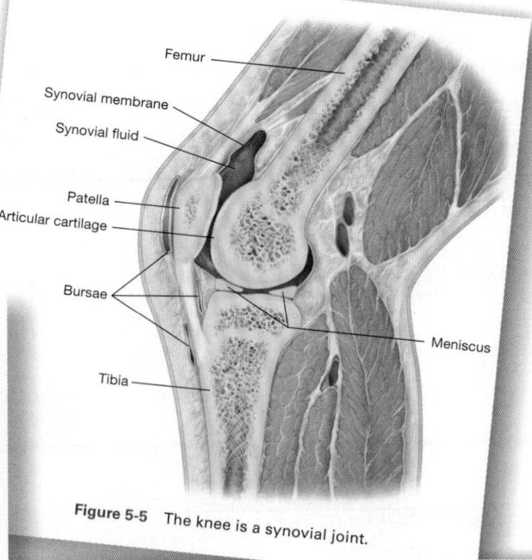

Figure 5-5 The knee is a synovial joint.

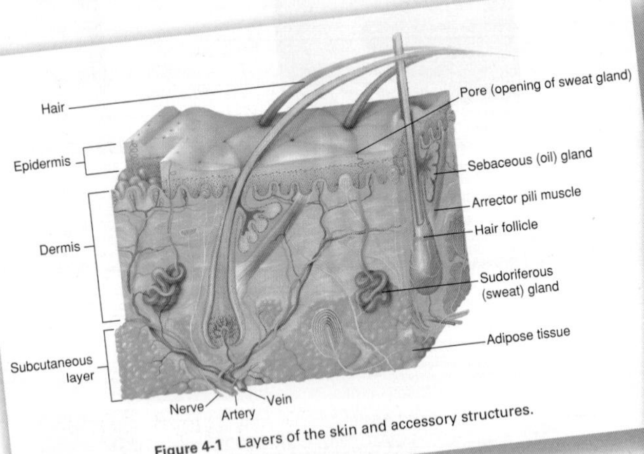

Figure 4-1 Layers of the skin and accessory structures.

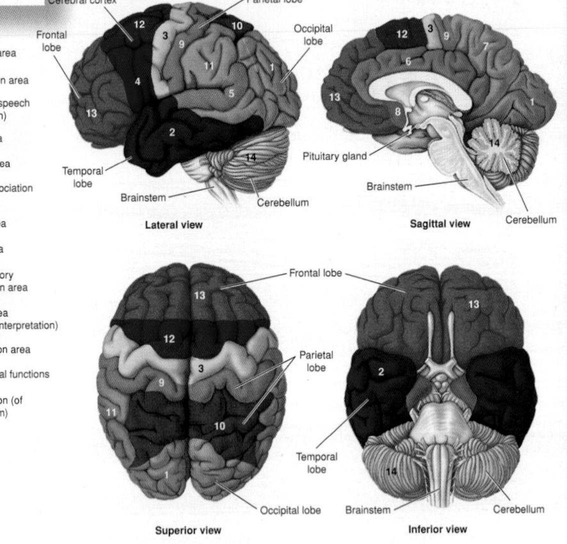

Figure 6-2 Different views of the brain identifying specific areas for various functions.

Study Tip

Adduction, abduction, supination, pronation: When distinguishing abduction from adduction, remember the common word abduct, meaning to take away. Adduction has the word "add," meaning to bring toward. To remember the difference between supination and pronation, think about your hand position when carrying a bowl of soup: in order to carry soup, the hand must be *supinated,* and the opposite of supinated is *pronated.*

Special Features include Study Tips and Extra! Extra! boxes. Use the Study Tips as memory joggers to help you learn or spell potentially confusing terms. Read the Extra! Extra! boxes to expand your knowledge of topics related to key concepts.

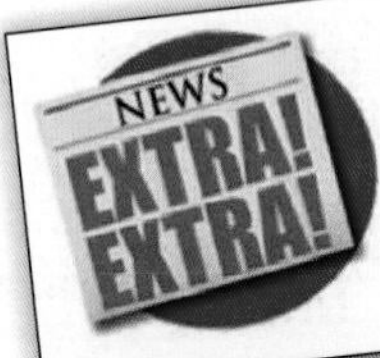

CAUDA EQUINA The name cauda equina is Latin for "horse's tail." This name was given because the spinal nerves end at various levels and branch off from the end of the spinal cord, giving the appearance of a horse's tail.

Case Reports and Medical Records present samples of clinical reports commonly encountered in health care settings. Use these real-world examples to see terms in context and help you learn and remember terminology. Read through each case report and medical record to get a general sense of the clinical situation. Do not stop to decode new terms; underline them and continue reading. Then go back and use context clues to help analyze the meaning of any unfamiliar terms. If necessary, use your medical dictionary.

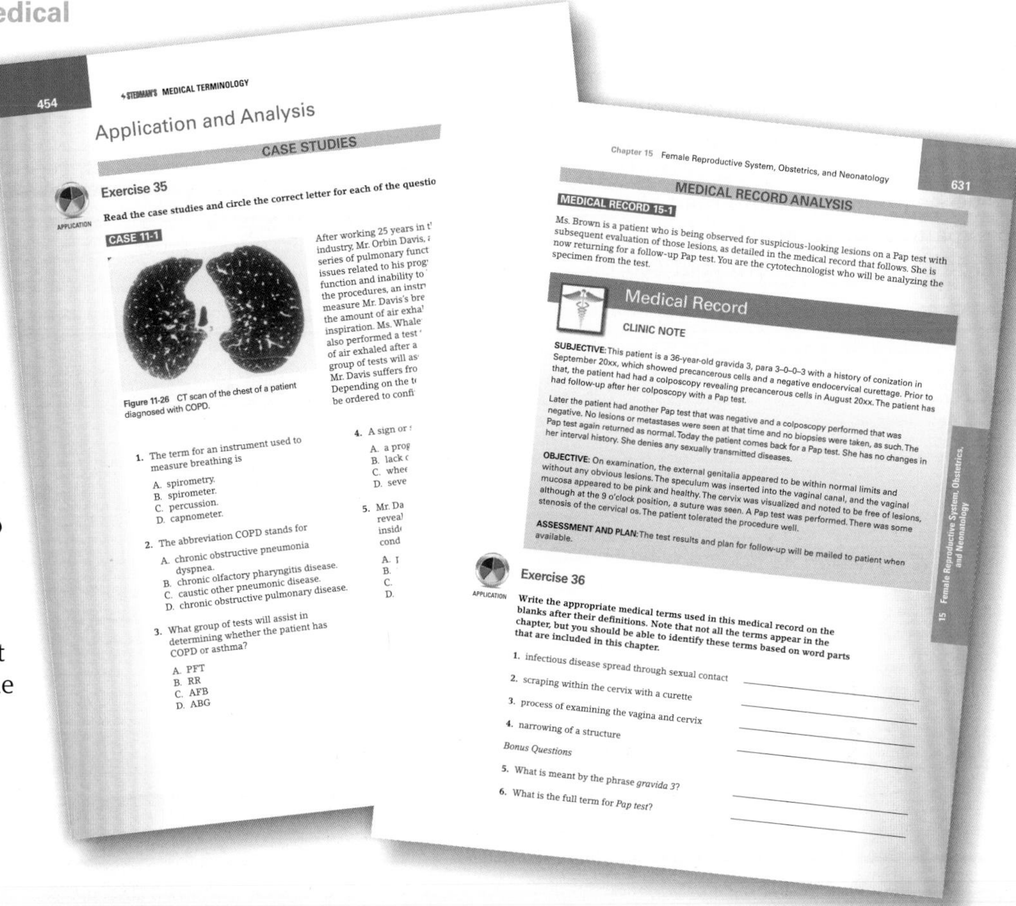

454 STEDMAN'S MEDICAL TERMINOLOGY

Application and Analysis

CASE STUDIES

Exercise 35

Read the case studies and circle the correct letter for each of the questio

CASE 11-1

Figure 11-26 CT scan of the chest of a patient diagnosed with COPD.

After working 25 years in t industry, Mr. Orbin Davis, a series of pulmonary funct issues related to his prog function and inability to the procedures, an instr measure Mr. Davis's bre the amount of air exha inspiration. Ms. Whale also performed a test of air exhaled after a group of tests will as Mr. Davis suffers fro Depending on the t be ordered to confi

1. The term for an instrument used to measure breathing is
A. spirometry.
B. spirometer.
C. percussion.
D. capnometer.

2. The abbreviation COPD stands for
A. chronic obstructive pneumonia dyspnea.
B. chronic olfactory pharyngitis disease.
C. caustic other pneumonic disease.
D. chronic obstructive pulmonary disease.

3. What group of tests will assist in determining whether the patient has COPD or asthma?
A. PFT
B. RR
C. AFB
D. ABG

4. A sign or
A. a prog
B. lack c
C. whee
D. seve

5. Mr. Da reveal insid cond
A. I
B.
C.
D.

Chapter 15 Female Reproductive System, Obstetrics, and Neonatology 631

MEDICAL RECORD ANALYSIS

MEDICAL RECORD 15-1

Ms. Brown is a patient who is being observed for suspicious-looking lesions on a Pap test with subsequent evaluation of those lesions, as detailed in the medical record that follows. She is now returning for a follow-up Pap test. You are the cytotechnologist who will be analyzing the specimen from the test.

Medical Record

CLINIC NOTE

SUBJECTIVE: This patient is a 36-year-old gravida 3, para 3-0-0-3 with a history of conization in September 20xx, which showed precancerous cells and a negative endocervical curettage. Prior to that, the patient had had a colposcopy revealing precancerous cells in August 20xx. The patient has had follow-up after her colposcopy with a Pap test.

Later the patient had another Pap test that was negative and a colposcopy performed that was negative. No lesions or metastases were seen at that time and no biopsies were taken, as such. The Pap test again returned as normal. Today the patient comes back for a Pap test. She has no changes in her interval history. She denies any sexually transmitted diseases.

OBJECTIVE: On examination, the external genitalia appeared to be within normal limits and without any obvious lesions. The speculum was inserted into the vaginal canal, and the vaginal mucosa appeared to be pink and healthy. The cervix was visualized and noted to be free of lesions, although at the 9 o'clock position, a suture was seen. A Pap test was performed. There was some stenosis of the cervical os. The patient tolerated the procedure well.

ASSESSMENT AND PLAN: The test results and plan for follow-up will be mailed to patient when available.

Exercise 36

Write the appropriate medical terms used in this medical record on the blanks after their definitions. Note that not all the terms appear in the chapter, but you should be able to identify these terms based on word parts that are included in this chapter.

1. infectious disease spread through sexual contact ____
2. scraping within the cervix with a curette ____
3. process of examining the vagina and cervix ____
4. narrowing of a structure ____

Bonus Questions

5. What is meant by the phrase *gravida 3*? ____
6. What is the full term for *Pap test*? ____

15 Female Reproductive System, Obstetrics, and Neonatology

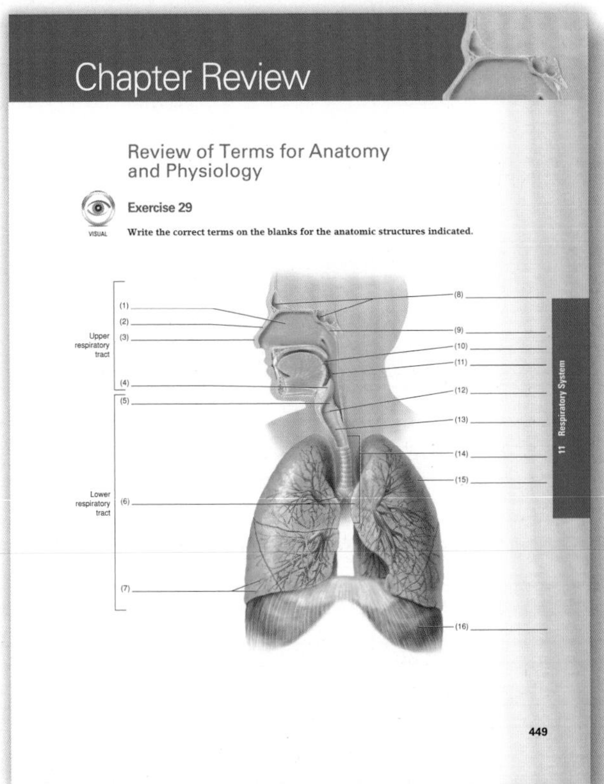

Chapter Review

Review of Terms for Anatomy and Physiology

Exercise 29

Write the correct terms on the blanks for the anatomic structures indicated.

11 Respiratory System

449

Chapter Review exercises test your knowledge of terminology presented in the chapter. Illustration exercises are also included to help you connect terms to related anatomy, while Pronunciation activities help you practice correct pronunciation. Complete all of the exercises to ensure a thorough review of the material, and then check your answers to assess your understanding.

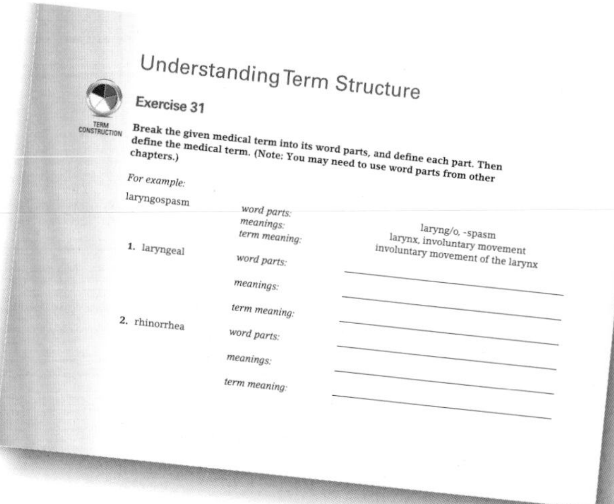

Understanding Term Structure

Exercise 31

Break the given medical term into its word parts, and define each part. Then define the medical term. (Note: You may need to use word parts from other chapters.)

For example:

laryngospasm — *word parts:* laryng/o, -spasm; *meanings:* larynx, involuntary movement; *term meaning:* involuntary movement of the larynx

1. laryngeal — *word parts:* ____ *meanings:* ____ *term meaning:* ____

2. rhinorrhea — *word parts:* ____ *meanings:* ____ *term meaning:* ____

Media Connection is located at the end of each Chapter Review section. It offers a checklist of activities you will find on the electronic Student Resources. Animations and information on relevant health professions are also available. Complete the interactive exercises for further practice and to test your learning. View the animations and read about potential careers to expand your knowledge. As a final review, take the Chapter Quiz and record your score.

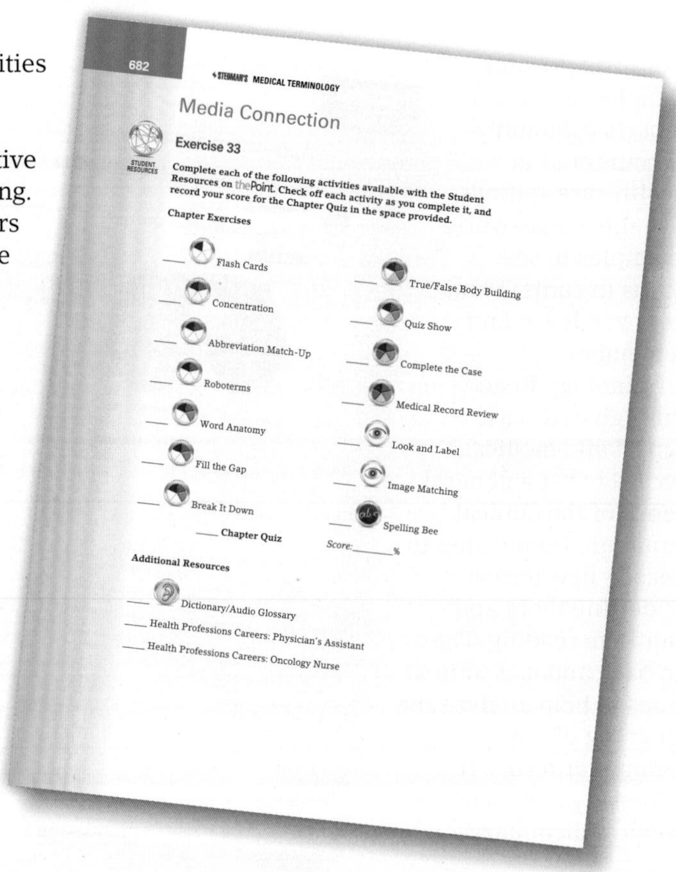

Media Connection

STUDENT RESOURCES

Exercise 33

Complete each of the following activities available with the Student Resources on thePoint. Check off each activity as you complete it, and record your score for the Chapter Quiz in the space provided.

Chapter Exercises

___ Flash Cards
___ Concentration
___ Abbreviation Match-Up
___ Roboterms
___ Word Anatomy
___ Fill the Gap
___ Break It Down
___ True/False Body Building
___ Quiz Show
___ Complete the Case
___ Medical Record Review
___ Look and Label
___ Image Matching
___ Spelling Bee

___ **Chapter Quiz** *Score:* ___%

Additional Resources

___ Dictionary/Audio Glossary
___ Health Professions Careers: Physician's Assistant
___ Health Professions Careers: Oncology Nurse

ACKNOWLEDGMENTS

Thanks to the many people who have shepherded this book from pages to publishing. Topping the list is my editor, Jonathan Joyce, who first brought this project to my attention. After our first meeting, I knew this was going to be a good venture. His support, candor, and ability to bring the second edition to fruition are greatly appreciated. A round of gratitude goes to my project manager, Staci Wolfson. Staci came on board midstream, amidst the hectic schedule; however, she stepped in, got to work, and ensured this book would meet our goals. I am always thankful for the students, instructors, and users of this textbook. Candid reviews and helpful suggestions from them shaped this second edition. Aspiring author, Kelsey Lindsley, deserves special thanks for her skills and attention to detail during paging. Completing this series of recognition is my husband, Mike, who always supports whatever I do.

REVIEWERS

Vanessa Austin, RMA, AHI(AMT), MEd
Program Director
Medical Assistant Program
National American University
Indianapolis, Indiana

Sarah Bolmarcich, PhD
Multi-Year Lecturer
School of International Letters and Cultures
Arizona State University
Tempe, Arizona

Kari Cook, MSRS
Assistant Professor
School of Allied Health
Northwestern State University
Alexandria, Louisiana

Stephanie Counts, PharmD, MEd
Associate Professor
Pharmacy Practice
Midwestern University - Glendale
Glendale, Arizona

Jamie Cuda, MS
Assistant Professor
Health & Life Sciences, Allied Health
Mohawk Valley Community College
Utica, New York

Steven Goldschmidt, DC
Instructor
Health care Management
Inver Hills Community College
Inver Grove Heights, Minnesota

Timothy Jones, MA
Adjunct Professor
Health Professions
Oklahoma City Community College
Oklahoma City, Oklahoma

Amie Mayhall, MBA, CCA
Lead Instructor
Medical Office
Olney Central College
Olney, Illinois

Pele Rich, PhD
Instructor
Biology
North Hennepin Community College
Brooklyn Park, Minnesota

Kim Rumley, BSHSA, AASMA, RMA(AMT), PN
Program Coordinator
Medical Assisting
National American University
Independence, Missouri

Gina Stephens, BSN
Assistant Dean
Business Administrative Technologies
Georgia Northwestern Technical College
Rome, Georgia

Monica Taylor, MSN
Professor
Associate Degree Nursing
San Jacinto College
Pasadena, Texas

■ CONTENTS

Preface. v
Steps to Success: How to Use Stedman's Medical Terminology ix
Acknowledgments xv
Reviewers xvii

Chapter 1	Introduction to Medical Terminology	1
Chapter 2	Prefixes, Suffixes, and Abbreviations	21
Chapter 3	Terms Related to the Whole Body	41
Chapter 4	Integumentary System	71
Chapter 5	Musculoskeletal System	109
Chapter 6	Nervous System and Mental Health	163
Chapter 7	Special Senses	209
Chapter 8	Endocrine System	271
Chapter 9	Blood and Immune System	309
Chapter 10	Cardiovascular and Lymphatic Systems	351
Chapter 11	Respiratory System	409
Chapter 12	Digestive System	461
Chapter 13	Urinary System	507
Chapter 14	Male Reproductive System	549
Chapter 15	Female Reproductive System, Obstetrics, and Neonatology	583
Chapter 16	Oncology	637
Appendix A	Glossary of Prefixes, Suffixes, and Combining Forms	683
Appendix B	Word Part Lookup by Meaning	690
Appendix C	Laboratory Tests and Values	697
Appendix D	Abbreviations	701
Appendix E	Complementary and Alternative Medicine Terms	706
Appendix F	Rules for Forming Plurals	709
Appendix G	Health-Related Websites	710
Appendix H	Key English-to-Spanish Health Care Phrases	719
Appendix I	Metric Measurements	725

Answers to Exercises 727
Figure Credits 763
Stedman's Anatomy Atlas 767
Index 783

Introduction to Medical Terminology

1

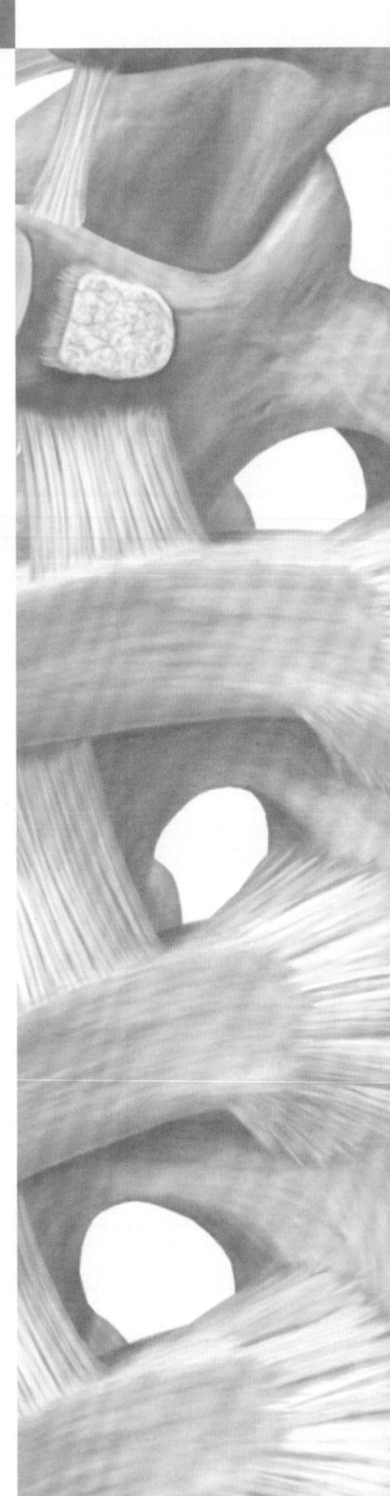

Chapter Outline

Introduction, 2

Derivation of Medical Terms, 3

Understanding Terms through Their Parts, 3

Word Roots, 3

Prefixes, 5

Suffixes, 6

Combining Vowels Added to Roots, 8

Putting the Parts Together, 9

Plural Endings, 10

Rules for Making Plural Medical Terms, 10

Pronunciation Key, 12

Understanding Terms through Analysis, 14

Building Terms, 16

Wrapping Up, 16

Chapter Review, 17

Learning Outcomes

After completing this chapter, you should be able to:

1. Explain why it is important to understand medical terms.
2. Define each of the three basic word parts.
3. Explain how word parts are put together to make a medical term, and give examples.
4. Understand medical terms by analyzing their parts.
5. Understand how to add combining vowels and plural endings to medical terms.
6. Use the pronunciation key to learn how to pronounce medical terms.
7. Successfully complete all chapter exercises.
8. Successfully complete all exercises included with the companion Student Resources on thePoint.

INTRODUCTION

Every profession has a range of special terms used by practitioners in that field. As someone who may work in a health-related area, you will need to read, write, speak, and understand medical terms as they are used daily in medical fields. Understanding medical terms is also a gateway to learning about the human body. When learning medical terms, you are learning much more than just *words*—you are learning fundamental concepts about the body in health and disease.

Why use medical terms? Why not just use everyday language? For example, why not say *stomach ache* instead of *gastritis*? As you will soon see, medical terms are much more precise than everyday words. What you refer to as a stomach ache *might* be the pain caused by gastritis (stomach inflammation), but this general term could also refer to the symptoms of other conditions, such as a peptic ulcer (sore on the stomach lining), ulcerative colitis (inflammation of the colon with open sores), or peritonitis (inflammation of the peritoneum, the tissue that covers the abdominal organs). These medical terms mean very different things to health care professionals. There usually is no simple, word-for-word "plain English" translation of any medical term that conveys its full medical meaning. You have to learn the correct terms to fully understand medical conditions.

The good news, however, is that medical terminology is not nearly as difficult to learn as it may seem at first **(Figure 1-1)**. For example, did you notice that three of the medical terms for conditions causing stomach pain all end in *-itis*? Once you know that the word part *-itis* means *inflammation,* you are well on your way to understanding the meaning of those three terms. In fact, many common medical terms end in *-itis,* so learning that one word ending allows you to understand dozens of terms. Although you do need to memorize many word parts to understand medical terminology, after you learn how terms are built from common parts, your understanding will grow quickly. The focus of this text is to help you learn new terms and expand your vocabulary.

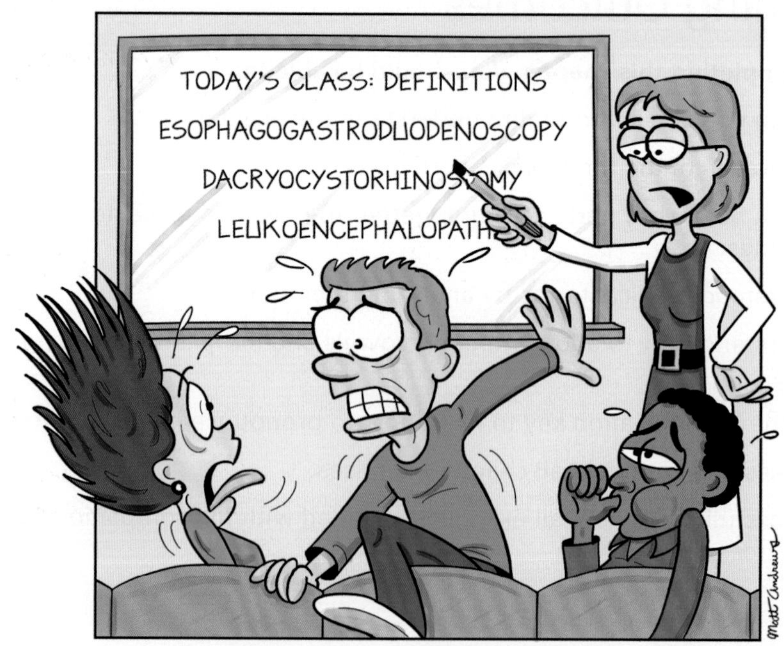

"WHO CAN DEFINE THE TERM 'ESOPHAGOGASTRODUODENOSCOPY?'"

Figure 1-1

DERIVATION OF MEDICAL TERMS

It's easier to learn medical terms when you understand where the basic word parts come from and how medical terms are derived. The earliest medical practitioners generally wrote, spoke, and read Greek and Latin, because these were the languages of science and education for more than 2000 years. Although few people in health care today study Greek or Latin, medical language is still based on these languages.

Most medical terms are built from word parts. In most cases, you will not learn the original Greek or Latin word but will instead learn a *word root*. This is the basic part of a term and is derived from a Greek or Latin word. For example, the word root *gastr* comes from the Greek word for belly or stomach, *gaster*. A few medical terms built from this word root are gastritis, gastrointestinal, gastroenteritis, gastroesophageal, and gastrostomy **(Figure 1-2)**. As you learn additional roots and word parts, you will find it easy to understand many medical terms.

Some medical terms are not built from word parts but instead have their origins in modern languages. This happens when new technology or treatments are developed. Other terms derive from the name of the person who first identified a condition or developed a procedure. These terms are called **eponyms.** An example of an eponym is *Kaposi sarcoma,* a skin cancer named for Hungarian dermatologist Moritz Kaposi, who originally described the condition in 1872.

UNDERSTANDING TERMS THROUGH THEIR PARTS

As you have already learned, most medical terms are built by combining different word parts. Basic word parts include roots, prefixes, and suffixes. These word parts are discussed in detail in this chapter. When you put these parts together to build a medical term, the term's meaning will come from the meanings of its parts. The first medical practitioner to study and write about stomach inflammation, for example, may have been the first to coin the term *gastritis*. *Gastr-* refers to the stomach, and *-itis* refers to inflammation, so gastritis means inflammation of the stomach.

You can understand the meanings of terms by breaking them down into their parts. Suppose that you have never seen the term *gastrotomy* before. You already know that *gastr* refers to the stomach. If you also know that *-tomy* refers to an incision into something, you can easily figure out that a *gastrotomy* must be an incision made into the stomach.

After you know that *crani* refers to the skull (cranium), can you figure out what a craniotomy is? If you said a craniotomy is an incision into the skull, you are correct.

Word Roots

A **word root** is the core, or main part, of the medical term. Most medical terms have a word root. Think of a word root as the word stem without a prefix or suffix.

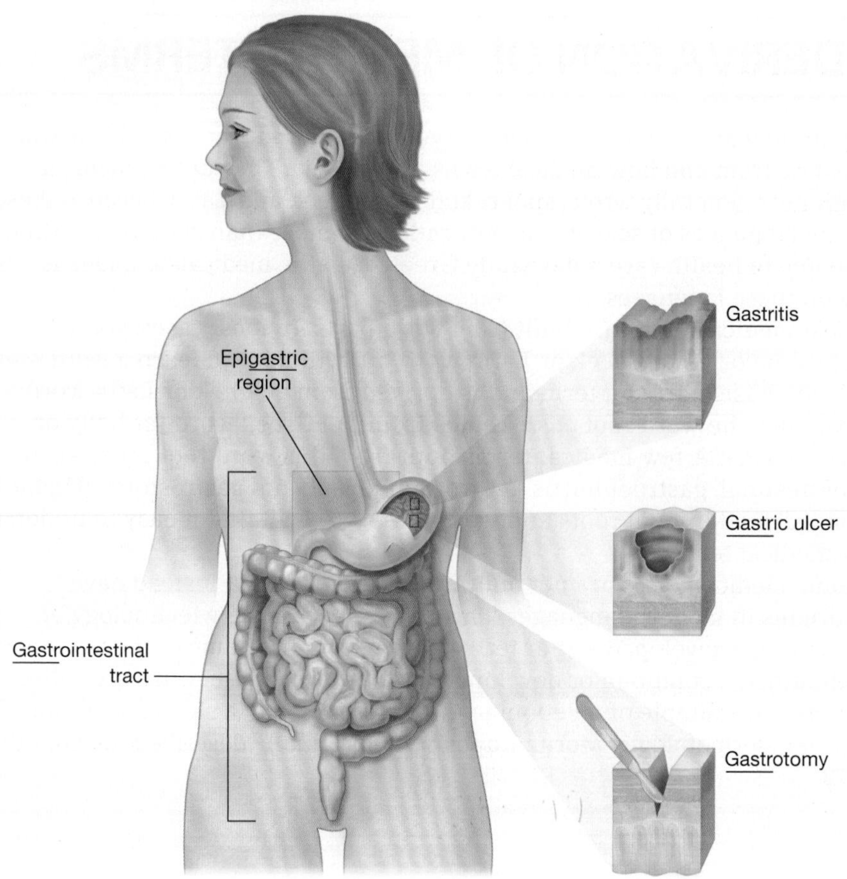

Figure 1-2 From one word root comes many different medical terms.

In many cases, you will have to memorize the meanings of word roots. You already know many common word roots, because some everyday words also are derived from them. Keep in mind that sometimes there are two or more word roots with the same meaning. Once you know what the root word means, you'll be able to understand many other words that contain the root word **(Figure 1-2)**. Memorize the meanings of the following common word roots, and then complete the exercises that follow.

Word Root	Meaning
cardi	heart
cerebr	brain, cerebrum
colo, colon	colon (section of large intestine)
crani	cranium, skull
dermat	skin
gastr	stomach
nephr	kidney
neuron	nerve
ost	bone
pulmon	lung
ren	kidney
vas	vessel

Exercises: Word Roots

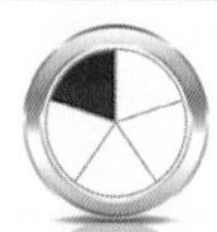

Exercise 1

Write the meaning of the word root given.

1. ost bone
2. cardi heart
3. cerebr brain
4. pulmon lung
5. dermat skin

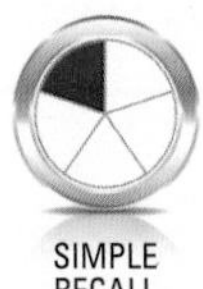

Exercise 2

Write the correct word root for the meaning given.

1. skull crani
2. heart cardi
3. stomach gastr
4. colon colo /colon
5. kidney ren

Prefixes

A **prefix** is the word part that comes *before the word root.* Many medical terms are built with prefixes. Prefixes usually add to the meaning of a term by adjusting or qualifying the meaning of the root word.

In this text, hyphens are used to signify prefixes, suffixes, and combining forms to indicate the placement of the word part when used to form a medical term. For example, a hyphen placed after the word part, as in *hypo-,* means the part is a prefix. If *hypo-* means below and *gastric* refers to the belly, what does *hypogastric* mean? Hypogastric means below the belly.

Here is another example. The prefix *post-* means after. *Post-* is the opposite of *pre-*. Thus, the term *postsurgical* refers to something that happens after surgery. For example, postsurgical medications are given after an operation.

Memorize the meanings of the following common prefixes, and then complete the exercises that follow.

Prefix	Meaning
a-, an-	without, not
dys-	painful, difficult, abnormal
inter-	between, among
intra-	inside, within
peri-	around, surrounding
poly-	many, much
post-	after, behind
pre-	before
sub-, infra-	below, beneath
supra-, super-	above

Exercises: Prefixes

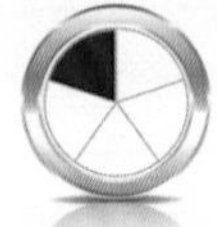

SIMPLE RECALL

Exercise 3

Write the meaning of the prefix given.

1. dys- painful/difficult/abnormal
2. intra- inside/within
3. peri- around
4. post- after
5. poly- many

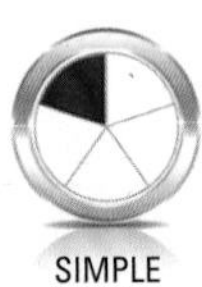

SIMPLE RECALL

Exercise 4

Write the correct prefix for the meaning given.

1. before pre
2. between, among inter
3. without, not a/an
4. above supra
5. below, beneath sub/infra

Suffixes

Like prefixes, **suffixes** are attached to a word root, but they come after the root. A hyphen placed before the word part, as in *-ac,* means the part is a suffix. For example, the suffix *-ac* means "pertaining to." Therefore, *cardiac* simply means "pertaining to the heart." The suffix *-al* also means "pertaining to," so what do you think *cranial* means? Cranial means pertaining to the skull.

Many medical terms are built with suffixes. Suffixes contribute to the meaning of a term by simply adding the meaning of the suffix to the meaning of the word root (and to the meaning of the prefix when one is present).

Memorize the meanings of the following common prefixes, and then complete the exercises that follow.

Suffix	Meaning
-ac, -al, -ary, -ic, -ous	pertaining to
-algia	pain
-ectomy	excision, surgical removal
-gram	record, recording
-ism, -ia	condition of
-itis	inflammation
-ium	pertaining to body region, structure
-logy	study of
-oma	tumor
-tomy	incision

Exercise: Suffixes

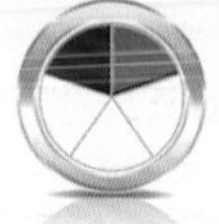

ADVANCED RECALL

Exercise 5

Match each suffix with its meaning.

-tomy	-ism	-oma	-ectomy	-al
-ium	-gram	-algia	-itis	-logy

1. incision -tomy
2. pertaining to body region, structure -ium
3. record, recording -gram
4. pertaining to -ac, -al, -ary, -ic, -ous
5. study of -logy
6. pain -algia
7. inflammation -itis
8. surgical removal -ectomy
9. condition of -ism + -ia
10. tumor -oma

Combining Vowels Added to Roots

Combining vowels are used between word parts. Unlike word roots, prefixes, and suffixes, combining vowels do not have meanings on their own. A **combining vowel** is a vowel (usually o, and sometimes i or e) that is added to the word root to make the term easier to pronounce. Combining vowels are used when attaching a suffix that begins with a consonant to a word root that ends in a consonant. For example, if you add the suffix *-logy* (study of) directly to the word root *dermat* (skin), you would get "dermatlogy"—something that would sound very odd if you tried to say it. For ease of pronunciation, a combining "o" is added to form the word "dermatology." Compare the pronunciation of *dermatlogy* with *dermatology.*

A **combining form** describes the word root with its associated combining vowel. It is often easier to learn combining forms (word root + combining vowel), so this text uses combining forms rather than word roots. For example, instead of learning just the word root *cardi,* you will learn the combining form *cardi/o.* The slash is used to indicate that use of the combining vowel varies depending on the other word part following the word root. Note the difference in the following terms:

peri- + cardi/o + ium = pericardium (tissue around the heart)—the "o" is not used

cardi/o + -logy = cardiology (study of the heart)—the "o" is used

If you tried to put in the combining vowel when it is not needed, you would see the problem when you tried to pronounce the word. For example, using the combining vowel in the term *pericardioum* results in having too many vowels! Similarly, if you left out the combining vowel when it is needed, you would hear the problem when you tried to pronounce the resulting term. For example, spelling *cardilogy* without the combining vowel results in too few vowels!

You may have noticed something about the formation of the term *pericardium* in the first example above. The combining form in this word is *cardi/o,* and the suffix is *-ium.* If you were to simply join the two, you would have two "i"s in the middle, since the word root ends with "i" and the suffix begins with "i." The result would be "pericardiium"—but how would that be pronounced? In cases like this, the rules of language favor common sense for ease of pronunciation. The rule in this case is simple: If a word root (without the optional vowel) ends with the same vowel with which the suffix begins, then the second instance of the vowel is dropped to prevent repetition.

Fortunately, there are only a few rules to learn about how terms are spelled when word parts are put together. We will look at those rules in the next section.

Memorize the spellings of the following common combining forms. Remember that the slash before the combining vowel is used to indicate that the vowel may be used when the combining form is joined to a following word part.

Combining Form	Meaning
cardi/o	heart
cerebr/o	brain, cerebrum
col/o, colon/o	colon (section of large intestine)
crani/o	cranium, skull
dermat/o	skin
gastr/o	stomach
nephr/o, ren/o	kidney
neur/o	nerve, nerve tissue
oste/o	bone
pulmon/o	lung

Exercise: Combining Forms

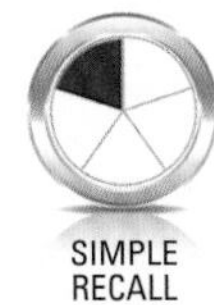

Exercise 6

Write the correct combining form for the meaning given.

1. nerve, nerve tissue neur/o
2. stomach gastr/o
3. kidney nephr/o, ren/o
4. heart cardi/o
5. cranium, skull crani/o
6. bone oste/o
7. lung pulmon/o
8. brain, cerebrum cerebr/o
9. skin dermat/o
10. colon colon/o

Putting the Parts Together

Medical terms are made up of combining forms together with prefixes and/or suffixes. The rules for when to include the combining vowel in forming a term are usually simple:

1. Use the combining vowel when a combining form is joined to a suffix that does not begin with a vowel:

   nephr/o (kidney) + -logy (study of) = nephrology (study of the kidneys)

2. Do not use the combining vowel when a combining form is joined to a suffix that begins with a vowel:

   arthr/o (joint) + -itis (inflammation) = arthritis (no *o*) (joint inflammation)

3. If the suffix begins with the *same* vowel with which the combining form ends, do not repeat the vowel:

   cardi/o + -itis = carditis (heart inflammation)

4. Use the combining vowel when two combining forms are joined together:

   my/o (muscle) + cardi/o (heart) + -al = myocardial (pertaining to the heart muscle)

   Note that this rule holds true usually even if the second combining form already begins with a vowel:

   oste/o (bone) + arthr/o (joint) + -itis = osteoarthritis (inflammation of bone and joint)

There are a few other special cases where the rules may vary slightly, but these are individual exceptions you will learn later on. Because these rules are generally based on how terms are spelled for ease of pronunciation, get in the habit of saying terms aloud as you see them in this text. Very soon, you will naturally know whether or not to use the combining vowel based on how a term sounds.

Exercise: Putting the Parts Together

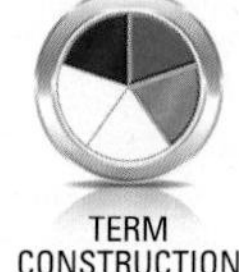
TERM CONSTRUCTION

Exercise 7

With the word parts given, write the medical term that matches the given meaning. Be mindful of the spelling of the term.

1. intra- + crani/o + -al = intracranial (pertaining to within the skull)
2. sub- + pulmon/o + -ary = subpulmonary (pertaining to below the lungs)
3. cardi/o + -gram = cardiogram (record of heart activity)
4. oste/o + -algia = ostealgia (pain in a bone)
5. gastr/o + -tomy = gastrotomy (incision into the stomach)

PLURAL ENDINGS

Most nouns in the English language become plural by adding an -s or -es at the end; for example, the plural of *student* is *students*. Some medical terms also add an -s or -es to make a plural, but many do not. They have special endings related to their origins in Greek or Latin. For example, if the singular noun ends in *a* (as in vertebra, referring to one bone in the spine), then the plural ends in *ae* (as in vertebrae, referring to multiple bones in the spine).

The following table shows some of the special plural endings common in medical terms. Note that these special plurals do not occur with *all* terms ending in those letters. For example, the plural of sinus is sinuses. In most cases, you have to learn the plural form when you learn the term.

Rules for Making Plural Medical Terms

Singular Ending	Rule	Plural Ending	Example
a	keep -a and add -e	ae	vertebra (a spinal bone)→vertebrae
en	drop -en and add -ina	ina	foramen (hole)→foramina
ex	drop -ex and add -ices	ices	pollex (thumb)→polices
ion	drop -ion and add -ia	ia	ganglion (group of nerve cell bodies)→ganglia
is	drop -is and add -es	es	ankylosis (stiff joint)→ankyloses testis (male reproductive gland)→testes
on	drop -on and add -a	a	phenomenon (occurrence or object perceived)→phenomena spermatozoon (male sex cell)→spermatozoa
ix	drop -ix and add -ices	ices	appendix→appendices
ium	drop -ium and add -ia	ia	epithelium (tissue type)→epithelia
um	drop -um and add -a	a	diverticulum (pouch within an organ)→diverticula atrium (upper heart chamber)→atria
us	drop -us and add -i	i	nucleus (structure within a cell)→nuclei embolus (blood clot)→emboli
x	drop -x and add -ges	ges	phalanx (finger bone)→phalanges
y	drop -y and add -ies	ies	biopsy (tissue sample)→biopsies

Exercise: Plural Endings

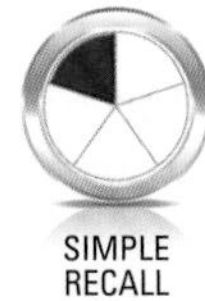

SIMPLE RECALL

Exercise 8

Write the correct plural form of the singular term given.

1. glomerulus (capillary cluster in nephron of kidney) glomerul __________
2. varicosis (swollen vein) __________
3. ovum (egg cell) ov __________
4. larynx (voice box) laryn __________
5. ulcer __________

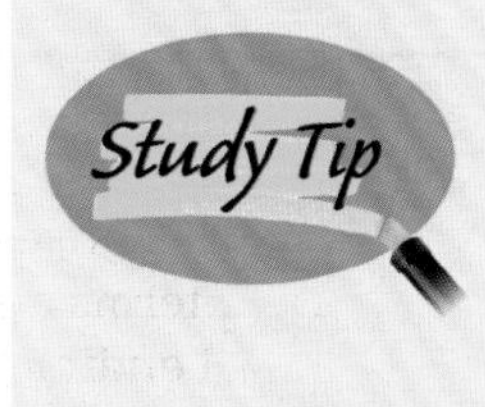

Spelling: Spelling medical terms correctly in health care is vital **(Figure 1-3)**. For example, misspelling a term in a patient's record could cause confusion or even a dangerous situation if another health care worker misunderstands what you have written. Many terms look nearly alike and may even be pronounced the same. For example, *ileum* (part of the small intestine) and *ilium* (hip bone) look similar and sound alike, but these terms designate two very different parts of the body. Therefore, take the time to learn correct spellings. Complete the spelling exercises in these chapters, being sure to write out the terms in all exercises.

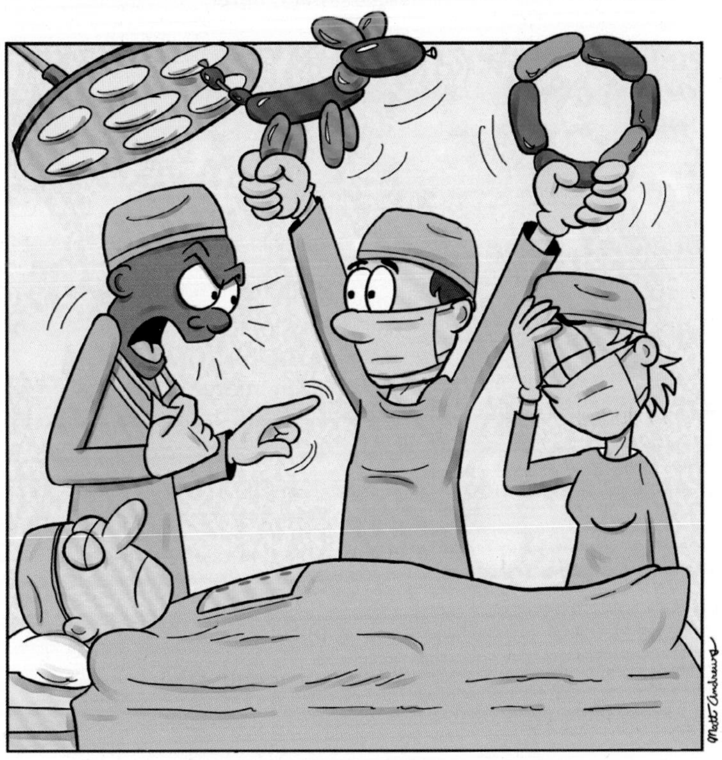

"JENKINS, YOU FOOL! I SAID 'BALLOON STENT,' NOT 'BALLOON STUNT!'"

Figure 1-3

PRONUNCIATION KEY

Pronunciations are given for medical terms throughout this text. It is best to learn the pronunciation at the same time you learn the term. Saying each term aloud will help you remember its meaning and spelling.

The pronunciation is indicated with letters of the alphabet and stress marks (′) that indicate which syllable (or syllables) should be accented. Following is a typical example of how stress marks are used to help with pronunciation:

nucleus   nū′klē-ŭs

If you are not familiar with stress marks, think of them as the guide to which syllable to say more forcefully when you pronounce the word. Nucleus is pronounced like this: NU-cle-us. It is not pronounced like this: nu-cle-US.

Here is the key to the different vowel sounds used in pronunciations.

Symbol	Sound as in:
ā	day
a	mat, far
ă	about
ah	father
aw	raw, fall
ē	beet, here
e	bed
ĕ	system
ī	island
i	hip
ĭ	pencil
ō	go, form
o	got
ŏ	oven, motor
ow	cow
oy	boy, oil
ū	prune
yū	cube
u	put
ŭ	up, tough

Here is a key to the sounds of consonants used in pronunciations.

Symbol	Sound as in:
b	bad, tab
ch	child, itch
d	dog, good
f	fit, defect, phase
g	got, bag
h	hit, behold
j	jade, gender, rigid, edge
k	cut, tic
ks	extra, tax
kw	quick, aqua
l	law, kill
m	me, bum
n	no, run
ng	ring
p	pain, top
r	rot, tar
s	so, mess, center
sh	show, wish
t	ten, put
th	thin, with
v	vote, nerve
w	we, tow
y	yes
z	zero, disease, xiphoid
zh	vision, measure

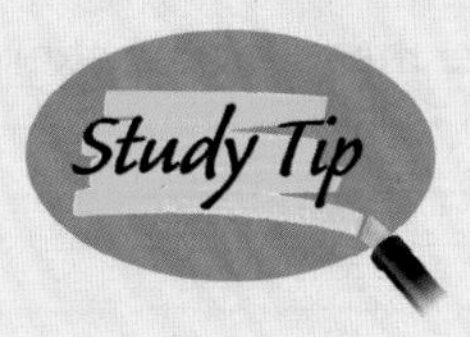

Read, Write, Speak, Listen: Scientists have discovered that using your senses (sight, hearing, touch) reinforces learning and assists in memory. Do not just passively read the terms on the page as you use this text. Practice saying them aloud, listen to their correct pronunciations using the Audio Glossary in the Student Resources on thePoint, and write them (or their meanings) in the spaces provided in the exercises.

The following exercise gives some practice in using the pronunciation key to learn how to pronounce unfamiliar words.

Exercise: Pronunciation

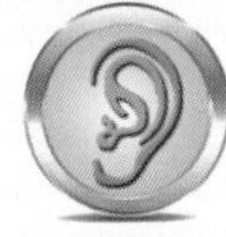
AUDITORY

Exercise 9

Listen to the pronunciations of the following terms using the Dictionary/ Audio Glossary included with the Student Resources on thePoint. Practice pronouncing each term, referring to the pronunciation guide as needed.

1. varicosis	var′i-kō′sis
2. diverticulum	dī′vĕr-tik′yū-lŭm
3. ankylosis	ang′ki-lō′sis
4. pulmonary	pul′mŏ-nār-ē
5. arthralgia	ahr-thral′jē-ă
6. osteoma	os-tē-ō′mă
7. nephritis	nĕ-frī′tis
8. craniopathy	krā′nē-op′ă-thē
9. gastrectomy	gas-trek′tŏ-mē
10. cardiopulmonary	kahr′dē-ō-pul′mŏ-nār-ē

UNDERSTANDING TERMS THROUGH ANALYSIS

Remember that the meaning of a medical term comes from the meaning of the different word parts that together make that term. There is little value in trying to memorize each and every medical term separately. It is much easier to learn the meanings of the parts and then apply those meanings to the many terms that use the same parts.

Analyzing word parts to understand the larger meaning is also useful when you encounter a medical term for the first time and do not have a dictionary or your textbook available. Quite often, you can figure out the meaning of a new term if you know the meaning of its separate word parts.

For example, you already know that the suffix *-itis* means inflammation. Earlier you saw the word *diverticulum,* which is a pouch or sac within an organ—such as diverticula that may occur within the large intestine. Its combining form is *diverticul/o*. From this information, can you make an educated guess what *diverticulitis* means?

Diverticulitis is the inflammation of a diverticulum.

To define a term based on its word parts, complete the following steps in order:

1. Analyze the meaning of the suffix.
2. Analyze the meaning of the prefix.
3. Analyze the meaning of the root or roots.

For example:

intra- (within) + *cerebr/o* (brain) + *-al* (pertaining to)

2 3 1

means pertaining to within the brain

The following exercise will give you more practice understanding terms by analyzing their word parts. As you learn more word parts through studying the chapters of this text, you will find that this becomes a natural process.

■ Exercise: Term Analysis

Exercise 10

TERM CONSTRUCTION

For example:

nephrectomy	*word parts:*	nephr/o, -ectomy
	meanings:	kidney; excision, surgical removal
	term meaning:	surgical removal of kidney
1. arthritis	*word parts:*	arthr/o , -itis
	meanings:	
	term meaning:	
2. pulmonary	*word parts:*	pulmon/o , -ary
	meanings:	
	term meaning:	
3. colonitis	*word parts:*	colon/o , -itis
	meanings:	
	term meaning:	
4. osteal	*word parts:*	oste/o , -al
	meanings:	
	term meaning:	
5. cardiotomy	*word parts:*	cardi/o , -tumy
	meanings:	
	term meaning:	

BUILDING TERMS

You can learn terms by breaking them apart and analyzing the meanings of their parts. It also helps to learn how to put word parts together—to build terms. In the real world, these medical terms almost always already exist, but building them on your own will help you learn more efficiently.

For example, you learned earlier that *cardi/o* is the combining form that means heart. Let's say you wanted to build a medical term that means inflammation of the heart. From what you have learned already, you should be able to build this term and write it here:

____

The answer, of course, is *carditis.* (Did you remember not to repeat the "i"?) If you look in your medical dictionary, you will find that it is a real medical term. You shouldn't be surprised to learn that it means inflammation of the heart.

The following exercise will give you more practice building terms.

Exercise: Building Terms

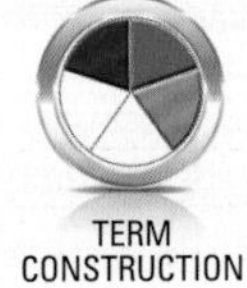

TERM CONSTRUCTION

Exercise 11

Using word parts found anywhere in this chapter, construct medical terms for the meanings given. Then, check your medical dictionary to see whether you are correct and have spelled the term correctly.

1. inflammation of the skin ____________________
2. pertaining to the area around the heart ____________________
3. study of nerves ____________________
4. tumor of bone ____________________
5. pertaining to the kidney ____________________

WRAPPING UP

- Medical terms include the following basic parts:

  Word root: main part of the word (*crani*)
  Prefix: word part added *before* the root (*intra-*)
  Suffix: word part added *after* the root (*-al*)

  intra- + crani + -al = intracranial

- A combining form is a word root with a combining vowel that makes it easier to pronounce the word when a suffix is added to the word root:

  cardi/o (combining form) + -logy (suffix) = cardiology

- To understand a medical term, first analyze its parts. You can usually figure out what the term means from the meanings of its parts.
- To build medical terms, use your knowledge of the definitions of word roots, prefixes, and suffixes to combine these parts into a word.

Chapter Review

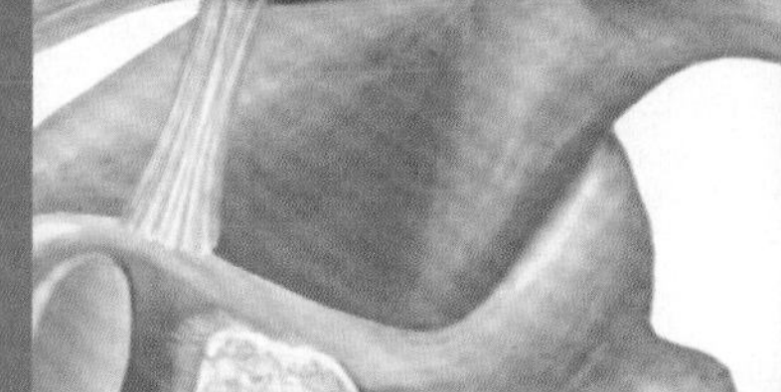

Review of Terms

In the following exercises, you will encounter a few medical terms you have not seen in this chapter. Nonetheless, you should be able to answer these questions based on the word parts used in these terms. Review the earlier tables of word part meanings if needed.

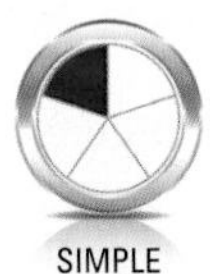

SIMPLE RECALL

Exercise 12

Complete each sentence by writing in the correct word.

1. The cerebral cortex is a part of the brain. A subcortical tumor would therefore be located below the cortex.
2. A tumor that grows from bone tissue is called a(n) osteoma.
3. Given that the suffix *-scopy* means visual examination using an instrument, the term for such an examination of the colon is colonoscopy.
4. A dermatologist is a specialist physician who treats skin disorders.
5. A gastric ulcer seems most likely to cause bleeding inside the stomach.
6. An intervertebral disk is located between two vertebrae (bones of spine).
7. The term *cardiac* means pertaining to the heart.
8. A physician specializing in cardiopulmonary diseases might often require x-rays of a patient's heart and lungs.
9. The prefix *an-* means without/not.
10. A tumor in lymph tissue (combining form: *lymph/o*) is called a(n) lymphoma.

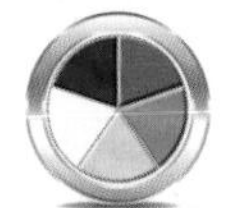

COMPREHENSION

Exercise 13

Circle the letter of the best answer in the following questions.

1. Which term refers to surgical removal of the stomach?
   A. gastrotomy
   B. gastrostomy
   C. gastrology
   D. gastrectomy

2. Given that the combining form *my/o* means muscle, which of the following refers to muscle pain?
   A. myogram
   B. myalgia
   C. myocardium
   D. myoma

3. The term *renal* means
   A. pertaining to the kidney.
   B. pertaining to the skull.
   C. pertaining to the lung.
   D. pertaining to the skin.

4. A patient who is having difficulty breathing may have what kind of problem?
   A. cerebral
   B. gastric
   C. cardiac
   D. pulmonary

5. Referring to surgery, an intraoperative procedure is carried out
   A. before the surgery begins.
   B. during the surgery.
   C. after the surgery.
   D. at any time.

6. Which of the following best defines the term *abacterial*?
   A. full of bacteria
   B. not pertaining to bacteria
   C. eaten by bacteria
   D. resulting from bacterial presence

7. The medical term *dysuria* is most likely to mean
   A. painful urination.
   B. frequent urination.
   C. infrequent urination.
   D. normal urination.

8. The medical term *polyuria* is most likely to mean
   A. painful urination.
   B. frequent urination.
   C. infrequent urination.
   D. normal urination.

9. A patient with a cerebral hemorrhage is experiencing bleeding inside the
   A. kidney.
   B. lungs.
   C. brain.
   D. heart.

10. Even if you have never seen the term *angiogram* (an x-ray record of blood vessels), you can assume the combining form used to make this term is
   A. ang/i.
   B. angi/o.
   C. angiogr/a.
   D. angiogra/o.

Spelling

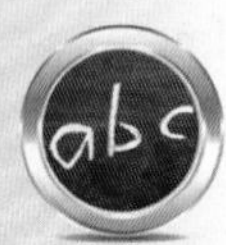

SPELLING

Exercise 14

Circle the correctly spelled term.

1.	cardioitis	cardiitis	carditis
2.	phenomena	phenomenons	phenomeni
3.	pericardial	perocardial	pericardiol
4.	gastroctomy	gastrectomy	gastroectomy
5.	nucleuses	nuclae	nuclei
6.	ostearthritis	osteoarthritis	ostarthriti
7.	cardigraphy	cardography	cardiography
8.	vertebrae	vertebraes	vertebriae
9.	dermatitis	dermatoitis	dermatotis
10.	cardipulmonary	cardiopulmonary	cardopulmonary

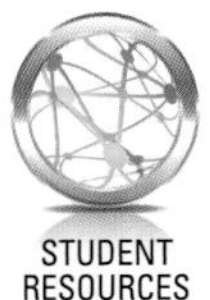
STUDENT RESOURCES

Additional spelling exercises for this and all chapters in the text are included as Spelling Bee activities in the Student Resources on thePoint.

Media Connection

Exercise 15

Complete each of the following activities available with the Student Resources. Check off each activity as you complete it, and record your score for the Chapter Quiz in the space provided.

Chapter Exercises

____ Flash Cards

____ Concentration

____ Roboterms

____ Word Anatomy

____ True/False Body Building

____ Quiz Show

____ Complete the Case

____ Spelling Bee

____ **Chapter Quiz** *Score:* ________%

Additional Resources

____ Dictionary/Audio Glossary

Prefixes, Suffixes, and Abbreviations

2

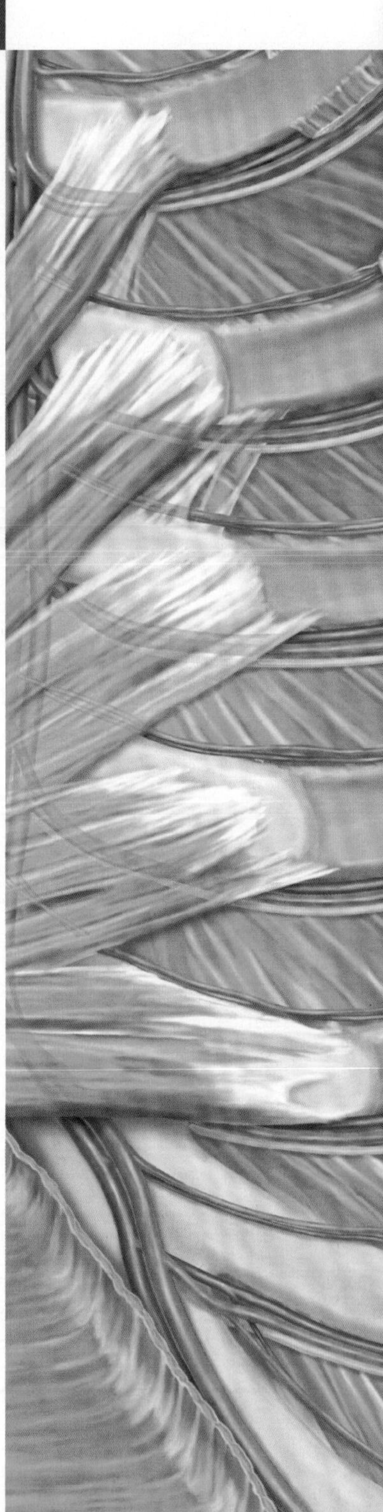

Chapter Outline

Introduction, 22

Common Prefixes, 22
- Prefixes Involving Number, 22
- Prefixes Involving Negation, 23
- Prefixes Involving Position, Time, or Direction, 24
- Prefixes Involving Relative Characteristics, 25
- Other Prefixes, 27

Common Suffixes, 27
- Suffixes Related to Conditions or Diseases, 27
- Suffixes Related to Surgery, 28
- Other Suffixes, 29

Common Abbreviations, 31

Wrapping Up, 34

Chapter Review, 35

Learning Outcomes

After completing this chapter, you should be able to:

1. Define common prefixes used in medical terms.
2. Define common suffixes used in medical terms.
3. Understand medical terms by analyzing their prefixes and suffixes.
4. Correctly spell and pronounce medical terms built with common prefixes and suffixes.
5. Understand common abbreviations used in health care.
6. Successfully complete all chapter exercises.
7. Successfully complete all exercises included with the companion Student Resources on thePoint.

INTRODUCTION

As you learned in Chapter 1, prefixes and suffixes are basic word parts used in many medical terms **(Figure 2-1)**. This chapter includes the most common prefixes and suffixes. Learning these now will pave the way for learning medical terms related to the body systems in later chapters.

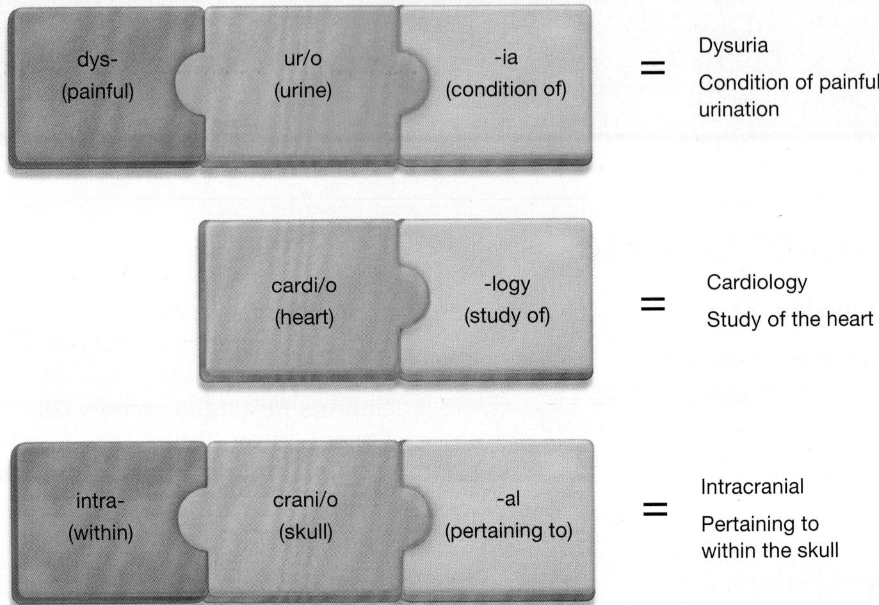

Figure 2-1 Word parts fit together like jigsaw puzzle pieces to form medical terms.

COMMON PREFIXES

A prefix modifies the meaning of the word root or combining form to which it is joined. Prefixes can be learned in groups based on number or based on similar or opposite meanings, as seen in the following tables.

Prefixes Involving Number

Prefix	Meaning	Example
uni-	one	unilateral (relating to one side of the body)
mono-	one	mononeural (supplied by one nerve)
bi-	two	bilateral (relating to two sides)
di-	two	diarthric (relating to two joints)
tri-	three	trimester (three months; one-third the length of pregnancy)
quad-, quadri-	four	quadruplets (four infants born together)
hemi-	half	hemiplegia (paralysis of one side of the body)
semi-	half, partly	semirecumbent (position of half sitting up in bed)
multi-	many	multicellular (composed of many cells)
poly-	many, much	polyarteritis (inflammation of several arteries)

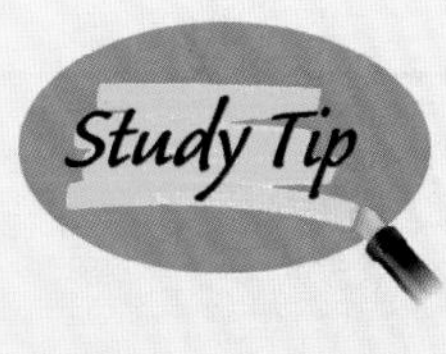

Prefixes with the Same Meaning: Several prefixes have the same basic meaning; however, they are not interchangeably used with a given word root. For instance, *bi-* and *di-* both mean two, but it would be incorrect to use the prefix *di-* with the word *lateral* to indicate both sides. The correct term is *bilateral.* Unfortunately, there are no rules on the usage of prefixes with the same meaning; however, you will learn which prefix goes with each word root as you encounter the actual medical terms in later chapters.

Exercises: Prefixes Involving Number

Exercise 1

SIMPLE RECALL

Write the correct prefix for the meaning given.

1. one: uni or mono
2. two: bi or di
3. three: tri
4. four: quad or quadri
5. many: multi or poly

Exercise 2

SIMPLE RECALL

Write the meaning of the prefix given.

1. semi- half / partly
2. hemi- half
3. poly- many / much
4. uni- one
5. quadr- four

Prefixes Involving Negation

Prefix	Meaning	Example
a-, an-	without, not	afebrile (without fever), anaerobic (without oxygen)
anti-, contra-	against	antibacterial (active against bacteria) contraception (prevention of conception or pregnancy)
de-	away from, cessation, without	deaminase (enzyme that takes away an amino group from a compound)
dis-	separate	disarticulate (separate bones at the joint)
im-, in-, non-	not	impotent (not able to perform sexual intercourse), incompetent (not capable) noninfectious (not able to spread disease)

Exercise: Prefixes Involving Negation

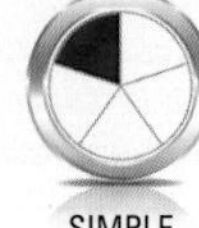

Exercise 3

SIMPLE RECALL

Write the meaning of the prefix given.

1. contra- against
2. im- not
3. de- without/away from
4. an- without/not
5. dis- seperate

Prefixes Involving Position, Time, or Direction

Prefix	Meaning	Example
ab-	away from	abduct (move a limb away from the body's midline)
ad-	to, toward	adduct (move a limb toward the body's midline)
ect-, ecto-	outer, outside	ectoderm (outer layer of cells in the embryo)
en-, end-, endo-	in, within	endemic (present within a region or group) endocardium (innermost layer of the heart)
ex-, exo-	out of, away from	exhale (to breathe out) exoenzyme (enzyme that functions outside the cell)
infra-	below, beneath	infrasplenic (below the spleen)
inter-	between	intercostal (between the ribs)
intra-	within	intra-articular (within the cavity of a joint)
per-	through	percutaneous (passage of a substance through unbroken skin)
peri-	around, surrounding	pericarditis (inflammation of the membrane around the heart)
post-	after, behind	postmortem (occurring after death)
pre-	before (in time or space)	precancerous (lesion that has not yet become cancerous)
sub-	below, beneath	subcutaneous (beneath the skin)
super-, supra-	above	superinfection (a new infection beyond the one that is already present) suprarenal (above the kidney)
sym-, syn-	together, with	symphysis (type of joint where bones come together) synapse (where one nerve cell meets another)
trans-	across, through	transection (cutting across)

Exercises: Prefixes Involving Position, Time, or Direction

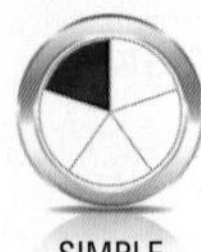

Exercise 4

SIMPLE RECALL

Write the correct prefix for the meaning given.

1. between Inter
2. after, behind post

3. through ___trans___ or ___per___

4. above ___super___ or ___supra___

5. within ___intra___ or ___endo___

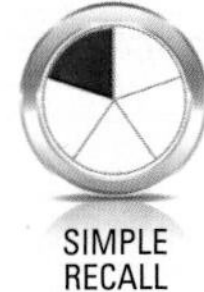
SIMPLE RECALL

Exercise 5

Write the meaning of the prefix given.

1. ecto- ___outside___
2. ab- ___away from___
3. pre- ___before___
4. sub- ___below___
5. syn- ___together, with___

Prefixes Involving Relative Characteristics

Many prefixes express a characteristic that is relative to something else. *Relative* means there is a relationship to something else or something can be compared to something else. You have already seen some relative prefixes in the preceding categories, including prefixes involving time (this happened *before* that) or space (this is located *beneath* that).

Often, these prefixes describe a quality or characteristic of something compared to a normal situation **(Figure 2-2)**.

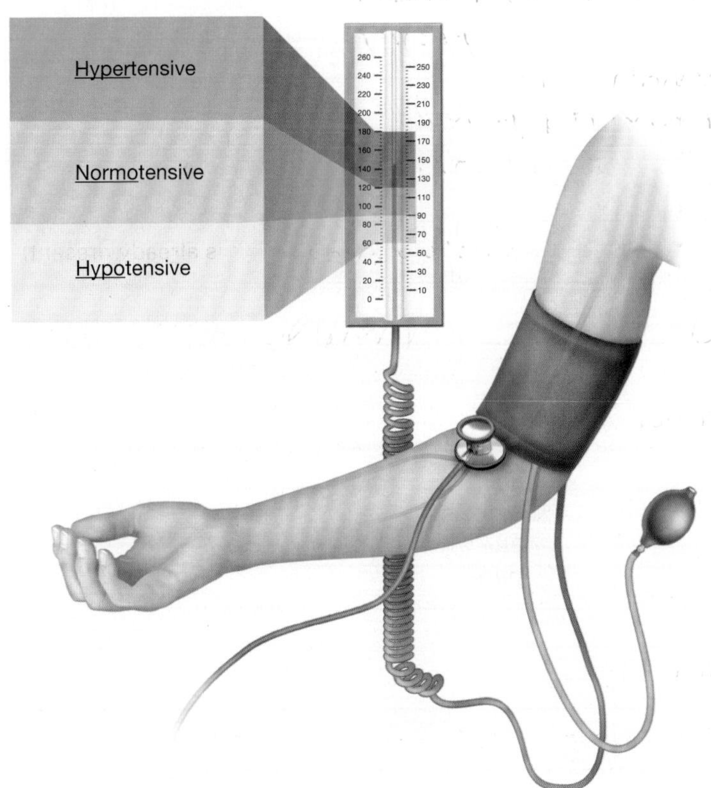

Figure 2-2 Different prefixes used with the same word root and suffix can change the word meaning, and the patient's care, dramatically.

Prefixes Involving Relative Characteristics

Prefix	Meaning	Example
dys-	painful, difficult, abnormal	dyspepsia (having impaired gastric function)
eu-	good, normal	eupeptic (having good digestion)
hetero-	other, different	heterogeneous (made up of elements with different properties)
homo-, homeo-	same, alike	homogeneous (of uniform structure throughout) homeometric (the same size)
hyper-	above normal, excessive	hypertension (high blood pressure)
hypo-	below normal, deficient	hypoglycemia (below normal blood sugar)
iso-	equal, alike	isomorphous (having the same form or shape)
macro-	large, long	macrosomia (abnormally large body)
mega-, megalo-	large, oversize	megadose (larger-than-normal dose) megalosplenia (enlarged spleen)
micro-	small	microcardia (abnormally small heart)
normo-	normal, usual	normotensive (normal blood pressure)
pan-	all, entire	panlobar (pertaining to the entire lung lobe)
ultra-	excess, beyond	ultrasonograph (diagnostic instrument that uses very high sound frequencies)

Exercises: Prefixes Involving Relative Characteristics

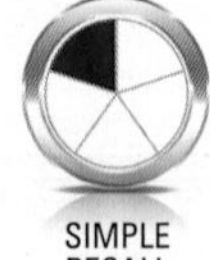
SIMPLE RECALL

Exercise 6

Write the correct prefix for the meaning given.

1. other, different hetero
2. normal eu / normo
3. large mega ______, ______, or megalo
4. good, normal eu
5. alike homo or homeo
6. small micro or hypo

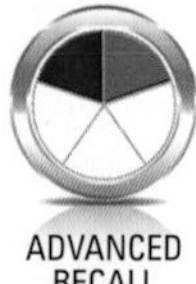
ADVANCED RECALL

Exercise 7

Match each prefix with its meaning.

hypo-	iso-	eu-
dys-	hyper-	pan-

1. painful, difficult, abnormal dys
2. good, normal eu
3. above normal, excessive hyper

4. all, entire pan

5. equal, alike iso

6. below normal, deficient hypo

Other Prefixes

Prefix	Meaning	Example
brady-	slow	bradycardia (a slow heartbeat)
neo-	new	neonate (a newborn infant)
pseudo-	false	pseudomalignancy (benign, noncancerous tumor that appears to be malignant cancer)
re-	again, backward	reactivate (to activate again)
tachy-	rapid, fast	tachycardia (a rapid heartbeat)

■ Exercise: Other Prefixes

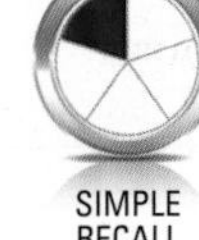

SIMPLE RECALL

Exercise 8

Write the meaning of the prefix given.

1. tachy- rapid / fast
2. neo- new
3. brady- slow
4. re- again
5. pseudo- false

■ COMMON SUFFIXES

Like a prefix, a suffix modifies the meaning of the word root to which it is joined. Suffixes can be learned in groups based on similar or opposite meanings, as seen in the following tables. Many medical terms have a suffix. A suffix and a combining form together usually form a noun or adjective.

Suffixes Related to Conditions or Diseases

Suffix	Meaning	Example
-algia	pain	myalgia (pain in one or more muscles)
-emia	blood (condition of)	hypoxemia (condition of abnormally low oxygen in arterial blood)
-ia	state or condition	pneumonia (condition involving inflammation in the lung)
-ism	condition, disease, or disorder	albinism (disorder resulting in a lack of skin pigment)
-itis	inflammation	gastritis (inflammation of the stomach)

(continued)

Suffixes Related to Conditions or Diseases *(continued)*

Suffix	Meaning	Example
-megaly	large, enlargement	cardiomegaly (enlargement of the heart)
-oma	tumor	osteoma (bone tumor)
-osis	abnormal condition	osteoporosis (brittle bone condition)
-pathy	disease	craniopathy (disease involving the cranial bones)
-rrhea	flow, discharge	diarrhea (frequent discharge of semisolid or fluid feces)

Exercises: Suffixes Related to Conditions or Diseases

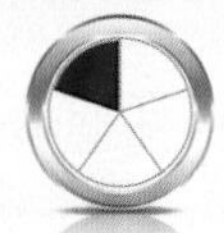

SIMPLE RECALL

Exercise 9

Write the meaning of the prefix given.

1. -megaly large
2. -osis abnormal condition
3. -ism condition/disease
4. -ia state or condition
5. -rrhea discharge/flow

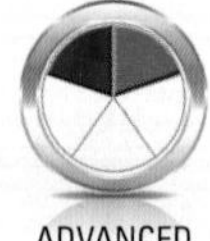

ADVANCED RECALL

Exercise 10

Match each suffix with its meaning.

-itis	-emia	-pathy
-algia	-oma	-rrhea

1. pain algia
2. inflammation itis
3. flow, discharge rrhea
4. blood (condition of) emia
5. tumor oma
6. disease pathy

Suffixes Related to Surgery

Suffix	Meaning	Example
-centesis	puncture to remove fluid	amniocentesis (needle puncture of amniotic sac in a pregnant woman to remove fluid for diagnosis)
-ectomy	surgical removal	appendectomy (surgical removal of the appendix)

Suffixes Related to Surgery

Suffix	Meaning	Example
-plasty	surgical repair, reconstruction	abdominoplasty (surgical repair of the abdominal wall)
-rrhaphy	suturing	cystorrhaphy (suture of a wound in the urinary bladder)
-stomy	surgical opening	colostomy (surgical creation of an outside opening into the colon)
-tomy	incision, cutting	gastrotomy (incision into the stomach)

■ Exercises: Suffixes Related to Surgery

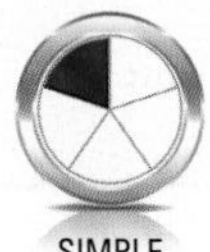

Exercise 11

Write the meaning of the suffix given.

1. -centesis puncture to remove fluid
2. -ectomy surgical removal
3. -stomy surgical opening
4. -plasty surgical repair

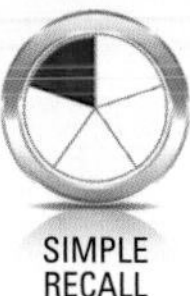

Exercise 12

Write the correct suffix for the meaning given.

1. incision, cutting -tomy
2. suturing -rrhaphy
3. surgical opening -stomy
4. surgical removal -ectomy

Other Suffixes

Suffix	Meaning	Example
-al	pertaining to	cranial (pertaining to the skull)
-ar	pertaining to	articular (pertaining to a joint)
-ary	pertaining to	pulmonary (pertaining to the lungs)
-ic, -ac	pertaining to	cardiac (pertaining to the heart)
-ous	pertaining to, characterized by	edematous (characterized by edema, which is a type of swelling)
-genic, -genesis	produced by, formed by	carcinogenic (causing cancer)
		osteogenesis (the formation of bone)

(continued)

Other Suffixes *(continued)*

Suffix	Meaning	Example
-gram	record, recording	cystogram (x-ray of the bladder)
-graphy	process of recording	radiography (x-ray studies)
-ium	tissue, structure	myocardium (heart muscle tissue)
-logist, -ist	one who specializes in	dermatologist (physician who treats skin conditions) dentist (doctor who treats conditions of the teeth)
-logy	study of	dermatology (study of skin conditions)
-meter	instrument for measuring	thermometer (instrument to measure heat)
-oid	resembling	lymphoid (resembling lymph)
-scope	instrument for examination	microscope (instrument for examining very small things)
-scopy	process of examining, examination	endoscopy (examination of the interior of a structure using a special instrument)

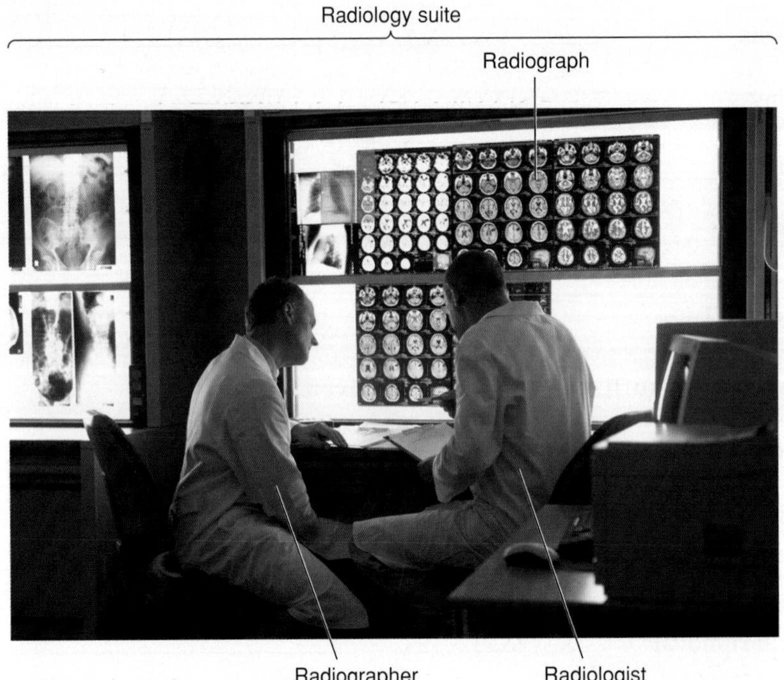

Figure 2-3 Different suffixes combined with the same word root help distinguish terms within the same specialty.

Once you understand a single root word, you can begin adding prefixes or suffixes to further clarify the root word **(Figure 2-3)**. Even though the terms are related to the same specialty, because they share the same root word, they have very different meanings based on the prefixes and suffixes that are added.

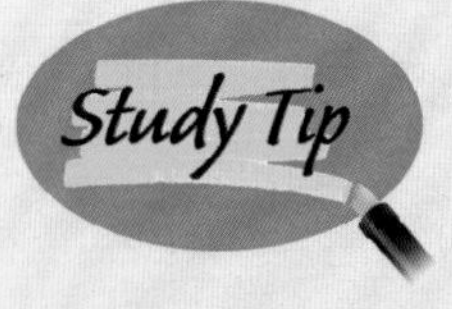

***-scope* and *-scopy*:** Some suffixes are very closely related and easily confused. For example, *-scope* means an instrument for examination, whereas *-scopy* means the process of examination. A gastroscope is an instrument used for examining the stomach, while *gastroscopy* refers to the actual examination using the gastroscope. There are many medical terms with these suffixes, so a good understanding of them now will lead to less confusion and easier memorization later.

Exercises: Other Suffixes

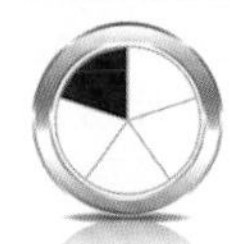

SIMPLE RECALL

Exercise 13

Write the meaning of the suffix given.

1. -meter instrument for measuring
2. -graphy process of recording
3. -al pertaining to
4. -scopy examination
5. -gram record
6. -ary pertaining to
7. -logy study of
8. -ic pertaining to

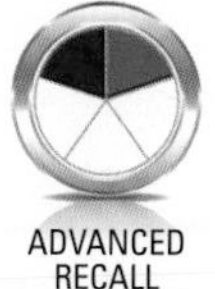

ADVANCED RECALL

Exercise 14

Match each suffix with its meaning.

-genic	-scope	-oid
-ary	-logist	-ium

1. specialist -logist
2. resembling -oid
3. tissue -ium
4. pertaining to -ary
5. produced by, formed by -genic
6. instrument for examination -scope

COMMON ABBREVIATIONS

Abbreviations are commonly used in health care, particularly in handwritten notes, where they save time by allowing busy practitioners to skip writing out a full term or expression. You will learn commonly used abbreviations throughout this text. Following are a few examples of common abbreviations. Appendix D contains a fuller listing of medical abbreviations.

Although using abbreviations is convenient, keep in mind that some abbreviations are prone to misinterpretation, which can lead to dangerous medical errors.

To avoid this problem, the Joint Commission has developed an official "Do Not Use" list of abbreviations that health care workers must never use. These are given in Appendix D. Of course, your health care facility may have its own list of abbreviations that should be avoided or that are acceptable to use; review this information carefully, and follow the guidelines in your daily practice.

Abbreviation	Meaning
	Diagnosis and Treatment
Dx	diagnosis
H&P	history and physical (examination)
Hx	history
pt	patient
Px	prognosis
Rx	prescription
Sx	symptom
Tx, Tr	treatment
	Practice Areas and Specialists
CAM	complementary and alternative medicine
DC	doctor of chiropractic medicine
DDS	doctor of dental surgery
ENT	ears, nose, throat
ER, ED	emergency room, emergency department
ICU	intensive care unit
MD	doctor of medicine
OB/GYN	obstetrics/gynecology
OD	doctor of optometry
PA	physician's assistant
Peds	pediatrics
PT	physical therapy, physical therapist
	Units of Measurement
C	Celsius, centigrade (temperature)
cc	cubic centimeter
F	Fahrenheit (temperature)
g or gm, mg, kg	gram, milligram, kilogram
L, mL	liter, milliliter
m, cm, mm	meter, centimeter, millimeter
oz	ounce
	Prescriptions
b.i.d.	twice a day (Latin, *bis in die*)
noct.	night (Latin, *nocte*)
p.c.	after meals (Latin, *post cibum*)
p.r.n.	as needed (Latin, *pro re nata*)
q.i.d.	four times a day (Latin, *quater in die*)

Abbreviation	Meaning
Other Abbreviations	
ADL	activities of daily living
AP	anteroposterior (from front to back)
BP	blood pressure
CT	computed tomography (type of x-ray)
Ht	height
lab	laboratory
MRI	magnetic resonance imaging
NPO, npo	nothing by mouth (don't eat or drink) (Latin, *non per os*)
P	pulse rate
postop, post-op	postoperative (after surgery)
preop, pre-op	preoperative (before surgery)
R	respiratory rate
RBC	red blood cell
STAT, stat	immediately
T	temperature
VS	vital signs
WBC	white blood cell
Wt	weight

Exercises: Common Abbreviations

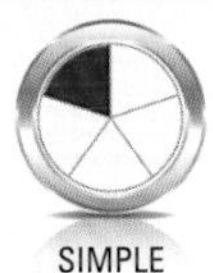

SIMPLE RECALL

Exercise 15

Write the meaning of each abbreviation.

1. ICU intensive care unit
2. RBC red blood cell
3. P pulse rate
4. H&P history & physical (examination)
5. ADL activities of daily living
6. ED emergency department
7. L liter
8. Tx treatment
9. ENT ears, nose, throat
10. lab laboratory

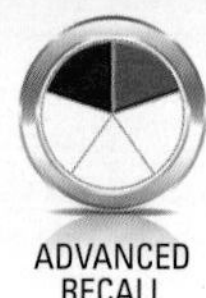

Exercise 16

Match each abbreviation with its meaning.

Rx	R	STAT	VS
PT	Sx	Hx	BP
p.r.n.	noct.	Ht	Dx

1. symptom Sx
2. vital signs VS
3. diagnosis Dx
4. height Ht
5. immediately STAT
6. as needed p.r.n
7. respiratory rate R
8. blood pressure BP
9. prescription Rx
10. night noct.
11. physical therapy PT
12. history Hx

WRAPPING UP

- Medical terminology uses common prefixes, suffixes, and abbreviations.
- Prefixes describe: numbers, negation, position, time, direction, or relative characteristics.
- Suffixes describe: conditions, diseases, surgery.
- These word parts will help you understand nearly every medical term you encounter.
- Abbreviations are commonly used in health care notes for convenience, and learning these will help you understand shorthand.

Chapter Review

In the following exercises, you will encounter a few medical terms you have not seen in this chapter. Nonetheless, you should be able to answer these questions based on the word parts used in these terms. Review the earlier tables of prefix and suffix meanings if needed.

Review of Prefixes and Suffixes

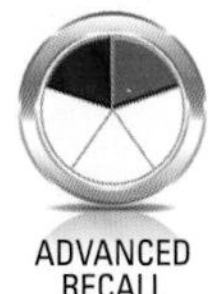

Exercise 17

Match each prefix with its meaning.

hypo-	hetero-	dys-	im-	intra-
hemi-	ad-	exo-	per-	poly-

1. not ______ im
2. toward ______ ad
3. many ______ poly
4. through ______ per
5. within ______ intra
6. outside ______ exo
7. half ______ hemi
8. different ______ hetro
9. below normal ______ hypo
10. painful ______ dys

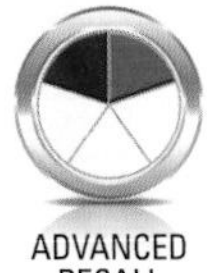

Exercise 18

Match each suffix with its meaning.

-plasty	-pathy	-ium	-emia	-gram
-graphy	-ar	-osis	-tomy	-rrhaphy

1. abnormal condition ______ osis
2. suturing ______ rrhaphy
3. record, recording ______ gram

4. incision tomy
5. blood (condition of) emia
6. disease pathy
7. pertaining to ar
8. surgical repair plasty
9. recording process graphy
10. tissue ium

Meaning Recognition

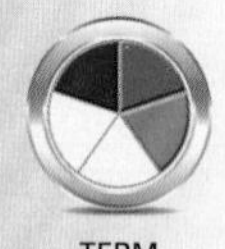

TERM CONSTRUCTION

Exercise 19

Match each word with its meaning. Because you have not yet learned some of the combining forms used in some of these terms, you may have to guess the meanings based on the meanings of the prefixes or suffixes in the terms.

bisect	polyarthritis	semiconscious	submandibular	panarthritis
cardiotomy	endoscope	cavitary	psychology	thrombosis

1. cut in two parts bisect
2. beneath the mandible (lower jaw) submandibular
3. pertaining to a cavity cavitary
4. incision of heart wall cardiotomy
5. study of mental processes psychology
6. instrument for examining inside an organ endoscope
7. inflammation of several joints polyarthritis
8. condition of having a blood clot thrombosis
9. inflammation of all the joints in body panarthritis
10. drowsy, partially conscious semiconscious

Term Building

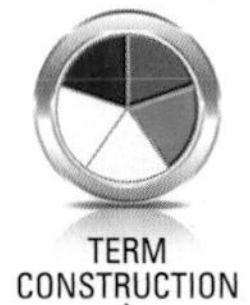

Exercise 20

Using the given combining form and a prefix or suffix (and sometimes both) from this chapter, build a medical term for the meaning given.

Use Combining Form	Meaning of Medical Term	Medical Term
myos/o + suffix	inflammation of muscle	1. ______
lob/o + suffix	surgical removal of lobe	2. ______
cardi/o + suffix	disease of the heart	3. ______
prefix + cost/o (rib) + suffix	pertaining to between the rib	4. ______
prefix + nas/o (nose) + suffix	pertaining to behind the nose	5. ______
prefix + bi/o + suffix	one who specializes in the study of very small life forms	6. ______
lymph/o + suffix	tumor of lymph tissue	7. ______
dermat/o + suffix	resembling skin	8. ______
crani/o + suffix	surgical repair of the skull	9. ______
ten/o (tendon) + suffix	suture of a tendon	10. ______

Spelling and Pronunciation

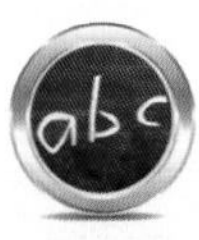

Exercise 21

Circle the correctly spelled term.

1. mononeural	monaneura	mononueral
2. hemopleiga	hemaplegia	hemiplegia
3. ectiderm	ectoderm	ectaderm
4. infrisonic	infrosonic	infrasonic
5. pericarditis	perocarditis	perecarditis
6. megalaspenia	megalesplenia	megalosplenia
7. hetrogeneous	heterogeneous	hetarogeneous
8. bradycardia	bradcardia	braydcardia

9. diarhea	diarrhea	diareah
10. hetrogenic	hetarogenic	heterogenic
11. mylgia	myolgia	myalgia
12. cystorhraphy	cystorrhaphy	cystorhaphry
13. osteogenesis	osteogenisis	osteoginesis
14. edematuos	edematous	edematus
15. gastrotomy	gastrotomomy	gastrotommy

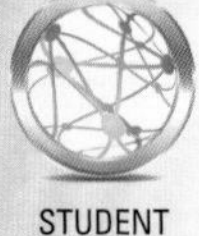
STUDENT RESOURCES

Additional spelling exercises for this and all chapters in the text are included as Spelling Bee activities in the Student Resources on thePoint.

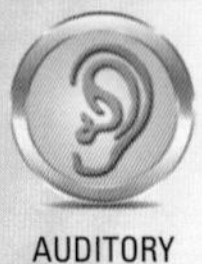
AUDITORY

Exercise 22

Listen to the pronunciations of the following terms in the Dictionary/ Audio Glossary on the Student Resources, and practice pronouncing each, referring to the pronunciation guide as needed.

1. quadruplets	kwahd-rūp′letz
2. abacterial	ā′bak-tēr′ē-ăl
3. suprarenal	sū′pră-rē′năl
4. hypoglycemia	hī′pō-glī-sē′mē-ă
5. diarthric	dī-ahr′thrik
6. dyspeptic	dis-pep′tik
7. neonate	nē′ō-nāt
8. osteoma	os-tē-ō′mă
9. cardiomegaly	kahr′dē-ō-meg′ă-lē
10. articular	ahr-tik′yū-lăr
11. edematous	e-dēm′ă-tŭs
12. antisepsis	an′ti-sep′sis
13. bradycardia	brad′ē-kahr′dē-ă
14. myocardium	mī′ō-kahr′dē-ŭm
15. amniocentesis	am′nē-ō-sen-tē′sis
16. tachycardia	tak′i-kahr′dē-ă
17. polyarteritis	pol′ē-ahr-tĕr-ī′tis
18. symphysis	sim′fi-sis
19. gastrotomy	gas-trot′ŏ-mē
20. subcutaneous	sŭb′kyū-tā′nē-ŭs

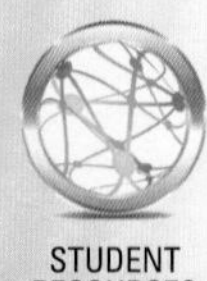
STUDENT RESOURCES

Study the correct punctuation of terms in this and all chapters with the Dictionary/ Audio Glossary in the Student Resources on thePoint.

Media Connection

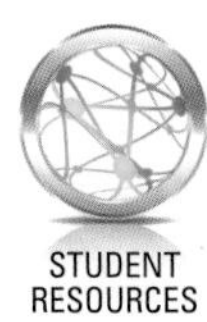

STUDENT RESOURCES

Exercise 23

Complete each of the following activities available with the Student Resources. Check off each activity as you complete it, and record your score for the Chapter Quiz in the space provided.

Chapter Exercises

____ Flash Cards	____ Break It Down
____ Concentration	____ True/False Body Building
____ Abbreviation Match-Up	____ Quiz Show
____ Roboterms	____ Complete the Case
____ Word Anatomy	____ Spelling Bee
____ Fill the Gap	

____ **Chapter Quiz** *Score:* ______%

Additional Resources

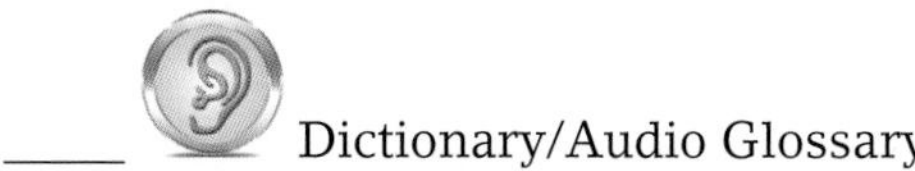

____ Dictionary/Audio Glossary

Terms Related to the Whole Body

3

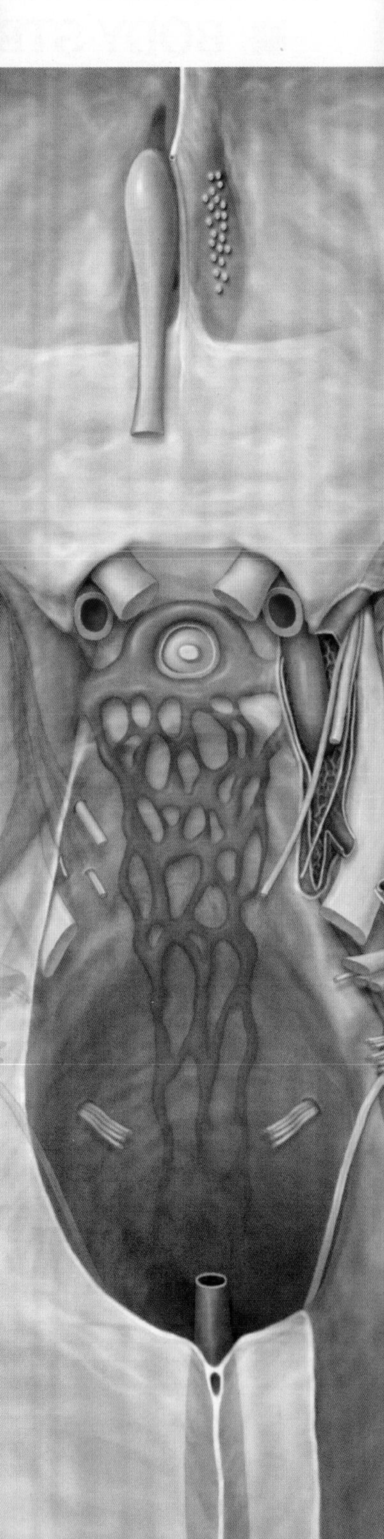

Chapter Outline

Introduction, 42

Body Structures in Health and Disease, 42
- Word Parts Related to Body Structures in Health and Disease, 42
- Terms Related to Body Structures in Health and Disease, 44
- Levels of Organization, 45

Body Areas, Cavities, and Abdominopelvic Divisions, 47
- Combining Forms Related to Body Areas, Cavities, and Abdominopelvic Divisions, 47
- Terms Related to Body Areas, Cavities, and Abdominopelvic Divisions, 48

Anatomic Directions, Positions, and Planes, 51
- Word Parts Related to Anatomic Directions, Positions, and Planes, 51
- Terms Related to Anatomic Directions, Positions, and Planes, 53

Colors, 57
- Combining Forms Related to Colors, 57
- Terms Related to Colors, 58

Introduction to Medical Records, 58

Introduction to Body Systems, 60

Wrapping Up, 61

Chapter Review, 62

Learning Outcomes

After completing this chapter, you should be able to:

1. Define word parts related to body structures, regions, and cavities.
2. Define terms related to body structures and regions, directions and positions, and colors.
3. Spell and pronounce medical terms built with common combining forms, prefixes, and suffixes related to the body as a whole.
4. Describe the common types of medical records used in the health care setting.
5. Explain what a body system is and why it is useful to learn medical terminology by body system.
6. Successfully complete all chapter exercises.
7. Successfully complete all exercises included with the companion Student Resources on thePoint.

INTRODUCTION

This chapter continues to build on word parts learned in Chapters 1 and 2. The focus now expands to include common terms used to refer to the body as a whole, rather than specific body systems, which will be covered in later chapters.

BODY STRUCTURES IN HEALTH AND DISEASE

A healthy state is one in which the body functions optimally without any sign of disease or abnormality. In such a state, the body is in *homeostatic balance*. When an imbalance exists, disease or disorder results. This section introduces you to word parts related to body structures in health and disease.

Word Parts Related to Body Structures in Health and Disease

Combining Form	Meaning	Combining Form	Meaning
aden/o	gland	morph/o	form, shape
blast/o	immature cell	my/o, myos/o	muscle
cyt/o	cell	necr/o	death
fibr/o	fiber	neur/o	nerve
gluc/o, glyc/o	glucose, sugar	nucle/o	nucleus
hem/o, hemat/o	blood	oste/o	bone
hist/o	tissue	path/o	disease
hydr/o	water, watery fluid	sarc/o	flesh
lei/o	smooth	troph/o	nourishment
lip/o	fat	viscer/o	internal organs

Suffix	Meaning
-cyte	cell
-oma	tumor
-osis	abnormal condition
-pathy	disease
-plasia	formation (especially of cells), growth
-stasis	stopping, standing still

Exercises: Word Parts Related to Body Structures in Health and Disease

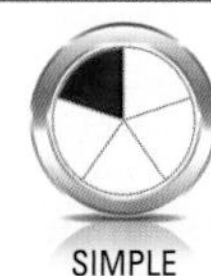
SIMPLE RECALL

Exercise 1

Write the meaning of the word part given.

1. fibr/o fiber
2. necr/o death
3. my/o muscle
4. -oma tumor
5. hydr/o water
6. path/o disease
7. neur/o nerve
8. hem/o blood
9. lei/o smooth
10. morph/o form/shape

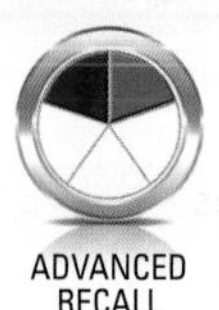
ADVANCED RECALL

Exercise 2

Match each word part with its meaning.

oste/o	hist/o	-osis	lip/o	-cyte
blast/o	-pathy	viscer/o	gluc/o	aden/o

1. glucose gluc/o
2. immature cell blast/o
3. internal organs viscer/o
4. tissue hist/o
5. disease -pathy
6. abnormal condition -osis
7. bone oste/o
8. fat lip/o
9. cell -cyte
10. gland aden/o

Terms Related to Body Structures in Health and Disease

Term	Pronunciation	Meaning
body system	bod'ē sis'tĕm	group of organs with related functions; organ system
cell	sel	smallest independent unit of a living structure
chromosome	krō'mō-sōm	structure in the cell nucleus that carries information in the form of genes
cytoplasm	sī'tō-plazm	substance of a cell excluding the nucleus
gene	jēn	sequence of DNA on a chromosome that determines heredity
nucleus	nū'klē-ŭs	central structure in a cell that contains chromosome
cytology	sī-tol'ŏ-jē	study of cells
histology	his-tol'ŏ-jē	study of cells and tissues
homeostasis	hō'mē-ō-stā'sis	state of equilibrium
metabolism	mĕ-tab'ŏ-lizm	sum of the normal chemical and physical changes occurring in tissue
organ	ōr'găn	grouping of two or more tissues that are integrated to perform a specific function
organ system	ōr'găn sis'tĕm	group of organs with related functions; body system
somatic	sō-mat'ik	pertaining to the body
systemic	sis-tem'ik	pertaining to the body as a whole
tissue	tish'ū	grouping of similar cells that perform a specific function
visceral	vis'ĕr-ăl	pertaining to the internal organs
Terms Related to Conditions and Disease		
acute	ă-kyūt'	referring to a disease of sudden onset and brief course
chronic	kron'ik	referring to a persistent disease or illness
etiology	ē'tē-ol'ŏ-jē	study of the cause of disease

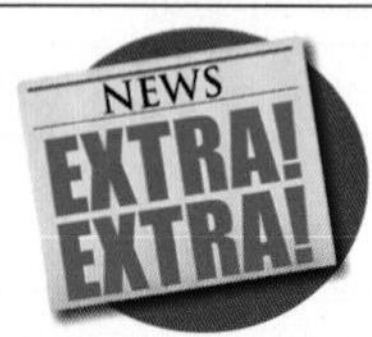

ETIOLOGY The term **etiology** is sometimes used to refer to a specific cause of a disease. For example, you could say that the etiology of an infection is a certain bacteria.

Term	Pronunciation	Meaning
exacerbation	eg-zas'ĕr-bā'shŭn	an increase in the severity of a disease or symptoms
hyperplasia	hī'pĕr-plā'zē-ă	excessive growth of tissue
idiopathic	id'ē-ō-path'ik	related to a disease of unknown cause
inflammation	in'flă-mā'shŭn	localized physical changes in tissue characterized by redness, heat, pain, and swelling, in response to an injury
lesion	lē'zhŭn	a pathologic change in tissue resulting from a wound or injury
necrosis	nĕ-krō'sis	pathologic death of cells or tissue
pathogen	path'ō-jĕn	any virus, microorganism, or other substance that causes disease
remission	rē-mish'ŭn	lessening in severity of disease symptoms

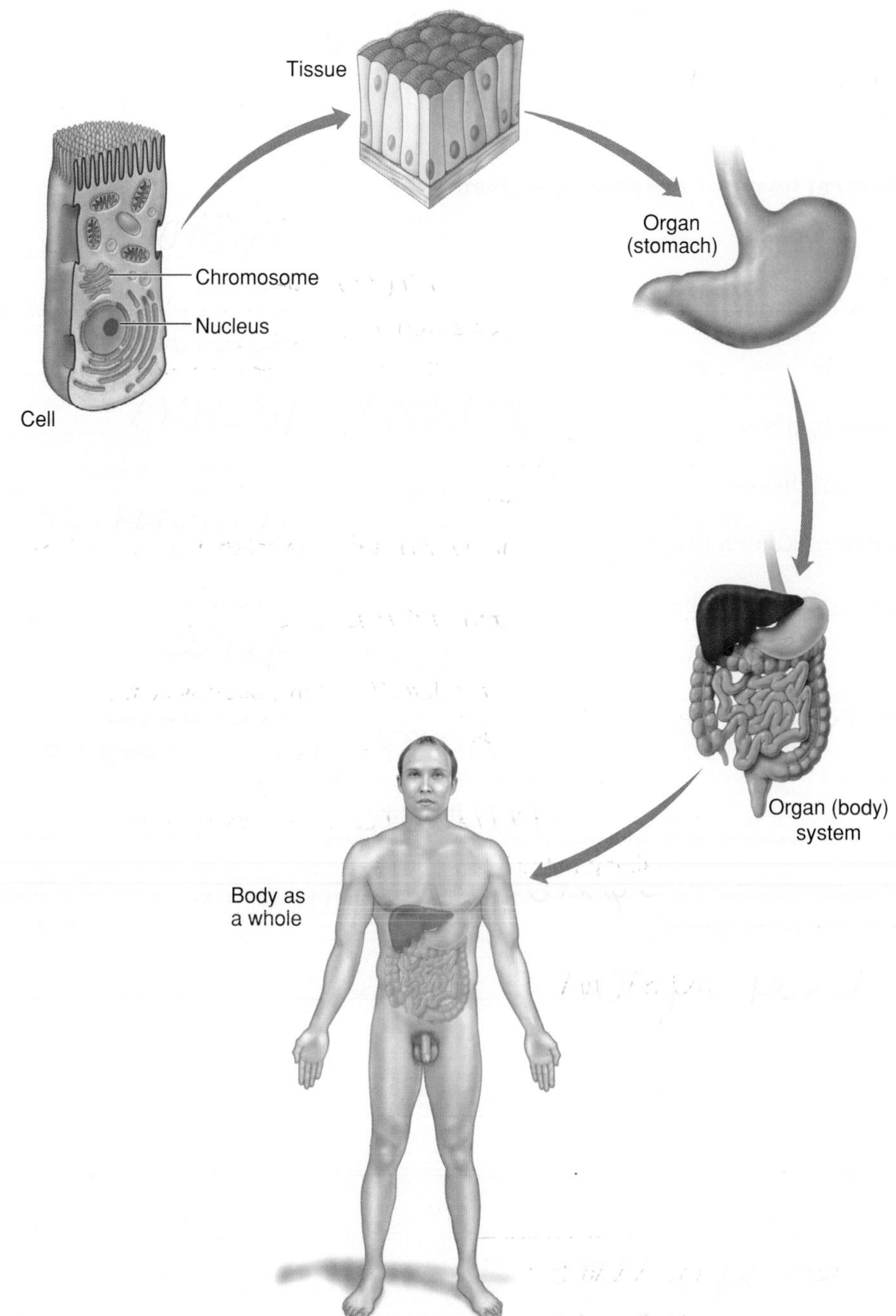

Figure 3-1 Levels of organization in the body.

Levels of Organization

To better understand the human body, it has been divided into different levels of organization **(Figure 3-1)**. Cells are the smallest independent units and compose the first level. Many similar cells together form tissues, tissues make up an organ, organs make up an organ (body) system, and all the organ systems form the body as a whole. Each level is more complex than the last. It is important to understand what each level is and how the levels are interrelated.

Exercises: Terms Related to Body Structures in Health and Disease

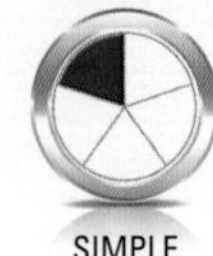

Exercise 3

SIMPLE RECALL

Write the correct medical term for the meaning given.

1. study of cells and tissues histology
2. increase in severity of disease exacerbation
3. pertaining to the body somatic
4. a pathologic change in tissue lesion
5. referring to persistent disease chronic
6. related to disease of unknown cause idiopathic
7. referring to disease of sudden onset acute
8. sequence of DNA on a chromosome that determines heredity gene
9. pathologic death of cells or tissues necrosis
10. state of equilibrium homeostasis

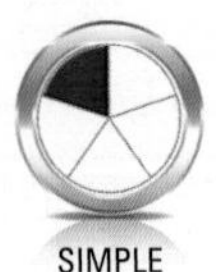

Exercise 4

SIMPLE RECALL

Write the meaning of the term given.

1. organ system body system
2. inflammation ______
3. pathogen ______
4. remission ______
5. visceral ______
6. cytology study of cells
7. etiology ______
8. organ ______
9. metabolism ______
10. hyperplasia ______

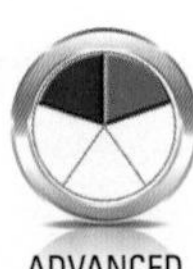

Exercise 5

ADVANCED RECALL

Circle the term that is appropriate for the meaning of the sentence.

1. The patient's chronic disease was often well controlled, but he had periods of (*remission, exacerbation, homeostasis*) when his symptoms became much worse.
2. Chromosomes are located within the (*cytology, nucleus, pathogen*) of the cell.

3. Some drugs affect only a specific organ or body area, whereas others may have (*chronic, idiopathic, systemic*) effects causing changes throughout the body.

4. A grouping of similar cells performing a specific function is termed (*a gene, tissue, a body system*).

5. Because physicians were unable to determine the cause of her symptoms, her disorder was considered (*idiopathic, visceral, systemic*).

6. The substance of a body cell excluding the nucleus is called the (*hyperplasia, chromosome, cytoplasm*).

7. Because the surgeon thought the lesion might be cancerous, he sent a sample of cells to the (*cytology, inflammation, somatic*) lab for analysis.

8. Her physician determined that the lesion on her skin was the result of infection by a (*gene, viscera, pathogen*).

BODY AREAS, CAVITIES, AND ABDOMINOPELVIC DIVISIONS

To pinpoint areas with universal precision, we divide the human body in different ways. Three commonly used ways to divide the body are body cavities, abdominopelvic regions, and abdominopelvic quadrants. This helps practitioners localize structures and enables health care workers to identify exact locations. For example, if a person has a pain in the hypogastric region, it may be an indication of appendicitis (inflammation of the appendix). A **region** is a portion of the body. This section covers combining forms and terms related to body areas, cavities, and abdominopelvic divisions.

Combining Forms Related to Body Areas, Cavities, and Abdominopelvic Divisions

Combining Form	Meaning
abdomin/o	abdomen
acr/o	extremity, tip
brachi/o	arm
cervic/o	neck
lumb/o	lumbar region, lower back
ped/o, pod/o	foot
pelv/i	pelvis
thorac/o	thorax, chest

Exercises: Combining Forms Related to Body Areas, Cavities, and Abdominopelvic Divisions

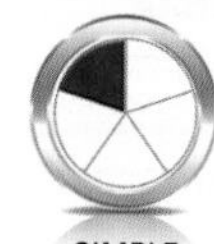
SIMPLE RECALL

Exercise 6

Write the meaning of the combining form given.

1. thorac/o thorax/chest

2. cervic/o 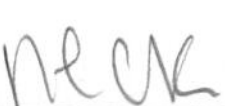 neck

3. lumb/o lower back

4. abdomin/o abdomen

5. pelv/i pelvis

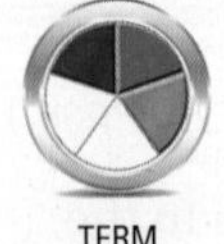
TERM CONSTRUCTION

Exercise 7

Using the given combining form and any of the following suffixes, build a medical term for the meaning given.

-meter	-ar	-centesis
-algia	-plasty	-ectomy

Combining Form	Meaning of Medical Term	Medical Term
abdomen/o	removal of abdominal fluid through puncture	1. -centesis
thorac/o	surgical repair of chest wall	2. -plasty
pelv/i	instrument for measuring the pelvis	3. -meter
lumb/o	pertaining to the lower back	4. -ar
cervic/o	surgical removal of the cervix	5. -ectomy
pod/o	pain in the foot	6. -algia

Terms Related to Body Areas, Cavities, and Abdominopelvic Divisions

Health care professionals use medical terminology to refer to specific areas of the body and to identify precise locations. The tables below introduce the terms used for different areas of the body, cavities within the body, and clinical divisions of the abdomen.

Terms Related to Body Areas

Term	Pronunciation	Meaning
Body Areas		
abdomen (abdominal region)	ab'dŏ-mĕn (ab-dom'i-năl rē'jŭn)	the section of the trunk between the pelvis and chest
cranium	krā'nē-ŭm	skull
diaphragm	dī'ă-fram	muscle between the abdominal and thoracic cavities
extremity	eks-trem'i-tē	limb
pelvis (pelvic region)	pel'vis (pel'vik rē'jŭn)	area of the pelvis below (inferior to) the abdomen
thorax	thō'raks	chest; upper part of the trunk

Terms Related to Body Cavities and Abdominopelvic Divisions

Term	Pronunciation	Meaning
Cavities (Figure 3-2)		
abdominal cavity	ab-dom'ĭ-năl kav'i-tē	space within the abdomen occupied by the digestive and other organs
cranial cavity	krā'nē-ăl kav'i-tē	space within the skull occupied by the brain
pelvic cavity	pel'vik kav'i-tē	space within the pelvis occupied by certain reproductive, urinary, and digestive organs
spinal cavity (vertebral canal)	spī'năl kav'i-tē ver'tĕ-brăl kă-nal'	space within the vertebrae occupied by the spinal cord
thoracic cavity	thōr-as'ik kav'i-tē	space within the chest occupied by the lungs, heart, and other organs
Abdominopelvic Divisions		
abdominopelvic regions	ab-dom'i-nō-pel'vik rē'jŭnz	nine specific anatomic areas of the abdominopelvic cavity **(Figure 3-3)**
epigastric region	ep'i-gas'trik rē'jŭn	abdominal region above (superior to) the umbilical region
hypochondriac region (left and right)	hī'pō-kon'drē-ak rē'jŭn	abdominal regions to the left and right of the epigastric region
hypogastric region	hī'pō-gas'trik rē'jŭn	abdominal region below (inferior to) the umbilical region; also called the suprapubic region
iliac region (left and right)	il'ē-ak rē'jŭn	abdominal regions to the left and right of the hypogastric region
lumbar region (left and right)	lŭm'bahr rē'jŭn	abdominal regions to the left and right of the umbilical region
umbilical region	ŭm-bil'i-kăl rē'jŭn	central abdominal region
abdominopelvic quadrants	ab-dom'i-nō-pel'vik kwahd'rănts	four divisions of the abdominopelvic cavity: left upper quadrant (LUQ), left lower quadrant (LLQ), right upper quadrant (RUQ), and right lower quadrant (RLQ) **(Figure 3-4)**

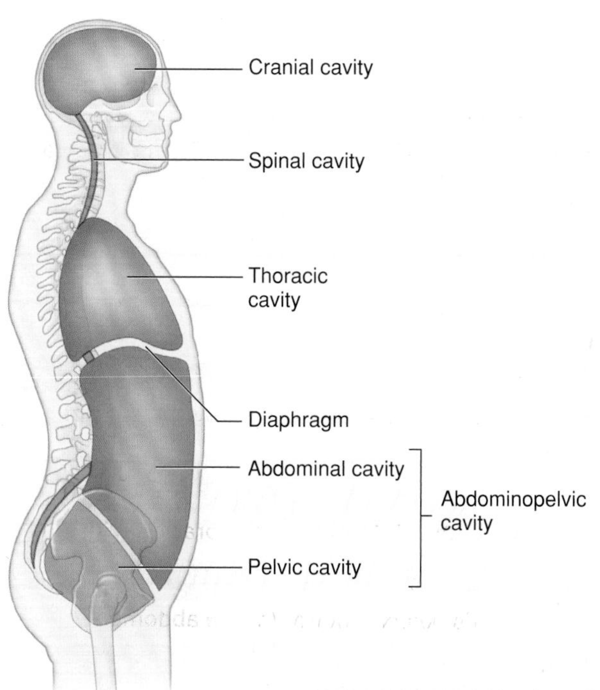

Figure 3-2 The different body cavities shown in the lateral view.

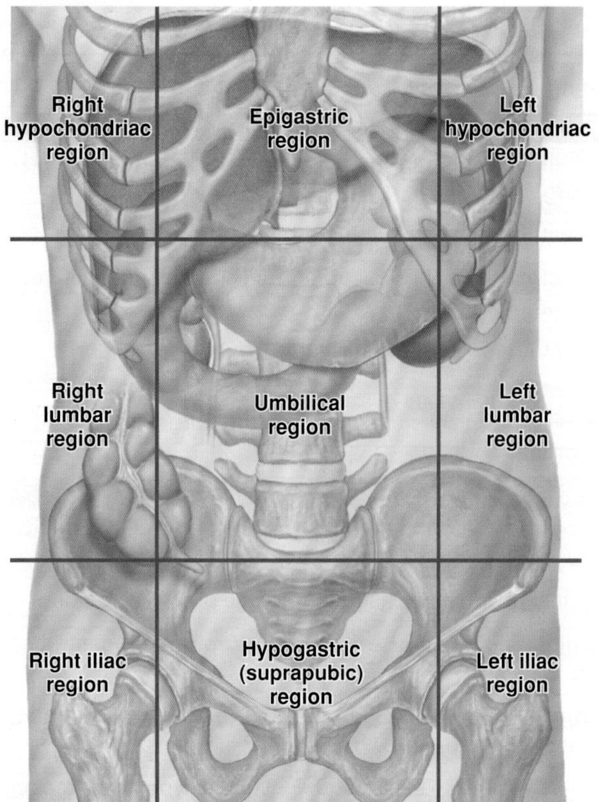

Figure 3-3 The nine abdominopelvic regions.

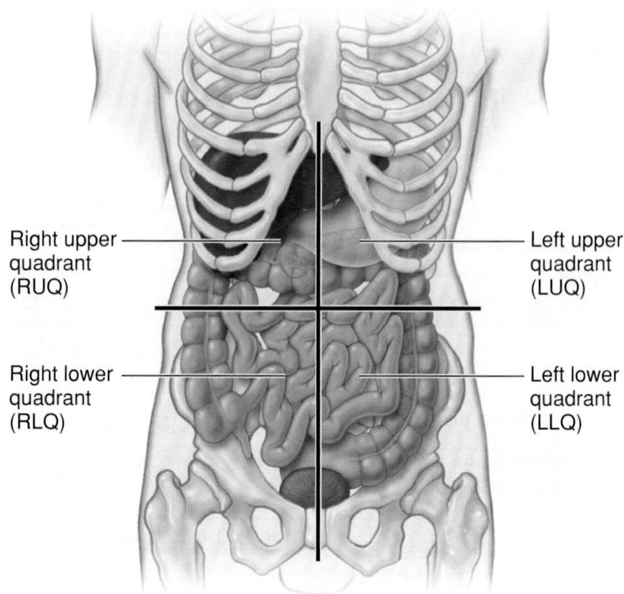

Figure 3-4 The abdominopelvic region can also be divided into four quadrants by one horizontal and one vertical line.

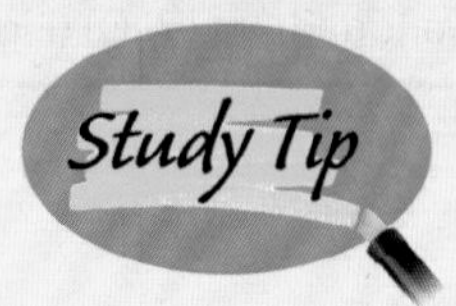

Abdominopelvic Regions: Think of the abdominopelvic regions as a tic-tac-toe board with two horizontal lines and two vertical lines dividing the area into nine regions.

Exercises: Terms Related to Body Areas, Cavities, and Abdominopelvic Divisions

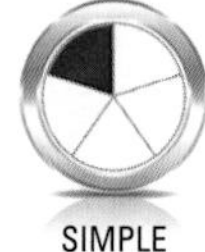

SIMPLE RECALL

Exercise 8

Write the correct medical term for the meaning given.

1. chest thorax
2. space occupied by the spinal cord spinal cavity
3. central abdominal region umbilical region
4. section of the trunk between the pelvis and chest abdomen
5. skull cranium

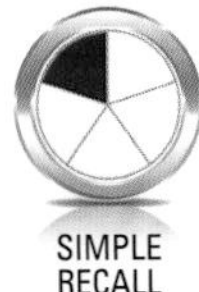

SIMPLE RECALL

Exercise 9

Write the meaning of the term given.

1. extremity limb
2. epigastric region ______
3. thoracic cavity ______
4. diaphragm ______
5. iliac region ______

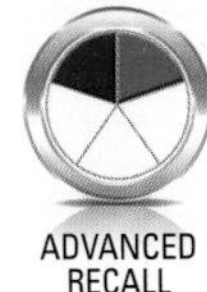

ADVANCED RECALL

Exercise 10

Circle the term that is appropriate for the meaning of the sentence.

1. Most digestive organs are located within the (*pelvic, thoracic, abdominal*) cavity.
2. To the left and right of the epigastric region are the (*hypochondriac, iliac, lumbar*) regions.
3. The abdominopelvic quadrants divide the abdominopelvic area of the body into (*four, six, nine*) regions.
4. The brain surgeon operated to remove a bullet lodged within the (*thoracic, cranial, pelvic*) cavity.
5. The diaphragm is located between the abdominal and (*pelvic, thoracic, spinal*) cavities.

■ ANATOMIC DIRECTIONS, POSITIONS, AND PLANES

When referring to a direction or a position on the body, it is important that health care professionals use consistent terminology to ensure that the correct meaning is understood. To that end, practitioners use directional terms to indicate the relationship of one body part to another. For example, *superior* means upward, and *inferior* means downward. The nose is superior to the chin. A **plane** is an imaginary flat surface used to divide the body or organs into distinct areas. Planes allow professionals to study and visualize the structure and arrangement of various organs, especially when viewing x-rays or CT scans. This section introduces word parts and terminology used to visualize the body and talk about specific locations.

Word Parts Related to Anatomic Directions, Positions, and Planes

Combining Forms and Terms	Meaning
caudal	tail
cephal/o	head
dorsal	back
inferior	below
medi/o	middle

(continued)

Word Parts Related to Anatomic Directions, Positions, and Planes *(continued)*

Prefixes	Meaning
antero-	front
circum-	around
epi-	on, following
infra-	below, beneath
inter-	between
intra-	within
latero-	side
peri-	around, surrounding
postero-	back
proximo-	near point of origin
retro-	backward, behind
sub-	below, beneath
super-	above
supra-	above
ventro-	belly

Exercises: Word Parts Related to Anatomic Directions, Positions, and Planes

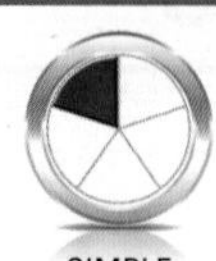

Exercise 11

Write the meaning of the word part given.

1. inferior below
2. intra- within
3. caudal tail
4. postero- back
5. antero- front
6. epi- on
7. latero- side
8. cephal/o head
9. circum- around
10. dorsal back

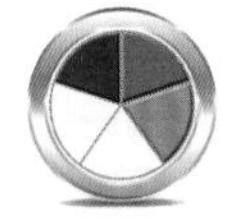
TERM CONSTRUCTION

Exercise 12

Considering the meanings of the word parts from which the medical term is made, write the meaning of the medical term given. (You have not yet learned many of these terms, but you can build their meanings from the word parts.)

Combining Form	Meaning	Medical Term	Meaning of Term
vertebr/o	vertebra	intervertebral	1. ______
cardi/o	heart	pericardiac	2. ______
cec/o	cecum	retrocecal	3. ______
carp/o	carpal bone	mediocarpal	4. ______
numer/o	number	supernumerary	5. ______

Terms Related to Anatomic Directions, Positions, and Planes

Terms in this table are grouped by opposite meanings.

Term	Pronunciation	Meaning
Directional Terms (Figure 3-5)		
cephalad	sef′ă-lad	toward the head
caudad	kaw′dad	toward the tail (opposite of cephalad)
superior	sŭ-pēr′ē-ŏr	above or upward
inferior	in-fēr′ē-ŏr	below or downward (opposite of superior)
anterior	an-tēr′ē-ŏr	toward the front of the body
posterior	pos-tēr′ē-ŏr	toward the back of the body (opposite of anterior)
ventral	ven′trăl	pertaining to the belly, front
dorsal	dōr′săl	pertaining to the back (opposite of ventral)
lateral	lat′ĕr-ăl	pertaining to the side
medial	mē′dē-ăl	pertaining to the middle (opposite of lateral)
unilateral	yū′ni-lat′ĕ-răl	pertaining to one side only
bilateral	bī-lat′ĕr-ăl	pertaining to both sides (opposite of unilateral)
proximal	prok′si-măl	closest to the trunk or attachment point
distal	dis′tăl	away from the trunk or attachment point (opposite of proximal)
superficial	sū′pĕr-fish′ăl	near the surface
deep	dēp	away from the surface (opposite of superficial)
anteroposterior	an′tĕr-ō-pos-tēr′ē-ŏr	from front (anterior) to back (posterior)

(continued)

Terms Related to Anatomic Directions, Positions, and Planes *(continued)*

Term	Pronunciation	Meaning
Positional Terms		
anatomic position	an'ă-tŏm'ik pŏ-zish'ŏn	body in standard reference position: standing erect, arms at the sides, palms facing forward **(Figure 3-6)**
decubitus	dē-kyū'bi-tŭs	lying down
dorsal recumbent	dōr'săl rē-kŭm'bĕnt	lying on back with legs bent and feet flat
Fowler position	fowl'ĕr pŏ-zish'ŏn	lying on back with head of bed raised 45 degrees
semirecumbent	sem'ē-rē-cŭm'bĕnt	synonymous with Fowler position
lateral recumbent	lat'ĕr-ăl rĕ-kŭm'bĕnt	lying on the side
prone	prōn	lying face down
supine	sū'pīn	lying face up
Body Planes (Figure 3-7)		
plane	plān	an imaginary surface that extends through two definite points
frontal plane	frŏn'tăl plān	vertical plane dividing the body into anterior and posterior halves
coronal plane	kōr'ŏ-năl plān	synonymous with frontal plane
sagittal plane	saj'i-tăl plān	vertical plane dividing the body into left and right halves
transverse plane	trans-vĕrs' plān	horizontal plane dividing the body into upper (superior) and lower (inferior) halves

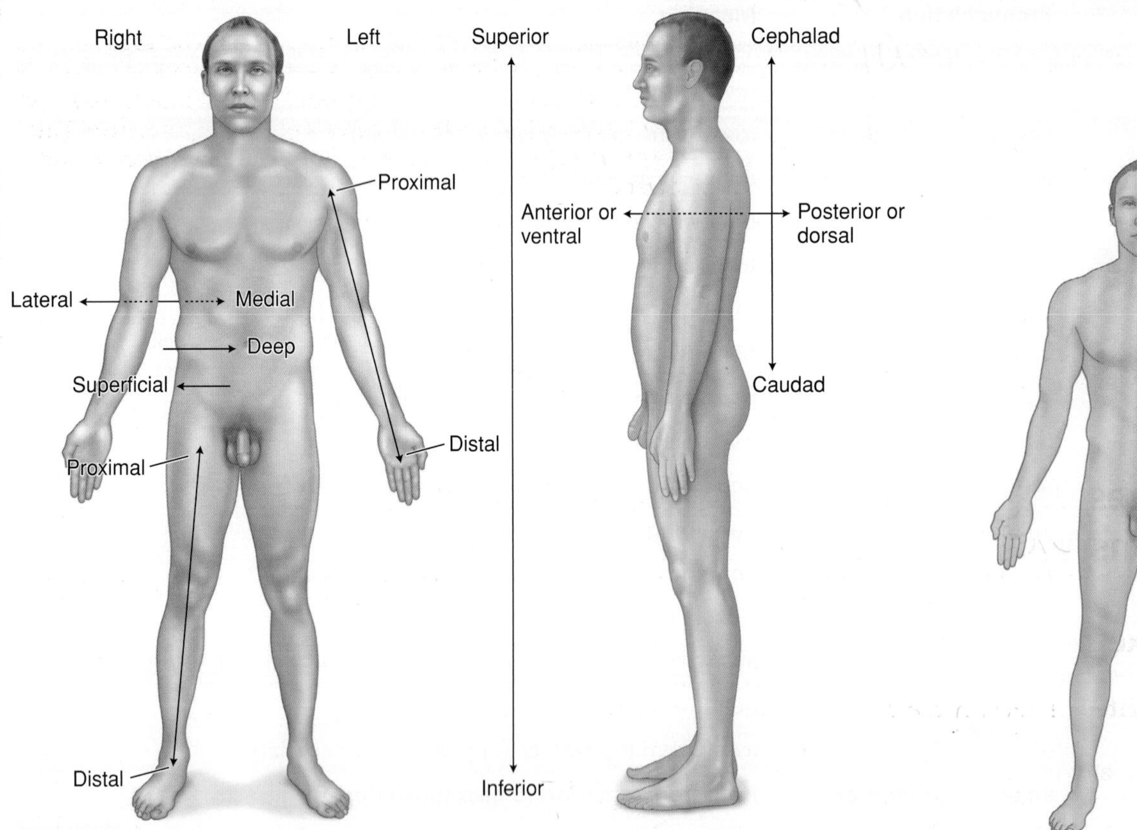

Figure 3-5 Directional terms describe the location of a body part in relationship to another.

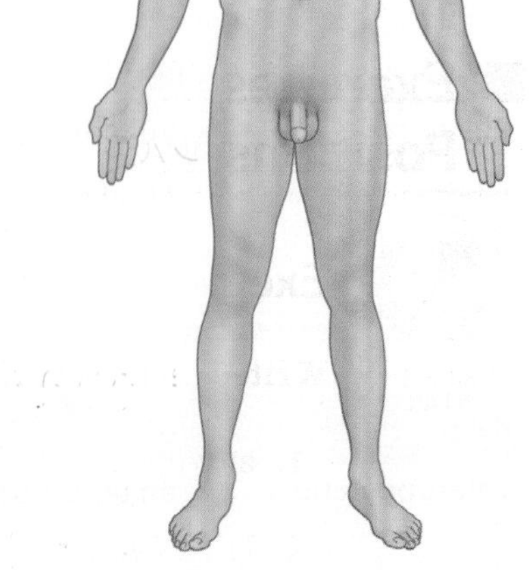

Figure 3-6 The anatomic position.

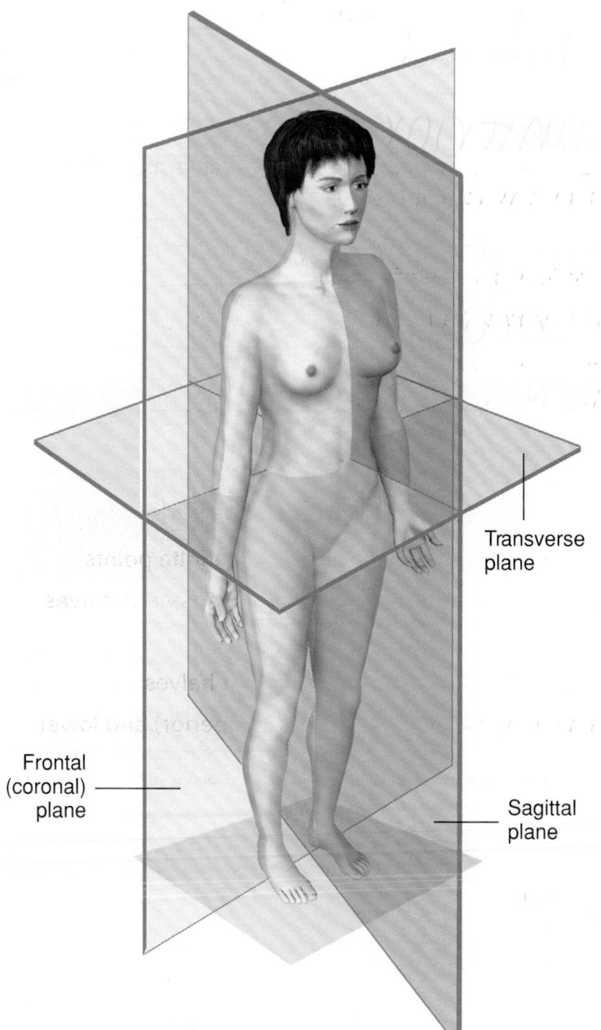

Figure 3-7 Body planes divide the body into halves in different ways for reference purposes. The frontal (coronal) plane divides the body into anterior and posterior halves. The sagittal plane divides the body into left and right halves. The transverse plane divides the body into upper (superior) and lower (inferior) halves.

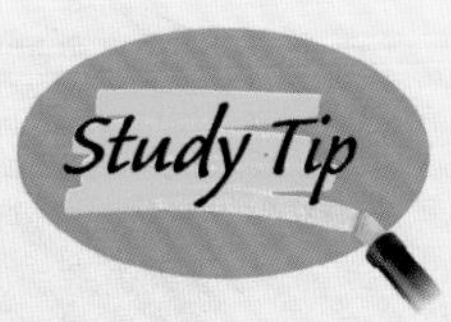

Planes of the Body: Think of a plane as an invisible, flat surface dividing parts of the body. The frontal and sagittal planes are positioned in a vertical (up and down) direction in relation to the body or parts of the body, whereas the transverse plane runs in a horizontal direction across the body.

Exercises: Terms Related to Anatomic Directions, Positions, and Planes

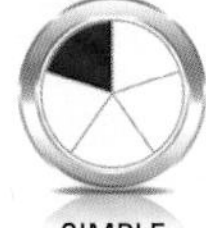

SIMPLE RECALL

Exercise 13

Write the correct medical term for the meaning given.

1. away from the trunk distal
2. lying face up supine
3. above or upward superior

4. near the surface superficial
5. pertaining to the side lateral
6. toward the front of the body anterior
7. from front to back anteroposterior
8. pertaining to the belly, front ventral
9. toward the head cephalad
10. lying on back with head of bed raised Fowler position

Exercise 14

SIMPLE RECALL

Write the meaning of the term given.

1. supine ______
2. inferior ______
3. frontal plane ______
4. proximal ______
5. caudad ______
6. transverse plane ______
7. bilateral ______
8. anatomic position ______
9. medial ______
10. dorsal ______

Exercise 15

ADVANCED RECALL

Complete each sentence by providing the correct medical term.

1. A patient in the lateral recumbent position is lying on his or her side.
2. The sagital plane divides the body vertically into left and right halves.
3. An internal organ that is away from the surface of the body is said to be ______.
4. A disease that affects only one side of the body is unilateral.
5. The opposite of anterior is posterior.
6. The ankle is located distal (away from the trunk) from the knee.
7. The palm is the ______ (front) surface of the hand.

8. The stomach is located superior (above) to the intestines.

9. The general term for lying down (not specifically face up or down) is decubitus.

10. The knee is located proximal (toward the trunk) to the ankle.

ANIMATION

View the animation "Terms Related to the Body as a Whole" on the Student Resources on thePoint for an in-depth overview of terminology related to direction and position, planes, positions, regions, and cavities.

COLORS

Many word parts indicate colors. For example, an erythrocyte is another term for a red blood cell; this term is derived from the word parts *erythro-* for red and *-cyte* for cell. This table lists some of the most common combining forms related to colors.

Combining Forms Related to Colors

Combining Form	Meaning
chlor/o	green
chrom/o	color
cyan/o	blue
erythr/o	red
leuk/o	white
melan/o	black, dark
xanth/o	yellow

Exercise: Combining Forms Related to Colors

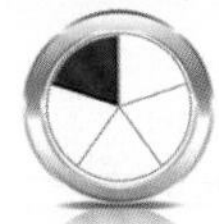
SIMPLE RECALL

Exercise 16

Write the meaning of the combining form given.

1. melan/o black/dark
2. cyan/o blue
3. xanth/o yellow
4. chlor/o green
5. leuk/o white
6. erythr/o red
7. chrom/o color

Terms Related to Colors

Term	Pronunciation	Meaning
chloroma	klōr-ō′mă	abnormal mass of green cells
chromaturia	krō′mă-tyūr′ē-ă	abnormal coloration of urine
cyanosis	sī′ă-nō′sis	bluish discoloration of the skin and other tissues
erythrocyte	ĕ-rith′rŏ-sīt	red blood cell
leukocyte	lū′kō-sīt	white blood cell
melanoma	mel′ă-nō′mă	tumor characterized by dark appearance
xanthoderma	zan′thō-dĕr′mă	yellow discoloration of the skin

■ Exercise: Terms Related to Colors

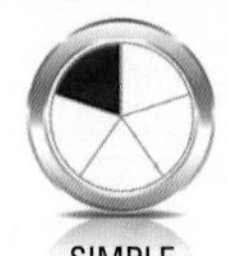
SIMPLE RECALL

Exercise 17

Write the correct medical term for the meaning given.

1. red blood cell — erythrocyte
2. yellow discoloration of skin — xanthoderma
3. tumor that is dark — melanoma
4. abnormal coloration of urine — Chromaturia
5. white blood cell — leukocyte
6. cyanosis — blue discoloration

■ INTRODUCTION TO MEDICAL RECORDS

In health care settings, medical terminology is used in both spoken and written communication. The primary form of written communication is the patient's medical record. Because you will likely encounter different types of medical records in your work, later chapters in this text frequently include medical records so that you can become familiar with the different formats and experience real-life uses of medical terminology.

The following are common types of medical records:

- **Hospital and clinic records,** sometimes simply called the patient's record, typically are collections of all written documents related to a patient's examination, diagnosis, and care.
- **History and physical (H&P) examinations** are a record of the patient's medical history. These may include forms the patient fills out and the health care provider's examination of the patient. This is usually a standardized report, because the examination is performed in a standard, systematic manner.
- **Consent forms** are signed by the patient to give permission for health care to be provided; these forms may include special forms for surgery and other procedures.

- **Health care provider patient care notes** are written into the patient record whenever a physician, nurse, or other health care provider gives the patient any form of care. Generally, health care providers document all diagnostic treatments and procedures along with observations, test results, and consultations with other specialists.
- **Laboratory and diagnostic test reports** may come from sources outside the primary care team, such as blood test results from an outside laboratory or a pathology report, or from another department within the health care facility.
- **Other specialty reports** include reports from other caregivers (such as a physical therapist or an anesthesiologist during surgery) and discharge reports when the patient leaves a hospital.

The following is a section of a follow-up note for a patient who has undergone treatment for lung cancer. As you read this record, underline all medical terms that you do not understand.

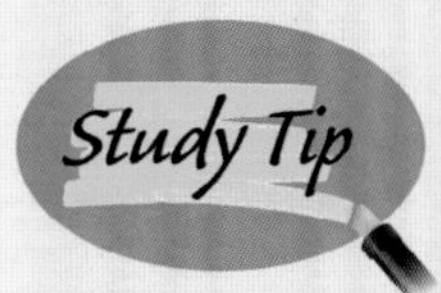

Reading Medical Records: When reading a medical record the first time, do not stop to puzzle out every new term you encounter. Instead, read the record all the way through to gain a general sense of its meaning. You will find it easier to understand specific terms once you are familiar with the overall context. If you are still unsure of some terms, however, consult your medical dictionary.

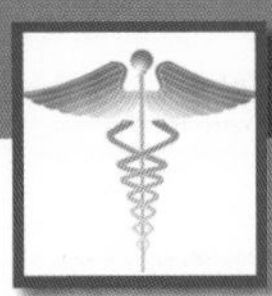

Medical Record

FOLLOW-UP NOTE

The patient is a 46-year-old white female with a diagnosis of stage IIB (T2, N1, M0) large cell carcinoma of the right upper lung lobe post right upper lobectomy. She received a course of postoperative radiation therapy directed to the mediastinum, receiving a total dose of 5,040 rads with completion of treatment on April 13, 20XX. She was last seen in follow-up on July 28, 20XX, and returns today for a routine four month follow-up. She was recently seen by Dr. Smith.

Chest x-ray was obtained on October 14, 20XX. This was compared with previous one of June 15, 20XX. The left lung remains completely clear. There is a slight increase in interstitial markings around the left hilar area. This is within the prior radiation therapy field. This most likely represents radiation-induced scarring.

She is feeling well overall. Her appetite has been good. She has occasional chest discomfort with occasional cough. She denies any pain referable to the thoracotomy site. She has no hemoptysis. She denies any bone pain. She has no bowel or bladder complaints. She remains active and is feeling well.

PHYSICAL EXAMINATION: Blood pressure is 110/74, pulse 72, and respirations 20. Weight is 153 lb, up 4½ lb since last being seen. Today on HEENT examination, extraocular movements are intact. Pupils are equal, round, and reactive to light and accommodation. Normocephalic. She has no palpable cervical, supraclavicular, axillary, or inguinal lymphadenopathy. The heart beats with a regular rate and rhythm. Lungs are clear to auscultation and percussion. The right thoracotomy incisional site is well healed. There are no palpable abnormalities. The abdomen is soft and nontender, with no mass or organomegaly. Extremities reveal no edema, cyanosis, or clubbing.

ASSESSMENT: We are pleased with the patient's condition with no evidence of recurrent, residual, or metastatic disease.

PLAN: She is scheduled to see Dr. Smith in January. We have asked her to return for routine follow-up in six months. We have requested a chest x-ray at that time. We will keep you informed of her progress.

Note: Many doctors do not write the appropriate units for tests, except for weight, because it is important to know pounds (lb) versus kilograms (kg).

Exercise: Medical Records

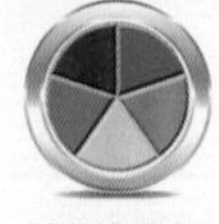
APPLICATION

Exercise 18

For each of the following medical terms used in this medical record, write the definition. Most of these terms are built from word parts used in this or the preceding chapters (or are provided here). Keep in mind that a term's meaning may not be precisely the sum of the meaning of its parts.

Term	Meaning
1. lobectomy (*lobos* = lobe of an organ)	______________
2. postoperative	______________
3. thoracotomy	______________
4. supraclavicular (*clavicular* = pertaining to the clavicle [collar bone])	______________
5. lymphadenopathy (lymph/o = lymph)	______________
6. organomegaly (organ/o = organ)	______________
7. cyanosis	______________

INTRODUCTION TO BODY SYSTEMS

A **body system** is a group of organs with related functions. It is also called an organ system. For example, the respiratory system includes the lungs and all the air passages from the nose and mouth to the lungs. The primary function of the respiratory system is the exchange of gases. We inhale (breathe in) oxygen from the air we breathe for delivery to our cells, and we exhale (breathe out) carbon dioxide, a waste product of cellular metabolism.

Human anatomy (structure of body parts) and disease are usually learned in relation to body systems. It helps to learn about different organs that work together with a related body system function rather than to study every organ by itself. Because many diseases affect single body systems, understanding health and health care by body system also makes sense. Since much medical terminology involves anatomy or health care by body systems, it also makes sense to learn medical terminology by body systems.

The main portion of this text is organized by body systems. Note that because many organs and body functions overlap, body systems can be organized in somewhat different ways. For example, the skeletal system (bones, ligaments) and the muscular system (muscles, tendons) work very closely together to move the body. Therefore, these systems are often combined as the musculoskeletal system. Similarly, because the lymph system drains into the cardiovascular system, these are often studied together. The following are the body systems covered in this text:

- Integumentary system (skin and related structures)
- Musculoskeletal system (muscles and bones)
- Nervous system (brain, spinal cord, and nerves)

- Special senses (eye, ear)
- Endocrine system (glands and hormones)
- Blood and immune system
- Cardiovascular and lymph systems (heart, blood vessels, and lymphatic vessels)
- Respiratory system (lungs and air passages)
- Digestive system (stomach, intestines, and related organs)
- Urinary system (kidneys, ureters, bladder, and urethra)
- Male reproductive system (penis, testes, and related structures)
- Female reproductive system (breasts, ovaries, uterus, vagina, and related structures)

Many diseases involve primarily one system, so medical specialties often focus on individual body systems. The following are a few examples:

- Dermatologists diagnose and treat skin conditions.
- Orthopedists diagnose and treat conditions of the musculoskeletal system.
- Neurologists diagnose and treat conditions of the nervous system.
- Endocrinologists diagnose and treat conditions of the endocrine system.

You will learn more about these medical specialties and the health conditions they care for in the chapters on specific body systems.

WRAPPING UP

- There are many terms used to describe body structures, show the levels of organization, and indicate color.
- The body can be divided by body cavities, abdominopelvic regions, and abdominopelvic quadrants.
- To orient the human body, we use anatomic directions, positions, and planes.
- Medical records come in many forms and provide valuable information.
- So far we have looked at terminology to describe any part of the body. The upcoming chapters will look at different body (organ) systems, which all function together to form the whole body.

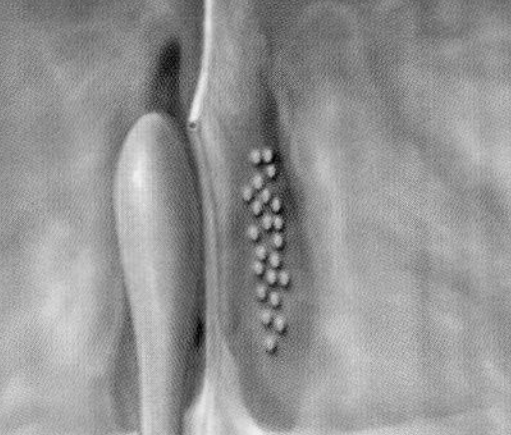

Chapter Review

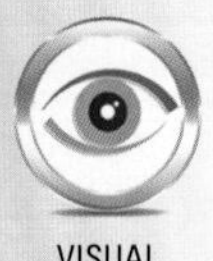

VISUAL

Exercise 19

Write the correct term for the body cavities and structure indicated.

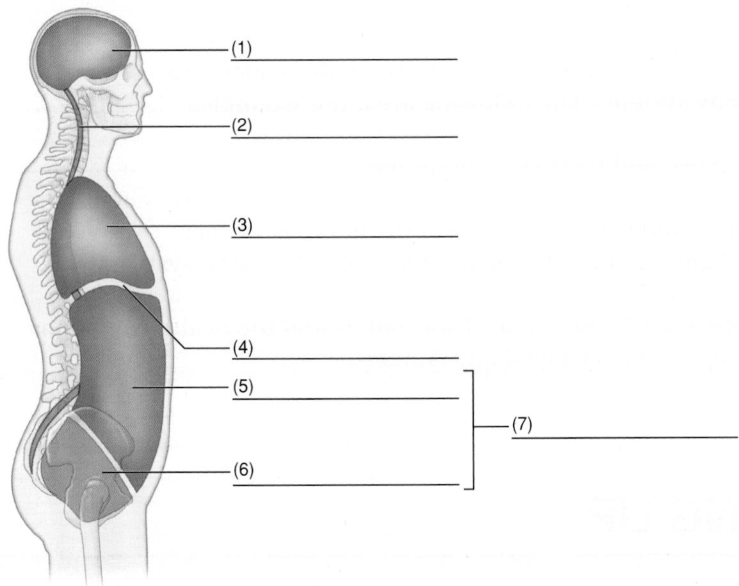

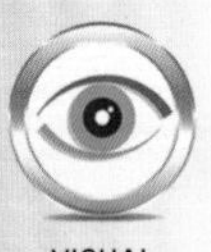

VISUAL

Exercise 20

Write the correct term for the abdominopelvic regions indicated.

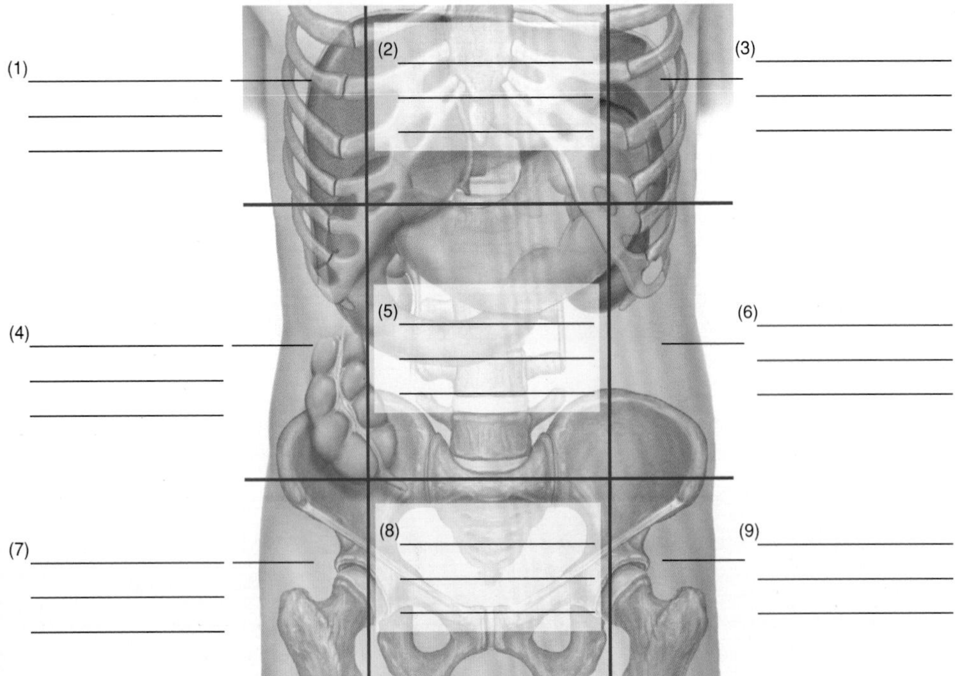

Understanding Term Structure

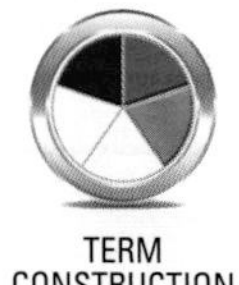
TERM CONSTRUCTION

Exercise 21

Break the given medical term into its word parts and define each part. Then define the medical term. (Note: You may need to use word parts from previous chapters.)

Example:

arthritis *word parts:* arthr/o, -itis
meanings: joint, inflammation
term meaning: inflammation of a joint

1. fibrosis *word parts:* ____________
meanings: ____________
term meaning: ____________

2. pathogenic *word parts:* ____________
meanings: ____________
term meaning: ____________

3. hemostasis *word parts:* ____________
meanings: ____________
term meaning: ____________

4. neuroblast *word parts:* ____________
meanings: ____________
term meaning: ____________

5. osteonecrosis *word parts:* ____________
meanings: ____________
term meaning: ____________

6. cervicobrachial *word parts:* ____________
meanings: ____________
term meaning: ____________

7. craniocerebral *word parts:* ____________
meanings: ____________
term meaning: ____________

8. superolateral — *word parts:* ______
meanings: ______
term meaning: ______

9. visceromegaly — *word parts:* ______
meanings: ______
term meaning: ______

10. hyperglycemia — *word parts:* ______
meanings: ______
term meaning: ______

Comprehension Exercises

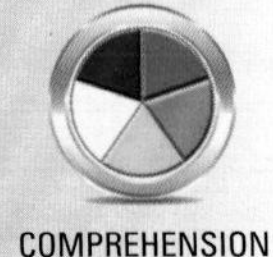
COMPREHENSION

Exercise 22

Fill in the blank with the correct term.

1. Excessive growth of tissue is termed ______.
2. Even if you do not recognize the term *acidosis,* from knowing the suffix -osis you can understand that this term likely refers to a(n) ______ condition.
3. Based on its two word parts, the term *morphology* means ______.
4. Based on its word parts, the term *lipemia* likely refers to ______.
5. After weeks of treatment, the patient no longer had symptoms. Although his chronic disease was still present, his physician said the disease was in ______.
6. The patient felt a sharp pain on the side of her abdomen, just left of her navel, in the ______ region.
7. The x-ray unit was positioned in front of the patient such that the x-rays passed through him in a(n) ______ direction.
8. The patient was lying supine in bed until the nurse raised the head of the bed 45 degrees to put the patient in the ______ position.
9. Because of a severe breathing problem, the patient was experiencing cyanosis, and her lips were turning ______. (color)
10. An increase in the severity of a disease or symptoms is called ______.

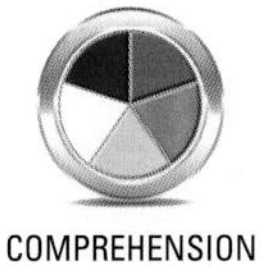
COMPREHENSION

Exercise 23

Write a short answer for each of the following.

1. When speaking of a skin lesion on the arm, describe the location of the most *proximal* edge of the lesion. ______

2. Describe the appearance of someone in the anatomic position. ______

3. What is a body system? ______

4. What part of a body cell is not considered part of the cytoplasm? ______

5. When is a disease considered *chronic*? ______

6. Strictly speaking, what does *etiology* mean? ______

7. Describe a body cavity. ______

8. Describe the *dorsal* surface of the hand. ______

9. Describe the appearance of someone with xanthoderma. ______

10. If an illness of the mind is called a psychic condition, what is an illness of the body called? ______

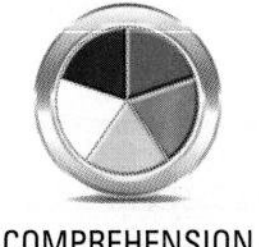
COMPREHENSION

Exercise 24

Circle the letter of the best answer to each of the following questions.

1. If the fluid taken into the body equals the fluid lost from the body, this balance can be described as a state of

   A. hyperplasia.
   B. homeostasis.
   C. necrosis.
   D. inflammation.

2. The lungs are located within the

   A. thoracic cavity.
   B. abdominal cavity.
   C. pelvic cavity.
   D. spinal cavity.

3. The abdominal region located inferior to (below) the umbilical region is the
   A. epigastric region.
   B. iliac region.
   C. hypochondriac region.
   D. hypogastric region.

4. After a stroke, the patient had partial paralysis of only his left side, a condition said to be
   A. idiopathic.
   B. sagittal.
   C. unilateral.
   D. metastatic.

5. The study of cells and tissues is called
   A. histology.
   B. etiology.
   C. cytology.
   D. morphology.

6. A xanthoma is generally what color?
   A. red
   B. yellow
   C. black
   D. blue

7. An *acute* illness is
   A. fatal.
   B. persistent.
   C. malignant.
   D. brief.

8. A toxin may cause symptoms throughout the body. Thus, it is said to have what kind of effects?
   A. metabolic
   B. idiopathic
   C. systemic
   D. inflammatory

9. Which of these terms may apply to an injury?
   A. cytoplasm
   B. hyperplasia
   C. proximal
   D. lesion

10. The diaphragm is a
   A. cavity.
   B. muscle.
   C. tumor.
   D. quadrant.

Application and Analysis

MEDICAL RECORD EXERCISE

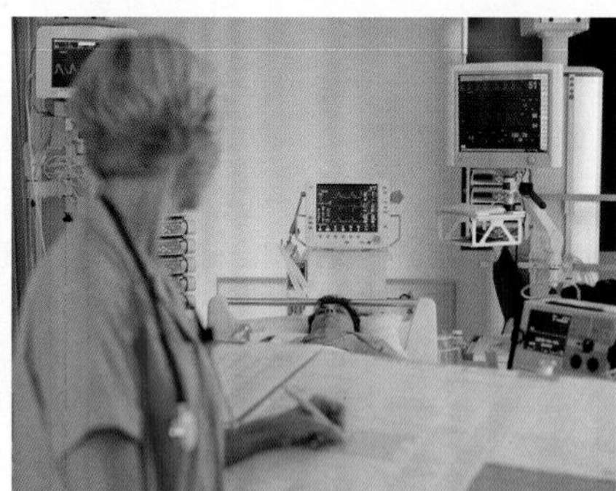

A registered nurse attends to a patient in the intensive care unit (ICU).

Following is the operative report for Mr. Stern, who has been diagnosed with bronchogenic carcinoma of the lung. As a registered nurse (RN) specializing in critical care, you are reviewing the patient's medical record to understand the procedure that was performed.

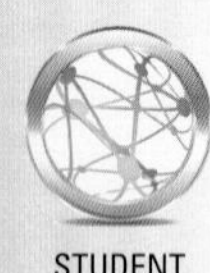

STUDENT RESOURCES

Learn more about careers in nursing and the other health professions highlighted in this text in the Additional Resources section of the Student Resources on thePoint.

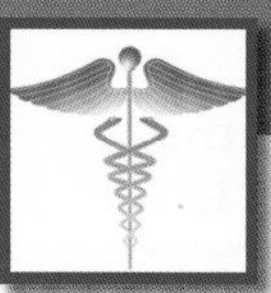

Medical Record

OPERATIVE REPORT

BRONCHOGENIC CARCINOMA EXCISION

PREOPERATIVE DIAGNOSIS: Solitary pulmonary nodule with bronchogenic carcinoma.

POSTOPERATIVE DIAGNOSIS: Solitary pulmonary nodule with bronchogenic carcinoma.

PROCEDURES PERFORMED

1. Bronchoscopy
2. Right thoracotomy
3. Lateral segmentectomy of right middle lobe, followed by completion of right middle lobectomy
4. Mediastinal lymphadenectomy

ANESTHESIA: General endotracheal

DESCRIPTION OF PROCEDURE: After successful induction of general endotracheal anesthesia, the patient was placed in the supine position and bronchoscopy was performed via the endotracheal tube. The left upper lingular lobes, right upper and lower lobes, were unremarkable. The bronchoscopy tube was well situated within the left main stem bronchus. Then the patient was positioned, prepped, and draped in the usual sterile fashion and underwent a right lateral thoracotomy.

The thorax was entered. The pleura was unremarkable. The lung was explored. There was a nodule present within the lateral segment of the right middle lobe. The dissection was carried down to the artery, which was doubly tied proximally and distally and divided, and this segment was then stapled off and sent for frozen section. The frozen section was consistent with a squamous cell carcinoma. Consequently, the lobectomy was completed, and lymph nodes were harvested.

A chest tube was brought out through a separate stab incision. The intercostal membranes were closed. The muscles, subcutaneous tissue, and skin were closed. A Dermabond dressing was applied. The chest tube was attached to drainage. The sponge, needle, and lap counts were correct ×3, and the patient was taken to the recovery room in stable condition.

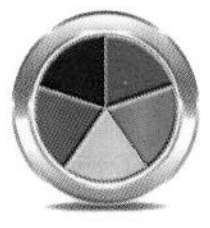

APPLICATION

Exercise 25

Write the appropriate medical terms used in this medical record on the blanks after their definitions. You should be able to identify these terms based on word parts included in this or the preceding chapters.

1. pertaining to the lungs ____________________
2. incision into the thorax ____________________
3. surgical removal of a lobe ____________________
4. pertaining to the side ____________________
5. closest to the trunk or attachment point ____________________
6. away from the trunk or attachment point ____________________

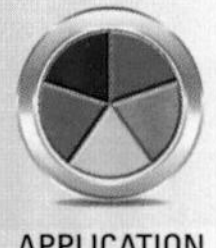
APPLICATION

Exercise 26

Write the appropriate medical terms used in this medical record on the blanks after their definitions. The meaning of new combining forms is provided to help you build medical terms that may be new to you.

1. originating in the bronchus (bronch/o) ______________
2. surgical removal of a segment ______________
3. surgical removal of lymph nodes ______________
4. within the trachea (trache/o) ______________
5. examination by instrument inside the bronchus (bronch/o) ______________
6. between the ribs (cost/o) ______________
7. beneath the skin (cutane/o) ______________

Pronunciation and Spelling

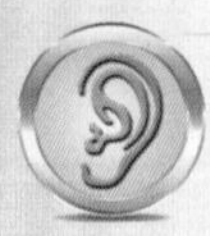
AUDITORY

Exercise 27

Review the Chapter 3 terms in the Dictionary/Audio Glossary in the Student Resources on thePoint, and practice pronouncing each term, referring to the pronunciation guide as needed.

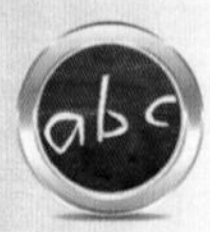
SPELLING

Exercise 28

Circle the correctly spelled term.

1. chromosome	chromosone	chronosome
2. diafragm	diaphragm	diphragm
3. homostasis	homeostesis	homeostasis
4. cepholad	cephalad	cepadad
5. cytoplasm	cyteplasm	cyteplazm
6. erythrocyte	erthrocyte	erythracyte
7. decubitus	decubetus	decubitous
8. umbilical	umbillical	umobilical
9. pathegen	pathogen	pathagen
10. luekocyte	lukeocyte	leukocyte
11. inflamation	inflammation	enflamation

12. citology	cytology	cytolagy
13. matabolism	matebolism	metabolism
14. cyenosis	cyanosis	cyonasis
15. nuclei	nucli	nuklei

Media Connection

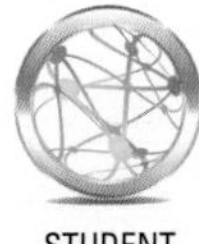
STUDENT RESOURCES

Exercise 29

Complete each of the following activities available with the Student Resources on thePoint. Check off each activity as you complete it, and record your score for the Chapter Quiz in the space provided.

Chapter Exercises

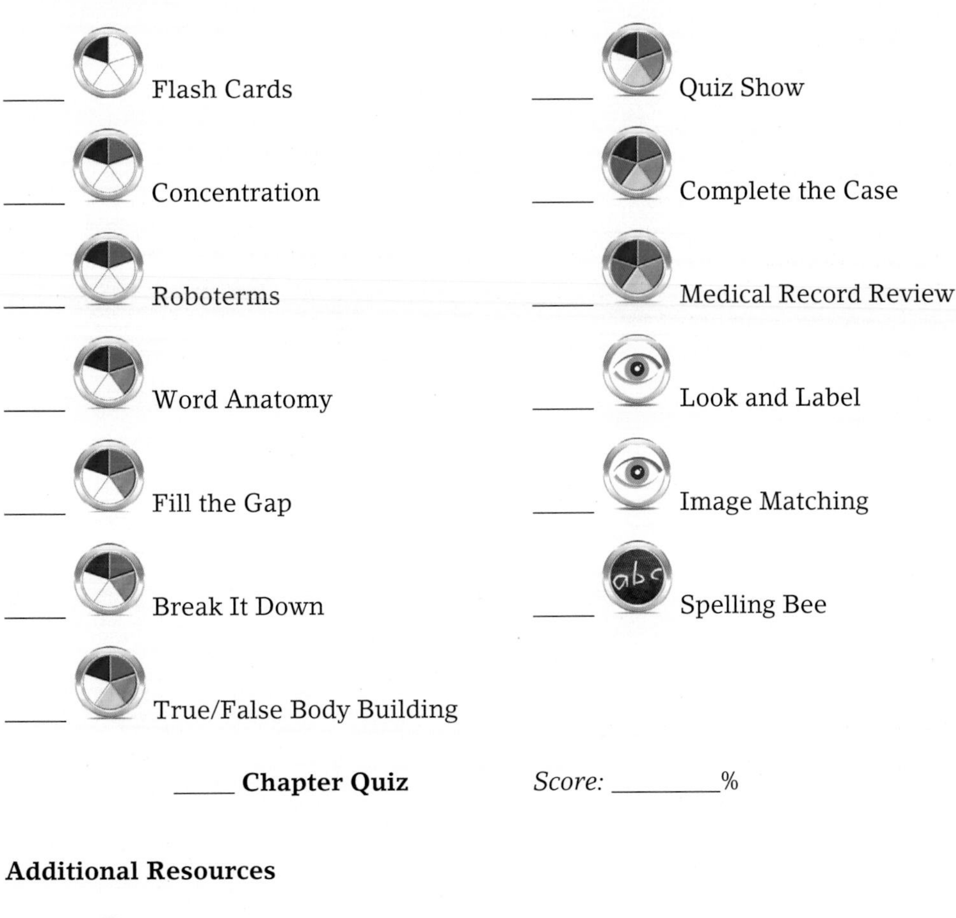

____ Flash Cards

____ Concentration

____ Roboterms

____ Word Anatomy

____ Fill the Gap

____ Break It Down

____ True/False Body Building

____ Quiz Show

____ Complete the Case

____ Medical Record Review

____ Look and Label

____ Image Matching

____ Spelling Bee

____ **Chapter Quiz** *Score:* ________%

Additional Resources

____ Animation: Terms Related to the Body as a Whole

____ Dictionary/Audio Glossary

____ Health Professions Careers: Registered Nurse

Integumentary System

4

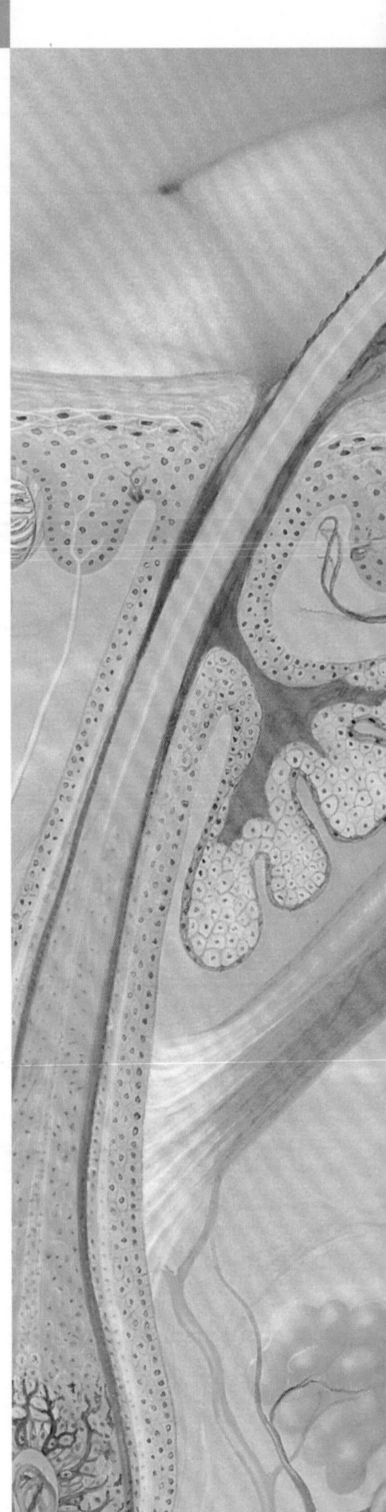

Chapter Outline

Introduction, 72

Anatomy and Physiology, 72
- Structures, 72
- Functions, 72
- Terms Related to the Integumentary System, 72

Word Parts, 75
- Combining Forms, 75
- Prefixes, 75
- Suffixes, 76

Medical Terms, 80
- Adjectives and Other Related Terms, 80
- Medical Conditions, 82
- Tests and Procedures, 90
- Surgical Interventions and Therapeutic Procedures, 91
- Medications and Drug Therapies, 94
- Specialties and Specialists, 94
- Abbreviations, 95

SOAP Notes, 96

Wrapping Up, 96

Chapter Review, 97

Learning Outcomes

After completing this chapter, you should be able to:

1. List the structures and functions of the skin.
2. Define terms related to the layers and the accessory structures of the skin.
3. Define combining forms, prefixes, and suffixes related to the integumentary system.
4. Define common medical terminology related to the integumentary system, including adjectives and related terms; signs, symptoms, and medical conditions; tests and procedures; surgical interventions and therapeutic procedures; medications and drug therapies; and medical specialties and specialists.
5. Define common abbreviations related to the integumentary system.
6. Successfully complete all chapter exercises.
7. Explain terms used in case studies and medical records involving the integumentary system.
8. Successfully complete all exercises included with the companion Student Resources on thePoint.

INTRODUCTION

The skin, sometimes called the **cutaneous membrane** or **integument**, is a protective covering. *Cutaneous* means relating to the skin. Consisting of two layers, an outer epidermis and an inner dermis, the skin is the body's first line of defense against environmental hazards, such as bacteria and viruses. The **integumentary system** includes the skin and its accessory structures. This chapter covers the anatomy and physiology of the skin, word parts related to the skin, and medical terms associated with the integumentary system.

ANATOMY AND PHYSIOLOGY

The skin is considered an organ because two or more tissues combine to perform specialized functions. Epithelial tissue and connective tissue are the two main types of tissue that make up the skin.

Structures

- The skin is the largest organ in the body.
- The skin is composed of two layers: the outer epidermis and the layer beneath the epidermis called the dermis.
- The accessory structures of the integumentary system are the hair, nails, sudoriferous glands (sweat glands), and sebaceous glands (oil glands).

Functions

- Protecting the body from harmful microorganisms
- Protecting underlying structures from the harmful effects of ultraviolet (UV) radiation
- Protecting the body from dehydration
- Producing vitamin D
- Regulating body temperature
- Housing sensory nerve endings

Terms Related to the Integumentary System (Figure 4-1)

Term	Pronunciation	Meaning
		Layers of the Skin
epidermis	ep'i-dĕrm'is	outer layer of skin; waterproof layer that functions as protection and contains melanocytes that secrete melanin
dermis	dĕr'mis	deep layer of skin that contains the sweat and oil glands; also contains tiny muscles attached to the hair follicles
subcutaneous layer	sŭb'kyū-tā'nē-ŭs lā'ĕr	layer of loose connective tissue that connects the skin to the surface muscles; contains the blood vessels and fat; also called the hypodermis

Terms Related to the Integumentary System

Term	Pronunciation	Meaning
Accessory Structures		
adipocytes	ad′i-pō-sītz	fat cells that make up most of the subcutaneous layer
arrector pili muscles	ă-rek′tŏr pī′lī	tiny muscles that attach to the hair follicle

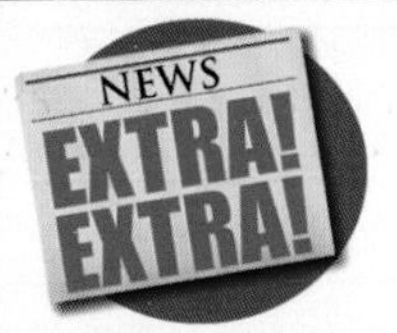

ARRECTOR PILI MUSCLES Goose bumps are made when the arrector pili muscles contract, an action that causes the hair to stand straight up.

Term	Pronunciation	Meaning
hair	hār	keratinized fibers that arise from hair follicles
hair follicle	hār fol′i-kĕl	area from which hair grows; located in the dermis
keratin	ker′ă-tin	protein found in the hair and nails that promotes hardness
keratinocytes	ke-rat′i-nō-sītz	cells found in the epidermal layer of skin that secrete keratin and assist in waterproofing the body
melanocytes	mel′ă-nō-sītz	cells that give color to skin, eyes, and hair by secreting the pigment melanin; located in the dermis
nail	nāl	translucent plate made of keratin that covers and protects the ends of the fingers and toes
sebaceous glands	sĕ-bā′shŭs	glands that secrete oil (sebum) into the hair follicle and onto the epidermis
sebum	sē′bŭm	oily secretion of the sebaceous gland
sudoriferous glands	sū′dōr-if′ĕr-ŭs	glands that secrete sweat and assist in body temperature regulation

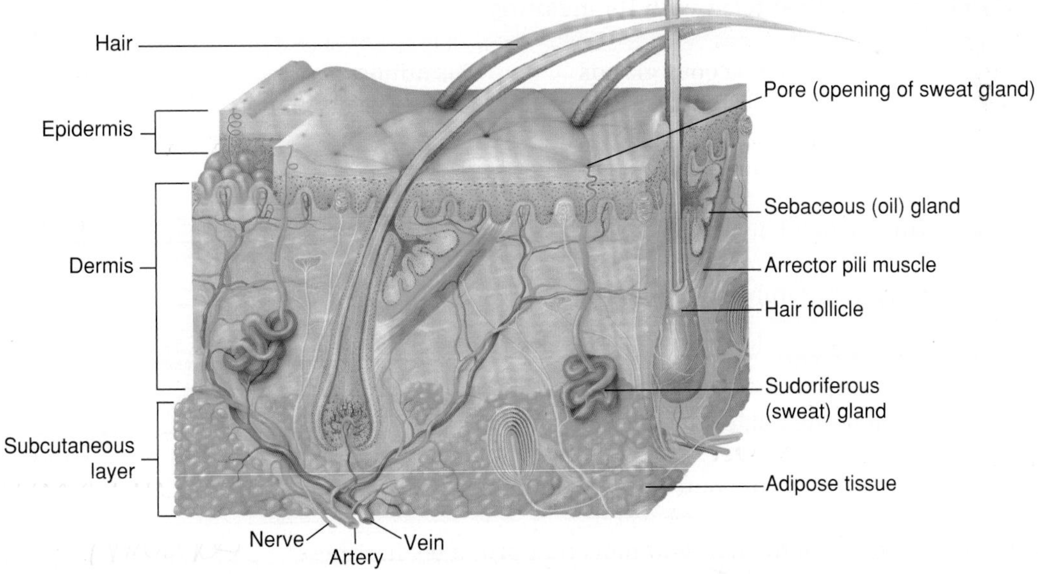

Figure 4-1 Layers of the skin and accessory structures.

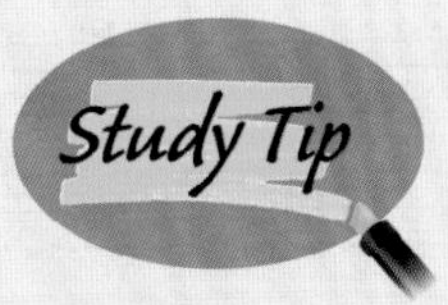

Epidermis: Remember that the prefix *epi-* means upon or on; therefore, the epidermis is the layer of skin on top of the dermis.

Exercises: Anatomy and Physiology

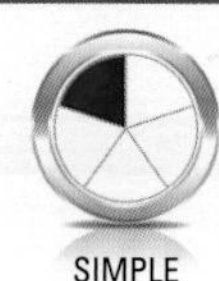

SIMPLE RECALL

Exercise 1

Write the correct anatomic structure or related term for the meaning given.

1. outer layer of skin that contains melanocytes epidermis
2. sweat glands sudoriferous glands
3. largest organ of the body skin
4. oil glands sebaceous glands
5. skin layer that contains blood vessels subcutaneous
6. tiny muscle attached to the hair follicle arrector pili muscles
7. deep layer of the skin dermis
8. skin layer that provides protection epidermis
9. keratinized fibers hair
10. oily secretion of the sebaceous gland sebum

ADVANCED RECALL

Exercise 2

Match each medical term with its meaning.

adipocytes	sebaceous glands	keratinocytes	nail
keratin	hair follicle	sudoriferous glands	melanocytes

1. translucent plate made of keratin nail
2. area from which hair grows hair follicle
3. assist in temperature regulation sudoriferous glands
4. give skin its color melanocytes
5. secrete oil to the epidermal layer of skin sebaceous glands
6. cells that make up the outermost layer of skin keratinocytes
7. protein found in the hair and nails that promotes hardness keratin
8. fat cells that make up most of the subcutaneous layer adipocytes

WORD PARTS

The following tables list word parts related to the integumentary system.

Combining Forms

Combining Form	Meaning
adip/o	fat
cry/o	cold
cyan/o	blue
derm/o, dermat/o, cutane/o	skin
electr/o	electric, electricity
erythr/o	red
hidr/o	sweat
kerat/o	hard
lip/o	fat
melan/o	black, dark
myc/o	fungus
necr/o	death
onych/o	nail
pachy/o	thick
py/o	pus
rhytid/o	wrinkle
scler/o	hard
seb/o	sebum (an oily secretion)
trich/o	hair
xanth/o	yellow
xer/o	dry

Prefixes

Prefix	Meaning
a-, an-	without, not
bio-	life
epi-	on, following
intra-	within
para-	beside
per-	through
sub-	below, beneath
trans-	across, through

Suffixes

Suffix	Meaning
-cide	substance that kills
-derma	skin
-ectomy	excision, surgical removal
-genic	originating, producing
-itis	inflammation
-logist	one who specializes in
-logy	study of
-malacia	softening
-pathy	disease
-phagia	eating
-plasia	formation, growth
-plasty	surgical repair, reconstruction
-rrhea	flowing, discharge
-tome	cutting instrument

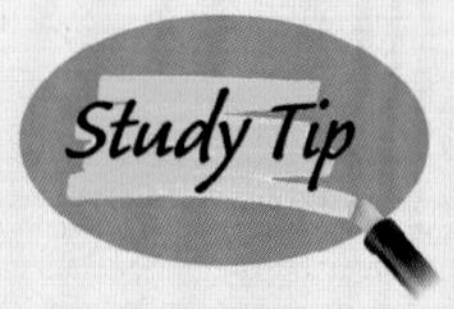

Spelling: Remember the difference between *hidr/o* and *hydr/o. Hidr/o* is the combining form that means sweat, as in hidroschesis (suppression of sweating). *Hydr/o* is the combining form that means water, as in fire hydrant.

Exercises: Word Parts

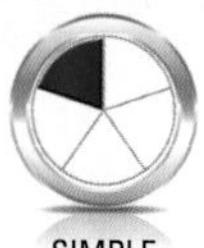

SIMPLE RECALL

Exercise 3

Write the meaning of the combining form given.

1. trich/o hair
2. rhytid/o wrinkle
3. onych/o nail
4. cutane/o ______
5. lip/o fat
6. seb/o sebum
7. xer/o dry
8. dermat/o skin

9. scler/o hard

10. erythr/o red

11. hidr/o sweat

12. cry/o cold

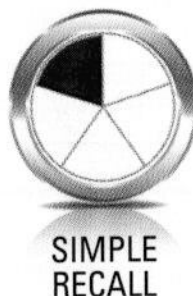

SIMPLE RECALL

Exercise 4

Write the correct combining form for the meaning given.

1. yellow xanth/o
2. sebum seb/o
3. blue cyan/o
4. skin derm/o
5. electric electr/o
6. red erythr/o
7. thick pachy/o
8. pus py/o
9. fungus myc/o
10. black, dark melan/o
11. death necr/o
12. sweat hidr/o
13. hard kerat/o

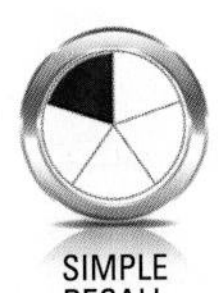

SIMPLE RECALL

Exercise 5

Write the meaning of the prefix or suffix given.

1. -malacia softening
2. sub- below
3. -pathy disease
4. -itis inflamation
5. per- through
6. para- beside

7. -tome cutting instrument

8. -phagia eating

9. intra- within

10. -rrhea discharge

11. trans- through

12. -plasia formation

13. bio- life

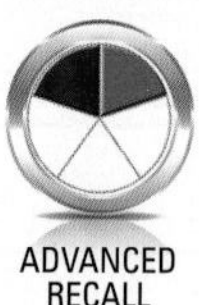

ADVANCED RECALL

Exercise 6

Considering the meanings of the word parts from which the medical terms are made, and write the meanings of the medical terms given. (You have not yet learned many of these terms but can build their meanings from the word parts.)

Combining Form	Meaning	Medical Term	Meaning of Term
dermat/o	skin	dermatitis	1. skin inflammation
py/o	pus	pyorrhea	2. pus discharge
myc/o	fungus	mycology	3. study of fungus
hidr/o	sweat	hidrosis	4. sweat abnormal condition
onych/o	nail	onychectomy	5. surgical removal of nail

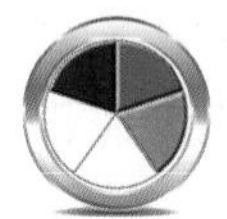

TERM CONSTRUCTION

Exercise 7

Given their meanings, build a medical term from an appropriate combining form and suffix.

Use Combining Form for	Use Suffix for	Term
dry	skin condition	1. xeroderma
skin	cutting instrument	2. dermatome
skin	one who specializes in	3. dermatologist
wrinkle	surgical repair, reconstruction	4. rhytidoplasty
death	abnormal condition	5. necrosis
nail	softening	6. onychomalacia
black, dark	cell	7. melanocyte

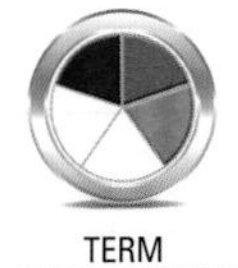
TERM CONSTRUCTION

Exercise 8

Break the given medical term into its word parts and define each part. Then define the medical term.

For example:

dermatitis	*word parts:*	dermat/o, -itis
	meanings:	skin, inflammation
	word meaning:	inflammation of the skin

1. anhidrosis	*word parts:*	______
	meanings:	______
	term meaning:	______
2. erythroderma	*word parts:*	______
	meanings:	______
	term meaning:	______
3. scleroderma	*word parts:*	______
	meanings:	______
	term meaning:	______
4. seborrhea	*word parts:*	______
	meanings:	______
	term meaning:	______
5. onychophagia	*word parts:*	______
	meanings:	______
	term meaning:	______
6. rhytidectomy	*word parts:*	______
	meanings:	______
	term meaning:	______
7. transdermal	*word parts:*	______
	meanings:	______
	term meaning:	______
8. epidermal	*word parts:*	______
	meanings:	______
	term meaning:	______

9. subcutaneous *word parts:* ______

meanings: ______

term meaning: ______

10. mycosis *word parts:* ______

meanings: ______

term meaning: ______

11. keratogenic *word parts:* ______

meanings: ______

term meaning: ______

■ MEDICAL TERMS

The following table gives adjective forms and terms used to describe the skin and its conditions.

Adjectives and Other Related Terms

Term	Pronunciation	Meaning
adipose	ad′i-pōs	fat, fatty
atypical	ā-tip′i-kăl	unusual
circumscribed	sĭr′kŭm-skrībd	contained to a specific area
cyanosis	sī′ă-nō′sis	blue discoloration of the skin and other tissues
diaphoresis	dī′ă-fŏr-ē′sis	profuse sweating
dysplasia	dis-plā′zē-ă	abnormal growth of tissue
erythematous	er′i-them′ă-tŭs	condition of being red
eschar	es′kahr	blackened area of burned tissue
exfoliation	eks′fō-lē-ā′shŭn	shedding of dead skin cells
hyperplasia	hī′pĕr-plā′zē-ă	excessive growth of tissue
indurated	in′dūr-ā-tĕd	pertaining to an area of hardened tissue
integumentary	in-teg′yū-men′tăr-ē	pertaining to the skin and accessory structures
pallor	pal′ŏr	abnormally pale skin coloration
pruritic	prūr-it′ik	pertaining to itching
purulent	pyūr′ū-lĕnt	containing pus
sebaceous	sĕ-bā′shŭs	pertaining to sebum
sudoriferous	sū′dōr-if′ĕr-ŭs	pertaining to sweat
turgor	tŭr′gŏr	state of turgidity (fullness) of cells due to fluid absorption

Exercises: Adjectives and Other Related Terms

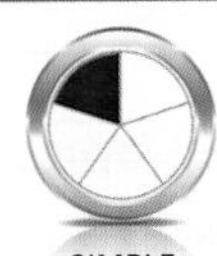
SIMPLE RECALL

Exercise 9

Write the correct medical term for the meaning given.

1. excessive growth of tissue hyperplasia
2. unusual atypical
3. containing pus purulent
4. pertaining to an area of hard tissue indurated
5. pertaining to the skin and accessory structures integumentary
6. abnormal growth of tissue dysplasia
7. contained in a specific area circumscribed
8. fat, fatty adipose

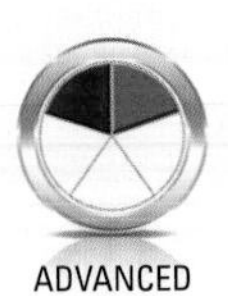
ADVANCED RECALL

Exercise 10

Circle the term that is most appropriate for the meaning of the sentence.

1. After working in the bright sun all day without applying sunscreen, Mr. Lee noticed his (*eschar, cyanosis, erythematous*) skin.
2. The physician diagnosed Mrs. Diaz with dehydration, which can lead to loss of skin fullness or (*turgor, pallor, hyperplasia*).
3. The patient's (*erythematous, pallor, cyanosis*), a bluish discoloring of the skin, was likely caused by lack of oxygenated blood to the body's peripheral areas.
4. Mrs. Davis was seen in the physician's office for extreme fatigue and (*eschar, pallor, turgor*), which is abnormally pale skin.
5. The dermatologist informed the patient that (*indurated, exfoliation, diaphoresis*) is the process of ridding the skin's surface of dead cells.
6. The deeply burned area on Mr. Botta's arm developed a thick black layer of dead tissue known as (*necrosis, eschar, purulent*).
7. The poison ivy patch that Mr. DeCostas stumbled into caused his skin to become (*sebaceous, pruritic, indurated*).
8. The physician explained that, along with chest pain, nausea, and vomiting, another sign of a possible heart attack is profuse sweating, known medically as (*dysplasia, exfoliation, diaphoresis*).

Medical Conditions

Term	Pronunciation	Meaning
abrasion	ă-brā′zhŭn	injury resulting in removal or disturbance of the superficial layer of the skin
abscess	ab′ses	a circumscribed collection of pus caused by a bacterial infection
acne	ak′nē	inflammatory disease of sebaceous glands and hair follicles marked by papules (pimples) and pustules (pimples with pus)
albinism	al′bi-nizm	a group of inherited disorders with deficiency of pigment in the skin, hair, and eyes **(Figure 4-2)**
burn	bŭrn	injury to the skin caused by heat or other means **(Figure 4-3)**
superficial burn	sū′pĕr-fish′ăl bŭrn	a burn involving only the epidermis; causes redness and swelling but no blisters (e.g., most cases of sunburn); commonly called a first-degree burn
partial-thickness burn	pahr′shăl-thik′nĕs bŭrn	a burn involving the epidermis and dermis; usually involves blisters; commonly called a second-degree burn
full-thickness burn	ful-thik′nĕs bŭrn	a burn involving destruction of the entire skin; extends into subcutaneous fat, muscle, and/or bone and often causes severe scarring; commonly called a third-degree burn
carbuncle	kahr′bŭng-kĕl	collection of large localized abscesses usually arising in hair follicles and typically infected with staphylococcus bacteria
cellulitis	sel′yū-lī′tis	inflammation of the subcutaneous connective tissue **(Figure 4-4)**
cicatrix	sik′ă-triks	the fibrous tissue replacing normal tissues destroyed by disease or injury; commonly called a scar
comedo	kom′ĕ-dō	a plug of sebum in the hair follicle that becomes darkened; commonly called a blackhead

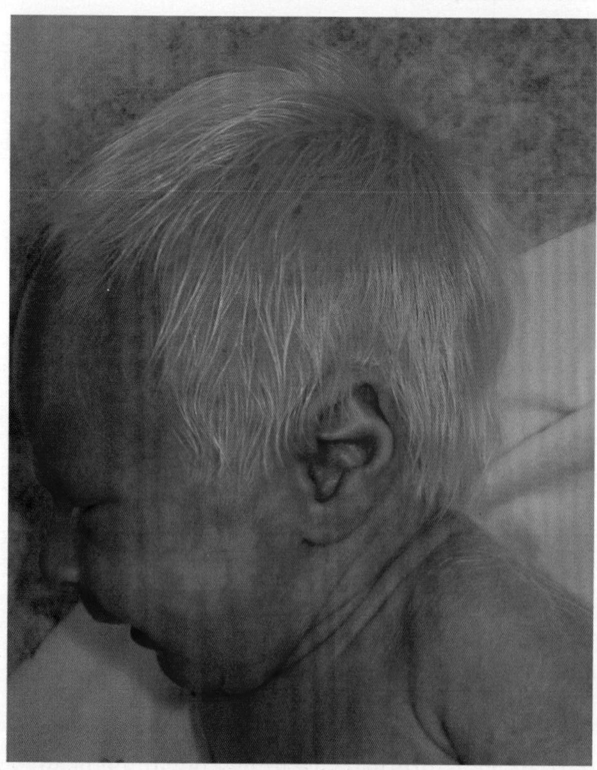

Figure 4-2 Albinism.

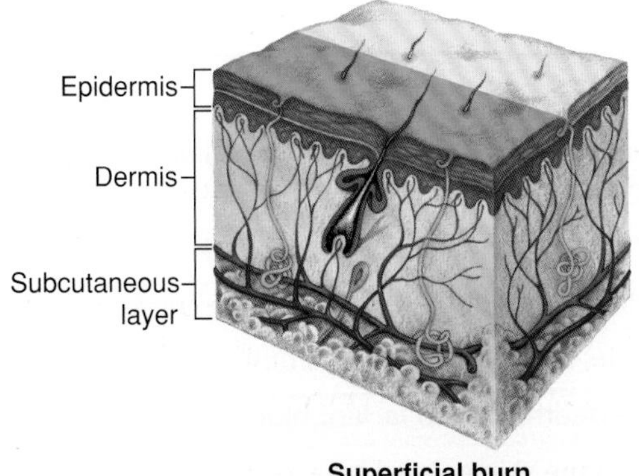

Superficial burn

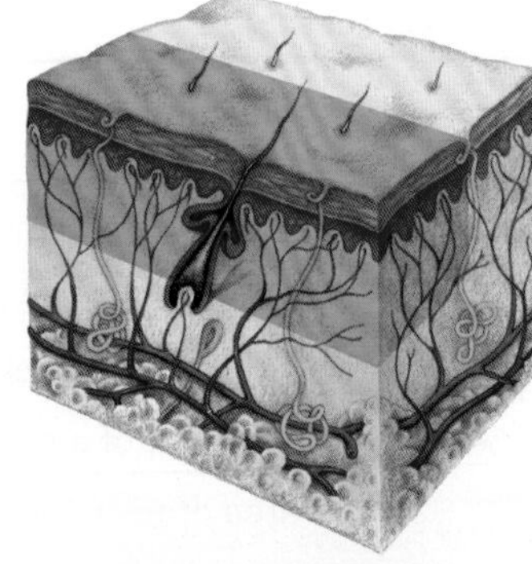

Partial-thickness burn

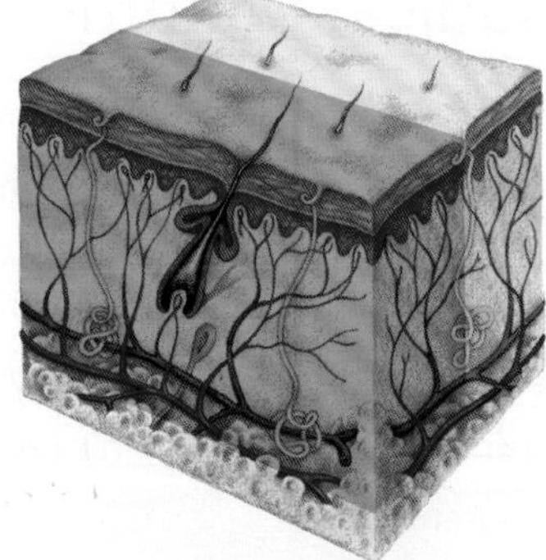

Full-thickness burn (after skin graft)

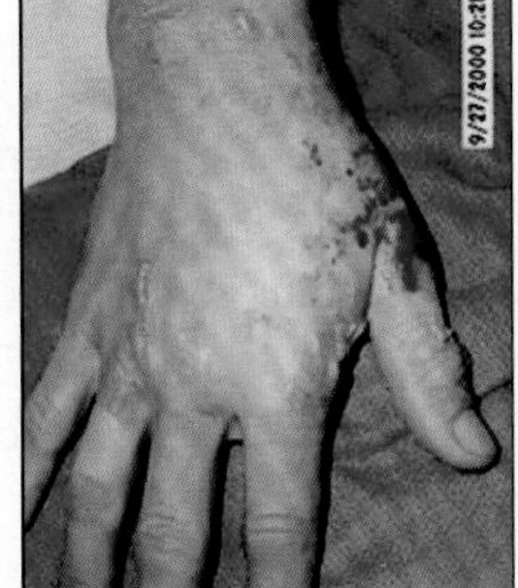

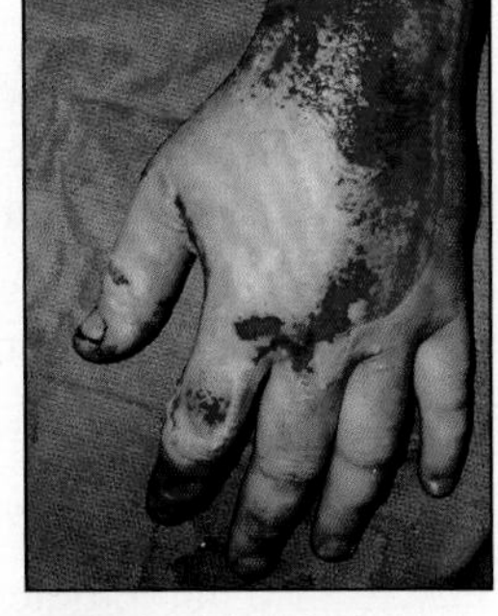

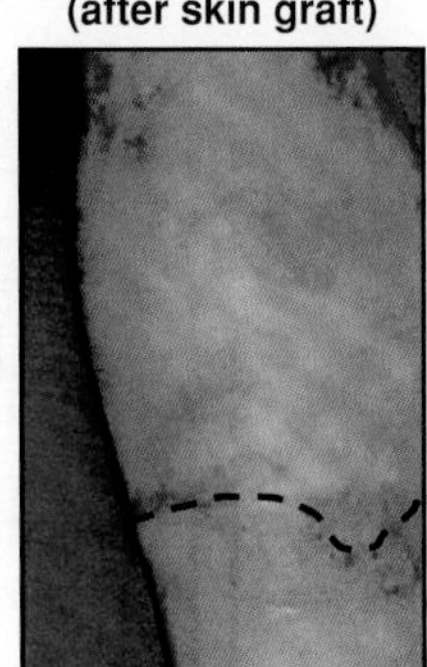

Figure 4-3 Degrees of burns.

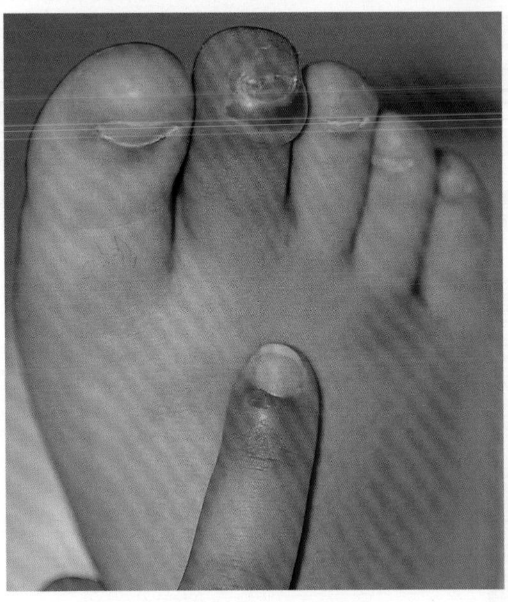

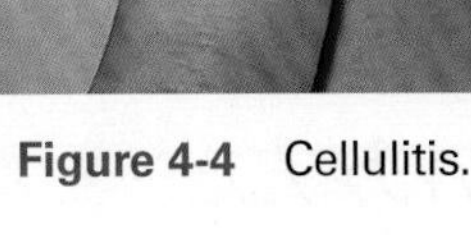

Figure 4-4 Cellulitis.

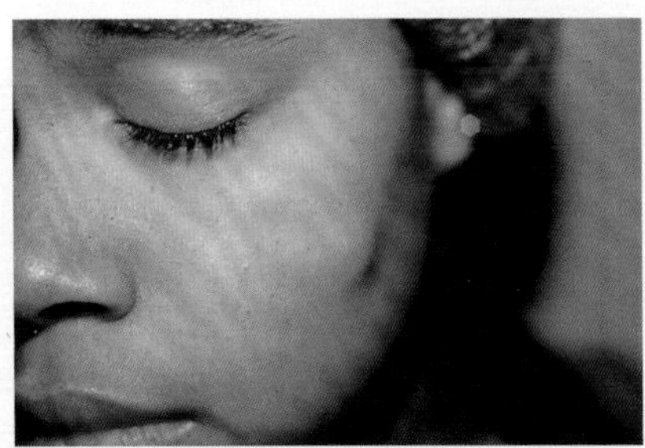

Figure 4-5 Cyst.

Medical Conditions

Term	Pronunciation	Meaning
contusion	kŏn-tū'zhŭn	injury producing discoloration and swelling without causing a break in the skin; commonly called a bruise
cyst	sist	a closed sac that contains liquid or semisolid material **(Figure 4-5)**
decubitus ulcer	dē-kyū'bi-tŭs ŭl'sĕr	a pressure sore of the skin and underlying tissues; commonly called a bedsore (see later **Figure 4-27**)
dermatome	der'mă-tōm	area of skin supplied by peripheral nerves

(continued)

Medical Conditions *(continued)*

Term	Pronunciation	Meaning
eczema	ek'sĕ-mă	inflammatory condition causing patchy redness, scales, blisters, itchiness, and burning **(Figure 4-6)**
excoriation	eks-kōr'ē-ā'shŭn	a scratch mark on the skin
fissure	fish'ŭr	a deep furrow, cleft, slit, or tear in the skin **(Figure 4-7)**
furuncle	fŭr-ŭng'kĕl	infection of a hair follicle; commonly called a boil
gangrene	gang'-grēn	area of necrosis (tissue death) due to lack of blood flow
herpes simplex	her'pēz sim'pleks	an eruption of blisters on the skin caused by a local infection of the herpes virus; known as cold sores when they appear on the lips
herpes zoster	hĕr'pēz zos'tĕr	an infection caused by the herpesvirus (varicella-zoster virus) characterized by an eruption of blisters that follows the course of affected peripheral nerves (dermatomes); commonly called shingles **(Figure 4-8)**
impetigo	im-pĕ-tī'gō	a contagious bacterial skin infection typically occurring on the face in children **(Figure 4-9)**
jaundice	jawn'dis	abnormal yellowing of the skin caused by bile accumulation
keloid	kē'loyd	an overgrowth of scar tissue **(Figure 4-10)**
lesion	lē'zhŭn	a pathologic change in tissue resulting from disease or injury
macula	mak'yū-lă	a small, flat discolored spot on the skin (see later **Figure 4-25**)
nevus	nē'vŭs	a birthmark or mole on the skin, especially one that is raised and red colored
nodule	nod'jūl	solid raised area located in any layer of the skin **(Figure 4-11)**
papule	pap'yūl	a small, raised, solid circumscribed area of the skin **(Figure 4-12)**
paronychia	par-ō-nik'ē-ă	inflammation and infection around the nail due to bacteria or fungi **(Figure 4-13)**

(continued)

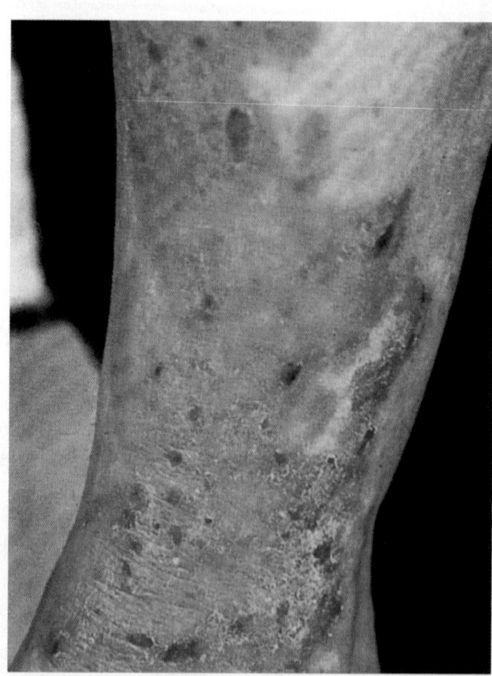

Figure 4-6 Eczema.

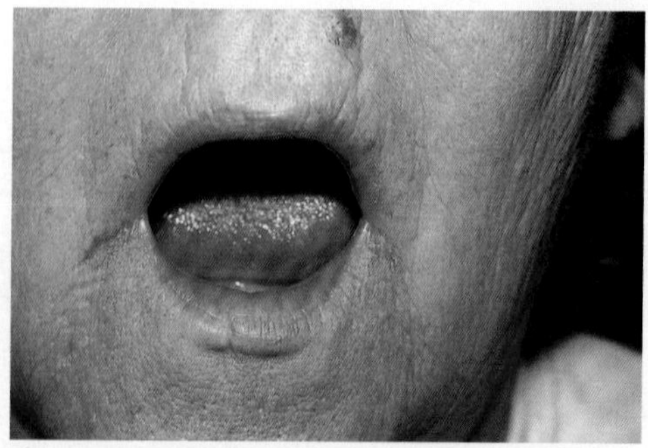

Figure 4-7 Fissure.

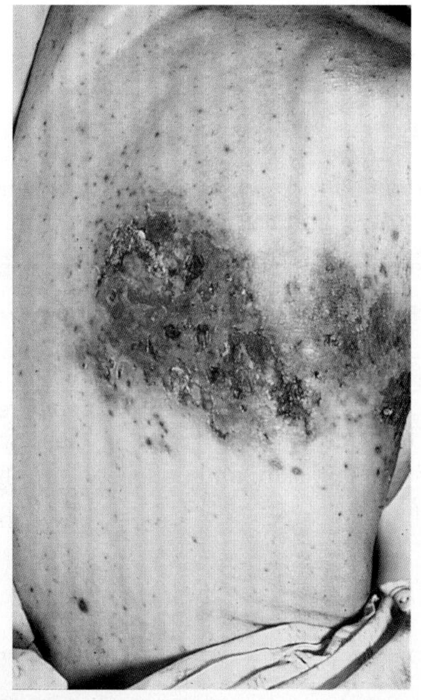

Figure 4-8 Herpes zoster (shingles).

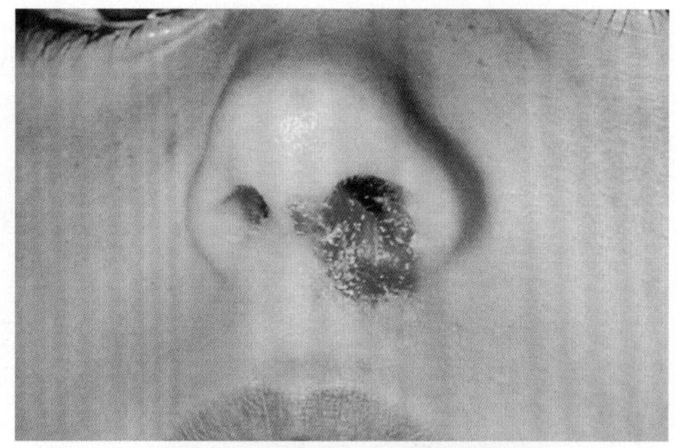

Figure 4-9 Impetigo.

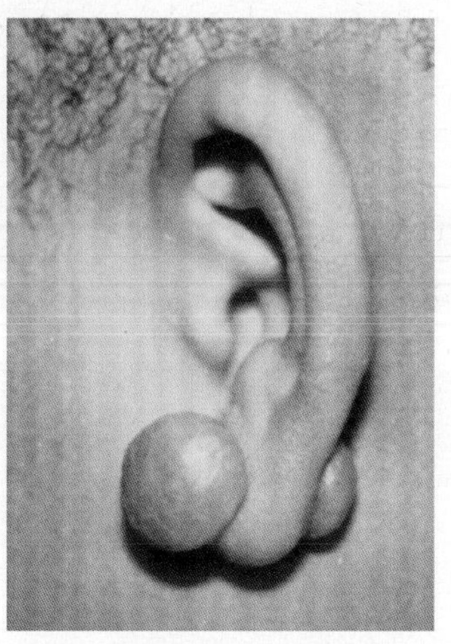

Figure 4-10 Keloid on site of earlobe piercing.

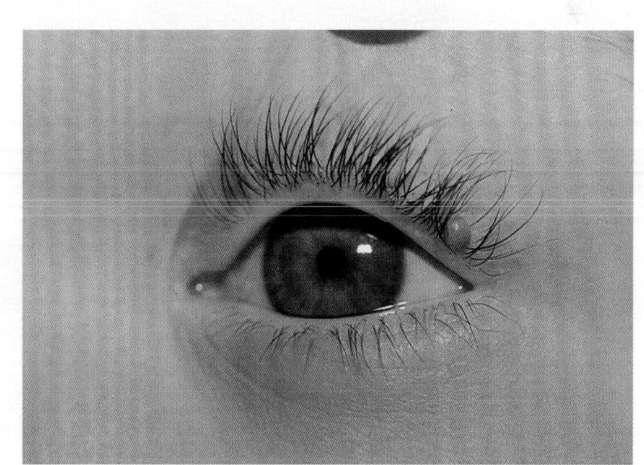

Figure 4-11 Nodule.

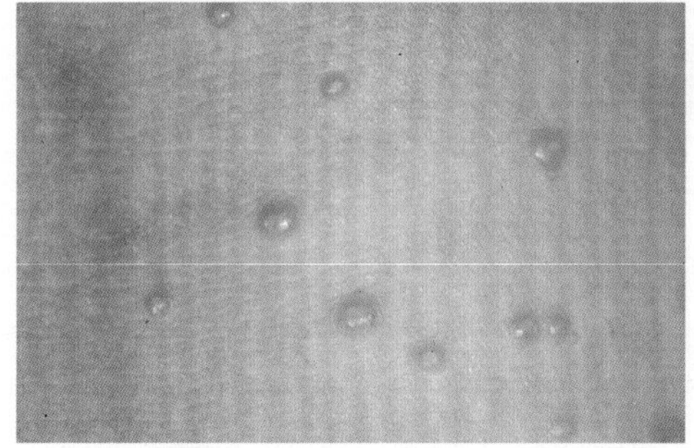

Figure 4-12 Papules.

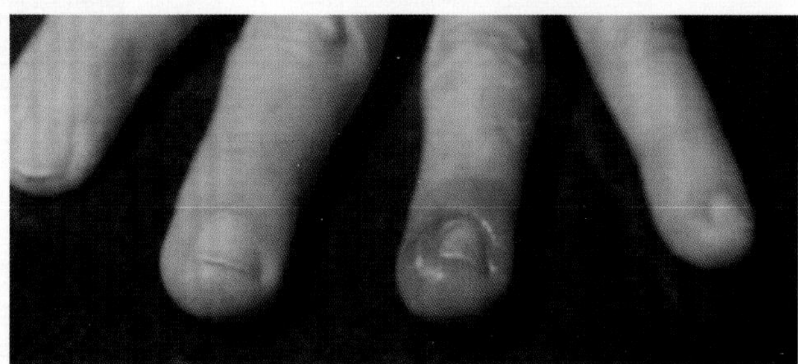

Figure 4-13 Paronychia.

Medical Conditions *(continued)*

Term	Pronunciation	Meaning
pediculosis	pĕ-dik-yū-lō′sis	an infestation of lice
psoriasis	sōr-ī′ă-sis	skin condition marked by red, itchy scaly patches primarily on the scalp, knees, elbows, and trunk **(Figure 4-14)**
pustule	pŭs′chūl	a small circumscribed elevation of the skin containing pus **(Figure 4-15)**
rosacea	rō-sā′shă	chronic disorder of the skin causing erythematous (red areas), papules, pustules, and increased sebum production; usually occurs on the face
scabies	skā′bēz	skin disease with eruptions and itching caused by mites **(Figure 4-16)**
tinea	tin′ē-ă	fungal infection of the hair, skin, and nails; commonly called ringworm **(Figure 4-17)**

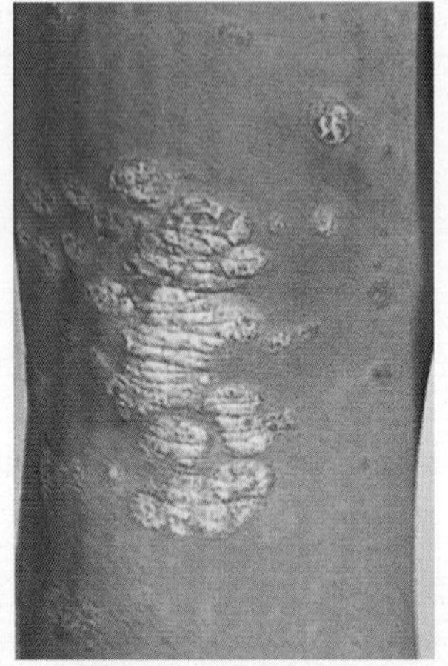

Figure 4-14 Psoriasis.

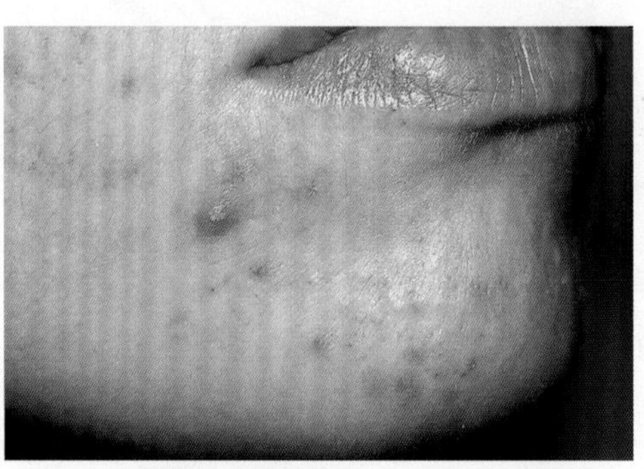

Figure 4-15 Pustule.

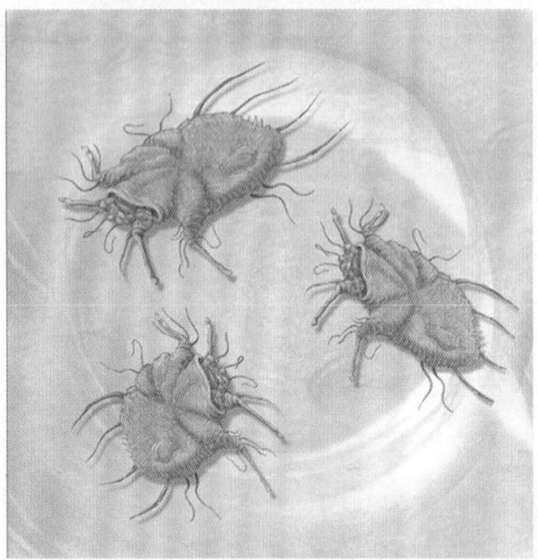

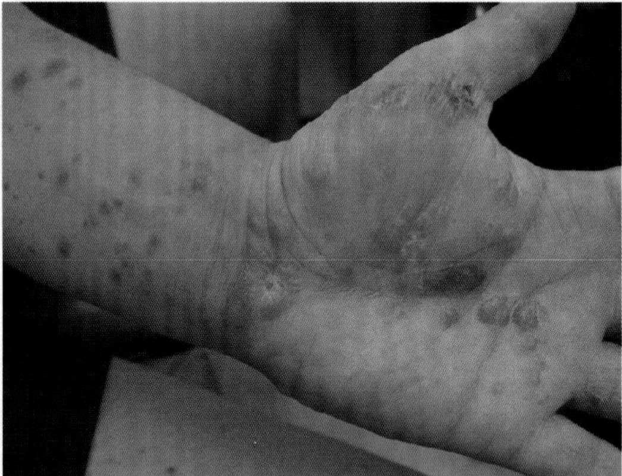

Figure 4-16 Scabies mites and infestation.

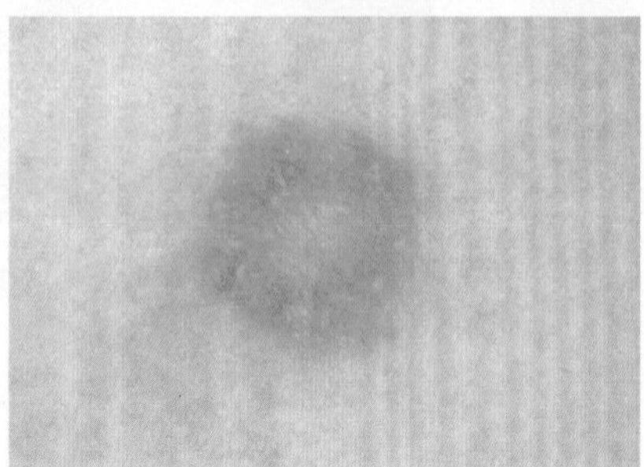

Figure 4-17 Tinea on the arm.

Medical Conditions

Term	Pronunciation	Meaning
tinea capitis	tin′ē-ă kap′i-tis	fungal infection of the scalp
tinea pedis	tin′ē-ă ped′is	fungal infection of the feet; commonly called athlete's foot
urticaria	ŭr′ti-kar′ē-ă	an eruption of itchy round, red welts (wheals) usually related to an allergy; commonly called hives
varicella	var′i-sel′ă	an acute contagious disease caused by the varicella-zoster virus and producing various skin eruptions; commonly known as chicken pox
verruca	vĕr-ū′kă	contagious and sometimes painful wart commonly caused by the human papillomavirus (HPV)
vesicle	ves′i-kĕl	a clear, fluid-filled, raised lesion; commonly called a blister **(Figure 4-18)**
vitiligo	vit′i-lī′gō	areas of skin that do not have melanocytes, appearing as white patches on otherwise normal skin **(Figure 4-19)**
wheal	wēl	a raised reddish lesion that often changes size and shape and extends into adjacent areas; usually associated with an allergen **(Figure 4-20)**
xanthoderma	zan′thō-dĕr′mă	any yellow coloration of the skin

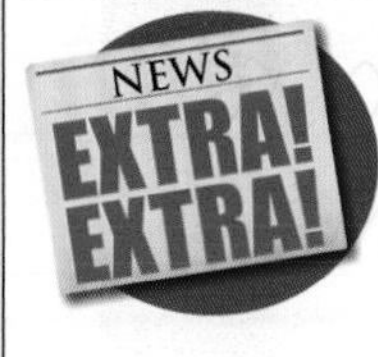

XANTHODERMA Several conditions, including hepatitis and eating foods high in beta-carotene, can cause yellowing of the skin. Hepatitis is characterized by liver inflammation and can lead to bile accumulation in the blood, causing the skin to appear yellow. Excessive consumption of food rich in beta-carotene, such as carrots, squash, and sweet potatoes, can lead to yellowing of the skin. This yellowing occurs because carotene is a lipochrome that can accumulate in the skin, making it appear yellow. It is important to determine the difference between xanthoderma caused by a disease process and that caused by dietary intake.

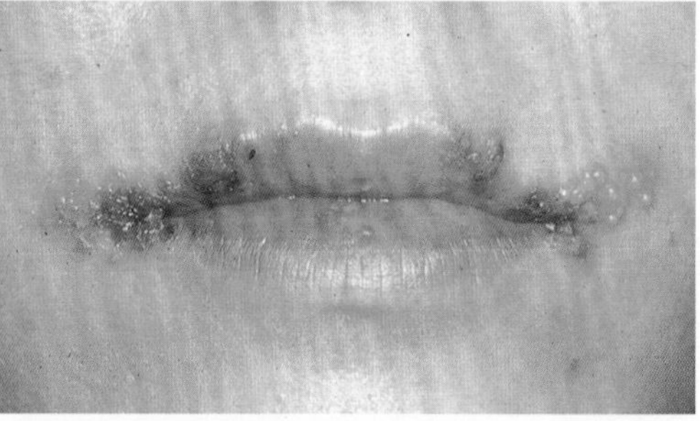

Figure 4-18 Vesicles.

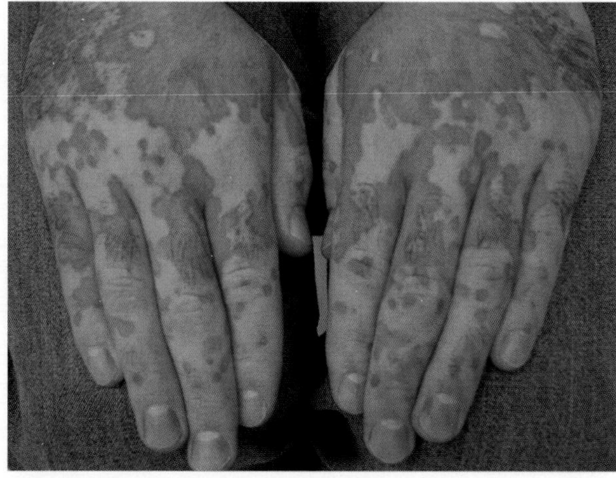

Figure 4-19 Vitiligo.

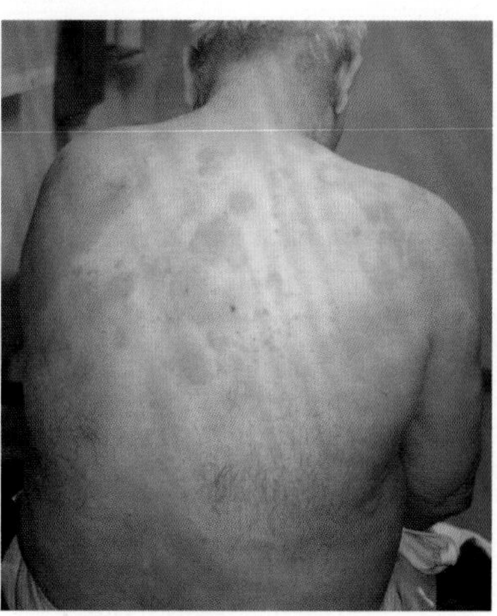

Figure 4-20 Wheals.

Exercises: Medical Conditions

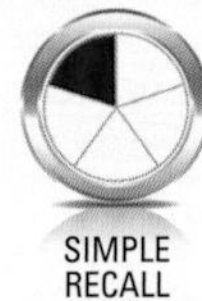
SIMPLE RECALL

Exercise 11

Write the correct medical term for the meaning given.

1. burn involving destruction of the entire skin ______ full-thickness burn
2. small, raised, circumscribed area of the skin ______ papule
3. small elevation of the skin containing pus ______ pustule
4. acute contagious disease causing skin eruptions ______ varicella
5. burn involving only the epidermis ______ superficial burn
6. inflammation of the subcutaneous connective tissue ______ cellulitis
7. viral infection affecting peripheral nerves ______ herpes zoster
8. skin condition marked by red, itchy, scaly patches ______ psoriasis
9. inflammatory condition causing patchy redness and scales ______ eczema
10. condition caused by local infection of herpesvirus ______
11. overgrowth of scar tissue ______
12. abnormal yellowing of the skin due to bile accumulation ______
13. pathologic change in tissue ______
14. injury resulting in removal of superficial skin layer ______

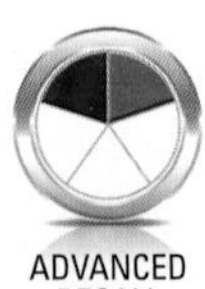
ADVANCED RECALL

Exercise 12

Circle the term that is most appropriate for the meaning of the sentence.

1. After examination, the medical assistant noted that the raised, reddish lesion on the anterior side of the patient's forearm could be a (*fissure, wheal, carbuncle*).
2. The physician examined the circumscribed malformation of the skin, or (*nevus, excoriation, furuncle*), for signs of cancer.
3. After lying in the same position for several hours, the patient developed a pressure sore of the skin, called a (*decubitus ulcer, keloid, comedo*), on the posterior aspect of his ankle.
4. Mary felt a solid raised area, called a (*tinea, nodule, paronychia*), while performing her monthly breast self-exam.

5. Several children at the day care center contracted (*psoriasis, scabies, verruca*), a condition that is caused by mites and were advised not to return to the center until 24 hours after treatment.

6. After cardiac surgery, Mr. Henry developed a scar or (*comedo, cicatrix, wheal*) on his chest where the incision had been made.

7. The patient's erythematous face was diagnosed as (*rosacea, tinea, vitiligo*).

8. Because of a lack of blood flow, an area of (*eczema, gangrene, pediculosis*) developed on the patient's leg.

9. Missy landed on her hip when she fell off her bicycle and developed an area of discoloration and swelling, called a (*contusion, verruca, cyst*).

10. After stepping out of the locker room shower, Mike noticed a fungal infection between his toes called (*tinea pedis, tinea capitis, scabies*).

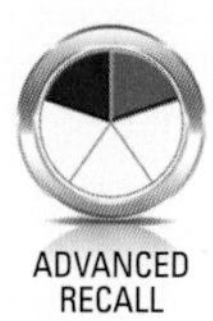
ADVANCED RECALL

Exercise 13

Match each medical term with its meaning.

urticaria	pediculosis	impetigo	macule
cyst	comedo	paronychia	vesicle
burn	tinea capitis	verruca	abscess

1. fluid-filled, raised lesion ___cyst___
2. flat area of skin that is changed in color ___macule___
3. wart ___verruca___
4. an infestation of lice ___pediculosis___
5. fungal infection of the scalp ___tinea capitis___
6. blackhead ___comedo___
7. hives ___urticaria___
8. inflammation and infection around the nail ___paronychia___
9. semisolid material within a closed sac ___vesicle___
10. contagious bacteria infection seen on the face in children ___imeptigo___
11. injury to skin by heat ___burn___
12. circumscribed collection of pus ___abscess___

Tests and Procedures

Term	Pronunciation	Meaning
biopsy (Bx)	bī'op-sē	process of removing tissue from living patients for microscopic examination
culture and sensitivity (C&S)	kŭl'chŭr and sen'si-tiv'i-tē	growing of an organism from a specimen from the body to determine its susceptibility to particular medications
frozen section (FS)	frō'zĕn sek'shŭn	a thin slice of tissue cut from a frozen specimen used for rapid microscopic diagnosis
scratch test	skrach test	type of allergy test in which an antigen (foreign substance) is applied through a scratch in the skin
tuberculosis skin test; *syn.* Mantoux test, purified protein derivative (PPD) test	tū-bĕr'kyū-lō'sis skin test; mahn-tū' test, prō'tēn dĕ-riv'ă-tiv test	an intradermal test to determine whether a patient has tuberculosis or has been exposed to the disease

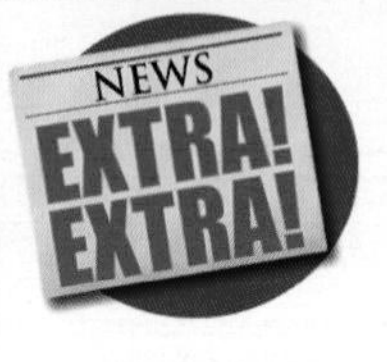

TUBERCULOSIS TESTING An older version of the tuberculosis skin test is the tuberculosis tine test. The skin was pricked evenly with a four- or six-pronged device coated with the tuberculin antigen. Studies have ultimately proven that the current PPD test, which is given as a single-puncture injection, gives more accurate results than the older tine test, so the tine test is not often used today.

Exercise: Tests and Procedures

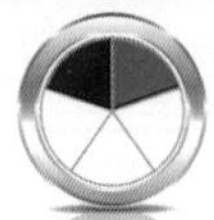

ADVANCED RECALL

Exercise 14

Circle the term that is most appropriate for the meaning of the sentence.

1. Every year, all medical office personnel at Central Hospital undergo a (*Mantoux test, biopsy, scratch test*) to determine whether they have been exposed to the tuberculosis bacterium, *Myobacterium tuberculosis.*

2. To determine the specific triggers for his allergies, Mr. Sabatino had a (*needle biopsy, scratch test, culture and sensitivity*).

3. The young man had a (*biopsy, tuberculosis skin test, scratch test*), which involved the removal of tissue for microscopic examination.

4. The physician ordered a (*biopsy, culture and sensitivity, frozen section*) to determine which medication was needed to treat the patient's infected hand.

5. The surgeon ordered a (*culture and sensitivity, scratch test, frozen section*) of the tissue specimen for rapid microscopic diagnosis.

Surgical Interventions and Therapeutic Procedures

Term	Pronunciation	Meaning
cauterization	kaw′tĕr-īz-ā′shŭn	the use of heat, cold, electric current, or caustic chemicals to destroy tissue
cryosurgery	krī′ō-ser′jer-ē	the use of freezing temperatures to destroy tissue **(Figure 4-21)**
debridement	dā-brēd-mawn[h]′	the removal of any necrotic skin or foreign matter from a wound
dermabrasion	dĕrm′ă-brā′zhŭn	the removal of acne scars from the skin with sandpaper, rotating brushes, or other abrasive materials
dermatoautoplasty; *syn.* autograft	dĕr′mă-tō-aw′to-plas-tē; aw′tō-graft	skin grafting using the patient's own skin
dermatoheteroplasty; *syn.* xenograft	dĕr′mă-tō-het′ĕr-ō-plas-tē; zen′ō-graft	skin grafting using skin from another species
dermatome	dĕr′mă-tōm	instrument used for cutting thin slices of skin for grafting or excising small lesions **(Figure 4-22)**
dermatoplasty	dĕr′mă-tō-plas-tē	surgical repair of the skin
electrodesiccation and curettage (ED&C)	ĕ-lek′trō-des-i-kā′shŭn and kūr′ĕ-tahzh′	burning off of skin growths using electrical currents
excision	ek-sizh′ŭn	the act of cutting out
incision	in-sizh′ŭn	the act of cutting into (surgically)
incision and drainage (I&D)	in-sizh′ŭn and drān′ăj	a sterile cut into the skin to release fluid
irrigation	ir′i-gā′shŭn	washing out an area with fluid
rhytidectomy	rit′i-dek′tō-mē	surgical removal of wrinkles
rhytidoplasty	rit′i-dō-plas-tē	surgical repair of wrinkles **(Figure 4-23)**
suture	sū′chŭr	to unite two surfaces by sewing **(Figure 4-24)**

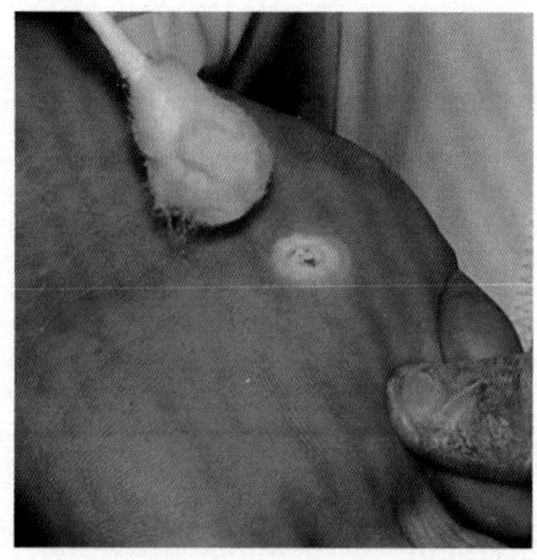

Figure 4-21 Cryosurgery with liquid nitrogen.

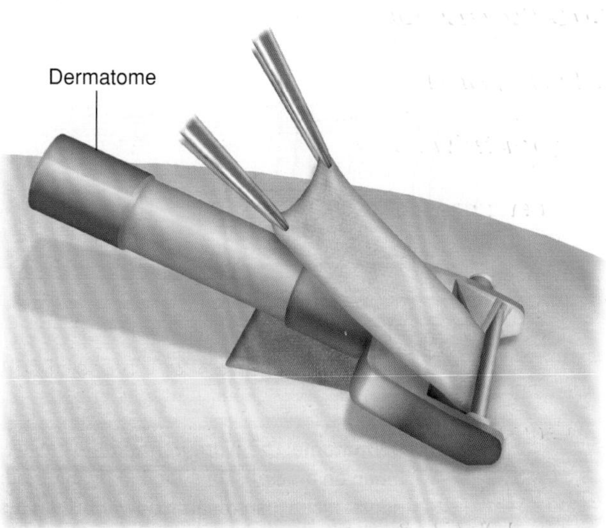

Figure 4-22 Dermatome preparing skin for grafting.

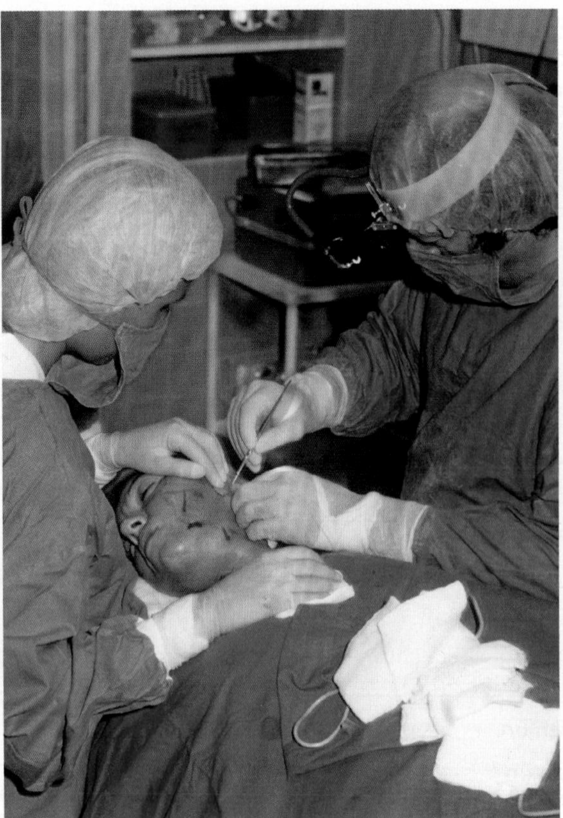

Figure 4-23 Rhytidoplasty.

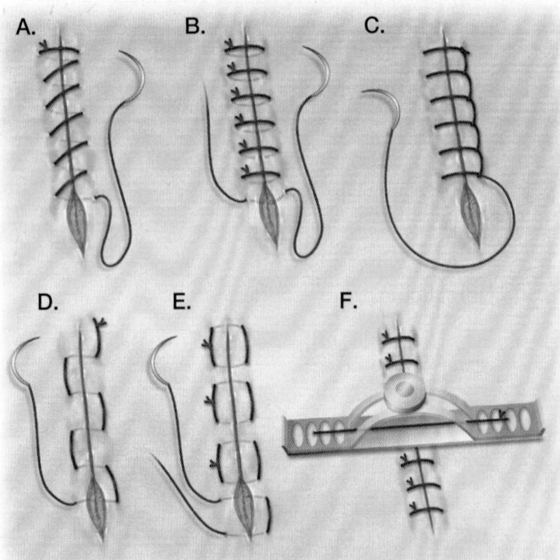

A. Plain continuous

B. Plain interrupted

C. Lock-stitch continuous

D. Mattress continuous

E. Mattress interrupted

F. Retention suture bridge

Figure 4-24 Types of sutures.

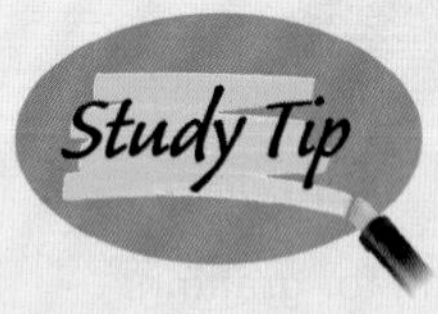

Dermatome: The word *dermatome* has two distinct meanings. Dermatome can mean an area of skin supplied by cutaneous branches of a single cranial or spinal nerve. It can also mean a power-driven instrument used to cut thin sections of epidermis or dermis for grafting purposes. The context of the sentence provides clues for understanding.

For example, the banding seen with shingles (herpes zoster) infection follows a dermatome. Or, the physician used a dermatome to cut thin sections of skin for grafting.

Exercises: Surgical Interventions and Therapeutic Procedures

SIMPLE RECALL

Exercise 15

Write the meaning of the term given.

1. dermatoplasty ____________________
2. cauterization ____________________
3. dermatoheteroplasty ____________________
4. excision ____________________

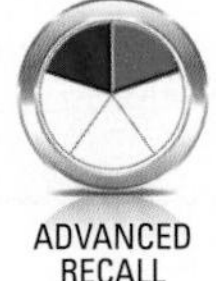

ADVANCED RECALL

Exercise 16

Circle the term that is most appropriate for the meaning of the sentence.

1. The physician diagnosed the infected condition as a furuncle and treated it with (*incision and drainage, punch biopsy, suturing*) to release fluid.
2. The surgeon had to make a(n) (*incision, excision, suture*) into the patient's skin to remove the lodged bullet.
3. Saline solution was used for (*cauterization, irrigation, punch biopsy*) to wash out the grass and dirt from the patient's laceration.
4. The child had a long, gaping wound on the posterior aspect of his leg that needed to be closed, or (*excised, sutured, incised*).
5. When the young man was brought into the emergency department after his motorcycle accident, his wounds had to be (*cauterized, debrided, excised*) to remove foreign matter and debris before other treatment.
6. After suffering severe burns, Mr. Simone had several skin grafts, including (*dermatoautoplasty, dermatoheteroplasty, dermatoplasty*), which involved a graft using his own skin.

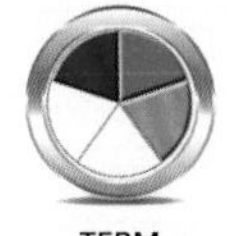

TERM CONSTRUCTION

Exercise 17

Write the combining form used in the medical term, followed by the meaning of the combining form.

Term	Combining Form	Combining Form Meaning
1. rhytidoplasty	rhytid/o	
2. dermabrasion	derm/a	
3. cryosurgery	cry/o	
4. electrodesiccation	electr/o	
5. rhytidectomy		
6. dermatome		

Medications and Drug Therapies

Term	Pronunciation	Meaning
antifungal	an'tē-fŭng'găl	drug used to kill fungi
antiinfective	an'tē-in-fek'tiv	drug used to decrease or remove infection
antiinflammatory	an'tē-in-flam'ă-tōr-ē	drug used to decrease inflammation
antipruritic	an'tē-prūr-it'ik	drug used to relieve itching
intralesional injection	intra-lē'zhŭn-al in-jek'shŭn	injection of medications into a lesion or scar
liquid nitrogen	lik'wid nī'trŏ-jĕn	nitrogen in a liquid state used in cryosurgery to remove a verruca or other lesion
pediculicide	pĕ-dik'yū-li-sīd	medication used to kill lice
scabicide	skā'bi-sīd	medication used to kill mites associated with scabies
steroid	ster'oyd	class of organic drug used to treat many inflammatory skin conditions

■ Exercise: Medications and Drug Therapies

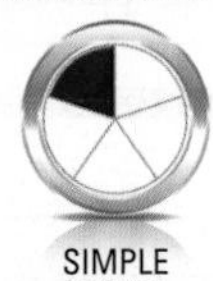

SIMPLE RECALL

Exercise 18

Write the correct medication or drug therapy term for the meaning given.

1. class of organic drug used to treat inflammatory skin conditions steroid
2. decreases or removes infection antiinfective
3. kills fungi antifungal
4. kills lice pediculicide
5. decreases inflammation antiinflammatory
6. liquid gas used in cryosurgery for verruca or other lesions liquid nitrogen
7. relieves itching antipruritic
8. injection of medications into a lesion intrausional injection
9. kills mites that cause scabies scabicide

Specialties and Specialists

Term	Pronunciation	Meaning
dermatology	dĕr'mă-tol'ŏ-jē	a medical specialty focusing on the study of skin and treatment of skin disorders
dermatologist	dĕr'mă-tol'ŏ-jist	physician who specializes in dermatology
medical aesthetician	med'i-kăl es-thet'i-shun	licensed professional specializing in skincare, especially facial skincare

Exercise: Specialties and Specialists

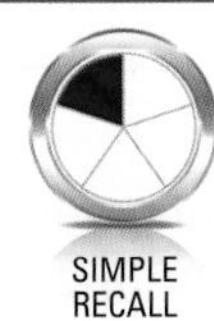
SIMPLE RECALL

Exercise 19

Write the correct medical term for the meaning given.

1. licensed professional specializing in skincare medical aesthetician
2. physician specializing in the study of skin dermatologist
3. specialty focusing on the study of skin and treatment of skin disorders dermatology

Abbreviations

Abbreviation	Meaning
Bx	biopsy
C&S	culture and sensitivity
ED&C	electrodesiccation and curettage
FS	frozen section
I&D	incision and drainage
PPD	purified protein derivative of tuberculin

Exercises: Abbreviations

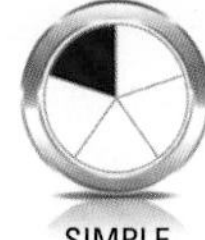
SIMPLE RECALL

Exercise 20

Write the meaning of each abbreviation.

1. PPD ______
2. C&S ______
3. I&D ______

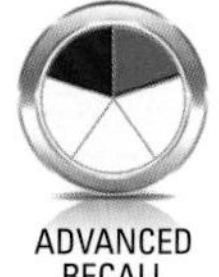
ADVANCED RECALL

Exercise 21

Match each abbreviation with the appropriate description.

ED&C Bx FS

1. slice of tissue from a frozen specimen FS
2. removing tissue for microscopic examination Bx
3. burning off of skin growths ED&C

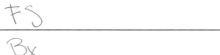

■ SOAP NOTES

SOAP notes are a type of documentation used by all types of health care professions. SOAP is an acronym for subjective, objective, assessment, and plan. This type of note is used to quickly summarize patient information and outline the treatment plan. An example of a SOAP note is shown on page 104 as the Medical Record exercise. This should begin to familiarize you with what a SOAP note looks like and how to find information from it.

■ WRAPPING UP

- The integumentary system is made up of the skin, which is divided into two layers, and its different structures.
- There are root words, prefixes, and suffixes that relate to the integumentary system.
- Various conditions affect the skin, and several pictures were included to easily identify and differentiate these conditions.
- Many tests, procedures, surgeries, medications, and specialties are specific to the skin.

Chapter Review

Review of Terms for Anatomy and Physiology

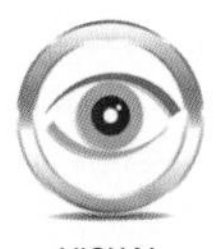

VISUAL

Exercise 22

Write the correct terms on the blanks for the anatomic structures indicated.

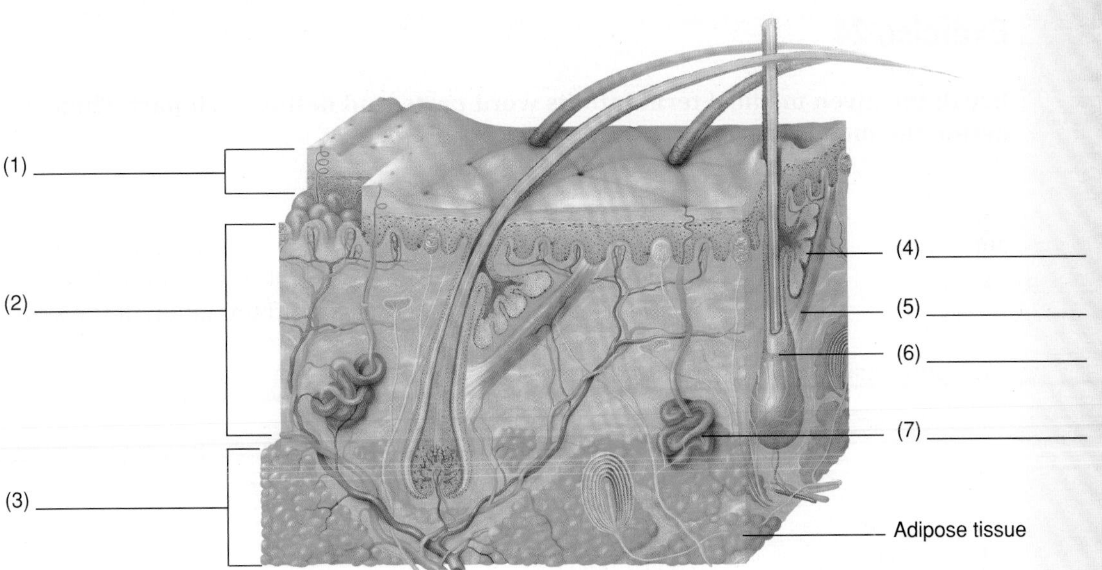

Understanding Term Structure

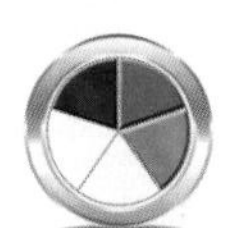

TERM CONSTRUCTION

Exercise 23

Write the combining form used in the medical term, followed by the meaning of the combining form.

Term	Combining Form	Combining Form Meaning
1. hidrosis	______	______
2. keratosis	______	______
3. cryosurgery	______	______
4. dermatology	______	______
5. scleroderma	______	______

6. onychomycosis ____________ ____________
7. rhytidectomy ____________ ____________
8. pyosis ____________ ____________
9. lipectomy ____________ ____________
10. seborrhea ____________ ____________
11. dermatomycosis ____________ ____________
12. subcutaneous ____________ ____________

TERM CONSTRUCTION

Exercise 24

Break the given medical term into its word parts, and define each part. Then define the medical term.

For example:

dermatitis	*word parts:*	dermat/o, -itis
	meanings:	skin, inflammation of
	term meaning:	inflammation of the skin

1. anhidrosis *word parts:* ____________
meanings: ____________
term meaning: ____________

2. erythrocyanosis *word parts:* ____________
meanings: ____________
term meaning: ____________

3. trichopathy *word parts:* ____________
meanings: ____________
term meaning: ____________

4. pyoderma *word parts:* ____________
meanings: ____________
term meaning: ____________

5. paronychia *word parts:* ____________
meanings: ____________
term meaning: ____________

6. dermatologist	*word parts:*	______________________
	meanings:	______________________
	term meaning:	______________________
7. transdermal	*word parts:*	______________________
	meanings:	______________________
	term meaning:	______________________
8. dermatoheteroplasty	*word parts:*	______________________
	meanings:	______________________
	term meaning:	______________________
9. pachyderma	*word parts:*	______________________
	meanings:	______________________
	term meaning:	______________________
10. onychomalacia	*word parts:*	______________________
	meanings:	______________________
	term meaning:	______________________
11. cyanosis	*word parts:*	______________________
	meanings:	______________________
	term meaning:	______________________
12. onychophagia	*word parts:*	______________________
	meanings:	______________________
	term meaning:	______________________
13. intradermal	*word parts:*	______________________
	meanings:	______________________
	term meaning:	______________________
14. xeroderma	*word parts:*	______________________
	meanings:	______________________
	term meaning:	______________________

Comprehension Exercises

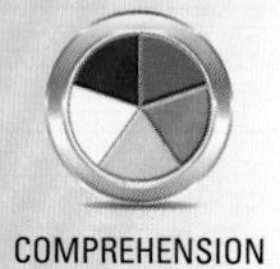
COMPREHENSION

Exercise 25

Fill in the blank with the correct term.

1. The three layers of skin are the ____________________, the ____________________, and the ____________________.
2. Contraction of the ____________________ muscles causes hairs to stand up straight.
3. The filling of a dilated hair follicle with bacteria and sebum causes a(n) ____________________.
4. The ____________________ glands assist in body temperature regulation.
5. A licensed professional specializing in skincare is called a(n) ____________________.
6. A bacterial infection that includes a collection of pus is called a(n) ____________________.
7. A facelift is the surgical repair of wrinkles, also known as ____________________.
8. Fat cells known as ____________________ and blood vessels make up the subcutaneous layer of the skin.
9. When reading the tuberculosis skin test, the medical assistant determines the amount of ____________________ (or hardened) tissue around the site of the injection.
10. White patches of various sizes on the skin caused from a lack of melanocytes indicate a condition called ____________________.
11. ____________________, a fungal infection of the hair, skin, and nails, causes ring-like lesions on the skin.
12. A(n) ____________________ develops when the skin surface is scratched.
13. A(n) ____________________ is caused by infection of a hair follicle.
14. Gangrene results from the ____________________ of tissue due to lack of blood flow.
15. Athlete's foot is a type of fungal infection called ____________________.
16. A child born without pigment in the skin, eyes, and hair would be diagnosed with ____________________.
17. A(n) ____________________ occurs when a tear extends deep into the dermis.

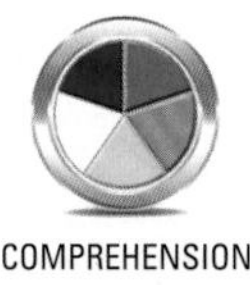

COMPREHENSION

Exercise 26

Circle the letter of the best answers to the following questions.

1. The type of burn that involves the dermis and epidermis is a
   A. superficial burn.
   B. partial-thickness burn.
   C. full-thickness burn.
   D. subcutaneous burn.

2. What is the medical term for a contagious and sometimes painful wart commonly caused by the human papillomavirus?
   A. papule
   B. purpura
   C. verruca
   D. comedo

3. When normal tissue is replaced by fibrous tissue it is called a(n)
   A. contusion.
   B. cicatrix.
   C. abscess.
   D. fissure.

4. Which involves secretions from the sudoriferous glands?
   A. keratosis
   B. alopecia
   C. diaphoresis
   D. pruritus

5. What is the medical term for what may form after a partial-thickness burn occurs?
   A. piloerections
   B. nodules
   C. melanocytes
   D. vesicles

6. Which layer of skin is affected in a superficial burn?
   A. dermis
   B. subdermis
   C. dermal layer
   D. epidermis

7. Which combining form refers to the secretions that come from the sebaceous gland?
   A. seb/o
   B. sudor/o
   C. hidr/o
   D. hydr/o

8. The medical term for a mole is a
   A. sarcoma.
   B. carbuncle.
   C. nevus.
   D. cyst.

9. A raised reddish lesion that may be caused by an allergen is called a
   A. macule.
   B. wheal.
   C. keratin.
   D. dermatome.

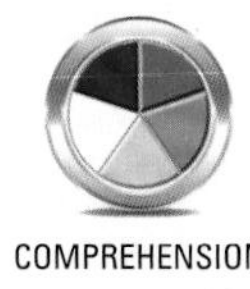

COMPREHENSION

Exercise 27

Fill in the blank with the correct term.

1. A treatment for acne scars that involves the use of abrasive material is known as __________.
2. A lesion that is contained within a certain area is said to be __________.
3. A surgical procedure that is used to remove gangrenous tissue is called __________.
4. A(n) __________ is a collection of abscesses in a group of hair follicles.
5. The fungal infection that can affect various areas of the body is called __________.

6. An infection that is commonly found in children and involves the face is known as

_______________.

7. Itchy wheals related to an allergy are known as hives or _______________.

8. The condition that involves fungi around the nail is called _______________.

9. The physician who performs an allergy test on the skin may call it a(n)

_______________ test.

10. An instrument called a(n) _______________ is used as a part of a skin graft procedure.

Application and Analysis

CASE STUDIES

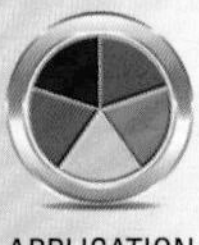

APPLICATION

Exercise 28

Read the case studies, and circle the correct letter for each of the questions.

CASE 4-1

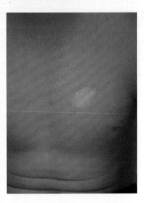

Figure 4-25 Macular rash on chest.

A young man visited his dermatologist because he noticed a macular rash on his chest **(Figure 4-25)**. The rash had been present for several weeks and was pruritic.

1. The term *macular* means that the rash is

   A. marked by a distinct spot.
   B. raised.
   C. purulent.
   D. the same color as the surrounding skin.

2. Because the rash was pruritic, what type of medication do you think the physician prescribed?

   A. scabicide
   B. anti-itch
   C. steroid
   D. antiinfective

3. The suffix *-logist* means

   A. study of.
   B. softening.
   C. disease.
   D. one who specializes in.

CASE 4-2

A class of preschool students experienced a scabies outbreak. All afflicted children presented with erythematous areas on their hands and on other areas where clothing was tight. All the affected areas also showed excoriations due to the extreme pruritus.

4. The excoriations are known commonly as

A. bruises.
B. scabs.
C. scratches.
D. warts.

5. Scabies is caused by

A. a fungus.
B. poison ivy.
C. lice.
D. mites.

6. Treatment to eradicate scabies includes the use of a(n)

A. scabicide.
B. antimite tablet.
C. antipruritic medication.
D. antifungal.

CASE 4-3

When the patient arrived in the clinic, the medical assistant noticed a group of verrucae on the lateral aspect of the patient's ankle. She informed the physician, and they prepared to remove the verrucae with electrodesiccation and curettage.

7. Verrucae is the plural form of the medical term more commonly known as

A. hives.
B. warts.
C. comedos.
D. papules.

8. As the medical assistant prepared the patient for the procedure, she informed him that the physician would

A. use cryosurgery to remove the verrucae.
B. use ultraviolet radiation to remove the verrucae.
C. give the patient an antifungal to use when he got home.
D. use electrical current to remove the verrucae.

MEDICAL RECORD ANALYSIS

MEDICAL RECORD 4-1

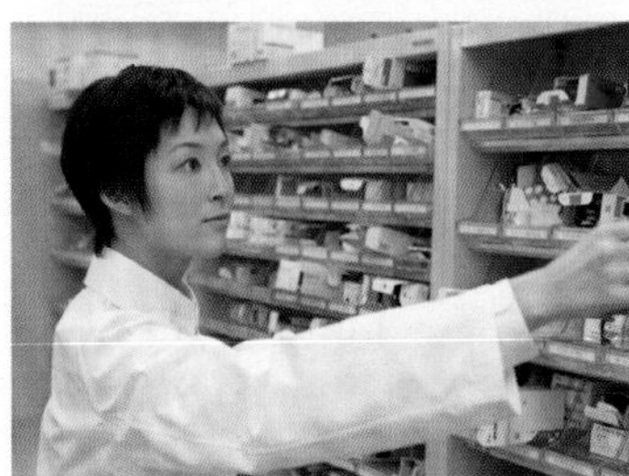

Figure 4-26 A pharmacy technician helps dispense prescriptions to patients.

A patient was seen in the emergency room this afternoon for an accidental burn. A pharmacy technician, are assisting the pharmacist in dispensing a prescription for acetaminophen with codeine as prescribed by the emergency room physician **(Figure 4-26)**.

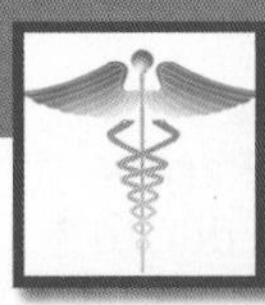

Medical Record

SUPERFICIAL AND PARTIAL-THICKNESS BURNS

SUBJECTIVE: This is an emergency visit for a 20-year-old man who accidentally knocked over a pot of boiling water onto his left leg and foot. He is complaining of extreme pain. He stated that he used some aloe on his leg and foot immediately after the accident occurred. Because of the continued pain, he presented to the office to ensure that the burn was nothing more than superficial.

OBJECTIVE: BP 130/76; P 98; T 98.6°F. This is a well-developed, well-nourished young man who presents with a reddened and blistered area on the anterior aspect of his left leg and on the dorsum of the left foot. Some of the blisters have broken and are weeping.

ASSESSMENT: Superficial and partial-thickness burns on the anterior aspect of the left lower leg and dorsum of the left foot.

PLAN: The patient was prescribed acetaminophen with codeine to take one every four hours p.r.n. for pain. The area was treated with silver sulfadiazine for possible infection. The patient was instructed to change the dressing daily and was given supplies to do this. He was instructed to return in three days for a recheck.

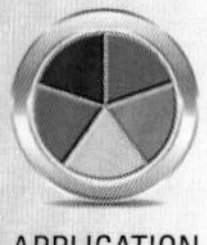

APPLICATION

Exercise 29

Read the medical record, and circle the correct letter for each of the questions.

1. What type of medication is silver sulfadiazine?

A. antipruritic
B. antifungal
C. antiinfective
D. antibiotic

2. A superficial burn involves the

A. dermis and the epidermis.
B. dermis and subcutaneous layer.
C. dermis, epidermis, and subcutaneous layer.
D. epidermis.

3. A partial-thickness burn involves the

A. dermis and the epidermis.
B. dermis and subcutaneous layer.
C. dermis, epidermis, and subcutaneous layer.
D. epidermis.

Bonus Question

4. Recalling the meaning of the word part *dors/o,* where is the dorsum of the foot?

____

MEDICAL RECORD 4-2

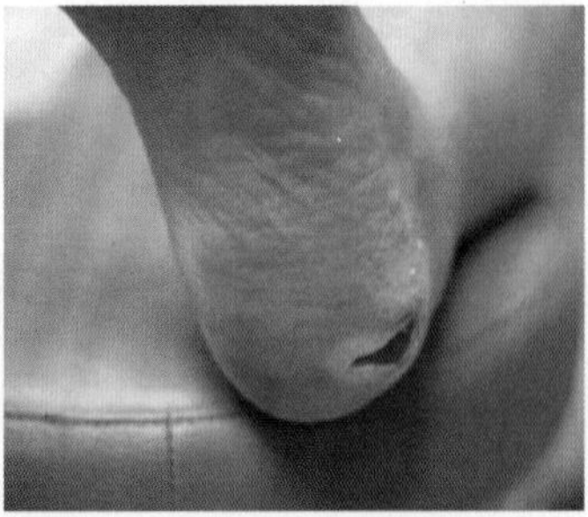

Figure 4-27 Stage II decubitus ulcer on heel.

You are a nursing assistant (NA) in a long-term care facility. One of your assignments is to reposition patients who are unable to move on their own. As you are moving a patient from the supine position onto her right side, you notice an area on her heel that you report to the physician **(Figure 4-27)**. The physician examines the patient and writes the following note.

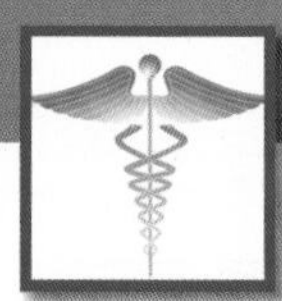

Medical Record

DECUBITUS ULCER

SUBJECTIVE: Nursing assistant noticed an area of broken skin on the right heel of the patient.

OBJECTIVE: This 83-year-old female is cachectic from her long-standing Alzheimer disease and refusal to take in sufficient nutrition. She is fed by way of nasogastric tube, which she has been known to pull out. Her weight is 110 lb. Her skin turgor is poor, and the area of broken skin is erythematous and shiny. Some areas of blackness are noted around the edges.

ASSESSMENT: C&S will be performed on a swab from the area in question. It appears to be a stage II, starting into stage III decubitus ulcer. At this point, it has not developed to the point where there is any necrotic tissue that needs to be debrided.

PLAN: The patient will be turned on a more frequent basis. The time frame will be increased from every two hours to every hour. Her tube feedings will have increased calories and protein to promote wound healing. The wound will be cleaned with normal saline. If the C&S comes back positive, the patient will be started on antibiotics. The heel area will be placed on an egg crate mattress when she is in the supine position.

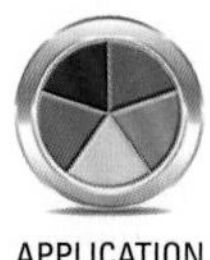

APPLICATION

Exercise 30

Read the medical record and circle the correct letter for each of the questions.

1. The area of broken skin on the right heel of the patient appears to be a(n)

   A. fissure.
   B. decubitus ulcer.
   C. excoriation.
   D. necrosis.

2. C&S is the abbreviation used when the physician wants

   A. to find out if there is infection.
   B. to perform a surgical procedure.
   C. to bill for more tests.
   D. to increase tube feeding times.

3. Necrotic tissue is

   A. red and full of turgor.
   B. red but has no turgor.
   C. black due to lack of blood flow.
   D. black and full of turgor.

Bonus Question

4. The combining form *nas/o* means nose. Based on this meaning and the word parts learned in previous chapters, define the term nasogastric.

____

Pronunciation and Spelling

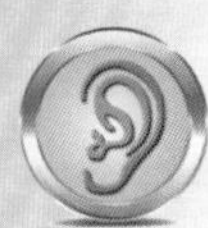
AUDITORY

Exercise 31

Review the Chapter 4 terms in the Dictionary/Audio Glossary in the Student Resources on thePoint and practice pronouncing each term, referring to the pronunciation guide as needed.

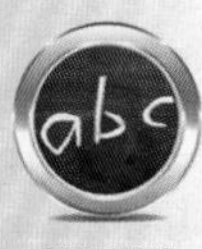

SPELLING

Exercise 32

Circle the correctly spelled term.

1.	anhydrosis	anhidrosis	enhydrosis
2.	sicatricks	cixatrix	cicatrix
3.	dermatomycosis	dermotamycosis	dermatomicosis
4.	onychofagia	unicoophagia	onychophagia
5.	erticareia	urtycaria	urticaria
6.	soriasis	psoriasis	psoryasis
7.	gangreen	ganrene	gangrene
8.	tinyea	tinia	tinea
9.	dysplasia	displazia	dysplasai
10.	puritic	pureitic	pruritic
11.	keritogenic	kerratagenic	keratogenic
12.	zeraderma	xeraderma	xeroderma
13.	jawndice	jaundice	jandice
14.	erythematous	erathematus	eryathematous
15.	arrector pili muscles	arector pili muscles	erector pili muscles

Media Connection

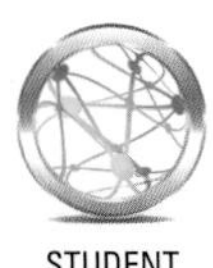

STUDENT RESOURCES

Exercise 33

Complete each of the following activities available with the Student Resources on thePoint. Check off each activity as you complete it, and record your score for the Chapter Quiz in the space provided.

Chapter Exercises

____ Flash Cards

____ Concentration

____ Abbreviation Match-Up

____ Roboterms

____ Word Anatomy

____ Fill the Gap

____ Break It Down

____ True/False Body Building

____ Quiz Show

____ Complete the Case

____ Medical Record Review

____ Look and Label

____ Image Matching

____ Spelling Bee

____ **Chapter Quiz** *Score:*________%

Additional Resources

____ Dictionary/Audio Glossary

____ Health Professions Careers: Pharmacy Technician

____ Health Professions Careers: Nursing Assistant

Musculoskeletal System

5

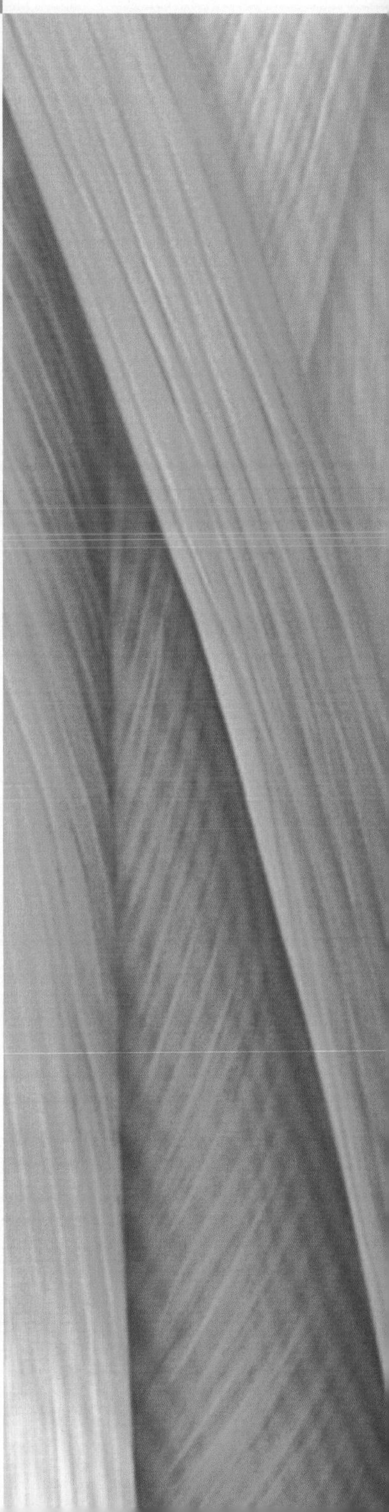

Chapter Outline

Introduction, 110

Anatomy and Physiology, 110
- Structures, 110
- Functions, 110
- Terms Related to Bone Structure, 110
- Terms Related to the Skeleton and Bones, 111
- Joints and Joint Movements, 114
- Terms Related to Joints and Joint Movements, 114
- Muscles, 115
- Terms Related to Muscles, 116

Word Parts, 121
- Combining Forms, 121
- Prefixes, 123
- Suffixes, 123

Medical Terms, 126
- Adjectives and Other Related Terms, 126
- Medical Conditions, 128
- Tests and Procedures, 136
- Surgical Interventions and Therapeutic Procedures, 140
- Medications and Drug Therapies, 146
- Specialties and Specialists, 146
- Abbreviations, 147

Wrapping Up, 149

Chapter Review, 150

Learning Outcomes

After completing this chapter, you should be able to:

1. List the structures and functions of the musculoskeletal system.
2. Describe the location of key bones and muscles in the body.
3. Define terms related to bone structure, joints, joint movements, and muscles.
4. Define combining forms, prefixes, and suffixes related to the musculoskeletal system.
5. Define common medical terminology related to the integumentary system, including the following: adjectives and related terms; signs, symptoms, and medical conditions; tests and procedures; surgical interventions and therapeutic procedures; medications and drug therapies; and medical specialties and specialists.
6. Define common abbreviations related to the musculoskeletal system.
7. Successfully complete all chapter exercises.
8. Explain terms used in case studies and medical records involving the musculoskeletal system.
9. Successfully complete all exercises included with the companion Student Resources on thePoint.

INTRODUCTION

The musculoskeletal system is composed of two organ systems that are closely related: the muscular system and the skeletal system. Skeletal muscle attaches to the bones of the skeleton. Because muscles insert into bones, we can move about. The musculoskeletal system also maintains body posture, protects vital organs, stores minerals (in bones), and generates heat (muscle contractions). This chapter discusses bones, joints, and muscles.

ANATOMY AND PHYSIOLOGY

Structures

- The body has 206 bones divided into the axial skeleton (bones of the head, neck, and trunk) and the appendicular skeleton (bones of the arms, legs, and girdles).
- The body has more than 700 muscles.
- Bones articulate (meet) at joints where muscle contractions allow for different types of joint movements.

Functions

- Supporting body structures
- Moving body structures
- Protecting internal organs
- Storing calcium and other minerals (bones)
- Producing blood cells (red bone marrow)
- Producing heat (muscles)

Terms Related to Bone Structure (Figure 5-1)

Term	Pronunciation	Meaning
bone marrow	bōn ma′rō	soft tissue within bone; has multiple functions including blood cell production in the red bone marrow
compact bone	kŏm-pakt′ bōn	harder, denser bone; noncancellous bone **(Figure 5-2)**
diaphysis	dī-af′i-sis	the shaft of a long bone
endosteum	en-dos′tē-ŭm	membrane lining the central medullary cavity
epiphysis	e-pif′i-sis	the wider ends of a long bone
epiphysial plate	ep′i-fiz′ē-ăl plāt	the growth area of a long bone
medullary cavity	med′ŭ-lar′ē kav′i-tē	space within a long bone's shaft filled with bone marrow
metaphysis	mĕ-taf′i-sis	section of a long bone between the diaphysis and epiphysis
osteoblast	os′tē-ō-blast	bone-forming cell
osteoclast	os′tē-ō-klast	bone-destroying cell
osteocyte	os′tē-ō-sīt	mature bone cell
periosteum	per′ē-os′tē-ŭm	fibrous membrane surrounding a bone
spongy bone; *syn.* cancellous bone or trabecular bone	spŏn′jē bōn; kan′sĕ-lŭs bōn tră-bek′yū-lăr bōn	mesh-like bone tissue **(Figure 5-2)**

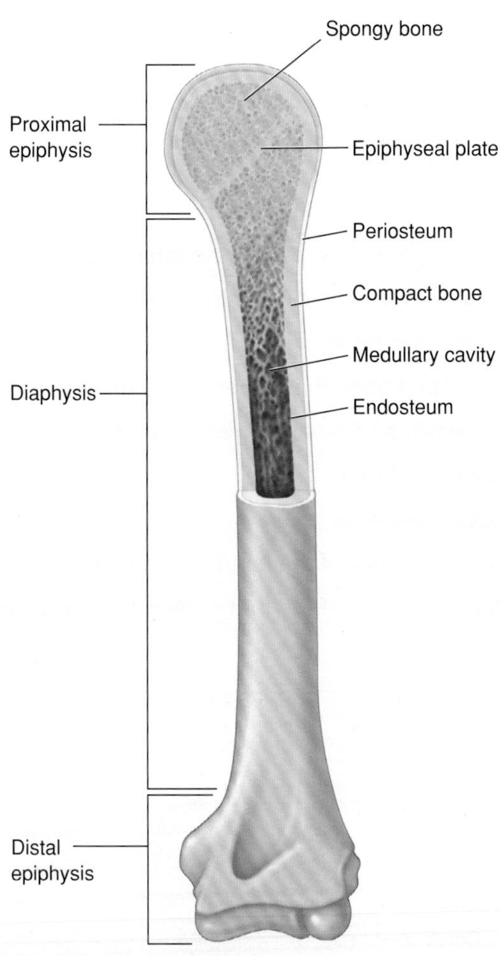

Figure 5-1 Major parts of a long bone.

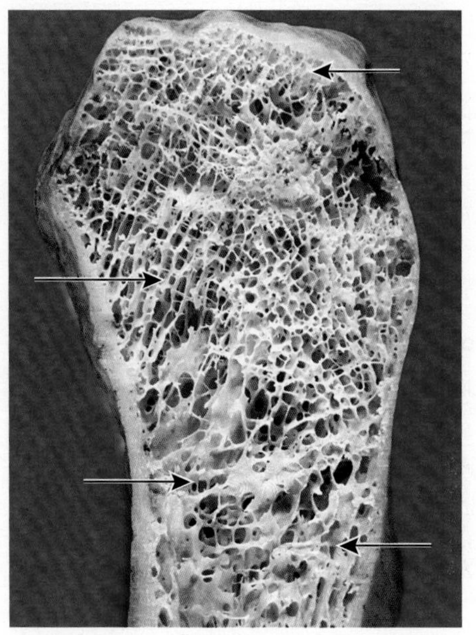

Figure 5-2 Types of bone tissue. Spongy bone makes up most of the epiphysis of this long bone (*arrows*). A thin layer of compact bone is seen at the surface.

Terms Related to the Skeleton and Bones (Figure 5-3)

Term	Pronunciation	Meaning
The Skeleton		
axial skeleton	ak′sē-ăl skel′ĕ-tŏn	bones of the head, vertebral column, and thorax
appendicular skeleton	ap′ĕn-dik′yŭ-lăr skel′ĕ-tŏn	bones of the upper and lower limbs and shoulder and pelvic girdles
thorax	thō′raks	the chest
Bones		
acetabulum	as-ĕ-tab′yū-lŭm	the socket of the hip bone where the femur articulates
acromion	ă-krō′mē-on	lateral upper section of the scapula that articulates with the clavicle
calcaneus	kal-kā′nē-ŭs	heel bone
carpal bones	kahr′păl bōnz	the eight bones of the wrist
clavicle	klav′i-kĕl	collar bone
cranium	krā′nē-ŭm	the skull; composed of eight bones excluding the face bones
femur	fē′mŭr	thigh bone
fibula	fib′yū-lă	smaller, lateral bone of the lower leg

(continued)

Terms Related to the Skeleton and Bones *(continued)*

Term	Pronunciation	Meaning
hip bone; *syn.* pelvic bone	hip bōn; pel′vik bōn	large flat bone composed of three fused bones (ilium, ischium, and pubis) on each side
ilium	il′ē-ŭm	superior broad part of the hip bone
ischium	is′kē-ŭm	inferior, rearmost part of the hip bone
pubis	pyū′bis	anterior lower section of the hip bone; pubic bone
humerus	hyū′mĕr-ŭs	upper arm bone
hyoid	hī′oyd	U-shaped bone that supports the tongue
lamina	lam′i-nă	posterior section of the vertebral arch
mandible	man′di-bĕl	lower jawbone
maxilla	mak-sil′ă	upper jawbone
metacarpal bones	met′ă-kahr′păl bōnz	the five bones of the hand between the wrist and fingers
metatarsal bones	met′ă-tahr′săl bōnz	the five bones of the foot between the ankle and toes
patella	pă-tel′ă	kneecap
phalanges	fă-lan′-jēz	the bones of the fingers and toes; there are 14 in each hand and foot

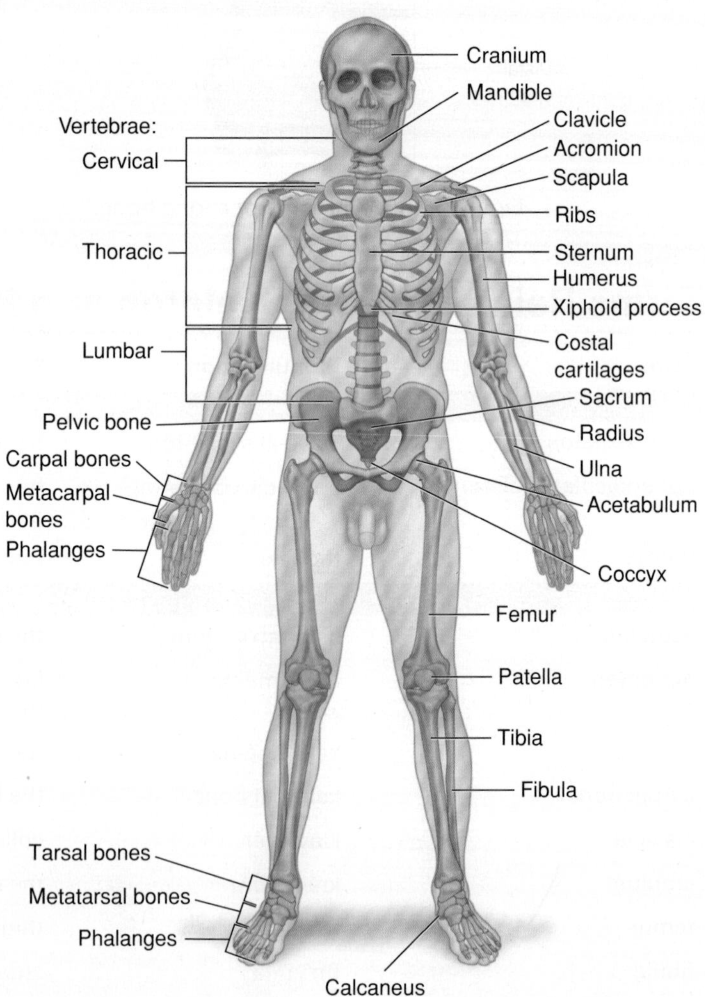

Figure 5-3 An anterior view of the skeleton with major bones identified.

Terms Related to the Skeleton and Bones

Term	Pronunciation	Meaning
radius	rā′dē-ŭs	outer forearm bone
ribs	ribz	long curved bones that form the bony walls of the chest
scapula	skap′yū-lă	shoulder blade
sternum	stĕr′nŭm	anterior bone of thorax; breast bone
tarsal bones	tahr′săl bōnz	the seven bones of the ankle
tibia	tib′ē-ă	larger inner bone of the lower leg; shin bone
ulna	ŭl′nă	inner forearm bone
vertebra	vĕr′tĕ-bră	bone of the vertebral column (spine) **(Figure 5-4)**
cervical vertebrae (C1–C7)	sĕr′vi-kăl vĕr′tĕ-brā	the seven bones of the vertebral column in the neck
thoracic vertebrae (T1–T12)	thōr-as′ik vĕr′tĕ-brā	the 12 bones of the vertebral column (midspine)
lumbar vertebrae (L1–L5)	lŭm′bahr vĕr′tĕ-brā	the five bones of the vertebral column (lower back)
sacrum	sā′krŭm	triangular bone consisting of five fused vertebrae inferior to the lumbar spine
coccyx	kok′siks	three to five fused vertebrae at the inferior end of the spine; tailbone
xiphoid process	zī′foyd pro′ses	lower section of the sternum

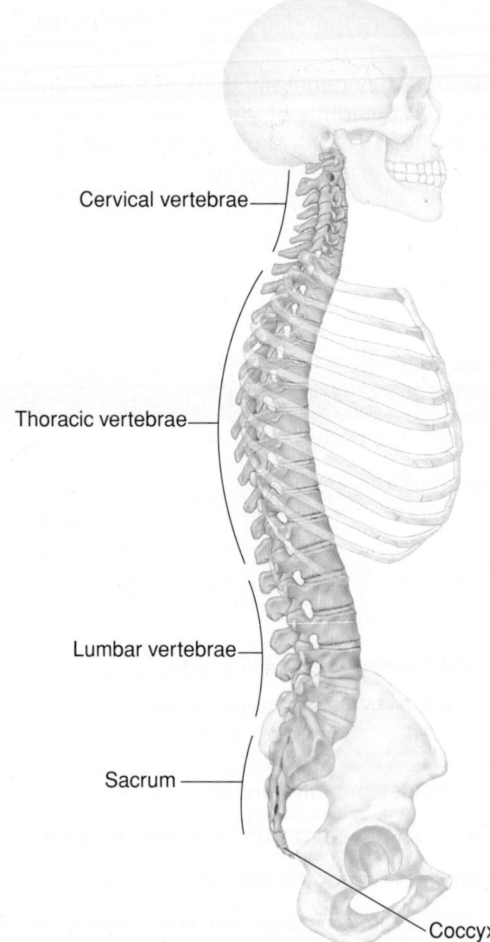

Figure 5-4 The vertebral column showing the locations of vertebrae.

ANIMATION

View the "Vertebral Disc" video on the Student Resources on thePoint to learn more about the structure of the bones of the vertebral column (spine).

Joints and Joint Movements

- Joints, also called *articulations,* occur wherever bones come together.
- Joints are categorized by their movements.
- Terms for joint movements are based on the type and direction of movement.

Terms Related to Joints and Joint Movements

Term	Pronunciation	Meaning
	Joints	
articulation	ahr-tik′yū-lā′shŭn	the site where bones come together; joint
bursa	bŭr′să	a fluid-filled fibrous sac within some joints
cartilage	kahr′ti-lăj	dense connective tissue attached to bone in many joints
synovial joint; *syn.* diarthrosis	si-nō′vē-ăl joynt; dī′ahr-thrō′sis	a joint that moves freely and contains synovial fluid in its cavity **(Figure 5-5)**
intervertebral disc	in′tĕr-vĕr′tĕ-brăl disk	mass of fibrocartilage between adjacent vertebrae
ligament	lig′ă-mĕnt	band of strong connective tissue that connects bones or cartilage at a joint
meniscus	mĕ-nis′kŭs	cartilage structure in the knee
suture	sū′chŭr	immovable fibrous joint found joining the skull bones

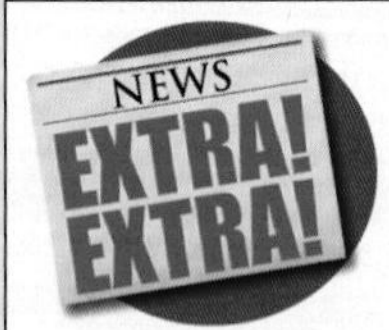

SUTURE When you think of joints, you may generally think of those joints that move. The skull also has joints, but the joints of the skull do not move. These joints, called sutures, hold the bones of the skull together, just as surgical sutures (or "stitches") hold two surfaces together.

Term	Pronunciation	Meaning
symphysis	sim′fi-sis	joint that moves only slightly
synovial fluid	si-nō′vē-ăl flū′id	lubricating fluid in a freely movable joint
tendon	ten′dŏn	band of fibrous connective tissue attaching a muscle to a bone
	Joint Movements (Figure 5-6)	
abduction	ab-dŭk′shŭn	moving away from the body's midline
adduction	ă-dŭk′shŭn	moving toward the body's midline
circumduction	sĭr′kŭm-dŭk′shŭn	moving in a circular manner, as when throwing a ball
inversion	in-vĕr′zhŭn	turning the foot sole inward
eversion	ē-vĕr′zhŭn	turning the foot sole outward
dorsiflexion	dōr-si-flek′shŭn	bending the foot upward toward the tibia
plantar flexion	plan′tahr flek′shŭn	bending the foot downward to point the toes
extension	eks-ten′shŭn	motion that increases the joint angle
flexion	flek′shŭn	motion that decreases the joint angle
pronation	prō-nā′shŭn	turning the palm downward or the foot sole outward
supination	sū′pi-nā′shŭn	turning the palm upward or the foot sole upward
rotation	rō-tā′shŭn	moving in circular direction around an axis, as when turning a doorknob

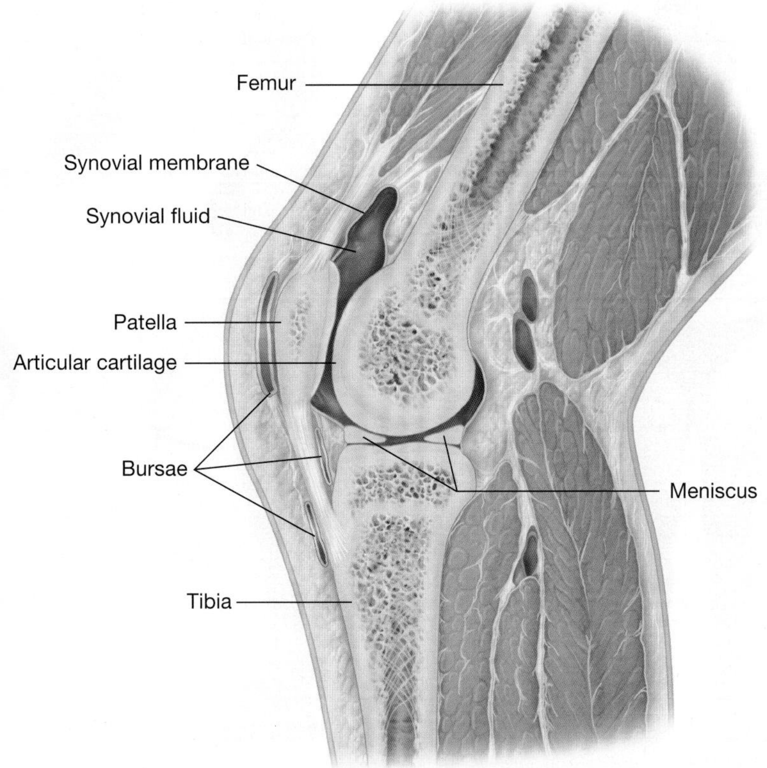

Figure 5-5 The knee is a synovial joint.

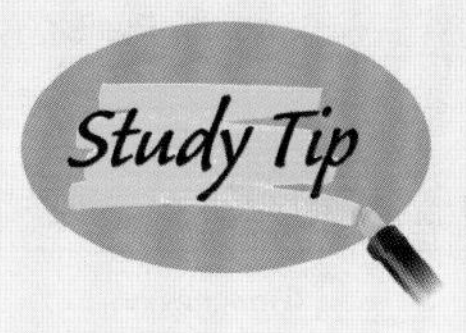

Adduction, abduction, supination, pronation: When distinguishing abduction from adduction, remember the common word abduct, meaning to take away. Adduction has the word "add," meaning to bring toward. To remember the difference between supination and pronation, think about your hand position when carrying a bowl of soup: in order to carry soup, the hand must be *supinated,* and the opposite of supinated is *pronated.*

ANIMATION

View the animation titled "Muscle Extension and Flexion" for a demonstration of muscles at work.

Muscles

- The three types of muscle tissue in the body are skeletal muscle, smooth muscle, and cardiac muscle.
- Muscles are composed of bundles of muscle fibers along with other tissues.
- Tendons attach muscles to bones.

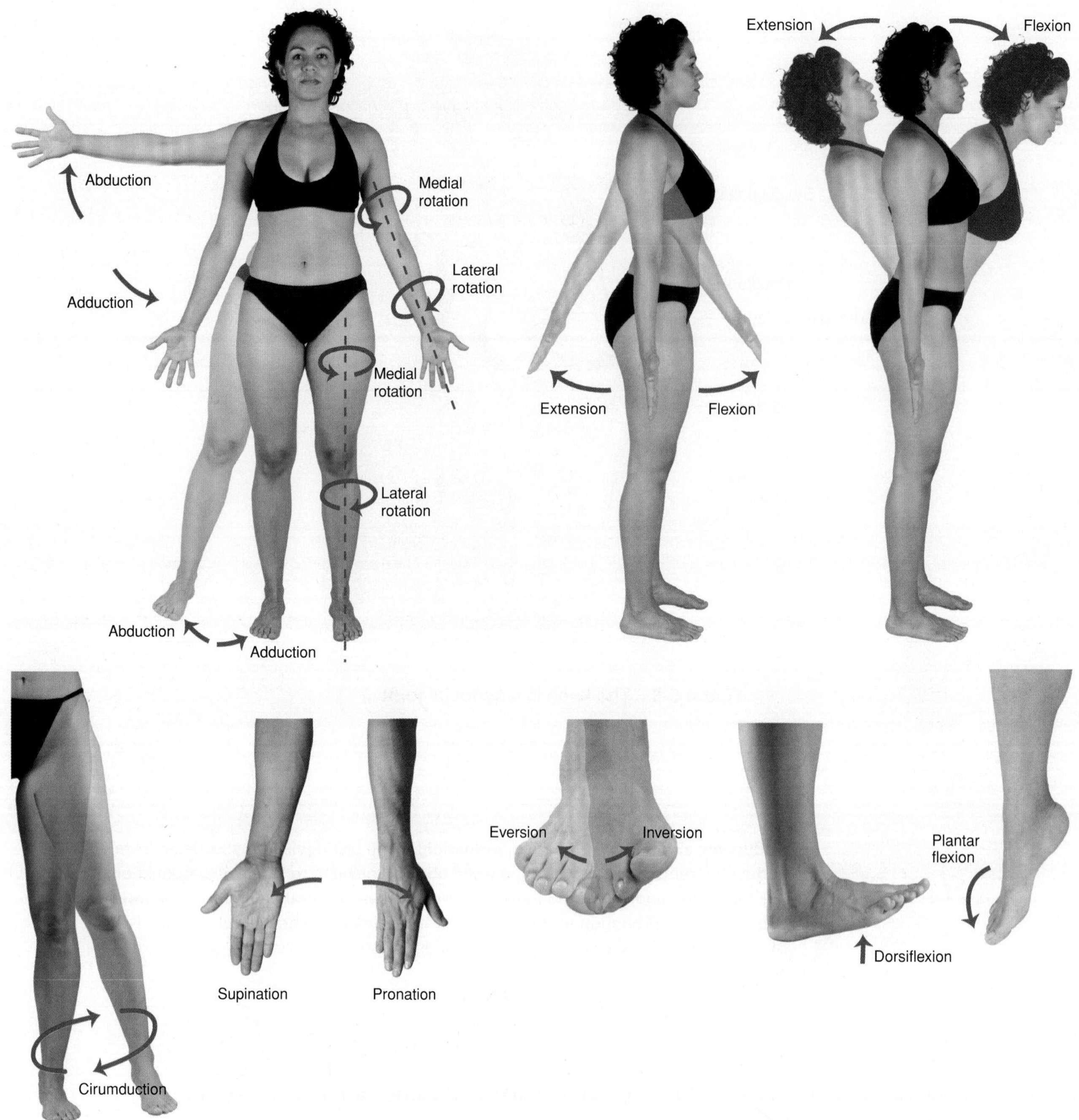

Figure 5-6 Movements at joints.

Terms Related to Muscles (Figure 5-7)

Term	Pronunciation	Meaning
agonist	ag′ŏn-ist	skeletal muscle that creates a movement by contracting; prime mover
antagonist	an-tag′ŏ-nist	skeletal muscle that opposes an agonist muscle and relaxes when the agonist contracts
cardiac muscle	kahr′dē-ak mŭs′ĕl	heart muscle **(Figure 5-8)**
fascia	fash′ē-ă	sheet of connective tissue covering a muscle

Terms Related to Muscles

Term	Pronunciation	Meaning
fascicle	fas′i-kĕl	bundle of muscle fibers (see later **Figure 5-10**)
insertion of muscle	in-sĕr′shŭn mŭs′ĕl	end of muscle attached to bone that moves during contraction (**Figure 5-10**)
origin of muscle	ōr′i-jin mŭs′ĕl	end of muscle attached to bone that does not move during contraction
smooth muscle	smūth mŭs′ĕl	nonstriated, voluntary muscle tissue lining organs and blood vessels (**Figure 5-8**)
skeletal muscle	skel′ĕ-tăl mŭs′ĕl	striated, voluntary muscle tissue attached to bones (the term "striated" refers to light and dark bands in muscle fibers) (**Figures 5-8** and **5-9**)
tonicity	tō-nis′i-tē	muscle tone; tonus

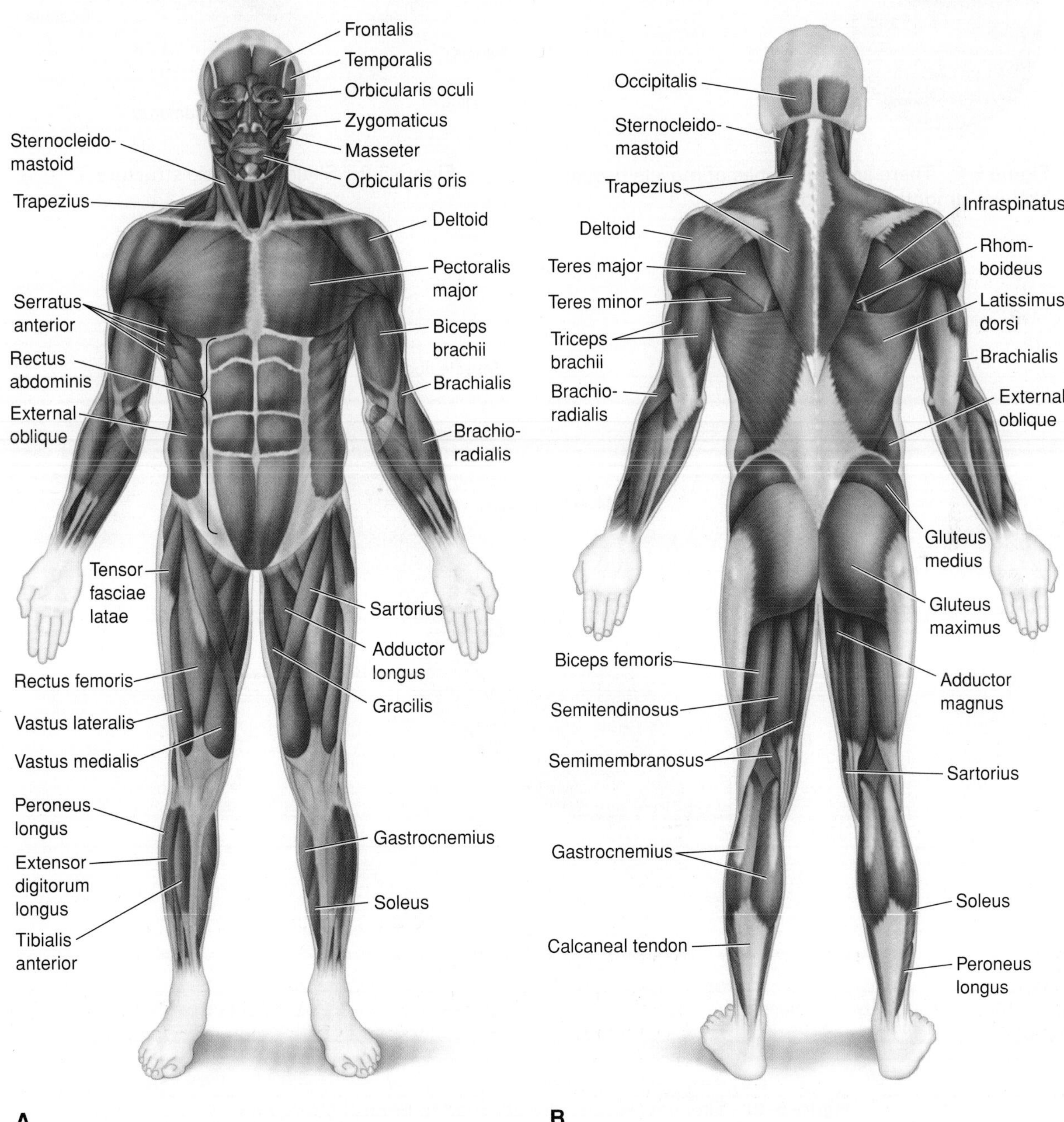

Figure 5-7 Skeletal muscles of the body. **A.** Anterior view. **B.** Posterior view.

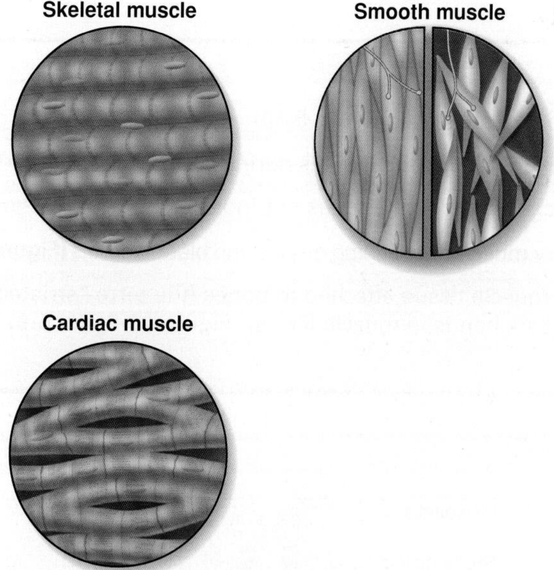

Figure 5-8 There are three types of muscle tissue: skeletal, smooth, and cardiac.

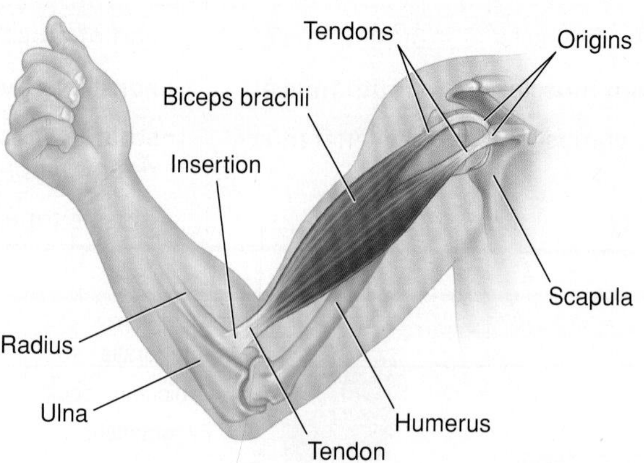

Figure 5-9 Skeletal muscle structure.

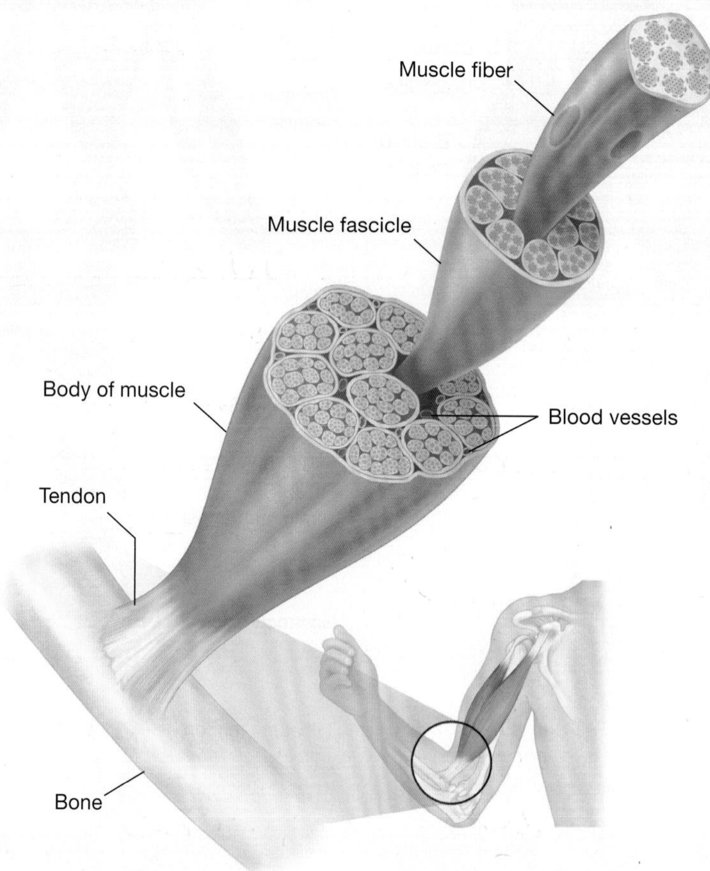

Figure 5-10 Skeletal muscles are attached to bones by tendons.

Exercises: Anatomy and Physiology

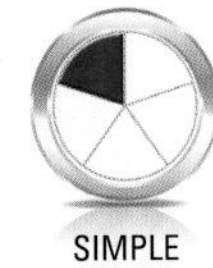
SIMPLE RECALL

Exercise 1

Write the correct anatomic structure for the definition given.

1. upper arm bone humerus
2. bones of the hand between the wrist and fingers metacarpal
3. shoulder blade scapula
4. breast bone sternum
5. shaft of long bone diaphysis
6. attaches muscle to bone tendon
7. bundle of muscle fibers ______
8. heel bone calcaneus
9. bones of the head, vertebral column, and thorax axial skeleton
10. bone of the vertebral column (spine) vertebra

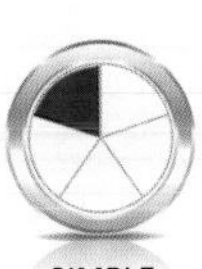
SIMPLE RECALL

Exercise 2

Write the meaning of the term given.

1. abduction moving away
2. ligament connects bone or cartilage at joint
3. articulation joint
4. dorsiflexion bending foot upward
5. acetabulum socket of hip bone
6. cranium skull
7. mandible lower jaw
8. synovial joint joint that moves freely
9. maxilla upper jaw
10. cartilage dense connective tissue
11. epiphysial plate growth area of long bone
12. tonicity muscle tone

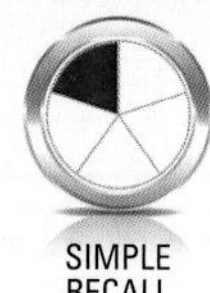

Exercise 3

SIMPLE RECALL

Circle the term that is most appropriate for the meaning of the sentence.

1. A severe injury to the kneecap may involve a fractured (*cerebellum, patella, scapula*).
2. The cartilage structure in the knee is called the (*synovium, meniscus, bursa*).
3. Muscle tissue present in internal organs is (*unstriated, agonist, fascial*).
4. (*Synovial fluid, Endosteum, Fascia*) is a sheet of connective tissue covering a muscle.
5. The smaller bone in the lower leg is the (*femur, ulna, fibula*).
6. The (*epiphysis, ilium, patella*), or superior broad part of the hip bone, connects with the ischium and pubis.
7. The (*tibia, sacrum, lamina*) is a part of each vertebra.
8. The (*clavicle, metaphysis, radius*) articulates with the acromion at one end and the top of the sternum at the other end.
9. Between the diaphysis and the epiphysis of a long bone is the (*metaphysis, meniscus, diarthrosis*).
10. The large inner bone of the lower leg is the (*tibia, ulna, radius*).
11. A (*tendon, fascia, bursa*) is a fluid-filled fibrous sac within some joints.
12. The (*ischium, ilium, pubis*) is the inferior rearmost part of the hip bone, whereas the (*ischium, ilium, pubis*) is the anterior lower section of the hip bone.
13. The plural of vertebra is (*vertebrum, vertebras, vertebrae*).
14. The metatarsal bones are just distal to the (*tarsal, carpal, phalangeal*) bones.
15. Movement that decreases the joint angle is termed (*extension, flexion, inversion*).

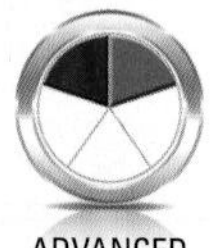

Exercise 4

ADVANCED RECALL

Match each medical term with its meaning.

spongy bone	ulna	carpal bones	endosteum	sacrum
intervertebral disc	radius	compact bone	epiphyseal plate	osteocyte

1. membrane within the medullary cavity endosteum
2. strong solid bone tissue compact bones
3. outer bone in forearm radius
4. eight bones of the wrist carpal bones
5. cancellous bone sacrum
6. triangular bone composed of fused vertebrae intervertebral disk
7. connective tissue between vertebrae spongy bone

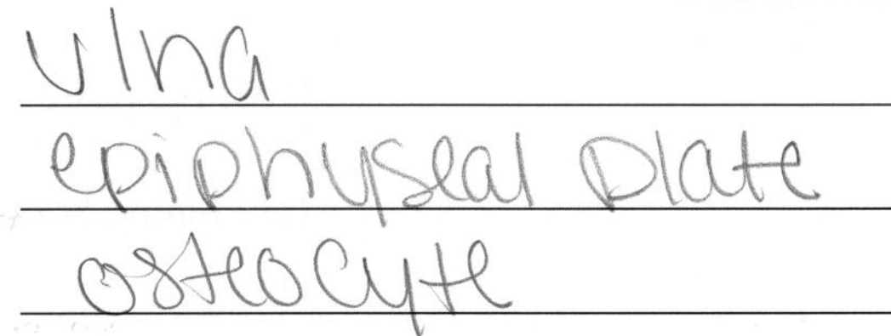

8. inner bone in the forearm ulna

9. growth area of a long bone epiphyseal plate

10. bone cell osteocyte

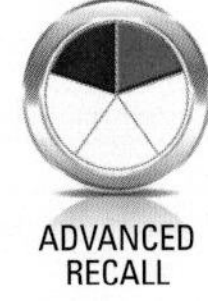

ADVANCED RECALL

Exercise 5

Complete each sentence by writing in the correct medical term.

1. A patient with a broken collar bone has a fracture of the __________.

2. A fracture of the upper arm bone, the humerus, is generally painful.

3. Bone tissue that is spongy and meshlike is called spongy bone.

4. A(n) __________ is a band of strong connective tissue that joins bones together at a joint.

5. The end of a muscle attached to bone that moves with contraction is called the __________ of the muscle.

6. A(n) __________ is a skeletal muscle that opposes a prime mover.

7. Skeletal muscle is __________, whereas smooth muscle is __________.

8. A freely moving joint is lubricated by synovial fluid.

9. The movement of turning the foot outward is called eversion.

10. The type of immovable joint connecting skull bones is a(n) __________.

11. Bones in many types of joints are by __________, a dense connective tissue.

12. Just superior to the coccyx is the bone called the __________.

■ WORD PARTS

The following tables list word parts related to the musculoskeletal system.

Combining Forms

Combining Form	Meaning
ankyl/o	stiff
arthr/o, articul/o	joint
burs/o	bursa
carp/o	carpal (wrist) bones
chondr/o	cartilage
clavic/o, clavicul/o	clavicle

(continued)

Combining Forms *(continued)*

Combining Form	Meaning
cervic/o	neck
cost/o	rib
crani/o	cranium, skull
disc/o	disc or disk
fasci/o	fascia, band
femor/o	femur
fibul/o	fibula
humer/o	humerus
ili/o	ilium
ischi/o	ischium
kinesi/o, kinet/o	movement
kyph/o	humpback
lei/o	smooth
lamin/o	lamina (plate)
lord/o	curved, bent
lumb/o	lumbar region, lower back
mandibul/o	mandible (lower jawbone)
maxill/o	maxilla (upper jawbone)
menisc/o	meniscus
my/o, mys/o, muscul/o	muscle
myel/o	bone marrow, spinal cord
oste/o	bone
patell/o	patella (kneecap)
pelv/i, pelv/o	pelvis, pelvic cavity
phalang/o	phalanges (bones of digits)
pub/o	pubis
rachi/o	spine
radi/o	radius
rhabd/o	striated muscle
sacr/o	sacrum
scapul/o	scapula (shoulder blade)
scoli/o	crooked, twisted
stern/o	sternum (breast bone)
synovi/o	synovial joint or fluid
tars/o	tarsal bones
ten/o, tend/o, tendin/o	tendon
thorac/o	thorax, chest
ton/o	tone, tension
uln/o	ulna
vertebr/o, spondyl/o	vertebra

Prefixes

Prefix	Meaning
inter-	between
intra-	within
supra-	above
sub-	below, beneath
sym-, syn-	together, with

Suffixes

Suffix	Meaning
-algia	pain
-asthenia	weakness
-centesis	puncture to aspirate
-clasia, -clasis, -clast	to break
-ectomy	excision, surgical removal
-itis	inflammation
-osis	abnormal condition
-physis	growth
-plasty	surgical repair, reconstruction
-porosis	pore, passage
-rrhaphy	suture
-schisis	to split
-trophy	development, nourishment

Exercises: Word Parts

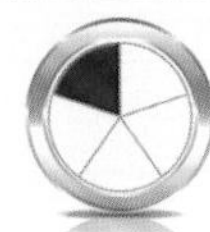

SIMPLE RECALL

Exercise 6

Write the meaning of the combining form given.

1. crani/o cranium/skull
2. lumb/o lower back
3. scoli/o crooked, twisted
4. oste/o bone
5. stern/o sternum
6. maxill/o maxilla

7. chondr/o cartilage
8. carp/o carpal
9. ten/o, tend/o tendon
10. spondyl/o vertebra
11. fasci/o fascia, band
12. my/o, mys/o muscle
13. mandibul/o mandible
14. sacr/o sacrum
15. femor/o femur

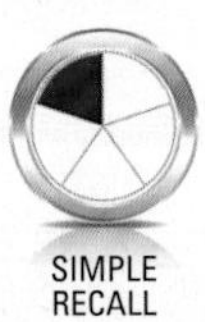
SIMPLE RECALL

Exercise 7

Write the correct combining form for the meaning given.

1. rib cost/o
2. tarsal bones tars/o
3. smooth kyph/o
4. fibula fibul/o
5. bursa burs/o
6. joint arthr/o
7. pelvis pelv/i or pelv/o
8. chest thorac/o
9. ischium ili/o
10. collar bone
11. lamina lamin/o
12. neck cervic/o
13. meniscus menisc/o
14. phalanges phalang/o

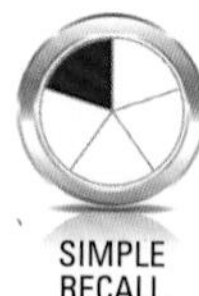
SIMPLE RECALL

Exercise 8

Write the meaning of the prefix or suffix given.

1. -plasty repair
2. -asthenia weakness
3. sub- below
4. -trophy development
5. -ectomy removal
6. -physis growth
7. -rrhaphy suture
8. sym- together
9. -schisis split
10. -clasis break

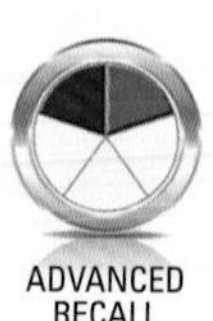
ADVANCED RECALL

Exercise 9

Considering the meanings of the word parts from which the medical terms are made, write the meanings of the medical terms given. (You have not yet learned many of these terms but can build their meanings from the word parts.)

Combining Form	Meaning	Medical Term	Meaning of Term
oste/o	bone	osteitis	1. bone inflammation
lord/o	bent (forward)	lordosis	2. curved condition
my/o	muscle	myalgia	3. muscle pain
burs/o	bursa	bursitis	4. bursa inflammation
maxill/o	maxilla	maxillitis	5. maxilla inflammation
scapul/o	scapula	subscapular	6. below scapula
pelv/i	pelvis	pelvic	7. pertaining to pelvis
tend/o	tendon	tendonitis	8. tendon inflamation
vertebr/o	vertebra	intervertebral	9. between vertebra
arthr/o	joint	arthroplasty	10. surgical repair of joint

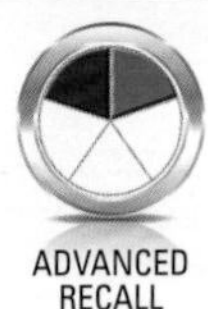
ADVANCED RECALL

Exercise 10

Using the given combining form and a word part from the earlier tables, build a medical term for the meaning given.

Combining Form	Meaning of Medical Term	Medical Term
mys/o	inflammation of muscle	1. ______
crani/o	surgical repair of skull	2. ______
patell/o	excision of patella	3. ______
ten/o	suture of tendon	4. ______
arthr/o	pain in a joint	5. ______
crani/o	pertaining to within the skull	6. ______
tars/o	excision of tarsal bone	7. ______
menisci/o	inflammation of a meniscus	8. ______
disc/o	excision of intervertebral disc	9. ______
chondr/o	surgical repair of cartilage	10. ______

MEDICAL TERMS

The following table gives adjective forms and terms used in describing the musculoskeletal system and its conditions.

Adjectives and Other Related Terms

Term	Pronunciation	Meaning
carpal	kahr′păl	pertaining to the carpal bones
costovertebral	kos′tō-vĕr′tĕ-brăl	pertaining to the ribs and thoracic vertebrae
cranial	krā′nē-ăl	pertaining to the skull
femoral	fem′ŏr-ăl	pertaining to the femur
humeral	hyū′mĕr-ăl	pertaining to the humerus
iliofemoral	il′ē-ō-fem′ŏr-ăl	pertaining to the ilium and femur
intercostal	in′tĕr-kos′tăl	pertaining to the area between the ribs
intervertebral	in′tĕr-vĕr′tĕ-brăl	pertaining to the area between vertebrae
intracranial	in-tră-krā′nē-ăl	pertaining to the area within the skull
ischiofemoral	is′kē-ō-fem′ŏr-ăl	pertaining to the ischium and femur

Adjectives and Other Related Terms

Term	Pronunciation	Meaning
lumbar	lŭm′bahr	pertaining to the lower back
lumbocostal	lŭm′bō-kos′tăl	pertaining to the lumbar vertebrae and ribs
lumbosacral	lŭm′bō-sā′krăl	pertaining to the lumbar vertebrae and sacrum
osseous	os′ē-ŭs	pertaining to bone
pelvic	pel′vik	pertaining to the pelvis or pelvic cavity
sacral	sā′krăl	pertaining to the sacrum
sacrovertebral	sā′krō-vĕr′tĕ-brăl	pertaining to the sacrum and the vertebrae above
sternoclavicular	stĕr′nō-klă-vik′yū-lăr	pertaining to the sternum and clavicle
sternoid	stĕr′noyd	resembling the sternum
subcostal	sŭb-kos′tăl	pertaining to the area below a rib or below the ribs
submandibular	sŭb′man-dib′yū-lăr	pertaining to the area below the mandible
submaxillary	sŭb-mak′si-lar-ē	pertaining to the area below the maxilla
subscapular	sŭb-skap′yū-lăr	pertaining to the area below the scapula
substernal	sŭb-stĕr′năl	pertaining to the area below the sternum
suprapatellar	sū′pră-pă-tel′ăr	pertaining to the area above the patella
suprascapular	sū′pră-skap′yū-lăr	pertaining to the area above the scapula
synovial	si-nō′vē-ăl	pertaining to, containing, or consisting of synovial fluid

Exercises: Adjectives and Other Related Terms

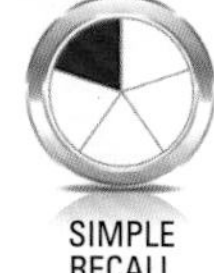

SIMPLE RECALL

Exercise 11

Circle the term that is most appropriate for the meaning of the sentence.

1. An (*iliofemoral, ischiopubic, intercostal*) wound is located between the ribs.
2. A broken upper leg bone is called a (*humeral, cranial, femoral*) fracture.
3. A herniated (*intervertebral, carpal, sternoclavicular*) disc involves an injury to the discs between the vertebrae.
4. The (*ischiofemoral, lumbocostal, subscapular*) area includes both the ischium and femur.
5. Diagnosing a knee condition may require a needle puncture to withdraw (*submaxillary, sternoid, synovial*) fluid for testing.
6. A(n) (*substernal, pelvic, osseous*) examination includes all of the organs in the pelvis.
7. The area below (inferior to) the shoulder blade is called the (*subcostal, pubofemoral, subscapular*) region.
8. A wrist injury may involve a (*carpal, subcostal, sternoid*) fracture.

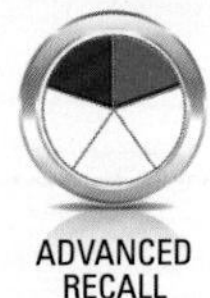

ADVANCED RECALL

Exercise 12

Match each medical term with its meaning.

substernal	costovertebral	intracranial	intervertebral
lumbar	submandibular	suprapatellar	sacral
humeral	lumbosacral	intercostal	cranial

1. pertaining to the humerus humeral
2. pertaining to the area between ribs intercostal
3. pertaining to the area below the sternum substernal
4. pertaining to the area above the patella suprapatellar
5. pertaining to the skull cranial
6. pertaining to the sacrum sacral.
7. pertaining to the area between vertebrae intervertebral
8. pertaining to the area within the skull intracranial
9. pertaining to the lower back lumbar
10. pertaining to the ribs and thoracic vertebrae costovertebral
11. pertaining to the area below the mandible submandibular
12. pertaining to the lumbar vertebrae and sacrum lumbosacral

Medical Conditions

Term	Pronunciation	Meaning
ankylosing spondylitis	ang'ki-lōs-ing spon'di-lī'tis	arthritis of the spine
ankylosis	ang'ki-lō'sis	abnormal condition of stiffening or fixation of a joint
arthralgia	ahr-thral'jē-ă	pain in a joint
arthritis	ahr-thrī'tis	inflammation of a joint **(Figure 5-11)**
arthrochondritis	ahr'thrō-kon-drī'tis	inflammation of an articular cartilage
atrophy	at'rŏ-fē	wasting of tissues, organs, or the entire body
bradykinesia	brad'ē-kin-ē'sē-ă	condition of decreased movement
bunion	bŭn'yŏn	swelling at the metatarsophalangeal joint caused by inflammatory bursa
bursitis	bŭr-sī'tis	inflammation of a bursa
bursolith	bŭr'sō-lith	a calculus (stone) formed in a bursa
carpal tunnel syndrome (CTS)	kahr'păl tŭn'ĕl sin'drōm	entrapment of the median nerve at the wrist causing pain
carpoptosis; *syn.* wrist-drop	kar'pop-tō'sis; rist drop	paralysis of wrist and finger muscles

Medical Conditions

Term	Pronunciation	Meaning
chondromalacia	kon′drō-mă-lā′shē-ă	softening of any cartilage
cranioschisis	krā′nē-os′ki-sis	congenital malformation of incomplete closure of the skull
curvature of the spine	kŭr′vă-chŭr of the spīn	curving of the spine in one or more directions **(Figure 5-12)**
kyphosis	kī-fō′sis	abnormal forward curvature; humpback
lordosis	lōr-dō′sis	abnormal backward curvature
scoliosis	skō′lē-ō′sis	abnormal lateral curvature
dyskinesia	dis′ki-nē′sē-ă	difficulty performing voluntary movements
dystrophy	dis′trŏ-fē	abnormal development or growth of a tissue or organ, often resulting from nutritional deficiency

(continued)

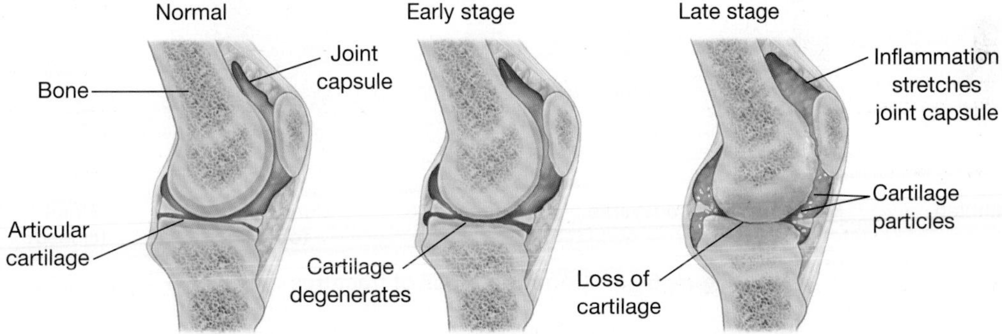

Figure 5-11 Progressive joint changes seen in knee arthritis.

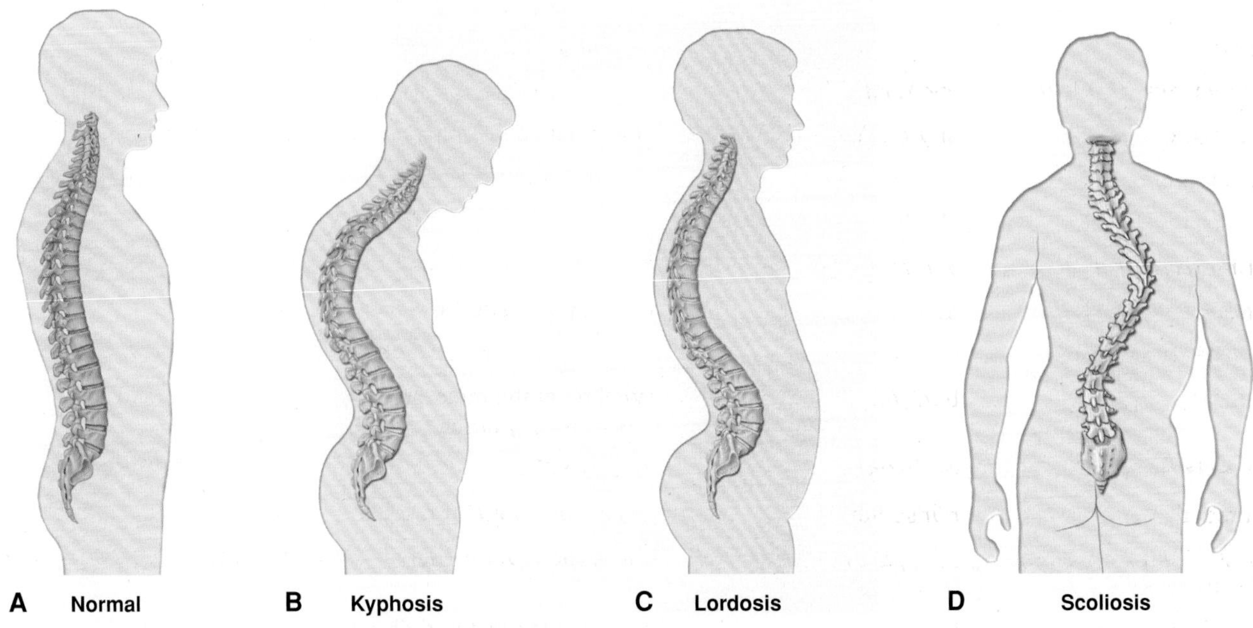

Figure 5-12 Abnormal curvatures of the spine can cause pain and disfigurement.

Medical Conditions *(continued)*

Term	Pronunciation	Meaning
exostosis	eks′os-tō′sis	bony projection that develops from cartilage
fibromyalgia	fī′brō-mī-al′jē-ă	condition of chronic aching and stiffness of muscles and soft tissues of unknown cause
fracture (fx)	frak′shŭr	a break in a bone or cartilage **(Figures 5-13** and **5-14)**
gout	gowt	metabolic disorder involving painful deposits of uric acid crystals in connective tissue and articular cartilage

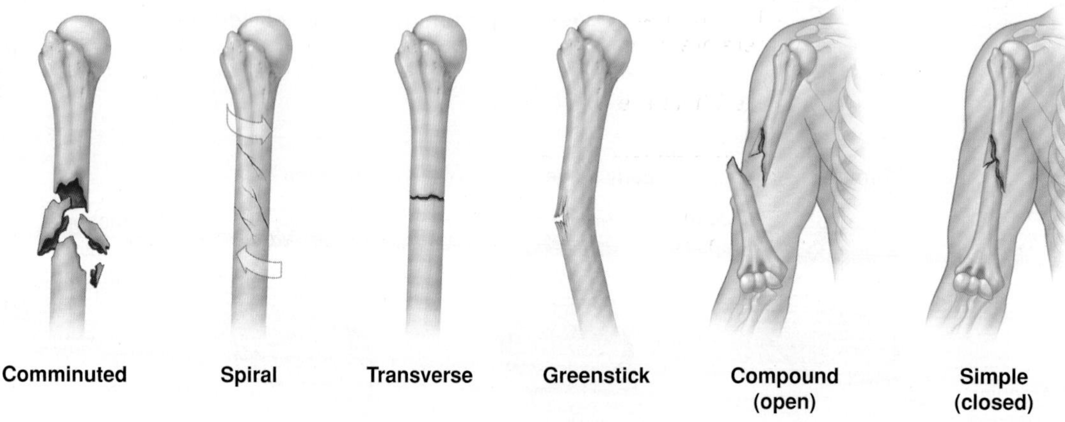

Figure 5-13 Common types of fractures.

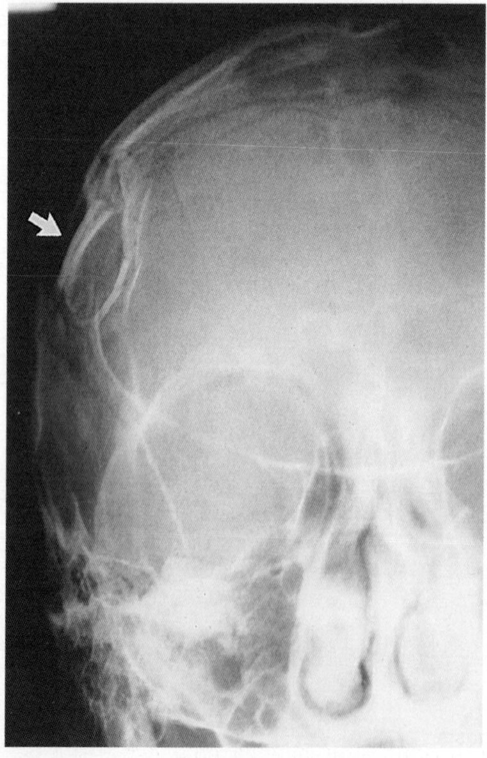

Figure 5-14 Depressed skull fracture.

Medical Conditions

Term	Pronunciation	Meaning
herniated disc	hĕr′nē-ā-tĕd disk	protrusion of nucleus pulposus of intervertebral disc into the vertebral canal **(Figure 5-15)**
hyperkinesia	hī′pĕr-ki-nē′zē-ă	condition of excessive muscular movements
hypertrophy	hī-pĕr′trō-fē	increased development of a part or organ not caused by a tumor
maxillitis	mak′si-lī′tis	inflammation of the maxilla
meniscitis	men-i-sī′tis	inflammation of a meniscus
muscular dystrophy (MD)	mŭs′kyū-lăr dis′trō-fē	hereditary condition causing progressive degeneration of skeletal muscles

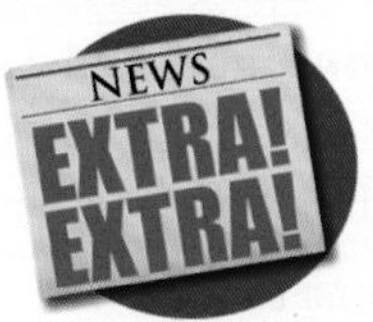

MUSCULAR DYSTROPHY While there are several variations of muscular dystrophy, there are two prominent types. They are called Becker and Duchenne. Both of these are X-linked, which means the gene is found on the X chromosome. There are two chromosomes, X and Y. Muscular dystrophy affects more boys (XY) than girls (XX).

Term	Pronunciation	Meaning
myalgia	mī-al′jē-ă	condition of muscular pain
myasthenia gravis (MG)	mī-as-thē′nē-ă gra′vis	neuromuscular disorder causing weakness and fatigue of voluntary muscles

(continued)

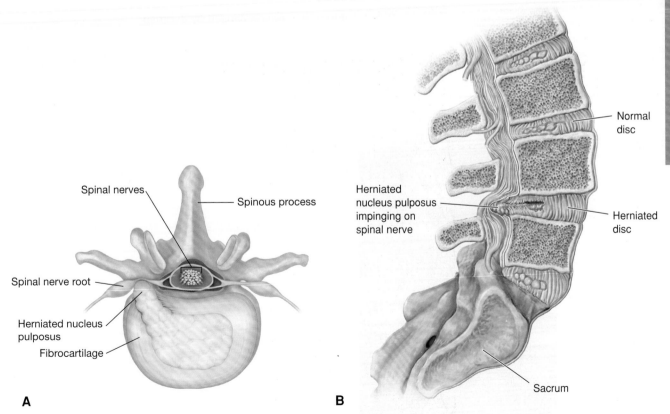

Figure 5-15 Views of a herniated disc showing protrusion of the gelatinous central portion called the nucleus pulposus. **A.** Cross-sectional view. **B.** Lateral view.

Medical Conditions *(continued)*

Term	Pronunciation	Meaning
myositis	mī-ō-sī'tis	inflammation of a muscle
osteitis	os-tē-ī'tis	inflammation of bone
osteoarthritis (OA)	os'tē-ō-ahr-thrī'tis	joint inflammation involving erosion and inflammation of articular cartilage
osteochondritis	os'tē-ō-kon-drī'tis	inflammation of a bone and its articular cartilage
osteomalacia	os'tē-ō-mă-lā'shē-ă	condition of bone softening
osteomyelitis	os'tē-ō-mī-ĕ-lī'tis	inflammation of bone marrow
osteonecrosis	os'tē-ō-nĕ-krō'sis	death of bone tissue
osteoporosis	os'tē-ō-pŏr-ō'sis	age-related disorder of decreased bone mass and weakening **(Figure 5-16)**
polymyositis	pol'ē-mī'ō-sī'tis	inflammation of multiple voluntary muscles
rachischisis	ră-kis'ki-sis	embryologic failure of vertebral arches to fuse
rheumatoid arthritis (RA)	rū'mă-toyd ahr-thrī'tis	disease causing progressive destructive changes and inflammation in multiple joints, especially in the hands and feet **(Figure 5-17)**
rickets	rik'ĕts	disease caused by vitamin D deficiency during childhood, involving skeletal deformities and muscular weakness
spondylarthritis	spon'dil-ahr-thrī'tis	inflammation of intervertebral articulations
sprain	sprān	injury of a ligament caused by abnormal or excessive forces on a joint
strain	strān	injury of a muscle caused by overuse
tendonitis, tendinitis	ten'dŏ-nī'tis, ten'di-nī'tis	inflammation of a tendon
tenodynia	ten-ō-din'ē-ă	condition of pain in a tendon
tenosynovitis	ten'ō-sin-ō-vī'tis	inflammation of a tendon and its sheath

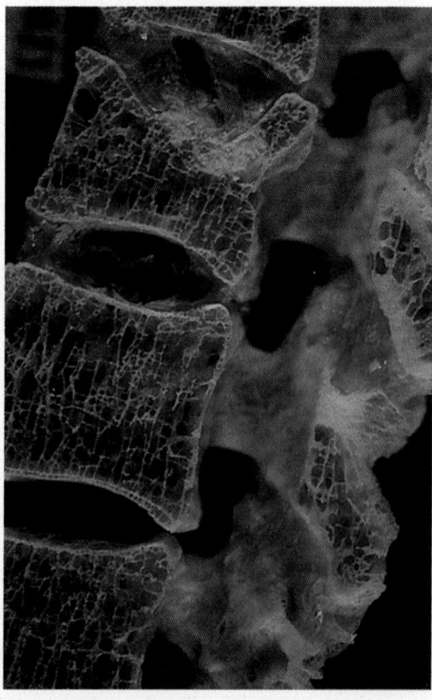

Figure 5-16 Bone becomes less dense in osteoporosis.

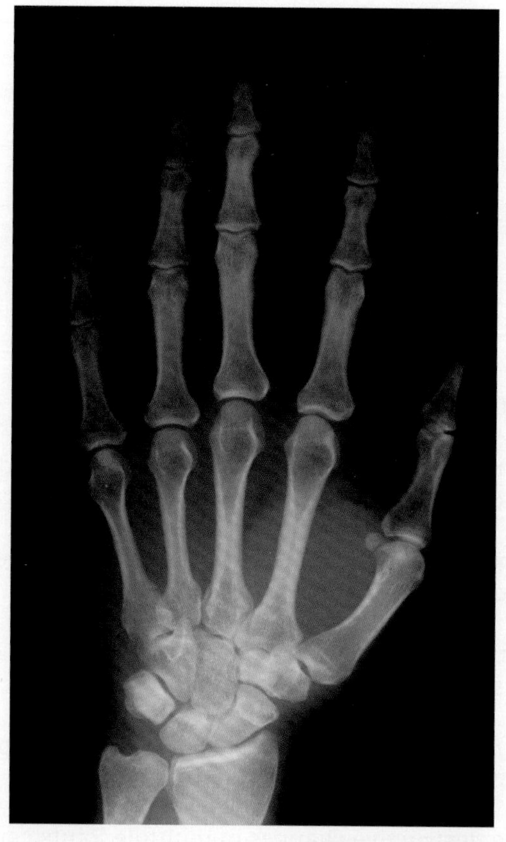

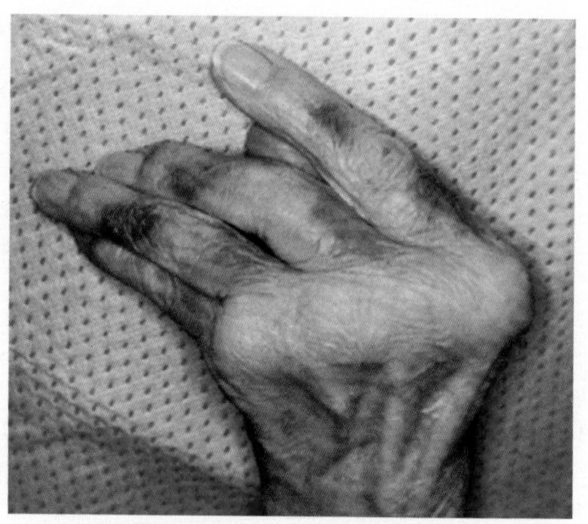

Figure 5-17 The changes of severe rheumatoid arthritis. **A.** X-ray of normal hand. **B.** Hand severely deformed from rheumatoid arthritis.

Exercises: Medical Conditions

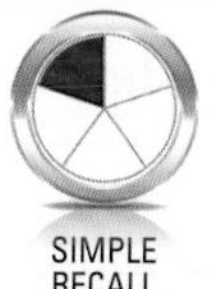

SIMPLE RECALL

Exercise 13

Write the correct medical term for the definition given.

1. abnormal lateral curvature of the spine ____________________
2. inflamed tendon ____________________
3. break in a bone ____________________
4. softening of cartilage ____________________
5. inflamed bursa ____________________
6. decreased bone mass ____________________
7. disease caused by vitamin D deficiency ____________________
8. pain in a tendon ____________________
9. inflamed intervertebral articulations ____________________

10. arthritis of the spine ______________________

11. abnormal forward curvature of the spine ______________________

12. pain in a joint ______________________

13. inflammation of a joint ______________________

14. bone softening ______________________

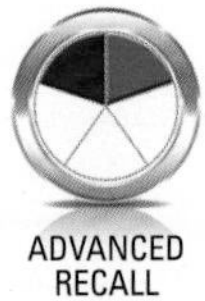
ADVANCED RECALL

Exercise 14

Circle the term that is most appropriate for the meaning of the sentence.

1. Mrs. Jones presented with weakness and fatigue in her voluntary muscles; after clinical study, her physician diagnosed her condition as (*myasthenia, myalgia, myositis*) gravis.

2. Mr. Carelton was seen in a follow-up for his condition of inflammation of multiple voluntary muscles, also called (*polymyositis, carpal tunnel syndrome, atrophy*).

3. Dr. Gonzalez informed Mr. Lawson that when (*gout, fibromyalgia, osteitis*) occurs, uric acid crystals are deposited in connective tissue and articular cartilage.

4. Young Bridget LaRoux suffered a(n) (*sprain, strain, atrophy*) to her calf muscle and a(n) (*sprain, strain, atrophy*) to one of her ligaments.

5. Mrs. Anderson suffers from progressive destructive changes in multiple joints caused by (*muscular dystrophy, rheumatoid arthritis, myasthenia gravis*).

6. After spending years in chronic pain without a known cause, the patient was diagnosed with (*fibromyalgia, gout, hypertrophy*).

7. After his x-ray report showed a stone in his elbow area, the patient was told that he had a(n) (*bunion, bursolith, exostosis*).

8. Miss Gabbi developed (*atrophy, hypertrophy, dystrophy*) of her lower limbs after spending many years in a wheelchair.

9. The physician diagnosed Ms. Allen with (*carpal, metacarpal, tarsal*) tunnel syndrome when she complained of pain in her wrist after many years of repetitive work.

10. Mr. Kowalski suffered from (*osteitis, dyskinesia, exostosis*) after his stroke.

11. After reporting pain in his throwing arm, the baseball player was diagnosed with inflammation of a tendon and its sheath, also called (*tenosynovitis, tenodynia, osteochondritis*).

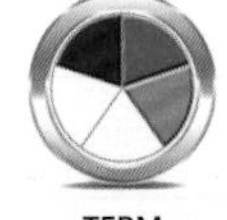
TERM CONSTRUCTION

Exercise 15

Given their meanings, build a medical term from an appropriate combining form and suffix.

Use Combining Form for	Use Suffix for	Term
joint	inflammation	1. ______________
joint	pain	2. ______________

spine	split	3. ______
maxilla	inflammation	4. ______
tendon	pain	5. ______
bursa	inflammation	6. ______
muscle	pain	7. ______
joint and cartilage	inflammation	8. ______
bone	softening	9. ______

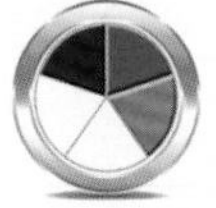

TERM CONSTRUCTION

Exercise 16

Break the given medical term into its word parts and define each part. Then define the medical term. (Note: This exercise uses some previously learned suffixes.)

For example:

arthritis
word parts: arthr/o, -itis
meanings: joint, inflammation
term meaning: inflammation of a joint

1. hypertrophy
word parts: ______
meanings: ______
term meaning: ______

2. scoliosis
word parts: ______
meanings: ______
term meaning: ______

3. cranioschisis
word parts: ______
meanings: ______
term meaning: ______

4. carpoptosis
word parts: ______
meanings: ______
term meaning: ______

5. ankylosis
word parts: ______
meanings: ______
term meaning: ______

6. bursolith *word parts:* ______________________

meanings: ______________________

term meaning: ______________________

7. atrophy *word parts:* ______________________

meanings: ______________________

term meaning: ______________________

8. osteitis *word parts:* ______________________

meanings: ______________________

term meaning: ______________________

9. bradykinesia *word parts:* ______________________

meanings: ______________________

term meaning: ______________________

10. polymyositis *word parts:* ______________________

meanings: ______________________

term meaning: ______________________

Tests and Procedures

Term	Pronunciation	Meaning
Laboratory Tests		
creatine kinase (CK)	krē′ă-tin kī′nās	test for the presence of the enzyme creatine kinase in the blood, which may indicate conditions that can cause muscle weakness or pain
erythrocyte sedimentation rate (ESR)	ĕ-rith′rō-sīt sed′i-mĕn-tā′shŭn rāt	time measurement of red blood cells settling in a test tube over one hour; increased rates are associated with anemia or inflammatory conditions
rheumatoid factor (RF)	rū′mă-toyd fak′tŏr	blood test used to help diagnose rheumatoid arthritis
synovial fluid analysis	si-nō′vē-ăl flū′id ă-nal′i-sis	test for the presence of crystals caused by some conditions, such as arthritis, and the presence of signs of joint infection
uric acid test	yūr′ik as′id	test for elevated presence of uric acid in the blood, indicating gout
Diagnostic Procedures		
arthrography	ahr-throg′ră-fē	x-ray imaging of a joint using a contrast dye
arthroscopy	ahr-thros′kŏ-pē	endoscopic examination of the interior of a joint **(Figure 5-18)**
bone densitometry	dens′i-tom′ĕ-trē	x-ray technique for determining density of bone
bone scan	bōn skan	nuclear medicine imaging of bone used to diagnose bone disorders **(Figure 5-19)**

(continued)

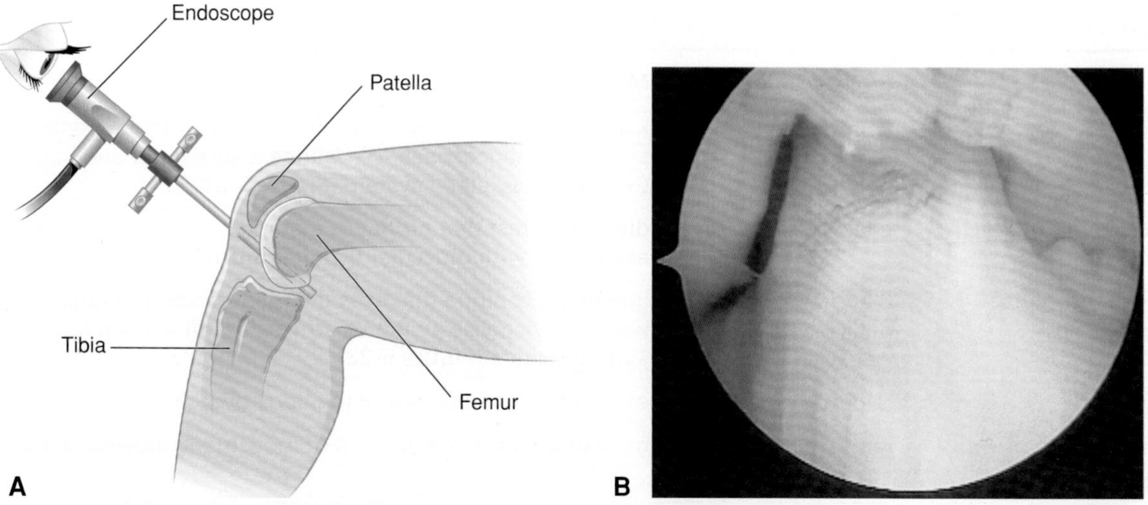

Figure 5-18 **A.** Arthroscopic examination of the knee. **B.** Endoscopic view of joint interior.

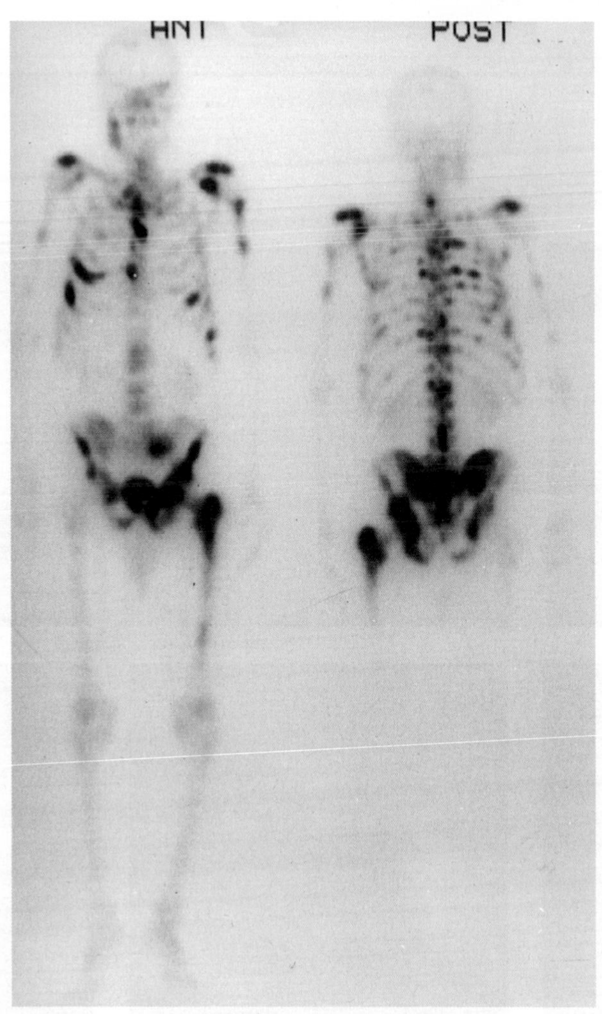

Figure 5-19 Whole body nuclear medicine bone scan.

Tests and Procedures *(continued)*

Term	Pronunciation	Meaning
computed tomography (CT)	kŏm-pyū′tĕd tō-mog′ră-fē	x-ray technique that produces computer-generated cross-sectional images; used to evaluate disorders of and injuries to the musculoskeletal system **(Figure 5-20)**
electromyogram (EMG)	ĕ-lek′trō-mī′ō-gram	diagnostic test that produces a graphic record of electric currents associated with muscular action **(Figure 5-21)**
magnetic resonance imaging (MRI)	mag-net′ik rez′ō-năns im′ăj-ing	imaging technique that uses magnetic fields and radiofrequency waves to visualize anatomic structures; often used to diagnose joint disorders **(Figure 5-22)**
radiography	rā′dē-og′ră-fē	examination of any part of the body by x-rays
range of motion (ROM) testing	rānj uv mō′shŭn	measurement of the amount of movement allowed in a joint

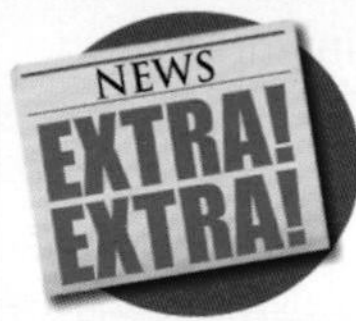

RANGE OF MOTION Range of motion testing is used to assess a patient's joint motion, and range of motion exercises are used to preserve or increase the amount of movement in a joint. An instrument called a goniometer measures the arc, or range of motion, of a joint.

A, B

C

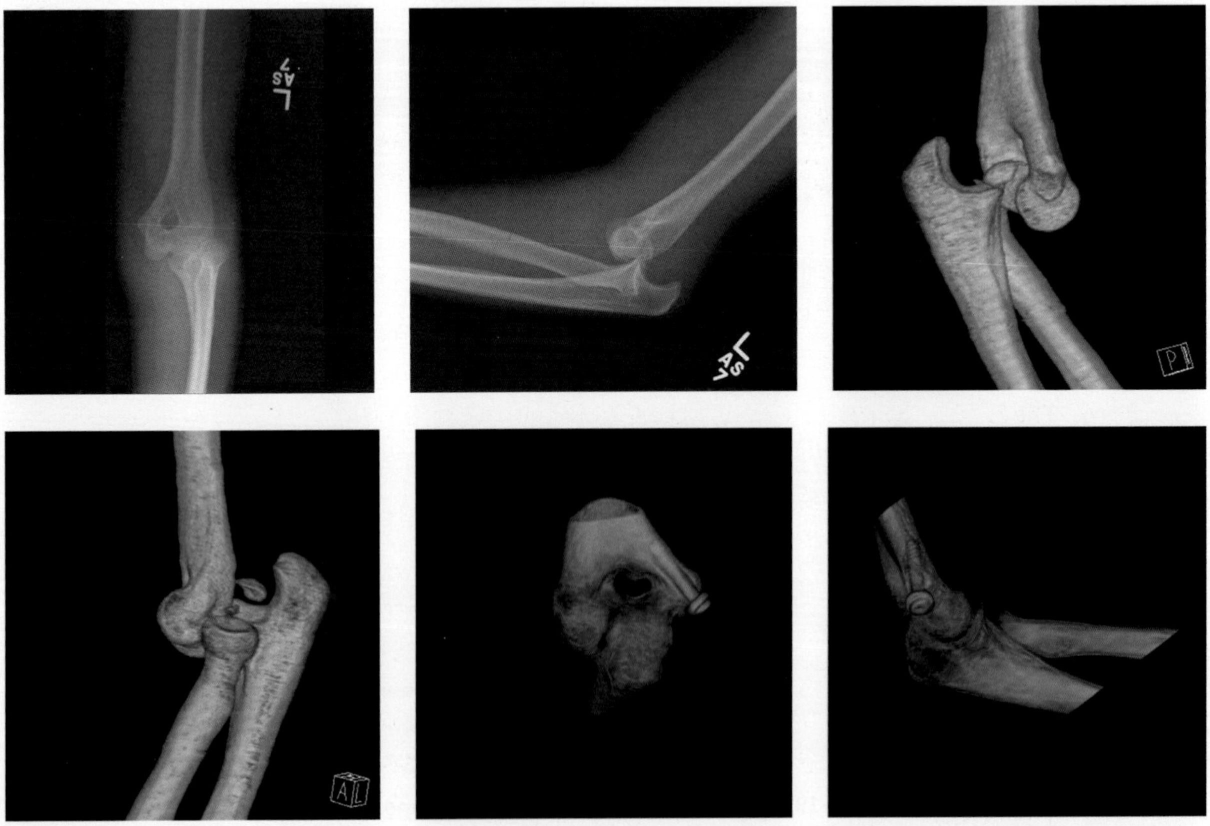

D, E

F

Figure 5-20 **A–D.** Computed tomography (CT) scan showing posterolateral elbow dislocation in a 13-year-old boy. **E, F.** Show the position of the screw and washer 4 months after surgery. The fracture is now completely healed.

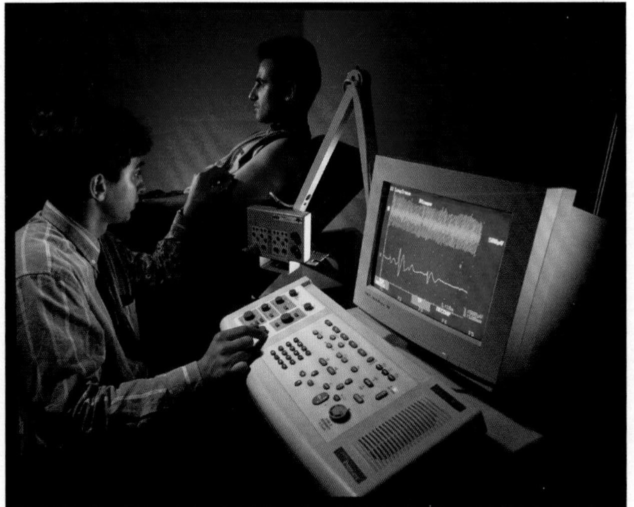

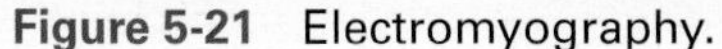

Figure 5-21 Electromyography.

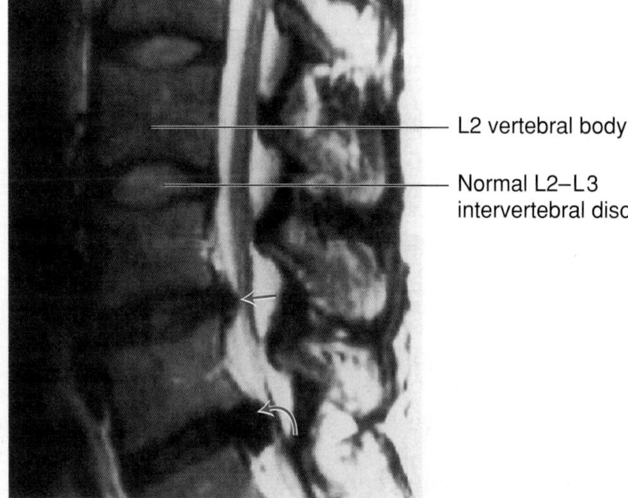

Figure 5-22 Magnetic resonance imaging (MRI) of a herniated intervertebral disc (*arrows*).

Exercises: Tests and Procedures

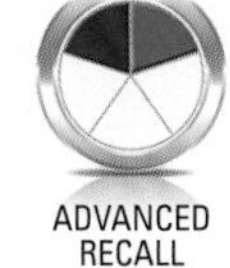

ADVANCED RECALL

Exercise 17

Circle the term that is most appropriate for the meaning of the sentence.

1. Wanting a cross-sectional view of the lateral meniscus, the orthopedist ordered a procedure using (*computed tomography, arthroscopy, range of motion testing*).
2. A record of the electrical currents associated with muscular action is called a(n) (*arthrogram, radiograph, electromyogram*).
3. (*Magnetic resonance imaging, Arthroscopy, Arthrography*) is a radiographic technique for imaging a joint, usually after administering a contrast dye.
4. A bone scan is produced with (*nuclear medicine imaging, endoscopy, arthrography*).
5. The examination of any part of the body by x-ray is called (*radiography, electromyography, computed tomography*).
6. The laboratory test for (*creatine kinase, rheumatoid factor, uric acid*) may help diagnose conditions that cause muscle weakness and pain.
7. (*Rheumatoid factor, Uric acid, Creatine kinase*) is the laboratory test that indicates gout.
8. The laboratory test that will help determine the presence of rheumatoid arthritis is called (*erythrocyte sedimentation rate, uric acid, rheumatoid factor*).

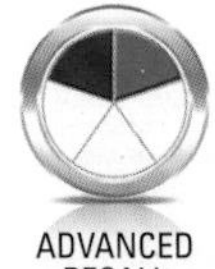

ADVANCED RECALL

Exercise 18

Complete each sentence by writing in the correct medical term.

1. The radiographic technique used to determine bone density is called ______________________.
2. The amount of movement a joint allows can be determined by ______________________.

3. The use of nuclear medicine imaging of bone to diagnose bone disorders is called a(n) ____________.

4. An interior joint space can be viewed through an endoscope in ____________.

5. The diagnostic modality based on the effects of a magnetic field on body tissues is called ____________.

6. The laboratory test that can indicate anemia or inflammatory conditions in the body is called ____________.

7. The laboratory test that may detect crystals caused by certain conditions and signs of joint infection is called ____________.

Surgical Interventions and Therapeutic Procedures

Term	Pronunciation	Meaning
arthrocentesis	ahr'thrō-sen-tē'sis	needle puncture to remove fluid from a joint **(Figure 5-23)**
arthroclasia	ahr'thrō-klā'zē-ă	surgical breaking of adhesions (abnormal unions of membranes) in ankylosis
arthrodesis	ahr-throd'ĕ-sis	surgical artificial stiffening of a joint
arthroplasty	ahr'thrō-plas-tē	surgical restoration of joint function or creation of an artificial joint (such as a total hip or knee replacement)
bursectomy	bŭr-sek'tŏ-mē	excision of a bursa
carpectomy	kahr-pek'tŏ-mē	excision of part or all of the carpal bones
chondrectomy	kon-drek'tŏ-mē	excision of cartilage
chondroplasty	kon'drō-plas-tē	surgical repair of cartilage
costectomy	kos-tek'tŏ-mē	excision of a rib
cranioplasty	krā'nē-ō-plas-tē	surgical repair of the skull
craniotomy	krā'nē-ot'ŏ-mē	surgical creation of an opening (incision) into the skull
discectomy	disk-ek'tŏ-mē	surgical removal of part or all of an intervertebral disc **(Figure 5-24)**
laminectomy	lam'i-nek'tŏ-mē	excision of a vertebral lamina
laminotomy; *syn.* rachiotomy	lam-i-not'ŏ-mē; rā'kē-ot'ŏ-mē	enlargement of the intervertebral foramen by excision of a portion of the lamina to relieve spinal nerve root pressure
maxillotomy	mak'si-lot'ŏ-mē	surgical sectioning of the maxilla to allow movement in all or part of the maxilla
meniscectomy	men'i-sek'tŏ-mē	excision of a meniscus, usually from the knee joint
myoplasty	mī'ō-plas-tē	surgical repair of muscular tissue
myorrhaphy	mī-ōr'ă-fē	suture of a muscle
open reduction, internal fixation (ORIF)	ō'pĕn rē-duk'shŭn, in-tĕr'năl fik-sā'shŭn	surgical repair of a fracture by making an incision into the skin and muscle at the site of the fracture, manually moving the bones into alignment, and fixing the bones in place with surgical wires, screws, pins, rods, or plates
ostectomy	os-tek'tŏ-mē	excision of bone tissue

Surgical Interventions and Therapeutic Procedures

Term	Pronunciation	Meaning
osteoclasis	os-tē-ok'lă-sis	intentional fracture of a bone to correct deformity
osteoclast	os'tē-ō-klast	surgical instrument used to fracture a bone to correct a deformity
patellectomy	pat-ĕ-lek'tŏ-mē	excision of the patella
phalangectomy	fal-an-jek'tŏ-mē	excision of one or more phalanges of the hand or foot
reduction	rĕ-dŭk'shŭn	manipulative or surgical procedure to restore a part to its normal position, such as by reducing a fracture (putting bone ends back in place)
spondylosyndesis	spon'di-lō-sin-dē'sis	surgical procedure to create ankylosis between two or more vertebrae **(Figure 5-25)**; also called spinal fusion

(continued)

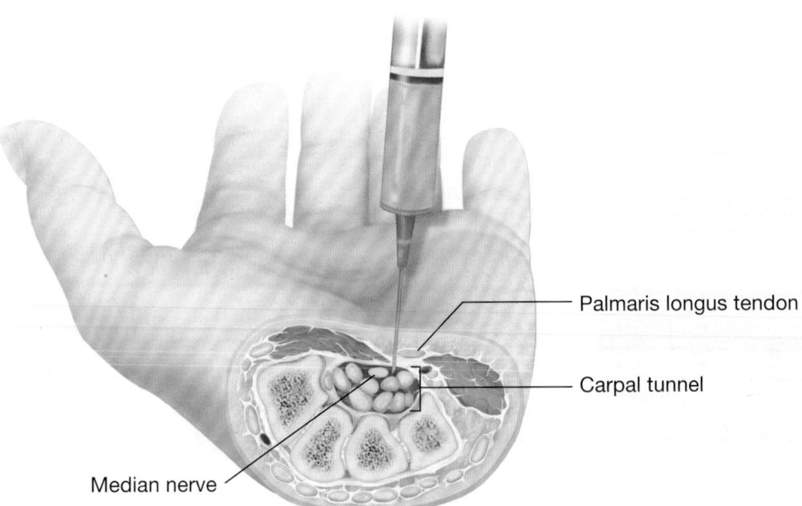

Figure 5-23 Using arthrocentesis, synovial fluid is aspirated from the wrist joint to reduce inflammation.

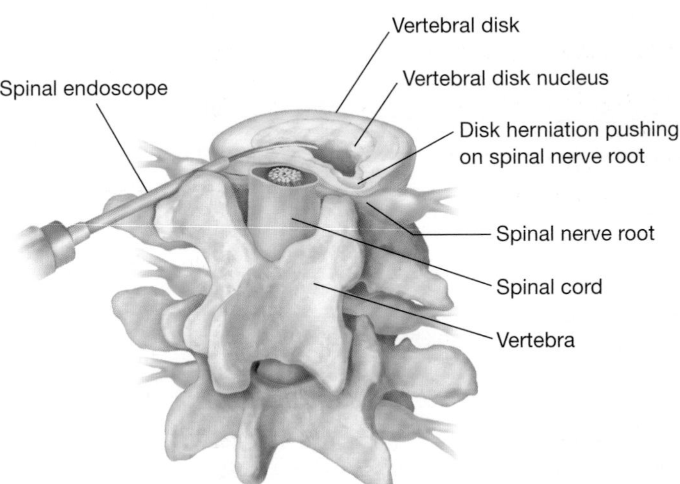

Figure 5-24 Surgical excision of tissue from a herniated disc (discectomy).

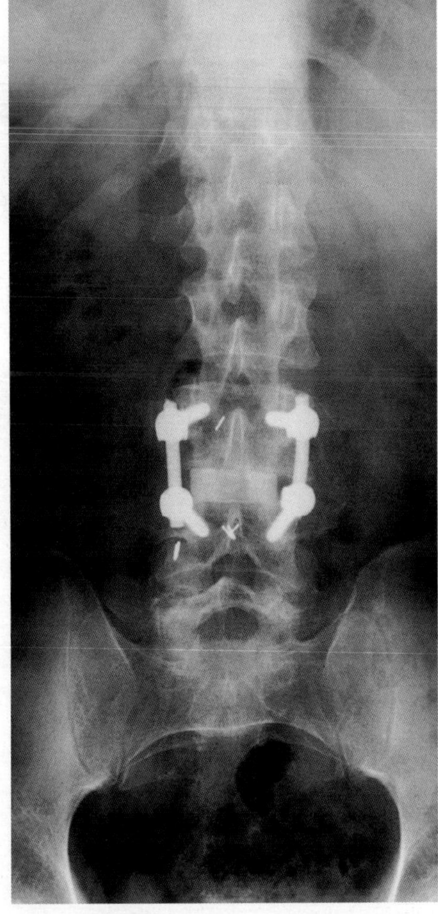

Figure 5-25 Surgical fixation is done to produce spinal fusion (spondylosyndesis) and limit movement along the spinal column.

Surgical Interventions and Therapeutic Procedures *(continued)*

Term	Pronunciation	Meaning
synovectomy	sin′ō-vek′tŏ-mē	excision of part or all of a joint's synovial membrane
tarsectomy	tahr-sek′tŏ-mē	excision of part or all of the tarsal bones
tenorrhaphy	te-nōr′ă-fē	suture of the divided ends of a tendon **(Figure 5-26)**
traction	trak′shŭn	a pulling force exerted on a limb or other part of the body to maintain a desired position for healing **(Figure 5-27)**
Related Terms		
orthosis	ōr-thō′sis	external orthopedic device, such as a brace or splint **(Figure 5-28)**
prosthesis	pros-thē′sis	artificial body part, such as a leg, used to replace a damaged or missing structure

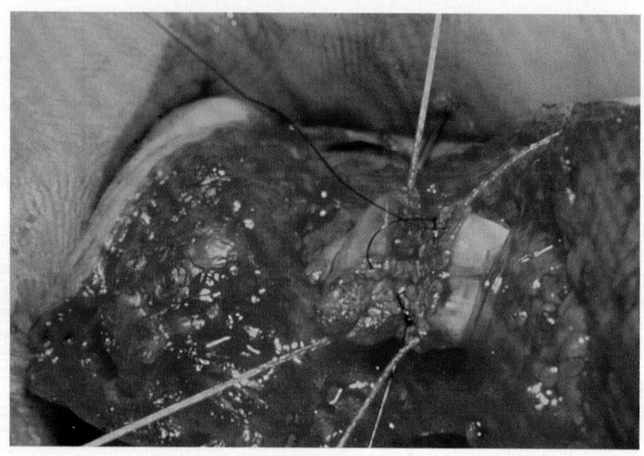

Figure 5-26 Suturing a torn tendon (tenorrhaphy).

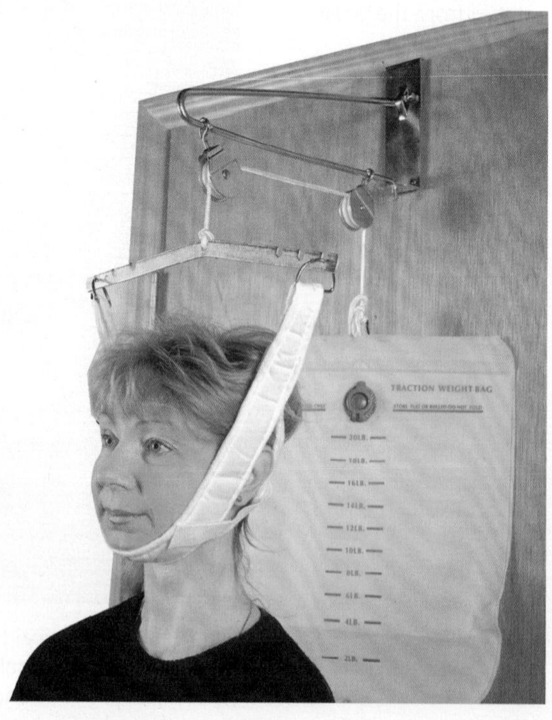

Figure 5-27 Cervical traction.

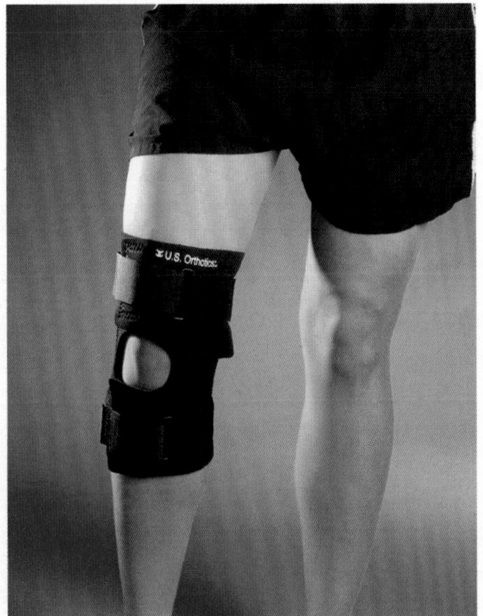

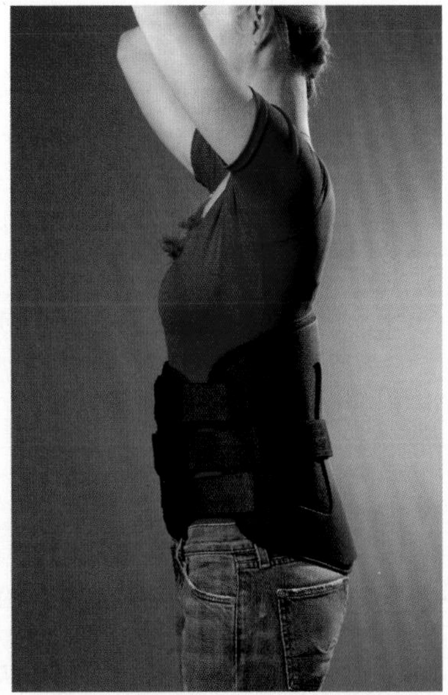

A B

Figure 5-28 Orthopedic devices (orthoses). **A.** Knee brace. **B.** Back brace.

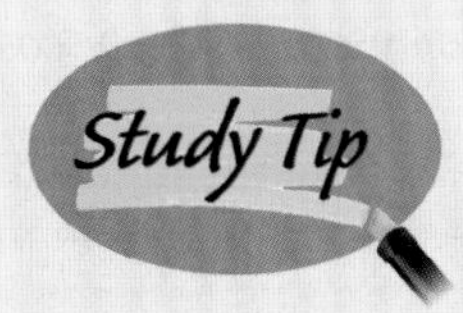

Osteoclast: "Osteoclast" has two meanings in medicine: (1) a body cell that helps remove osseous tissue and (2) a surgical instrument used to fracture a bone to correct a deformity. The correct definition depends on the context in which it is used. For example, the first definition might be used in a laboratory report, and the second definition might be used in an operative report.

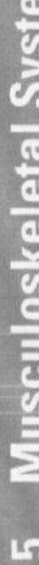

Exercises: Surgical Interventions and Therapeutic Procedures

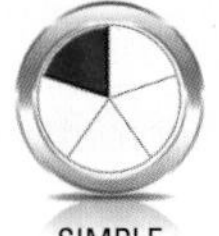

SIMPLE RECALL

Exercise 19

Write the correct medical term for the definition given.

1. excision of some or all of a synovial membrane ____________
2. putting bone ends back in their proper places ____________
3. suture of a muscle ____________
4. excision of cartilage ____________
5. surgical breaking of adhesions in ankylosis ____________
6. surgical removal of an intervertebral disc ____________
7. pulling force exerted on a limb ____________
8. surgical repair of the skull ____________
9. spinal fusion ____________
10. intentional fracture to correct bone deformity ____________

11. excision of the patella ____________________

12. surgical instrument used to break a bone ____________________

13. surgical repair of cartilage ____________________

14. excision of a meniscus ____________________

15. surgical sectioning of the maxilla ____________________

16. surgical creation of an artificial joint ____________________

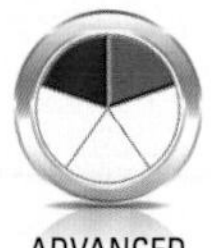

ADVANCED RECALL

Exercise 20

Circle the term that is most appropriate for the meaning of the sentence.

1. Mrs. Yin required a(n) (*cranioplasty, arthrodesis, ostectomy*) to excise a cancerous bone growth.
2. Mr. Behringer had a very painful bursa but was reluctant to undergo (*arthroplasty, bursectomy, laminectomy*) to remove it.
3. The first step of surgery for Ms. Barbosa's brain tumor was a (*craniotomy, cranioplasty, costectomy*).
4. Following surgical removal of a sarcoma that had spread through his vastus medialis muscle, Mr. McCarty required extensive (*tenorrhaphy, myoplasty, arthrodesis*) to repair the muscle.
5. To brace her leg and provide support while healing occurred, Mrs. Ahern needed to wear a custom (*osteoclasis, arthrodesis, orthosis*) at all times.
6. After breaking her arm, Mrs. Latta had a(n) (*meniscectomy; open reduction, internal fixation; osteoclast*) to repair the fracture.
7. Mr. Karposky's surgery for a herniated intervertebral disc included (*carpectomy, tarsectomy, laminectomy*).
8. During surgery for the skier's injured knee, Dr. Tanaka discovered a tendon that had completely divided; he therefore had to perform (*phalangectomy, tenorrhaphy, arthroclasia*).
9. With (*arthrocentesis, arthrodesis, chondrectomy*), the orthopedic surgeon aspirated synovial fluid from Mrs. Updike's severely swollen shoulder joint.
10. Within months of the emergency amputation of her gangrenous left leg, Ms. Pappas was adapting well to walking using a (*spondylosyndesis, prosthesis, traction*).

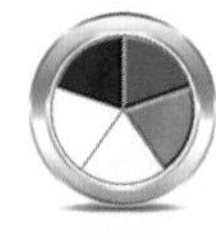

TERM CONSTRUCTION

Exercise 21

Using the given suffix, build a medical term for the meaning given.

Suffix	Meaning of Medical Term	Medical Term
-plasty	surgical repair of muscle	1. ____________
-ectomy	excision of cartilage	2. ____________

-desis	surgical fixation or binding of a joint	3. ______
-rrhaphy	suture of divided ends of a tendon	4. ______
-tomy	incision into the skull	5. ______

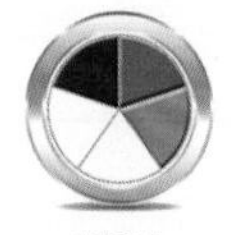

TERM CONSTRUCTION

Exercise 22

Break the given medical term into its word parts and define each part. Then define the medical term.

For example:

arthritis	*word parts:*	arthr/o, -itis
	meanings:	joint, inflammation
	term meaning:	inflammation of a joint

1. osteoclasis	*word parts:*	______
	meanings:	______
	term meaning:	______
2. myorrhaphy	*word parts:*	______
	meanings:	______
	term meaning:	______
3. arthroplasty	*word parts:*	______
	meanings:	______
	term meaning:	______
4. phalangectomy	*word parts:*	______
	meanings:	______
	term meaning:	______
5. rachiotomy	*word parts:*	______
	meanings:	______
	term meaning:	______
6. discectomy	*word parts:*	______
	meanings:	______
	term meaning:	______
7. chondroplasty	*word parts:*	______
	meanings:	______
	term meaning:	______

8. arthrocentesis *word parts:* ______________

meanings: ______________

term meaning: ______________

9. synovectomy *word parts:* ______________

meanings: ______________

term meaning: ______________

10. ostectomy *word parts:* ______________

meanings: ______________

term meaning: ______________

Medications and Drug Therapies

Term	Pronunciation	Meaning
analgesic	an′ăl-jē′zik	a drug that relieves pain without producing anesthesia
corticosteroid	kōr′ti-kō-ster′oyd	a drug that reduces inflammation around joints
nonsteroidal antiinflammatory drug (NSAID)	non′ster-oy′dăl an′tī-in-flam′ă-tōr-ē drŭg	a drug (such as aspirin or ibuprofen) with antiinflammatory action (and usually analgesic and antipyretic effects as well); used to treat joint and muscle conditions
skeletal muscle relaxant	skel′ĕ-tăl mŭs′ĕl rē-lak′sănt	a drug that relaxes skeletal muscle spasms and spasticity

Exercise: Medications and Drug Therapies

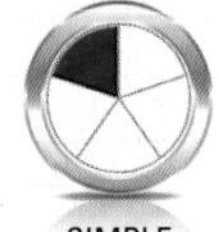

SIMPLE RECALL

Exercise 23

Write the correct medication or drug therapy term for the definition given.

1. relaxes skeletal muscles ______________
2. relieves pain without anesthesia ______________
3. reduces inflammation around joints ______________
4. reduces inflammation without the use of steroids ______________

Specialties and Specialists

Term	Pronunciation	Meaning
chiropractic	kī′rō-prak′tik	health care discipline involving physical manipulation of musculoskeletal structures
chiropractor	kī′rō-prak′tŏr	one who specializes in chiropractic health care

Specialties and Specialists

Term	Pronunciation	Meaning
orthopedics, orthopaedics	ōr′thō-pē′diks	medical specialty focusing on diagnosis and treatment of disorders of the musculoskeletal system
orthopedist, orthopaedist	ōr′thō-pē′dist	physician who specializes in orthopedics
orthotics	ōr-thot′iks	the science of making and fitting orthopedic devices
orthotist	ōr-thŏt′ist	one who makes and fits orthopedic appliances
osteopathy	os′tē-op′ă-thē	school of medicine emphasizing manipulative measures in addition to techniques of conventional medicine
osteopath	os′tē-ō-path	physician who specializes in osteopathy
podiatry	pō-dī′ă-trē	medical specialty focusing on diagnosis and treatment of foot disorders
podiatrist	pō-dī′ă-trist	practitioner who specializes in podiatry
rheumatology	rū′mă-tol′ŏ-jē	medical specialty focusing on the study, diagnosis, and treatment of joint conditions
rheumatologist	rū′mă-tol′ŏ-jist	physician who specializes in rheumatology

Exercise: Specialties and Specialists

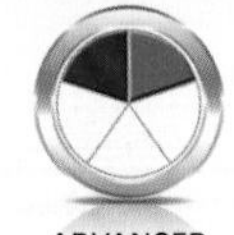

ADVANCED RECALL

Exercise 24

Match each medical specialist with the description of the specialty.

podiatrist chiropractor orthopedist
rheumatologist osteopath orthotist

1. physical manipulation of musculoskeletal structures ________
2. diagnosis and treatment of foot disorders ________
3. making and fitting orthopedic devices ________
4. school of medicine emphasizing manipulative measures ________
5. diagnosis and treatment of joint conditions ________
6. diagnosis and treatment of disorders of the musculoskeletal system ________

Abbreviations

Abbreviation	Meaning
C1–C7	cervical vertebrae 1–7
CK	creatine kinase
CT	computed tomography
CTS	carpal tunnel syndrome

(continued)

Abbreviations *(continued)*

Abbreviation	Meaning
EMG	electromyogram
ESR	erythrocyte sedimentation rate
Fx	fracture
L1–L5	lumbar vertebrae 1–5
MD	muscular dystrophy
MG	myasthenia gravis
MRI	magnetic resonance imaging
NSAID	nonsteroidal antiinflammatory drug
OA	osteoarthritis
ORIF	open reduction, internal fixation
RA	rheumatoid arthritis
RF	rheumatoid factor
ROM	range of motion
T1–T12	thoracic vertebrae 1–12

Exercises: Abbreviations

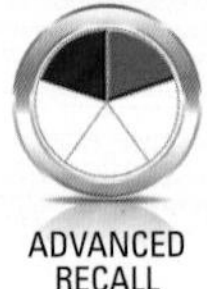
ADVANCED RECALL

Exercise 25

Write the meaning for the abbreviation(s) used in each sentence.

1. Mr. de la Cruz had an **MRI** to assist with the diagnosis of a herniated intervertebral disc.

 ____

2. Because of her **MG,** Ms. Hart frequently felt fatigued after walking even a short distance.

 ____

3. After her car accident, it was found on radiography that Mrs. Stegner had a fracture of **C2.**

 ____

4. **MD** is a hereditary degenerative disease.

 ____

5. Because of pain resulting from severe osteoarthritis, Mr. Springer has limited **ROM** in his shoulder.

 ____

6. An **ORIF** was performed to repair Mr. Harrell's fracture of the femur.

 ____

7. An **EMG** was obtained to help diagnose the nerve damage in Mr. Dura's arm.

____

8. Ms. Dhalaya told her orthopedist that she was sure her **CTS** resulted from all the typing she did at work.

____

9. Mr. Murphy's medical record indicated **RA** diagnosed at age 55.

____

10. Mrs. Helmsley's physician wanted her to try an **NSAID** for her arthritis before prescribing a different drug.

____

11. To test for musculoskeletal problems, Mr. Kapur was scheduled for the following lab tests: **ESR, RF,** and **CK.**

____

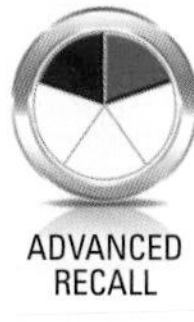
ADVANCED RECALL

Exercise 26

Match each abbreviation with the appropriate description.

CT	OA	T4
L3	Fx	MRI

1. fourth thoracic vertebra _______________
2. injury of osseous tissue _______________
3. radiographic cross-section _______________
4. located inferior to the ribs _______________
5. imaging of magnetic effects _______________
6. involving articular cartilage _______________

WRAPPING UP

- Skeletal muscles attach to bones and function together as the musculoskeletal system to cause movement.
- A joint is where two bones come together. There are different types of joints, which are categorized by how they move.
- You learned the names of many bones and skeletal muscles, word parts relating to the musculoskeletal system, prefixes, suffixes, tests, surgeries, medications, specialists, and abbreviations that all relate to skeletal muscles, bones, and joints.

Chapter Review

Review of Terms for Anatomy and Physiology

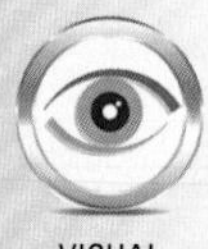

Exercise 27

Give the names of the bones as indicated.

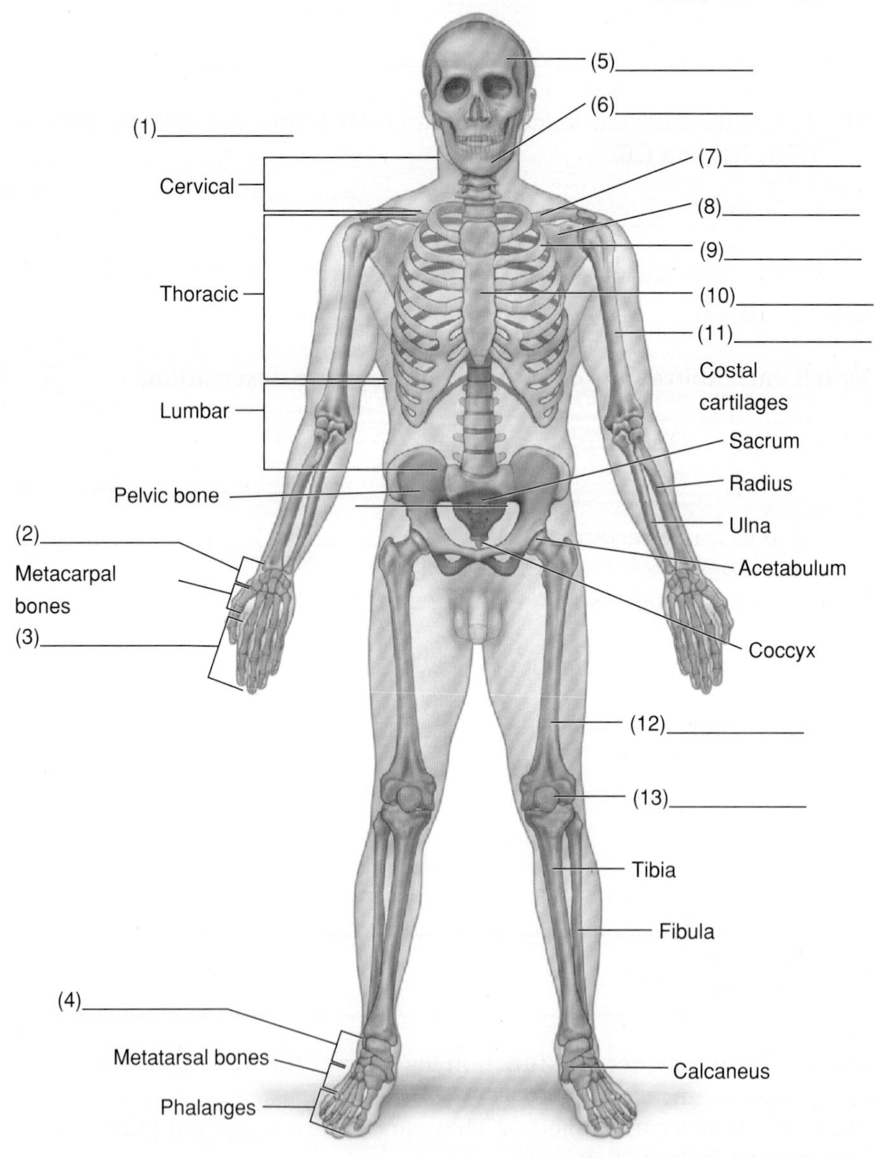

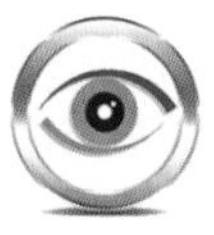

VISUAL

Exercise 28

Give the name of the muscle or combining form as indicated.

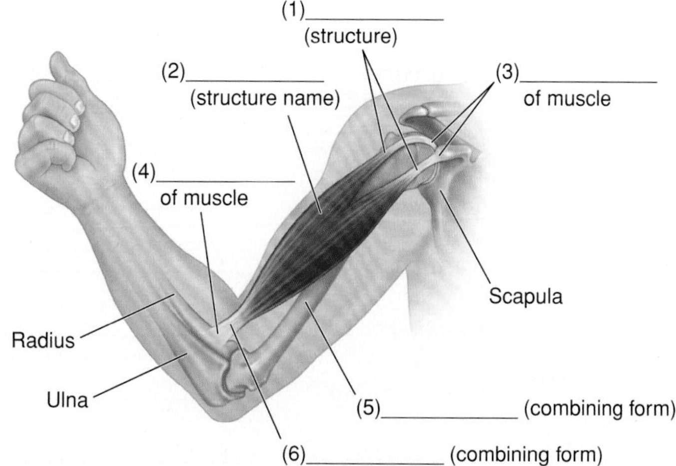

Understanding Term Structure

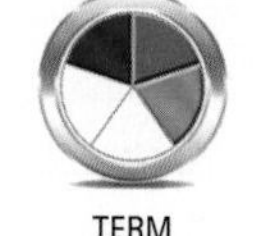

TERM CONSTRUCTION

Exercise 29

Break the given medical term into its word parts and define each part. Then define the medical term. (Note: You may need to use word parts from other chapters.)

For example:

arthritis	*word parts:*	arthr/o, -itis
	meanings:	joint, inflammation
	term meaning:	inflammation of a joint
1. ankylosis	*word parts:*	___________
	meanings:	___________
	term meaning:	___________
2. carpoptosis	*word parts:*	___________
	meanings:	___________
	term meaning:	___________
3. electromyogram	*word parts:*	___________
	meanings:	___________
	term meaning:	___________

4. myositis *word parts:* ______

meanings: ______

term meaning: ______

5. kyphosis *word parts:* ______

meanings: ______

term meaning: ______

6. intracranial *word parts:* ______

meanings: ______

term meaning: ______

7. polymyositis *word parts:* ______

meanings: ______

term meaning: ______

8. suprapatellar *word parts:* ______

meanings: ______

term meaning: ______

9. tenodynia *word parts:* ______

meanings: ______

term meaning: ______

10. arthrocentesis *word parts:* ______

meanings: ______

term meaning: ______

11. chondrectomy *word parts:* ______

meanings: ______

term meaning: ______

12. costovertebral — *word parts:* ______
meanings: ______
term meaning: ______

13. submandibular — *word parts:* ______
meanings: ______
term meaning: ______

14. osteoarthritis — *word parts:* ______
meanings: ______
term meaning: ______

15. myorrhaphy — *word parts:* ______
meanings: ______
term meaning: ______

16. osteomalacia — *word parts:* ______
meanings: ______
term meaning: ______

17. arthroscopy — *word parts:* ______
meanings: ______
term meaning: ______

18. myalgia — *word parts:* ______
meanings: ______
term meaning: ______

19. spondylarthritis — *word parts:* ______
meanings: ______
term meaning: ______

Comprehension Exercises

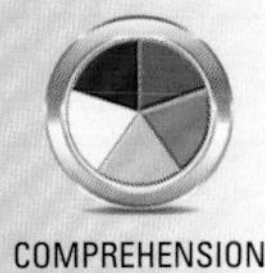
COMPREHENSION

Exercise 30

Fill in the blank with the correct term.

1. Movement of an arm or leg toward the midline of the body is called ____________________.
2. ____________________ is the science of making and fitting orthopedic devices.
3. The general term for the surgical restoration of joint function or creation of an artificial joint is ____________________.
4. A(n) ____________________ is one who specializes in the diagnosis and treatment of disorders of the foot.
5. An artificial leg is an example of a(n) ____________________.
6. ____________________ is caused by nerve entrapment in the wrist that produces pain.
7. The type of bone tissue that is solid and strong is called ____________________.
8. A bony projection that develops from cartilage is called ____________________.
9. ____________________ is a condition of chronic aching and stiffness of muscles and soft tissues of unknown cause.
10. ____________________ is movement that increases the joint angle.
11. Nuclear medicine imaging can produce an image of the body's bones, called a(n) ____________________, to diagnose possible bone disorders.
12. Muscular ____________________ is a hereditary condition causing progressive degeneration of skeletal muscles.
13. Progressive destructive changes and inflammation in multiple joints, especially in the hands and feet, may be caused by ____________________.
14. The amount of movement at a joint is termed its ____________________.
15. Excessive muscular activity is termed ____________________.
16. ____________________ is a health care discipline that involves physical manipulation of musculoskeletal structures.
17. ____________________ is the joint movement that bends the foot upward toward the tibia.
18. The medical specialty focusing on diagnosis and treatment of disorders of the musculoskeletal system is ____________________.

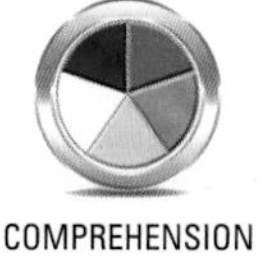

Exercise 31

Write a short answer for each question.

1. What kind of joint is a suture? ______

2. A ligament attaches what structures together? ______

3. Where in the body are the metacarpal bones? ______

4. What does it mean to say a tissue is osseous? ______

5. How is the practice of an osteopath different from that of other physicians? ______

6. In what situation might a tenorrhaphy be done? ______

7. Rickets may result from a deficiency of what? ______

8. Arthrodesis performed during spinal surgery does what to a spinal joint? ______

9. What is deposited in joint tissue that causes pain to someone with gout? ______

10. What kind of diagnostic image is produced with arthrography? ______

11. Which end of a muscle is its insertion? ______

12. Where is the xiphoid process located? ______

13. In addition to skeletal (striated, voluntary) and smooth (unstriated, involuntary) muscle tissue, what other type of muscle tissue is found in the body? ______

14. What is another term for a laminotomy? ______

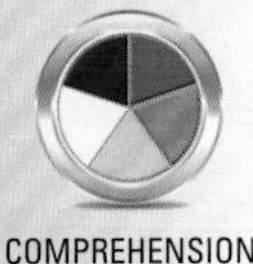

Exercise 32

COMPREHENSION

Circle the letter of the best answer in the following questions.

1. The term that most specifically applies to inflammation of an articular cartilage is

A. osteitis.
B. chondritis.
C. arthrochondritis.
D. arthritis.

2. The clavicle articulates with the

A. femur.
B. fibula.
C. ilium.
D. sternum.

3. A diarthrosis

A. moves freely.
B. causes pain.
C. requires surgery.
D. is herniated.

4. An exostosis may develop from

A. bone marrow.
B. a sarcoma.
C. a herniated disc.
D. cartilage.

5. Hypertrophy of an organ means it is

A. increased in size.
B. malignant.
C. gouty.
D. necrotic.

6. Dyskinesia generally refers to difficulty in

A. hyperextending the wrist.
B. embryonic fusing of vertebra.
C. obtaining a clear radiographic image.
D. performing voluntary movements.

7. Even if you had never heard of this condition, you might assume that chondromalacia refers to

A. hardening of cartilage.
B. softening of cartilage.
C. hardening of bone.
D. softening of bone.

8. An example of circumduction is

A. movement at the shoulder joint when the arm is moved in circles.
B. movement at cervical spinal joints when the head is turned right and left.
C. movement at the wrist when the hand is turned from palm down to palm up.
D. movement at the wrist when the hand is turned from palm up to palm down.

9. A patient with ankylosing spondylitis is most likely to feel pain when

A. typing at a computer keyboard.
B. bending down to tie his or her shoes.
C. waving hello to someone at a distance.
D. chewing gum.

10. A traumatic injury that fractures the patella might also injure

A. the humerus.
B. a suture.
C. the pubis.
D. a meniscus.

11. Which of the following vertebrae is closest to the sacrum?

A. L5
B. T12
C. T1
D. C7

12. Which kind of tissue is in closest proximity to periosteal tissue?

A. bone
B. muscle
C. ligament
D. bone marrow

13. Tenodynia is most likely to occur with

A. rickets.
B. tarsectomy.
C. tenosynovitis.
D. bursitis.

14. In scoliosis, the spinal column curves

A. laterally from side to side.
B. from forward to backward in the lumbar area.
C. from forward to backward in the cervical area.
D. from backward to forward.

Application and Analysis

CASE STUDIES

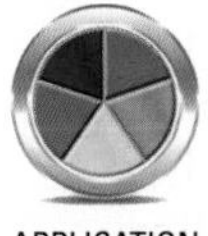

Exercise 33

Read the case studies and circle the correct letter for each of the questions.

CASE 5-1

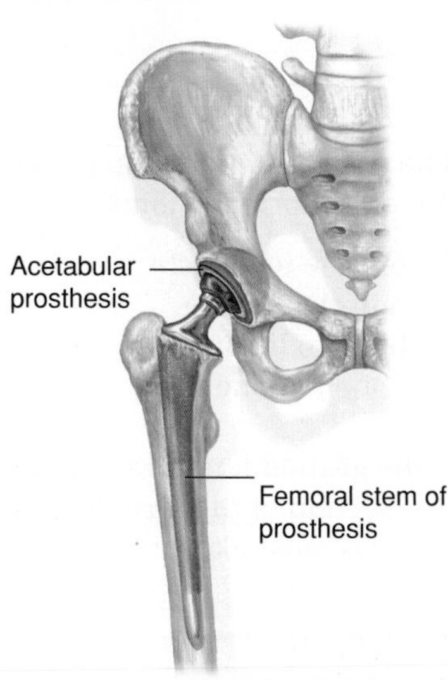

Figure 5-29 Total hip replacement with the prosthesis in place.

Because of severe osteoarthritis, Mr. Hughes is undergoing total hip replacement. During this surgery, the proximal end of his femur will be resected, and the stem of a metal prosthesis will be inserted into the femur. Damaged bone in the acetabulum will be excised, and a plastic cup–shaped prosthetic piece will be cemented into the bone. The ball on top of the femoral prosthesis fits within this cup. Together, these components will compose his new hip joint **(Figure 5-29)**.

1. The acetabulum is part of what bone?

A. the hip (pelvic) bone
B. the femur
C. the coccyx
D. the ilium

2. The new hip is called a prosthesis because it is

A. a surgical correction.
B. inside the body.
C. an orthopedic device.
D. an artificial replacement joint.

3. Resection of the proximal end of the femur means

A. it is filed down to a smooth surface.
B. it is surgically removed.
C. a new osseous section will be transplanted there.
D. surgical reconstruction.

4. The stem of the femoral prosthesis will extend down into

A. the pubis.
B. the patella.
C. the femur's medullary cavity.
D. the epiphysis of the tibia.

5. In Mr. Hughes' new hip, the metallic femoral ball will articulate with

A. the ischium.
B. the acetabular prosthesis.
C. the femoral periosteum.
D. spongy bone.

6. This total hip replacement is an example of a(n)

A. chondroplasty.
B. discectomy.
C. arthroplasty.
D. arthroclasia.

CASE 5-2

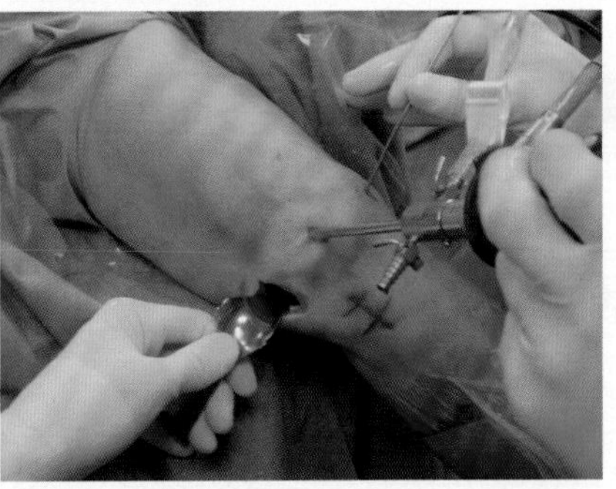

Figure 5-30 Arthroscopic knee surgery.

Mr. Bhatnagar suffered a tear of his anterior cruciate ligament (ACL) during a football game, causing significant pain and instability of the joint. The diagnosis was made with x-rays, MRI scans, and a stress test of the ligament. Arthroscopic reconstructive surgery of the knee joint is to be performed. The ACL will be reconstructed using a harvested section of the central third of the patellar tendon in a graft. The entire procedure will be performed arthroscopically **(Figure 5-30)**.

7. The ACL joins

A. muscle to muscle.
B. muscle to bone.
C. bone to muscle.
D. bone to bone.

8. An arthroscope is an instrument that

A. allows viewing inside a joint.
B. forms an image based on tissue effects of magnetism.
C. is used to create radiographic images.
D. involves administration of radionuclides.

9. Which suffix most likely is used in the term for the procedure for creating an opening into the knee joint?

A. -physis
B. -desis
C. -clasia
D. -tomy

10. The patellar tendon harvested for use in the graft normally joins

A. muscle to muscle.
B. muscle to bone.
C. bone to ligament.
D. bone to bone.

11. If the grafted tendon section is sutured to a section of the torn ligament, which suffix is most likely used in the term for that procedure?

A. -rrhaphy
B. -physis
C. -ectomy
D. -centesis

MEDICAL RECORD ANALYSIS

MEDICAL RECORD 5-1

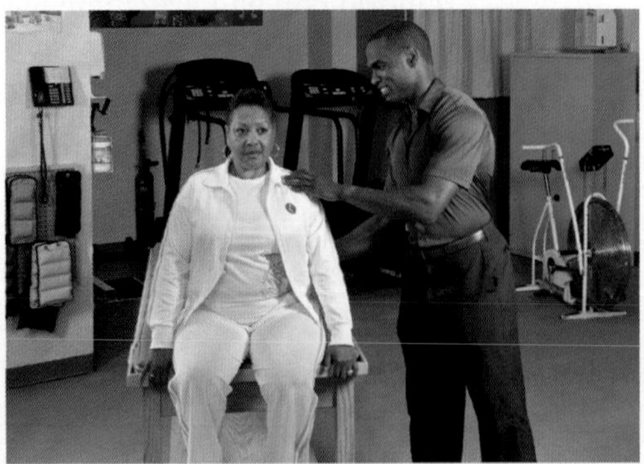

Physical therapy assistant working with a patient.

You are a physical therapy assistant working in a physical therapy clinic. It is your job to help assess patients and develop individualized treatment programs under the guidance of the physical therapist. Ms. Jackson's primary physician referred her to your clinic because of a history of chronic back pain. You review this medical record from her physician so you may assist in her care.

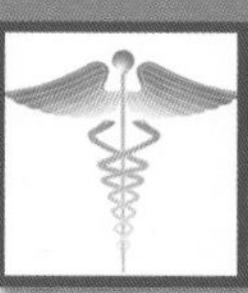

Medical Record

LOW BACK PAIN

SUBJECTIVE: The patient came to my office with chief complaints of chronic back pain radiating down to the right more than left buttock and the thigh area. This pain increases with walking, standing, and rotating the back. She is taking Ambien (zolpidem) and Lodine (etodolac) at this time. She is a known hypertensive with low back pain and left foot pain. She denies any new family or social history. She was on Vioxx (rofecoxib) and stopped when changed to etodolac. On review of systems, she reports some weight loss. She denies any heart pain, skin problems, eye problems, ear problems, hearing problems, swallowing problems, abdominal problems, diarrhea, constipation, or bowel/bladder incontinence.

OBJECTIVE: On examination, the patient is a moderately built, well-nourished female. She appears to be comfortable. Her blood pressure is 136/69, heart rate 63, temperature 98.6°F. Her current weight is 200 lb. She is awake, alert, and oriented. Pupils are equal and reacting. Scleras are anicteric. Oropharynx is clear. The neck is supple. Carotid pulses are felt well. Trachea is midline. Breath sounds are heard. The abdomen is soft. The breath sounds are easily heard. The heart has a regular rate and rhythm. Upper extremity sensation reveals motor power within normal limits. The back has an old surgical scar. There is severe myofascial tenderness noted, paraspinal region in the lower lumbar and upper sacral area. Lower extremities are symmetrical. There is mild edema noted, more so in the ankles. There is decreased range of motion in the hips secondary to pain. Sensation is intact to light touch. Gait is slow and stable. She walks with a single-point cane. Sensation is intact.

ASSESSMENT: This is a patient with chronic low back pain, bilateral total knee replacement, and a prior low back surgery. She continues to have pain.

PLAN: The previous injection significantly helped the patient with her pain for about three months. I will consider her for a repeat L5–S1 foraminal block under fluoroscopy in the next two to three weeks. I have advised the patient to continue the current medications and have ordered a physical therapy consultation.

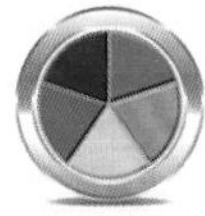

APPLICATION

Exercise 34

Write the appropriate medical terms used in this medical record on the blanks after their definitions. Note that not all the terms appear in the chapter, but you should be able to identify these terms based on word parts that are included in this chapter.

1. pertaining to area beside or around the spine ____________
2. pertaining to location of fused vertebrae inferior to lumbar vertebrae ____________
3. pertaining to muscle and fascia ____________
4. amount of movement in a joint ____________

Bonus Question

5. Which joint in this patient has undergone past arthroplasty? ____________

MEDICAL RECORD 5-2

Mrs. Formosa, a patient who suffers from rheumatoid arthritis, has returned to the physician's office where you work as a phlebotomist. You are responsible for drawing blood samples from Mrs. Formosa to be used for the CBC and sedimentation rate tests ordered by the physician.

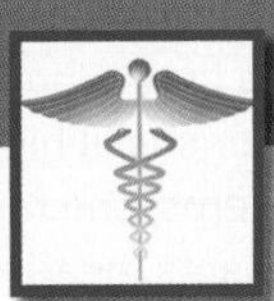

Medical Record

RHEUMATOID ARTHRITIS FOLLOW-UP NOTE

HISTORY OF PRESENT ILLNESS: The patient is a 38-year-old woman who has an illness of about three to four years, characterized by myalgia, (1) _______________, and arthritis located in the MCP joints, PIP joints, wrists, and ankles. In addition, the patient has had intermittent Raynaud, mild hair loss, and a transient rash located on the face and the neck. Other problems are sleep abnormalities and problems with equilibrium that are under evaluation by neurology. In our initial evaluation, we considered that the patient may have an undifferentiated connective tissue disease, and the possibilities were rheumatoid arthritis, lupus, or scleroderma. A trial of prednisone 15 mg was initiated. Two days after the patient started taking prednisone, she felt an impressive improvement that she describes as a miracle. The chronic sensation of fatigue was almost eliminated, and the (2) _______________ is very mild, as well as the arthritis. The patient has not had episodes of (3) _______________ since. The patient has been unusually active at work with energy and is able to do gardening. There is no significant change in morning stiffness, and this is still about 30 minutes in duration.

PERTINENT PHYSICAL FINDINGS: The general examination is benign. There is no hair loss. There is very mild erythema on the neck with fine telangiectasis that was mentioned before. There are no other skin lesions, and there are no mucosal lesions either. Musculoskeletal examination shows a motor power of 5/5 in all four extremities, (4) _______________ is normal in all joints, and there is no evidence of synovitis at any level. X-rays of hands show only mild osteopenia around the MCP and PIP joints. There are no erosions.

ASSESSMENT/PLAN: The patient is a 38-year-old woman with an undifferentiated inflammatory polyarthritis. Considering the family history of a father and a brother with rheumatoid arthritis, it is possible that the patient is at the stage of an early (5) _______________, which is seronegative. Given the presence of Raynaud and fine telangiectasis, we have to keep in mind the possibility of this illness evolving to scleroderma. We do not have serologic evidence of lupus, and there is no biochemical evidence of myositis. Our plan at the moment is initiation of high-dose chloroquine at 400 mg once daily, evaluation by an ophthalmologist, and a slow reduction of prednisone to 10 mg in one month and then 1 mg per week. We are scheduling an appointment in two months and requesting a CBC and sedimentation rate for the next visit.

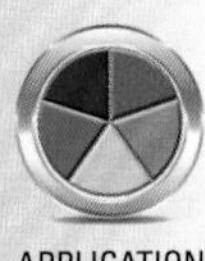

APPLICATION

Exercise 35

Fill in the blanks in the medical record above with the correct medical terms. The definitions of the missing terms are listed below.

1. joint pain

2. muscle pain

3. joint inflammation

4. degree of movement in a joint

5. disease that causes progressive destructive changes in multiple joints

Bonus Question

6. Although this chapter does not define the term "polyarthritis," used in the Assessment/Plan section of the record, you should be able to define it from its word parts. What is the definition of this term?

____

Pronunciation and Spelling

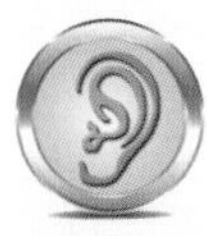
AUDITORY

Exercise 36

Review the Chapter 5 terms in the Dictionary/Audio Glossary in the Student Resources on thePoint, and practice pronouncing each term, referring to the pronunciation guide as needed.

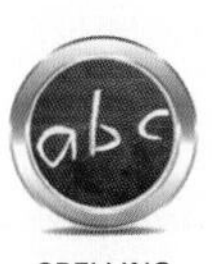
SPELLING

Exercise 37

Circle the correctly spelled term.

1.	laminectomy	laminotomy	lamanotomy
2.	ostoarthritis	ostioarthritis	osteoarthritis
3.	rheumatology	rhuematology	rheumetology
4.	tenodyne	tenodyna	tenodynia
5.	osseis	osseous	oseous
6.	clavicle	clavicel	clavecle
7.	myorhaphy	myorrhapphy	myorrhaphy
8.	vertebrea	vertebrae	vertabrae
9.	fibromyalgia	fibrilmyalgia	fibromyolgia
10.	dorseflexion	dorsaflexion	dorsiflexion
11.	ankelosis	ankylosis	ankylesis
12.	polimyositis	polymyositis	polymiositis
13.	faisca	fasckia	fascia
14.	osteoporosis	ostioporosis	osteoporesis
15.	intervertebrel	intervertabral	intervertebral

Media Connection

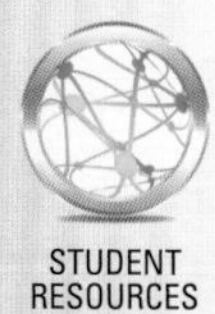

Exercise 38

Complete each of the following activities available with the Student Resources on thePoint. Check off each activity as you complete it, and record your score for the Chapter Quiz in the space provided.

Chapter Exercises

____ Flash Cards

____ Concentration

____ Abbreviation Match-Up

____ Roboterms

____ Word Anatomy

____ Fill the Gap

____ Break It Down

____ True/False Body Building

____ Quiz Show

____ Complete the Case

____ Medical Record Review

____ Look and Label

____ Image Matching

____ Spelling Bee

____ **Chapter Quiz** *Score:*________%

Additional Resources

____ Video: Vertebral Disc

____ Animations: Muscle Flexion and Extension; Bone Growth

____ Dictionary/Audio Glossary

____ Health Professions Careers: Physical Therapy Assistant

____ Health Professions Careers: Phlebotomist

Nervous System and Mental Health

6

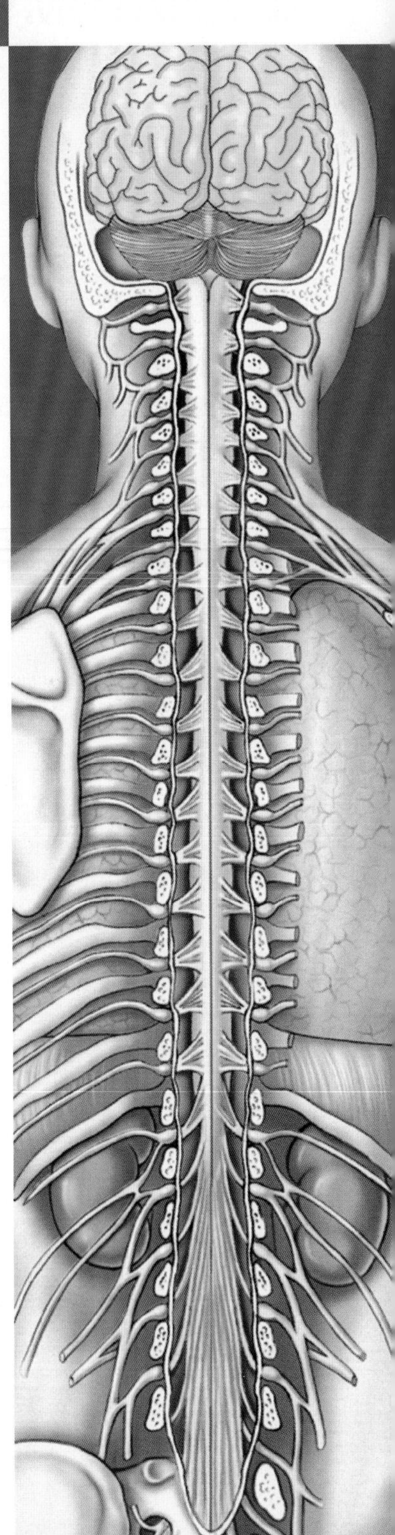

Chapter Outline

Introduction, 164

Anatomy and Physiology, 164
- Structures, 164
- Functions, 165
- Terms Related to the Nervous System, 165

Word Parts, 170
- Combining Forms, 170
- Prefixes, 171
- Suffixes, 171

Medical Terms, 175
- Adjectives and Other Related Terms, 175
- Medical Conditions, 176
- Diagnostic Procedures, 187
- Surgical Interventions and Therapeutic Procedures, 190
- Medications and Drug Therapies, 192
- Specialties and Specialists, 193
- Abbreviations, 194

Wrapping Up, 196

Chapter Review, 197

Learning Outcomes

After completing this chapter, you should be able to:

1. List the structures and functions of the nervous system.
2. Describe the locations of the main structures in the nervous system.
3. Define terms related to the central and peripheral nervous systems.
4. Define combining forms, prefixes, and suffixes related to the nervous system and mental health.
5. Define common medical terminology related to the nervous system and mental health, including adjectives and related terms; signs, symptoms, and medical conditions; tests and procedures; surgical interventions and therapeutic procedures; medications and drug therapies; and medical specialties and specialists.
6. Define common abbreviations related to the nervous system and mental health.
7. Successfully complete all chapter exercises.
8. Explain terms used in case studies and medical records involving the nervous system and mental health.
9. Successfully complete all exercises included with the companion Student Resources on thePoint.

INTRODUCTION

The nervous system is a complex network that plays a role in nearly every body function. It is composed of two main divisions: the central nervous system (brain and spinal cord) and the peripheral nervous system (cranial nerves and spinal nerves). Nerves and their associated structures are vital to maintaining homeostasis and also making us who we are. This chapter focuses on the nervous system and provides a brief lesson on terms related to mental health.

ANATOMY AND PHYSIOLOGY

Structures

- The nervous system is divided into two parts: the central nervous system and the peripheral nervous system (**Figure 6-1**).

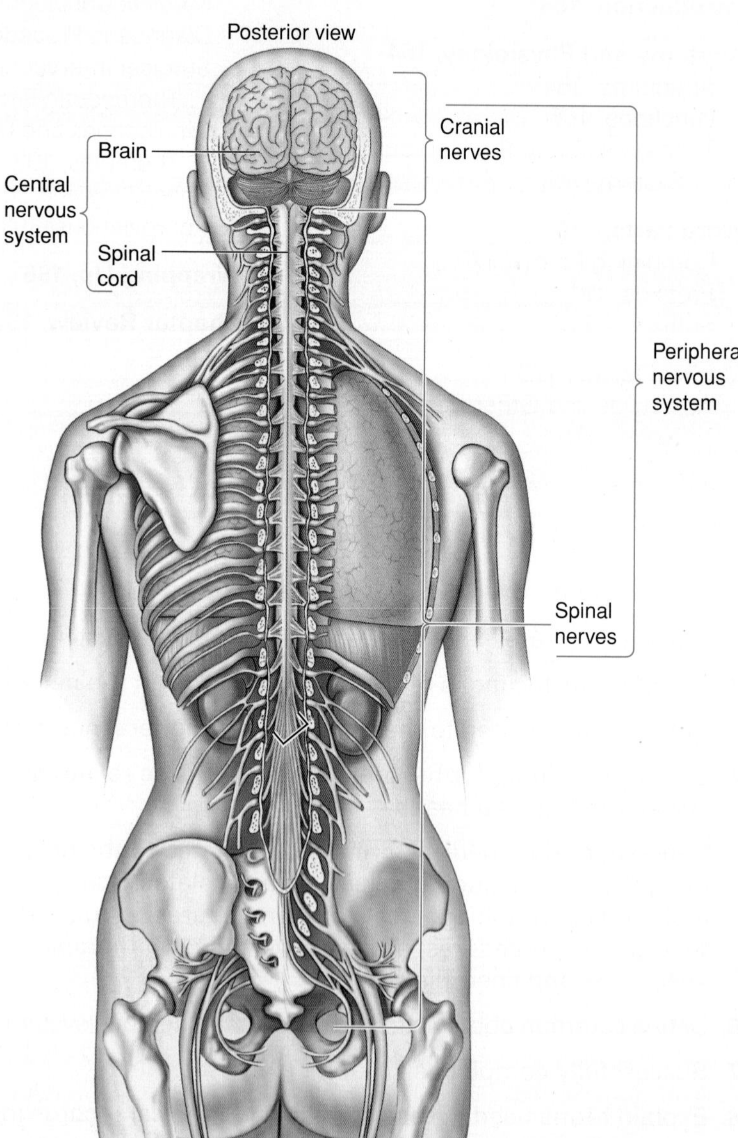

Figure 6-1 The two divisions of the nervous system.

- The central nervous system consists of the brain and the spinal cord.
- The brain consists of four main parts: the cerebrum, the diencephalon, the brainstem, and the cerebellum.
- The spinal cord begins at the medulla oblongata in the brainstem and tapers to an end at the first and second lumbar vertebrae.
- The terminal ends of the spinal nerves taper into a structure called the cauda equina.
- The peripheral nervous system consists of all of the other nerves throughout the body.
- Each nerve ends with two roots. The dorsal (posterior) root carries sensory impulses *to* the spinal cord, and the ventral (anterior) root carries motor impulses *away from* the spinal cord to muscles or glands.

Functions

- Carrying impulses between the brain, neck, head, and spinal nerves
- Releasing chemicals called neurotransmitters
- Controlling voluntary and involuntary body functions

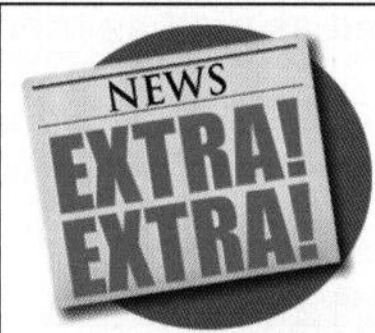

CAUDA EQUINA The name cauda equina is Latin for "horse's tail." This name was given because the spinal nerves end at various levels and branch off from the end of the spinal cord, giving the appearance of a horse's tail.

Terms Related to the Nervous System

Term	Pronunciation	Meaning
	Terms Related to the Central Nervous System	
central nervous system (CNS)	sen′trăl nĕr′vŭs sis′tĕm	The brain and the spinal cord
brain	brān	the part of the central nervous system contained within the cranium **(Figure 6-2)**
basal ganglia	bā′săl gang′glē-ă	group of nerve cell bodies linked to the thalamus, involved with coordination and movement
brainstem	brān′stem	connects the brain to the spinal cord; assists in breathing, heart rhythm, vision, and consciousness; composed of the midbrain, pons, and medulla oblongata
midbrain; *syn.* mesencephalon	mid′brān; mes′en-sef′ă-lon	part of the brainstem that contains reflex centers associated with eye and head movements
pons	ponz	part of the brainstem between the medulla and midbrain that is a relay station from the peripheral nerves to the brain
medulla oblongata	mĕ-dŭl′ă ob-long-gah′tă	part of the brainstem that connects the brain and the spinal cord and contains reflex centers for the heart, blood vessels, and breathing
cerebellum; *syn.* hindbrain	ser-ĕ-bel′ŭm; hīnd′brān	posterior portion of the brain that coordinates the voluntary muscles and maintains balance and muscle tone

(continued)

Terms Related to the Nervous System *(continued)*

Term	Pronunciation	Meaning
cerebrum	ser′ĕ-brŭm	largest and uppermost portion of the brain; divided into right and left halves (called cerebral hemispheres) and subdivided into lobes
cerebral cortex	ser′ĕ-brăl kōr′teks	outer layer of the cerebrum; controls higher mental functions
frontal lobe	frŏn′tăl lōb	front portion of the cerebrum that is involved with voluntary muscle movement and emotions
gyrus	jī′rŭs	elevated ridge (raised convolution) on the surface of the cerebrum
occipital lobe	ok-sip′i-tăl lōb	posterior portion of the cerebrum involved with vision
parietal lobe	pă-rī′ĕ-tăl lōb	middle-top portion of the cerebrum; involved in perception of touch, temperature, and pain
sulcus	sŭl′kŭs	groove or depression on the surface of the brain
temporal lobe	tem′pŏr-ăl lōb	portion of the cerebrum below the frontal lobe; involved with the senses of hearing and smell as well as memory, emotion, speech, and behavior

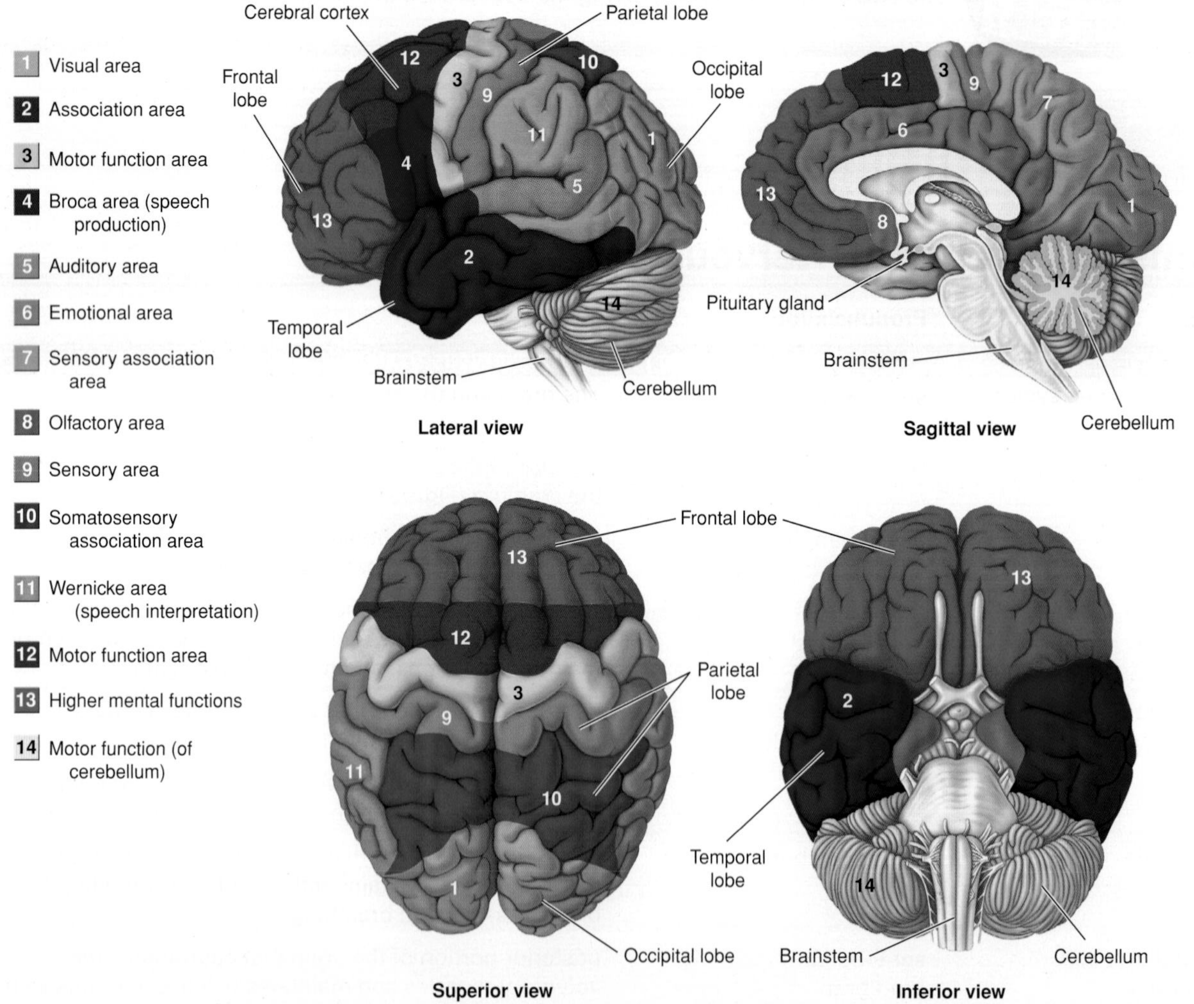

Figure 6-2 Different views of the brain identifying specific areas for various functions.

Terms Related to the Nervous System

Term	Pronunciation	Meaning
diencephalon	dī′en-sef′ă-lon	area deep within the brain that contains the thalamus and hypothalamus and is the link between the cerebral hemispheres and the brainstem; responsible for directing sensory information to the cortex
cerebrospinal fluid (CSF)	ser′ĕ-brō-spī′năl flū′id	colorless liquid that circulates in and around the brain and spinal cord and transports nutrients
meninges	mĕ-nin′jēz	three membranous coverings of the brain and spinal cord **(Figure 6-3)**
dura mater	dūr′ă mā′tĕr	tough, fibrous outermost layer of the meninges
arachnoid mater	ă-rak′noyd mā′tĕr	delicate fibrous membrane forming the middle layer of the meninges
pia mater	pī′ă mā′tĕr	thin inner layer of the meninges that attaches directly to the brain and spinal cord
spinal cord	spī′năl kōrd	portion of the central nervous system contained in the vertebral canal that conducts nerve impulses to and from the brain and body
ventricle	ven′tri-kĕl	one of four interconnected cavities within the brain that secrete cerebrospinal fluid

(continued)

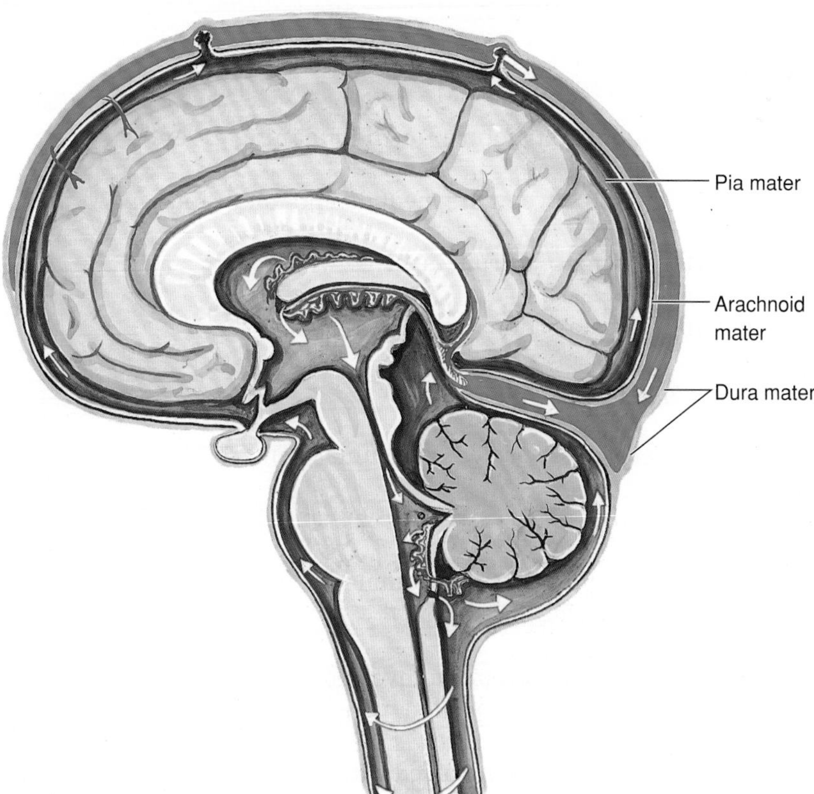

Figure 6-3 The meninges protect the brain and spinal cord. Arrows indicate the flow of cerebrospinal fluid (CSF).

Terms Related to the Nervous System *(continued)*

Term	Pronunciation	Meaning
Terms Related to the Peripheral Nervous System		
peripheral nervous system	pĕr-if′ĕr-ăl nĕr′vŭs sis′tĕm	part of the nervous system external to the brain and spinal cord that consists of all other nerves throughout the body
nerve	nĕrv	whitish cord-like structure that transmits stimuli from the central nervous system to another area of the body or from the body to the central nervous system
ganglion	gang′glē-ŏn	group of nerve cell bodies located along the pathway of a nerve
neuroglia; *syn.* glia	nūr-og′lē-ă; glī′ă	cells that support and protect nervous tissue

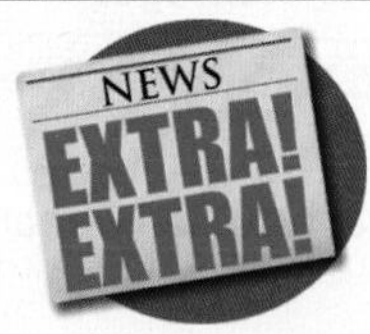

GLIAL CELLS Glial cells support and protect neurons, or nerve cells, the other main type of cell in the nervous system. They are considered the "glue" of the nervous system. The Greek word for glue is *glio*.

Term	Pronunciation	Meaning
neuron	nūr′on	nerve cell; cell that makes up the basic structure of the nervous system and conducts impulses
cranial nerves	krā′nē-ăl nĕrvz	12 pairs of nerves that emerge from the brain
spinal nerves	spī′năl nĕrvz	31 pairs of nerves that emerge from the spinal cord

Exercises: Anatomy and Physiology

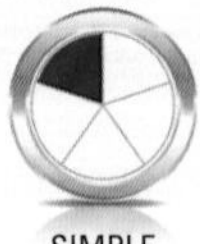
SIMPLE RECALL

Exercise 1

Write the correct anatomic structure for the meaning given.

1. part of the brainstem between the medulla and midbrain ______
2. posterior portion of the cerebrum involved with vision ______
3. largest and uppermost portion of the brain ______
4. the brain and spinal cord, collectively ______
5. portion of the brain that coordinates voluntary muscles ______
6. cavity within the brain that secretes cerebrospinal fluid ______
7. portion of the cerebrum below the frontal lobe involved with the senses of hearing and smell ______
8. middle-top portion of the cerebrum involved in perception of touch, temperature, and pain ______
9. front portion of the cerebrum involved with voluntary muscle movement and emotions ______
10. connects the brain to the spinal cord ______

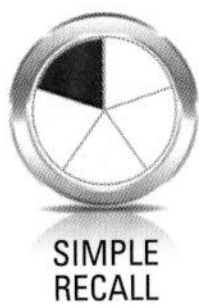
SIMPLE RECALL

Exercise 2

Write the meaning of the term given.

1. spinal cord ______
2. cerebral cortex ______
3. nerve ______
4. sulcus ______
5. pia mater ______
6. peripheral nervous system ______
7. midbrain ______
8. cranial nerves ______
9. brain ______
10. meninges ______

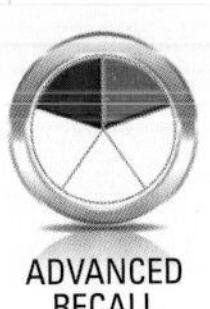
ADVANCED RECALL

Exercise 3

Match each medical term with its meaning.

gyrus	arachnoid mater	ganglion
dura mater	neuron	diencephalon
spinal nerves	cerebrospinal fluid	neuroglia

1. group of nerve cell bodies along the pathway of a nerve ______
2. 31 pairs of nerves emerging from the spinal cord ______
3. cell that conducts impulses ______
4. the middle layer of the meninges ______
5. colorless liquid in and around the brain and spinal cord ______
6. convolution on the surface of the cerebrum ______
7. cells that support and protect nervous tissue ______
8. tough, fibrous outermost layer of the meninges ______
9. area deep within the brain responsible for directing sensory information to the cortex ______

WORD PARTS

The following tables list word parts related to the nervous system and mental health.

Combining Forms

Combining Form	Meaning
	Related to the Nervous System
cerebell/o	cerebellum (little brain)
cerebr/o	brain, cerebrum
cortic/o	outer portion of an organ, cortex (as in cerebral cortex)
crani/o	cranium, skull
dur/o	hard, dura mater
encephal/o	brain
esthesi/o	sensation, perception
gangli/o, ganglion/o	ganglion
gli/o	glue, neuroglia
mening/o, meningi/o	meninges
myel/o	bone marrow, spinal cord
narc/o	stupor, numbness, sleep
neur/o	nerve
phas/o	speech
poli/o	gray matter
radicul/o	nerve root
somn/o, somn/i	sleep
spin/o	spine
spondyl/o	vertebra
thalam/o	thalamus
ventricul/o	ventricle
vertebr/o	vertebra
	Related to Mental Health
anxi/o	fear, worry
hallucin/o	to wander in one's mind
hypn/o	sleep, hypnosis
ment/o	mind, mental
phren/o	mind
psych/o	mind, mental
schiz/o	split
soci/o	social, society
thym/i, thym/o	mind, soul, emotion

Prefixes

Prefix	Meaning
Related to the Nervous System	
epi-	on, upon, following
hemi-	half
hyper-	above, excessive
hypo-	below, deficient
para-	beside
poly-	many, much
quadri-	four
Related to Mental Health	
bi-	two, twice
de-	away from, cessation, without
eu-	good, normal

Suffixes

Suffix	Meaning
Related to the Nervous System	
-al, -ar	pertaining to
-gram	record, recording
-ia	condition of
-ictal	relating to or caused by a stroke or seizure
-lepsis, -lepsy	seizure
-logist	one who specializes in
-paresis	partial or incomplete paralysis
-phrenia	the mind
-plegia	paralysis
-tomy	incision
Related to Mental Health	
-iatrist	one who specializes in
-mania	excited state, obsession
-phile, -philia	attraction to
-phobia	abnormal fear of, aversion to, sensitivity to

Exercises: Word Parts

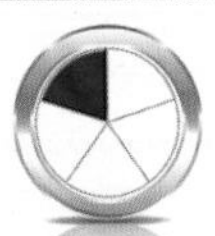

Exercise 4

Write the meaning for the combining form given.

1. encephal/o ______________________
2. gli/o ______________________

3. cerebr/o ______
4. neur/o ______
5. dur/o ______
6. meningi/o ______
7. cerebell/o ______
8. radicul/o ______
9. somn/i ______
10. ment/o ______
11. gangli/o ______
12. thalam/o ______
13. crani/o ______
14. esthesi/o ______
15. phas/o ______
16. spondyl/o ______
17. myel/o ______
18. spin/o ______
19. psych/o ______
20. poli/o ______

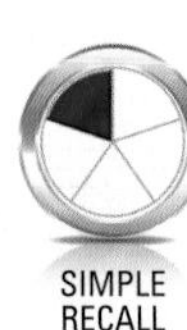

Exercise 5

SIMPLE RECALL

Write the correct combining form for the meaning given.

1. glue ______
2. ventricle ______
3. brain ______
4. fear, worry ______
5. spinal cord ______
6. cerebellum ______
7. cortex ______
8. ganglion ______

9. thalamus ______

10. split ______

11. spine ______

12. mind, soul, emotions ______

13. cerebrum ______

14. mind ______

15. vertebra ______

16. sensation, perception ______

17. hard, dura mater ______

18. to wander in one's mind ______

19. stupor, numbness, sleep ______

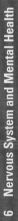

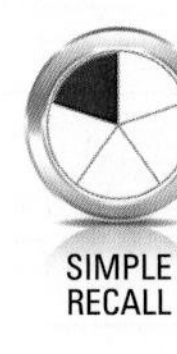

SIMPLE RECALL

Exercise 6

Write the meaning of the prefix or the suffix given.

1. -iatrist ______

2. hemi- ______

3. -phile, -philia ______

4. -mania ______

5. -phobia ______

6. poly- ______

7. quadri- ______

8. -ia ______

9. -tomy ______

10. hyper- ______

11. -paresis ______

12. hypo- ______

13. -plegia ______

14. epi- ______

15. -ictal ______

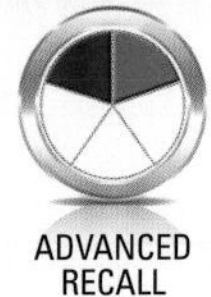

ADVANCED RECALL

Exercise 7

Considering the meaning of the combining form from which the medical term is made, write the meaning of the medical term.

Combining Form	Meaning	Medical Term	Meaning of Term
encephal/o	brain	encephalitis	**1.** ________________
crani/o	cerebrum, skull	craniotomy	**2.** ________________
myel/o	spinal cord	myelogram	**3.** ________________
gli/o	glue, neuroglia	glial	**4.** ________________
phas/o	speech	dysphasia	**5.** ________________
spin/o	spine	spinal	**6.** ________________
cerebell/o	cerebellum	cerebellar	**7.** ________________
psych/o	mind	psychologist	**8.** ________________
schiz/o; phren/o	split; mind	schizophrenia	**9.** ________________
esthesi/o	sensation	anesthesia	**10.** ________________
radicul/o	nerve root	radiculopathy	**11.** ________________
neur/o	nerve	polyneuropathy	**12.** ________________

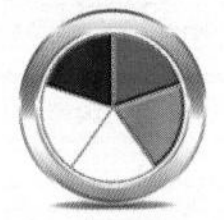

TERM CONSTRUCTION

Exercise 8

Using the given combining forms and word parts from the earlier tables, build medical terms for the meanings given.

Combining Form	Meaning of Medical Term	Medical Term
myel/o	inflammation of the spinal cord	**1.** ________________
crani/o	incision into the skull	**2.** ________________
neur/o	disease of the nerves	**3.** ________________
gli/o	tumor of the glial cells	**4.** ________________
crani/o	pertaining to the skull	**5.** ________________
esthesi/o	condition of painful sensation	**6.** ________________
meningi/o	inflammation of the membranes of the spinal cord	**7.** ________________
dur/o	pertaining to deep in the dura mater	**8.** ________________
meningi/o	tumor of the membranes of the spinal cord	**9.** ________________
encephal/o	disease of the brain	**10.** ________________

MEDICAL TERMS

The following table gives adjective forms and terms used in describing the nervous system and mental conditions.

Adjectives and Other Related Terms

Term	Pronunciation	Meaning
bipolar	bī-pō′lăr	having two ends or extremes
cerebral	ser′ĕ-brăl	pertaining to the cerebrum
cerebellar	ser-ĕ-bel′ăr	pertaining to the cerebellum
cranial	krā′nē-ăl	pertaining to the cranium or skull
dural	dūr′ăl	pertaining to the dura mater
epidural	ep′i-dūr′ăl	pertaining to on or outside the dura mater
glial	glī′ăl	pertaining to the glia
ictal	ik′tăl	pertaining to or caused by a stroke or seizure
ischemic	is-kē′mik	pertaining to a lack of blood flow
meningeal	men′in-jē′ăl	pertaining to the meninges
mental	men′tăl	pertaining to the mind
neural	nūr′ăl	pertaining to the nerves or any structure composed of nerves
postictal	pōst-ik′tăl	following a seizure
radicular	ră-dik′yū-lăr	pertaining to a nerve root
subdural	sŭb-dūr′ăl	deep in the dura mater

Exercises: Adjectives and Other Related Terms

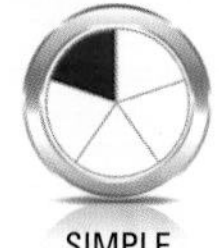

SIMPLE RECALL

Exercise 9

Write the meaning of the term given.

1. meningeal ____________________
2. cranial ____________________
3. epidural ____________________
4. cerebral ____________________
5. ischemic ____________________
6. radicular ____________________
7. mental ____________________

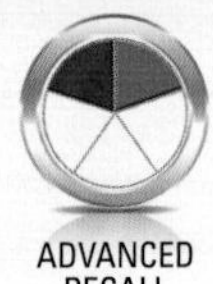

Exercise 10

Match each medical term with its meaning.

neural	cerebellar	bipolar
postictal	subdural	ischemic
ictal	glial	dural

1. having two ends or extremes __________
2. pertaining to the dura mater __________
3. pertaining to the nerves or any structure composed of nerves __________
4. pertaining to the glia __________
5. pertaining to or caused by a stroke or seizure __________
6. following a seizure __________
7. pertaining to the cerebellum __________
8. pertaining to a lack of blood flow __________
9. deep in the dura mater __________

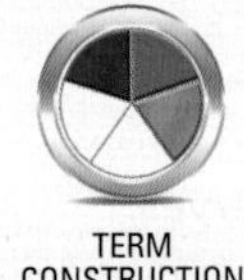

Exercise 11

Write the combining form used in the medical term, and then write the meaning of the combining form.

Term	Combining Form	Combining Form Meaning
1. cerebral	__________	__________
2. radicular	__________	__________
3. mental	__________	__________
4. epidural	__________	__________
5. spinal	__________	__________
6. cerebellar	__________	__________

Medical Conditions

Term	Pronunciation	Meaning
Related to the Nervous System		
Alzheimer disease	awlts'hī-mĕr di-zēz'	a progressive degenerative brain disease that results in memory impairment and dementia **(Figure 6-4)**
amnesia	am-nē'zē-ă	loss of memory
amyotrophic lateral sclerosis (ALS); *syn.* Lou Gehrig disease	ă-mī'ō-trō'fik lat'ĕr-ăl skler-ō'sis; lū ger'ig di-zēz'	fatal degenerative disease of the motor neurons marked by muscle weakness and atrophy **(Figure 6-5)**

(continued)

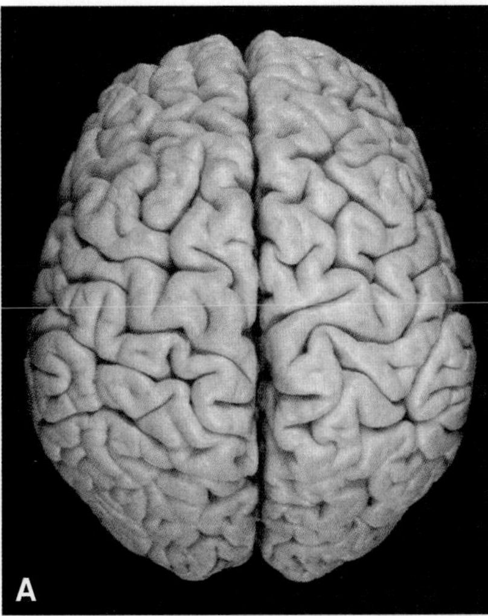

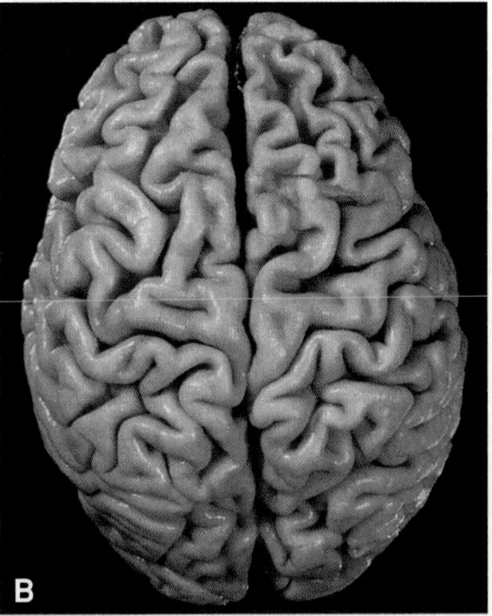

Figure 6-4 Alzheimer disease. **A.** Normal brain. **B.** The brain of a person with Alzheimer disease shows cortical atrophy, characterized by slender gyri and widened sulci.

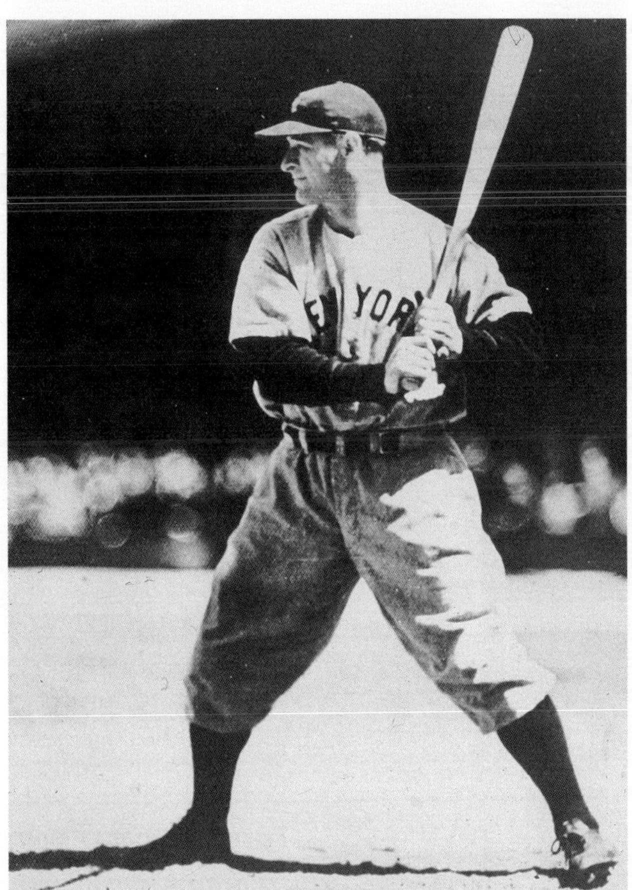

Figure 6-5 Amyotrophic lateral sclerosis (ALS) is also called Lou Gehrig disease after Gehrig, a major league baseball player who was diagnosed with the disease in 1939.

Medical Conditions *(continued)*

Term	Pronunciation	Meaning
aphasia	ă-fā'zē-ă	impaired comprehension or formulation of speech, reading, or writing caused by damage to the brain
ataxia	ă-tak'sē-ă	lack of muscle coordination; may involve the limbs, head, or trunk
Bell palsy	bel pawl'zē	paralysis of facial muscles, usually on one side of the face, caused by dysfunction of the facial nerve (cranial nerve VII) **(Figure 6-6)**

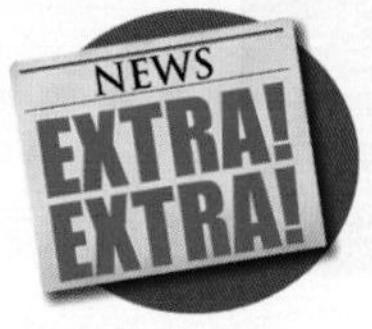

BELL PALSY Bell palsy is paralysis of the facial muscles caused by dysfunction of the facial nerve (cranial nerve VII). It is probably due to a viral infection, and the diagnosis is made by ruling out stroke or other infections, such as Lyme disease or herpes.

Term	Pronunciation	Meaning
cerebral aneurysm	ser'ĕ-brăl an'yūr-izm	widening of a blood vessel in the brain, usually due to a weakness in the wall of the artery
cerebral embolism	ser'ĕ-brăl em'bŏ-lizm	obstruction or occlusion of a vessel in the brain by an embolus (blood clot, air bubble, or fat deposit in a blood vessel) **(Figure 6-7)**
cerebral palsy (CP)	ser'ĕ-brăl pawl'zē	term for various types of nonprogressive movement dysfunction present at birth or in early childhood
cerebral thrombosis	ser'ĕ-brăl throm-bō'sis	thrombus (blood clot) within a blood vessel of the brain **(Figure 6-7)**

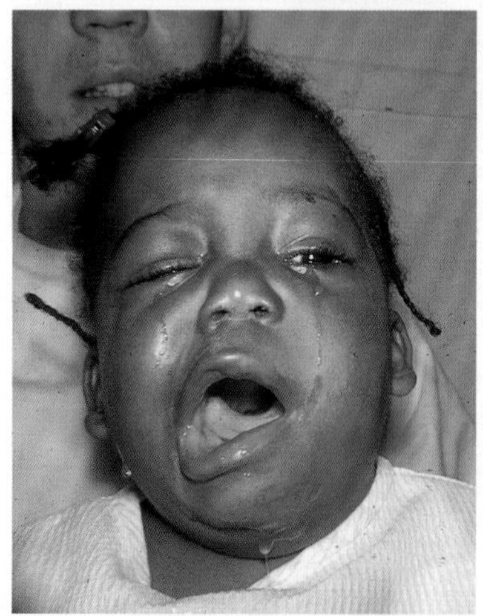

Figure 6-6 Bell palsy caused by dysfunction of the facial nerve, leading to facial paralysis on the affected side.

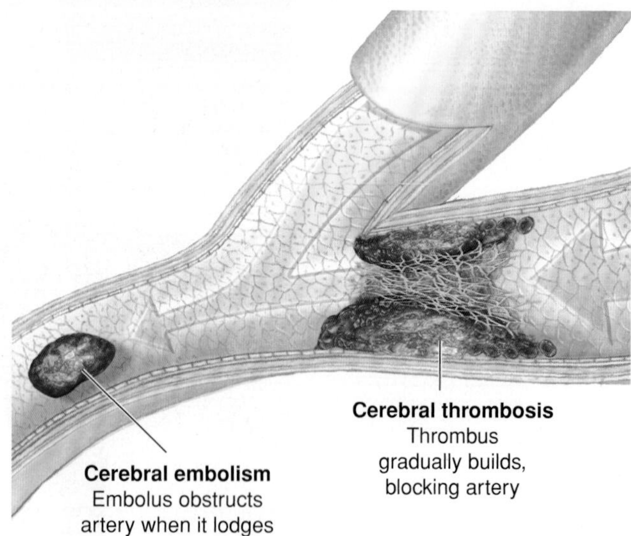

Figure 6-7 Cerebral embolism and cerebral thrombosis.

Medical Conditions

Term	Pronunciation	Meaning
cerebrovascular accident (CVA); *syn.* stroke	ser′ĕ-brō-vas′kyū-lăr ak′si-dĕnt; strōk	damage to the brain caused by an interruption of blood supply to a region of the brain **(Figure 6-8)**

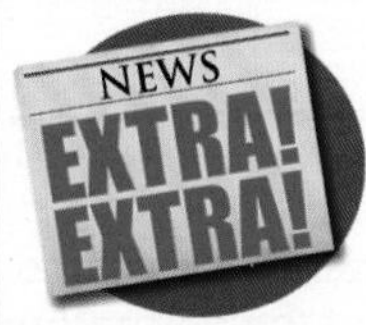

FAST FAST is an acronym to remember the signs of a stroke. **F** is for **f**ace drooping, **A** is for **a**rm weakness, **S** is for **s**peech difficulty, and **T** is for **t**ime to call 9-1-1.

Term	Pronunciation	Meaning
clonus	klō′nŭs	repeated muscular spasms seen with seizure disorders
coma	kō′mă	prolonged state of deep unconsciousness
concussion	kŏn-kŭsh′ŭn	injury to the brain resulting from violent shaking or a blow to the head
disorientation	dis-ōr′ē-ĕn-tā′shŭn	loss of sense of familiarity with one's surroundings (time, place, and self)

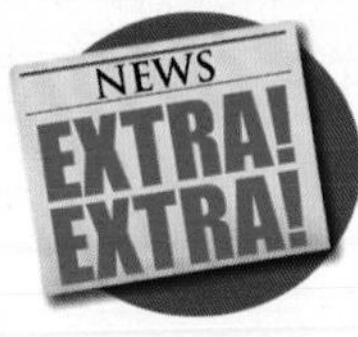

"ORIENTED ×3" When trying to determine if a person is aware of his or her surroundings, usually after an accident or a temporary loss of consciousness, medical personnel will typically ask the victim if he or she knows his or her name; where he or she is; and the day, week, month, or year. In so doing, the professional can determine if the patient is awake, alert, and oriented to person, place, and time. This is known as *orientation times 3.* It is charted as A&O ×3, which means "alert and oriented ×3."

(continued)

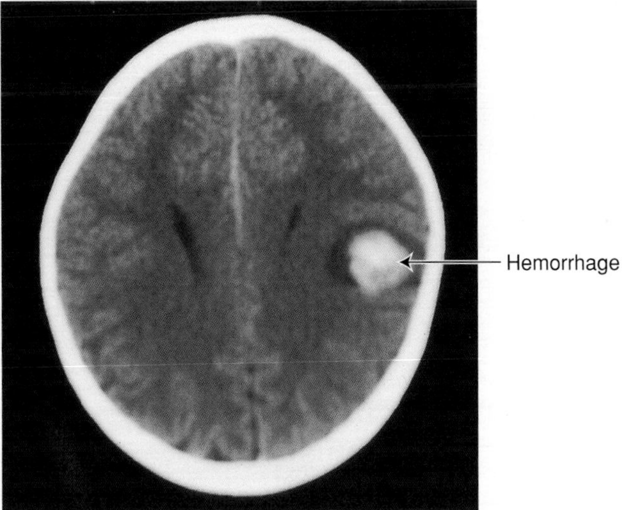

Figure 6-8 Cerebrovascular accident (stroke). Computed tomography scan of the brain showing a large hemorrhage in the brain of a 4-year-old boy.

Medical Conditions *(continued)*

Term	Pronunciation	Meaning
encephalitis	en-sef′ă-lī′tis	inflammation of the brain
epilepsy	ep′i-lep′sē	disorder of the central nervous system that is usually characterized by seizure activity and some alteration of consciousness
hemiparesis	hem′ē-pă-rē′sis	partial or incomplete paralysis affecting one side of the body **(Figure 6-9)**
herpes zoster; *syn.* shingles	hĕr′pēz zos′tĕr; shing′gĕlz	painful viral infection that affects the peripheral nerves and causes an eruption of blisters that follow the path of the dermatome of the affected nerves; closely related to varicella **(Figure 6-10)**
hydrocephalus	hī′drō-sef′ă-lŭs	a condition involving increased cerebrospinal fluid; leads to enlargement of the cerebral ventricles and an increase in intracranial pressure; commonly known as "water on the brain" **(Figure 6-11)**
incoherence	in′kō-hēr′ens	confusion; denoting unconnected speech or thoughts
lethargy	leth′ăr-jē	a feeling of sluggishness or stupor
meningitis	men′in-jī′tis	inflammation of the meninges
meningomyelocele	mĕ-ning′gō-mī′ĕ-lō-sēl	protrusion of the meninges and spinal cord through a defect in the vertebra **(Figure 6-12)**

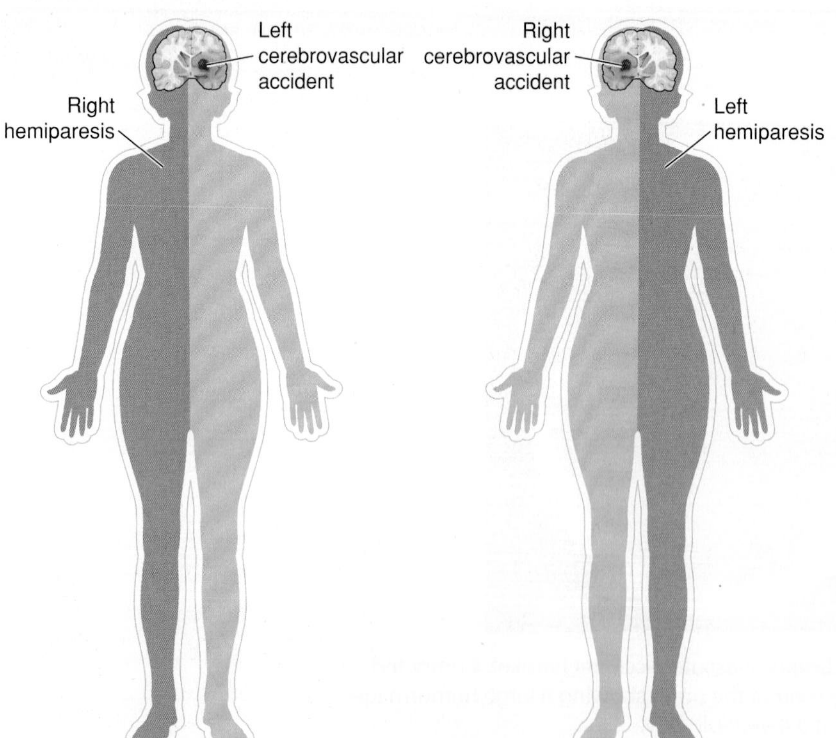

Figure 6-9 Right and left hemiparesis caused by CVA.

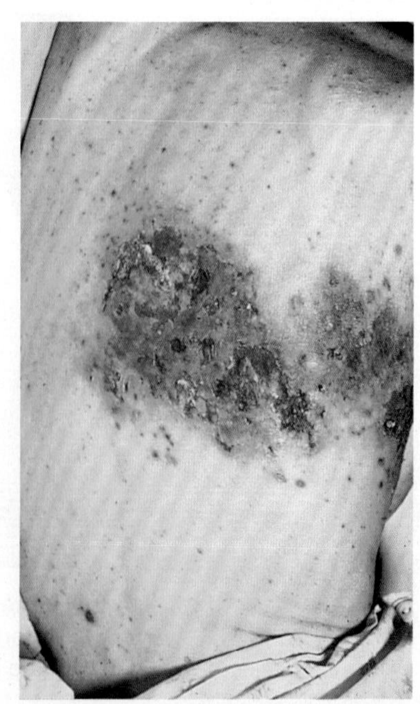

Figure 6-10 An outbreak of shingles with the primary skin lesions following the path of a dermatome.

Medical Conditions

Term	Pronunciation	Meaning
migraine	mī′grān	recurrent syndrome characterized by unilateral head pain, vertigo, nausea, and sensitivity to light
multiple sclerosis (MS)	mŭl′ti-pĕl skler-ō′sis	demyelinating disorder of the central nervous system that causes sclerotic patches (plaques) in the brain and spinal cord; symptoms may include visual loss, weakness, paresthesias, bladder abnormalities, and mood alterations
narcolepsy; *syn.* excessive sleep disorder	nahr′kō-lep-sē; eks-es′iv slēp dis-ōr′dĕr	sleep disorder characterized by recurring episodes of sleep during the day and disrupted sleep at night
neuralgia	nūr-al′jē-ă	pain in a nerve
neuritis	nūr-ī′tis	inflammation of a nerve
neuropathy	nūr-op′ă-thē	disease of the nerves
paraplegia	par′ă-plē′jē-ă	paralysis of the legs and lower part of the body
paresthesia	par-es-thē′zē-ă	an abnormal sensation, such as numbness, tingling, or "pins and needles"
parkinsonism; *syn.* Parkinson disease	pahr′kin-sŏn-izm; pahr′kin-sŏn di-zēz′	degenerative disorder resulting from deterioration of dopamine-producing neurons in the brain that causes impaired speech and motor function; characterized by tremors of the limbs

(continued)

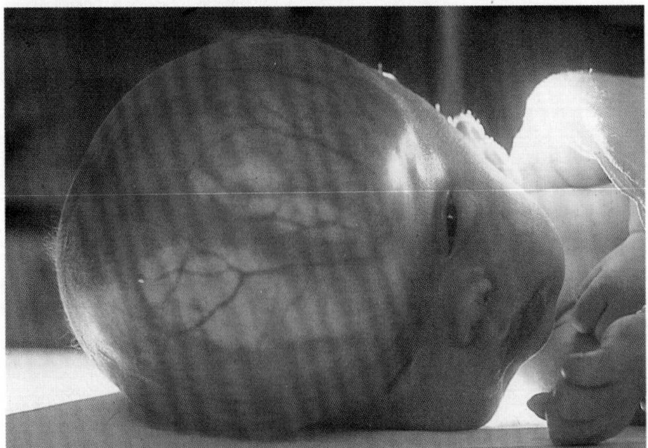

Figure 6-11 An enlargement of the cerebral ventricles leads to hydrocephalus, as seen in this infant.

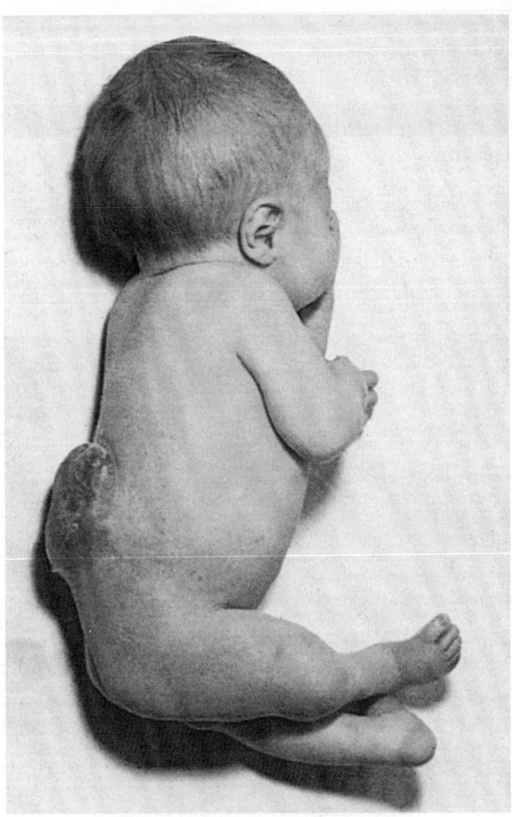

Figure 6-12 Meningomyelocele.

Medical Conditions *(continued)*

Term	Pronunciation	Meaning
poliomyelitis	pō′lē-ō-mī-ĕ-lī′tis	severe infectious viral disease that inflames the gray matter of the spinal cord and can lead to paralysis and muscle wasting; also called polio **(Figure 6-13)**
polyneuropathy	pol′ē-nū-rop′ă-thē	inflammation of a number of peripheral nerves; also called polyneuritis
radiculopathy	ră-dik′yū-lop′ă-thē	disorder of the spinal nerve roots; also called radiculitis
seizure	sē′zhŭr	violent spasm or series of jerky movements of the face, trunk, or limbs
sleep apnea	slēp ap′nē-ă	disorder marked by interruptions of breathing during sleep
stupor	stū′pŏr	state of impaired consciousness in which the person shows a marked reduction in reactivity to environmental stimuli
subdural hematoma	sŭb-dūr′ăl hē′mă-tō′mă	a collection of blood deep in the dura mater resulting from a broken blood vessel, usually due to trauma **(Figure 6-14)**
syncope; *syn.* syncopal episode	sing′kŏ-pē; sing′kŏ-păl ep′i-sōd	fainting, or an episode of fainting, usually due to lack of blood supply to the cerebrum
tic	tic	sudden, rapid, recurrent, nonrhythmic, involuntary motor movement or vocalization
tonic–clonic seizure	ton′ik-klon′ik sē′zhŭr	seizure characterized by successive phases of tonic and clonic spasms (repeated contractions and relaxations of muscles); "grand mal" seizure
Tourette syndrome	tūr-et′ sin′drōm	tic disorder characterized by intermittent motor and vocal manifestations; begins in childhood
transient ischemic attack (TIA)	tran′sē-ĕnt is-kē′mik ă-tak′	sudden, brief, and temporary cerebral dysfunction; usually caused by interruption of blood flow to the brain
Related to Mental Health		
anxiety	ang-zī′ĕ-tē	feeling of fear, worry, uneasiness, or dread
attention deficit hyperactivity disorder (ADHD)	ă-ten′shŭn def′i-sit hī′pĕr-ak-tiv′i-tē dis-ōr′dĕr	condition that begins in childhood and is characterized by short attention span, rapid boredom, impulsive behavior, and hyperactivity

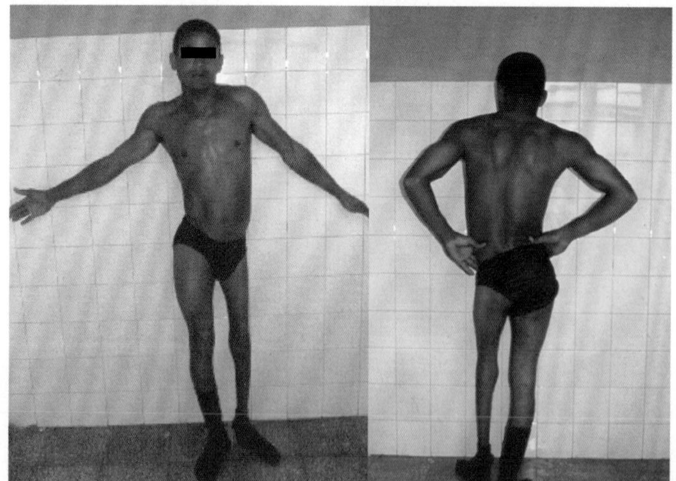

Figure 6-13 The deformed leg of the young boy is due to poliomyelitis.

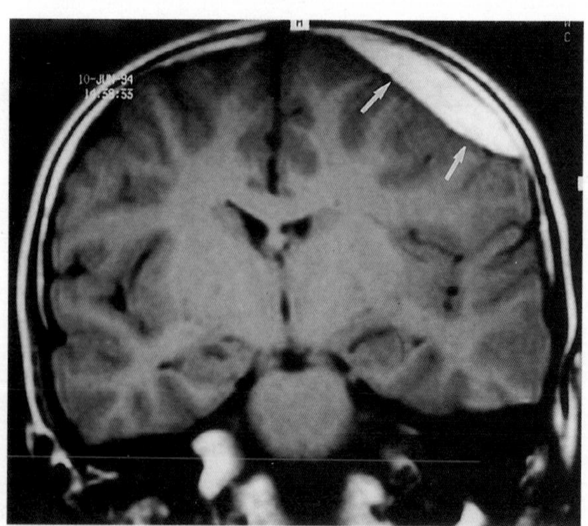

Figure 6-14 Magnetic resonance image (MRI) showing a subdural hematoma (*arrows*).

Medical Conditions

Term	Pronunciation	Meaning
agoraphobia	ag′ŏr-ă-fō′bē-ă	type of mental disorder with an irrational fear of leaving home and going out into the open; usually associated with panic attacks
autism	aw′tizm	disorder of unknown cause consisting of self-absorption, withdrawal of social contacts, repetitive movements and other mannerisms; severity varies from mild (functional) to severe (catatonic)
bipolar disorder	bī-pō′lăr dis-ōr′dĕr	disorder characterized by the occurrence of alternating periods of euphoria (mania) and depression
catatonia	kat′ă-tō′nē-ă	a phase of schizophrenia in which the patient is unresponsive, sometimes remaining in a fixed position without moving or talking
claustrophobia	klaw′strō-fō′bē-ă	fear of being shut in or enclosed
compulsion	kŏm-pŭl′shŭn	uncontrollable impulse to perform an act, often repetitively, to relieve anxiety; if the compulsive act is prevented, the anxiety becomes fully manifested
delirium	dĕ-lir′ē-ŭm	an altered state with confusion, distractibility, hallucinations, and overactivity; caused by medication or a metabolic disorder
delusion	dĕ-lū′zhŭn	a false belief or decision that is strongly held and remains unchanged regardless of any outside factors
dementia	dĕ-men′shē-ă	usually progressive loss of cognitive and intellectual functions, without impairment of perception or consciousness; most commonly associated with structural brain disease
depression	dĕ-presh′ŭn	mental state characterized by profound feelings of sadness, emptiness, hopelessness, and lack of interest or pleasure in activities
euphoria	yū-fōr′ē-ă	an exaggerated feeling of well-being
hallucination	hă-lū′si-nā′shŭn	false perception unrelated to reality or external stimuli; can be visual, auditory, or related to the other senses
mania	mā′nē-ă	emotional disorder characterized by euphoria or irritability as well as rapid speech, decreased need for sleep, distractibility, and poor judgment; usually occurs in bipolar disorder
neurosis	nūr-ō′sis	psychologic or behavioral disorder characterized by excessive anxiety
obsessive-compulsive disorder (OCD)	ob-ses′iv-kŏm-pŭl′siv dis-ōr′dĕr	condition associated with recurrent and intrusive thoughts, images, and repetitive behaviors performed to relieve anxiety
panic disorder	pan′ik dis-ōr′dĕr	form of anxiety disorder marked by episodes of intense fear of social or personal situations
paranoia	par′ă-noy′ă	mental state characterized by jealousy, delusions of persecution, or perceptions of threat or harm
phobia	fō′bē-ă	extreme persistent fear of a specific object or situation
posttraumatic stress disorder (PTSD)	pōst′traw-mat′ik stres dis-ōr′dĕr	persistent emotional disturbances that follow exposure to life-threatening catastrophic events such as trauma, abuse, natural disasters, or war
psychosis	sī-kō′sis	mental disorder extreme enough to cause gross misperception of reality with delusions and hallucinations
schizophrenia	skits′ō-frē′nē-ă	common type of psychosis, characterized by abnormalities in perception, content of thought, hallucinations and delusions, and withdrawn or bizarre behavior

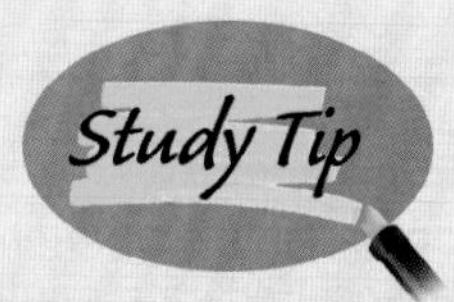

Aphasia Versus Aphagia: Avoid confusing these sound-alike terms. *Aphasia* means loss of the ability to understand or express speech and is caused by brain damage. *Aphagia* means difficulty eating and is derived from the word part *phago,* to eat. To prevent mix-ups, use this hint: Aphasia has an "s" (as in speech), and aphagia has a "g" (as in gut, which is related to eating).

Exercises: Medical Conditions

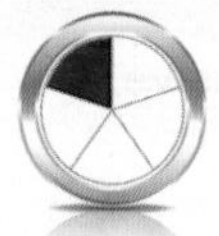

Exercise 12

SIMPLE RECALL

Write the correct medical term for the meaning given.

1. injury to the brain resulting from violent shaking or a blow to the head ________________
2. state of impaired consciousness in which the person shows a marked reduction in reactivity to environmental stimuli ________________
3. a state of impaired unconsciousness ________________
4. disorder resulting from deterioration of dopamine-producing neurons in the brain ________________
5. loss of sense of familiarity with one's surroundings ________________
6. damage to the brain caused by an interruption of blood supply to a region of the brain ________________
7. demyelinating disorder of the central nervous system that causes sclerotic patches (plaques) in the brain and spinal cord ________________
8. widening of a blood vessel in the brain ________________
9. obstruction or occlusion of a vessel in the brain ________________
10. loss of memory ________________
11. fatal disease marked by progressive deterioration of motor neurons ________________
12. paralysis of the legs and lower part of the body ________________

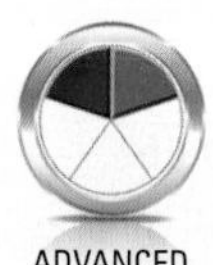

Exercise 13

ADVANCED RECALL

Complete each sentence by writing in the correct medical term.

1. A person who repeatedly washes household items that are already clean because of an intrusive fear they will get infected with germs is suffering from a condition called ________________.

2. A person who worries or is overly fearful about a situation may be diagnosed as having _______________.

3. Children and adults who cannot focus on their tasks without being easily distracted and who display impulsive behavior may be diagnosed with _______________.

4. A person with _______________ experiences persistent emotional disturbances following exposure to life-threatening catastrophic events.

5. Patients suffering from _______________ feel persecuted and think that others are out to cause them harm.

6. Individuals who strongly hold a false belief that remains unchanged despite outside factors may be diagnosed with _______________.

7. Someone with an uncontrollable impulse to gamble at every opportunity may be exhibiting a(n) _______________ for the activity.

8. Patients who have profound feelings of sadness, emptiness, hopelessness, and lack of interest or pleasure in activities are often diagnosed with _______________.

9. The phase of schizophrenia in which a patient is unresponsive is called _______________.

10. Patients with _______________ have difficulty leaving their home because of an irrational fear of going out in the open.

11. Children who suffer from _______________ withdraw from social contacts and exhibit repetitive movements.

12. A patient who is in an altered state with confusion, distractibility, hallucinations, and overactivity might be suffering from _______________.

Exercise 14

TERM CONSTRUCTION

Break the given medical term into its word parts, and define each part. Then define the medical term. (Note: This exercise uses some word parts learned previously in this text.)

For example:

neuritis	*word parts:*	neur/o, -itis
	meanings:	nerve, inflammation of
	term meaning:	inflammation of a nerve

1. polyneuritis

word parts: _______________

meanings: _______________

term meaning: _______________

2. radiculopathy *word parts:* ____________________
meanings: ____________________
term meaning: ____________________

3. aphasia *word parts:* ____________________
meanings: ____________________
term meaning: ____________________

4. meningomyelocele *word parts:* ____________________
meanings: ____________________
term meaning: ____________________

5. encephalitis *word parts:* ____________________
meanings: ____________________
term meaning: ____________________

6. hemiparesis *word parts:* ____________________
meanings: ____________________
term meaning: ____________________

7. neuralgia *word parts:* ____________________
meanings: ____________________
term meaning: ____________________

8. schizophrenia *word parts:* ____________________
meanings: ____________________
term meaning: ____________________

9. subdural *word parts:* ____________________
meanings: ____________________
term meaning: ____________________

10. poliomyelitis *word parts:* ____________________
meanings: ____________________
term meaning: ____________________

Diagnostic Procedures

Term	Pronunciation	Meaning
Babinski sign	bă-bin′skē sīn	reflex action in which the big toe remains extended when the sole of the foot is stroked; neurologic test performed on the sole of the foot to indicate injury to the brain or spinal nerves **(Figure 6-15)**
cerebral angiography	ser′ĕ-brăl an′jē-og′ră-fē	radiography of blood vessels in the brain after injection of radiopaque contrast dye
deep tendon reflex (DTR)	dēp ten′dŏn rē′fleks	evaluation of the response of a muscle to stimuli to provide information on the integrity of the central and peripheral nervous systems; generally, lively or exaggerated reflexes indicate a problem with the *central* nervous system, and decreased reflexes indicate a problem with the *peripheral* nervous system
electroencephalography (EEG)	ē-lek′trō-en-sef′ă-log′ră-fē	electrical recording of brain activity **(Figure 6-16)**

(continued)

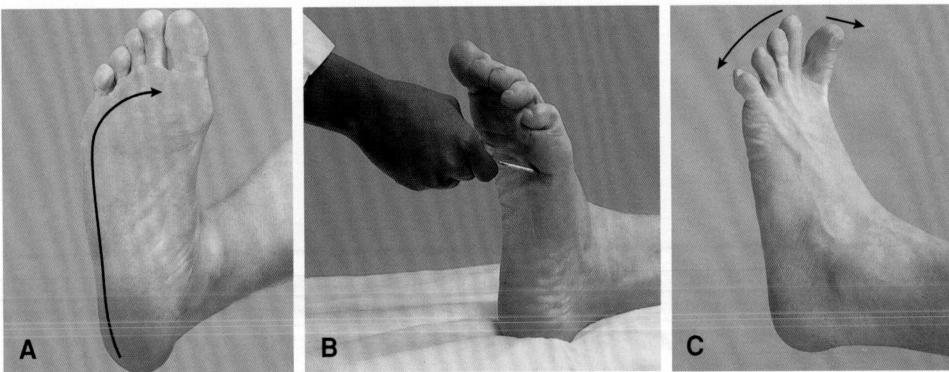

Figure 6-15 Babinski sign. **A.** The physician uses an instrument to stroke the sole of the patient's foot, beginning at the heel and curving upward. **B.** Toe flexion (absent Babinski sign). **C.** Toes that fan outward (present Babinski sign) may indicate injury to the brain or spinal nerves.

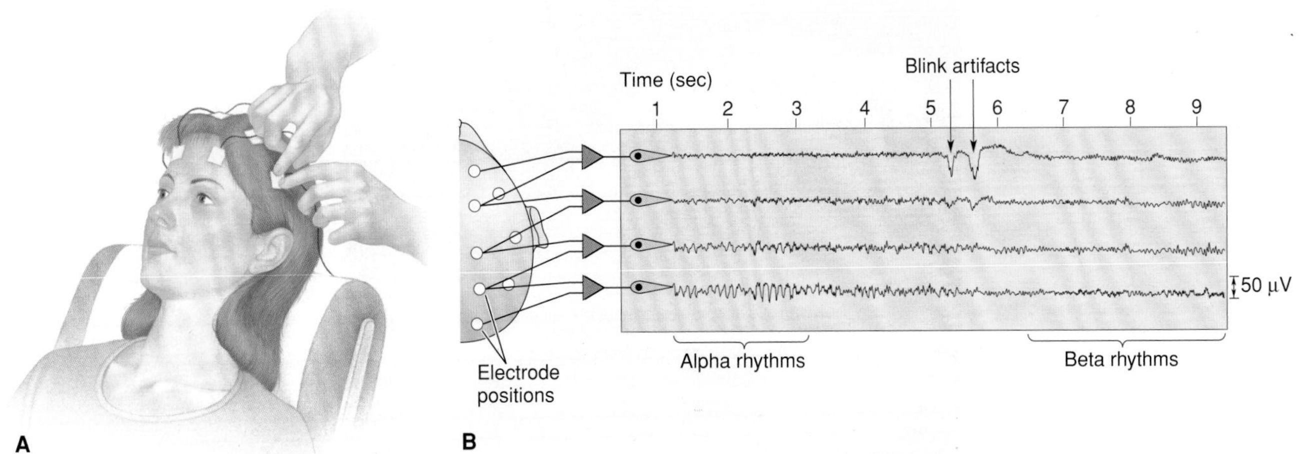

Figure 6-16 Electroencephalography. **A.** Using an electroencephalograph to monitor brain activity. **B.** A normal EEG.

Diagnostic Procedures *(continued)*

Term	Pronunciation	Meaning
evoked potential studies	ē-vōkt′ pŏ-ten′shăl stŭd′ēz	diagnostic tests that use an EEG to record changes in brain waves during various stimuli
Glasgow coma scale (GCS)	glas′gō kō′mă skāl	a neurologic scale used to assess level of consciousness **(Figure 6-17)**
lumbar puncture (LP)	lŭm′bahr pungk′shŭr	the process of inserting a needle into the subarachnoid space of the lumbar spine to obtain cerebrospinal fluid for analysis **(Figure 6-18)**

Glasgow Coma Scale	Best possible total score 15	Worst possible total score 3
Monitored performance	**Reaction**	**Score**
Eye opening	Spontaneous	4
	Open when spoken to	3
	Open at pain stimulus	2
	No reaction	1
Verbal performance	Coherent	5
	Confused, disoriented	4
	Disconnected words	3
	Unintelligible sounds	2
	No verbal reaction	1
Motor responsiveness	Follows instructions	6
	Intentional pain-avoidance	5
	Large motor movement	4
	Flexor synergism	3
	Extensor synergism	2
	No reaction	1

Figure 6-17 The Glasgow Coma Scale (GCS). The GCS is scored between 3 and 15, with 3 being the worst score and 15 being the best score.

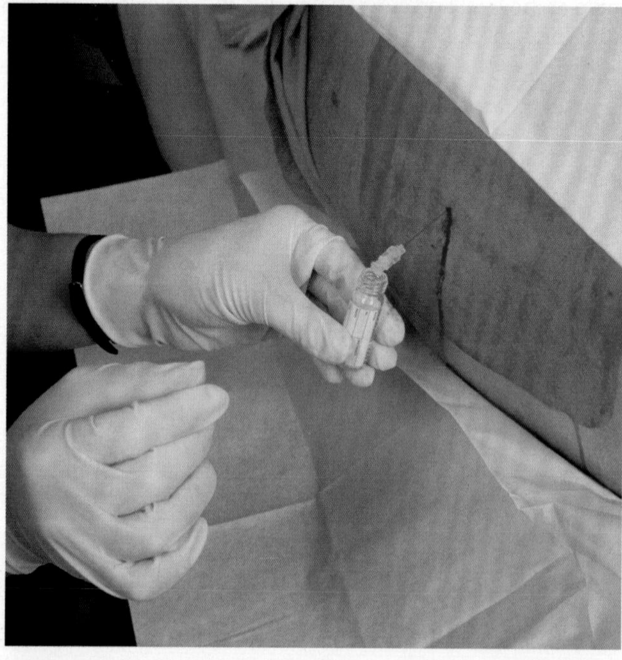

Figure 6-18 Obtaining a sample of cerebrospinal fluid after a lumbar puncture.

Diagnostic Procedures

Term	Pronunciation	Meaning
magnetic resonance imaging (MRI)	mag-net'ik rez'ŏ-năns im'ăj-ing	imaging technique that uses magnetic fields and radiofrequency waves to visualize anatomic structures; often used for evaluating soft tissue **(Figure 6-19)**
myelogram	mī'ĕ-lō-gram	radiographic contrast study of the spinal subarachnoid space and its contents
polysomnography	pol'ē-som-nog'ră-fē	monitoring and recording of normal and abnormal activity during sleep to diagnose sleep disorders
positron emission tomography (PET)	poz'i-tron ĕ-mish'ŭn tŏ-mog'ră-fē	a nuclear medicine procedure that shows metabolic activity in the brain that can correspond to various types of brain activity **(Figure 6-20)**

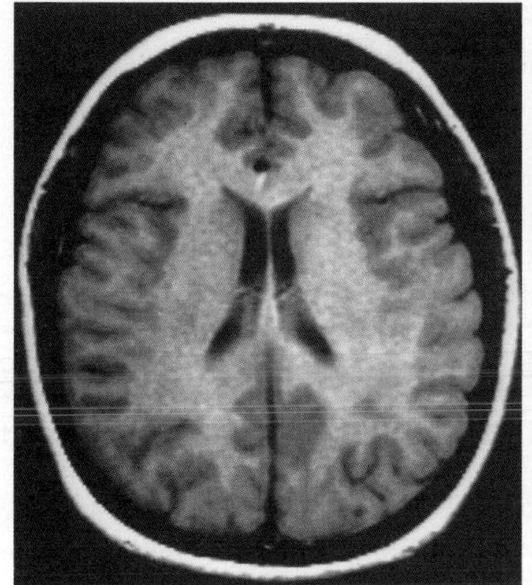

Magnetic resonance image, normal brain, horizontal view

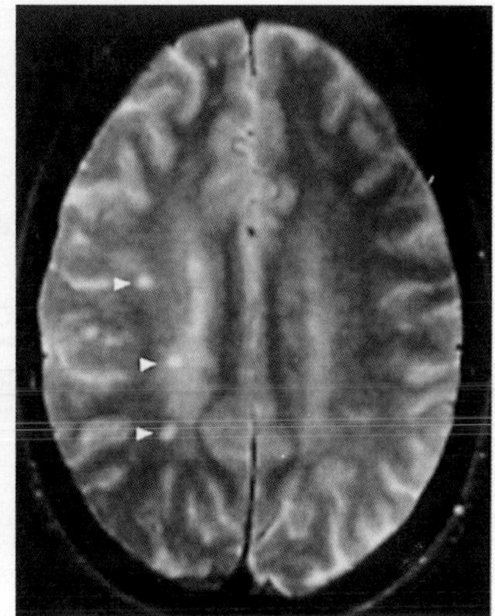

Magnetic resonance image, multiple sclerosis, horizontal view

Figure 6-19 Magnetic resonance imaging of the brain.

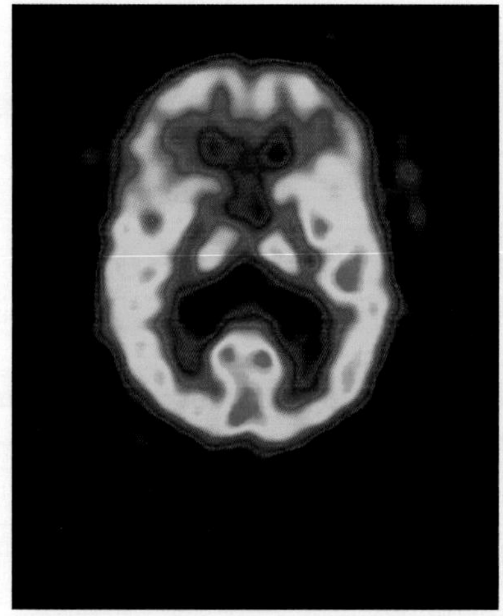

PET scan of healthy brain

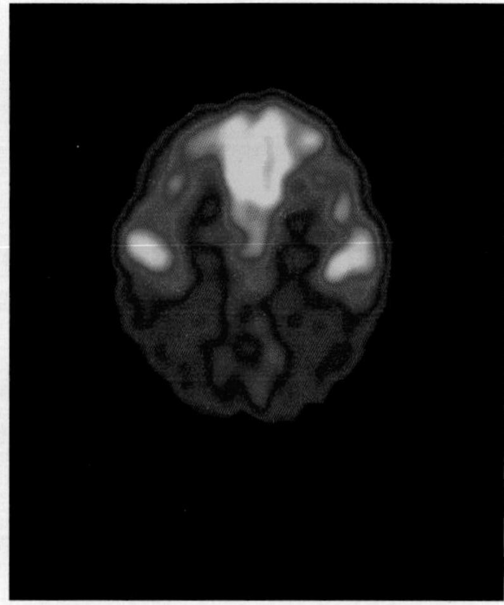

PET scan of Alzheimer brain

Figure 6-20 Positron emission tomography (PET) scans of the brain.

Exercises: Diagnostic Procedures

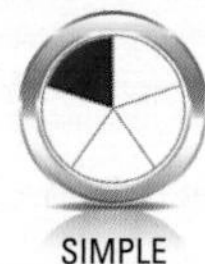
SIMPLE RECALL

Exercise 15

Write the correct medical term for the meaning given.

1. neurologic scale to assess level of consciousness ____________________
2. group of tests to record changes in brain waves ____________________
3. result of neurologic test performed on the sole of the foot ____________________
4. test that shows metabolic activity in the brain corresponding to brain activity ____________________
5. radiography of blood vessels in the brain after injection of radiopaque contrast dye ____________________

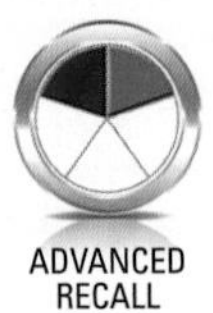
ADVANCED RECALL

Exercise 16

Complete each sentence by writing the correct medical term.

1. The process of inserting a needle into the low back area to extract a small amount of cerebrospinal fluid for analysis is called a(n) ____________________.
2. During ____________________, various aspects of sleep are recorded to diagnose sleep disorders.
3. Before undergoing ____________________, which generates images by using a magnetic field, patients are thoroughly questioned to determine if they have any metal within their bodies.
4. The test that evaluates how a muscle responds to stimuli is called ____________________.
5. The procedure in which sensors are applied to a patient's head to produce an electrical recording of brain activity is called a(n) ____________________.
6. A(n) ____________________ is a type of contrast study that allows visualization of the spinal subarachnoid space and its contents.

Surgical Interventions and Therapeutic Procedures

Term	Pronunciation	Meaning
craniectomy	krā'nē-ek'tŏ-me	excision of part of the skull, without replacement of bone, to access the brain **(Figure 6-21)**
cranioplasty	krā'nē-ō-plas'tē	operation to correct cranial defects, which may include bone grafts
craniotomy	krā'nē-ot'ŏ-mē	opening into the skull allowing access to the brain **(Figure 6-21)**
ganglionectomy	gang'glē-ō-nek'tŏ-mē	excision of a ganglion
laminectomy	lam'i-nek'tŏ-mē	excision of the thin plate (lamina) of the vertebra to relieve pressure on the spinal cord

Surgical Interventions and Therapeutic Procedures

Term	Pronunciation	Meaning
neurolysis	nūr-ol′i-sis	separation of a nerve from inflammatory adhesions
neuroplasty	nūr′ō-plas-tē	surgical repair of the nerves
psychotherapy	sī′kō-thār′ă-pē	the general term for an interaction in which a trained mental health professional tries to help a patient resolve emotional and mental distress
rhizotomy; *syn.* radicotomy	rī-zot′ō-mē; rad′i-kot′ō-mē	incision into the spinal nerve roots to relieve pain or spastic paralysis

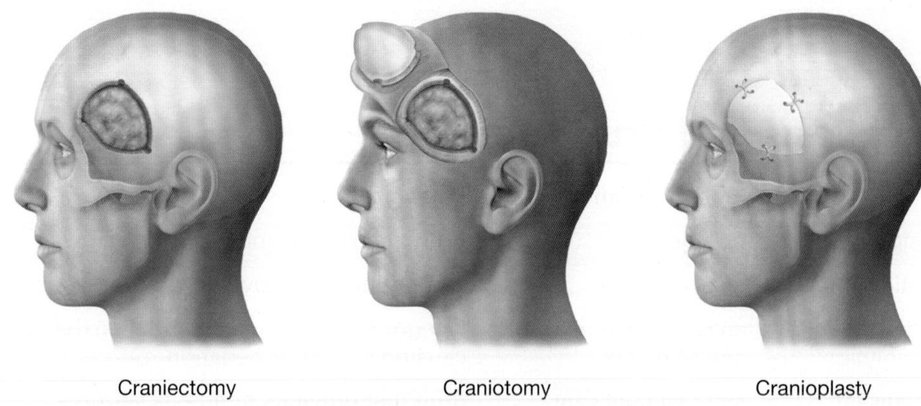

Figure 6-21 Surgeries of the skull.

Exercises: Surgical Interventions and Therapeutic Procedures

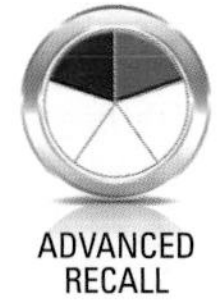
ADVANCED RECALL

Exercise 17

Match each medical term with its meaning.

neuroplasty, craniectomy, neurolysis, ganglionectomy, craniotomy, radicotomy, laminectomy, psychotherapy

1. surgical repair of the nerves ____________
2. excision of part of the skull ____________
3. removal of the thin plate of the vertebra ____________
4. incision into the skull ____________
5. incision into the spinal nerve roots ____________
6. separation of a nerve from inflammatory adhesions ____________
7. excision of a ganglion ____________
8. intervention to help a patient deal with emotional distress ____________

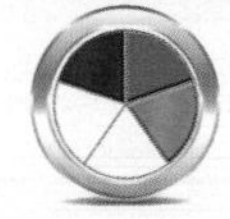

Exercise 18

TERM CONSTRUCTION

Build a medical term from an appropriate combining form and suffix given their meanings.

Use Combining Form for	Use Suffix for	Medical Term
nerve	surgical repair	1. ______
ganglion	excision	2. ______
nerve root	incision	3. ______
cranium	excision	4. ______

Medications and Drug Therapies

Term	Pronunciation	Meaning
analgesic	an′ăl-jē′zik	drug that relieves pain
anesthetic	an′es-thet′ik	compound that provides temporary loss of sensation
antianxiety agent; *syn.* anxiolytic	an′tē-ang-zī′ĕ-tē ā′jĕnt; ang′zē-ō-lit′ik	category of drugs used to treat anxiety without causing excessive sedation
anticonvulsant	an′tē-kŏn-vŭl′sănt	drug that prevents or arrests seizures
antidepressant	an′tē-dĕ-pres′ănt	drug used to treat depression
antiinflammatory	an′tē-in-flam′ă-tōr-ē	drug that reduces inflammation
epidural injection	ep′i-dūr′ăl in-jek′shŭn	injection of an analgesic into the epidural space
hypnotic	hip-not′ik	drug that promotes sleep
neuroleptic	nūr′ō-lep′tik	class of psychotropic drugs used to treat psychosis, particularly schizophrenia
psychotropic	sī′kō-trō′pik	drug used to treat mental illnesses
sedative	sed′ă-tiv	drug that quiets nervous excitement

Exercises: Medications and Drug Therapies

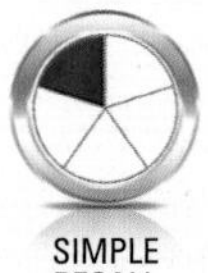

Exercise 19

SIMPLE RECALL

Write the correct medication or drug therapy term for the meaning given.

1. a drug that prevents or arrests seizures ______
2. a drug used to treat depression ______
3. a category of drugs used to treat anxiety ______

4. a drug that reduces inflammation ______________________

5. a drug that quiets nervous excitement ______________________

6. a drug that relieves pain ______________________

7. a class of psychotropic drugs used to treat psychosis ______________________

8. injection of an analgesic into the epidural space ______________________

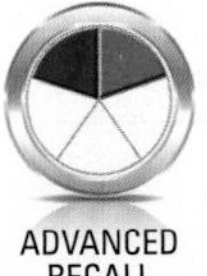

ADVANCED RECALL

Exercise 20

Considering the meaning of the combining form from which the medication or drug therapy is made, write the meaning of the term.

Combining Form	Meaning	Medical Term	Meaning of Term
anxi/o	anxiety	anxiolytic	1. ______________
psych/o	mind, mental	psychotropic	2. ______________
esthesi/o	sensation	anesthetic	3. ______________
hypn/o	sleep, hypnosis	hypnotic	4. ______________

Specialties and Specialists

Term	Pronunciation	Meaning
electroencephalography (EEG) technician	ĕ-lek′trō-en-sef′ă-log′ră-fē tek-nish′ŭn	a person who is trained to set up and perform electroencephalograms (EEGs) (tests that evaluate the electrical functions of the brain)
neurology	nūr-ol′ŏ-jē	medical specialty concerned with the study and treatment of conditions involving the nervous system
neurologist	nūr-ol′ŏ-jist	physician who specializes in neurology
psychiatry	sī-kī′ă-trē	medical specialty concerned with the diagnosis and treatment of mental disorders as practiced by a licensed medical doctor who may prescribe medications
psychiatrist	sī-kī′ă-trist	physician who specializes in psychiatry
psychology	sī-kol′ŏ-jē	medical specialty concerned with the study and treatment of mental processes, behaviors, and abnormal/irregular mood disorders as practiced by a trained professional who is not a medical doctor and is not authorized to prescribe medications
psychologist	sī-kol′ŏ-jist	one who specializes in psychology

Exercise: Specialties and Specialists

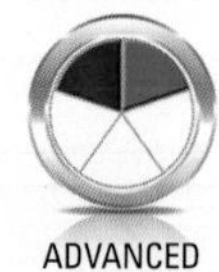
ADVANCED RECALL

Exercise 21

Match each medical specialty or specialist with its description.

psychologist	psychology	neurology	psychiatry
psychiatrist	neurologist	EEG technician	

1. professional who specializes in psychology ________
2. study and treatment of nervous system conditions ________
3. specialty concerned with the diagnosis and treatment of mental disorders as practiced by a licensed medical doctor who may prescribe medications ________
4. physician who specializes in psychiatry ________
5. specially trained person who performs tests that evaluate the electrical currents of the brain ________
6. medical specialty concerned with the study and treatment of mental processes, behaviors, and abnormal or irregular mood disorders as practiced by a trained professional who is not a medical doctor and is not authorized to prescribe medications ________
7. physician who specializes in the nervous system ________

Abbreviations

Abbreviation	Meaning
ADHD	attention deficit hyperactivity disorder
ALS	amyotrophic lateral sclerosis
CNS	central nervous system
CP	cerebral palsy
CSF	cerebrospinal fluid
CVA	cerebrovascular accident
DTR	deep tendon reflex
EEG	electroencephalogram
LP	lumbar puncture
MRI	magnetic resonance imaging
MS	multiple sclerosis
OCD	obsessive-compulsive disorder
PET	positron emission tomography
PTSD	posttraumatic stress disorder
TIA	transient ischemic attack

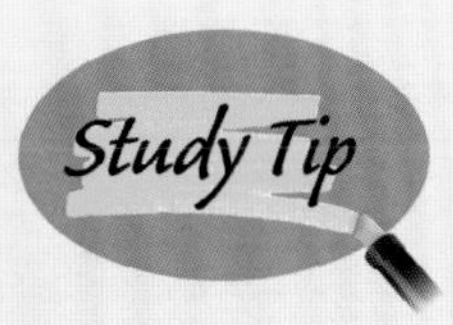

EEG Versus ECG or EKG: Be very careful when using EEG, the abbreviation for electroencephalogram. Do not confuse it with ECG or EKG, the abbreviations for **e**lectro**c**ardio**g**ram. The "K" in EKG is derived from the Greek term, *kardia,* meaning heart.

Exercises: Abbreviations

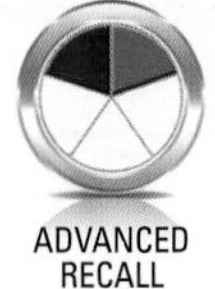

ADVANCED RECALL

Exercise 22

Write the meaning of each abbreviation used in these sentences.

1. The child was diagnosed with **CP** as a result of damage to the brain that occurred prenatally.

____

2. Mr. Jackowski was admitted with stroke-like symptoms, but testing revealed that he had suffered a **TIA**.

____

3. Mrs. Wu had to undergo an **LP** to check for bacteria in her cerebrospinal fluid.

____

4. Patients with **MS** may become weak and lethargic and may have problems with coordination.

____

5. **CSF** is normally clear without any evidence of cells or bacteria.

____

6. Mrs. Merriman received a written warning at work because she has **OCD** and was constantly in the ladies' room washing her hands.

____

7. The patient had an **MRI** to assess his injuries after a car accident.

____

8. The effects of a **CVA** can be either minimal with a short recovery period, or debilitating, requiring extensive rehabilitation.

____

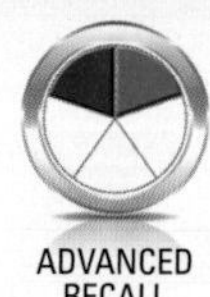

ADVANCED RECALL

Exercise 23

Match each abbreviation with the appropriate meaning.

PET	PTSD	ADHD	CNS
EEG	ALS	DTR	CVA

1. study that measures brain waves, function, and status ____________
2. condition that results in a stroke ____________
3. progressive deterioration of motor neurons ____________
4. persistent emotional disturbances that follow exposure to life-threatening catastrophic events ____________
5. condition characterized by an inability to sit still, a lack of focus, and easy distraction ____________
6. procedure that shows metabolic activity in the brain ____________
7. the brain and the spinal cord system, collectively ____________
8. assessment of reflexes by tapping or stimulating at certain points ____________

WRAPPING UP

- The nervous system has 2 major divisions: the central nervous system and the peripheral nervous system.
- There are many parts of the brain and each has specific functions.
- You learned words associated with the nervous system and mental health including word parts, adjectives, conditions, diagnostic criteria, surgical options, medications, specialists, and abbreviations.

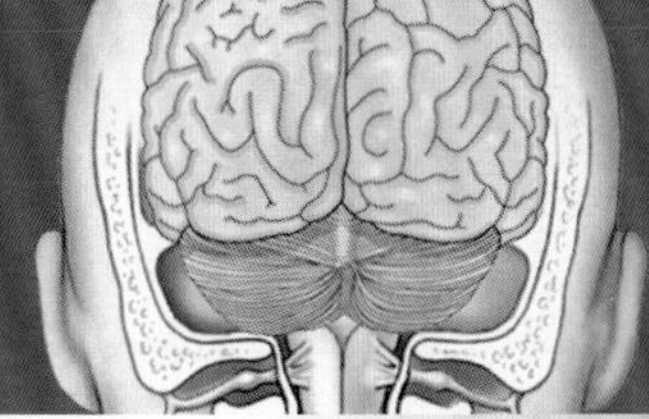

Review of Terms for Anatomy and Physiology

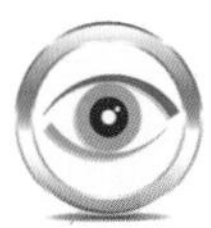
VISUAL

Exercise 24

Write the correct terms on the blanks for the anatomic structures indicated.

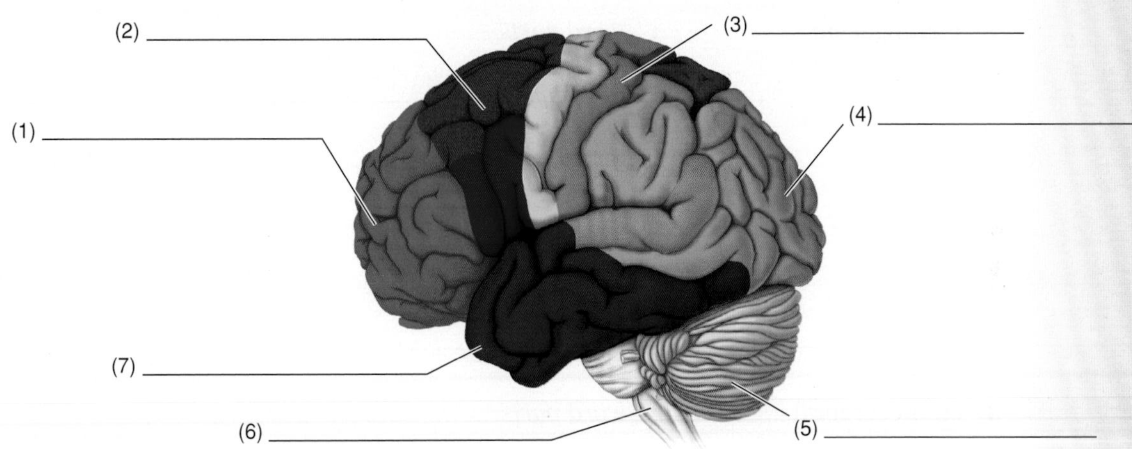

Lateral view

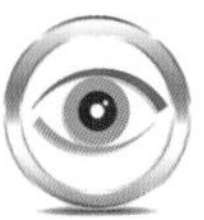
VISUAL

Exercise 25

Write the correct terms on the blanks for the anatomic structures indicated.

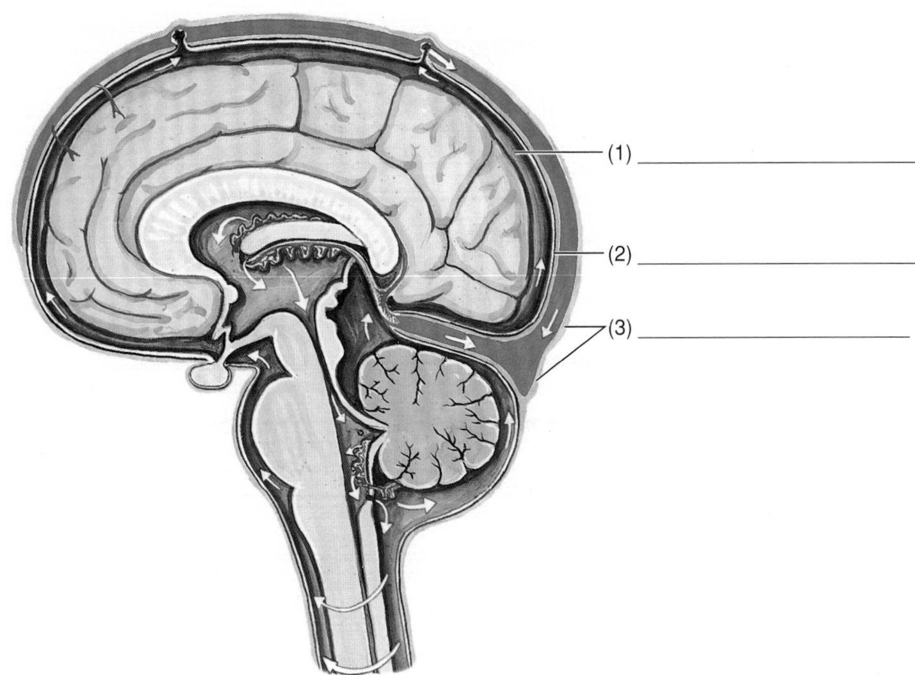

Understanding Term Structure

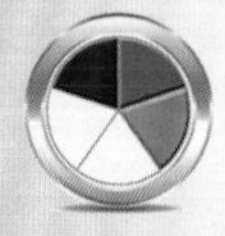
TERM CONSTRUCTION

Exercise 26

Break the given medical term into its word parts and define each part. Then define the medical term.

For example:

encephalitis	*word parts:*	encephal/o, -itis
	meanings:	brain, inflammation of
	term meaning:	inflammation of the brain

1. meningocyte
word parts: ______________________
meanings: ______________________
term meaning: ______________________

2. neuropathy
word parts: ______________________
meanings: ______________________
term meaning: ______________________

3. craniocerebral
word parts: ______________________
meanings: ______________________
term meaning: ______________________

4. quadriparesis
word parts: ______________________
meanings: ______________________
term meaning: ______________________

5. radiculomyelopathy
word parts: ______________________
meanings: ______________________
term meaning: ______________________

6. electroencephalography
word parts: ______________________
meanings: ______________________
term meaning: ______________________

7. encephaloscopy
word parts: ______________________
meanings: ______________________
term meaning: ______________________

8. poliodystrophy *word parts:* ____________________

meanings: ____________________

term meaning: ____________________

9. spondylosis *word parts:* ____________________

meanings: ____________________

term meaning: ____________________

10. ganglionectomy *word parts:* ____________________

meanings: ____________________

term meaning: ____________________

Comprehension Exercises

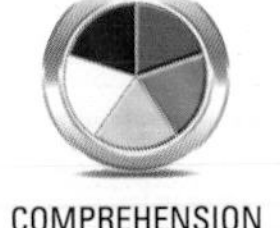
COMPREHENSION

Exercise 27

Fill in the blank with the correct term.

1. A patient with auditory and visual ____________________, or false perceptions unrelated to reality, may be admitted into the psychiatric ward of the hospital.
2. ____________________ is a feeling of sluggishness or a state of impaired consciousness.
3. The inability to walk because of a lack of muscle coordination is called ____________________.
4. The patient had ____________________, a condition involving paralysis on one side of the face.
5. The disorder that causes patients to stop breathing for short periods in their sleep is called ____________________.
6. A progressive degenerative brain disease that results in memory impairment and dementia is called ____________________.
7. Loss of sensation, usually caused by administration of a medication, is called ____________________.
8. An electrical recording of brain activity is called ____________________.
9. Herpes zoster, also known as ____________________, causes blisters along the course of affected nerves.
10. Patients with ____________________ constantly fear that they are going to be harmed.

11. ______________________ is the term for various types of nonprogressive movement dysfunction present at birth or in early childhood.

12. Inflammation of the membranous covering of the brain and spinal cord is called ______________________.

13. ______________________ is a disease of the nerve roots.

14. A patient experiencing a(n) ______________________ usually has pain on only one side of the head.

15. A(n) ______________________ impairs circulation to the brain due to a blood clot.

16. The ______________________ is the part of the brain that is divided into right and left hemispheres.

17. Prominent rounded elevations that form the cerebral hemispheres are called ______________________.

18. The ______________________ connects the brain to the spinal cord.

19. ______________________ is the medical term for fainting.

20. A neurologic disorder characterized by temporary loss of consciousness and violent spasms or series of jerky movements of the face, trunk, or limbs is called ______________________.

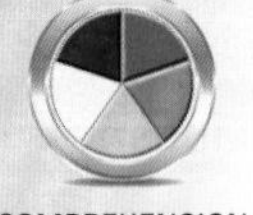
COMPREHENSION

Exercise 28

Circle the letter of the best answer in the following questions.

1. A patient who is having problems formulating thoughts into words is experiencing
   A. paraplegia.
   B. aphagia.
   C. ataxia.
   D. aphasia.

2. A person who exhibits involuntary vocal or motor dysfunctions in a tic-like manner suffers from
   A. a stroke.
   B. Alzheimer disease.
   C. Tourette syndrome.
   D. dementia.

3. A patient visits her physician complaining of a severe headache and nausea. She states that she must lie down in a darkened room. Her likely diagnosis is
   A. migraine.
   B. claustrophobia.
   C. myelitis.
   D. delusion.

4. Patients with diabetes who have long-term manifestations often have pain in the nerves of their feet. This is called
   A. neurology.
   B. neuralgia.
   C. stupor.
   D. amnesia.

5. A child was hit in the head by a foul ball at a baseball game. At the hospital, he was found to have a collection of blood under the skull, just inside the brain. The diagnosis was

A. neuritis.
B. a subdural hematoma.
C. a temporal lobe.
D. a frontal lobe.

6. A patient suddenly appears to be staring off into space. Her face droops slightly at the mouth, and she does not respond to verbal stimuli. After about 30 minutes, she appears fine and is speaking clearly and coherently. Her face no longer droops at the mouth. She most likely had a(n)

A. EEG.
B. TIA.
C. CNS.
D. CSF.

7. A sleep disturbance in which a person cannot sleep at night but can often fall asleep without notice is called

A. Alzheimer disease.
B. sleep apnea.
C. narcolepsy.
D. meningitis.

8. A patient suddenly has difficulty speaking and her right arm feels stiff and weak. Her face has a right-sided droop, and her speech is slurred. She most likely suffered a(n)

A. EEG.
B. LP.
C. CSF.
D. CVA.

9. In elderly patients, a progressive loss of thought processes without loss of awareness is called

A. sleep apnea.
B. meningitis.
C. dementia.
D. neuropathy.

10. Symptoms of this disorder mimic a stroke and are thought to be caused by a dysfunction of a nerve. This illness is called

A. shingles.
B. Bell palsy.
C. autism.
D. anxiety.

11. The accumulation of excessive fluid that circulates in and around the brain and spinal cord with resulting increased intracranial pressure is called

A. encephalitis.
B. hydrocephalus.
C. hydromeningitis.
D. hydrocraniosis.

12. A patient who lacks normal clarity of speech and also is confused is said to be suffering from

A. lethargy.
B. incoherence.
C. stupor.
D. phobia.

13. A patient complains of feeling "pins and needles." The medical term for this abnormal sensation is

A. paralysis.
B. hemiplegia.
C. paresthesia.
D. hydrocephalus.

14. A young man suddenly falls to the floor convulsing and appears unconscious. He is thought to be having a(n)

A. migraine.
B. autism.
C. seizure.
D. amnesia.

Application and Analysis

CASE STUDIES

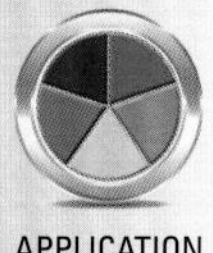

Exercise 29

APPLICATION

Read the case studies, and circle the correct letter for each of the questions.

CASE 6-1

Mr. Parker, age 78, was found somewhat confused and disoriented at home on the bathroom floor. He does not recall exactly what happened. He remembers going to the bathroom, talks about falling, and then speaks about moving things around that did not belong in the bathroom. When asked about the type of objects being moved, the patient was not able to name anything specific. Some expressive aphasia is noted during our discussion. It was determined he does not have a mental disorder. Neurologically, he is oriented to person (self) but not to time or place.

1. Based on the information provided in the case, what specialist might be called to see this patient?

A. psychiatrist
B. neurology
C. neurologist
D. psychologist

2. Aphasia is

A. the inability to walk.
B. the inability to swallow.
C. the inability to respond or communicate appropriately.
D. the inability to see.

3. Disorientation can include the loss of familiarity with

A. time.
B. place.
C. person (self).
D. all of the above

4. This patient might have had an episode of fainting, also called

A. syncope.
B. seizures.
C. lethargy.
D. ataxia.

CASE 6-2

A 16-year-old boy was riding his bike when he skidded on a patch of sand. The bike made a sudden turn, and the boy flipped over the handlebars, hitting his head in the street; he suffered lacerations, a concussion, and a hematoma. He was taken to the emergency room, where he was found to be disoriented, lethargic, and suffering from amnesia. A CT scan was done, and he was found to have an epidural hematoma **(Figure 6-22)**. He was immediately brought to the operating room for surgical intervention to open the skull and evacuate the blood clot.

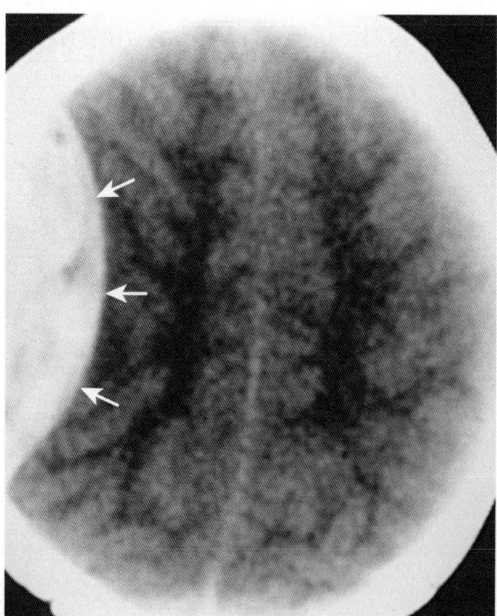

Figure 6-22 Computed tomography (CT) scan revealing epidural hematoma (*arrows*).

5. Where is the hematoma located?
   A. deep to the dura mater
   B. within the dura mater
   C. in the pia mater
   D. between the skull and the dura mater

6. A procedure to open the skull and remove the clot was performed. The medical term for "incision into the skull" is
   A. craniectomy.
   B. cranioplasty.
   C. craniotomy.
   D. craniocele.

7. A concussion is an injury to the
   A. spine.
   B. spinal cord.
   C. cranial nerves.
   D. brain.

8. The medical term for the loss of memory is
   A. ataxia.
   B. amnesia.
   C. aphasia.
   D. stupor.

MEDICAL RECORD ANALYSIS

MEDICAL RECORD 6-1

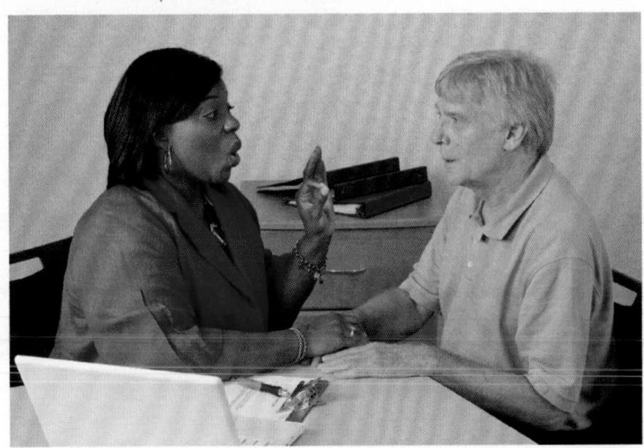

Speech therapists work with patients to improve or regain their speech.

The following is the admission history and physical for a patient who sustained a cerebrovascular accident (CVA) and is now undergoing rehabilitation. As a speech therapist, you will be working with the physician to develop a speech therapy plan for this patient. You take this opportunity to review the medical record.

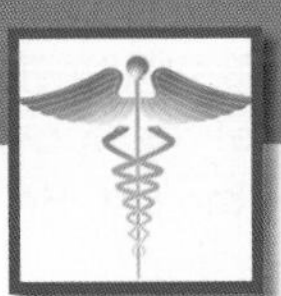

Medical Record

CEREBROVASCULAR ACCIDENT REHABILITATION HISTORY AND PHYSICAL

REASON FOR ADMISSION: Cerebrovascular accident (CVA), left hemiparesis, for advanced rehabilitation.

PATIENT GOAL: To be able to return home to live independently.

HISTORY OF PRESENT ILLNESS: This is a 64-year-old male. He developed sudden onset of left-sided weakness in early November. He was on the floor of his home approximately one week before being found. He was taken to the local hospital. In the emergency room, he was found to have a CPK of greater than 5,000, which was felt to be secondary to rhabdomyolysis from lying on the floor. He also had left-sided hemiparesis. CT scan of the head showed advance periventricular malacia, compatible with deep white matter ischemia. There was a superimposed edema to this infarct in the right basal ganglia. MRI of the head showed small vessel ischemic changes with an acute infarction of the right basal ganglia.

PAST MEDICAL HISTORY: Significant for hypertension.

ALLERGIES: He has no known drug allergies.

SOCIAL HISTORY: He lives at home alone. He has all of his arrangements on the first floor. The patient is right-handed.

HABITS: He admits to smoking cigarettes. He denies drinking alcohol or using illicit drugs.

FAMILY HISTORY: Significant for CVA, diabetes mellitus, and cancer.

REVIEW OF SYSTEMS

GENERAL: He denies weight gain, weight loss, chills, fevers, or night sweats. Head, ears, eyes, nose, and throat: Review is significant for mild dysphasia.

CARDIOVASCULAR: Significant for hypertension.

NEUROLOGIC: As above.

All other systems are negative.

PHYSICAL EXAMINATION

VITAL SIGNS: Temperature 98.8°F, pulse 78, respirations 20, blood pressure 150/98, weight 158 lb.

EXTREMITIES: His right upper and lower limbs have functional range of motion and strength.

PULMONARY: Chest is clear.

CARDIOVASCULAR: Heart has regular rate and rhythm.

ABDOMEN: Abdomen is soft with normal active bowel sounds. Foley catheter is in place.

NEUROLOGIC: This is a well-developed, thin male in no acute distress. He is alert and oriented ×3. Pupils are equal and reactive to light and accommodation. Pays attention bilaterally. Has left central facial weakness. Tongue deviates to the left. He has moderate dysphasia. His swallowing reflex appears intact. He has dense left hemiparesis without appreciable moving of the upper or lower extremity. Sensation remains intact on the left. Babinski sign is positive on the left. He has one to two beats of clonus at the left ankle.

IMPRESSION

1. Cerebrovascular accident, dense left hemiparesis
2. Rhabdomyolysis
3. Hypertension

PLAN: The patient will be admitted for a comprehensive inpatient rehabilitation program consisting of physical therapy, occupational therapy, speech therapy, recreational therapy, and case management support. Goals will be directed toward patient-and-family goals to allow the patient to return home to live independently or else to live with support.

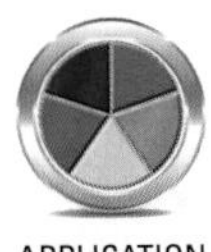

APPLICATION

Exercise 30

Read the medical record, and circle the correct letter for each of the questions. (Note: Although some of the medical terms do not appear in this chapter, you should understand them from their word parts.)

1. The patient had a CVA, or a cerebrovascular accident. What is another name for this medical problem?
   A. stupor
   B. stroke
   C. hallucination
   D. Alzheimer disease

2. The patient is admitted for rehabilitation because he has weakness only on his left side. This is called
   A. paraplegia.
   B. quadriplegia.
   C. hemiparesis.
   D. paraparesis.

3. A Babinski sign is a neurologic test performed on the
   A. top of the foot.
   B. sole of the foot.
   C. back of the calf.
   D. big toe.

4. What two radiologic tests were performed?
   A. echocardiogram and CPK
   B. MRI and CT scan
   C. CPK and CT scan
   D. MRI and echocardiogram

5. The patient has moderate dysphasia. This means that he has
   A. difficulty swallowing.
   B. difficulty walking.
   C. difficulty speaking.
   D. difficulty breathing.

MEDICAL RECORD 6-2

You are a physician working in an acute hospital setting; you are completing the discharge summary for an elderly patient. She will be discharged home with her daughter.

Medical Record

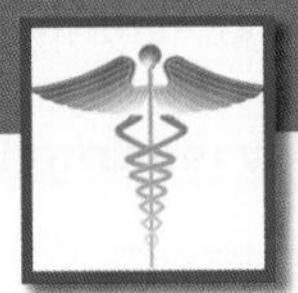

ACUTE SEIZURES DISCHARGE SUMMARY

CHIEF COMPLAINT: Mental status changes and expressive aphasia.

HISTORY OF PRESENT ILLNESS: This is an elderly white female who has a history of multiple hospitalizations in the past with the same complaint, who presented to the hospital with expressive (1)________________, mental status changes.

PAST MEDICAL HISTORY: Past medical history significant for the patient having similar episode with seizures, (2)__________________________, hypertension, CAD, CABG, CHF, atrial fibrillation, hypothyroidism, (3)________________________, respiratory arrest, UTI, right carotid endarterectomy, cholecystectomy, hysterectomy, CABG, and peripheral vascular disease.

HOSPITAL COURSE: On admission to the hospital, the patient had expressive aphasia. The whole time she was alert and oriented ×1. She could move all four extremities well. She was seen by the neurologist, who recommended that we maintain her Dilantin 100 mg t.i.d. and also recommended increasing the Lamictal to 200 mg b.i.d. She tolerated the increase of the Lamictal with no problems. Her expressive aphasia improved while she was in the hospital. Her mentation was good, and she was alert and oriented ×1.

Also on admission she was noted to have atrial fibrillation, RVR. She was seen by a cardiologist, who recommended increasing her sotalol and decreasing the metoprolol. Her heart rate came down. She was also continued on Coumadin while she was in the hospital.

She was running a low-grade temperature on admission. UA was positive for UTI, and she was put on Macrobid. She had defervescence of her fever.

The (4)____________________ was positive for (5)____________________ disorder. Again, we felt that her expressive aphasia and mental status changes were probably secondary to acute seizures. She had no evidence of any tonic–clonic seizures. At this point she is alert and essentially back to baseline.

DISCHARGE DIAGNOSES: Acute seizures, history of cerebrovascular accident, atrial fibrillation, rapid ventricular response, hypertension, coronary artery bypass graft, and urinary tract infection.

DISCHARGE MEDICATIONS: Sotalol 80 mg b.i.d. for atrial fibrillation, Macrobid 100 mg b.i.d. for UTI, metoprolol 50 mg once a day for hypertension, Lamictal 100 mg 2 tablets b.i.d. for seizures, Dilantin 100 mg t.i.d. for seizures. She is also to continue her Lasix, Lipitor, Cozaar, Coumadin, Synthroid, and Trental.

FOLLOW-UP CARE: See the doctor in one week. Have a Coumadin check once a week.

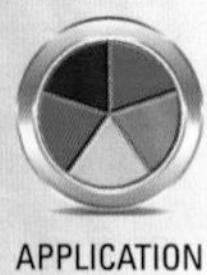

APPLICATION

Exercise 31

Fill in the blanks in the medical report with the correct medical terms. The meanings of the missing terms are listed below.

1. impaired comprehension or formulation of speech, reading, or writing caused by damage to the brain
2. damage to the brain caused by an interruption of blood supply to a region of the brain
3. a sudden, brief, and temporary cerebral dysfunction usually caused by interruption of blood flow to the brain
4. an electrical recording of the activity of the brain
5. violent spasm or series of jerky movements of the face, trunk, or limbs

Bonus Questions

6. Which two medications prescribed to the patient on discharge are anticonvulsants?

____

7. Using what you have learned about other body systems, what procedure did the patient have that removed the plaque from the main artery in her neck?____________________

Pronunciation and Spelling

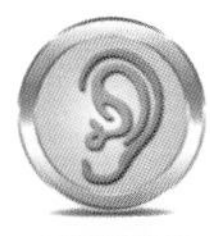

AUDITORY

Exercise 32

Review the Chapter 6 terms in the Dictionary/Audio Glossary in the Student Resources on thePoint, and practice pronouncing each term, referring to the pronunciation guide as needed.

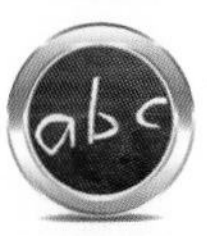

SPELLING

Exercise 33

Circle the correctly spelled term.

1.	cerebrum	cerebrim	ceribrum
2.	encephalopithy	encepholopathy	encephalopathy
3.	temporil	temporal	temperal
4.	delusiun	delusion	delusian
5.	Alzheirmer	Alazheimer	Alzheimer
6.	schizophrenia	scziophrenia	schzerphrenia
7.	radiculopithy	radicolopathy	radiculopathy
8.	catatonia	catotonia	catitonia
9.	cerebelum	cerebellum	cerabellum
10.	mylopathy	myeleopathy	myelopathy
11.	anathesia	anestesia	anesthesia
12.	nuropathy	niropathy	neuropathy
13.	paraital	parietal	perietal
14.	hallucination	hallocination	hellucination
15.	siezure	seizure	sizeure

Media Connection

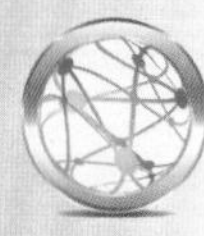

Exercise 34

Complete each of the following activities available with the Student Resources on thePoint. Check off each activity as you complete it, and record your score for the Chapter Quiz in the space provided.

Chapter Exercises

____ Flash Cards

____ Concentration

____ Abbreviation Match-Up

____ Roboterms

____ Word Anatomy

____ Fill the Gap

____ Break It Down

____ True/False Body Building

____ Quiz Show

____ Complete the Case

____ Medical Record Review

____ Image Matching

____ Spelling Bee

____ **Chapter Quiz** *Score:*________%

Additional Resources

____ Dictionary/Audio Glossary

____ Health Professions Careers: Speech Therapist

____ Health Professions Careers: Physician

Special Senses

7

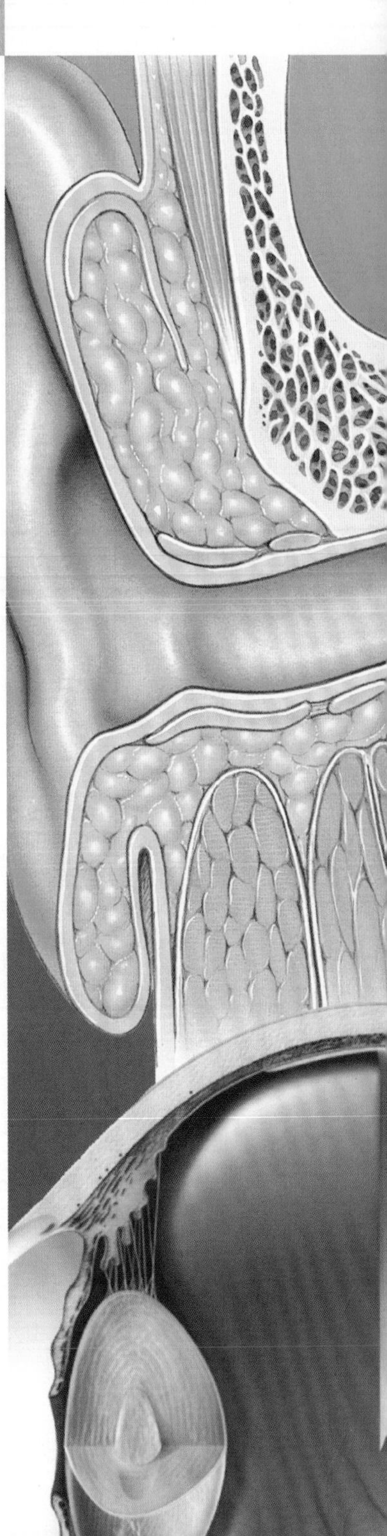

Chapter Outline

Introduction, 210

Anatomy and Physiology of the Eye, 210
- Structures, 210
- Functions, 210
- Terms Related to the Eye, 210

Word Parts for the Eye, 213
- Combining Forms, 213
- Prefixes, 214
- Suffixes, 214

Medical Terms Related to the Eye, 218
- Adjectives and Other Related Terms, 218
- Medical Conditions, 220
- Tests and Procedures, 227
- Surgical Interventions and Therapeutic Procedures, 231
- Medications and Drug Therapies, 233
- Specialties and Specialists, 234
- Abbreviations, 235

Anatomy and Physiology of the Ear, 236
- Structures, 236
- Functions, 236
- Terms Related to the Ear, 237

Word Parts for the Ear, 240
- Combining Forms, 240
- Prefixes, 240
- Suffixes, 240

Medical Terms Related to the Ear, 242
- Adjectives and Other Related Terms, 242
- Medical Conditions, 244
- Tests and Procedures, 247
- Surgical Interventions and Therapeutic Procedures, 249
- Medications and Drug Therapies, 252
- Specialties and Specialists, 252
- Abbreviations, 253

Wrapping Up, 254

Chapter Review, 255

Learning Outcomes

After completing this chapter, you should be able to:

1. List the structures and functions of the eyes and ears.
2. Define terms related to the eyes and ears.
3. Define combining forms, prefixes, and suffixes related to the eyes and ears.
4. Define common medical terminology related to the eyes and ears, including adjectives and related terms; signs, symptoms, and medical conditions; tests and procedures; surgical interventions and therapeutic procedures; medications and drug therapies; and medical specialties and specialists.
5. Define common abbreviations for terms related to the eyes and ears.
6. Successfully complete all chapter exercises.
7. Explain terms used in case studies and medical records involving the eyes and ears.
8. Successfully complete all exercises included with the companion Student Resources on thePoint.

INTRODUCTION

Special senses are those senses that have organs devoted to them: sight, hearing, balance, smell, and taste. In this chapter, you will study word parts and terms related to the eyes (vision) and ears (hearing and balance). This chapter follows the nervous system, because these are specialized functions of that system.

ANATOMY AND PHYSIOLOGY OF THE EYE

Structures

- Each eye is located in a bony cavity (socket) in the skull called the orbit.
- Upper and lower movable folds of skin called the eyelids protect the eyes.
- Tears secreted by the lacrimal gland lubricate the eyes.

Functions

- Observing light, perceiving depth, and serving as the organ of vision
- Maintaining balance by detecting changes in posture when we move

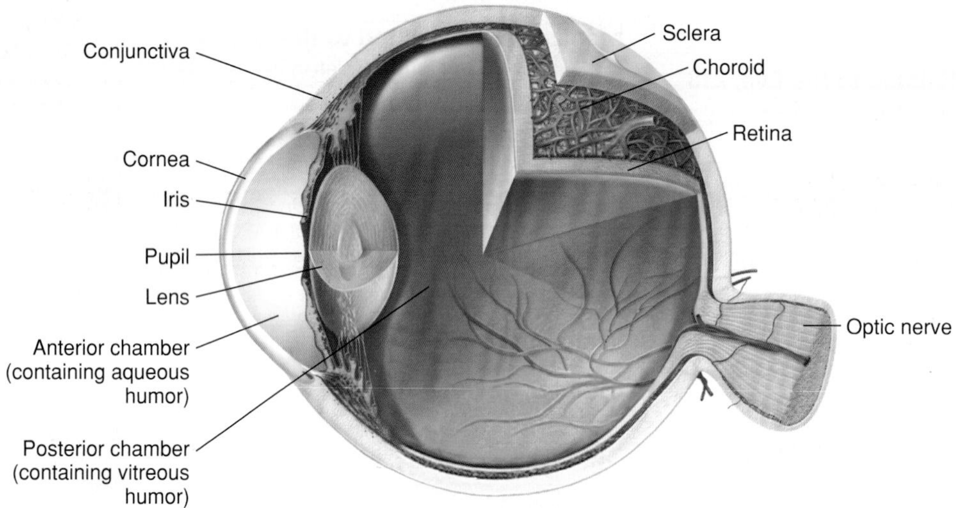

Figure 7-1 Structures of the eye.

Terms Related to the Eye

Term	Pronunciation	Meaning
conjunctiva	kon′jŭnk-tī′vă	mucous membrane that lines the eyelids and outer surface of the eyeball (**Figure 7-1**)
orbit	ōr′bit	bony cavity of the skull that encases the eye
lacrimal glands	lak′ri-măl glandz	glands that secrete tears (**Figure 7-2**)
lacrimal ducts	lak′ri-măl dŭktz	channels that carry tears to the eyes (**Figure 7-2**)

Terms Related to the Eye

Term	Pronunciation	Meaning
nasolacrimal ducts	nā′zō-lak′ri-măl dŭktz	ducts that carry tears from the lacrimal glands to the nose (**Figure 7-2**)

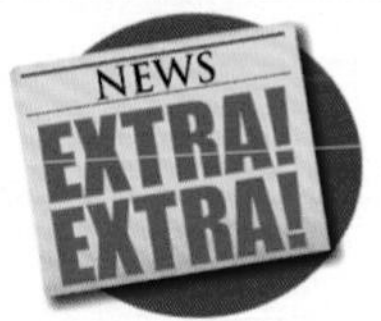

NASOLACRIMAL DUCTS Do you know why your nose runs when you cry? The reason is because the nasolacrimal ducts carry tears that are released from the tear glands directly into your nose.

Term	Pronunciation	Meaning
tarsal glands; *syn.* meibomian glands	tahr′săl glandz; mī-bō′mē-ăn glandz	oil glands along the edges of the eyelids that lubricate the eye (**Figure 7-2**)
Outer Layer of the Eye (Figure 7-1)		
aqueous humor	ā′kwē-ŭs hyū′mŏr	watery fluid that fills the anterior chamber of the eye between the lens and the cornea
cornea	kōr′nē-ă	transparent outer covering of the anterior portion of the eye
iris	ī′ris	colored muscular part of the eye located behind (posterior to) the cornea that allows light to pass through
sclera	sklē′ră	tough fibrous outer layer of the eye (the white of the eye) that extends from the cornea to the optic nerve
Middle Layer of the Eye (Figure 7-1)		
choroid	kor′oyd	middle layer of the eye that contains blood vessels
lens	lenz	transparent structure behind (posterior to) the pupil that bends and focuses light rays
pupil	pyū′pil	opening in the middle of the iris through which light passes
vitreous humor	vit′rē-ŭs hyū′mŏr	jelly-like fluid that fills the posterior chamber of the eye between the lens and the retina
Inner Layer of the Eye (Figure 7-1)		
fundus	fŭn′dŭs	posterior portion of the interior of the eyeball, visible through the ophthalmoscope
optic nerve (CN I)	op′tik nerv	cranial nerve I that carries impulses from the retina to the brain to provide the sense of sight
retina	ret′i-nă	innermost layer of the eye that contains visual receptors (rods and cones)

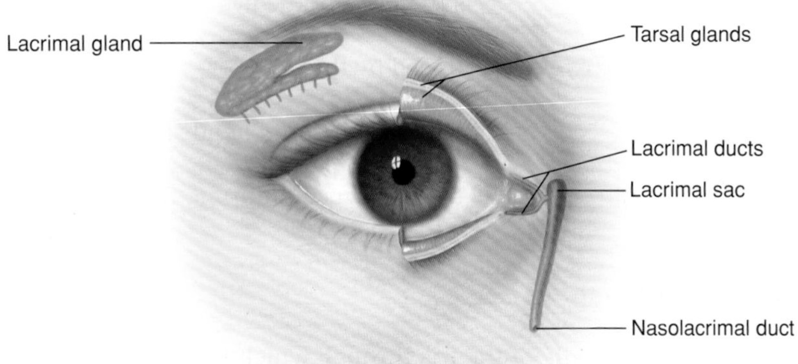

Figure 7-2 Right lacrimal gland and ducts.

Exercises: Anatomy and Physiology of the Eye

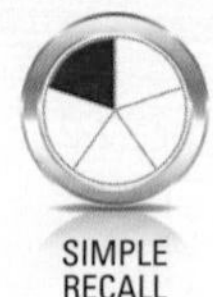

Exercise 1

Write the correct anatomic structure for the definition given.

1. part of the eye that bends and focuses light rays ______________
2. jelly-like fluid in the posterior chamber of the eye ______________
3. layer of the eye that contains blood vessels ______________
4. bony cavity of the skull that encases the eye ______________
5. colored muscular part of the eye ______________
6. mucous membrane that lines the eyelids and eye surface ______________
7. opening in the iris through which light passes ______________
8. transparent outer covering of the anterior eye ______________
9. cranial nerve (CN I) that carries impulses to the brain to provide sight ______________
10. ducts that carry tears from the lacrimal glands to the nose ______________

ADVANCED RECALL

Exercise 2

Complete each sentence by writing in the correct medical term.

1. The ______________ is the part of the eye that contains visual receptors.
2. The ______________ is the white outer layer of the eye.
3. Tears are carried through the______________ to the eye.
4. The ______________ is the layer of the eye that contains blood vessels.
5. Oil that lubricates the eyes is produced by the______________.
6. The ______________ is behind the pupil and bends and focuses light rays.
7. The ______________ is the mucous membrane that lines the eyelid and eye surface.
8. Tears are secreted by the ______________.
9. The opening in the middle of the iris through which light passes is the ______________.
10. The ______________ is a watery fluid filling the anterior chamber of the eye.

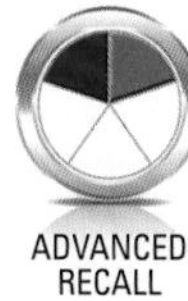

Exercise 3

Match each medical term with its meaning.

vitreous humor	retina	iris
lacrimal glands	cornea	aqueous humor
optic nerve	sclera	tarsal glands

1. oil-producing glands of the eye ____________
2. layer of the eye that contains visual receptors ____________
3. watery fluid in the anterior chamber of the eye ____________
4. nerve that carries vision impulses to the brain ____________
5. transparent outer covering of the anterior portion of the eye ____________
6. jelly-like fluid in the posterior chamber of the eye ____________
7. tear-producing glands of the eye ____________
8. colored part of the eye behind the cornea ____________
9. tough, white outer layer of the eye ____________

WORD PARTS FOR THE EYE

The following tables list word parts related to the eye.

Combining Forms

Combining Form	Meaning
blephar/o	eyelid
conjunctiv/o	conjunctiva
cor/e, cor/o	pupil (of the eye)
corne/o	cornea
cry/o	cold
dacry/o	tears, lacrimal (tear) duct
dipl/o	double, two
ir/o, irid/o	iris
kerat/o	cornea
lacrim/o	tears, lacrimal (tear) duct
ocul/o	eye
ophthalm/o	eye

(continued)

Combining Forms *(continued)*

Combining Form	Meaning
opt/o	vision, eye
phot/o	light
presby/o	related to aging
pupill/o	pupil (of the eye)
retin/o	retina
scler/o	hard, sclera
ton/o	tension, pressure

Prefixes

Prefix	Meaning
bi-, bin-	two, twice
choroido-	the choroid
ictero-	jaundice (yellow)

Suffixes

Suffix	Meaning
-ectasia, -ectasis	dilation, stretching
-lysis	destruction, breakdown, separation
-malacia	softening
-meter	instrument for measuring
-metry	measurement of
-opia, -opsia	vision
-pexy	surgical fixation
-phobia	abnormal fear of, aversion to, sensitivity to
-plasty	surgical repair, reconstruction
-plegia	paralysis
-ptosis	prolapse, drooping, sagging
-rrhea	flow, discharge
-scopy	process of examining, examination
-spasm	involuntary movement
-trophia	to turn

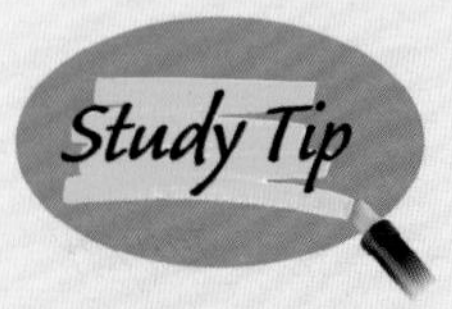

Spelling: The combining form for the eye, *ophthalm/o,* can be tricky to spell. To avoid errors, check that you have an "h" before *and* after the "t."

Exercises: Word Parts Related to the Eye

SIMPLE RECALL

Exercise 4

Write the meaning of the combining form given.

1. ocul/o ____________________
2. lacrim/o ____________________
3. ir/o ____________________
4. cor/o ____________________
5. dacry/o ____________________
6. kerat/o ____________________
7. ophthalm/o ____________________
8. pupill/o ____________________
9. corne/o ____________________
10. blephar/o ____________________

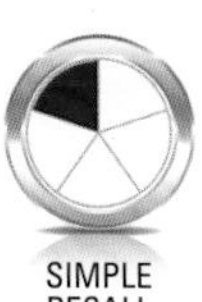

SIMPLE RECALL

Exercise 5

Write the correct combining form for the meaning given.

1. conjunctiva ____________________
2. hard, sclera ____________________
3. light ____________________
4. eyelid ____________________
5. tension, pressure ____________________
6. related to aging ____________________
7. double ____________________
8. vision ____________________
9. iris ____________________
10. retina ____________________

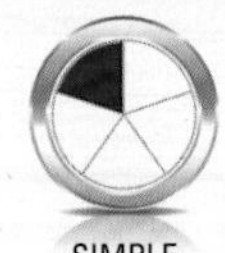

SIMPLE RECALL

Exercise 6

Write the meaning of the prefix or suffix given.

1. -plegia ______
2. -opia ______
3. -ptosis ______
4. bin- ______
5. -lysis ______
6. -rrhea ______
7. -pexy ______
8. -malacia ______
9. -plasty ______
10. -scopy ______
11. -ectasis ______
12. -phobia ______

ADVANCED RECALL

Exercise 7

Match each combining form with its meaning.

scler/o	retin/o	pupill/o
corne/o	ir/o	conjunctiv/o

1. colored muscular part of the eye ______
2. innermost layer of the eye ______
3. opening in the middle of the iris ______
4. mucous membrane that lines the eyelids ______
5. tough outer layer of the eye ______
6. outer covering of the anterior portion of the eye ______

TERM CONSTRUCTION

Exercise 8

Using the given combining form and a word part learned previously, build a medical term for the meaning given.

Combining Form	Meaning of Medical Term	Medical Term
conjunctiv/o	inflammation of the conjunctiva	1. ______
dipl/o	double vision	2. ______

blephar/o	drooping of the eyelid	3. ______
pupill/o	instrument for measuring the pupil	4. ______
phot/o	extreme sensitivity to light	5. ______
retin/o	disease of the retina	6. ______
irid/o	paralysis of the iris	7. ______
kerat/o	surgical repair of the cornea	8. ______
scler/o	incision into the sclera	9. ______
ophthalm/o	one specialized in the study of the eye	10. ______

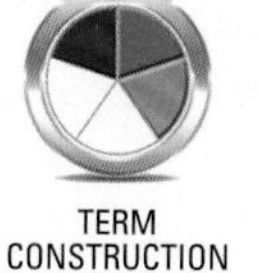

TERM CONSTRUCTION

Exercise 9

For each term, first write the meaning of the term. Then write the meaning of the word parts in that term.

1. ophthalmoscope ______
   ophthalm/o ______
   -scope ______
2. optometry ______
   opt/o ______
   -metry ______
3. blepharospasm ______
   blephar/o ______
   -spasm ______
4. dacryorrhea ______
   dacry/o ______
   -rrhea ______
5. presbyopia ______
   presby/o ______
   -opia ______

6. retinopexy ______

retin/o ______

-pexy ______

7. corectasia ______

cor/e ______

-ectasia ______

8. iritis ______

ir/o ______

-itis ______

9. tonometer ______

ton/o ______

-meter ______

10. keratopathy ______

kerat/o ______

-pathy ______

MEDICAL TERMS RELATED TO THE EYE

The following table gives adjective forms and terms used in describing the eye and its conditions.

Adjectives and Other Related Terms

Term	Pronunciation	Meaning
accommodation	ă-kom′ŏ-dā′shŭn	ability of the eye to adjust focus on near objects
binocular	bin-ok′yū-lăr	pertaining to both eyes
blepharal	blef′ă-răl	pertaining to the eyelid
conjunctival	kon′jŭnk-tī′văl	pertaining to the conjunctiva
corneal	kōr′nē-ăl	pertaining to the cornea
intraocular	in′tră-ok′-lăr	within or inside the eye

Adjectives and Other Related Terms

Term	Pronunciation	Meaning
iridal, iridial	ī′ri-dăl, ir′i-dăl, ī-rid′ē-ăl	pertaining to the iris
lacrimal	lak′ri-măl	pertaining to tears
ocular	ok′yū-lăr	pertaining to the eye
ophthalmic	of-thal′mik	pertaining to the eye
optic	op′tik	pertaining to vision
pupillary	pyū′pi-lār′ē	pertaining to the pupil
retinal	ret′i-năl	pertaining to the retina
scleral	sklē′răl	pertaining to the sclera

■ Exercises: Adjectives and Other Related Terms

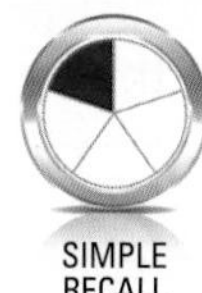
SIMPLE RECALL

Exercise 10

Write the meaning of the term given.

1. ocular ______________________
2. lacrimal ______________________
3. optic ______________________
4. intraocular ______________________
5. iridal ______________________
6. conjunctival ______________________
7. ophthalmic ______________________
8. scleral ______________________
9. accommodation ______________________

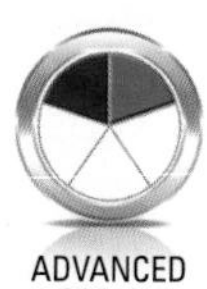
ADVANCED RECALL

Exercise 11

Match each medical term with its meaning.

retinal	pupillary	intraocular	iridial
blepharal	binocular	corneal	optic

1. within the eye ______________________
2. pertaining to both eyes ______________________
3. pertaining to the eyelids ______________________

4. pertaining to the pupil ______________________________
5. pertaining to the retina ______________________________
6. pertaining to vision ______________________________
7. pertaining to the cornea ______________________________
8. pertaining to the iris ______________________________

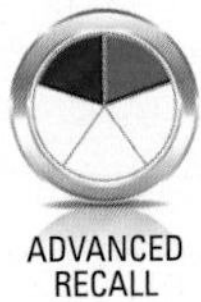
ADVANCED RECALL

Exercise 12

Circle the term that is most appropriate for the meaning of the sentence.

1. The (*binocular, dacryocyst, ophthalmic*) artery supplies blood to the right eye.
2. The red spots in the patient's eye were due to a(n) (*lacrimal, conjunctival, optic*) hemorrhage, or a hemorrhage in the mucous membrane that lines the outer surface of the eyeball.
3. Mr. Kendrick's vision was blurred due to inflammation of his (*iridial, binocular, optic*) nerve.
4. The physician checked the patient's (*intraocular, lacrimal, blepharal*) pressure, or the pressure within each eye.
5. After the wind blew sand into Mr. Lin's eye, he suffered a (*corneal, retinal, lacrimal*) abrasion on the outside surface of the eye.
6. The child's left eyelid was red and swollen due to a (*corneal, blepharal, papillary*) infection.
7. The physician used a (*retinal, corneal, binocular*) microscope to make it possible for both her eyes to focus on the specimen.

Medical Conditions

Term	Pronunciation	Meaning
amblyopia	am′blē-ō′pē-ă	poor vision, usually in only one eye, caused by abnormal development of the visual areas; also known as "lazy eye"
astigmatism	ă-stig′mă-tizm	distorted, blurry vision caused by abnormal curvature of the cornea and/or lens
blepharitis	blef′ă-rī′tis	inflammation of the eyelid
blepharoptosis	blef′ă-rop′tōsis	drooping of the eyelids; also shortened to ptosis (**Figure 7-3**)
blepharospasm	blef′ă-rō-spazm	contraction of the muscles surrounding the eye, causing uncontrolled blinking
cataract	kat′ă-rakt	clouding of the lens of the eye, causing poor vision (**Figure 7-4**, see later **Figure 7-8B**)
chalazion; *syn.* meibomian cyst	ka-lā′zē-on; mī-bō′mē-ăn sist	inflammation of the eyelid from a blocked tarsal gland (**Figure 7-5**)
color blindness	kŭl′ŏr blīnd′nes	deficiency in distinguishing some colors

Medical Conditions

Term	Pronunciation	Meaning
conjunctivitis	kon-jŭnk′ti-vī′tis	highly contagious inflammation of the conjunctiva; commonly known as pinkeye
dacryoadenitis	dak′rē-ō-ad′ĕ-nī′tis	inflammation of a lacrimal gland
dacryocystitis	dak′rē-ō-sis-tī′tis	inflammation of the lacrimal sac
dacryolith	dak′rē-ō-lith	stone in the lacrimal sac or lacrimal ducts
dacryorrhea	dak′rē-ō-rē′ă	excessive discharge of tears
detached retina	dē-tacht′ ret′i-nă	separation of the retina from the choroid in the back of the eye; can be caused by injury, tumor, or hemorrhage (**Figures 7-6** and **7-10E**)
diabetic retinopathy	dī′ă-bet′ik ret′i-nop′ă-thē	degenerative changes of the retina caused by diabetes mellitus; may lead to blindness (see later **Figures 7-8C** and **7-10D**)
diplopia	di-plō′pē-ă	double vision

(continued)

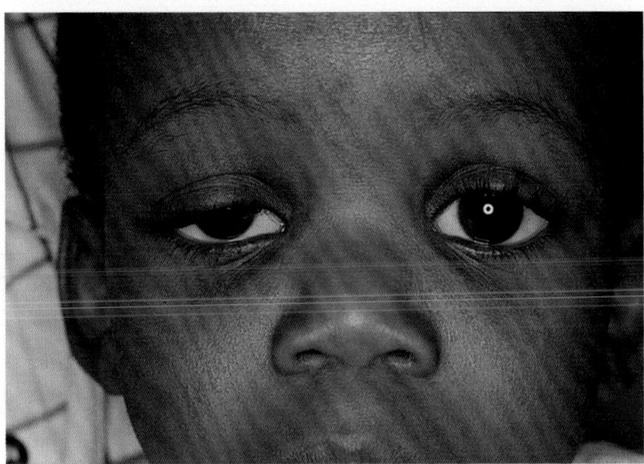

Figure 7-3 Blepharoptosis.

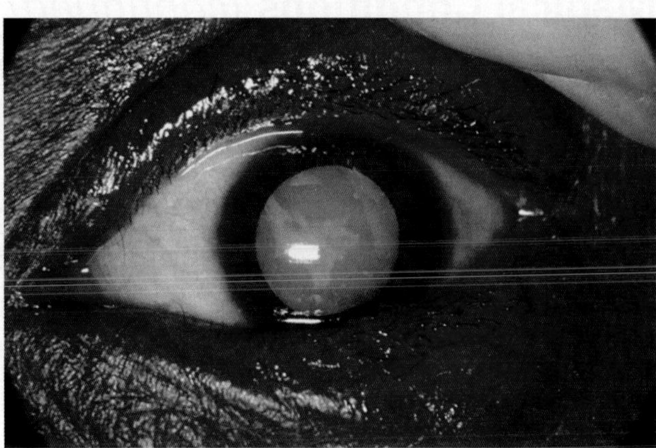

Figure 7-4 Cataract.

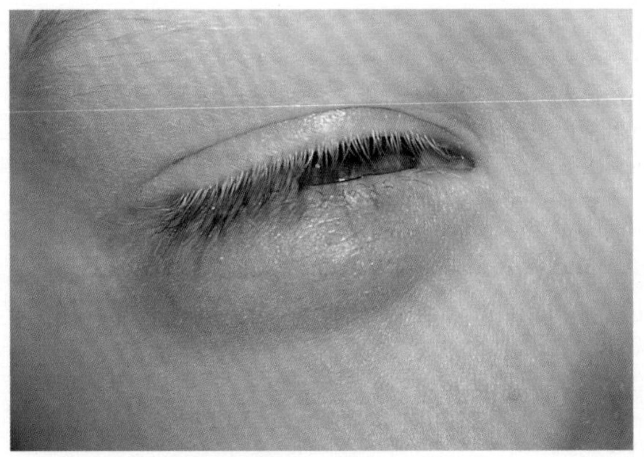

Figure 7-5 Chalazion.

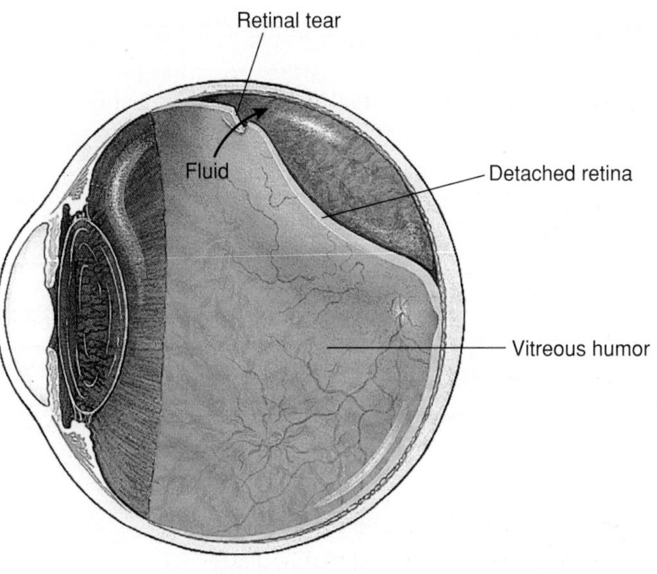

Figure 7-6 Detached retina.

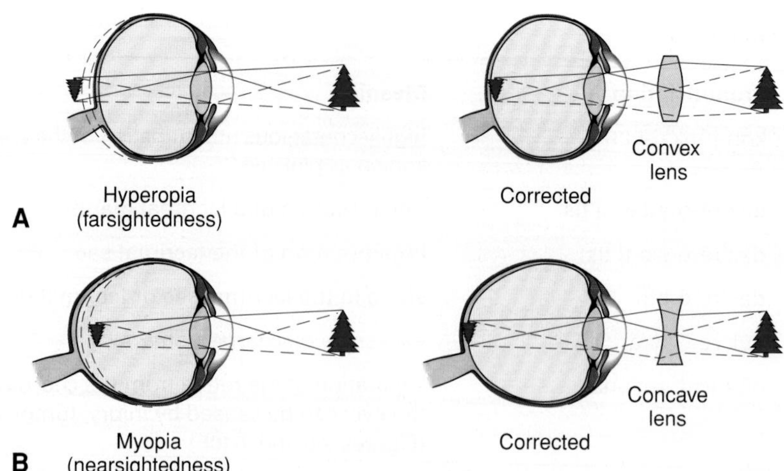

Figure 7-7 Vision problems and corrections. **A.** Hyperopia. **B.** Myopia.

Medical Conditions *(continued)*

Term	Pronunciation	Meaning
exophthalmos; *syn.* exophthalmus	eks′of-thal′mos; eks′of-thal′mŭs	abnormal protrusion of one or both eyeballs
glaucoma	glaw-kō′mă	group of diseases of the eye characterized by increased intraocular pressure that damages the optic nerve (see later **Figure 7-8D**)
hordeolum	hōr-dē′ō-lŭm	infection of an oil gland of the eyelid; commonly called a sty
hyperopia	hī′pĕr-ō′pē-ă	farsightedness (**Figure 7-7**)
iridomalacia	ir′i-dō-mă-lā′shē-ă	softening of the iris
iridoplegia	ir′i-dō-plē′jē-ă	paralysis of the iris
iritis	ī-rī′tis	inflammation of the iris
keratitis	ker′ă-tī′tis	inflammation of the cornea
keratomalacia	ker′ă-tō-mă-lā′shē-ă	softening of the cornea, usually associated with severe vitamin A deficiency
macular degeneration	mak′yū-lăr dē-jen′ĕr-ā′shŭn	deterioration of the macula (the central part of the retina), causing impaired central vision; most commonly related to advancing age (**Figure 7-8E**)
myopia	mī-ō′pē-ă	nearsightedness (**Figure 7-7**)
nyctalopia	nik-tă-lō′pē-ă	poor vision in reduced light or at night; commonly called night blindness
nystagmus	nis-tag′mŭs	involuntary rhythmic movements of the eye
ophthalmalgia	of′thal-mal′jē-ă	pain in the eye

NEWS EXTRA! EXTRA!

THE MATURING LENS As eyes age, the shape of the lens changes. In infancy, the lens is more spherical; and in the elderly, the lens is more flattened. This flattening of the lens is what causes the need for prescription lenses.

(continued)

A Normal vision

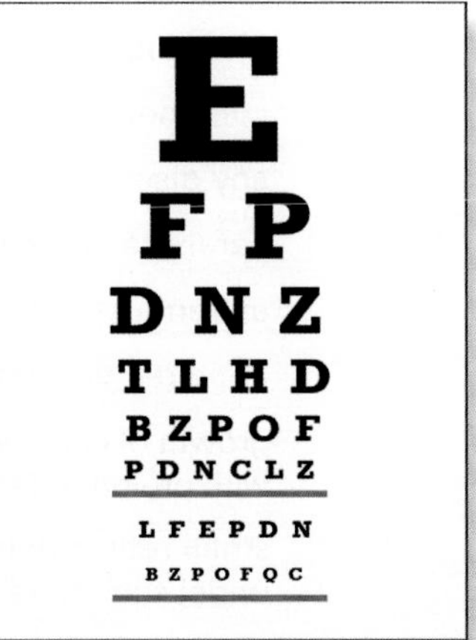

B Cataract
(hazy vision)

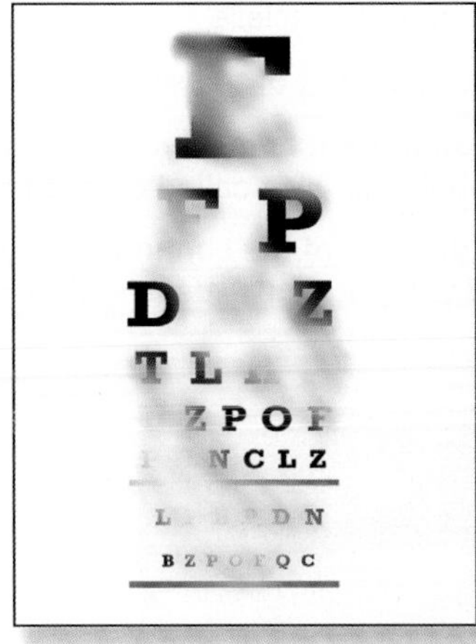

C Diabetic retinopathy
(retinal damage leads to blind spots)

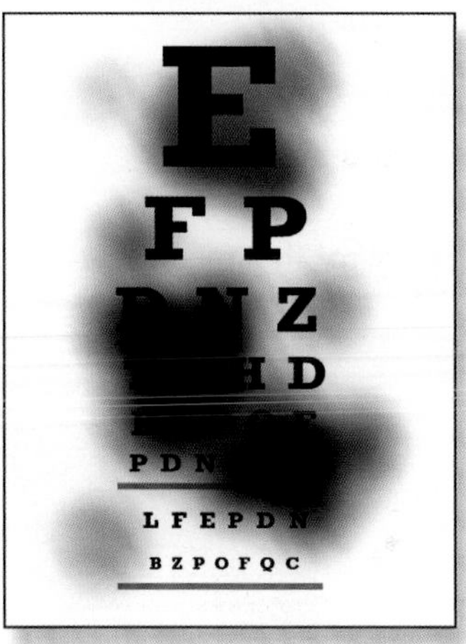

D Glaucoma
(loss of peripheral vision)

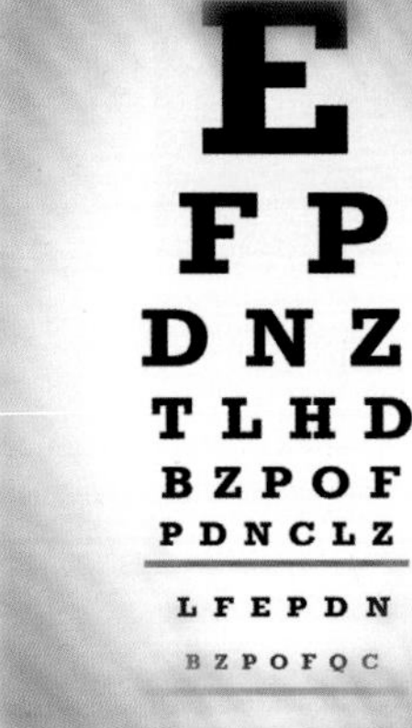

E Macular degeneration
(loss of central vision)

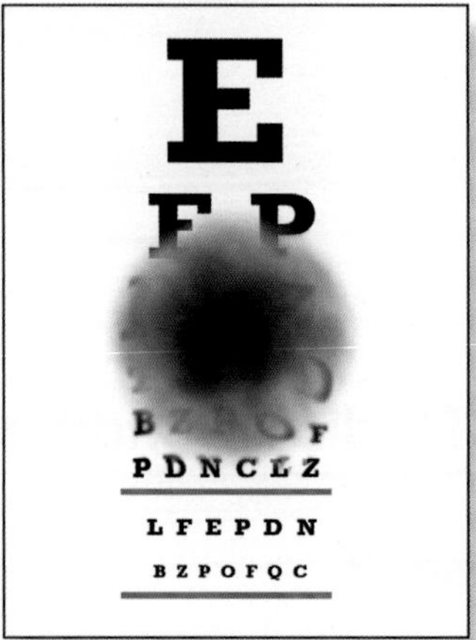

Figure 7-8 Simulated vision abnormalities.

Medical Conditions *(continued)*

Term	Pronunciation	Meaning
ophthalmia	of-thal′mē-ă	condition of the eye characterized by severe conjunctivitis
ophthalmopathy	of′thal-mop′ă-thē	any disease of the eyes
ophthalmoplegia	of-thal′mō-plē′jē-ă	paralysis of the eye muscle(s)
photophobia	fō′tō-fō′bē-ă	extreme sensitivity to light
presbyopia	prez′bē-ō′pē-ă	impaired vision caused by old age
pterygium	tĕ-rij′ē-ŭm	growth of conjunctival tissue over the cornea; usually associated with prolonged exposure to ultraviolet light (**Figure 7-9**)
retinal tear	ret′i-năl tār	small retinal detachment that allows vitreous fluid to seep under the retina (**Figure 7-6**)
retinitis pigmentosa	ret′i-nī′tis pig′men-to′să	hereditary progressive deterioration of the retina causing nyctalopia and impaired vision
retinopathy	ret′i-nop′ă-thē	any disease of the retina
scleritis	sklē-rī′tis	inflammation of the sclera
scleromalacia	sklē′rō-mă-lā′shē-ă	softening or thinning of the sclera
strabismus	stra-biz′mŭs	abnormal alignment of the eyes caused by intraocular muscle imbalance; also called crossed eyes
xerophthalmia	zē′rof-thal′mē-ă	excessive dryness of the conjunctiva and cornea, usually associated with vitamin A deficiency; dry eyes

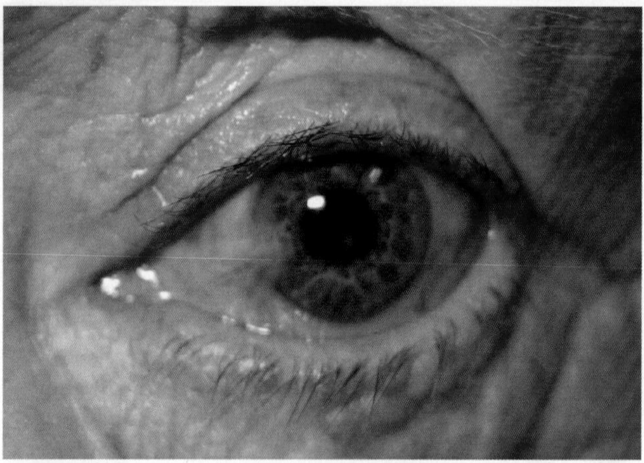

Figure 7-9 Pterygium.

Exercises: Medical Conditions

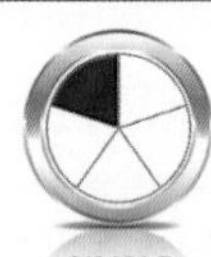

SIMPLE RECALL

Exercise 13

Write the meaning of the term given.

1. nystagmus ______________________
2. retinopathy ______________________
3. iridomalacia ______________________

4. blepharitis ______________________________

5. cataract ______________________________

6. exophthalmos ______________________________

7. dacryolith ______________________________

8. xerophthalmia ______________________________

9. glaucoma ______________________________

10. ophthalmopathy ______________________________

Exercise 14

ADVANCED RECALL

Complete each sentence by writing in the correct medical term.

1. Distorted blurry vision caused by abnormal curvature of the cornea and/or lens is called ______________________.

2. ______________________ is the medical term for farsightedness.

3. ______________________ is a deficiency in distinguishing some colors.

4. The medical term for poor vision, usually in one eye, commonly referred to as "lazy eye" is ______________________.

5. The medical term for double vision is ______________________.

6. Vision impairment caused by old age is called ______________________.

7. The term for poor vision in reduced light or at night (night blindness) is ______________________.

8. ______________________ is the medical term for nearsightedness.

9. The term for deterioration of the macula resulting in impaired central vision, most commonly caused by aging, is ______________________.

10. Extreme sensitivity to light is known as ______________________.

11. The term ______________________ refers to a condition of the eye characterized by severe conjunctivitis.

Exercise 15

ADVANCED RECALL

Match each medical term with its meaning.

hordeolum	ophthalmoplegia	chalazion	dacryocystitis
detached retina	diabetic retinopathy	pterygium	dacryoadenitis
retinitis pigmentosa	strabismus		

1. degenerative changes of the retina caused by diabetes mellitus ______________________________

2. paralysis of the eye muscle ______________________________

3. inflammation of a lacrimal gland ____________________

4. obstruction of an oil gland in the eye ____________________

5. inflammation of the tear sac ____________________

6. infection of an oil gland of the eyelid ____________________

7. growth of conjunctival tissue over the cornea ____________________

8. hereditary deterioration of the retina ____________________

9. abnormal alignment of the eyes caused by intraocular muscle imbalance ____________________

10. separation of the retina from the choroid ____________________

Exercise 16

TERM CONSTRUCTION

Break the given medical term into its word parts and define each part. Then define the medical term.

For example:

iritis	*word parts:*	ir/o, -itis
	meanings:	iris, inflammation of
	term meaning:	inflammation of the iris

1. scleromalacia
   word parts: ____________________
   meanings: ____________________
   term meaning: ____________________

2. keratitis
   word parts: ____________________
   meanings: ____________________
   term meaning: ____________________

3. iridoplegia
   word parts: ____________________
   meanings: ____________________
   term meaning: ____________________

4. dacryorrhea
   word parts: ____________________
   meanings: ____________________
   term meaning: ____________________

5. blepharospasm
   word parts: ____________________
   meanings: ____________________
   term meaning: ____________________

6. scleritis *word parts:* ______
meanings: ______
term meaning: ______

7. conjunctivitis *word parts:* ______
meanings: ______
term meaning: ______

8. ophthalmalgia *word parts:* ______
meanings: ______
term meaning: ______

9. blepharoptosis *word parts:* ______
meanings: ______
term meaning: ______

10. keratomalacia *word parts:* ______
meanings: ______
term meaning: ______

Tests and Procedures

Term	Pronunciation	Meaning
		Diagnostic Procedures
extraocular movement (EOM)	eks′tră-ok′yū-lăr mūv′mĕnt	movement of the upper eyelids and eyeballs through use of the extraocular muscles; assessed during clinical examination to screen for eye movement disorders

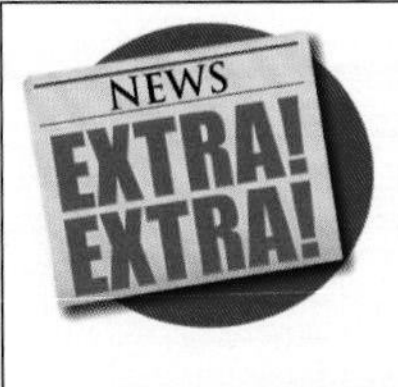

DOCUMENTATION INVOLVING THE EYES In a clinical examination, the physician checks the eyes as part of an overall review of the head, eyes, ears, neck, and throat (abbreviated as HEENT). Documentation of the physician's findings in the patient's medical record might look something like this:

EYES: Pupils equal, round, and reactive to light and accommodation. Conjunctivae are clear. Extraocular movements are intact bilaterally. Sclerae not icteric.

Term	Pronunciation	Meaning
fluorescein angiography	flōr-es′ē-in an′jē-og′ră-fē	visualization and photographic recording of the flow of an orange fluorescent dye through the blood vessels of the eye
keratometer	ker′ă-tom′ĕ-tĕr	instrument used for measuring the curvature of the cornea
ophthalmoscope	of-thal′mō-skōp	instrument used for examining the interior of the eye through the pupil (**Figure 7-10A**)
ophthalmoscopy	of′thal-mos′kŏ-pē	use of the ophthalmoscope to view the interior of the eye (**Figure 7-10B**)

(continued)

Tests and Procedures *(continued)*

Term	Pronunciation	Meaning
pupillometer	pyū'pi-lom'ĕ-tĕr	instrument used for measuring the diameter of the pupil
pupillometry	pyū'pi-lom'ĕ-trē	measurement of the pupil
refraction	rē-frak'shŭn	test using a manual refractor to determine an exact prescription for corrective lenses (**Figure 7-11**)
retinoscopy	ret'i-nos'kŏ-pē	examination of the retina
Snellen chart	snel'ĕn chart	chart containing letters that is used to test visual sharpness (acuity) (**Figure 7-12**)
tonometer	tō-nom'ĕ-tĕr	instrument used for measuring pressure within the eye
tonometry	tō-nom'ĕ-trē	use of the tonometer to measure intraocular pressure within the eye; done to diagnose glaucoma
visual acuity (VA) testing	vizh'yū-ăl ă-kyū'i-tē test'ing	testing for the sharpness (clarity) of distant vision, usually with a Snellen chart; normal visual acuity is 20/20
visual field (VF) testing	vizh'ū-ăl fēld test'ing	assessment of the range (area) visible to one eye without movement

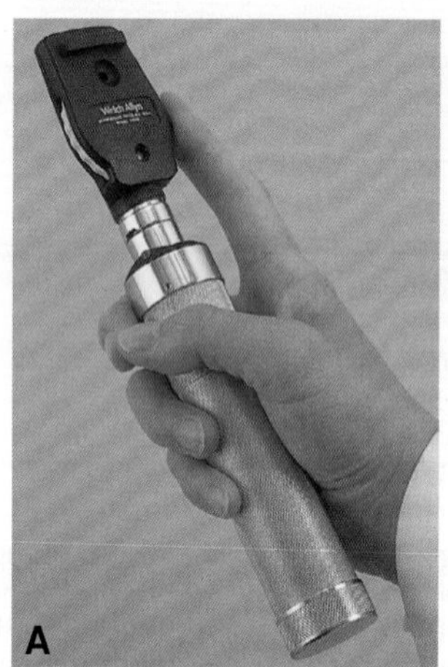

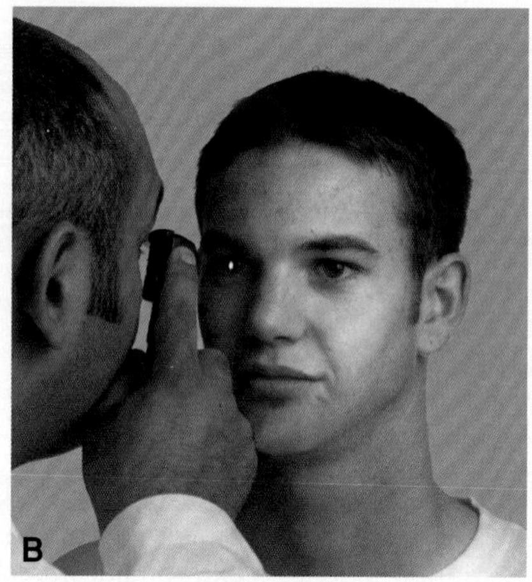

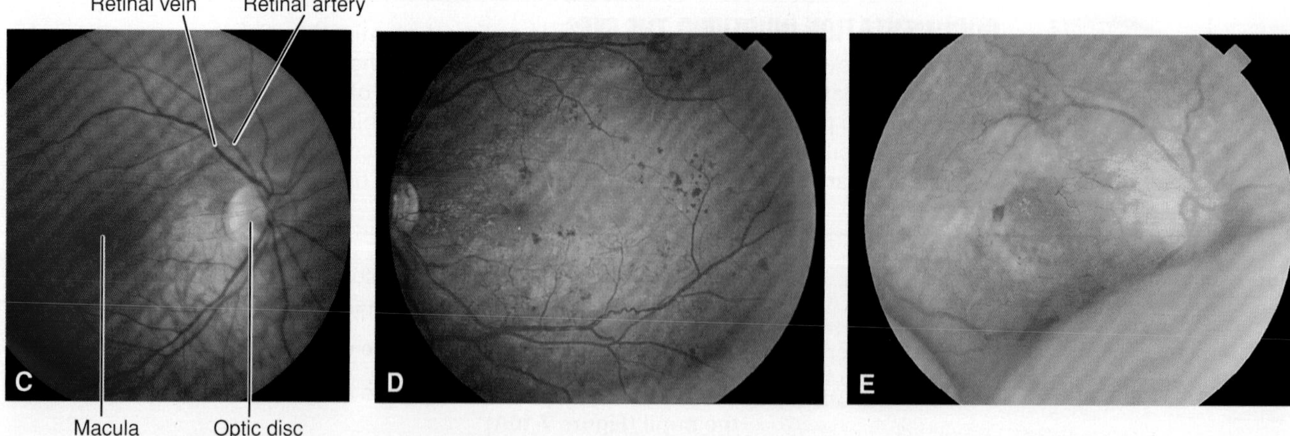

Figure 7-10 Using an ophthalmoscope **(A)** to perform ophthalmoscopy **(B)**. **C.** Normal retina. **D.** Aneurysms seen in diabetic retinopathy. **E.** Detached retina.

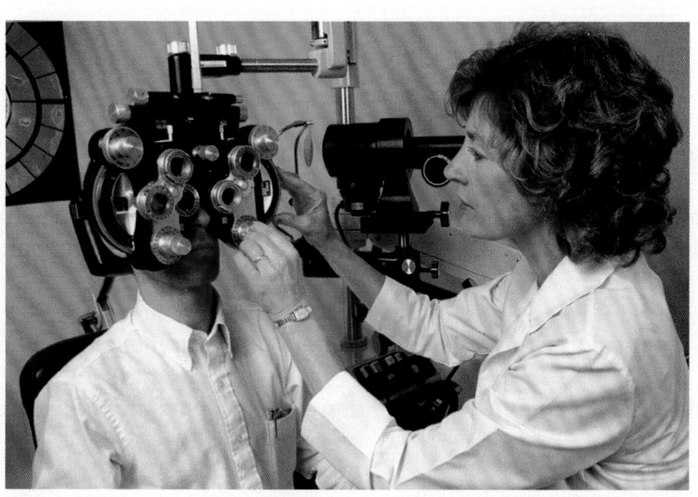

Figure 7-11 A manual refractor assists the health care professional in determining the exact vision correction.

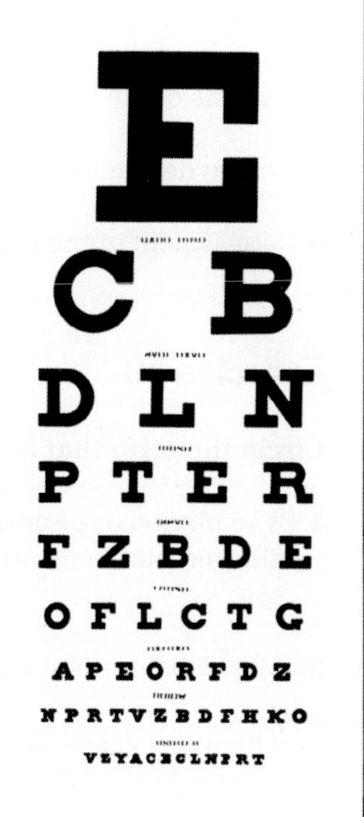

Figure 7-12 Snellen eye chart.

Exercises: Tests and Procedures

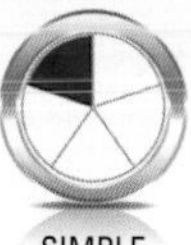

SIMPLE RECALL

Exercise 17

Write the meaning of the term given.

1. tonometer ____________________
2. ophthalmoscope ____________________
3. retinoscopy ____________________
4. keratometer ____________________
5. pupillometry ____________________

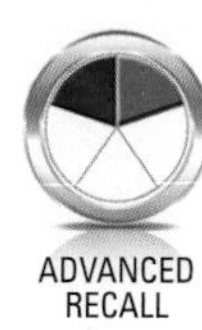

ADVANCED RECALL

Exercise 18

Match each medical term with its meaning.

visual field testing	pupillometry	extraocular movement assessment
Snellen chart	refraction	fluorescein angiography

1. measurement of the range of one eye ____________________
2. chart used to test visual acuity ____________________

3. measurement of the pupil ______________________

4. recording of the flow of a dye through the blood vessels of the eye ______________________

5. test to determine how to correct vision ______________________

6. assessment of the extraocular muscles working together ______________________

Exercise 19

ADVANCED RECALL

Circle the term that is most appropriate for the meaning of the sentence.

1. The physician performed (*tonometry, pupillometry, fluorescein angiography*), a procedure that allowed him to record the flow of fluorescent dye through the blood vessels in the patient's eye.

2. Mrs. Rina's retinal tear was diagnosed using (*tonometry, retinoscopy, pupillometry*).

3. The nurse asked Mr. Ketson to read a (*tonometer, refraction, Snellen chart*) so that she could test his visual acuity.

4. Dr. Pujabi performed (*retinoscopy, refraction, pupillometry*) to measure the degree of refractive errors and determine how to correct Mrs. Frank's vision.

5. The physician measured the amount of pressure in Mr. Johannson's eye using a(n) (*ophthalmoscope, keratometer, tonometer*) to rule out glaucoma.

6. The optometrist used a Snellen chart to measure the patient's (*visual acuity, visual field, extraocular movements*).

Exercise 20

TERM CONSTRUCTION

Break the given medical term into its word parts and define each part. Then define the medical term.

For example:

iritis	*word parts:*	ir/o, -itis
	meanings:	iris, inflammation of
	term meaning:	inflammation of the iris

1. pupillometer
   word parts: ______________________
   meanings: ______________________
   term meaning: ______________________

2. tonometry
   word parts: ______________________
   meanings: ______________________
   term meaning: ______________________

3. ophthalmoscopy *word parts:* __________

meanings: __________

term meaning: __________

4. keratometer *word parts:* __________

meanings: __________

term meaning: __________

5. retinoscopy *word parts:* __________

meanings: __________

term meaning: __________

6. ophthalmoscope *word parts:* __________

meanings: __________

term meaning: __________

Surgical Interventions and Therapeutic Procedures

Term	Pronunciation	Meaning
blepharoplasty	blef′ă-ro-plas′tē	surgical repair of the eyelid
cataract extraction	kat′ă-rakt eks-trak′shŭn	surgical removal of a cataract
cryoretinopexy	krī′ō-ret′i-nō-pek′sē	surgical fixation of a detached retina or retinal tear by using extreme cold (freezing) to seal the tear
dacryocystotomy	dak′rē-ō-sis-tot′ŏ-mē	incision into the lacrimal sac
enucleation	ē-nū′klē-ā′shŭn	removal of an eyeball
intraocular lens (IOL) implant	in′tră-ok′yū-lăr lenz im′plant	implantation of an artificial lens to replace a defective natural lens
iridectomy	ir′i-dek′tŏ-mē	excision of part of the iris
iridotomy	ir′i-dot′ŏ-mē	incision into the iris, usually with a laser, to allow drainage of aqueous humor in therapy for narrow-angle glaucoma
keratoplasty	ker′ă-tō-plas′tē	surgical repair of the cornea; corneal transplantation
laser-assisted in situ keratomileusis (LASIK)	lā′zĕr ă-sis′-ted in sī′tū ker′ă-tō-mī-lū′sis	procedure that uses a laser to create a corneal flap and reshape the corneal tissue; used to correct vision problems such as myopia, hyperopia, and astigmatism
phacoemulsification	fak′ō-ē-mŭl′si-fi-kā′shŭn	use of ultrasound to shatter and break up a cataract followed by aspiration and removal
photorefractive keratectomy (PRK)	fō′tō-rē-frak′tiv ker′ă-tek′tŏ-mē	procedure using a laser to reshape the cornea to correct vision

(continued)

Surgical Interventions and Therapeutic Procedures *(continued)*

Term	Pronunciation	Meaning
retinal photocoagulation	ret'i-năl fō'tō-kō-ag'yū-lā'shŭn	repair of a retinal detachment or tear by using a laser beam to coagulate the tissues to allow a seal to form
scleral buckling	sklē'răl bŭk-ling	repair of a retinal detachment by attaching a band (buckle) around the sclera to keep the retina from pulling away (**Figure 7-13**)
sclerotomy	sklē-rot'ŏ-mē	incision into the sclera
trabeculectomy	tră-bek'yū-lek'tŏ-mē	surgical procedure to create a drain to reduce pressure within the eye
vitrectomy	vi-trek'tŏ-mē	removal of all or part of the vitreous humor

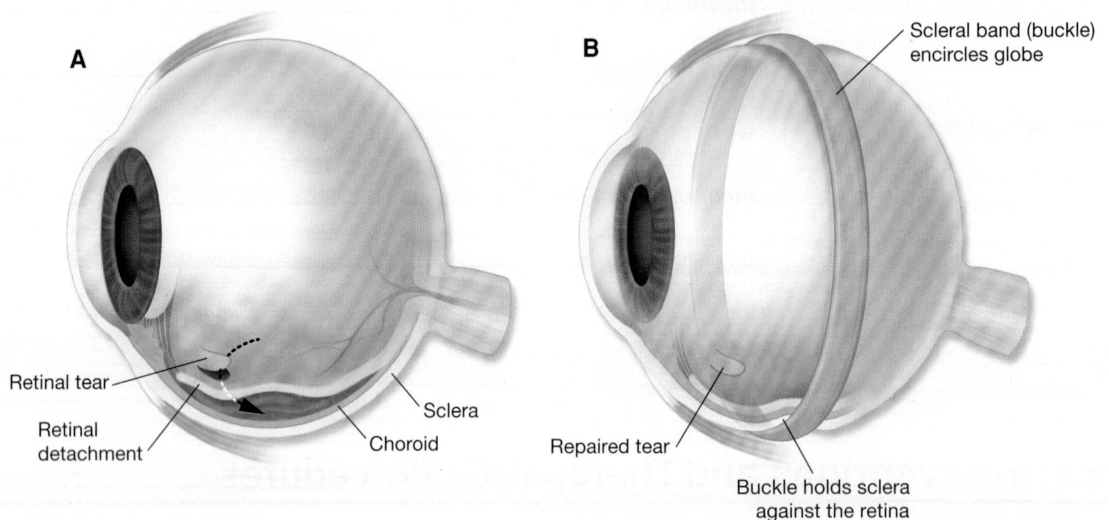

Figure 7-13 **A.** Detached retina. The *arrow* shows the movement of fluid. **B.** Scleral buckling. Repair of a retinal tear by attaching a band (buckle) around the sclera to keep the retina from pulling away.

Exercises: Surgical Interventions and Therapeutic Procedures

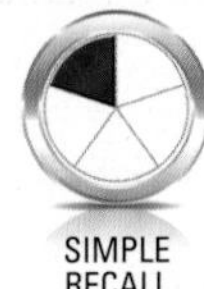

Exercise 21

Write the correct medical term for the definition given.

1. removal of an eyeball ______________________
2. repair of a detached retina using extreme cold ______________________
3. removal of all or part of the vitreous humor ______________________
4. laser vision correction by reshaping the cornea ______________________
5. surgical removal of a cataract ______________________
6. repair of a retinal detachment or tear using a laser beam ______________________
7. laser vision correction by creating a corneal flap and reshaping the corneal tissue ______________________

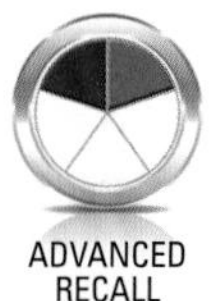
ADVANCED RECALL

Exercise 22

Complete each sentence by writing in the correct medical term.

1. ______________________ is the use of ultrasound to shatter and break up a cataract, followed by aspiration and removal.
2. The surgical procedure that creates a drain in the eye to reduce pressure within it is called a(n) ______________________.
3. Making an incision into the lacrimal sac is called ______________________.
4. When a physician repairs a retinal detachment by attaching a band around the sclera to keep it from pulling away, he or she is performing ______________________.
5. Corneal transplantation and repairing a cornea to alter its shape are both called ______________________.
6. The procedure to repair a drooping eyelid is ______________________.
7. A(n) ______________________ replaces a defective natural lens with an artificial one.

TERM CONSTRUCTION

Exercise 23

Write the remainder of the term for the meaning given.

1. incision into the sclera — sclero ______________________
2. surgical repair of the eyelid — ______________________ plasty
3. excision of part of the iris — irid ______________________
4. surgical repair of the cornea — ______________________ plasty
5. removal of the vitreous humor — vitr ______________________
6. incision into the iris — ______________________ tomy

Medications and Drug Therapies

Term	Pronunciation	Meaning
corticosteroid	kōr′ti-kō-ster′oyd	drug that reduces inflammation; used to treat swelling and itching of the eye
hypotonic	hī′pō-ton′ik	drug used to relieve dry irritated eyes
miotic	mī-ot′ik	drug used to constrict the pupil
mydriatic	mi-drē-at′ik	drug used to dilate the pupil
prostaglandin	pros′tă-glan′dĕn	drug that relaxes muscles in the eye's interior to allow better outflow of fluids

Exercise: Medications and Drug Therapies

Exercise 24

SIMPLE RECALL

Write the correct medication or drug therapy for the definition given.

1. dilates the pupil ______________________
2. treats swelling and itching of the eye ______________________
3. relaxes muscles in the eye's interior ______________________
4. constricts the pupil ______________________
5. relieves dry irritated eyes ______________________

Specialties and Specialists

Term	Pronunciation	Meaning
optician	op-tish'ăn	one who fills prescriptions for corrective lenses
optometry	op-tom'ĕ-trē	medical specialty concerned with examination of the eyes and related structures to determine vision problems and eye disorders and prescribe corrective treatment or lenses
optometrist	op-tom'ĕ-trist	one who practices optometry
ophthalmology	of'thal-mol'ŏ-jē	medical specialty concerned with the study of the eye, its diseases, and refractive errors
ophthalmologist	of'thal-mol'ŏ-jist	physician who specializes in ophthalmology

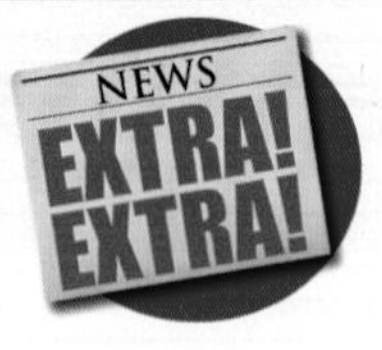

OPTOMETRIST VERSUS OPHTHALMOLOGIST What is the difference between an optometrist and an ophthalmologist? An optometrist is an OD, a Doctor of Optometry. Optometrists can evaluate vision problems, diagnose some eye conditions, and prescribe corrective treatments such as exercises or corrective lenses. Because optometrists are not medical doctors, however, they cannot perform eye surgery and are limited in the medical treatments they may give. An ophthalmologist is an MD, a Doctor of Medicine or a DO, an Osteopathic Doctor, who has completed medical school. Ophthalmologists can diagnose and treat any eye disease or vision problem as well as perform eye surgery.

Exercise: Specialties and Specialists

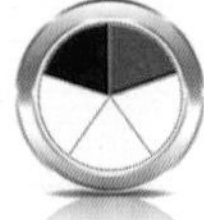

Exercise 25

ADVANCED RECALL

Match each medical term with its meaning.

ophthalmologist   optometrist   optician
optometry   ophthalmology

1. specialty in the measurement of vision and prescription of treatment ______________________
2. specialty in the study of the eye and its diseases ______________________

3. one who fills prescriptions for corrective lenses ______________________

4. physician who specializes in the study and treatment of eyes ______________________

5. one who practices optometry ______________________

Abbreviations

Abbreviation	Meaning
EOM	extraocular movement
IOL	intraocular lens
IOP	intraocular pressure
LASIK	laser-assisted in situ keratomileusis
OD	right eye (oculus dexter)
OS	left eye (oculus sinister)
OU	each eye; both eyes (oculus uterque)
PRK	photorefractive keratectomy
VA	visual acuity
VF	visual field

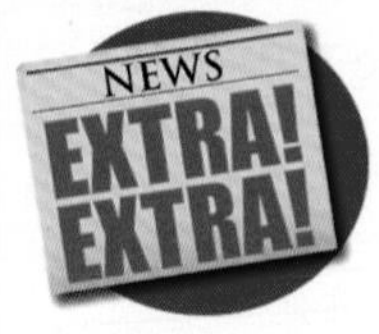

DANGEROUS ABBREVIATIONS RELATED TO THE EYE The abbreviations OD, OS, and OU are included on the list of "Error-Prone Abbreviations, Symbols, and Dose Designations" published by the Institute for Safe Medication Practices. According to the ISMP, these abbreviations are frequently confused for each other or for the abbreviations for right ear (AD), left ear (AS), or both ears (AU), which can lead to errors in patient care. For this reason, ISMP recommends eliminating use of these abbreviations. However, if you do encounter any of these abbreviations in practice, use special care to ensure proper interpretation to prevent errors.

Exercises: Abbreviations

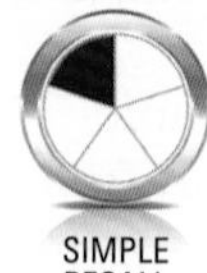

SIMPLE RECALL

Exercise 26

Write the meaning of each abbreviation.

1. OU ______________________

2. EOM ______________________

3. IOL ______________________

4. OS ______________________

5. VF ______________________

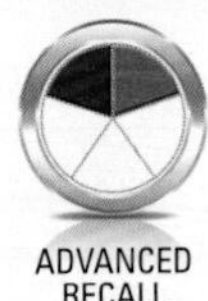

Exercise 27

Write the meaning of each abbreviation used in these sentences.

1. The patient's **VA** was 20/40 in the right eye without corrective lenses.

   ____

2. Mr. Friedman expressed interest in having **LASIK** surgery to correct his astigmatism.

   ____

3. The physician instructed Ms. Herrera to instill two drops of the ophthalmic drops **OD** for five days as therapy for her conjunctivitis.

   ____

4. Mr. Hall's vision was corrected using a laser to reshape his cornea, a process known as **PRK.**

   ____

5. Dr. Morgan's patient is scheduled to undergo a trabeculectomy to minimize the **IOP** in his left eye.

   ____

ANATOMY AND PHYSIOLOGY OF THE EAR

We now focus our attention on the special sense of hearing and balance and the organs that make it possible. This section will identify major anatomic structures and functions related to the ear as well as hearing and balance.

Structures

- The ear consists of three major parts: the outer (external) ear, middle ear, and inner (internal) ear.
- The outer ear consists of the pinna, external auditory canal, and tympanic membrane (eardrum). The tympanic membrane separates the outer ear from the middle ear.
- The middle ear consists of the auditory (pharyngotympanic) tube and the auditory ossicles: the malleus, incus, and stapes.
- The inner ear, also known as the labyrinth, consists of the cochlea, semicircular ducts (canals), and vestibule.

Functions

- Allowing hearing by translating sound waves into nerve impulses that are carried to the brain
- Assisting in maintaining equilibrium or balance

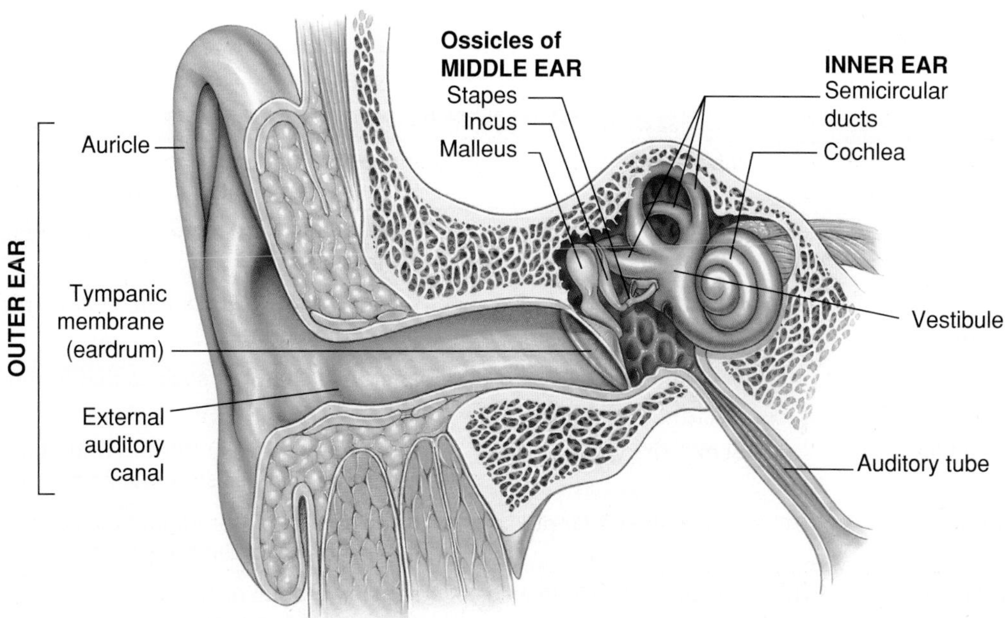

Figure 7-14 Structures of the outer, middle, and inner ear.

Terms Related to the Ear (Figure 7-14)

Term	Pronunciation	Meaning
Outer Ear (External Ear)		
auricle; *syn.* pinna	aw′ri-kl; pin′ă	external portion of the ear that directs sound waves
external auditory canal; *syn.* external auditory meatus	eks-ter′năl aw′di-tōr-ēkă-nal′, mē-ā′tŭs	passage leading inward from the auricle to the tympanic membrane (eardrum)
cerumen	sĕ-rū′men	waxy substance produced by glands of the external auditory canal; earwax
tympanic membrane (TM)	tim-pan′ik mem′brān	eardrum; a semitransparent membrane that vibrates to transmit sound waves to the ossicles; separates the external auditory canal from the middle ear cavity
Middle Ear		
mastoid cells	mas′toyd selz	numerous small interconnecting cavities in the mastoid process of the temporal bone
auditory tube; *syn.* pharyngotympanic tube, eustachian tube	aw′di-tōr-ē tūb; fă-ring′ō-tim-pan′ik tūb, yū-stā′shăn tūb	canal that connects the middle ear to the pharynx (throat)
auditory ossicles	aw′di-tōr-ē os′i-kĕlz	three small bones (malleus, incus, stapes) of the middle ear that transmit sound waves (**Figure 7-15**)
malleus	mal′ē-ŭs	largest auditory ossicle; shaped like a hammer or club
incus	ing′kŭs	middle auditory ossicle; shaped like an anvil
stapes	stā′pēz	smallest auditory ossicle; shaped like a stirrup

(continued)

Terms Related to the Ear *(continued)*

Term	Pronunciation	Meaning
Inner Ear (Internal Ear)		
labyrinth	lab′i-rinth	inner ear; made up of a series of semicircular ducts (canals), the vestibule, and the cochlea
cochlea	kok′lē-ă	a snail shell–shaped organ that contains the organ of hearing
spiral organ; *syn.* organ of Corti	spī′răl ōr′găn; ōr′găn of kōr′tē	receptor for hearing located within the cochlea; the organ of hearing
vestibule	ves′ti-byūl	anatomic chamber such as that found in the inner ear
semicircular canals	sem′ē-sir′kyū-lăr kă-nal′z	three bony tubes in the labyrinth that contain receptors that assist in maintaining balance
semicircular ducts	sem′ē-sir′kyū-lăr dŭktz	three small membranous tubes of the vestibular labyrinth within the bony semicircular canals
vestibulocochlear nerve (CN VIII)	ves-tib′yū-lō-kō′klē-ăr nerv	sensory cranial nerve within the labyrinth that consists of two branches, the vestibular nerve (for balance) and the cochlear nerve (for hearing)

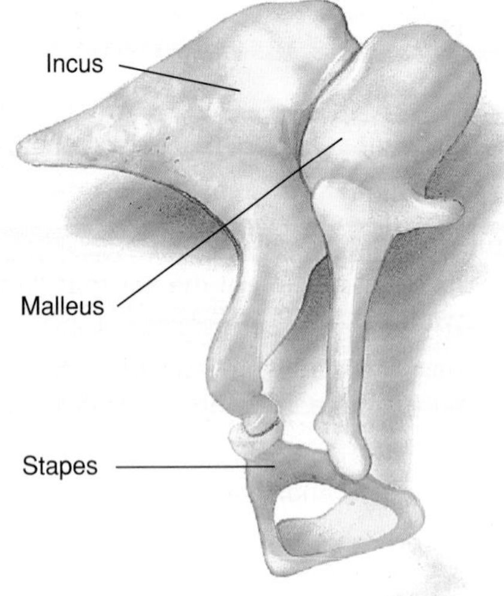

Figure 7-15 Ossicles of the middle ear.

Exercises: Anatomy and Physiology of the Ear

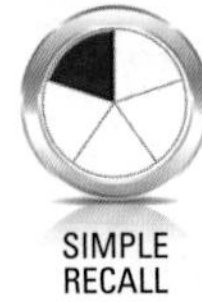

Exercise 28

Write the meaning of the anatomic structure given.

1. stapes ____________________

2. spiral organ ____________________

3. external auditory canal ____________________

4. incus ____________________

5. auricle ______________________

6. malleus ______________________

7. auditory ossicles ______________________

8. cerumen ______________________

9. labyrinth ______________________

ADVANCED RECALL

Exercise 29

Match each anatomic structure with its meaning.

vestibule	cochlea	tympanic membrane
auricle	auditory ossicles	auditory tube
semicircular canals	mastoid cells	external auditory canal

1. chamber such as that found in the inner ear ______________________
2. three bony tubes in the labyrinth that help with balance ______________________
3. three small middle ear bones ______________________
4. eardrum ______________________
5. canal that connects the middle ear to the pharynx (throat) ______________________
6. numerous small interconnecting cavities in the mastoid process of the temporal bone ______________________
7. external portion of the ear that directs sound waves ______________________
8. snail shell–shaped organ that contains the organ of hearing ______________________
9. passage leading inward from the auricle to the tympanic membrane (eardrum) ______________________

ADVANCED RECALL

Exercise 30

Complete each sentence by writing the correct medical term.

1. The middle ear bones are known as the ______________________.
2. Numerous small interconnecting cavities in the mastoid process of the temporal bone are called ______________________.
3. The ______________________ is the name for the inner ear, which is made up of semicircular canals, the vestibule, and the cochlea.
4. A waxy substance produced by glands in the external auditory canal (commonly known as earwax) is called ______________________.
5. The organ of hearing is known as the ______________________.

6. The three small membranous tubes of the vestibular labyrinth within the bony semicircular canals are called ____________.

7. A chamber, such as that of the inner ear, is called a(n) ____________.

8. The canal that connects the middle ear to the pharynx (throat) is the ____________.

9. The semitransparent membrane that vibrates to transmit sound waves is called the ____________.

WORD PARTS FOR THE EAR

The following tables list word parts related to the ear.

Combining Forms

Combining Form	Meaning
acous/o	hearing, sound
audi/o	hearing
aur/i, aur/o	ear
cochle/o	cochlea
labyrinth/o	labyrinth, inner ear
mastoid/o	mastoid cells, mastoid process
myring/o	tympanic membrane, eardrum
ot/o	ear
scler/o	hard, sclera
staped/o	stapes
tympan/o	tympanic membrane, eardrum
vestibul/o	vestibule

Prefixes

Prefix	Meaning
dys-	painful, difficult, abnormal
meato-	passage, external opening of a canal

Suffixes

Suffix	Meaning
-acousis, -acusis	hearing
-algia	pain
-ectomy	excision, surgical removal
-stomy	surgical opening

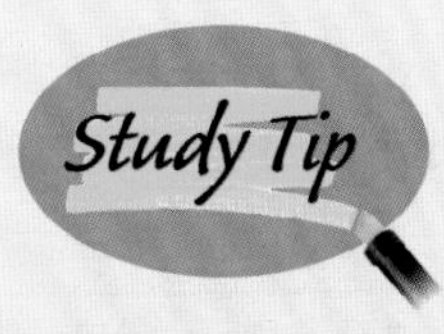

Myring/o Versus Tympan/o: When trying to decide whether to use *myring/o* or *tympan/o* for the tympanic membrane (eardrum), remember this hint: *Myring/o* usually refers only to the tympanic membrane. *Tympan/o,* however, usually refers to the tympanic membrane and/or the middle ear space. The space behind (posterior to) the tympanic membrane is referred to as the middle ear space or the tympanic cavity.

Exercises: Word Parts for the Ear

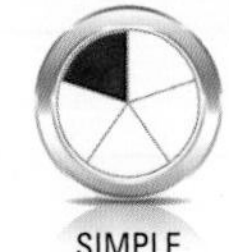

SIMPLE RECALL

Exercise 31

Write the meaning of the word part given.

1. -acousis ______
2. -algia ______
3. vestibul/o ______
4. aur/i ______
5. acous/o ______
6. scler/o ______
7. dys- ______
8. cochle/o ______

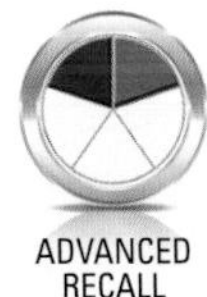

ADVANCED RECALL

Exercise 32

Match each word part with its meaning.

-stomy	dys-	-ectomy
labyrinth/o	scler/o	ot/o

1. labyrinth, inner ear ______
2. excision, surgical removal ______
3. surgical opening ______
4. hard ______
5. painful, difficult, abnormal ______
6. ear ______

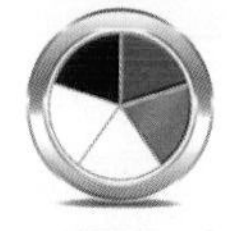

Exercise 33

TERM CONSTRUCTION

Considering the meaning of the combining form from which the medical term is made, write the meaning of the medical term.

Combining Form	Meaning	Medical Term	Meaning of Term
labyrinth/o	inner ear	labyrinthitis	1. ______
tympan/o	middle ear	tympanostomy	2. ______
mastoid/o	mastoid cells; mastoid process	mastoiditis	3. ______
ot/o	ear	otorrhea	4. ______
audi/o	hearing	audiometer	5. ______
myring/o	eardrum	myringotomy	6. ______
staped/o	stapes	stapedectomy	7. ______

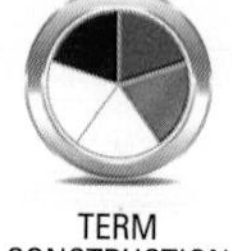

Exercise 34

TERM CONSTRUCTION

Using the given combining form, build a medical term for the meaning given.

Combining Form	Meaning of Medical Term	Medical Term
vestibul/o	incision into the vestibule	1. ______
aur/i	pertaining to the ear	2. ______
acous/o	pertaining to hearing or sound	3. ______
cochle/o	inflammation of the cochlea	4. ______
scler/o	abnormal condition of hardness	5. ______
ot/o	pain in the ear	6. ______
myring/o	inflammation of the eardrum	7. ______

MEDICAL TERMS RELATED TO THE EAR

The following table gives adjective forms and terms used in describing the ear.

Adjectives and Other Related Terms

Term	Pronunciation	Meaning
acoustic	ă-kūs′tik	pertaining to hearing or sound
auditory	aw′di-tōr-ē	pertaining to hearing

Adjectives and Other Related Terms

Term	Pronunciation	Meaning
aural	aw'răl	pertaining to the ear
cochlear	kok'lē-ăr	pertaining to the cochlea
labyrinthine	lab'i-rin'thīn	pertaining to the labyrinth or inner ear
mastoid	mas'toyd	pertaining to the mastoid cells
otic	ō'tik	pertaining to the ear
tympanic	tim-pan'ik	pertaining to the tympanic membrane or tympanic cavity
vestibular	ves-tib'yū-lăr	pertaining to a vestibule

Exercises: Adjectives and Other Related Terms

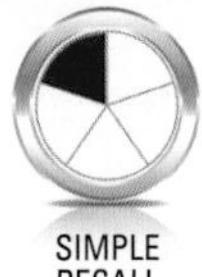
SIMPLE RECALL

Exercise 35

Write the meaning of the term given.

1. otic __________
2. acoustic __________
3. aural __________
4. tympanic __________
5. vestibular __________
6. auditory __________
7. cochlear __________

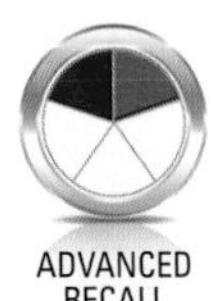
ADVANCED RECALL

Exercise 36

Match each medical term with its meaning.

vestibular	aural	labyrinthine
acoustic	tympanic	mastoid

1. pertaining to the ear __________
2. pertaining to the vestibule __________
3. pertaining to the tympanic membrane __________
4. pertaining to sound __________
5. pertaining to the labyrinth __________
6. pertaining to the mastoid cells __________

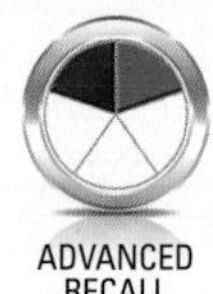
ADVANCED RECALL

Exercise 37

Circle the term that is most appropriate for the meaning of the sentence.

1. The school nurse used a(n) (*aural, mastoid, acoustic*) thermometer to take the child's temperature in his ear.
2. Mrs. Gallo had an inner ear or (*acoustic, mastoid, labyrinthine*) infection.
3. Helen claims that she is a(n) (*auditory, otic, tympanic*) learner, so she enjoys listening to educational lectures.
4. The physician showed Timmy's mother how to put (*labyrinthine, acoustic, otic*) drops in his ears.
5. The (*auditory, mastoid, vestibular*) infection was in the temporal bone behind the patient's left ear.
6. Fluid had accumulated in the middle ear behind the (*acoustic, otic, tympanic*) membrane.

Medical Conditions

Term	Pronunciation	Meaning
acoustic neuroma	ă-kūs′tik nū-rō′mă	a benign but life-threatening tumor that develops on the vestibulocochlear nerve (CN VIII); causes hearing loss and balance problems
cerumen impaction	sĕ-rū′men im-pak′shŭn	excessive buildup of earwax
cholesteatoma	kō′les-tē′ă-tō′mă	cyst-like tumor of skin in the middle ear behind the tympanic membrane that grows into the bone; usually caused by chronic otitis media (**Figure 7-16**)
conductive hearing loss	kon′dŭk-tiv′ hēr′ing los	hearing loss due to a lesion in the external auditory canal or middle ear
dysacusis; *syn.* dysacousia	dis′ă-kyū′sis; dis′ă-kyū′sē-ă	any hearing impairment involving difficulty in the processing of sound
labyrinthitis	lab′i-rin-thī′tis	inflammation of the inner ear
mastoiditis	mas′toy-dī′tis	inflammation of the air cell system of the mastoid process
Ménière disease; *syn.* Ménière syndrome	men-ē-ār′ di-zēz′	chronic disorder of the inner ear caused by fluid accumulation in the labyrinth and characterized by dizziness, tinnitus, hearing loss, and a sensation of pressure in the ear
myringitis	mir′in-jī′tis	inflammation of the tympanic membrane
otalgia	ō-tal′jē-ă	pain in the ear
otitis externa (OE)	ō-tī′tis eks-ter′nă	inflammation of the external auditory canal; also known as "swimmer's ear"
otitis media (OM)	ō-tī′tis mē′dē-ă	inflammation of the middle ear (**Figure 7-17**)
otomycosis	ō′tō-mī-kō′sis	fungal infection in the ear
otopyorrhea	ō-tō-pī′ō-rē′ă	discharge of pus from the ear
otorrhea	ō-tō-rē′ă	discharge from the ear
otosclerosis	ō′tō-sklĕ-rō′sis	hardening of the ossicles, particularly the stapes

Medical Conditions

Term	Pronunciation	Meaning
presbycusis	prez′bē-kū′sis	impaired hearing caused by old age
sensorineural hearing loss	sen′sŏ-rē-nū′răl hēr′ing los	hearing loss caused by damage to the inner ear or the cochlear branch of cranial nerve VIII
tinnitus	tin′i-tŭs	noises in the ear, such as ringing, buzzing, or humming
tympanic membrane perforation	tim-pan′ik mem′brān per′fō-rā′shŭn	a hole in or rupture of the eardrum
vertigo	ver-ti′gō	a spinning sensation; commonly used to mean dizziness

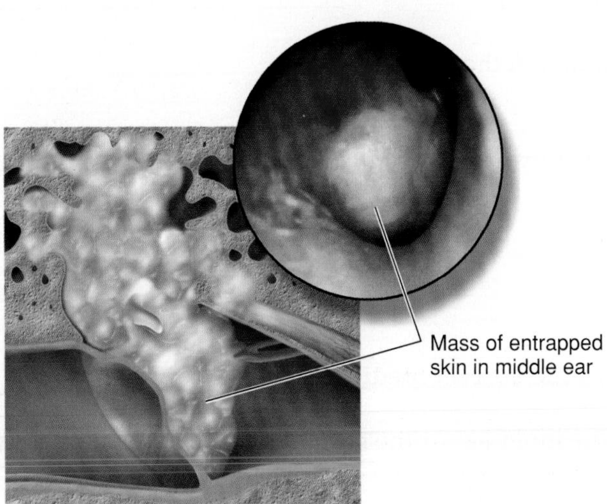

Figure 7-16 A cholesteatoma in the middle ear.

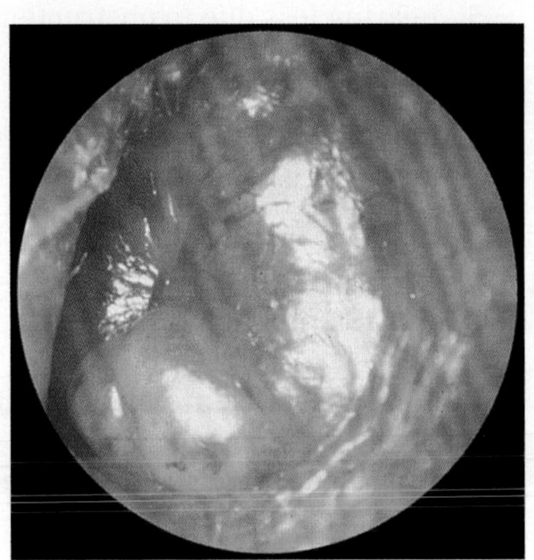

Figure 7-17 Otitis media.

Exercises: Medical Conditions

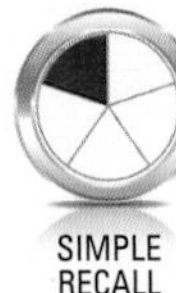

Exercise 38

Write the correct medical term for the definition given.

1. fungal infection in the ear
2. hardening of the ossicles, particularly the stapes ____________
3. noises within the ear ____________
4. cyst-like tumor of skin in the middle ear ____________
5. excessive buildup of earwax ____________
6. age-related hearing loss ____________
7. spinning sensation, dizziness ____________
8. a tumor that develops on the vestibulocochlear nerve ____________

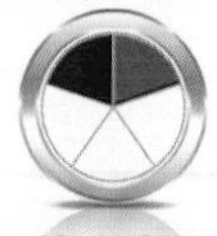

ADVANCED RECALL

Exercise 39

Match each medical term with its meaning.

presbycusis	conductive hearing loss	otitis externa
otitis media	sensorineural hearing loss	dysacusis

1. inflammation of the middle ear __________
2. hearing loss due to damage to the inner ear __________
3. age-related hearing loss __________
4. inflammation of the external auditory canal __________
5. hearing loss due to obstruction or lesion in the outer and/or middle ear __________
6. impairment of hearing involving difficulty in the processing of sound __________

ADVANCED RECALL

Exercise 40

Complete each sentence by writing in the correct medical term.

1. Hearing loss caused by damage to the inner ear or the cochlear branch of cranial nerve VIII is called __________.
2. __________ is inflammation of the external auditory canal.
3. Hearing loss due to an obstruction or lesion in the outer and/or middle ear is called __________.
4. __________ is a discharge of pus from the ear.
5. A chronic condition of the ear known as __________ is characterized by dizziness, tinnitus, hearing loss, and a sensation of pressure.
6. A hole or rupture of the eardrum is called a(n) __________.
7. Inflammation of the middle ear is called __________.

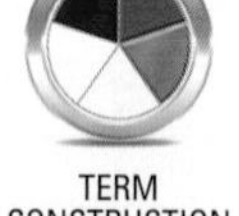

TERM CONSTRUCTION

Exercise 41

Build the correct medical term for the meaning given. Indicate the combining form and the suffix, and write the term in the space provided.

1. pain in the ear

   Combining form: __________

   Suffix: __________

   Term: __________

2. inflammation of the inner ear

Combining form: ______________

Suffix: ______________

Term: ______________

3. discharge from the ear

Combining form: ______________

Suffix: ______________

Term: ______________

4. inflammation of the mastoid cells

Combining form: ______________

Suffix: ______________

Term: ______________

5. inflammation of the tympanic membrane

Combining form: ______________

Suffix: ______________

Term: ______________

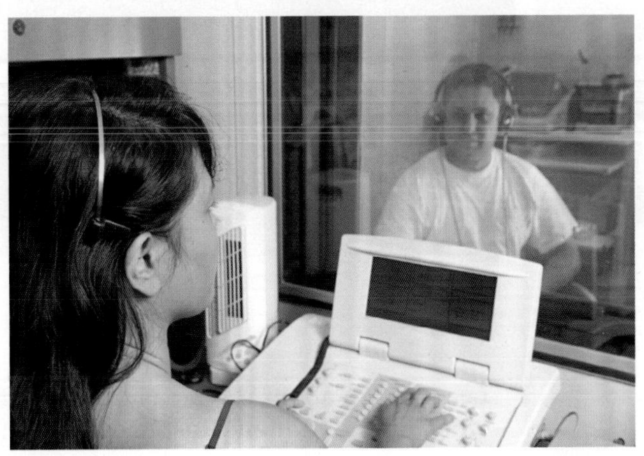

Figure 7-18 Patient undergoing audiometry.

Tests and Procedures

Term	Pronunciation	Meaning
		Diagnostic Procedures
audiogram	aw′dē-ō-gram	record of hearing (presented in graph form) (see later **Figure 7-22**)
audiometer	aw′dē-om′ĕ-ter	instrument for measuring hearing
audiometry	aw′dē-om′ĕ-trē	measurement of hearing (**Figure 7-18**)
decibel (dB)	des′i-bel	unit for expressing the intensity of sound

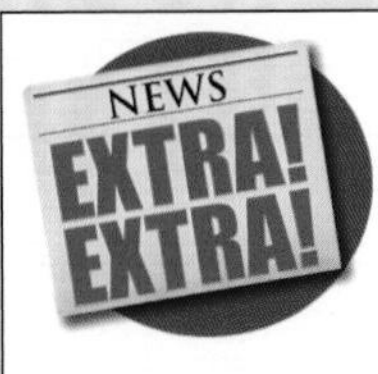

NOISE-INDUCED HEARING LOSS Sound is measured in decibels (dB). Noises that are greater than 80 dB are considered dangerous to your hearing. Exposure to this level of sound can cause permanent hearing damage. Examples of noises greater than 80 dB are chain saws, leaf blowers, loud car stereos, and airplanes at the point of takeoff. The use of earbuds with MP3 players is a potential hazard to hearing if the volume is kept too high.

(continued)

Tests and Procedures *(continued)*

Term	Pronunciation	Meaning
electronystagmography (ENG)	ē-lek'trō-nis'tag-mog'ră-fē	recording of eye movements in response to electrical impulses to diagnose balance problems
hertz (Hz)	herts	unit of measure of frequency or pitch of sound
otoscope	ō'tō-skōp	instrument for examining the ear (**Figure 7-19A**)
otoscopy	ō-tos'kŏ-pē	use of an otoscope to examine the external auditory canal and tympanic membrane (**Figure 7-19B**)
tympanogram	tim'pă-nō-gram	record of middle ear function (presented in graph form)
tympanometer	tim'pă-nom'ĕ-tĕr	instrument for measuring middle ear function
tympanometry	tim'pă-nom'ĕ-trē	measurement of middle ear function

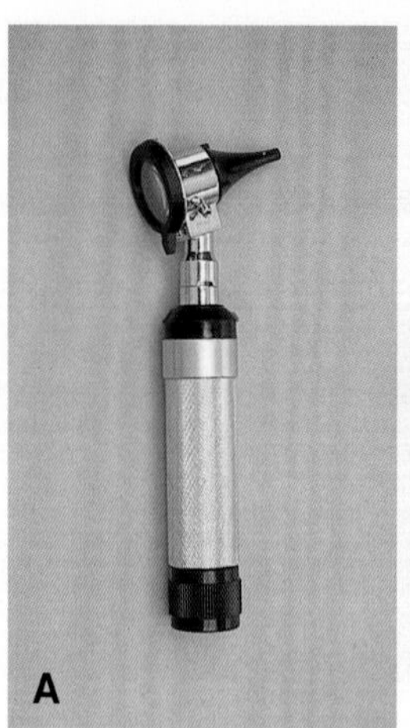

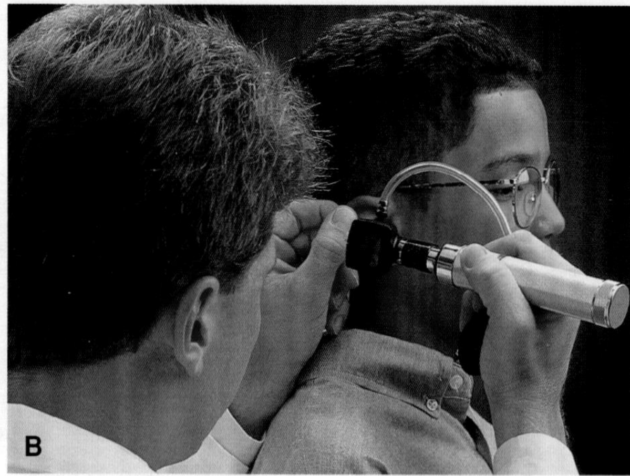

Figure 7-19 Using an otoscope **(A)** to perform otoscopy **(B)**.

Learn more about the measurement of hearing by viewing the "Audiometry" video on the Student Resources on thePoint.

Exercises: Tests and Procedures

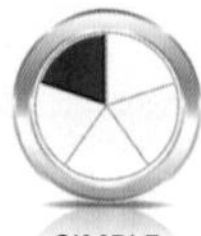

Exercise 42

Write the meaning of the term given.

1. hertz ____________________
2. audiogram ____________________
3. otoscopy ____________________
4. tympanometry ____________________
5. decibel ____________________
6. tympanogram ____________________

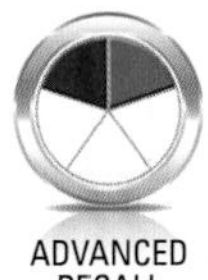

ADVANCED RECALL

Exercise 43

Circle the term that is most appropriate for the meaning of the sentence.

1. The physician used a(n) (*otoscope, audiometer, decibel*) to assess the patient's hearing.
2. Mr. Vladimir was referred to the (*tympanometry, electronystagmography, audiometry*) department to get a measurement of his hearing.
3. The results of Mrs. James' (*tympanogram, audiogram, electronystagmogram*) indicated that she had significant hearing loss in her right ear.
4. Dr. Davies measured Mrs. MacDonald's middle ear function using a(n) (*audiometer, otoscope, tympanometer*).

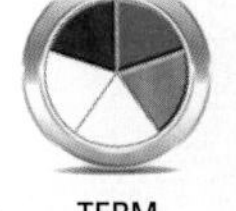

TERM CONSTRUCTION

Exercise 44

Using the given combining form, build a medical term for the meaning given.

Combining Form	Meaning of Medical Term	Medical Term
ot/o	instrument for examining the ear	1. ______________
tympan/o	record of middle ear function	2. ______________
audi/o	instrument for measuring hearing	3. ______________
ot/o	use of an otoscope to examine the ear	4. ______________
tympan/o	measurement of middle ear function	5. ______________
audi/o	record of hearing	6. ______________

Surgical Interventions and Therapeutic Procedures

Term	Pronunciation	Meaning
cochlear implant	kok'lē-ăr im'plant	an electronic device implanted in the cochlea to stimulate the cochlear (auditory) nerve and provide hearing sensations for the profoundly deaf (**Figure 7-20**)
ear lavage	ēr lă-vahzh'	irrigation of the ear to remove cerumen (wax) buildup
labyrinthectomy	lab'i-rin-thek'tō-mē	excision of part of the labyrinth
mastoidectomy	mas'toy-dek'tŏ-mē	excision of part of the mastoid process of the temporal bone and middle ear to drain or remove lesions
mastoidotomy	mas'toyd-ot' ŏ-mē	incision into the mastoid process of the temporal bone
myringotomy; *syn.* tympanostomy	mir'in-got'ŏ-mē; tim'pan-os'tŏ-mē	surgical incision (opening) into the tympanic membrane to drain fluid from the middle ear (usually done with subsequent tympanostomy tube placement) (**Figure 7-21**)
otoplasty	ō'tō-plas'tē	surgical repair of the external ear
stapedectomy	stā'pĕ-dek'tŏ-mē	removal of the stapes and replacement with a prosthesis; done to correct hearing loss from otosclerosis

(continued)

Surgical Interventions and Therapeutic Procedures *(continued)*

Term	Pronunciation	Meaning
tympanoplasty	tim′pă-nō-plas′tē	surgical repair of the tympanic membrane and/or middle ear
tympanostomy tube placement	tim′pan-os′tŏ-mē tūb plās′mĕnt	placement of a small tube through the tympanic membrane to relieve symptoms caused by fluid buildup

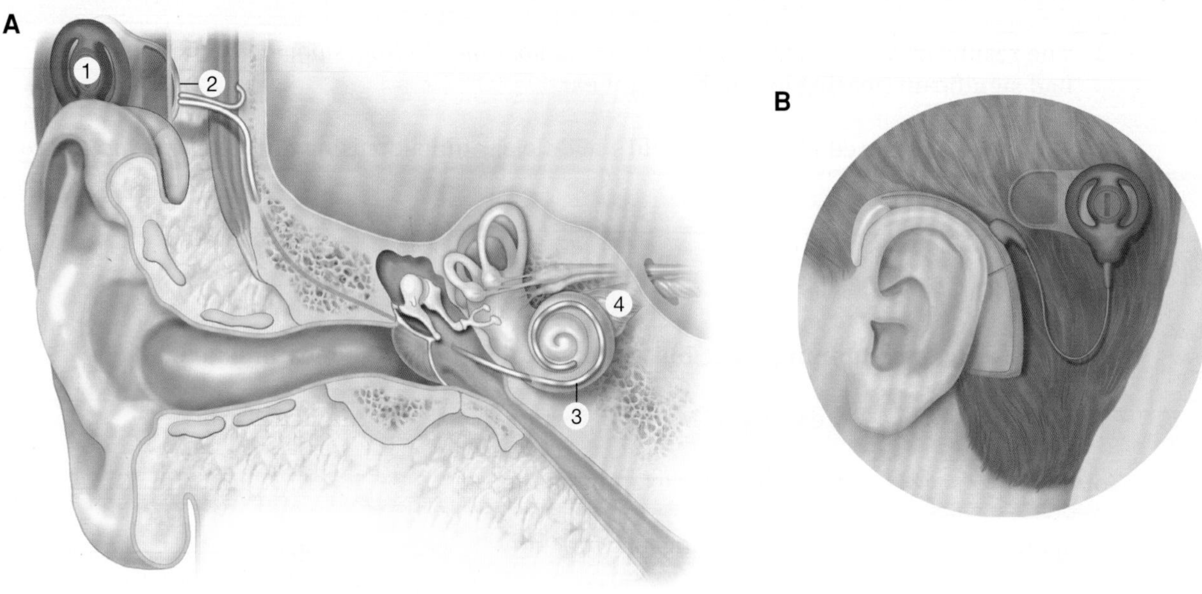

1. External speech processor captures sound and converts it into digital signals
2. Processor sends digital signal to internal implant
3. Internal implant converts signals into electrical energy, sending it to an electrode array inside the cochlea
4. Electrodes stimulate hearing nerve, bypassing damaged hair cells, and the brain perceives signals to hear sound

Figure 7-20 **A.** Function of a cochlear implant. **B.** Side view showing placement of external speech processor.

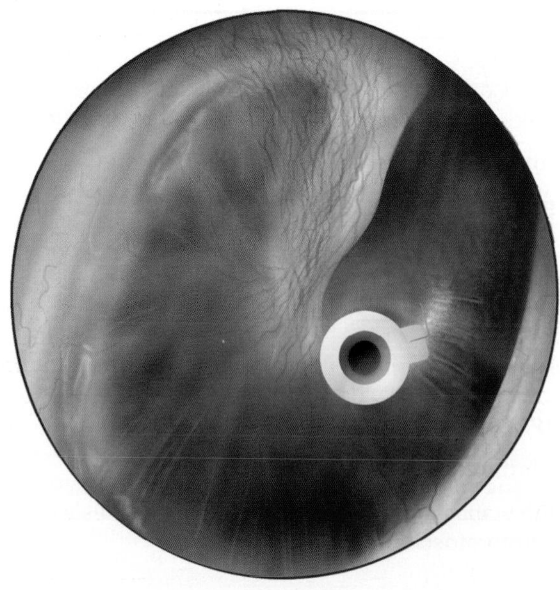

Figure 7-21 Tympanic membrane with tympanostomy tube in place as viewed through an otoscope.

Exercises: Surgical Interventions and Therapeutic Procedures

SIMPLE RECALL

Exercise 45

Write the correct medical term for the definition given.

1. excision of part of the labyrinth ______________________
2. incision into the mastoid process of the temporal bone ______________________
3. removal of the stapes ______________________
4. irrigation of the ear to remove cerumen ______________________
5. surgical repair of the external ear ______________________

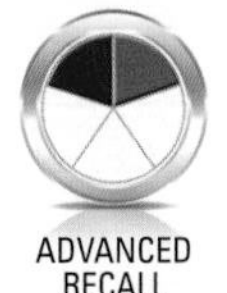

ADVANCED RECALL

Exercise 46

Complete each sentence by writing in the correct medical term(s).

1. Sammy was profoundly deaf, so the otologist recommended a(n) ______________________, which is an electronic device that stimulates the hearing nerves to provide hearing sensations.
2. Dr. Cole drained the fluid out of Kara's middle ear with a procedure called a(n) ______________________, in which he made an incision into her tympanic membrane.
3. Jenny had chronic otitis media, so the physician recommended a(n) ______________________ to create an opening into the middle ear and ______________________ with placement of a tube into the tympanic membrane to prevent further buildup of fluid.
4. Mr. Douglas's tympanic membrane perforation would not heal, so the physician performed a(n) ______________________ to repair the tympanic membrane.
5. The surgeon performed a(n) ______________________ to remove part of the mastoid process of the temporal bone.

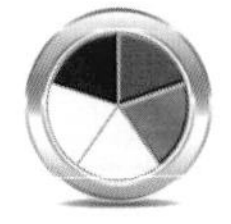

TERM CONSTRUCTION

Exercise 47

Using the given suffix, build a medical term for the meaning given.

Suffix	Meaning of Medical Term	Medical Term
-tomy	incision into the mastoid process	1. ______________
-ectomy	removal of the stapes	2. ______________
-stomy	surgical opening into tympanic membrane	3. ______________
-plasty	surgical repair of the tympanic membrane	4. ______________

Medications and Drug Therapies

Term	Pronunciation	Meaning
antibiotic	an'tē-bī-ot'ik	drug that acts against microorganisms; used to treat otitis media and other ear diseases caused by bacteria
ceruminolytic	sĕ-rū'mi-nō-lit'ik	a substance instilled into the external auditory canal to soften earwax
otic	ō'tik	any medication that can be instilled drop by drop into the ear

Exercise: Medications and Drug Therapies

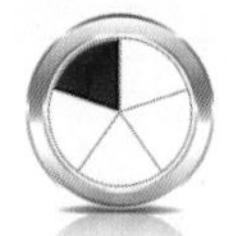
SIMPLE RECALL

Exercise 48

Write the correct medication or drug therapy term for the definition given.

1. medication that can be instilled drop by drop into the ear __________
2. drug used to treat ear diseases caused by bacteria __________
3. medication used to soften earwax __________

Specialties and Specialists

Term	Pronunciation	Meaning
audiology	aw'dē-ol'ō-jē	medical specialty concerned with the study and treatment of hearing disorders and fitting of hearing aids
audiologist	aw'dē-ol'ō-jist	one who specializes in audiology
otology	ō-tol'ō-jē	medical specialty concerned with the study of the ears and treatment of ear disease
otologist	ō-tol'ŏ-jist	one who specializes in otology
otorhinolaryngology	ō'tō-rī'nō-lar-in-gol'ŏ-jē	medical specialty concerned with diseases of the ear, nose, and throat (pharynx and larynx)
otorhinolaryngologist	ō'tō-rī'nō-lar-in-gol'ŏ-jist	physician who specializes in otorhinolaryngology, or disorders of the ears, nose, and throat

Exercise: Specialties and Specialists

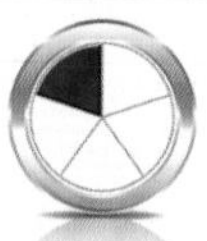
SIMPLE RECALL

Exercise 49

Write the correct medical term for the definition given.

1. medical specialty concerned with the study of the ears and treatment of ear diseases __________
2. one who specializes in audiology __________
3. medical specialty concerned with diseases of the ear, nose, and throat __________

4. medical specialty concerned with the study and treatment of hearing disorders and fitting of hearing aids ______

5. one who specializes in otology ______

6. physician who specializes in otorhinolaryngology ______

Abbreviations

Abbreviation	Meaning
AD	right ear (auris dexter)
AS	left ear (auris sinister)
AU	each ear, both ears (auris utraque)

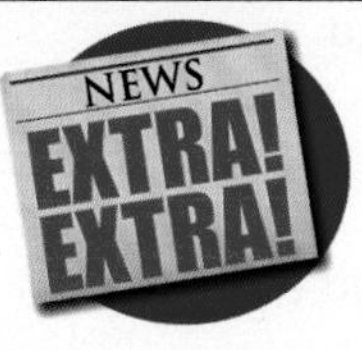

DANGEROUS ABBREVIATIONS RELATED TO THE EAR The Institute on Safe Medication Practices includes the abbreviations AD, AS, and AU on their list of "Error-Prone Abbreviations, Symbols, and Dose Designations" and recommends that they not be used in any medical communications. See the box "Dangerous Abbreviations" on page 235 for more information.

Abbreviation	Meaning
dB	decibel
EENT	eyes, ears, nose, and throat
ENG	electronystagmography
ENT	ears, nose, and throat
HEENT	head, eyes, ears, neck, and throat
Hz	hertz
OE	otitis externa
OM	otitis media
TM	tympanic membrane

Exercises: Abbreviations

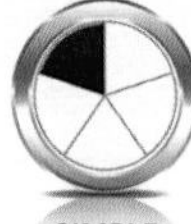
SIMPLE RECALL

Exercise 50

Write the definition of each abbreviation.

1. EENT ______
2. AU ______
3. Hz ______
4. OM ______
5. dB ______
6. AD ______

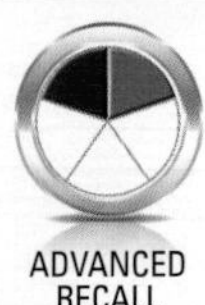
ADVANCED RECALL

Exercise 51

Write the definition of each abbreviation used in these sentences.

1. Sara's mother took her to an **ENT** physician because of her chronic otitis media.

____

2. The patient is a surfer and frequently suffers from **OE.**

____

3. Mr. Malach has severe hearing loss **AS.**

____

4. Ms. Tasara's physician recommended **ENG** to diagnose the cause of her vertigo.

____

5. The otologist diagnosed a ruptured **TM** as the cause of the patient's otalgia and otorrhea.

____

WRAPPING UP

- Sensory organs respond to external stimuli by conveying impulses to the sensory nervous system, which is made up of sensory receptors, neural pathways, and the brain.
- The eyes and ears are two sensory organs that allow us to see, hear, and maintain our balance.
- In this chapter, you learned medial terminology including word parts, prefixes, suffixes, adjectives, conditions, procedures, medications, specialties, and abbreviations related to both the eye and the ear.

Chapter Review

Review of Terms for Anatomy and Physiology

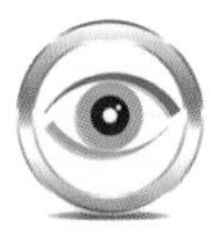

VISUAL

Exercise 52

Write the correct terms on the blanks for the anatomic structures indicated.

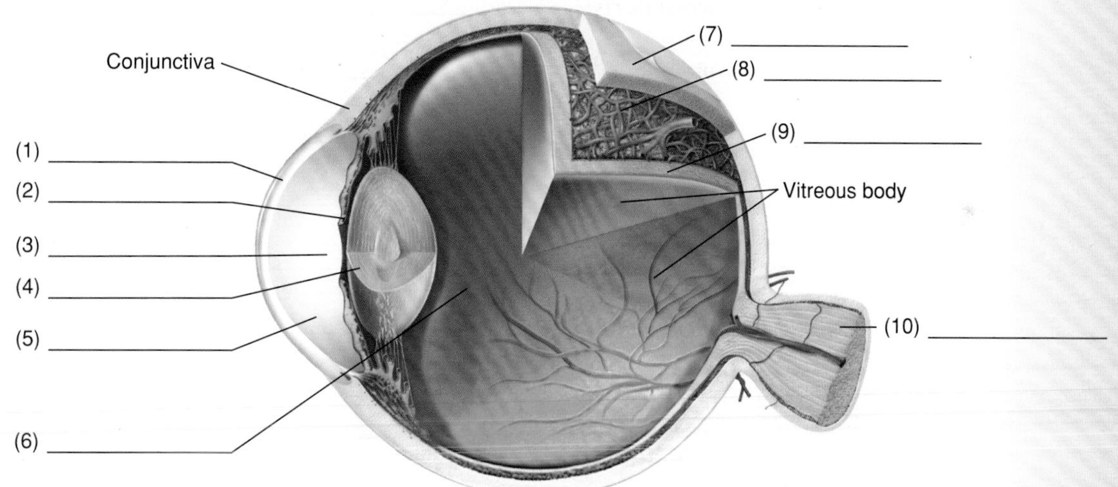

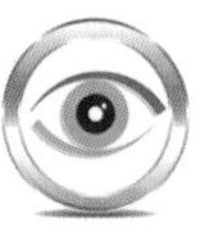

VISUAL

Exercise 53

Write the correct terms on the blanks for the anatomic structures indicated.

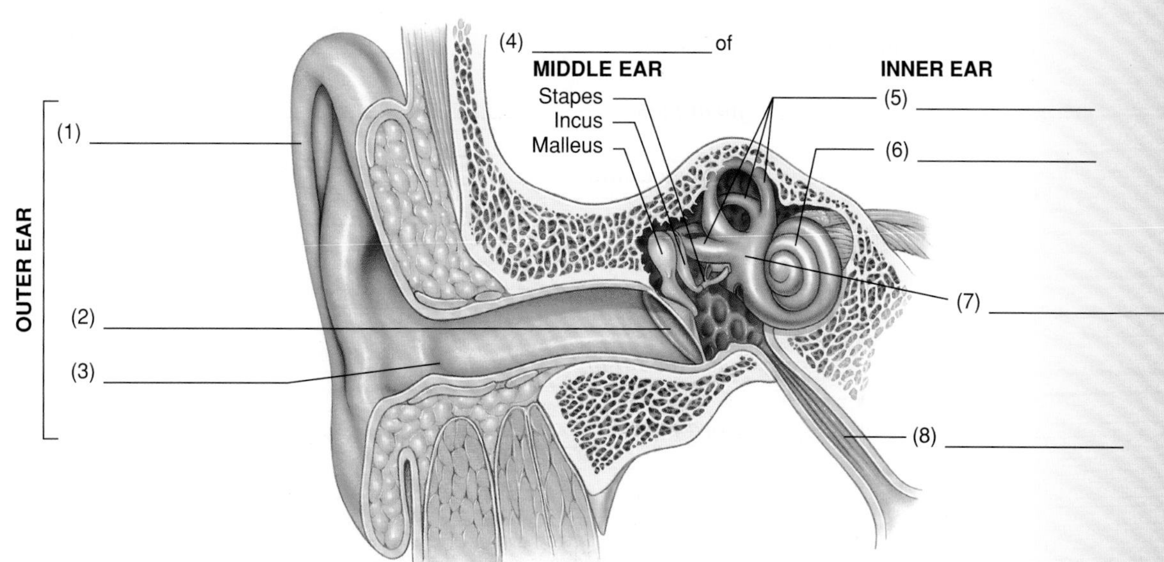

Understanding Term Structure

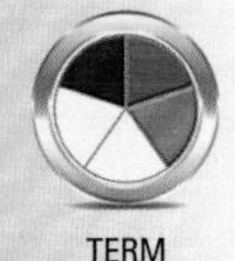
TERM CONSTRUCTION

Exercise 54

Break the given medical term into its word parts, and define each part. Then define the medical term.

For example:

mastoiditis	*word parts:*	mastoid/o, -itis
	meanings:	mastoid bone, inflammation of
	term meaning:	inflammation of the mastoid cells

1. ophthalmic
word parts: ______________________
meanings: ______________________
term meaning: ______________________

2. audiometer
word parts: ______________________
meanings: ______________________
term meaning: ______________________

3. blepharitis
word parts: ______________________
meanings: ______________________
term meaning: ______________________

4. tympanostomy
word parts: ______________________
meanings: ______________________
term meaning: ______________________

5. iridomalacia
word parts: ______________________
meanings: ______________________
term meaning: ______________________

6. labyrinthitis
word parts: ______________________
meanings: ______________________
term meaning: ______________________

7. retinopathy
word parts: ______________________
meanings: ______________________
term meaning: ______________________

8. acoustic *word parts:* ______

meanings: ______

term meaning: ______

9. pupillometer *word parts:* ______

meanings: ______

term meaning: ______

10. stapedectomy *word parts:* ______

meanings: ______

term meaning: ______

11. tonometer *word parts:* ______

meanings: ______

term meaning: ______

12. vestibular *word parts:* ______

meanings: ______

term meaning: ______

13. sclerotomy *word parts:* ______

meanings: ______

term meaning: ______

14. otoscopy *word parts:* ______

meanings: ______

term meaning: ______

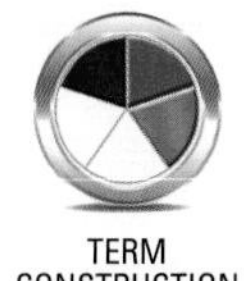

TERM CONSTRUCTION

Exercise 55

For each term, first write the meaning of the term. Then write the meaning of the word parts in that term.

1. otorrhea ______

ot/o ______

-rrhea ______

2. ophthalmoscopy ______

ophthalm/o ______

-scopy ______

3. optometry ______

opt/o ______

-metry ______

4. myringitis ______

myring/o ______

-itis ______

5. otopyorrhea ______

ot/o ______

py/o ______

-rrhea ______

6. dacryorrhea ______

dacry/o ______

-rrhea ______

7. aural ______

aur/o ______

-al ______

8. presbyopia ______

presby/o ______

-opia ______

9. audiogram ______

audi/o ______

-gram ______

10. mastoidectomy ______

mastoid/o ______

-ectomy ______

11. conjunctivitis ______
    conjunctiv/o ______
    -itis ______
12. tympanometry ______
    tympan/o ______
    -metry ______
13. keratoplasty ______
    kerat/o ______
    -plasty ______
14. presbycusis ______
    presby/o ______
    -cusis ______

Comprehension Exercises

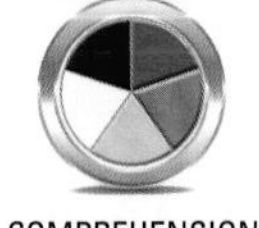
COMPREHENSION

Exercise 56

Match each medical specialist with the description of the specialty in which he or she works.

audiologist   optometrist   otologist
ophthalmologist   otorhinolaryngologist

1. diseases of the ears, nose, and throat ______
2. measurement of vision and prescription of corrective treatment or lenses ______
3. study and treatment of hearing disorders ______
4. study of the ears and treatment of ear disease ______
5. physician who studies the eye, its diseases, and refractive errors ______

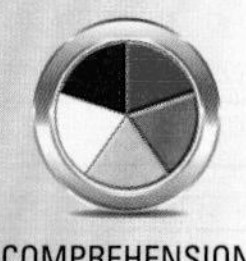
COMPREHENSION

Exercise 57

Fill in the blank with the correct term.

1. The snail shell–shaped organ that contains the spiral organ is the ________.
2. The ________ are the auditory bones that include the malleus, incus, and stapes.
3. The part of the eye that contains the vision receptors is the ________.
4. A buildup of a waxy substance produced by the glands in the external auditory canal is called a(n) ________.
5. The ________ lubricate the eyes by producing tears.
6. ________ is a chronic condition caused by fluid accumulation of the inner ear characterized by dizziness, tinnitus, and hearing loss.
7. The medical term for an inflammation of the external auditory canal, often referred to as "swimmer's ear," is ________.
8. ________ is blurry or distorted vision due to abnormal curvature of the cornea.
9. ________ is hearing loss that is related to aging.
10. An ophthalmologist might use ________ drops to dilate the pupils.
11. Medication used to relieve dry irritated eyes is called a(n) ________.
12. ________ is the term for separation of the retina from the choroid in the back of the eye.
13. The procedure that uses a laser to reshape the cornea to correct vision problems is called ________.
14. The term for dry eye is ________.
15. A photographic recording of the flow of a fluorescent dye through the blood vessels of the eye is called ________.
16. The procedure for irrigating the ear to remove earwax buildup is called ________.
17. A(n) ________ is a chart containing letters that is used to test visual acuity.
18. A(n) ________ is done to correct otosclerosis by removing the stapes and replacing it with a prosthesis.
19. ________ are medications that relax muscles in the eye's interior to allow better outflow of fluids.
20. ________ is the procedure in which extreme cold is used to repair a retinal tear.

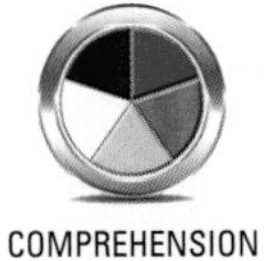
COMPREHENSION

Exercise 58

Write a short answer for each question.

1. What is the clinical term for nearsightedness? ____________________

2. Define vertigo. ____________________

____

3. What would an elderly patient with presbyopia experience? ____________________

____

4. What is the medical term for "seeing double?" ____________________

5. A patient asks you to dim the lights because she states that they are "too bright." What condition might this patient have? ____________________

6. How does hyperopia differ from myopia? ____________________

____

7. Why would a patient be given a ceruminolytic? ____________________

8. Which procedure usually occurs before placement of a tympanostomy tube? ____________________

____

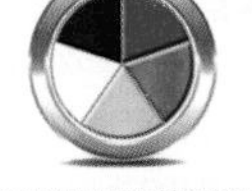
COMPREHENSION

Exercise 59

Circle the letter of the best answer in the following questions.

1. A chalazion involves obstruction of which of these?

   A. lacrimal glands
   B. ossicles
   C. tarsal glands
   D. dacryocyst

2. A clinical test used to diagnose glaucoma is

   A. tonometry.
   B. pupillometry.
   C. audiometry.
   D. tympanometry.

3. A person who has difficulty driving at night due to poor vision in reduced light probably has

   A. diplopia.
   B. amblyopia.
   C. presbyopia.
   D. nyctalopia.

4. Which of the following is located within the cochlea?

   A. pharyngotympanic tube
   B. mastoid process
   C. spiral organ
   D. vestibule

5. A patient with a hole in his or her eardrum has a ruptured

   A. cochlea.
   B. retina.
   C. pinna.
   D. tympanic membrane.

6. A construction worker who is out in the sun all day might develop a growth of conjunctival tissue over his cornea known as a

   A. pterygium.
   B. dacryolith.
   C. hordeolum.
   D. cataract.

7. The medical term for earwax is
   A. auricle.
   B. cerumen.
   C. vestibule.
   D. cholesteatoma.

8. A stapedectomy might be performed for which condition?
   A. otosclerosis
   B. cholesteatoma
   C. acoustic neuroma
   D. otomycosis

9. Which of these is *not* an ossicle?
   A. incus
   B. stapes
   C. labyrinth
   D. malleus

10. Patients who experience diabetic retinopathy due to chronically high, uncontrolled blood sugar are at an increased risk of
    A. glaucoma.
    B. presbyopia.
    C. conjunctivitis.
    D. blindness.

11. Children with poor vision in one eye have a condition commonly called "lazy eye." In clinical terms, this condition is called
    A. photophobia.
    B. amblyopia.
    C. myopia.
    D. retinitis pigmentosa.

12. Removal of a lesion from the middle ear might relieve which condition?
    A. sensorineural hearing loss
    B. conductive hearing loss
    C. presbycusis
    D. otopyorrhea

13. Which condition is usually caused by chronic otitis media?
    A. otitis externa
    B. acoustic neuroma
    C. otomycosis
    D. cholesteatoma

14. Which of the following conditions is caused by the aging process?
    A. diabetic retinopathy
    B. retinitis pigmentosa
    C. exophthalmos
    D. macular degeneration

15. What condition involves the eighth cranial nerve that connects the ear to the brain?
    A. acoustic neuroma
    B. cholesteatoma
    C. tympanic membrane perforation
    D. cerumen impaction

16. The condition that is known to be hereditary is
    A. hyperopia.
    B. retinitis pigmentosa.
    C. macular degeneration.
    D. detached retina.

17. The structure that runs from the middle ear space to the pharynx is called the
    A. ossicle.
    B. semicircular canal.
    C. vestibule.
    D. auditory (pharyngotympanic) tube.

18. The test that might be performed to diagnose balance problems is called
    A. Weber test.
    B. electronystagmography.
    C. tympanometry.
    D. Rinne test.

19. Children who appear "cross-eyed" have a condition of ocular misalignment called
    A. retinopathy.
    B. strabismus.
    C. amblyopia.
    D. nystagmus.

20. Which of these is *not* a procedure to repair a torn or detached retina?
    A. trabeculectomy
    B. cryoretinopexy
    C. scleral buckling
    D. retinal photocoagulation

Application and Analysis

CASE STUDIES

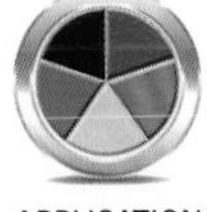

APPLICATION

Exercise 60

Read the case studies, and circle the correct letter for each of the questions.

CASE 7-1

Mr. Larson was working with a compressor when the hose broke loose and he was injured from the blast of air pressure that was released near the right side of his head. He suddenly could not hear out of his right ear. He was sent to an otorhinolaryngologist for evaluation. Mr. Larson described symptoms of vertigo as well as right-sided hearing loss. An audiogram revealed pronounced hearing loss at between 4,000 and 8,000 Hz (**Figure 7-22**). The diagnosis was sensorineural hearing loss due to blast injury with accompanying tinnitus.

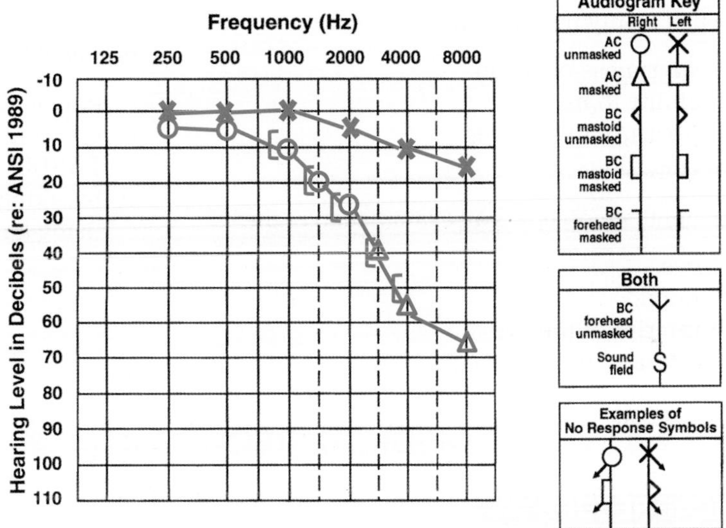

Figure 7-22 Audiogram revealing sensorineural hearing loss on the right side.

1. An otorhinolaryngologist, such as the one seen by Mr. Larson, specializes in

   A. eyes.
   B. ears, nose, and throat.
   C. vision.
   D. hearing aids.

2. Vertigo refers to which of these symptoms?

   A. hearing loss
   B. pressure sensation in the ears
   C. noise in the ears
   D. spinning sensation, dizziness

3. Tinnitus is defined as the perception of various noises in the ear, such as

   A. ringing.
   B. buzzing.
   C. humming.
   D. all of the above

4. The audiogram was a recording of

   A. eardrum movement.
   B. the middle ear space.
   C. hearing measurement.
   D. eye movements in response to electrical stimulation.

5. Hz is the abbreviation for a
   A. unit of measure of sound frequency.
   B. hearing test.
   C. unit for expressing the intensity of sound.
   D. two-pronged steel bar whose vibrations produce pure tones.

CASE 7-2

Mrs. Holtzinger failed the eye test when she tried to renew her driver's license. She went to an ophthalmologist for evaluation of her vision problem. Visual acuity testing was performed using a Snellen chart. Ophthalmoscopy was also performed. The diagnosis was cataracts in both eyes (OU). It was recommended that she be scheduled for phacoemulsification and lens replacement.

6. An ophthalmologist specializes in
   A. ears, nose, and throat.
   B. eyes.
   C. hearing.
   D. making corrective lenses.

7. Visual acuity testing is the testing for
   A. sharpness of vision.
   B. ability to hear.
   C. pressure in the eyes.
   D. chalazions.

8. An ophthalmoscopy is an examination of the
   A. eye.
   B. pupil.
   C. interior of the eye.
   D. sclera.

9. A cataract is
   A. increased pressure in the eye.
   B. clouding of the lens of the eye.
   C. detachment of the retina.
   D. hemorrhage of the choroid.

10. In phacoemulsification, a cataract is removed by
   A. enucleation.
   B. cryoretinopexy.
   C. LASIK.
   D. breaking up the lens by vibration using a needle probe.

MEDICAL RECORD ANALYSIS

MEDICAL RECORD 7-1

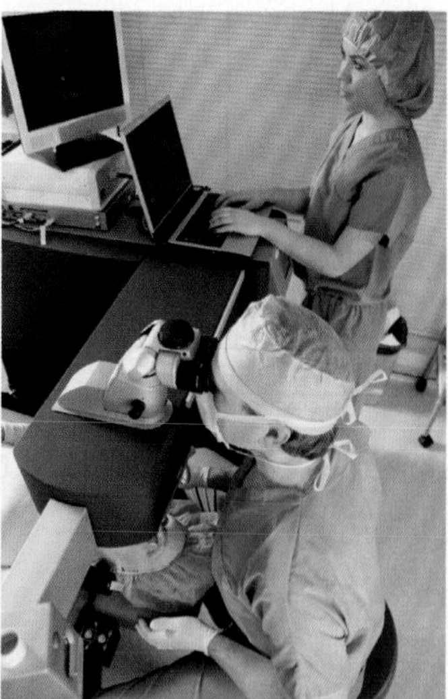

An ophthalmic technologist assists an ophthalmologist who is performing LASIK surgery.

You are the ophthalmic technologist for Dr. Brunner. Patient Nikita Stewart is here for a postoperative refraction after undergoing LASIK surgery two weeks ago. The operative report for her LASIK surgery, during which you served as Dr. Brunner's assistant, is as follows:

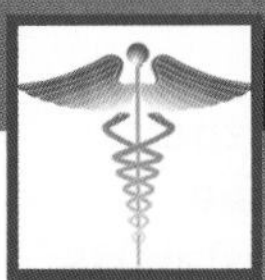

Medical Record

LASIK SURGERY REPORT

PREOPERATIVE DIAGNOSIS: Myopia, right eye

POSTOPERATIVE DIAGNOSIS: Myopia, right eye

OPERATION: LASIK, right eye

SURGEON: Thomas Brunner, MD

Refraction and preoperative testing were performed two weeks ago. At that time, the patient underwent computerized topographic analysis via video keratography to map the surface of the eye. Corneal thickness and corneal surface elevations were measured. Tonometry revealed normal intraocular pressure. Slitlamp biomicroscopy was performed to ensure that there were no contraindications for the procedure. The retina appeared normal. The patient signed an informed consent for the procedure after the risks and benefits were explained in detail. The patient was given Valium for preoperative sedation to be taken 30 minutes prior to surgery.

On arrival today, topographic analysis was repeated to confirm all measurements. Measurements were then entered into the laser's computer. Patient was brought into the operating room and placed in a supine position on the table. Ophthalmic anesthetic drops were instilled into the right eye, and the eye was disinfected. A speculum was placed in the right eye for lid retraction. Reference marks were made for laser alignment.

A suction ring was applied to the eye, and the cornea was flattened. A small incision was made using the microkeratome to create a flap. The flap was lifted to reveal the underlying stromal tissue. Using the excimer laser, the cornea was contoured to the predetermined measurements. The eye was then irrigated, and the flap was repositioned. The suction ring and speculum were removed.

The patient tolerated the procedure well. Postoperative instructions and medications were given to the patient, and she was discharged home in the care of her husband. She is to return in two weeks for postoperative follow-up and refraction.

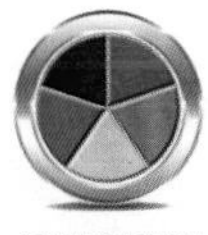

APPLICATION

Exercise 61

Read the medical report and circle the correct letter for each of the questions.

1. The term myopia means that the patient

A. is farsighted.
B. has presbyopia.
C. is nearsighted.
D. has macular degeneration.

2. The test done to measure the patient's intraocular pressure was

A. tonometry.
B. refraction.
C. topographic analysis.
D. keratography.

3. The term that means the patient's refractive errors were measured is

A. keratography.
B. refraction.
C. tonometry.
D. topographic analysis.

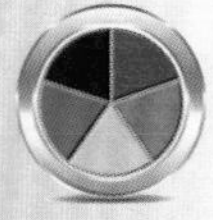

Exercise 62

Write the appropriate medical terms used in this medical record on the blanks after their definitions. Note that not all the terms appear in the chapter, but you should be able to identify these terms based on word parts that are included in this chapter.

1. relating to the cornea ____________________

2. inside the eye ____________________

3. instrument for making small cuts in the cornea ____________________

4. process of recording the cornea ____________________

Bonus Question

5. The term that describes an instrument that opens a body part for examination or procedures is ____________________

MEDICAL RECORD 7-2

You are an audiologist working in an otorhinolaryngology office. One month ago, a child was referred to your office by his pediatrician for an ear problem. You performed the audiometry test to assess the patient's hearing loss.

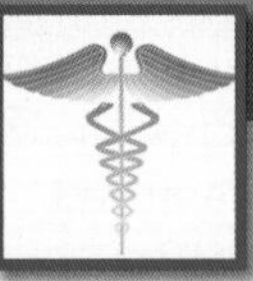

Medical Record

OTORHINOLARYNGOLOGY CONSULTATION REPORT

Thank you for your kind referral of Kenny Mason. Kenny was seen today because of a right tympanic membrane perforation noted by you on recent examination. Kenny previously had a perforation of the right ear in February of 20XX, after he had been hit on the ear with a ladder. This perforation healed spontaneously in several weeks. He had no postinjury infections or complications.

On questioning today, Kenny admits that he was hit in the right ear with a soccer ball about 1½ weeks ago and has had some tinnitus and dysacusis in the right ear since that time.

The medical history is unremarkable with the exception of bilateral tympanostomies with insertion of tympanostomy tubes at age 3 and a tonsillectomy at age 10. He is otherwise in good health.

Examination today is unremarkable with the exception of an anterior superior tympanic membrane perforation with purulent otorrhea in the right ear. Audiometry done in the office revealed a significant conductive hearing loss in the right ear. The left ear was normal.

I prescribed otic antibiotic drops to be instilled in the right ear q.i.d. I instructed Kenny's mother to make sure that his ear stays dry at all times. We will adopt an expectant attitude toward this perforation. I think that there is a good chance that it will heal on its own. I will see Kenny back for a recheck in one month. If it has not healed at that time, we will schedule him for a right tympanoplasty.

Thank you for referring this pleasant young man to me. I will keep you updated regarding his status.

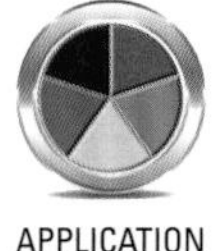
APPLICATION

Exercise 63

Write the appropriate medical terms used in this medical record on the blanks after their definitions.

1. measurement of hearing ____________________
2. discharge from the ear ____________________
3. pertaining to the ear ____________________
4. surgical repair of the eardrum ____________________
5. condition of impaired hearing ____________________
6. hole in the eardrum ____________________
7. pertaining to the tympanic membrane or cavity ____________________
8. ringing noise in the ear ____________________
9. surgical opening in the eardrums ____________________
10. hearing loss due to blockage of sound transmission through the external and middle ear ____________________

Bonus Questions

11. The record indicates that the patient has an *anterior superior* tympanic membrane perforation. Based on what you have learned previously, describe the location of the perforation on the tympanic membrane. ____________________

____

12. What did the results of Kenny's audiometry reveal? ____________________

____

Pronunciation and Spelling

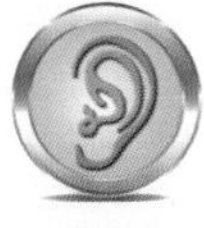
AUDITORY

Exercise 64

Review the Chapter 7 terms in the Dictionary/Audio Glossary in the Student Resources, and practice pronouncing each term, referring to the pronunciation guide as needed.

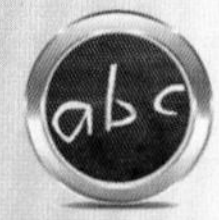

SPELLING

Exercise 65

Circle the correctly spelled term.

1.	tarsel	tarsal	tarrsal
2.	koroid	choroyd	choroid
3.	vitreous	vitrious	vitreus
4.	corneal	cornial	korneal
5.	ophthallmology	ophthalmology	ophtholmology
6.	chalazion	kalazion	calazion
7.	diploplia	diplopea	diplopia
8.	glawcoma	gluacoma	glaucoma
9.	nystagmus	nistagmus	nystagmis
10.	presbiopia	presbyopia	presbyopea
11.	pterygium	pterigium	pterygeum
12.	strabysmus	strabismus	strabismis
13.	florescien	flurescien	fluorescein
14.	refraction	refracshun	refraktion
15.	Snellin	Snelen	Snellen
16.	pupilometry	pupillometry	pupellometry
17.	aquity	acuwity	acuity
18.	catarect	catarract	cataract
19.	midreatic	mydriatic	midriatic
20.	optishun	optician	optishian

Media Connection

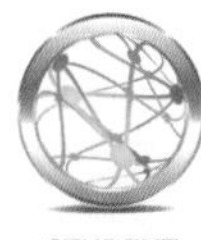
STUDENT RESOURCES

Exercise 66

Complete each of the following activities available with the Student Resources on thePoint. Check off each activity as you complete it, and record your score for the Chapter Quiz in the space provided.

Chapter Exercises

_____ Flash Cards
_____ Concentration
_____ Abbreviation Match-Up
_____ Roboterms
_____ Word Anatomy
_____ Fill the Gap
_____ Break It Down
_____ True/False Body Building
_____ Quiz Show
_____ Complete the Case
_____ Medical Record Review
_____ Look and Label
_____ Image Matching
_____ Spelling Bee

________ **Chapter Quiz** *Score:*________%

Additional Resources

_____ Video: Audiometry
_____ Dictionary/Audio Glossary
_____ Health Professions Careers: Ophthalmic Technologist
_____ Health Professions Careers: Audiologist

Endocrine System

8

Chapter Outline

Introduction, 272

Anatomy and Physiology, 272
- Structures, 272
- Functions, 272
- Terms Related to the Endocrine System, 272

Word Parts, 279
- Combining Forms, 279
- Prefixes, 279
- Suffixes, 279

Medical Terms, 282
- Adjectives and Other Related Terms, 282
- Medical Conditions, 283
- Tests and Procedures, 291
- Surgical Interventions and Therapeutic Procedures, 293
- Medications and Drug Therapies, 294
- Specialties and Specialists, 295
- Abbreviations, 296

Wrapping Up, 297

Chapter Review, 298

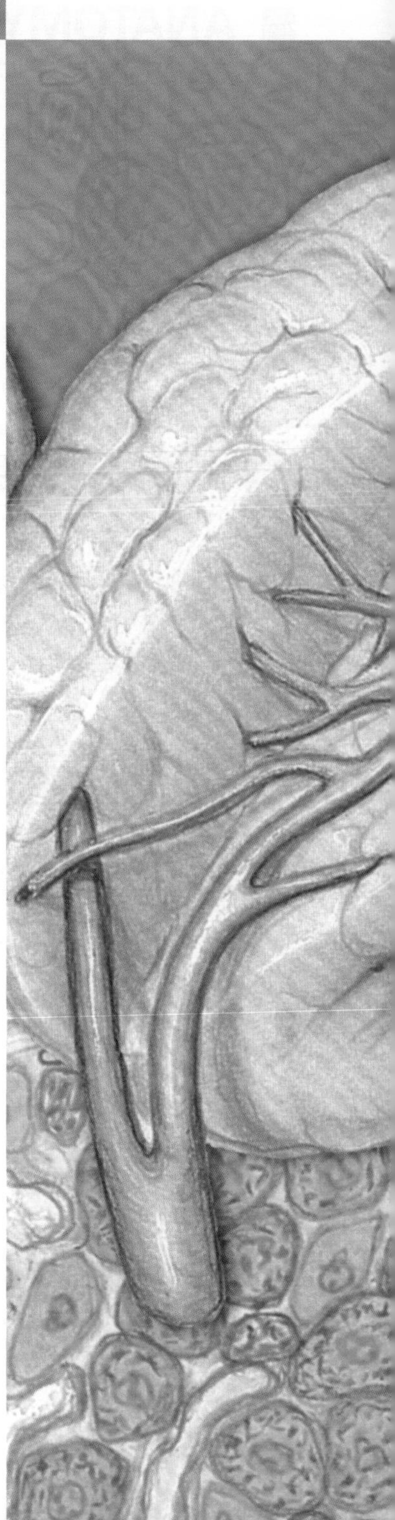

Learning Outcomes

After completing this chapter, you should be able to:

1. List the structures and functions of the endocrine system.
2. Describe the locations of main structures in the endocrine system.
3. Define terms related to the anatomy and physiology of the endocrine system.
4. Define combining forms, prefixes, and suffixes related to the endocrine system.
5. Define common medical terminology related to the endocrine system, including adjectives and related terms; signs, symptoms, and medical conditions; tests and procedures, surgical interventions and therapeutic procedures; medications and drug therapies; and medical specialties and specialists.
6. Define common abbreviations related to the endocrine system.
7. Successfully complete all chapter exercises.
8. Explain terms used in case studies and medical records involving the endocrine system.
9. Successfully complete all exercises included with the companion Student Resources on thePoint.

INTRODUCTION

The endocrine system, consisting of glands and hormones, is devoted to maintaining homeostasis. Organized masses of cells called glands have no ducts; they secrete their chemical products, called hormones, directly into the bloodstream. The nervous system works with the endocrine system; therefore, these systems are often referred to as the neuroendocrine system. The endocrine system affects all body systems, so its effects—both normal and abnormal—are widespread.

ANATOMY AND PHYSIOLOGY

Structures

- Endocrine glands are ductless glands that secrete hormones directly into the bloodstream.
- Glands and organs include the hypothalamus, pineal gland, pituitary gland, thyroid gland, parathyroid glands, thymus gland, adrenal glands, islets of Langerhans in the pancreas, ovaries in the female, and testes in the male.

Functions

- Producing, storing, and releasing hormones directly into the bloodstream for use by other organs
- Controlling and coordinating functions such as metabolism, reproduction, growth, and development

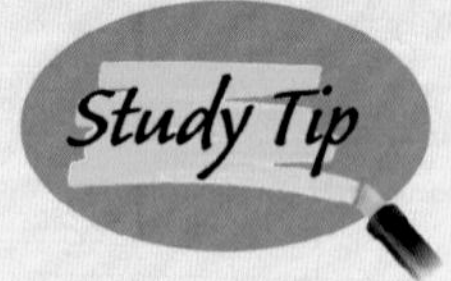

Endocrine: The word endocrine comes from the English prefix *endo-*, meaning within, and the Greek word *krinein,* meaning to secrete. The endocrine glands secrete directly into the bloodstream rather than through ducts.

Terms Related to the Endocrine System (Figure 8-1)

Term	Pronunciation	Meaning
Glands and Organs		
adrenal glands; *syn.* suprarenal glands	ă-drē′năl glandz; sū′pră-rē′năl glandz	triangular-shaped glands located above each kidney that secrete hormones that aid in metabolism, electrolyte balance, and stress reactions; each gland consists of an outer part called the adrenal cortex, and an inner part called the adrenal medulla
hypothalamus	hī′pō-thal′ă-mŭs	part of the brain located near the pituitary gland that secretes releasing hormones that control the release of other hormones by the pituitary gland
islets of Langerhans	ī′lets ov lahng′ĕr-hahnz	endocrine cells inside the pancreas that secrete hormones (glucagon and insulin) that aid carbohydrate (sugar) metabolism (**Figure 8-2**)
ovaries	ō′vă-rēz	paired female reproductive organs that produce hormones and release oocytes (egg cells)
parathyroid glands	par′ă-thī′royd glandz	four small glands embedded on the posterior surface of the thyroid gland that regulate calcium and phosphorus levels in the bloodstream

(continued)

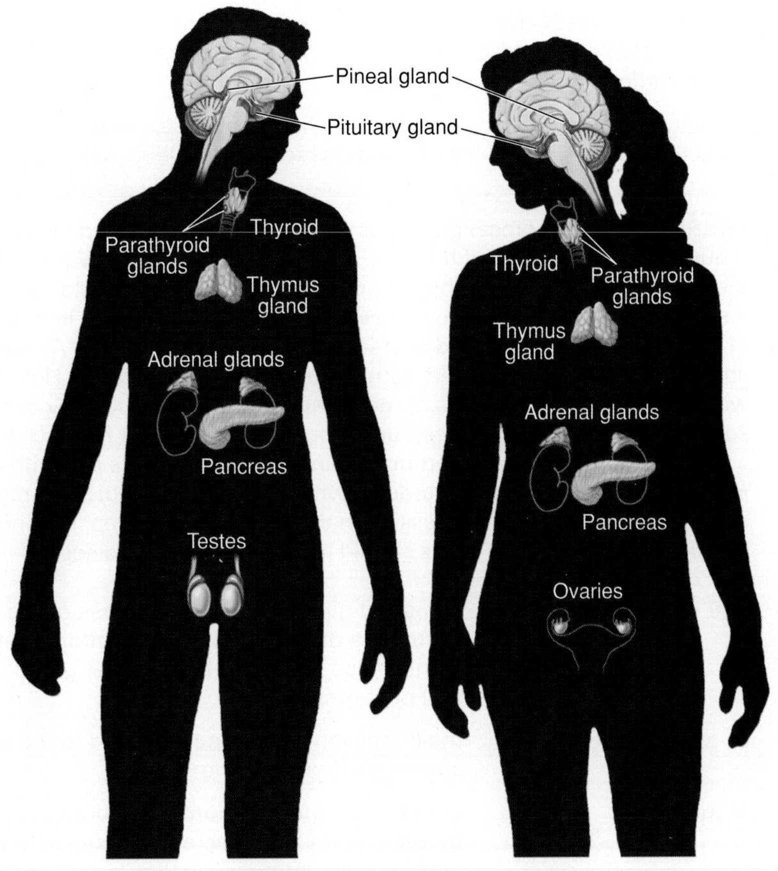

Figure 8-1 The endocrine system.

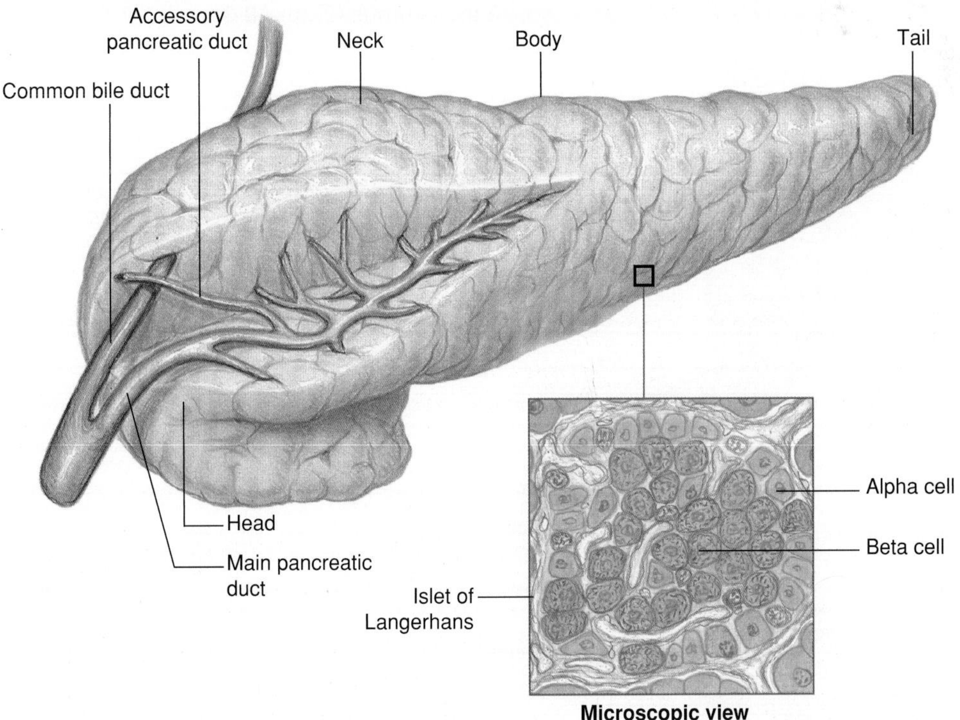

Figure 8-2 The pancreas, islets of Langerhans, and adjacent structures.

Terms Related to the Endocrine System *(continued)*

Term	Pronunciation	Meaning
pineal gland; *syn.* pineal body	pin′ē-ăl gland; pin′ē-ăl bod′ē	small, cone-shaped gland located in the brain that secretes melatonin, which affects sleep-wake cycles and reproduction

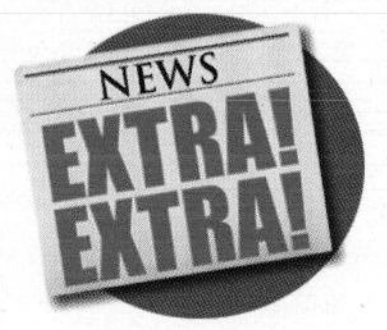

PINEAL GLAND The pineal gland sits deep inside the brain and was once thought to be the center of the soul. As research emerged, it was found that the only hormone secreted by the pineal gland is melatonin. Melatonin is instrumental in the circadian, or sleep-wake, cycle in the body. Increased levels of melatonin cause sleep and decreased levels cause alertness. As we age, the amount of melatonin secreted from the pineal gland decreases. However, when we are young, large amounts of melatonin are secreted. This may explain why some younger people can sleep until noon or later! Recent research has also linked light exposure from computers and computer tablets use with decreased levels of melatonin. College students who used their computers at night experienced melatonin suppression in the hours before sleep, leading to sleep disturbances. (Normally, levels should increase just before sleep.)

Term	Pronunciation	Meaning
pituitary gland	pi-tū′i-tār′ē gland	pea-sized gland located at the base of the brain that secretes hormones that stimulate the function of other endocrine glands; also known as the "master gland"; divided into anterior and posterior lobes
testes; *syn.* testicles	tes′tēz; tes′tĭ-kĕlz	male reproductive glands, located in the scrotum, that produce sperm and testosterone
thymus gland	thī′mŭs gland	gland in the mediastinum (membranous partition in the thoracic cavity) that secretes thymosin, a hormone that regulates the immune system
thyroid gland	thī′royd gland	bilobed gland located in the neck that secretes thyroid hormone that is needed for cell growth and metabolism; the largest endocrine gland; has two lobes connected by a tissue called the isthmus (**Figure 8-3**)

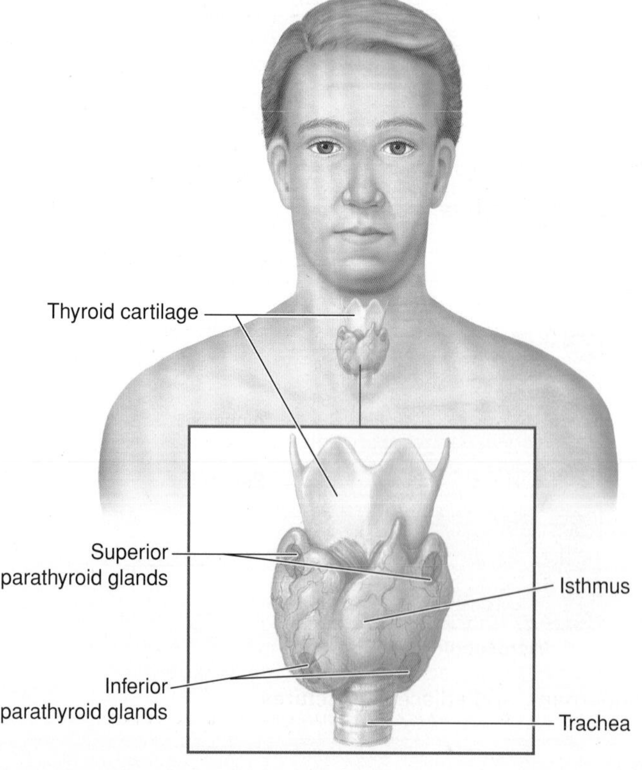

Figure 8-3 The thyroid gland, parathyroid glands, and adjacent structures. The parathyroid glands are on the posterior surface of the thyroid gland but are highlighted in this anterior view.

Terms Related to the Endocrine System

Term	Pronunciation	Meaning
Hormones (Figure 8-4)		
Anterior Pituitary Gland		
adrenocorticotropic hormone (ACTH)	ă-drē′nō-kōr′ti-kō-trō′pik hōr′mōn	targets the adrenal cortex; stimulates secretion of corticosteroids
follicle-stimulating hormone (FSH)	fol′i-kĕl-stim′yū-lā′ting hōr′mōn	targets the ovaries and testes; stimulates secretion of estrogen in females and testosterone in males
growth hormone (GH)	grōth hōr′mōn	targets bones and other tissues; stimulates protein synthesis and body growth
luteinizing hormone (LH)	lū′tē-in-ī-zing hōr′mōn	targets the ovaries and testes; stimulates secretion of progesterone in females and testosterone in males
prolactin	prō-lak′tin	targets breast tissue; stimulates milk production
thyroid-stimulating hormone (TSH)	thī′royd-stim′yū-lā′ting hōr′mōn	targets the thyroid gland; stimulates the production of thyroid hormones for regulating metabolism

(continued)

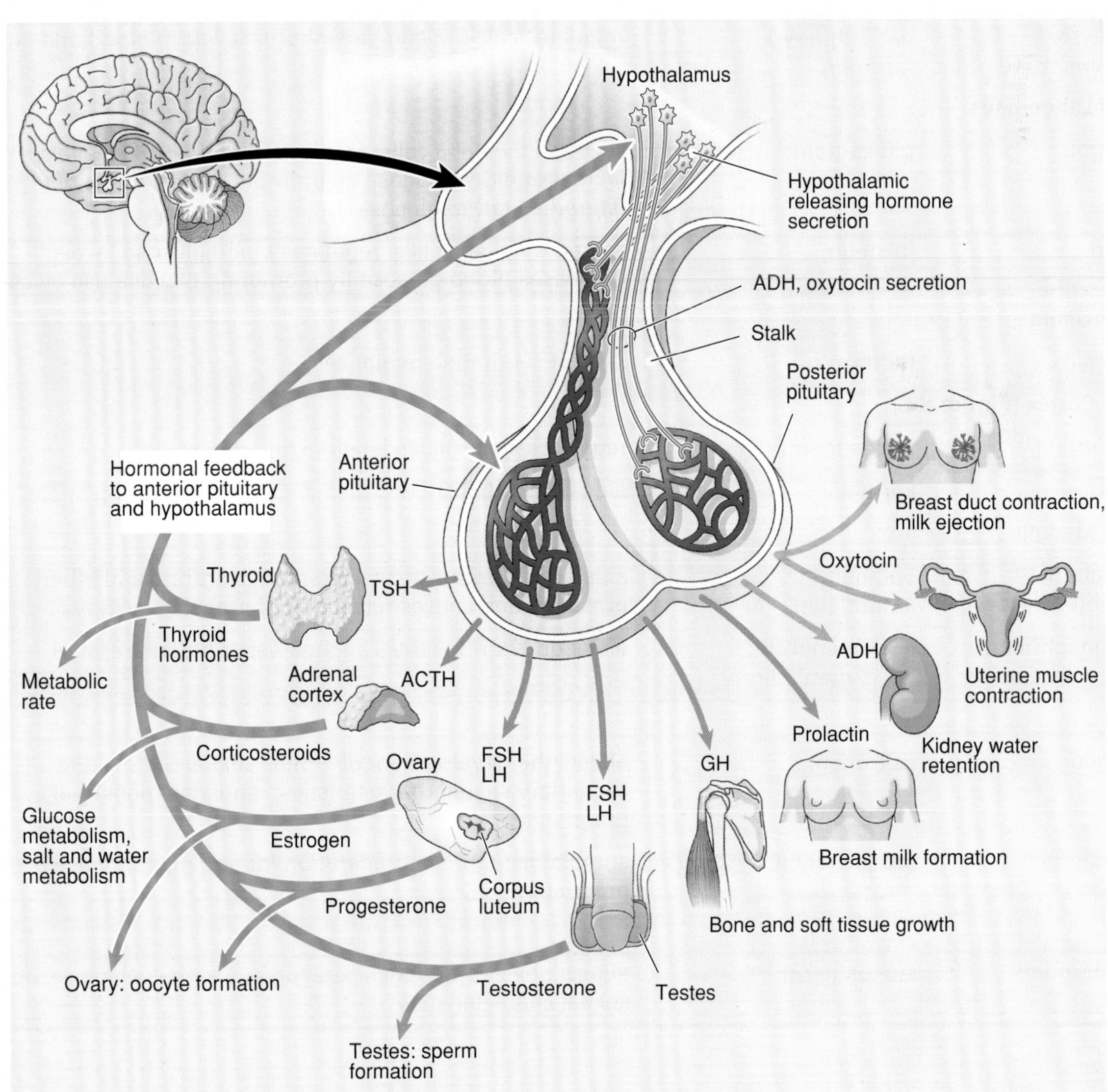

Figure 8-4 The hypothalamus, pituitary gland, and target organs and tissues. Arrows indicate targets and subsequent secretions.

Terms Related to the Endocrine System *(continued)*

Term	Pronunciation	Meaning
Posterior Pituitary Gland		
antidiuretic hormone (ADH); *syn.* vasopressin	an′tē-dī-yū-ret′ik hōr′mōn; vā′sō-pres′in	targets the kidneys; stimulates water reabsorption by the kidneys
oxytocin (OXT)	ok′sē-tō′sin	targets the uterus and breasts; stimulates uterine contractions and milk ejection from breasts
Pineal Gland		
melatonin	mel′ă-tōn′in	affects sleep-wake cycles and reproduction
Thyroid Gland		
thyroxine (T_4)	thī-rok′sēn	hormone that regulates metabolism by increasing metabolic rate
triiodothyronine (T_3)	trī′ī-ō′dō-thī′rō-nēn	hormone that regulates metabolism; similar to thyroxine but has greater potency
Parathyroid Glands		
parathyroid hormone (PTH)	par′ă-thī′royd hōr′mōn	regulates calcium and phosphorus levels in blood and bones
Islets of Langerhans		
glucagon	glū′kă-gon	secreted by alpha cells; regulates blood glucose levels; increases blood glucose by promoting breakdown of glycogen (stored sugar) to glucose
insulin	in′sŭ-lin	secreted by beta cells; regulates blood glucose levels; decreases blood glucose by promoting glucose use by cells
Thymus Gland		
thymosin	thī′mō-sin	regulates immune responses
Adrenal Cortex (Figure 8-5)		
aldosterone	al-dos′tĕr-ōn	regulates electrolytes (sodium and potassium)
cortisol	kōr′ti-sol	aids in metabolism and also aids the body during stress
Adrenal Medulla (Figure 8-5)		
epinephrine; *syn.* adrenaline	ep′i-nef′rin; ă-dren′ă-lin	aids body during stress, increases heart rate and blood pressure, and causes relaxation of bronchial airways
norepinephrine; *syn.* noradrenaline	nōr′ep-i-nef′rin; nor′ă-dren′ă-lin	aids body during stress and increases blood pressure
Ovaries		
estrogen	es′trō-jen	affects the development of female sexual organs and secondary sexual characteristics; regulates menstrual cycle and pregnancy
progesterone	prō-jes′tĕr-ōn	stimulates uterus in preparation for and maintenance of pregnancy
Testes		
testosterone	tes-tos′tĕ-rōn	affects development of sexual organs in males and secondary sexual characteristics

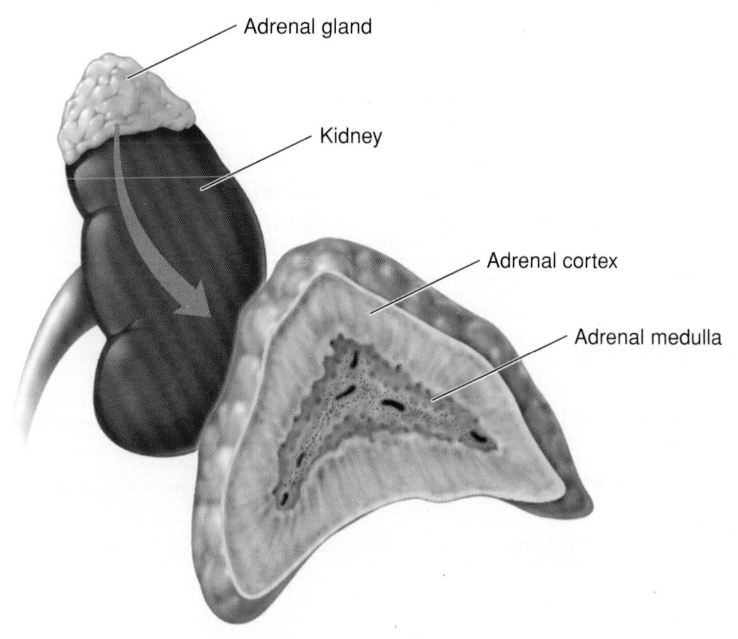

Figure 8-5 The adrenal glands are positioned above each kidney and have an inner medulla and an outer cortex.

Exercises: Anatomy and Physiology

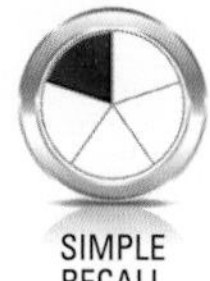

Exercise 1

Write the correct gland or organ for the meaning given.

1. pea-sized gland at the base of the brain pituitary gland
2. triangular-shaped glands above each kidney adrenal glands
3. endocrine cells inside the pancreas islets of Langerhans
4. bilobed endocrine gland located near the larynx thyroid gland
5. four small glands embedded in the thyroid parathyroid glands
6. cone-shaped gland in the brain pineal gland
7. part of the brain that controls the release of hormones by the pituitary gland ________
8. gland that affects the immune system ________
9. organs that secrete estrogen and progesterone ________

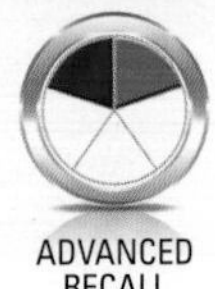

ADVANCED RECALL

Exercise 2

Match each medical term with its meaning.

thyroxine	prolactin	aldosterone
growth hormone	oxytocin	melatonin
parathyroid hormone	insulin	follicle-stimulating hormone

1. regulates body growth ____________________
2. regulates metabolism ____________________
3. regulates ovaries and testes ____________________
4. regulates calcium levels in blood ____________________
5. stimulates milk production ____________________
6. stimulates uterine contractions ____________________
7. regulates electrolyte levels ____________________
8. regulates sleep-wake cycles ____________________
9. regulates blood glucose levels ____________________

ADVANCED RECALL

Exercise 3

Complete each sentence by writing in the correct medical term(s).

1. The hormone that regulates calcium and phosphorus levels in the blood and bones is ____________________.
2. ____________________, the hormone secreted by the thymus gland, regulates immune responses.
3. ____________________ stimulates the adrenal cortex.
4. The secretion of progesterone in females and testosterone in males is stimulated by ____________________, the hormone secreted by the anterior pituitary gland.
5. The thyroid gland is stimulated by ____________________.
6. ____________________ and ____________________ are produced by the thyroid gland and help regulate metabolism.
7. The posterior pituitary gland secretes ____________________, the hormone that stimulates the kidneys to reabsorb water.
8. Testosterone is secreted by the ____________________.
9. The glands that produce the hormones that aid in regulating the menstrual cycle are the ____________________.
10. The adrenal cortex produces ____________________, which aids the body during stress.

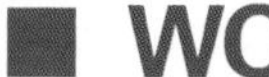

WORD PARTS

The following tables list word parts related to the endocrine system.

Combining Forms

Combining Form	Meaning
acr/o	extremity, tip
aden/o	gland
adren/o	adrenal glands
adrenal/o	adrenal glands
calc/i	calcium
cortic/o	cortex
crin/o	to secrete
dips/o	thirst
endocrin/o	endocrine
gluc/o, glucos/o	glucose, sugar
glyc/o, glycos/o	glucose, sugar
hormon/o	hormone
kal/i	potassium
natr/i	sodium
pancreat/o	pancreas
parathyroid/o	parathyroid glands
thym/o	thymus gland
thyr/o, thyroid/o	thyroid gland

Prefixes

Prefix	Meaning
eu-	good, normal
hyper-	above, excessive
hypo-	below, deficient
poly-	many, much

Suffixes

Suffix	Meaning
-al, -ic	pertaining to
-emia	blood
-ism	condition of
-megaly	enlargement

(continued)

Suffixes *(continued)*

Suffix	Meaning
-oid	resembling
-osis	abnormal condition
-penia	deficiency
-uria	urine, urination

Exercises: Word Parts

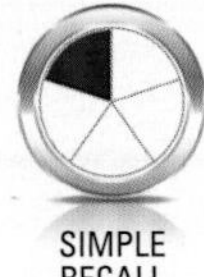

SIMPLE RECALL

Exercise 4

Write the meaning of the combining form given.

1. glucos/o ______
2. cortic/o ______
3. thyr/o ______
4. kal/i ______
5. crin/o ______
6. dips/o ______
7. gluc/o ______
8. natr/i ______

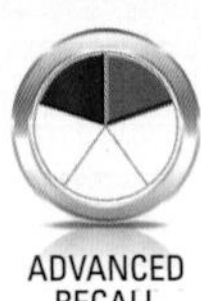

ADVANCED RECALL

Exercise 5

Considering the meaning of the suffix used in the medical term, write the meaning of the medical term.

Suffix	Meaning	Medical Term	Meaning of Term
-ectomy	excision, surgical removal	adrenalectomy	1. ______
-penia	deficiency	calcipenia	2. ______
-al	pertaining to	hormonal	3. ______
-megaly	enlargement	acromegaly	4. ______
-tomy	incision	thyroidotomy	5. ______
-itis	inflammation	thymitis	6. ______
-ectomy	excision, surgical removal	parathyroidectomy	7. ______
-logist	one who specializes in	endocrinologist	8. ______

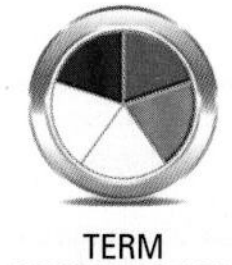
TERM CONSTRUCTION

Exercise 6

For each term, first write the meaning of the term. Then write the meaning of the word parts in that term.

1. hypothyroidism ______________________

hypo- ______________________

thyroid/o ______________________

-ism ______________________

2. pancreatic ______________________

pancreat/o ______________________

-ic ______________________

3. euthyroid ______________________

eu- ______________________

thyr/o ______________________

-oid ______________________

4. glycosuria ______________________

glyc/o ______________________

-uria ______________________

5. hyperglycemia ______________________

hyper- ______________________

glyc/o ______________________

-emia ______________________

6. adrenopathy ______________________

adren/o ______________________

-pathy ______________________

7. polydipsia ______________________

poly- ______________________

dips/o ______________________

-ia ______________________

8. adenosis ______________________

aden/o ______________________

-osis ______________________

■ MEDICAL TERMS

The following table gives adjective forms and terms used in describing the endocrine system and its conditions.

Adjectives and Other Related Terms

Term	Pronunciation	Meaning
cortical	kōr'ti-kăl	pertaining to the cortex
endogenous	en-doj'ĕ-nŭs	produced inside the body
euthyroid	yū'thī-royd	normal thyroid
exogenous	eks-oj'ĕ-nŭs	produced outside of the body
metabolism	mĕ-tab'ō-lizm	all physical and chemical changes that occur in tissues
pancreatic	pan'rē-at'ik	pertaining to the pancreas
postprandial	pōst-pran'dē-ăl	after a meal
thymic	thī'mik	pertaining to the thymus gland

■ Exercises: Adjectives and Other Related Terms

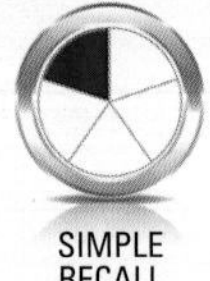
SIMPLE RECALL

Exercise 7

Write the correct medical term for the meaning given.

1. pertaining to the cortex ____________________
2. produced outside the body ____________________
3. pertaining to the pancreas ____________________
4. pertaining to the thymus gland ____________________
5. produced inside the body ____________________

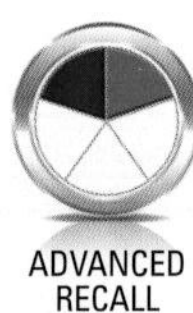
ADVANCED RECALL

Exercise 8

Complete each sentence by writing in the correct medical term.

1. The term that denotes a normal thyroid is ____________________.
2. A disease that is related to the pancreas is considered to be ____________________.
3. All physical and chemical changes that occur in tissues are called ____________________.
4. A hormonal change related to the thymus is ____________________.
5. Hormones that are not produced by the body are ____________________ hormones.

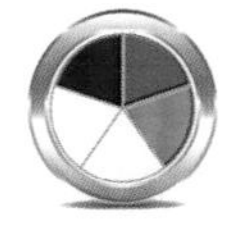

TERM CONSTRUCTION

Exercise 9

Write the combining form used in the medical term, followed by the meaning of the combining form.

Term	Combining Form	Combining Form Meaning
1. thymic	______	______
2. cortical	______	______
3. adrenal	______	______
4. euthyroid	______	______
5. pancreatic	______	______
6. hormonal	______	______

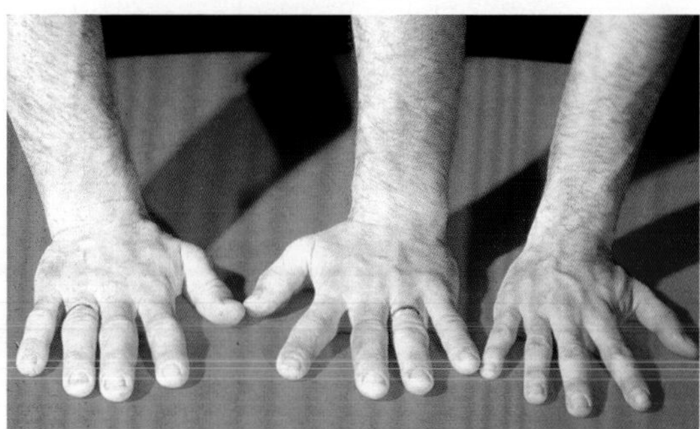

Figure 8-6 Comparison of patient with normal hand (far right) and hands of a patient with acromegaly.

Medical Conditions

Term	Pronunciation	Meaning
acidemia	as′i-dē′mē-ă	abnormally low blood pH (below 7.35)
acidosis	as′i-dō′sis	pathologic state characterized by an excessively acidic condition of the body fluids or tissues
acromegaly	ak′rō-meg′ă-lē	disorder caused by excessive growth hormone secretion in adulthood causing thick bones in the extremities, especially the hands and feet (**Figure 8-6**)
Addison disease	ad′i-sŏn di-zēz′	disorder in which the adrenal glands do not produce sufficient cortisol; characterized by skin darkening, weakness, and loss of appetite (**Figure 8-7**)
adenitis	ad′ĕ-nī′tis	inflammation of a lymph node or gland
adenomegaly	ad′ĕ-nō-meg′ă-lē	enlargement of a gland

(continued)

Medical Conditions *(continued)*

Term	Pronunciation	Meaning
adrenalitis	ă-drē-năl-ī′tis	inflammation of an adrenal gland
adrenomegaly	ă-drē-nō-meg′ă-lē	enlargement of an adrenal gland
adrenalopathy	ă-drē-nă-lop′ă-thē	disease of the adrenal gland
alkalemia	al-kă-lē′mē-ă	abnormally high blood pH (above 7.45)
autoimmune disease	aw′tō-i-mūn′ di-zēz′	disorder in which normal tissue is destroyed by the body's own immune system response
calcipenia	kal′si-pē′nē-ă	deficiency of calcium in tissues and body fluids
congenital hypothyroidism	kon-jen′i-tăl hī′pō-thī′royd-izm	condition that is present at birth and is caused by thyroid hormone deficiency due to absence or atrophy of the thyroid gland; leads to mental deficiency and dwarfism (formerly known as cretinism)
Cushing syndrome	kush′ing sin′drōm	disease caused by excessive cortisol production by the adrenal glands; characterized by fat pads in the chest and abdomen and a "moon face" appearance (**Figure 8-8**)
diabetes insipidus (DI)	dī′ă-bē′tēz in-sip′i-dŭs	disorder caused by deficiency of antidiuretic hormone production by the pituitary gland resulting in excessive urination and excessive thirst
diabetes mellitus (DM)	dī-ă-bē′tēz mel′i-tŭs	disorder caused by deficiency of insulin and/or insulin resistance causing poor carbohydrate metabolism and high blood glucose levels

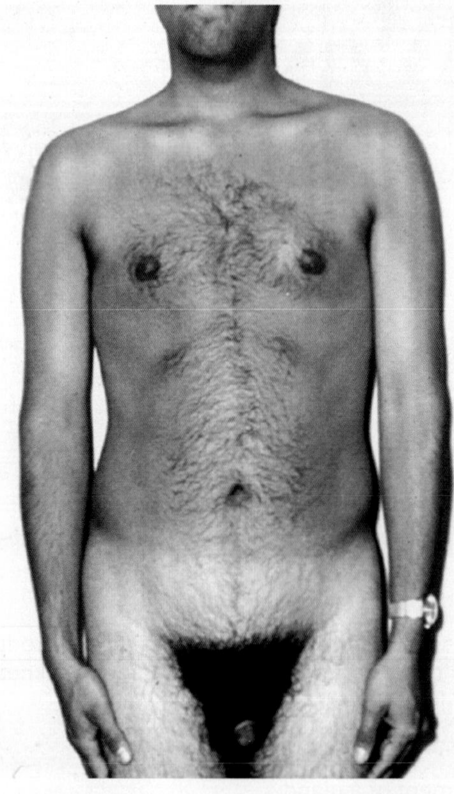

Figure 8-7 Darkening of the skin caused by Addison disease.

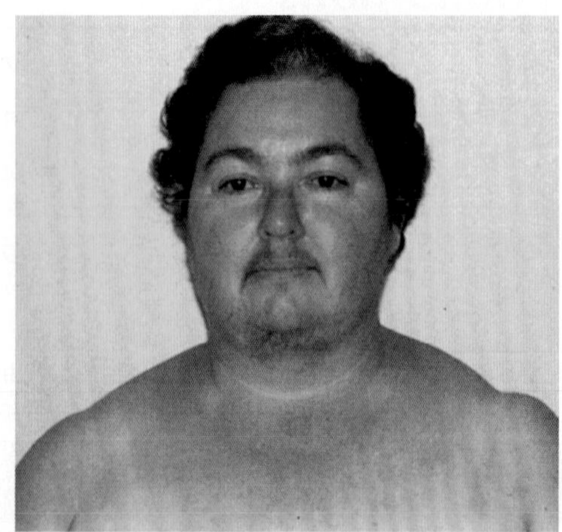

Figure 8-8 Patient with Cushing syndrome.

Medical Conditions

Term	Pronunciation	Meaning
Type 1 diabetes mellitus	tīp 1 dī-ă-bē'tēz mel'i-tŭs	diabetes caused by a total lack of insulin production; usually develops in childhood; patients require insulin replacement therapy to control the disorder
Type 2 diabetes mellitus	tīp 2 dī-ă-bē'tēz mel'i-tŭs	diabetes caused by either a lack of insulin or the body's inability to use insulin efficiently; usually develops in middle-aged or older adults; patients usually do not require insulin replacement therapy to control the disorder

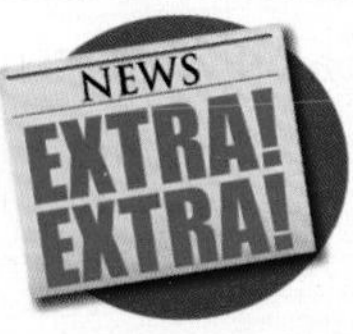

DIABETES MELLITUS The World Health Organization (WHO) calls the incidence of diabetes mellitus (DM) an epidemic and estimates that the number of people diagnosed with DM worldwide will double by the year 2030. In the United States, the high incidence of Type 2 DM is linked to an increase in obesity. The American Diabetes Association (ADA) recommends screening for DM for people with risk factors for Type 2 DM, which include the following:

- Obesity
- Age 45 years or older
- Family history of diabetes mellitus (parents or siblings with diabetes)
- Race/ethnicity (Black, Hispanic, Asian, Native American, Pacific Islanders)
- History of gestational diabetes
- Inactivity
- Smoking
- Cardiovascular disease
- Hypertension

Term	Pronunciation	Meaning
diabetic ketoacidosis (DKA)	dī'ă-bet'ik kē'tō-as'i-dō'sis	excessive ketones (compounds produced during fat metabolism) in blood due to breakdown of stored fats for energy; a complication of diabetes mellitus; if left untreated, can lead to coma and death
endocrinopathy	en'dō-kri-nop'ă-thē	disease of an endocrine gland
exophthalmos	ek'sof-thal'mos	protruding or bulging of eyes from their sockets (**Figure 8-9**)
gigantism; *syn.* giantism	jī-gan'tizm; jī'an-tizm	disorder caused by excessive growth hormone secretion before puberty; characterized by abnormally long bones (**Figure 8-10**)
glucosuria; *syn.* glycosuria	glū'kō-syū'rē-ă; glī'kō-syū'rē-ă	glucose (sugar) in the urine
goiter	goy'tĕr	enlargement of the thyroid gland (**Figure 8-11**)
Graves disease	grāvz di-zēz'	condition of excessive secretion of thyroid hormone, causing goiter and exophthalmos
Hashimoto thyroiditis; *syn.* Hashimoto disease	hah-shē-mō'tō thī'roy-dī'tis; hah-shē-mō'tō di-zēz'	autoimmune disease causing chronic thyroiditis

(continued)

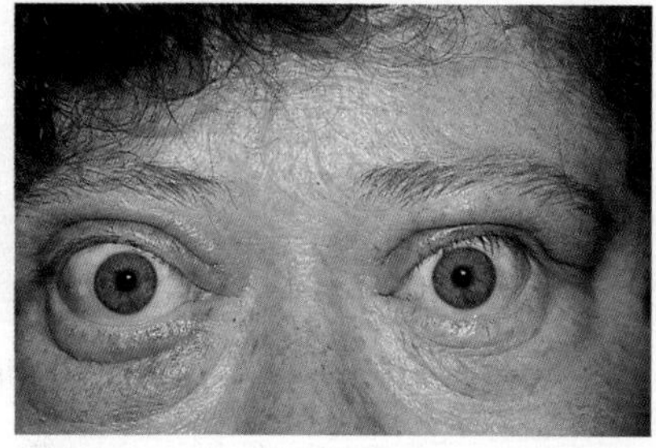

Figure 8-9 Patient with exophthalmos.

Medical Conditions *(continued)*

Term	Pronunciation	Meaning
hirsutism	hĭr′sū-tizm	excessive hair growth or hair growth in unusual places, especially in women (**Figure 8-12**)
hypercalcemia	hī′pĕr-kal-sē′mē-ă	high levels of calcium in the blood
hyperglycemia	hī′pĕr-glī-sē′mē-ă	high levels of glucose (sugar) in the blood
hyperkalemia	hī′pĕr-kă-lē′mē-ă	high levels of potassium in the blood
hypernatremia	hī′per-nă-trē′mē-ă	high levels of sodium in the blood
hyperparathyroidism	hī′pĕr-par′ă-thī′royd-izm	excessive hormone production by the parathyroid glands
hyperthyroidism	hī-per-thī′royd-izm	excessive hormone production by the thyroid gland
hypocalcemia	hī′pō-kal-sē′mē-ă	low levels of calcium in the blood
hypoglycemia	hī′pō-glī-sē′mē-ă	low levels of glucose (sugar) in the blood
hypokalemia	hī′pō-ka-lē′mē-ă	low levels of potassium in the blood
hyponatremia	hī′pō-nă-trē′mē-ă	low levels of sodium in the blood
hypoparathyroidism	hī′pō-par′ă-thī′royd-izm	deficient hormone production by the parathyroid glands

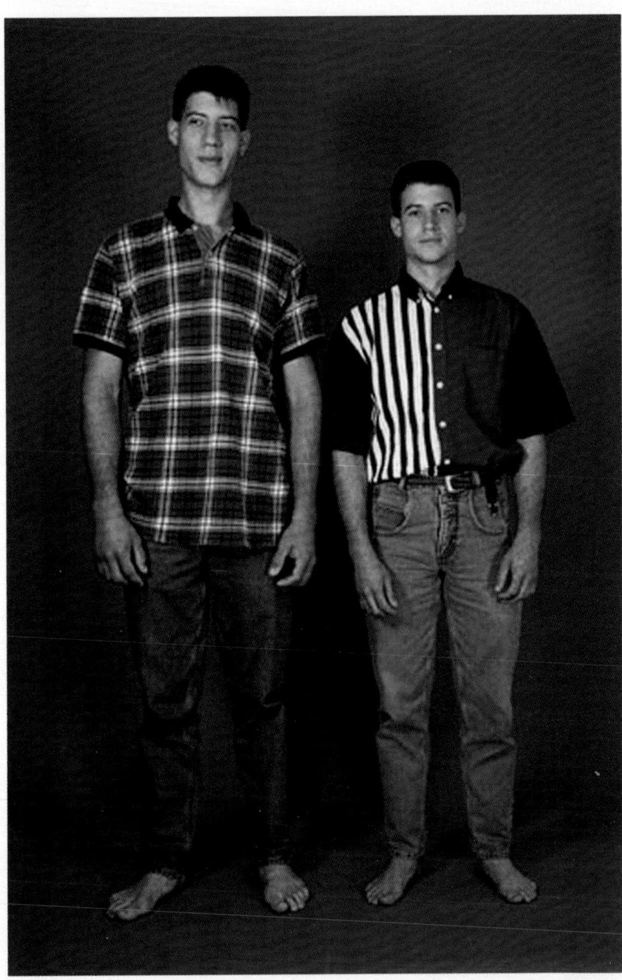

Figure 8-10 A 22-year-old man with gigantism due to excess growth hormone is shown next to his identical twin.

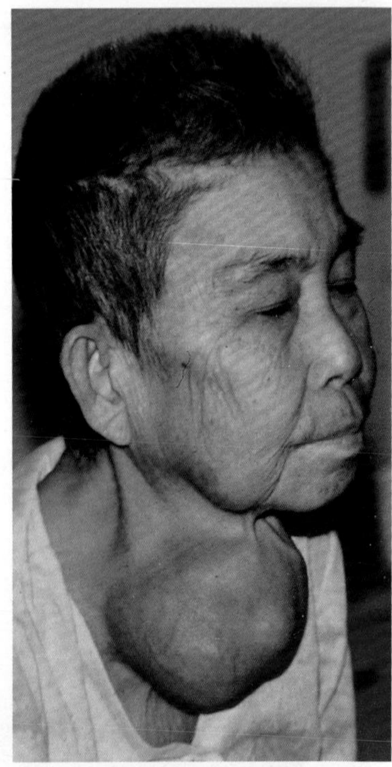

Figure 8-11 Patient with a goiter.

Medical Conditions

Term	Pronunciation	Meaning
hypothyroidism	hī′pō-thī′royd-izm	deficient hormone production by the thyroid gland
ketosis	kē-tō′sis	excessive ketones (compounds produced during fat metabolism) in the blood
myxedema	miks′e-dē′mă	severe hypothyroidism in an adult, characterized by pale dry skin, brittle hair, and sluggishness
pancreatitis	pan′krē-ă-tī′tis	inflammation of the pancreas
polydipsia	pol′ē-dip′sē-ă	excessive thirst
polyuria	pol′ē-yū′rē-ă	excessive and frequent urination
tetany	tet′ă-nē	spasms of nerves and muscles due to low levels of calcium in the blood caused by deficient production of parathyroid hormone
thyroiditis	thī′roy-dī′tis	inflammation of the thyroid gland
thyromegaly	thī′rō-meg′ă-lē	enlargement of the thyroid gland
thyrotoxicosis	thī′rō-tok′si-kō′sis	condition of excessively high levels of thyroid hormone (either endogenous or exogenous)

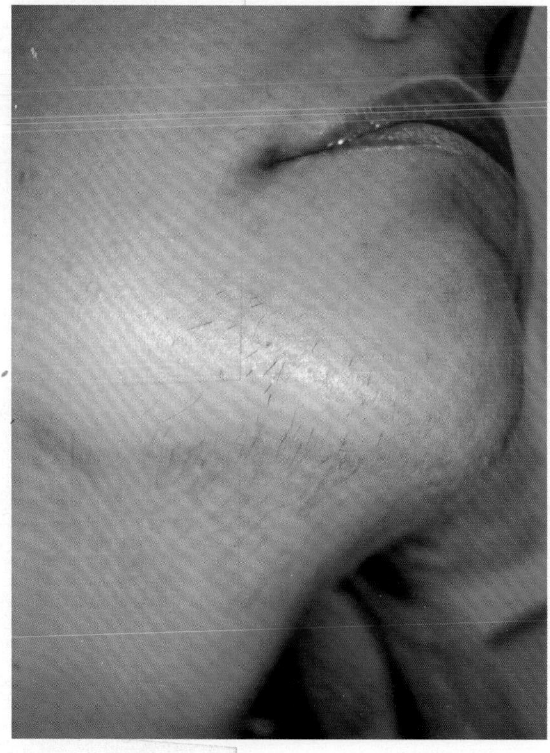

Figure 8-12 Patient with hirsutism. Note the excessive hair growth on this woman's chin.

ANIMATION

For a more in-depth look at diabetes, view the animation "Diabetes Mellitus" on the Student Resources on thePoint.

Exercises: Medical Conditions

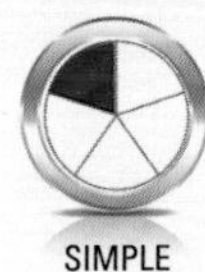
SIMPLE RECALL

Exercise 10

Write the correct medical term for the meaning given.

1. excessive thirst __________
2. autoimmune disease causing chronic thyroiditis __________
3. protruding eyes __________
4. abnormally low blood pH __________
5. excessively high levels of thyroid hormone __________
6. excessive hair growth or hair growth in unusual places __________
7. excessive ketones in the blood __________
8. disorder caused by total lack of insulin __________
9. severe hypothyroidism causing dry skin and hair __________
10. excessive urination __________
11. enlargement of a gland __________
12. excessive production of thyroid hormone __________
13. disorder caused by body's inability to use insulin efficiently __________

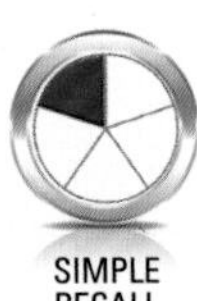
SIMPLE RECALL

Exercise 11

Circle the term that is most appropriate for the meaning of the sentence.

1. Excessive body growth due to overproduction of growth hormone before puberty can result in a condition called (*goiter, gigantism, tetany*).
2. (*Cushing syndrome, Diabetes insipidus, Addison disease*) is caused by a deficiency of adrenal gland hormone production.
3. Congenital absence of the thyroid gland can cause a condition known as (*myxedema, hirsutism, congenital hypothyroidism*).
4. Condition resulting in abnormally thick bones is known as (*goiter, hypokalemia, acromegaly*).
5. A blood test that shows low levels of thyroid hormone in the blood indicates that the patient has (*hypernatremia, hypokalemia, hypothyroidism*).
6. Excessive hormone production by the thyroid causing goiter and exophthalmos can result in a condition known as (*Graves disease, Cushing syndrome, gigantism*).

7. A patient with polyuria and polydipsia may have (*Cushing syndrome, diabetes insipidus, thyrotoxicosis*).

8. (*Hashimoto disease, Addison disease, Diabetic ketoacidosis*) is a condition in which there are excessive ketones in the blood due to breakdown of fats stored for energy.

9. A patient with fat pads on the chest and abdomen and a moon-shaped face may have (*myxedema, Hashimoto disease, Cushing syndrome*).

10. Inflammation of the adrenal gland is known as (*hyperthyroidism, adrenalitis, adenitis*).

11. (*Adenitis, Goiter, Ketosis*) is the name for enlargement of the thyroid gland.

12. Spasms of nerves and muscles caused by deficient parathyroid hormone production leads to a condition called (*Graves disease, Addison disease, tetany*).

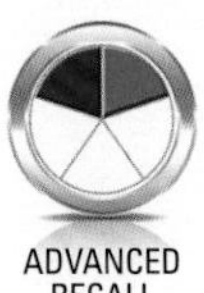
ADVANCED RECALL

Exercise 12

Match each medical term with its meaning.

hypercalcemia	polydipsia	hyponatremia
glycosuria	calcipenia	hyperkalemia
polyuria	hyperglycemia	hypocalcemia

1. low levels of sodium in the blood ______________________
2. high levels of potassium in the blood ______________________
3. high levels of calcium in the blood ______________________
4. excessive urination ______________________
5. glucose in the urine ______________________
6. high levels of glucose in the blood ______________________
7. deficiency of calcium ______________________
8. excessive thirst ______________________
9. low levels of calcium in the blood ______________________

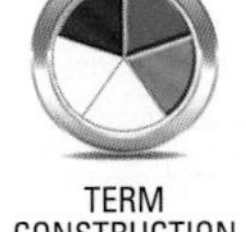
TERM CONSTRUCTION

Exercise 13

Build a medical term from an appropriate combining form and suffix given their meanings.

Use Combining Form for	Use Suffix for	Term
glucose, sugar	urine, urination	1. ______________________
endocrine gland	disease	2. ______________________

8 Endocrine System

extremity, tip	enlargement	**3.** ______________________
adrenal gland	enlargement	**4.** ______________________
thyroid gland	inflammation	**5.** ______________________
gland	inflammation	**6.** ______________________
pancreas	inflammation	**7.** ______________________
calcium	deficiency	**8.** ______________________
adrenal gland	disease	**9.** ______________________
thyroid gland	enlargement	**10.** ______________________

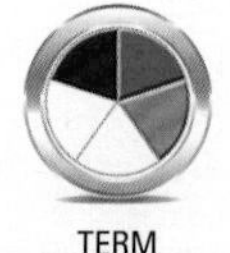

Exercise 14

TERM CONSTRUCTION

Write the meaning of the word parts used in each of the medical terms in the correct blanks (P = prefix, CF = combining form, S = suffix).

1. hyperparathyroidism ________ / ________ / ________
P CF S

2. hypoparathyroidism ________ / ________ / ________
P CF S

3. hypercalcemia ________ / ________ / ________
P CF S

4. hypocalcemia ________ / ________ / ________
P CF S

5. hyperglycemia ________ / ________ / ________
P CF S

6. hypoglycemia ________ / ________ / ________
P CF S

7. hypernatremia ________ / ________ / ________
P CF S

8. hyponatremia ________ / ________ / ________
P CF S

9. hyperkalemia ________ / ________ / ________
P CF S

10. hypokalemia ________ / ________ / ________
P CF S

Tests and Procedures

Term	Pronunciation	Meaning
Laboratory Tests		
blood glucose; *syn.* blood sugar	blŭd glū'kōs; blŭd shug'ăr	test to measure the amount of glucose in the blood (**Figure 8-13**)
electrolyte panel	ĕ-lek'trō-līt pan'ĕl	blood test to measure the amount of sodium, potassium, chloride, and carbon dioxide in the blood
fasting blood glucose (FBG)	fast'ing blŭd glū'kōs	blood test that measures the amount of glucose in the blood after fasting (not eating) for at least 8 hours
glucometer	glū-kom'ĕ-ter	device for measuring blood glucose levels from a drop of blood obtained by a finger stick (**Figure 8-14**)
glucose tolerance test (GTT)	glū'kos tol'ĕr-ăns test	blood test that measures the amount of glucose in the blood after administering a dose of glucose to the patient; used to gauge the body's ability to metabolize glucose
glycosylated hemoglobin (HbA_{1c})	glī-kō'si-lāt-ĕd hē'mō-glō-bin	blood test that indicates the amount of glucose in the blood over the previous few months; used to indicate how well diabetes mellitus is being controlled
thyroid function tests	thī'royd fŭnk'shŭn testz	blood tests that measure thyroid hormone levels in the blood
thyroid-stimulating hormone level	thī'royd-stim'yū-lā'ting hōr'mōn lev'ĕl	blood test that measures the amount of thyroid-stimulating hormone (TSH) in the blood; used to diagnosis hyperthyroidism or to monitor thyroid replacement therapy
thyroxine level	thī-rok'sēn lev'ĕl	blood test that measures the amount of thyroxine in the blood to diagnose hyperthyroidism or hypothyroidism
Diagnostic Procedures		
radioactive iodine uptake test (RAIU); *syn.* ^{131}I uptake test	rā'dē-ō-ak'tiv ī'ō-dīn ŭp'tāk test	test of thyroid function by measuring the uptake of iodine by the thyroid (**Figure 8-15**)
thyroid scan	thī'royd skan	scan of the thyroid gland using a radioactive dye, ultrasound, or computed tomography to show the size, shape, and position of the thyroid gland (**Figure 8-16**)

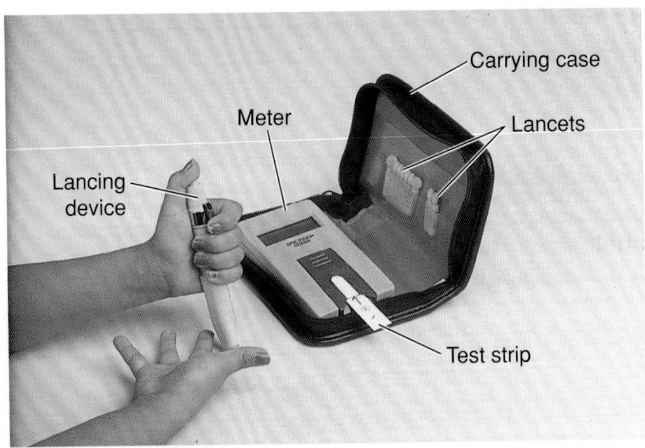

Figure 8-13 Materials for monitoring blood glucose.

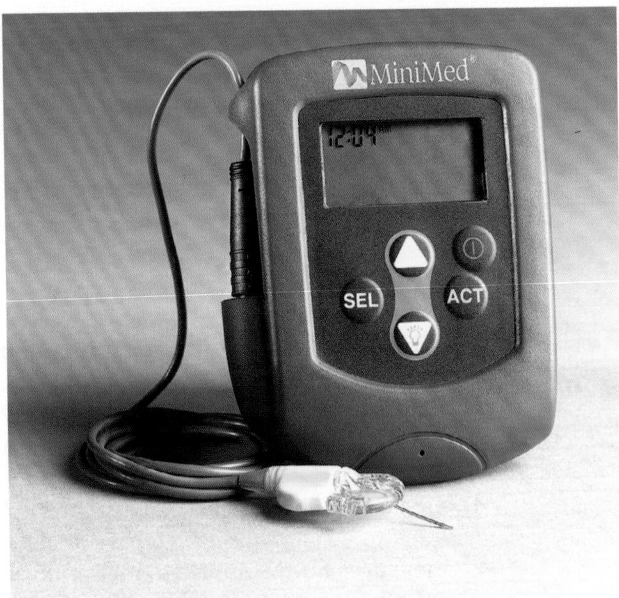

Figure 8-14 Glucometer.

8 Endocrine System

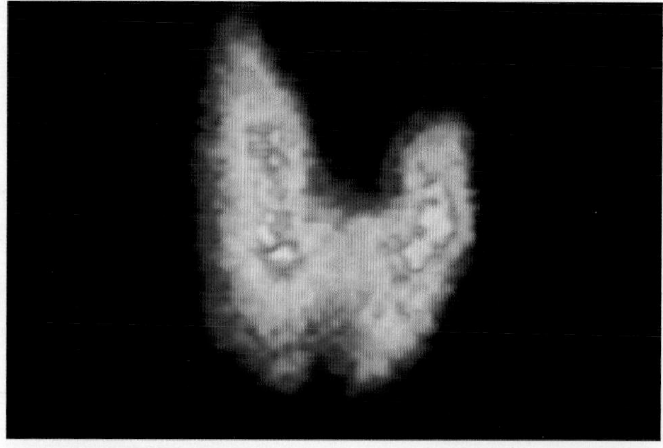

Figure 8-15 Image of an abnormal thyroid using radioactive iodine uptake test (RAIU). The right lobe (on the left) appears brighter and larger than the left lobe, indicating it has higher activity.

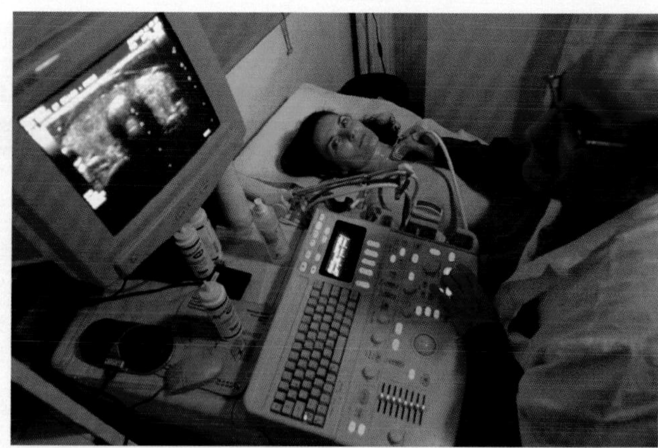

Figure 8-16 Ultrasound of the thyroid.

Exercises: Tests and Procedures

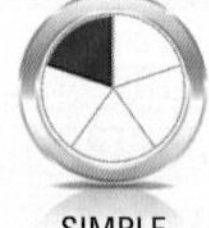

SIMPLE RECALL

Exercise 15

Write the correct medical term for the meaning given.

1. instrument for measuring blood glucose level from a drop of blood ____________________
2. measures thyroid hormone levels in the blood ____________________
3. test measuring glucose in the blood after administration of a dose of glucose ____________________
4. test of thyroid function by measuring thyroid's uptake of iodine ____________________
5. scan that shows size, shape, and position of thyroid ____________________
6. test that measures the amount of TSH in the blood ____________________

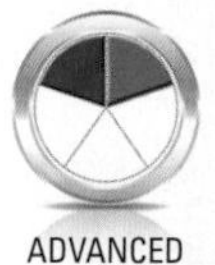

ADVANCED RECALL

Exercise 16

Match each medical term with its meaning.

glycosylated hemoglobin	electrolyte panel	fasting blood glucose
thyroxine level	blood glucose	glucose tolerance test

1. measures amount of thyroxine in the blood ____________________
2. measures body's ability to metabolize glucose ____________________
3. measures amount of glucose in the blood ____________________

4. measures glucose in the blood after a period of fasting ______________________

5. measures sodium, potassium, chloride, and carbon dioxide in blood ______________________

6. measures how well diabetes is being controlled ______________________

Surgical Interventions and Therapeutic Procedures

Term	Pronunciation	Meaning
adenectomy	ad′ĕ-nek′tŏ-mē	excision of a gland
adrenalectomy	ă-drē-năl-ek′tŏ-mē	excision of an adrenal gland
pancreatectomy	pan′krē-ă-tek′tŏ-mē	excision of the pancreas
parathyroidectomy	par′ă-thī-royd-ek′tŏ-mē	excision of a parathyroid gland
thymectomy	thī-mek′tŏ-mē	excision of the thymus gland
thyroidectomy	thī′roy-dek′tŏ-mē	excision of the thyroid gland
thyroidotomy	thī′roy-dot′ŏ-mē	incision into a thyroid gland
thyroparathyroidectomy	thī′rō-par′ă-thī′roy-dek′tŏ-mē	excision of the thyroid and parathyroid glands

■ Exercises: Surgical Interventions and Therapeutic Procedures

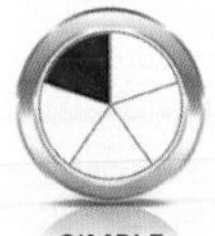
SIMPLE RECALL

Exercise 17

Write the meaning of the term given.

1. thyroidectomy ______________________
2. adrenalectomy ______________________
3. thymectomy ______________________
4. thyroparathyroidectomy ______________________

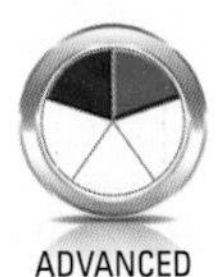
ADVANCED RECALL

Exercise 18

Circle the term that is most appropriate for the meaning of the sentence.

1. Mrs. Riley was hospitalized for a thyroidectomy, which involved removal of her (*thymus gland, thyroid gland, parathyroid glands*).

2. Mr. Ling has been diagnosed with a tumor on his adrenal gland and will require a(n) (*thyroidectomy, adenectomy, adrenalectomy*).

3. Part of Ms. Williamson's surgery will include a thyroidotomy, which is a(n) (*excision, removal, incision*) of her thyroid gland.

4. The surgeon performed a thyroparathyroidectomy, which includes excision of the (*thymus, thyroid, thyroxine*) gland.

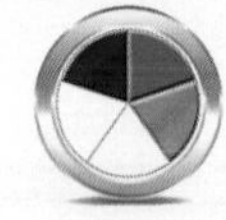

Exercise 19

Write the combining form used in the medical term, followed by the meaning of the combining form.

Term	Combining Form	Combining Form Meaning
1. pancreatectomy	______	______
2. thyroidotomy	______	______
3. adenectomy	______	______
4. parathyroidectomy	______	______
5. thymectomy	______	______

Medications and Drug Therapies

Term	Pronunciation	Meaning
antidiabetic	an′tē-dī-ă-bet′ik	drug used to treat diabetes mellitus by lowering glucose levels in the blood
antithyroid	an′tē-thī′royd	drug used to treat overproduction of thyroid hormone
continuous subcutaneous insulin infusion (CSII)	kon-tin′yū-ŭs sŭb′kyū-tā′nē-ŭs in′sŭ-lin in-fyū′zhŭn	infusion of insulin to subcutaneous tissues by a device worn on the body (**Figure 8-17**)
insulin pump	in′sŭ-lin pŭmp	device worn on the body to infuse insulin
insulin therapy	in′sŭ-lin thār′ă-pē	method used to treat diabetes mellitus by replacing natural insulin
hormone replacement therapy (HRT)	hōr′mōn rĕ-plās′mĕnt thār′ă-pē	treatment used to replace hormones that are normally produced by the body

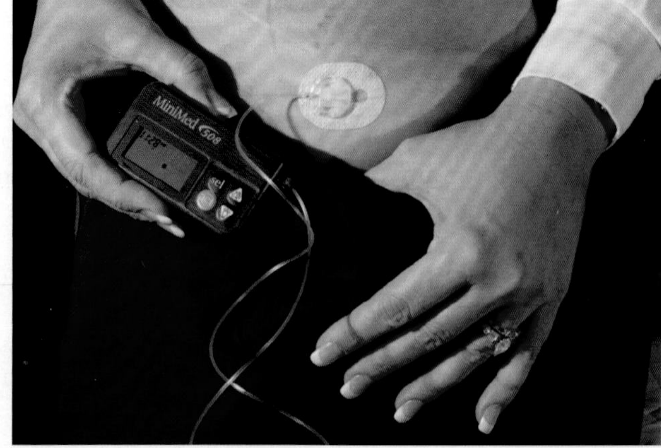

Figure 8-17 Continuous subcutaneous insulin infusion (CSII) pump.

Exercise: Medications and Drug Therapies

Exercise 20

SIMPLE RECALL

Write the correct medication or drug therapy term for the meaning given.

1. used to replace natural insulin __________
2. used to treat overproduction of thyroid hormone __________
3. used to replace natural hormones __________
4. used to lower glucose levels in the blood __________
5. device worn on the body to infuse insulin __________

Specialties and Specialists

Term	Pronunciation	Meaning
endocrinology	en′dō-kri-nol′ŏ-jē	medical specialty concerned with diagnosis and treatment of disorders of the endocrine system
endocrinologist	en′dō-kri-nol′ŏ-jist	physician who specializes in endocrinology

Exercise: Specialties and Specialists

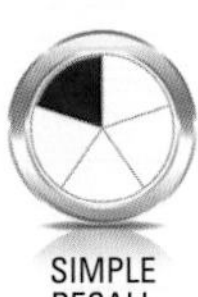

Exercise 21

SIMPLE RECALL

Write the correct medical term for the meaning given.

1. specialty concerned with the endocrine system __________
2. specialist in the endocrine system __________

Abbreviations

Abbreviation	Meaning
ACTH	adrenocorticotropic hormone
ADH	antidiuretic hormone
CSII	continuous subcutaneous insulin infusion
DI	diabetes insipidus
DKA	diabetic ketoacidosis
DM	diabetes mellitus
FBG	fasting blood glucose
FSH	follicle-stimulating hormone
GH	growth hormone
GTT	glucose tolerance test
HbA_{1c}	glycosylated hemoglobin alpha 1c
^{131}I	radioactive iodine
LH	luteinizing hormone
PTH	parathyroid hormone
RAIU	radioactive iodine uptake
T_3	triiodothyronine
T_4	thyroxine
TSH	thyroid-stimulating hormone

Exercises: Abbreviations

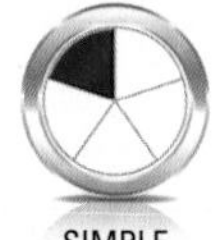

Exercise 22

Write the meaning of each abbreviation.

1. DI ______________________
2. TSH ______________________
3. FBG ______________________
4. ADH ______________________
5. PTH ______________________
6. GTT ______________________
7. RAIU ______________________
8. T_3 ______________________
9. HbA_{1c} ______________________

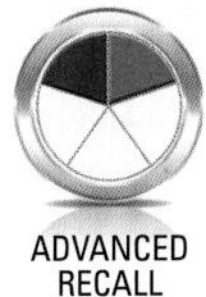

Exercise 23

Match each abbreviation with the appropriate description.

DI	DM	CSII
DKA	LH	T_4
GH	FSH	ACTH

1. hormone that stimulates the adrenal cortex ____________
2. disorder caused by deficiency of insulin ____________
3. regulates the ovaries and testicles ____________
4. regulates metabolism ____________
5. excessive ketones in the blood that can lead to coma or death ____________
6. device worn by patient to administer insulin subcutaneously ____________
7. disorder caused by deficiency of antidiuretic hormone ____________
8. regulates body growth ____________
9. stimulates secretion of progesterone in females ____________

WRAPPING UP

- The endocrine system consists of endocrine glands and the hormones these glands produce, which have specific target tissues.
- Endocrine glands are ductless, so they release their substances directly into the bloodstream, which carries the substance to target cells to exert its effects.
- In this chapter, you learned medical terminology including word parts, prefixes, suffixes, adjectives, conditions, tests, procedures, medications, specialties, and abbreviations related to the endocrine system.

Chapter Review

Review of Terms for Anatomy and Physiology

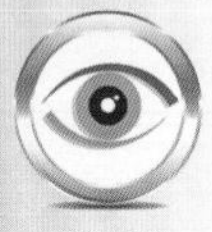

VISUAL

Exercise 24

Write the correct terms on the blanks for the anatomic structures indicated.

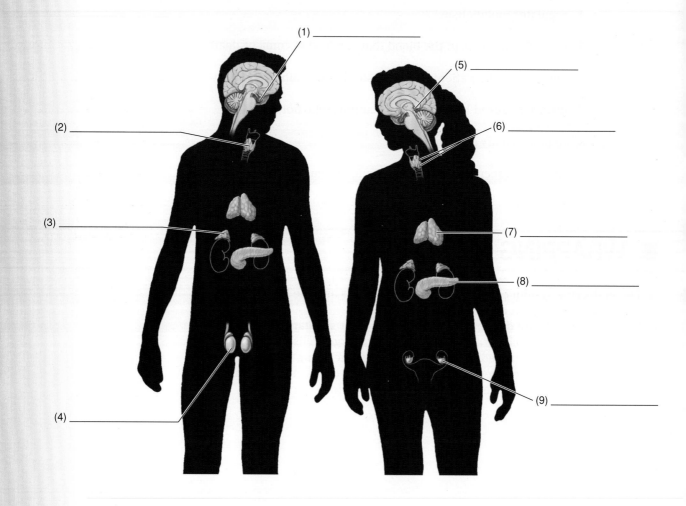

(1) ____________________

(2) ____________________

(3) ____________________

(4) ____________________

(5) ____________________

(6) ____________________

(7) ____________________

(8) ____________________

(9) ____________________

Understanding Term Structure

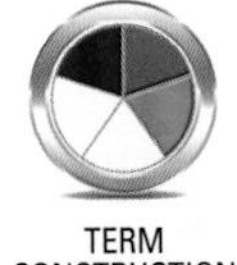
TERM CONSTRUCTION

Exercise 25

Break the given medical term into its word parts, and define each part. Then define the medical term.

For example:

thymitis	*word parts:*	thym/o, -itis
	meanings:	thymus, inflammation
	term meaning:	inflammation of the thymus gland

1. pancreatic
word parts: ____________________
meanings: ____________________
term meaning: ____________________

2. adrenalitis
word parts: ____________________
meanings: ____________________
term meaning: ____________________

3. glucosuria
word parts: ____________________
meanings: ____________________
term meaning: ____________________

4. acromegaly
word parts: ____________________
meanings: ____________________
term meaning: ____________________

5. cortical
word parts: ____________________
meanings: ____________________
term meaning: ____________________

6. calcipenia
word parts: ____________________
meanings: ____________________
term meaning: ____________________

7. thyroidotomy
word parts: ____________________
meanings: ____________________
term meaning: ____________________

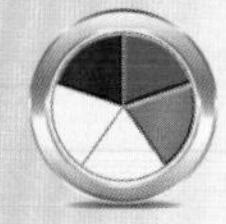

Exercise 26

TERM CONSTRUCTION

Write the combining form used in the medical term, followed by the meaning of the combining form.

Term	Combining Form	Combining Form Meaning
1. thymic	______	______
2. thyromegaly	______	______
3. hypokalemia	______	______
4. adrenalectomy	______	______
5. hypernatremia	______	______
6. endocrinopathy	______	______
7. pancreatitis	______	______
8. polydipsia	______	______

Comprehension Exercises

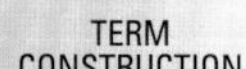

Exercise 27

COMPREHENSION

Fill in the blank with the correct term.

1. Excessive production of the T_3 and T_4 hormones can lead to a condition called ______.
2. The test that measures the glucose levels in the blood after administering a dose of glucose is called the ______.
3. A patient who had the surgical procedure known as a(n) ______ is no longer able to produce the hormone cortisol.
4. The hormone that keeps the body from accumulating excess water is called the ______.
5. ______ are endocrine cells that aid in glucose metabolism.
6. The opposite of anuria is ______.
7. The term for a thyroid with no functional problems is ______.
8. A patient who was born without a thyroid gland has ______.
9. The disease that includes signs and symptoms of both polydipsia and polyuria is ______.
10. A physician specializing in all types of thyroid disorders is called a(n) ______.

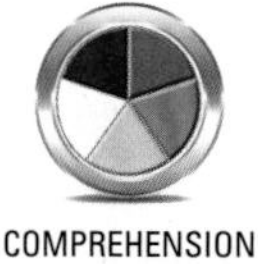

COMPREHENSION

Exercise 28

Circle the letter of the best answer in the following questions.

1. A patient who has hypothyroidism does not have enough __________ thyroxine.

A. endogenous
B. euthyroid
C. exogenous
D. cortical

2. The blood test used to measure how well diabetes is being controlled over a period of months is

A. thyroid function.
B. thyroid scan.
C. fasting blood sugar.
D. glycosylated hemoglobin.

3. The condition caused by severely deficient hormone production by the thyroid gland is called

A. tetany.
B. myxedema.
C. Cushing syndrome.
D. Graves disease.

4. An autoimmune disease that causes chronic inflammation of the thyroid is

A. Graves disease.
B. Cushing syndrome.
C. Addison disease.
D. Hashimoto disease.

5. Excessive hair growth on the face of a woman might be diagnosed as

A. hirsutism.
B. myxedema.
C. acromegaly.
D. hyperkalemia.

6. The test that measures the hormone made by the thyroid gland that helps to regulate metabolism is the

A. radioactive iodine uptake test.
B. thyroxine level test.
C. glycosylated hemoglobin test.
D. thyroid function test.

7. A hormone that might be used to induce labor is called

A. insulin.
B. oxytocin.
C. luteinizing hormone.
D. thymosin.

8. A patient with diabetes mellitus tests her blood sugar level using a(n)

A. electrolyte panel.
B. glucometer.
C. ketosis.
D. hirsutism.

9. A patient with fat pads on the chest and a "moon face" appearance may have

A. Hashimoto thyroiditis.
B. thyrotoxicosis.
C. Cushing syndrome.
D. goiter.

10. Enlargement of the thyroid gland is called

A. acromegaly.
B. goiter.
C. hyperglycemia.
D. myxedema.

Application and Analysis

CASE STUDIES

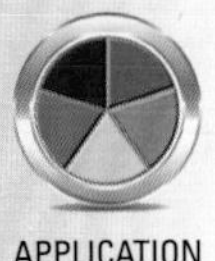

Exercise 29

APPLICATION

Read the case studies and circle the correct letter for each of the questions.

CASE 8-1

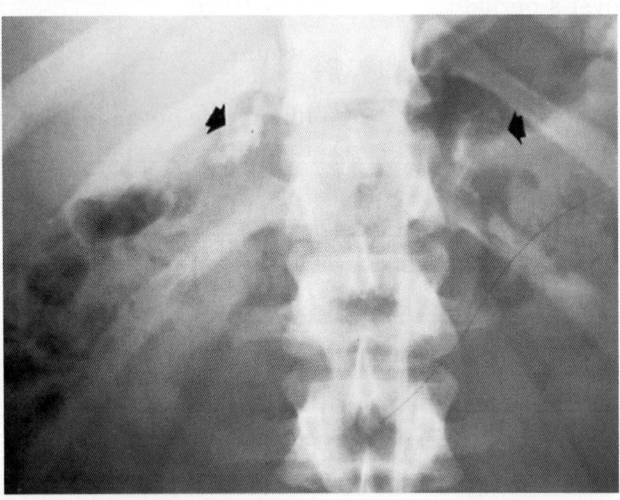

Figure 8-18 Computed tomography scan of a patient with possible Addison disease. The adrenal glands (*arrows*) appear small and with dense calcification.

Mrs. Brewer presented to the office today with a complaint of significant weight loss, worsening fatigue, anorexia, lethargy, and irregular menses. Examination revealed hyperpigmentation of her skin. A review of the patient's record from the previous visit revealed a weight loss of 20 lb over the past four months. A blood glucose level test was done; it revealed hypoglycemia. Lab tests including an FBG, electrolytes, and ACTH levels were ordered. A CT scan of the adrenal glands was also ordered (**Figure 8-18**). The patient will return after testing for follow-up.

1. The test that will measure the levels of sodium, potassium, chloride, and CO_2 in the patient's blood is

A. CT scan.
B. blood glucose.
C. electrolytes.
D. FBG.

2. The term that describes low blood glucose is

A. anorexia.
B. hypoglycemia.
C. hyperpigmentation.
D. lethargy.

3. The ACTH level test will measure the levels of both ________ and ________ in the blood.

A. thyroid hormone; adrenocorticotropic hormone
B. adrenocorticotropic hormone; cortisol
C. thyroid hormone; cortisol
D. cortisol; thymosin

4. Based on the patient's signs and symptoms and the workup ordered by the physician, which disease is most likely being considered for this patient?

A. Addison disease
B. Cushing syndrome
C. Hashimoto thyroiditis
D. Graves disease

CASE 8-2

Ms. Ramirez returned to her physician, Dr. Doray, for a follow-up visit for hyperthyroidism and a repeat of her thyroid tests. The results show that her TSH level remains suppressed below 0.04. Free T_4 and total T_4 remain in the upper limit of normal. A thyroid scan and uptake show predominantly active uptake in the left lobe. Based on these findings, Dr. Doray indicated that a diagnosis of multinodular toxic goiter was more likely than Graves disease. She discussed possible treatment options, including surgery, with the patient. Ms. Ramirez is inclined to undergo radioactive iodine treatment and understands that she will need to receive lifelong hormone replacement.

5. The term hyperthyroidism refers to

_______________ production of thyroid hormone.

A. inefficient
B. deficient
C. excessive
D. unacceptable

6. The abbreviation T_4 stands for

A. thyroid.
B. thyroxine.
C. triiodothyronine.
D. tetany.

7. A goiter is an enlargement of the

A. parathyroid gland.
B. endocrine gland.
C. adrenal gland.
D. thyroid gland.

8. A thyroid scan can indicate a thyroid's size, shape, and

A. functionality.
B. position.
C. color.
D. fullness.

MEDICAL RECORD ANALYSIS

MEDICAL RECORD 8-1

You are a nurse practitioner specializing in diabetes care. You have been asked to see Ms. Hayes to discuss her newly diagnosed diabetes mellitus, and you are reviewing the medical record from her physician prior to meeting with her.

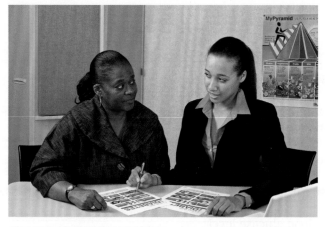

Nurse practitioners manage a patient's total health care, including treatment of chronic conditions such as diabetes or high blood pressure.

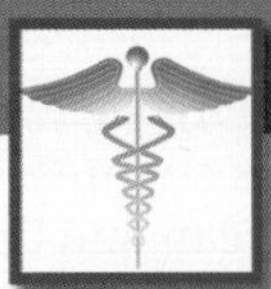

Medical Record

NEW ONSET DIABETES MELLITUS

SUBJECTIVE: The patient is seen today for complaints of an unusually large appetite as well as polydipsia and polyuria. She is concerned because she has had significant weight loss over the past few months despite her increased appetite. On questioning, she admits to increased fatigue as well as some irritability. The patient takes exogenous thyroxine for hypothyroidism. Medical history reveals a single episode of pancreatitis three years ago. It is otherwise noncontributory with the exception of gestational diabetes during her second pregnancy. Family history is positive for a mother and sister with diabetes mellitus. Her sister is under treatment with a continuous subcutaneous insulin infusion.

OBJECTIVE: General examination reveals an obese female in no acute distress. Blood pressure is elevated at 150/95. Physical examination was unremarkable. Inspection of skin was negative for rashes, lesions, or ulcerations. Snellen testing revealed 20/20 vision in both eyes.

Urinalysis was performed and revealed slight glycosuria. Blood glucose testing revealed a glucose level of 260 two hours postprandial.

ASSESSMENT: My impression is new-onset diabetes mellitus with a family history of DM.

PLAN: Laboratory testing has been ordered to include a GTT, electrolytes, glycosylated hemoglobin, and lipid panel. The patient has been counseled regarding dietary considerations. She was advised of the importance of blood glucose control and regular exercise. The patient was counseled at length about the risks associated with diabetes, including diabetic nephropathy, retinopathy, and peripheral vascular disease.

Patient will be referred to endocrinologist Dr. Tom Hong for further evaluation and workup as soon as insurance authorization can be procured. A copy of her laboratory results will be forwarded to Dr. Hong upon completion.

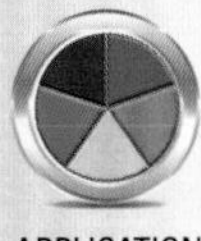

APPLICATION

Exercise 30

Write the appropriate medical terms used in this medical record on the blanks after their meanings.

1. produced inside the body ____________________
2. excessive urination ____________________
3. test of blood glucose level ____________________
4. inflammation of the pancreas ____________________
5. glucose in the urine ____________________

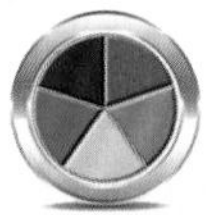

Exercise 31

APPLICATION **Read the medical report, and circle the correct letter for each of the questions.**

1. What test did the physician perform on the patient to check her vision?
   A. urinalysis
   B. glycosylated hemoglobin
   C. Snellen
   D. continuous subcutaneous insulin infusion

2. The glycosylated hemoglobin test will test for blood levels of
   A. thyroid hormone.
   B. glucose over the past few months.
   C. calcium.
   D. thyroxine.

3. The physician's impression is that the patient has a deficiency and/or resistance to insulin, which is called
   A. diabetes mellitus.
   B. nephropathy.
   C. peripheral vascular disease.
   D. diabetes insipidus.

4. The symptom polydipsia means that the patient is excessively
   A. overweight.
   B. hungry.
   C. thirsty.
   D. tired.

5. The abbreviation GTT stands for a test that measures
   A. blood levels of potassium.
   B. blood levels of glucose after administration of a measured dose of glucose.
   C. blood levels of thyroxine.
   D. amount of thyroid-stimulating hormone in the blood.

MEDICAL RECORD 8-2

Mirinda Maloney was admitted for a thyroidectomy after being diagnosed with hyperthyroidism. As a surgical technologist, you assisted in this patient's surgery by maintaining supplies, counting materials, and assisting in suturing. The resulting operative report is as follows.

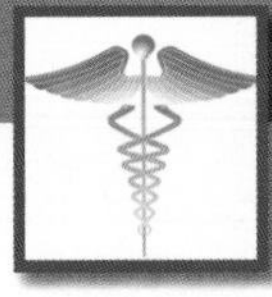

Medical Record

OPERATIVE REPORT: THYROIDECTOMY

PREOPERATIVE DIAGNOSIS: Primary (1) ____________________

POSTOPERATIVE DIAGNOSIS: Left thyroid tumor

OPERATION: Minimally invasive thyroidectomy

SURGEON: Joel Sugiwara, MD

ASSISTANT SURGEON: Tom Hansen, MD

ANESTHESIA: General

INDICATIONS: The patient is a 54-year-old female with a history of weight loss, fatigue, (2) ______________, and (3) ______________. A thyroxine level test revealed excessive levels of thyroxine and a(n) (4) ______________ showed a nodule in the left thyroid. The patient is brought to the operating room for minimally invasive (5) ______________.

PROCEDURE: The patient was taken to the operating room and placed in a supine position on the operating table. After satisfactory induction of general endotracheal anesthesia, the patient was positioned and draped for the procedure. The patient's recurrent laryngeal nerves were monitored throughout the operation using electromyography.

A small horizontal incision was made in the lower neck. Flaps were raised superiorly and inferiorly. The left thyroid was identified and separated from surrounding tissues. The blood supply to the left thyroid gland was clamped off. The gland was removed from the neck. The mass was sent for frozen section diagnosis and was determined to be nodular thyroid gland tissue. Hemostasis was obtained using bipolar cautery.

A Penrose drain was placed, and the wound was closed using layered closure. The patient was awakened from anesthesia.

Exercise 32

APPLICATION

Fill in the blanks in the medical record above with the correct medical terms. The meanings of the missing terms are listed below.

1. excessive hormone production by a thyroid gland
2. enlargement of the thyroid gland
3. bulging eyes
4. scan showing the size, shape, and position of the thyroid
5. excision of a thyroid gland

Bonus Questions

6. What term used in this record means to stop bleeding? ______________________________
7. The patient was placed in the supine position. Describe this position. ______________________________

____

Pronunciation and Spelling

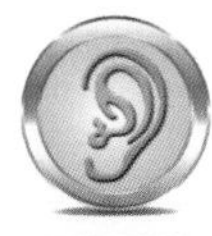
AUDITORY

Exercise 33

Review the Chapter 8 terms in the Dictionary/Audio Glossary in the Student Resources on thePoint, and practice pronouncing each term, referring to the pronunciation guide as needed.

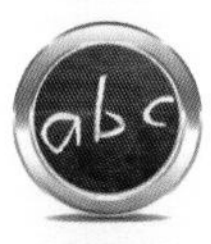
SPELLING

Exercise 34

Check the spelling of each term. If it is correct, check off the correct box. If incorrect, write the correct spelling on the line.

1. pituitery ☐ ______
2. pancrease ☐ ______
3. antidiuretic ☐ ______
4. metabolism ☐ ______
5. uthyroyd ☐ ______
6. diabeties ☐ ______
7. exopthalmos ☐ ______
8. hirutism ☐ ______
9. hyperkalemia ☐ ______
10. glycosuria ☐ ______
11. mixedema ☐ ______
12. thyromegaly ☐ ______
13. polydipsia ☐ ______
14. glycosilated ☐ ______
15. glucose ☐ ______

Media Connection

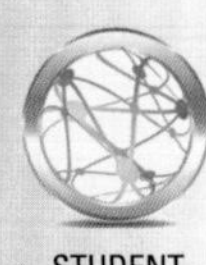

Exercise 35

Complete each of the following activities available with the Student Resources on thePoint. Check off each activity as you complete it, and record your score for the Chapter Quiz in the space provided.

Chapter Exercises

____ Flash Cards

____ Concentration

____ Abbreviation Match-Up

____ Roboterms

____ Word Anatomy

____ Fill the Gap

____ Break It Down

____ True/False Body Building

____ Quiz Show

____ Complete the Case

____ Medical Record Review

____ Look and Label

____ Image Matching

____ Spelling Bee

____ **Chapter Quiz** *Score:*________%

Additional Resources

____ Animation: Diabetes Mellitus

____ Dictionary/Audio Glossary

____ Health Professions Careers: Nurse Practitioner

____ Health Professions Careers: Surgical Assistant

Blood and Immune System

9

Chapter Outline

Introduction, 310

Anatomy and Physiology, 310
- Structures, 310
- Functions, 311
- Terms Related to Blood and the Immune System, 311

Word Parts, 318
- Combining Forms, 318
- Prefixes, 318
- Suffixes, 319

Medical Terms, 321
- Adjectives and Other Related Terms, 321
- Medical Conditions, 323
- Tests and Procedures, 327
- Surgical Interventions and Therapeutic Procedures, 331
- Medications and Drug Therapies, 334
- Specialties and Specialists, 335
- Abbreviations, 336

Wrapping Up, 337

Chapter Review, 338

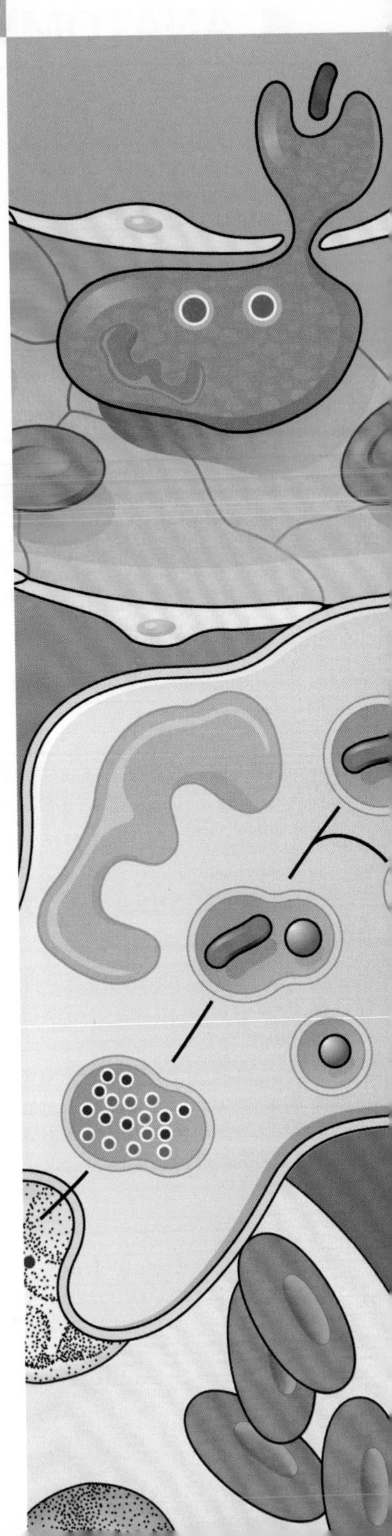

Learning Outcomes

After completing this chapter, you should be able to:

1. Describe the functions and main components of blood and the immune system.
2. Define terms related to the blood, blood cells, blood components, and the immune system.
3. Define combining forms, prefixes, and suffixes related to blood and the immune system.
4. Define common medical terminology related to blood and the immune system, including the following: adjectives and related terms; signs, symptoms, and medical conditions; tests and procedures; surgical interventions and therapeutic procedures; medications and drug therapies; and medical specialties and specialists.
5. Define common abbreviations related to blood and the immune system.
6. Successfully complete all chapter exercises.
7. Explain terms used in case studies and medical records involving blood and the immune system.
8. Successfully complete all exercises included with the companion Student Resources on thePoint.

INTRODUCTION

Blood plays a vital role in maintaining homeostasis (internal balance), because it is the medium in which nutrients and hormones are transported, gas exchange occurs, body temperature is regulated, pH levels are maintained, and immunity is provided. The immune system protects us from disease-causing agents known as pathogens. This chapter focuses on blood and the immune system.

ANATOMY AND PHYSIOLOGY

Structures

- Blood, the "circulating tissue" of the body, is classified as a connective tissue.
- Whole blood is made up of 45% formed elements (cells and cell fragments) and 55% plasma (liquid) (**Figure 9-1**).
- Formed elements are produced in bone marrow and include erythrocytes, leukocytes, and platelets (**Figure 9-2**).
- Erythrocytes, or red blood cells, are biconcave discs without a nucleus.
- Leukocytes, or white blood cells, are colorless cells that circulate in body fluids. There are 5 classes of leukocytes.
- Platelets (thrombocytes) are cell fragments without a nucleus.
- Plasma is the fluid matrix of blood and contains proteins and other solutes.
- Plasma proteins include albumin (the main protein), fibrinogen (blood clotter), and globulins (antibodies).
- Serum is plasma without fibrinogen.
- The immune system includes organs that provide defense, known as the immune response.

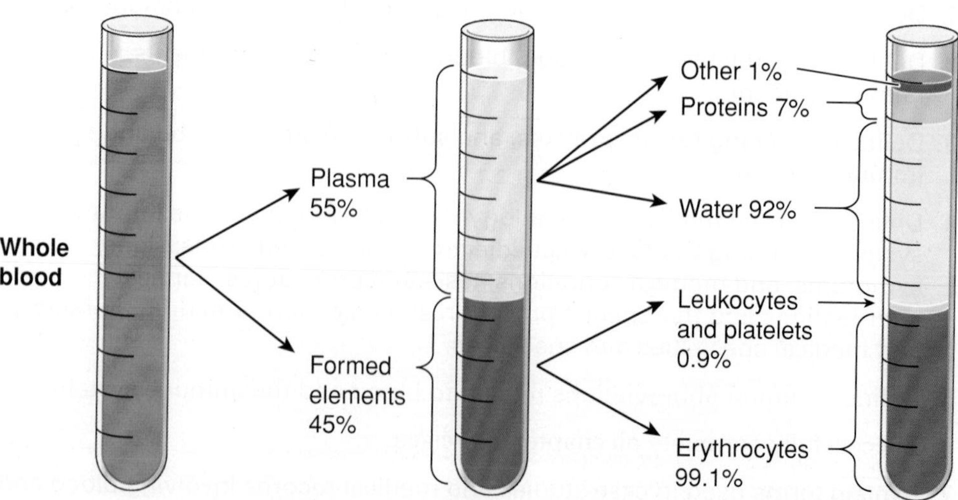

Figure 9-1 Composition of whole blood.

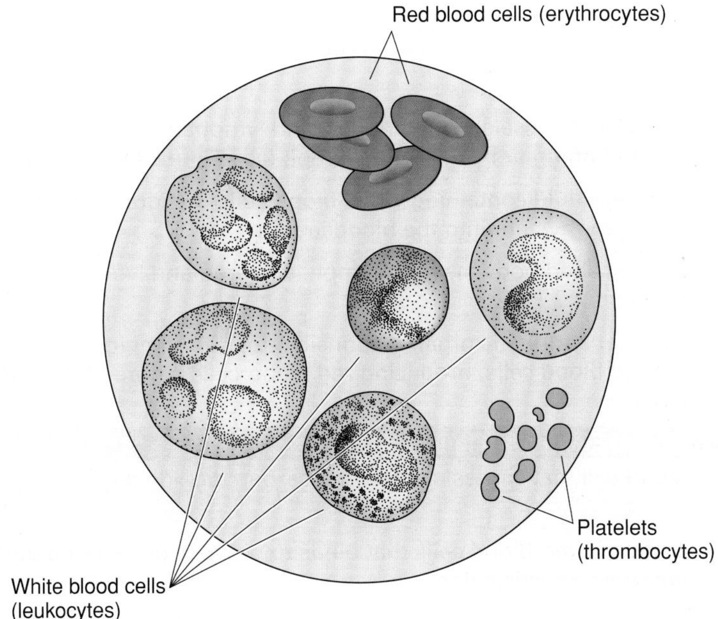

Figure 9-2 Blood components.

Functions

- Transporting oxygen, carbon dioxide, nutrients, electrolytes, vitamins, hormones, and wastes throughout the body
- Protecting the body with circulating white blood cells, antibodies of the immune system, and clotting factors
- Protecting the body by naturally and artificially acquired immunity
- Producing an immune response (the body's reaction to an antigen), such as producing antibodies as a reaction to the toxin or foreign substance.

Terms Related to Blood and the Immune System

Term	Pronunciation	Meaning
		Whole Blood and Specific Organs
blood	blŭd	fluid that circulates through the heart, arteries, capillaries, and veins, transporting oxygen, carbon dioxide, and nutrients to the tissues
formed elements	fōrmd el'ĕ-mĕnts	blood cells and cellular fragments
packed cell volume	pakt sel vol'yŭm	the volume of blood cells in a sample after it has been centrifuged; normally about 45% of the blood sample
plasma	plaz'mah	liquid portion of blood that carries formed elements, clotting factors, electrolytes, and proteins
serum	sēr'ŭm	liquid portion of blood left after removing the clotting factors and blood cells
bone marrow	bōn mar'ō	soft tissue within medullary cavities of bone, with multiple functions including the production of blood cells
erythropoietin (EPO)	ĕ-rith'rō-poy'ĕ-tin	hormone released by kidneys that stimulates red blood cell production in bone marrow
hemopoiesis; *syn.* hematopoiesis	hē'mō-poy-ē'sis; hē'mă-tō-poy-ē'sis	formation of various types of blood cells and other formed elements

(continued)

Terms Related to Blood and the Immune System *(continued)*

Term	Pronunciation	Meaning
lymphatic system	lim-fat′ik sis′tĕm	network of vessels, lymph nodes, and lymphatic organs that plays a role in immunity by collecting lymph (see **Figure 10-9**, Chapter 10)
lymph	limf	colorless fluid containing white blood cells that drains through the lymphatic system into the bloodstream
lymph node	limf nōd	bean-shaped body in which lymph is filtered and lymphocytes are formed
spleen	splēn	vascular lymphatic organ responsible for filtering blood, destroying old red blood cells, producing red blood cells before birth, and storing blood
Formed Elements (Figure 9-3)		
erythrocyte; *syn.* red blood cell (RBC)	ĕ-rith′rō-sīt; red blŭd sel	blood cell that carries oxygen and carbon dioxide **(Figure 9-4)**
hemoglobin (HGB, Hb, Hgb)	hē′mō-glō′bin	protein in red blood cells that binds to oxygen; gives red blood cells the characteristic color
iron (Fe)	ī′ŏrn	essential trace element necessary for hemoglobin to transport oxygen in red blood cells
macrocyte	mak′rō-sīt	a large red blood cell
Rh factor	ahr āch fak′tŏr	protein substance present in the red blood cells of most people (85%); it is capable of inducing intense antigenic reactions

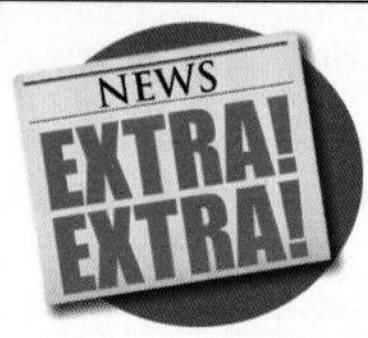

HEMOGLOBIN Millions of hemoglobin molecules in a red blood cell carry oxygen (O_2) to the cells of the body. Oxygen molecules bind to the hemoglobin protein and are released in body tissues during the appropriate conditions. The more oxygen carried by the hemoglobin, the brighter red the blood will be. Carbon dioxide (CO_2) is swapped for oxygen and carried back to the lungs to be "blown off." Carbon dioxide interferes with the ability of hemoglobin to bind oxygen. For example, smoking and air pollution can lead to higher-than-normal CO_2 levels and can have an adverse effect on your health.

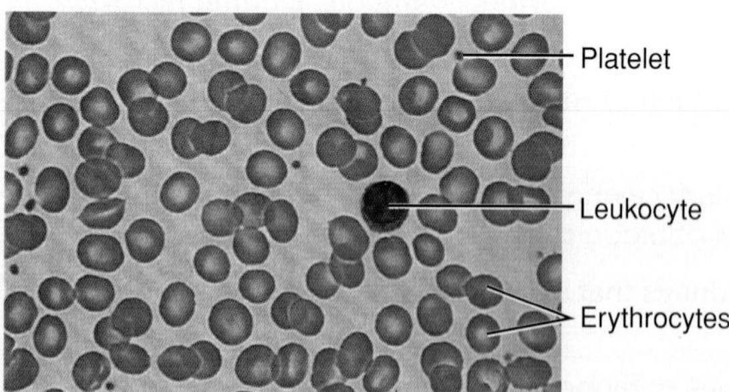

Figure 9-3 The three formed elements of blood as seen under a microscope.

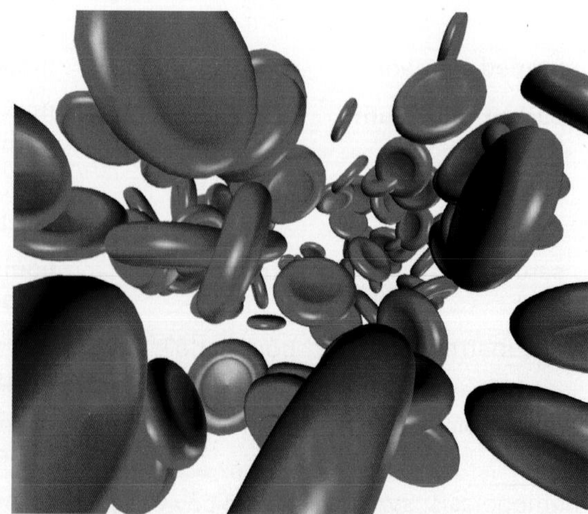

Figure 9-4 Three-dimensional shape of red blood cells showing thin centers and thick edges.

Terms Related to Blood and the Immune System

Term	Pronunciation	Meaning
leukocyte; *syn.* white blood cell (WBC)	lū′kō-sīt; wīt blŭd sel	largest blood cell; protects against pathogens, foreign substances, and cellular debris **(Figure 9-5)**
granulocyte	gran′yū-lō-sīt	white blood cell with visible granules; the three types of granulocytes are named according to the type of dye to which each is attracted
neutrophil	nū′trō-fil	type of granulocyte that fights against bacterial infections; stains a neutral pink; 60–70% of circulating WBCs
eosinophil	ē′ō-sin′ō-fil	type of granulocyte that functions in allergic reactions and against parasites; stains red; 2–4% of circulating WBCs
basophil	bā′sō-fil	type of granulocyte that releases histamine in allergic reactions and inflammatory responses; stains a dark blue with a basic dye; 0.5–1.0% of circulating WBCs
agranulocyte	ā-grăn′ŭ-lō-sīt	white blood cell without clearly visible granules
lymphocyte	lim′fō-sīt	type of agranulocyte that circulates in the lymphatic system and is active in immunity; 20–25% of circulating WBCs
B lymphocyte; *syn.* B cell	bē lim′fō-sīt; bē sel	white blood cell that, when in contact with a foreign antigen, produces antibodies to inactivate the antigen
T lymphocyte; *syn.* T cell	tē lim′fō-sīt; tē sel	white blood cell that matures in the thymus gland and specializes in creating an immune response
monocyte	mon′ō-sīt	largest type of white blood cell; 3–8% of circulating WBCs

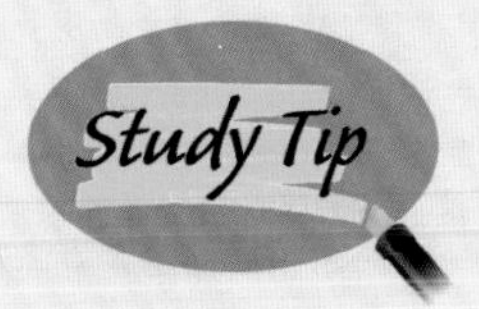

The White Blood Cells: To remember the types of white blood cells, think of the phrase, "**N**ever **l**et **m**onkeys **e**at **b**ananas," where the N stands for neutrophils, L for lymphocytes, M for monocytes, E for eosinophils, and B for basophils.

Term	Pronunciation	Meaning
macrophage	mak′rō-fāj	enlarged and matured monocyte active in phagocytosis (eating and destroying)
platelets (PLT); *syn.* thrombocytes	plāt′lĕts; throm′bō-sīts	cellular fragments in the blood that stick together, forming a clot **(Figure 9-6)**

(continued)

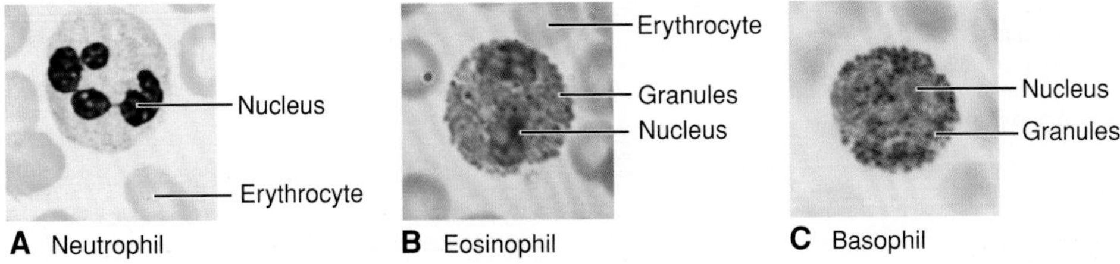

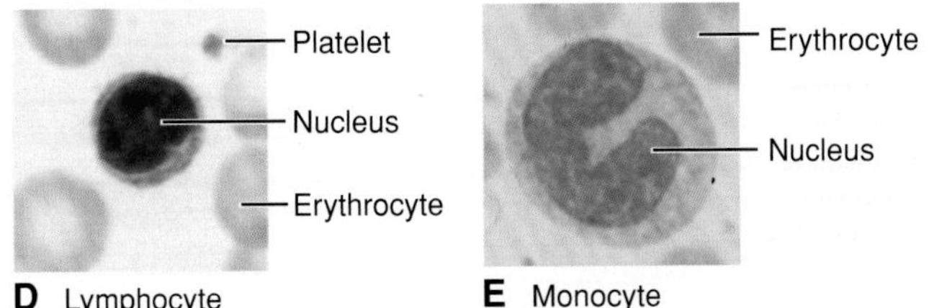

Figure 9-5 Leukocytes (white blood cells).

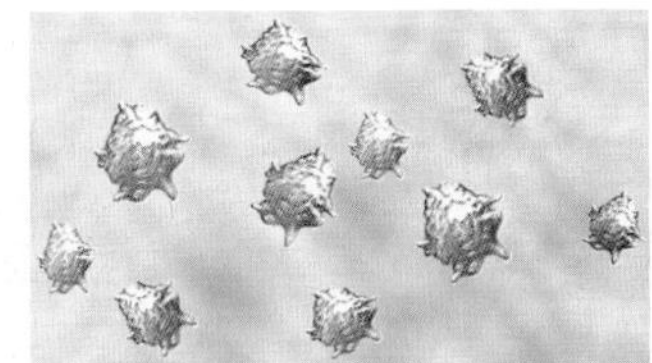

Figure 9-6 Platelets.

Terms Related to Blood and the Immune System *(continued)*

Term	Pronunciation	Meaning
Blood Clotting		
clotting factors	kloting fak'tŏrz	any of the various plasma components involved in the clotting process
coagulation	kō-ag'yū-lā'shŭn	clotting; changing from a liquid to a solid state
fibrin	fī'brin	elastic fiber protein needed in clotting and derived from fibrinogen
fibrinogen	fī-brin'ō-jen	plasma protein that is converted into solid threads called fibrin
The Immune System		
antibody (Ab)	an'ti-bod-ē	soldier-like protein that protects the body and inactivates antigens; provides immunity against specific substances and microorganisms **(Figure 9-7)**
antigen (Ag)	an'ti-jen	agent or substance that provokes an immune response
histamine	his'tă-mēn	substance released by damaged cells that increases blood flow to the area, causing an inflammatory response (inflammation) involving heat, redness, swelling, and pain
immune response	i-myūn' rē-spons'	the body's reaction to an antigen
immunity	i-myū'ni-tē	protection against disease
pathogen	path'ō-jĕn	any virus, microorganism, or other substance that causes disease
phagocytosis	fāg-ō-sī-tō'sis	cellular process of eating and destroying substances, usually by the neutrophils and macrophages **(Figure 9-8)**

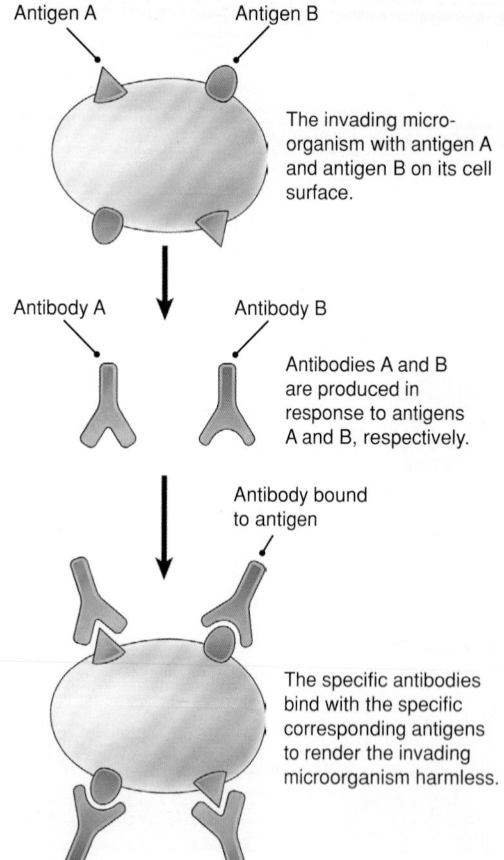
Antigen A
Antigen B
The invading micro-organism with antigen A and antigen B on its cell surface.
Antibody A
Antibody B
Antibodies A and B are produced in response to antigens A and B, respectively.
Antibody bound to antigen
The specific antibodies bind with the specific corresponding antigens to render the invading microorganism harmless.

Figure 9-7 Antibodies bind with antigens to provide immunity against specific microorganisms.

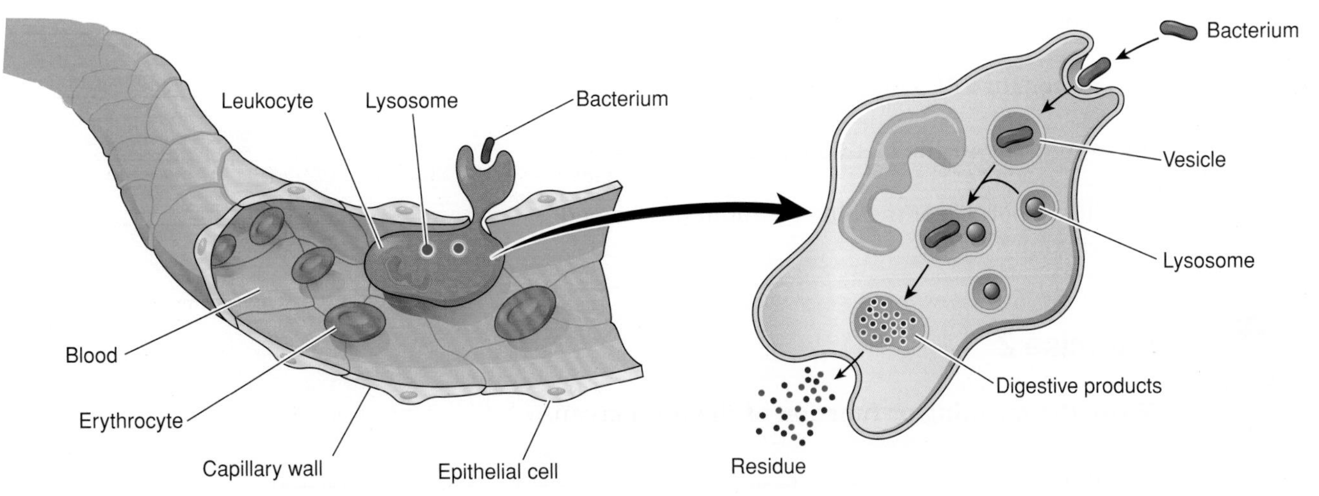

Figure 9-8 Phagocytosis.

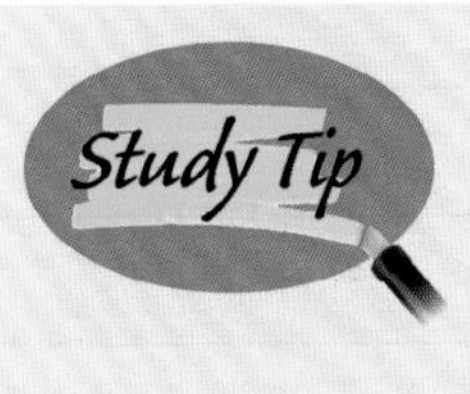

Phagocytosis: You may be familiar with a video arcade game called *Pac-Man,* featuring the titular round yellow character that goes around eating anything in his way. Phagocytosis is a process in which a particular type of white blood cell does a similar activity (*phag/o* = eating, *cyt/o* = cell, and *-osis* = process). Leukocytes ingest substances such as other cells, bacteria, foreign particles, and dead tissue. Visualizing a cell as resembling Pac-Man may help you to remember the process of phagocytosis.

Exercises: Anatomy and Physiology

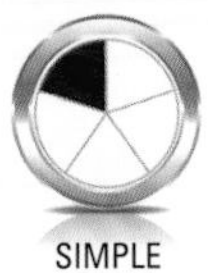

SIMPLE RECALL

Exercise 1

Write the correct anatomic term for the structure described.

1. largest blood cell that protects against pathogens __________
2. cell fragments in blood that form clots __________
3. fluid that circulates through the heart, arteries, capillaries, and veins __________
4. agranulocyte that circulates in the lymphatic system __________
5. liquid portion of blood that carries formed elements __________
6. vascular lymphatic organ __________
7. WBC with visible granules __________
8. WBC without visible granules __________
9. largest of the WBCs __________
10. WBC that stains red __________
11. WBC that stains dark blue __________

12. blood cell that carries oxygen and carbon dioxide ____________________

13. protein in RBCs that binds to oxygen ____________________

14. soft tissue inside medullary cavities of bones ____________________

15. liquid portion of the blood without the formed elements ____________________

SIMPLE RECALL

Exercise 2

Write the meaning or function of the term given.

1. iron ____________________
2. antibody ____________________
3. antigen ____________________
4. pathogen ____________________
5. immunity ____________________
6. erythropoietin ____________________
7. hemopoiesis ____________________
8. neutrophil ____________________
9. clotting factors ____________________
10. Rh factor ____________________

SIMPLE RECALL

Exercise 3

Circle the term that is most appropriate for the meaning of the sentence.

1. The most numerous type of blood cell is the (*leukocyte, erythrocyte, thrombocyte*).
2. (*Stain, Hemoglobin, Granulocytes*) give(s) erythrocytes their red color.
3. The blood cells are also referred to as (*formed elements, histamine, sera*).
4. (*Hemoglobin, Histamine, Fibrin*) is a substance released by damaged cells causing inflammation, redness, and pain.
5. Soldier-like proteins that protect the body are called (*antigens, antibodies, fibrins*).
6. Foreign invaders that can create an immune response are called (*antigens, antibodies, fibrins*).
7. Blood cell production takes place in the (*bone marrow, liver, spleen*).
8. The (*bone marrow, liver, spleen*) is responsible for filtering blood.

9. The kidneys release a hormone called (*erythropoietin, histamine, hematopoiesis*) that stimulates the production of RBCs in bone marrow.

10. The medical term for white blood cell is (*erythrocyte, leukocyte, thrombocyte*).

11. The monocyte that is active in phagocytosis in tissues is called a (*granulocyte, macrophage, monophage*).

12. The liquid portion of blood, without the clotting factors and blood cells, is called (*serum, plasma, formed elements*).

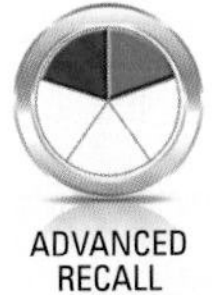

ADVANCED RECALL

Exercise 4

Match each term with its meaning.

phagocytosis	leukocyte	antibody
Rh factor	pathogen	fibrin
coagulation	hemoglobin	platelet

1. may induce intense antigenic reactions ____________________
2. clotting ____________________
3. soldier-like protein protecting the body ____________________
4. elastic fiber protein used in clotting ____________________
5. white blood cell ____________________
6. oxygen-binding protein found in RBCs ____________________
7. any disease-causing substance ____________________
8. thrombocyte ____________________
9. cellular process of eating and destroying ____________________

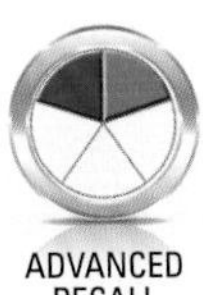

ADVANCED RECALL

Exercise 5

Fill in the blanks with the correct answers.

1. A white blood cell that produces antibodies to inactivate an antigen is called a(n) ____________________ lymphocyte.
2. A white blood cell that matures in the thymus gland and specializes in creating an immune response is called a(n) ____________________ lymphocyte.
3. The ____________________ is a lymphatic organ that filters out aging red blood cells.
4. The type of blood cell that carries oxygen and carbon dioxide is a(n) ____________________.
5. The elastic fiber protein needed in clotting is called ____________________.

6. A white blood cell with visible granules when stained is referred to as a(n) ______________________.

7. A large red blood cell is called a(n) ______________________.

8. ______________________ is the plasma protein that is converted into solid threads called fibrin.

9. The ______________________ is an enlarged and mature monocyte active in phagocytosis.

WORD PARTS

The following tables list word parts related to blood and the immune system.

Combining Forms

Combining Form	Meaning
chrom/o, chromat/o	color
cyt/o	cell
erythr/o	red
granul/o	granules
hem/o, hemat/o	blood
immun/o	immune, safe
leuk/o	white
lymph/o	lymph
neutr/o	neutral
nucle/o	nucleus
path/o	disease
phag/o	eat, swallow
phleb/o	vein
plas/o	formation, growth
thromb/o	blood clot

Prefixes

Prefix	Meaning
auto-	self, same
basi-, baso-	base
macro-	large, long
micro-	small
mono-	one
pro-	before, promoting
poly-	many, much

Suffixes

Suffix	Meaning
-cyte	cell
-emia	blood (condition of)
-sis	condition, process
-gen	origin, production
-lysis	destruction, breakdown, separation
-osis	abnormal condition
-penia	deficiency
-philia	attraction for, liking
-poiesis	production, formation
-rrhage	flowing forth
-y	condition of

Exercises: Word Parts

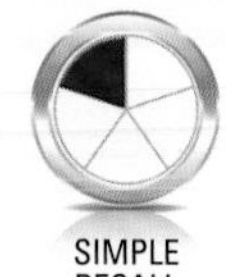
SIMPLE RECALL

Exercise 6

Write the meaning of the combining form given.

1. hem/o, hemat/o ______
2. path/o ______
3. thromb/o ______
4. immun/o ______
5. leuk/o ______
6. erythr/o ______
7. phag/o ______
8. granul/o ______
9. phleb/o ______
10. chrom/o, chromat/o ______
11. neutr/o ______
12. plas/o ______

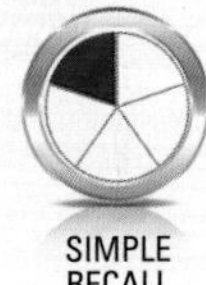

Exercise 7

Write the correct combining form for the meaning given.

1. blood clot ______
2. formation, growth ______
3. lymph ______
4. neutral ______
5. blood ______
6. red ______
7. white ______
8. eat, swallow ______
9. cell ______
10. nucleus ______

SIMPLE RECALL

Exercise 8

Write the meaning of the prefix or suffix given.

1. auto- ______
2. -rrhage ______
3. mono- ______
4. baso- ______
5. poly- ______
6. -philia ______
7. -penia ______
8. -lysis ______
9. -poiesis ______
10. macro- ______
11. micro- ______
12. -emia ______
13. -gen ______
14. -osis ______

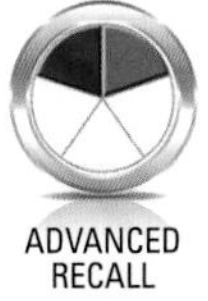

ADVANCED RECALL

Exercise 9

Considering the meaning of the combining form from which the medical term is made, write the meaning of the medical term. (You have not yet learned many of these terms, but you can build their meanings from the word parts.)

Combining Form	Meaning	Medical Term	Meaning of Term
phleb/o	vein	phlebology	1. ______
hem/o	blood	hemorrhage	2. ______
thromb/o	blood clot	thrombocyte	3. ______
erythr/o	red	erythrocyte	4. ______
neutr/o	neutral	neutrophil	5. ______

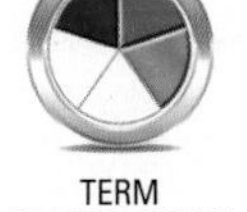

TERM CONSTRUCTION

Exercise 10

Write the remainder of the term for the meaning given.

Meaning	Medical Term
1. white (blood) cell	leuko______
2. destruction of a blood clot	lysis______
3. abnormal condition of a single nucleus	mono______osis
4. deficiency of all blood cells	______cytopenia
5. condition of many blood cells	______cythemia
6. formation of red (blood cells)	______poiesis
7. study of veins	phlebo ______

■ MEDICAL TERMS

The following table gives adjective forms and terms used in describing blood, the immune system, and conditions of the blood and immune system.

Adjectives and Other Related Terms

Term	Pronunciation	Meaning
autoimmunity	aw′tō-i-myū′ni-tē	pertaining to one's immune system attacking its own tissues or cells
cytopathic	sī′tō-path′ik	pertaining to a disease or disorder of a cell or cellular component
hemopoietic; *syn.* hematopoietic	hē′mō-poy-et′ik; hē′mă-tō-poy-et′ik	pertaining to the formation of blood cells
hemolytic	hē′mō-lit′ik	pertaining to the rupture or destruction of red blood cells

(continued)

Adjectives and Other Related Terms *(continued)*

Term	Pronunciation	Meaning
hemorrhagic	hem′ŏr-aj′ik	pertaining to profuse or excessive bleeding
hemostasis	hē′mō-stā′sis	stopping blood flow or arresting bleeding
hypersensitive	hī′per-sen′si-tiv	condition of excessive response or an exaggerated sensitivity to a stimulus
inflammatory	in-flam′ă-tōr-ē	pertaining to heat, redness, swelling, and pain in response to tissue injury
predisposition	prē′dis-pō-zish′ŭn	condition of being susceptible to disease
proliferative	prō-lif′ĕr-ă-tiv	growing and increasing in number of similar cells
rejection	rē-jek′shŭn	immunologic response of incompatibility to a transplanted organ or tissue
systemic	sis-tem′ik	pertaining to the whole body
virulent	vir′yū-lĕnt	denotes an extremely toxic pathogen

ANIMATION

To learn more about the inflammatory response and the role that it and phagocytosis play in healing wounds, view the animation "Wound Healing" included with the Student Resources on thePoint.

Exercises: Adjectives and Other Related Terms

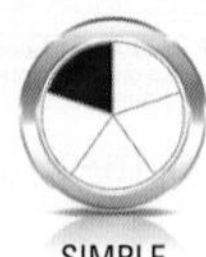
SIMPLE RECALL

Exercise 11

Circle the term that is most appropriate for the meaning of the sentence.

1. Hemophilia is a disorder characterized by a tendency to bleed excessively; this may also be called a(n) (*inflammatory, hemorrhagic, proliferative*) disease.

2. Lupus erythematosus is usually referred to as a (*systemic, hypersensitive, hemolytic*) disease because it can affect the body as a whole.

3. (*Autoimmunity, Predisposition, Rejection*) occurs when there is an incompatibility with transplanted tissue.

4. The condition of being susceptible to disease is called (*predisposition, rejection, autoimmunity*).

5. (*Hemorrhagic, Hemolytic, Hemostasis*) means pertaining to the rupture or destruction of red blood cells.

6. The term (*cytopathic, hematopoietic, systemic*) means pertaining to a disease or disorder of a cell or cellular component.

7. When a patient's immune system attacks its own tissues or cells, it is called (*cytopathic, autoimmunity, rejection*).

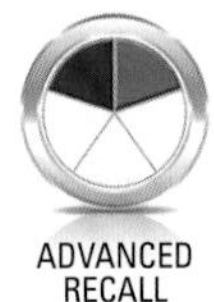

Exercise 12

Match each word with its meaning.

rejection	virulent	hemostasis	hypersensitive
inflammatory	systemic	hemopoietic	proliferative

1. stopping or arresting bleeding ______________________
2. immune response of incompatibility ______________________
3. growing and increasing in number of similar cells ______________________
4. pertaining to swelling, pain, and redness ______________________
5. denoting a very toxic pathogen ______________________
6. denoting an exaggerated response to a stimulus ______________________
7. pertaining to the formation of blood cells ______________________
8. pertaining to the whole body ______________________

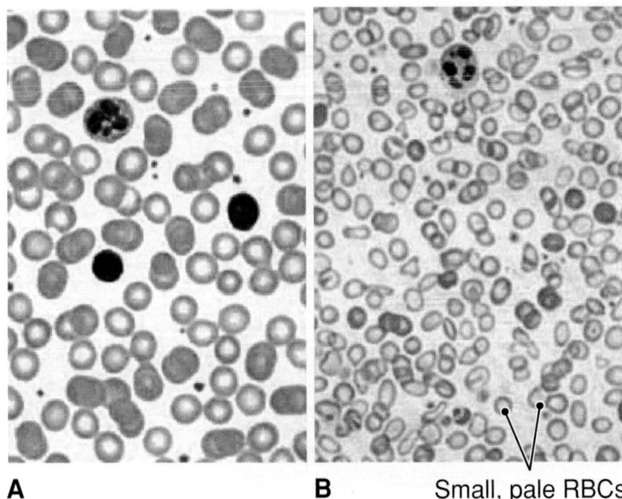

Figure 9-9 A blood smear showing normal red blood cells **(A)** compared with red blood cells in a patient with iron deficiency anemia **(B).** Iron-deficient red blood cells are small (microcytic) and pale (hypochromic).

Medical Conditions

Term	Pronunciation	Meaning
anemia	ă-nē′mē-ă	condition in which the number of red blood cells, hemoglobin, or packed cell volume is lower than normal
Types of Anemia due to Impaired Production of Red Blood Cells		
aplastic anemia	ā-plas′tik ă-nē′mē-ă	disorder in which the bone marrow does not produce enough red blood cells
iron deficiency anemia	ī′ŏrn dĕ-fish′ĕn-sē ă-nē′mē-ă	disorder in which hemoglobin is unable to transport oxygen due to a lack of iron **(Figure 9-9)**

(continued)

Medical Conditions *(continued)*

Term	Pronunciation	Meaning
pernicious anemia	pĕr-nish′ŭs ă-nē′mē-ă	disorder in which the number of red blood cells decreases with simultaneous enlargement of individual cells (i.e., macrocytes) due to an inability to absorb vitamin B12; usually in older adults **(Figure 9-10)**
Types of Anemia due to the Destruction or Loss of Red Blood Cells		
hemorrhagic anemia; *syn.* blood loss anemia	hem′ŏr-aj′ik ă-nē′mē-ă; blŭd laws ă-nē′mē-ă	disorder involving lack of red blood cells due to profuse blood loss
thalassemia	thal′ă-sē′mē-ă	disorder caused by a genetic defect resulting in low hemoglobin production
sickle cell anemia	sik′ĕl sel ă-nē′mē-ă	disorder caused by a genetic defect resulting in abnormal hemoglobin causing sickle-shaped red blood cells, which have difficulty moving through small capillary vessels **(Figure 9-11)**
autoimmune disease	aw′tō-i-myūn′ di-zēz′	condition in which the immune system attacks normal body tissues

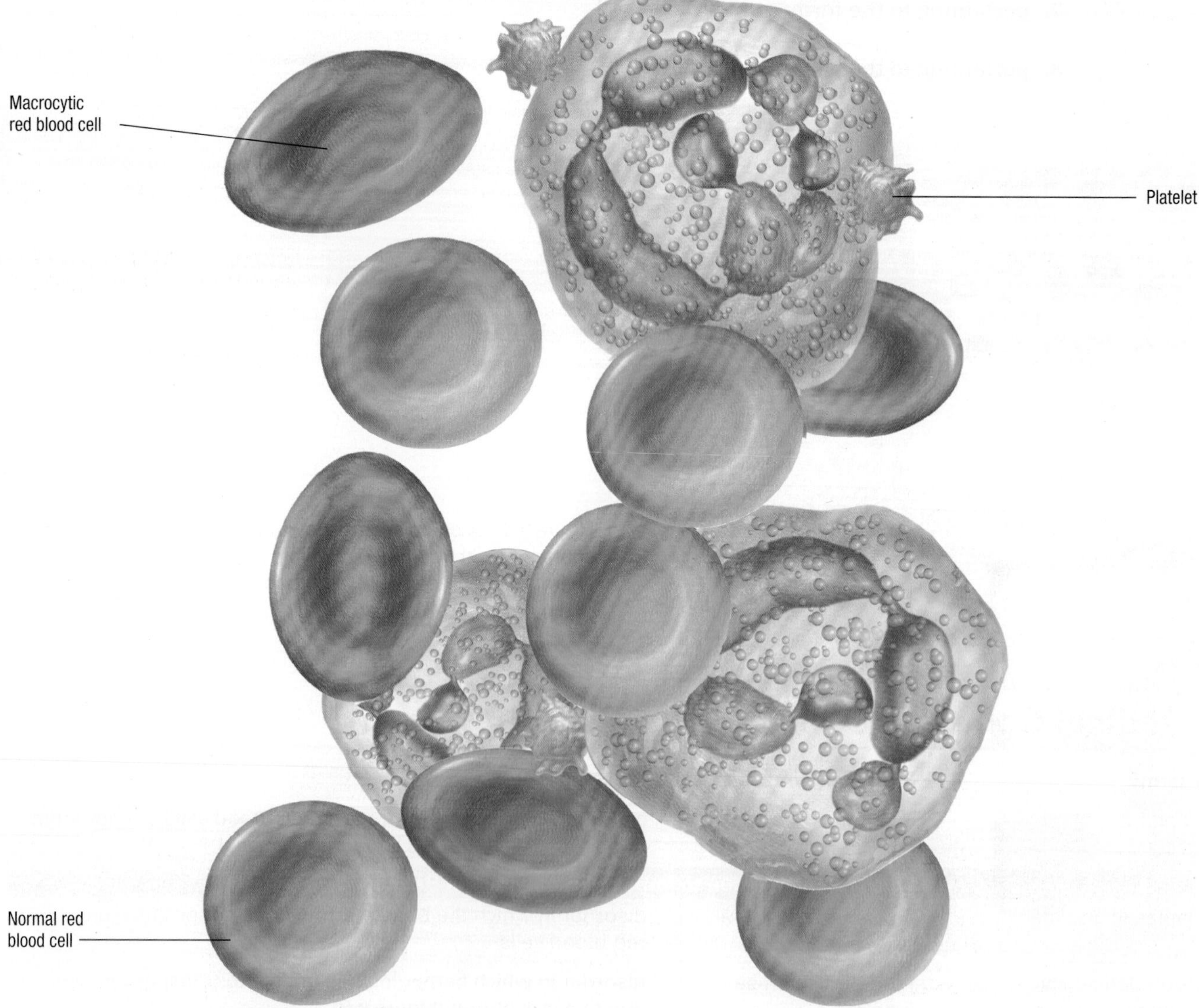

Figure 9-10 A blood smear showing pernicious anemia. Note the large (macrocytic) red blood cells.

Medical Conditions

Term	Pronunciation	Meaning
clotting disorder	klot′ing dis-ōr′dĕr	condition characterized by an inability of blood to coagulate
hemophilia	hē′mō-fil′ē-ă	bleeding disorder due to a deficiency of a clotting factor
thrombocytopenia	throm′bō-sī-tō-pē′nē-ă	disorder involving low levels of platelets in the blood
idiopathic thrombocytopenic purpura (ITP)	id′ē-ō-path′ik throm′bō-sī-tō-pē′nik pur′pyur-ă	disorder resulting from platelet destruction by macrophages characterized by bruising and bleeding from mucous membranes
von Willebrand disease (vWD)	vahn vil′ĕ-brahnt di-zēz′	bleeding disorder characterized by a tendency to bleed primarily from the mucous membranes due to a deficiency of a clotting factor
hemochromatosis	hē′mō-krō-mă-tō′sis	excessive absorption and storage of dietary iron in body tissues causing dysfunction
mononucleosis	mon′ō-nū-klē-ō′sis	increase of mononuclear leukocytes with symptoms of fever, enlarged cervical lymph nodes, and fatigue (Figure 9-12)
pancytopenia	pan′sī-tō-pē′nē-ă	deficiency in all types of blood cells
polycythemia	pol′ē-sī-thē′mē-ă	increase in number of red blood cells
rheumatoid arthritis (RA)	rū′mă-toyd ahr-thrī′tis	autoimmune disease causing progressive destructive changes and inflammation in multiple joints, especially in the hands and feet
septicemia	sep′ti-sē′mē-ă	spread of microorganisms or toxins through circulating blood
Sjögren syndrome	shōr′gren sin′drōm	chronic autoimmune disease characterized by degeneration of the salivary and lacrimal glands causing dryness of the mouth and eyes and other mucous membranes
systemic lupus erythematosus (SLE)	sis-tem′ik lū′pŭs ĕr-ith′ĕ-mă-tō′sŭs	inflammatory, autoimmune, connective tissue disease that can affect all organ systems
thrombosis	throm-bō′sis	abnormal presence of clotting within a blood vessel

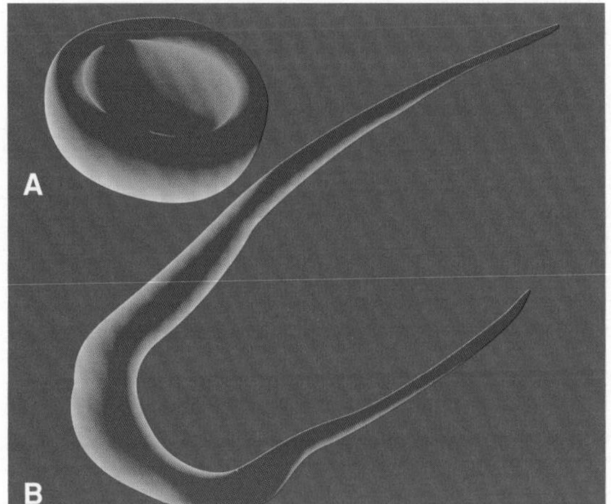

Figure 9-11 Sickle cell anemia. **A.** Normal-shaped red blood cell. **B.** Crescent-shaped sickle cell. A sickle cell crisis causes blood flow obstruction and pain.

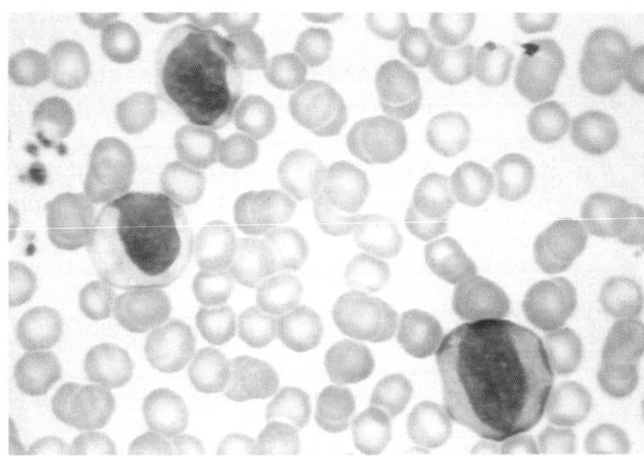

Figure 9-12 Mononucleosis with atypical lymphocytes.

Exercises: Medical Conditions

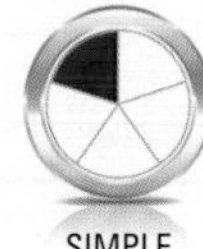

Exercise 13

SIMPLE RECALL

Select the best term to complete the meaning given.

1. hemophilia = tendency to (*bleed, clot*)
2. hemorrhagic anemia = low red blood cell count due to (*bleeding, clotting*)
3. thrombocytopenia = difficulty with clotting due to low (*RBCs, WBCs, platelets*)
4. iron deficiency anemia = inability of hemoglobin to (*produce, transport*) oxygen
5. hemochromatosis = excessive absorption of (*calcium, iron*)
6. aplastic anemia = inability of bone marrow to (*produce, transport*) red blood cells
7. pernicious anemia = (*destruction, increase*) of red blood cells due to inability to absorb vitamin B_{12}
8. von Willebrand disease = (*clotting, autoimmune*) disorder
9. polycythemia = (*decrease, increase*) of red blood cells
10. thalassemia = (*high, low*) hemoglobin production

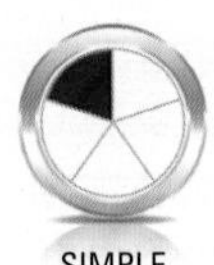

Exercise 14

SIMPLE RECALL

Circle the term that is most appropriate for the meaning of the sentence.

1. Idiopathic thrombocytopenic purpura is a disease due to a destruction of (*leukocytes, platelets, electrolytes*).
2. In (*aplastic, pernicious, virulent*) anemia, there is a decrease in the number of erythrocytes with an increase in their size.
3. The disease that affects mucous membranes is (*septicemia, SLE, Sjögren syndrome*).
4. Mononucleosis has the symptom of enlarged (*lymph nodes, erythrocytes, thrombocytes*).
5. The condition that causes abnormally shaped red blood cells is called (*aplastic anemia, sickle cell anemia, pernicious anemia*).
6. A condition in which the immune system attacks normal body tissues is called (*thrombocytopenia, sickle cell anemia, autoimmune disease*).
7. A clotting disorder is characterized by an inability of blood to (*form, coagulate, dissolve*).
8. An increase in red blood cells is called (*thrombosis, polycythemia, mononucleosis*).
9. Septicemia is the spread of toxins through circulating (*plasma, serum, blood*).
10. Systemic lupus erythematosus is a(n) (*autoimmune, inherited, cytopathic*) connective tissue disease.
11. Rheumatoid arthritis affects a patient's (*bones, organs, joints*).

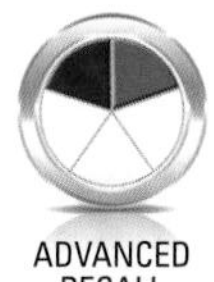
ADVANCED RECALL

Exercise 15

Considering the meaning of the combining form from which the medical term is made, write the meaning of the medical term. (You have not yet learned many of these terms, but you can build their meanings from the word parts.)

Combining Form	Meaning	Medical Term	Meaning of Term
cyt/o	cell	pancytopenia	1. ________
nucle/o	nucleus	mononucleosis	2. ________
plas/o	formation, growth	aplastic	3. ________
hem/o	blood	hemophilia	4. ________
arthr/o	joint	arthritis	5. ________

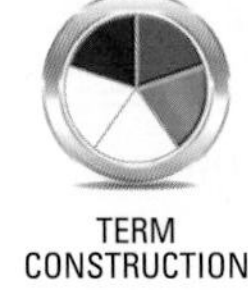
TERM CONSTRUCTION

Exercise 16

Given their meanings, build a medical term from the appropriate combining form and suffix.

Combining Form	Suffix	Term
blood; color	abnormal condition	1. ________
blood	attraction for	2. ________
blood clot; cell	deficiency	3. ________
blood clot	abnormal condition	4. ________
blood	flowing forth	5. ________

Tests and Procedures

Term	Pronunciation	Meaning
Laboratory Tests Related to Hematology		
albumin	al-bū′min	measurement of this protein level; used to diagnose liver or kidney problems, inflammation, malnutrition, or dehydration
bilirubin	bil′i-rū′bin	screen for liver disorders or anemia; bile, found in bilirubin, is a yellow pigment formed from hemoglobin, and excess is associated with jaundice (abnormal yellowing of the skin)
blood smear	blŭd smēr	evaluation of the appearance and number of blood cells and the different types of white blood cells **(Figure 9-13)**

(continued)

Tests and Procedures *(continued)*

Term	Pronunciation	Meaning
complete blood count (CBC); *syn.* hemogram	kŏm-plēt′ blŭd kownt; hē′mō-gram	automated count of all blood cells **(Figure 9-14)**
erythrocyte sedimentation rate (ESR)	ĕ-rith′rŏ-sīt sed′i-mĕn-tā′shŭn rāt	time measurement of red blood cells settling in a test tube over one hour; used to diagnose inflammation and anemias
hematocrit (HCT, Hct)	hē-mat′ō-krit	percentage of red blood cells in a sample of whole blood; used to diagnose various disorders including anemia **(Figure 9-15)**
hemoglobin (HGB, Hgb, Hb) test	hē′mō-glō′bin	test for the red blood cell protein responsible for binding oxygen; used to diagnose various disorders including anemia
platelet count (PLT)	plāt′lĕt kownt	number of platelets present; used to diagnose bleeding disorders or bone marrow disease
red blood cell count (RBC)	red blŭd sel kownt	number of erythrocytes present; used to diagnose various disorders including anemia
white blood cell count (WBC)	wīt blŭd sel kownt	number of leukocytes present; used to diagnose various disorders, including infections and diseases, and for monitoring treatment
crossmatching	kraws mach′ing	blood typing test for compatibility between donor and recipient blood
culture and sensitivity (C&S)	kŭl′chŭr sen′si-tiv′i-tē	growing a microorganism from a specimen taken from the body to determine its susceptibility to particular medications
prothrombin time (PT)	prō-throm′bin tīm	measurement of time for blood to clot
differential white blood count; *syn.* differential count	dif′ĕr-en′shăl wīt blŭd kownt	test that determines the number of each type of white blood cell in a blood sample **(Figure 9-14)**

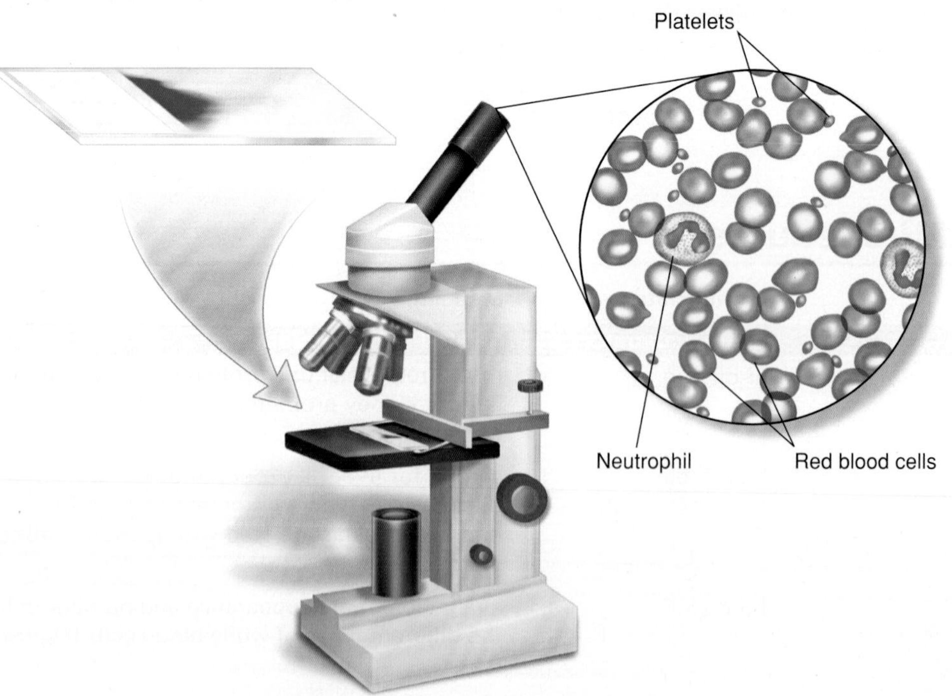

Figure 9-13 Preparation for a blood smear.

Tests and Procedures

Term	Pronunciation	Meaning
Laboratory Tests for Antibodies		
antinuclear antibody (ANA) test	an′tē-nū′klē-ăr an′ti-bod-ē test	assessment for autoimmune disorders such as systemic lupus erythematosus, rheumatoid arthritis, and others
Epstein–Barr virus (EBV) antibody test	ep′stīn bahr vī′rŭs an′ti-bod-ē test	diagnostic test for mononucleosis and evaluation of Epstein–Barr virus
mononucleosis spot test	mon′ō-nū-klē-ō′sis spot test	assessment for mononucleosis
rheumatoid factor test	rū′mă-toyd fak′tŏr test	test for rheumatoid arthritis and Sjögren syndrome

Complete Blood Count (CBC) with differential

Test	Result	Units	Reference Interval
White blood count	1.5 L	x $10^3/mm^3$	5.0–10.0
Red blood count	3.50 L	x $106/mm^3$	4.1–5.3
Hemoglobin	10.8 L	g/dL	12.0–18.0
Hematocrit	31.1 L	%	37.0–52.0
Platelets	302	x $10^3/mm^3$	150–400
Polys (neutrophils)	23 L	%	45–76
Lymphs	68 H	%	17–44
Monocytes	7	%	3–10
Eos	2	%	0–4
Basos	0.6	%	0.2
Polys (absolute)	.34 L	x $10^3/mm^3$	1.8–7.8
Lymphs (absolute)	1.0	x $10^3/mm^3$	0.7–4.5
Monocytes (absolute)	0.1	x $10^3/mm^3$	0.1–1.0
Eos (absolute)	0.1	x $10^3/mm^3$	0.0–0.4
Basos (absolute)	0.0	x $10^3/mm^3$	0.0–0.2

Figure 9-14 Complete blood count (CBC) report.

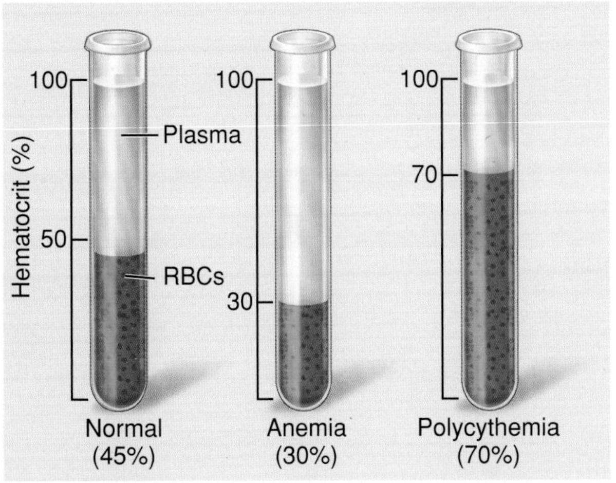

Figure 9-15 Hematocrit. The hematocrit can diagnose anemia or polycythemia.

Exercises: Tests and Procedures

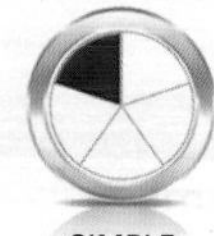

SIMPLE RECALL

Exercise 17

Circle the term that is most appropriate for the meaning of the sentence.

1. The rheumatoid factor test is used to help diagnosis rheumatoid arthritis and (*Epstein–Barr virus, Sjögren syndrome, anemia*).
2. The diagnostic test for mononucleosis and evaluation for Epstein–Barr virus is called the (*EBV antibody test, PLT count, ANA test*).
3. It is important for a blood donor and recipient to have had (*crossmatching, culture and sensitivity, prothrombin time*) tests done to assess compatibility.
4. A test designed to measure the clotting time of blood is a (*bilirubin, prothrombin time, blood smear*).
5. (*HCT, HGB, ESR*) is a test that measures the red blood cell protein responsible for carrying oxygen.
6. In the complete blood count, an increase in the erythrocyte sedimentation rate may signal (*hemophilia, inflammation, erythrocytes*) and/or anemia.
7. To evaluate the number of each type of leukocyte, a (*differential white blood count, white blood cell count, platelet count*) might be ordered.
8. A (*hemoglobin, complete blood count, hematocrit*) measures the percentage of red blood cells in a volume of blood.
9. A culture and sensitivity identifies a (*blood cell, donor, pathogen*) and tests its susceptibility to (*blood transfusion, antibiotic, gene therapy*) treatment.
10. To rule out an autoimmune disease, a physician may order a(n) (*ANA, ESR, BUN*).

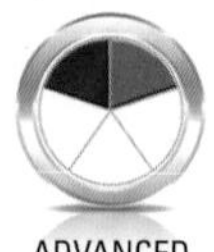

ADVANCED RECALL

Exercise 18

Match each laboratory test with its description.

platelet count	albumin	white blood cell count	blood smear
red blood cell count	hemogram	bilirubin	

1. evaluation of blood cells and different WBCs ____________________
2. number of erythrocytes ____________________
3. another name for complete blood count ____________________
4. diagnosis of bleeding disorders ____________________
5. measurement of protein level ____________________
6. screen for liver disorders or anemia ____________________
7. number of leukocytes ____________________

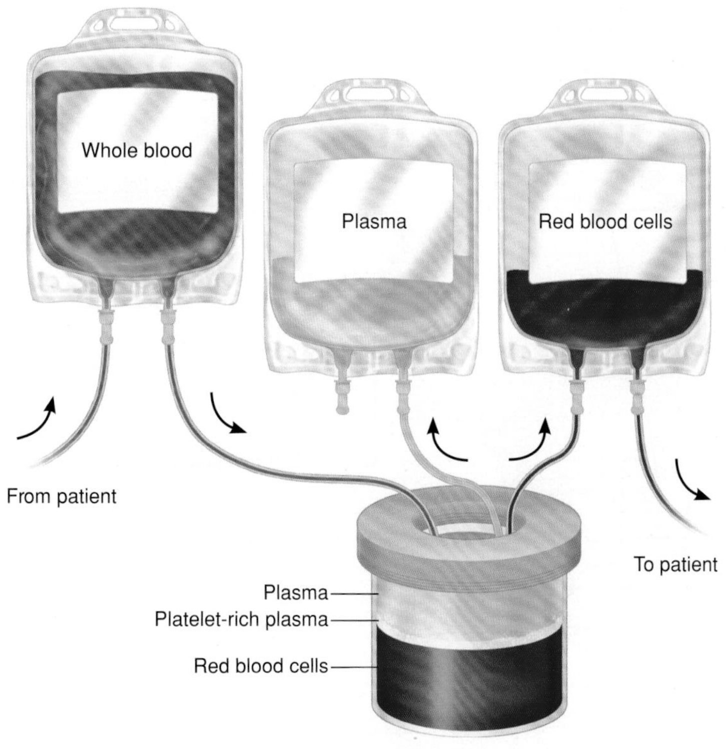

Figure 9-16 Apheresis.

Surgical Interventions and Therapeutic Procedures

Term	Pronunciation	Meaning
apheresis	ā-fĕr-ē'sis	infusion of a patient's own blood after certain cellular or fluid elements have been removed; used especially to remove antibodies in treating autoimmune disorders **(Figure 9-16)**
blood transfusion (BT)	blŭd trans-fyū'zhŭn	transfer of blood between compatible donor and recipient
autologous blood	aw-tol'ŏ-gŭs blud	blood donated for future use by same patient; usually presurgical
blood component therapy	blŭd kŏm-pō'nĕnt thār'ă-pē	transfusion of specific blood components such as packed red blood cells, plasma, or platelets
homologous blood	hŏ-mol'ō-gŭs blŭd	blood donated from same species for use by a compatible recipient
bone marrow aspiration (BMA)	bōn mar'ō as-pir-ā'shŭn	removal of a small amount of fluid and cells from inside the bone with a needle and syringe **(Figure 9-17)**
bone marrow transplant (BMT)	bōn mar'ō trans'plant	transfer of bone marrow from one person to another
immunization; *syn.* vaccination	im'myū-nī-zā'shŭn; vak'si-nā'shŭn	administration of a weakened or killed pathogen, or a protein of a pathogen, to cause the immune system to create antibodies for future protection **(Figure 9-18)**
immunosuppression	im'yū-nō-sŭ-presh'ŭn	use of chemotherapy or immunosuppressant drugs to interfere with immune responses; usually prescribed for autoimmune disorders
phlebotomy; *syn.* venipuncture, venotomy	fle-bot'ŏ-mē; ven'i-pŭngk'shŭr, vē-not'ŏ-mē	incision into a vein to inject a solution or withdraw blood **(Figure 9-19)**
plasmapheresis	plaz'mă-fĕr-ē'sis	removal and replacement of a patient's own blood after plasma has been removed and replaced with a plasma substitute
splenectomy	splē-nek'tŏ-mē	surgical removal of the spleen

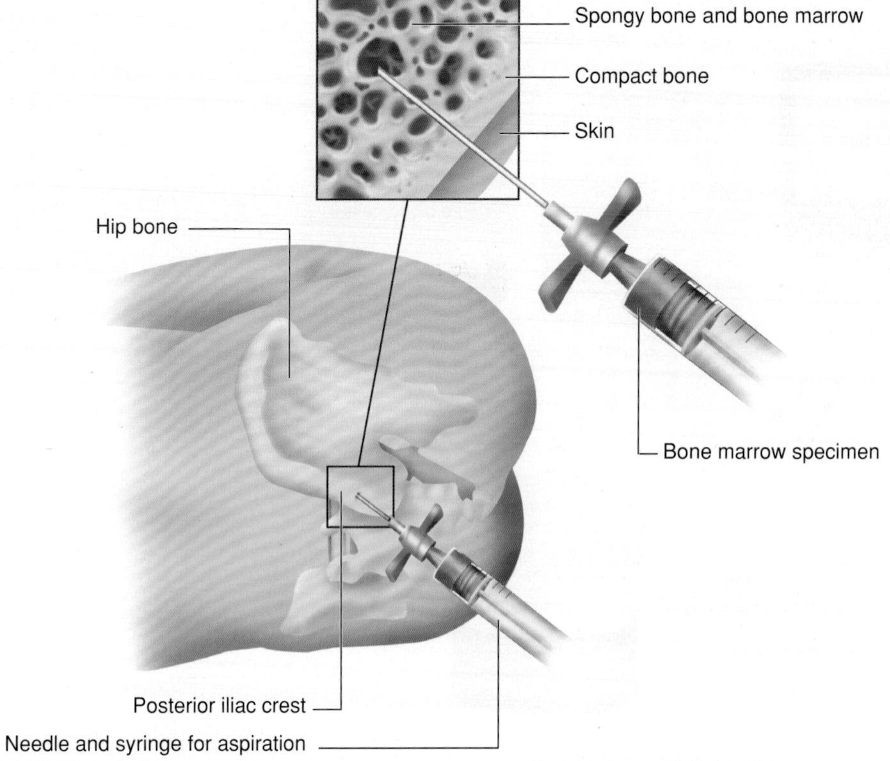

Figure 9-17 Bone marrow aspiration.

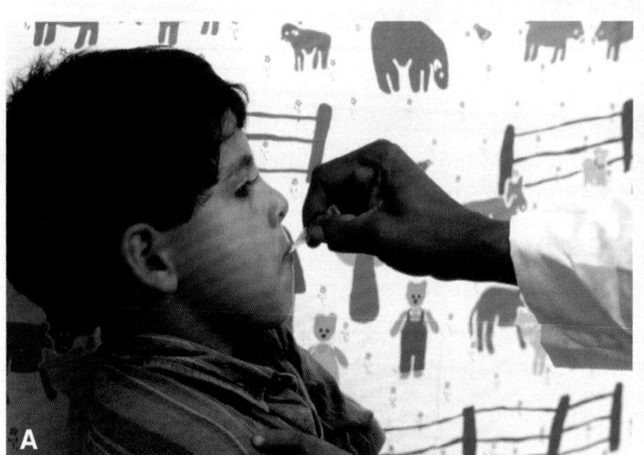

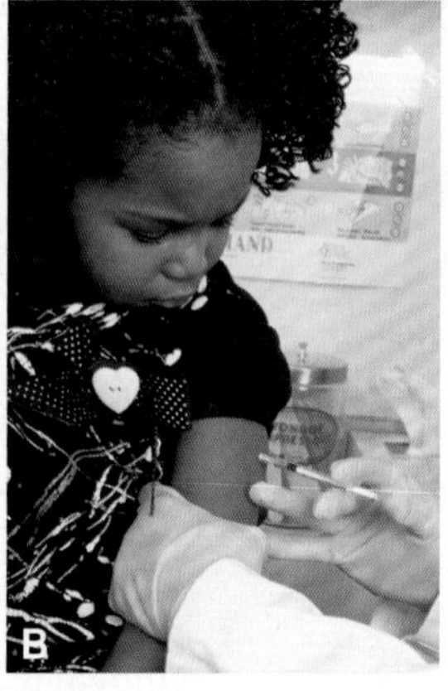

Figure 9-18 Forms of immunization. **A.** Oral administration of an immunization. **B.** Immunization by injection.

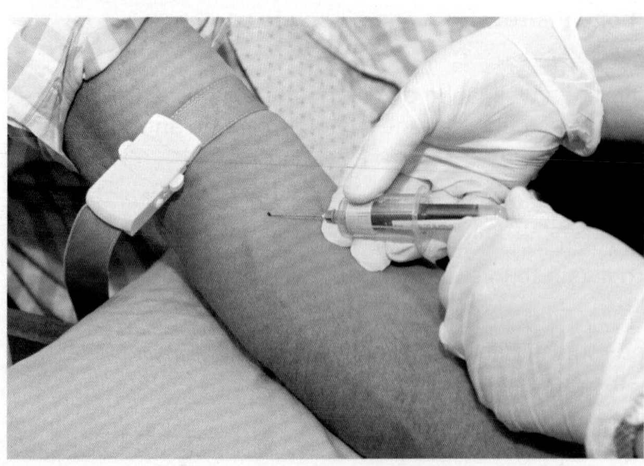

Figure 9-19 Phlebotomy to withdraw blood.

ANIMATION

View the video "Venipuncture" on the Student Resources on thePoint for a demonstration of a phlebotomist using a syringe to withdraw blood from a patient.

Exercises: Surgical Interventions and Therapeutic Procedures

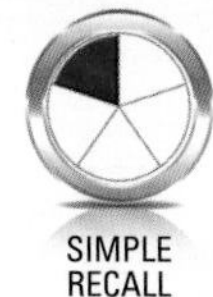
SIMPLE RECALL

Exercise 19

Write the correct medical term or procedure for the meaning given.

1. removal of plasma from the blood ____________________
2. bone marrow transfer from one person to another ____________________
3. removal of the spleen ____________________
4. transfer of blood between donor and recipient ____________________
5. transfusion of blood components ____________________
6. blood donated by same person for future use ____________________
7. blood donated by another person ____________________
8. removal and replacement of patient's own blood after removal of specific substances ____________________

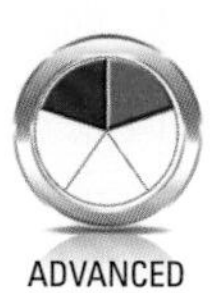
ADVANCED RECALL

Exercise 20

Circle the term that is most appropriate for the meaning of the sentence.

1. Mr. DeHaan was on the surgical schedule for a (*splenectomy, hepatectomy, bone marrow aspiration*), a removal of the immune system organ responsible for removing old blood cells.
2. Mrs. Chon wanted to be protected from pathogens while she traveled abroad, so her physician ordered a series of (*immunosuppressants, vaccinations, anticoagulants*).
3. The medical assistant is responsible for drawing blood from patients. This procedure is called (*phlebotomy, venectomy, splenectomy*).
4. The medical technologist who works in the clinical lab occasionally performs crossmatching tests for (*blood transfusions, bone marrow aspirations, vaccinations*).
5. The physician removed a small amount of fluid and cells from inside the bone with a needle and syringe; this procedure is called a bone marrow (*transplant, aspiration, biopsy*).
6. The child received (*apheresis, immunizations, transfusions*) to prevent future illnesses.
7. Dr. Adams prescribed (*immunization, immunosuppression, blood transfusion*) therapy to help treat the patient's autoimmune disease.

Medications and Drug Therapies

Term	Pronunciation	Meaning
antibiotic	an'tē-bī-ot'ik	drug that kills or inhibits the growth of microorganisms
anticoagulant	an'tē-kō-ag'yŭ-lănt	drug that prevents or inhibits blood clotting
antihistamine	an'tē-his'tă-mēn	drug used to stop the effects of histamine; used especially to treat allergies
hemostatic agent; *syn.* procoagulant	hē'mō-stat'ik ā'jĕnt; prō-kō-ag'yū-lant	drug that stops the flow of blood within vessels
immune serum; *syn.* antiserum	i-myūn' sēr'ŭm; an'tē-sē'rŭm	serum containing antibodies against specific antigens; used to treat specific diseases
immunosuppressant	im'yū-nō-sŭ-pres'ănt	drug used to suppress or reduce immune responses in organ transplant recipients or those with severe autoimmune diseases

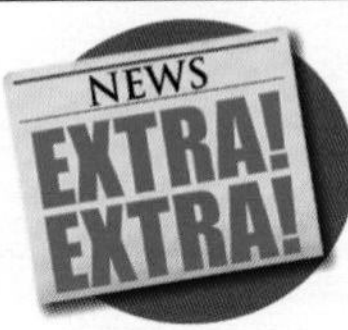

IMMUNOSUPPRESSANT DRUGS When a patient receives an organ transplant, the body treats the transplanted organ as if it were an invader or pathogen and attempts to fight it off. To protect the newly introduced organ from the recipient's own immune system, the patient is prescribed immunosuppressive drugs. These drugs suppress the person's immune system response, which in turn makes them susceptible to other diseases. It is important that patients receiving immunosuppressants see their physician regularly to screen for side effects that may lead to hypertension (high blood pressure) and kidney or liver issues.

Term	Pronunciation	Meaning
thrombolytic agent	throm'bō-lit'ik ā'jĕnt	drug that dissolves a blood clot
vaccine	vak-sēn'	preparation composed of a weakened or killed pathogen

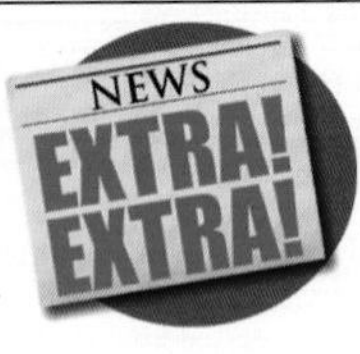

VACCINES AND COWS The Latin word *vaccinus* means relating to a cow. During the mid-1700s, it was known around the English countryside that milkmaids previously infected with the mild cowpox disease would not catch the more deadly smallpox disease. During the devastating smallpox outbreak in 18th-century Europe, Dr. Edward Jenner developed the first vaccination by injecting pus and lymph from a cowpox-infected cow into healthy people. These people never became afflicted with smallpox. This practice was widely successful and has contributed to the concept of vaccines today.

Exercise: Medications and Drug Therapies

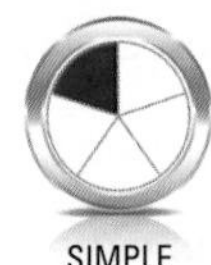

Exercise 21

Write the correct medication or drug therapy term for the meaning given.

1. drug that prevents or inhibits blood clotting ______________________
2. preparation that contains a weakened or killed pathogen ______________________
3. drug that acts against microorganisms ______________________
4. serum containing specific antibodies ______________________
5. drug that stops the flow of blood within blood vessels ______________________
6. drug used to suppress or reduce immune response ______________________

7. drug that stops the effects of histamine ____________

8. drug that dissolves a blood clot ____________

Specialties and Specialists

Term	Pronunciation	Meaning
allergology	al′er-gol′o-jē	medical specialty concerned with diagnosis and treatment of allergic conditions
allergist	al′er-jist	physician who specializes in the treatment of allergies
hematology	hē′mă-tol′o-jē	medical specialty concerned with diagnosis and treatment of disorders of the blood and blood-forming organs
hematologist	hē′mă-tol′o-jist	physician who specializes in hematology
immunology	im′yū-nol′o-jē	medical specialty concerned with immunity, allergy, and induced sensitivity
immunologist	im′yū-nol′o-jist	one who practices immunology
rheumatology	rū′mă-tol′o-jē	medical specialty concerned with diagnosis and treatment of rheumatic conditions (those affecting joints), arthritis, and autoimmune diseases
rheumatologist	rū′mă-tol′o-jist	a physician who specializes in rheumatology

Exercise: Specialties and Specialists

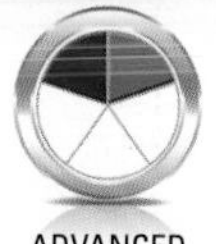

ADVANCED RECALL

Exercise 22

Match each medical specialty or specialist with its description.

hematology	rheumatology	allergology	immunology
hematologist	rheumatologist	allergist	immunologist

1. medical specialty concerned with diagnosis and treatment of allergic conditions ____________

2. physician who specializes in rheumatology ____________

3. physician who specializes in disorders of the blood ____________

4. medical specialty concerned with disorders of blood and blood-forming organs ____________

5. medical specialty concerning with immunity, allergy, and induced sensitivity ____________

6. physician who specializes in treatment of allergies ____________

7. physician who specializes in immunology ____________

8. medical specialty concerned with rheumatic conditions and autoimmune diseases ____________

Abbreviations

Abbreviation	Meaning
Ab	antibody
Ag	antigen
ANA	antinuclear antibody test
BMA	bone marrow aspiration
BMT	bone marrow transplant
BT	blood transfusion
CBC	complete blood count
C&S	culture and sensitivity
EBV	Epstein–Barr virus
EPO	erythropoietin
ESR	erythrocyte sedimentation rate
Fe	iron
HCT, Hct, ht	hematocrit
HGB, Hb, Hgb	hemoglobin
ITP	idiopathic thrombocytopenic purpura
PLT	platelet or platelet count
PT	prothrombin time
RA	rheumatoid arthritis
RBC	red blood cell; red blood cell count
SLE	systemic lupus erythematosus
vWD	von Willebrand disease
WBC	white blood cell; white blood cell count

Exercises: Abbreviations

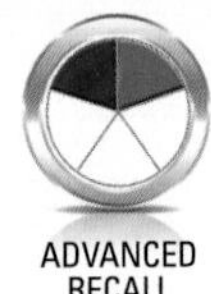
ADVANCED RECALL

Exercise 23

Write the meaning of each abbreviation used in these sentences.

1. Mr. Matthews must have a **PT** done once a month because he has **vWD,** a blood clotting disorder.

____

2. It was necessary to perform a **BMA** on the donor before scheduling the **BMT.**

____

3. Today, Ms. Tisha will be responsible for performing all **CBC** tests in the clinical lab.

____

4. An **ESR** test is used to diagnose inflammation.

____

5. Routinely, an **Hgb** and an **Hct** are performed together.

____

6. Two types of blood cells are **RBC**s and **WBC**s.

____

7. A patient with **ITP** will likely need several **BT**s in their lifetime.

____

8. An **Ab** is a cell that inactivates **Ag**s; this provides immunity against specific organisms.

____

9. A **C&S** is performed to identify a pathogen and determine antibiotic treatment.

____

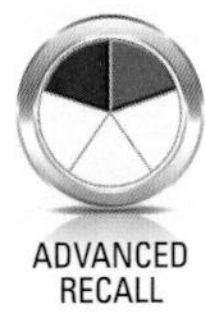
ADVANCED RECALL

Exercise 24

Match each abbreviation with the appropriate description.

PLT	SLE	Fe	RA
EPO	ESR	ANA	EBV

1. needed for oxygen transport by hemoglobin ______________
2. platelet count ______________
3. time measurement of RBCs settling in a test tube ______________
4. hormone that stimulates RBC production ______________
5. test for autoimmune diseases ______________
6. test for mononucleosis ______________
7. autoimmune connective tissue disease ______________
8. autoimmune disease causing inflammation in multiple joints ______________

WRAPPING UP

- The blood system consists of the organs, namely the red bone marrow and spleen, that make blood.
- The major organs of the immune system are the thymus and the lymph nodes, which protect the body against foreign microorganisms and abnormal native cells.
- In this chapter, you learned medical terminology including word parts, prefixes, suffixes, adjectives, conditions, tests, procedures, medications, specialties, and abbreviations related to both the blood and immune systems.

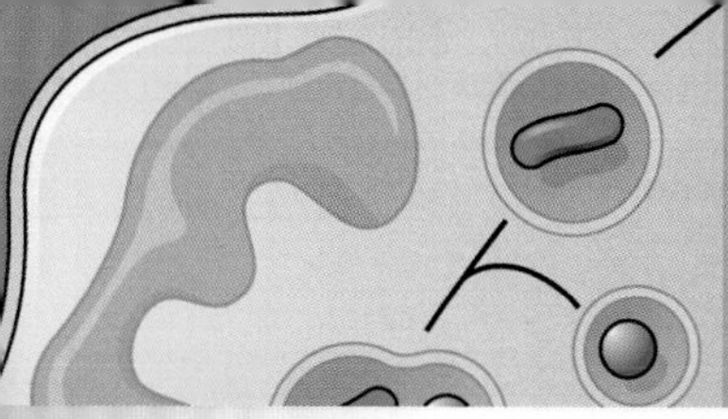

Chapter Review

Review of Terms for Anatomy and Physiology

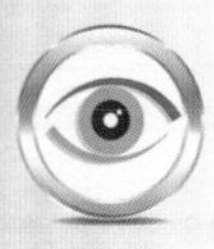

VISUAL

Exercise 25

Write the correct terms on the blanks for the blood cells indicated.

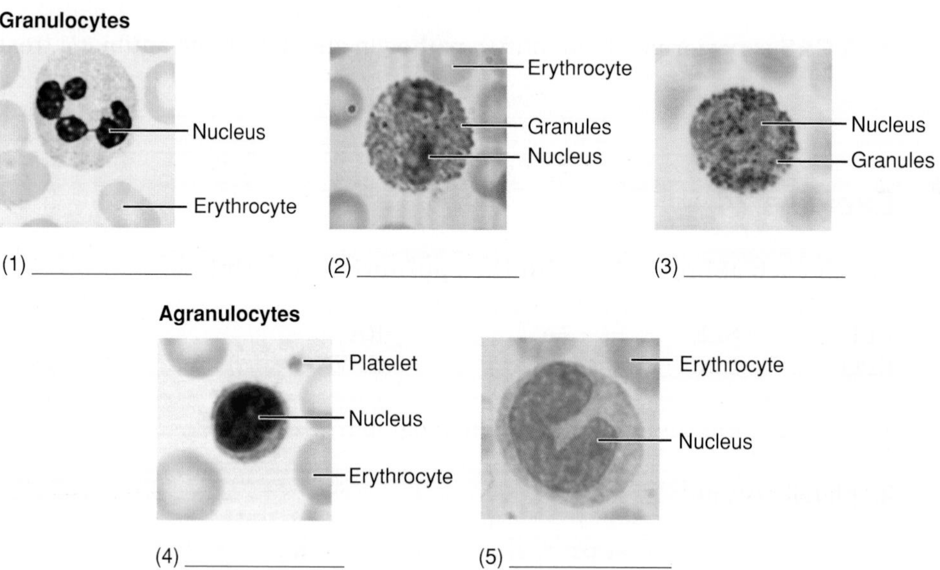

(1) ____________ (2) ____________ (3) ____________

(4) ____________ (5) ____________

Understanding Term Structure

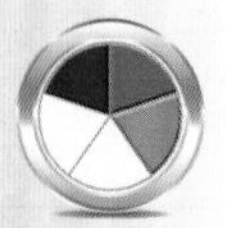

TERM CONSTRUCTION

Exercise 26

Break the given medical term into its word parts and define each part. Then define the medical term. (Note: You may need to use word parts from other chapters.)

For example:

granulocyte	*word parts:*	granul/o, -itis
	meanings:	granules, inflammation of
	term meaning:	cell with (visible) granules

1. hemostasis	*word parts:*	____________
	meanings:	____________
	term meaning:	____________

2. erythrocyte
word parts: ______
meanings: ______
term meaning: ______

3. hematopoiesis
word parts: ______
meanings: ______
term meaning: ______

4. thrombocytopenia
word parts: ______
meanings: ______
term meaning: ______

5. pathogen
word parts: ______
meanings: ______
term meaning: ______

6. cytopathic
word parts: ______
meanings: ______
term meaning: ______

7. aplastic
word parts: ______
meanings: ______
term meaning: ______

8. chromatic
word parts: ______
meanings: ______
term meaning: ______

9. anemia
word parts: ______
meanings: ______
term meaning: ______

10. hemochromatosis
word parts: ______
meanings: ______
term meaning: ______

11. hemophilia *word parts:* ______________________

meanings: ______________________

term meaning: ______________________

12. granulocyte *word parts:* ______________________

meanings: ______________________

term meaning: ______________________

13. lymphocytic *word parts:* ______________________

meanings: ______________________

term meaning: ______________________

14. hemorrhage *word parts:* ______________________

meanings: ______________________

term meaning: ______________________

15. mononucleosis *word parts:* ______________________

meanings: ______________________

term meaning: ______________________

Comprehension Exercises

Exercise 27

COMPREHENSION

Fill in the blank with the correct term.

1. Soldier-like cells that protect the body and inactivate antigens and also provide immunity against specific organisms are called ______________________.
2. ______________________ are agents or substances that induce an immune response.
3. A(n) ______________________ is the administration of a weakened pathogen for future protection.
4. ______________________ anemia results from blood loss.
5. ______________________ is the medical term for low number of blood platelets.
6. ______________________ is an immune system response causing heat, redness, pain, and swelling.
7. ESR stands for ______________________.
8. A differential count usually evaluates ______________________ blood cells.

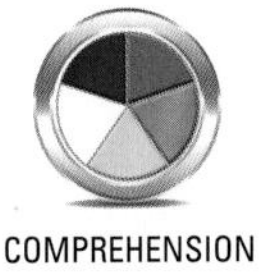

COMPREHENSION

Exercise 28

Write a phrase or short answer for each question.

1. Why would immunosuppressants be given to organ transplant recipients? ____________

2. List the three types of blood cells involved in pancytopenia. ____________

3. What type of drug would not be given to a patient with von Willebrand disease? ____________

4. What red blood cell test might indicate inflammation? ____________

5. What is the difference between an antigen and an antibody? ____________

6. In what process is fibrin needed? ____________

7. In idiopathic thrombocytopenic purpura, which of the three types of basic formed element is attacking the body? ____________

8. A positive mononucleosis spot test would indicate the increased presence of which type of blood cell? ____________

9. What type of transplant might be necessary to treat aplastic anemia? ____________

10. What type of blood transfusion does not require crossmatching? ____________

11. How do immunosuppressant drugs aid in the treatment of rheumatoid arthritis? ____________

12. What is the difference between a vaccine and a vaccination? ____________

13. Why is the term *systemic* included in the term *systemic lupus erythematosus*? ____________

14. Which blood test looks for a pathogen and possible treatment? ____________

15. Where does most hematopoiesis occur? ____________

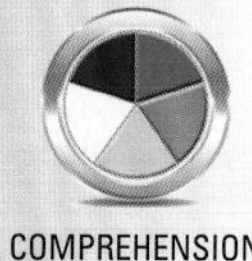

Exercise 29

COMPREHENSION

Circle the letter of the best answer in the following questions.

1. *Plas/o* is a combining form that means

A. chemistry.
B. immune.
C. immature.
D. formation.

2. The best definition for the word *pathogen* is a

A. treatment.
B. lab test.
C. virulent disease.
D. disease-causing agent.

3. An erythrocyte is also known as a

A. granule.
B. red blood cell.
C. hemoglobin cell.
D. membrane.

4. Thrombocytopenia is a condition of

A. too many leukocytes.
B. too few leukocytes.
C. too many platelets.
D. too few platelets.

5. The procedure for drawing blood from a vein is

A. plasmapheresis.
B. phlebotomy.
C. phagocytosis.
D. blood transfusion.

6. The word *cell* can be represented by the combining form *cyt/o,* or with the word part *-cyte,* which is a

A. combining vowel.
B. combining form.
C. suffix.
D. prefix.

7. The monocyte active in phagocytosis in tissue is called a(n)

A. macrophage.
B. eosinophil.
C. neutrophil.
D. macrocyte.

8. Hemoglobin transports oxygen in which type of blood cell?

A. erythrocyte
B. leukocyte
C. thrombocyte
D. eosinophil

9. The action of a hemostatic agent is to

A. prolong bleeding time.
B. prevent clotting.
C. promote clotting.
D. produce blood cells.

10. Cells with granules that are stainable with a basic dye are called

A. basophils.
B. eosinophils.
C. thrombocytes.
D. neutrophils.

11. An immunologist studies

A. immunity.
B. allergy.
C. induced sensitivity.
D. all of the above

12. EPO is an abbreviation for a hormone that stimulates production of

A. thrombocytes.
B. lymphocytes.
C. leukocytes.
D. erythrocytes.

Application and Analysis

CASE STUDIES

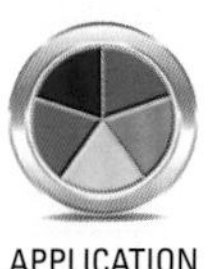
APPLICATION

Exercise 30

Read the case studies and circle the correct letter for each of the questions.

CASE 9-1

Mrs. Ryan is 46 years old and perimenopausal. Dr. Milban, her gynecologist, ordered a CBC after she complained about excessive fatigue for the past three months. The results showed a low RBC count of 3.67 (normal 4.00 to 5.00) and a low Hgb of 10.2 (normal 12.0 to 16.0). Mrs. Ryan explained she was currently having more frequent and heavier than normal menstrual periods. Dr. Milban suspected Mrs. Ryan was anemic due to blood loss. He instructed her to take an iron supplement and see her internist for a complete workup.

1. What is the medical term for anemia due to blood loss?

A. hemolytic anemia
B. hemorrhagic anemia
C. hemoglobinuria
D. hemoglobinemia

2. Which of the following statements does *not* apply to erythrocytes?

A. They transport oxygen.
B. They transport carbon dioxide.
C. They are disc-shaped with a depression on both sides.
D. Their main purpose is immunity.

3. Which of the following is *not* an indication of anemia?

A. low RBC
B. low Hgb
C. low clotting factor
D. low volume of packed cells

4. Which of the following tests would *not* be performed as part of a CBC lab test?

A. EBV
B. HGB
C. Lymphs
D. WBC

5. Which of the following is *not* an abbreviation for hemoglobin?

A. HGB
B. Hb
C. Hgb
D. Hg

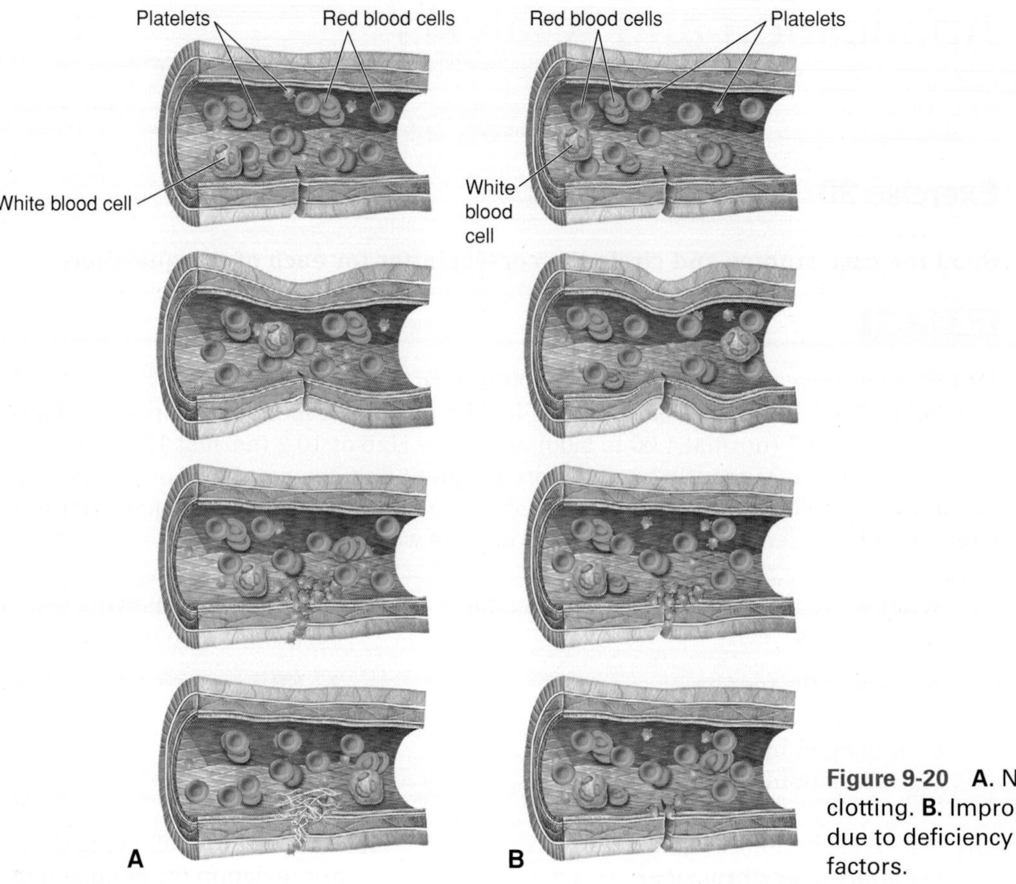

Figure 9-20 **A.** Normal clotting. **B.** Improper clotting due to deficiency in clotting factors.

CASE 9-2

Mr. Morozoff has a bleeding disorder that has affected his life since birth. His blood does not clot properly due to a deficiency in clotting factors **(Figure 9-20)**. The disease is genetically inherited and primarily affects males. As a child, he had to be careful to avoid injuries because even a small bruise could escalate into a life-threatening situation. He has regular lab tests to monitor his blood clotting time.

6. Based on the information in Case 9-2, what disease do you think Mr. Morozoff has?

A. hemophilia
B. hepatitis
C. hemochromatosis
D. septicemia

7. What is the medical term for clotting?

A. coagulopathy
B. hemolytic
C. coagulation
D. fibrinogen

8. What lab test would be used to diagnose a clotting disorder?

A. C&S
B. PT
C. ANA
D. HCT

9. Which drug, used to stop the flow of blood within vessels, may be prescribed for Mr. Morozoff's condition?

A. thrombolytic agent
B. vaccine
C. hemostatic agent
D. anticoagulant

10. Which procedure may be performed to transfer blood from a donor to a recipient in a life-threatening situation?

A. bone marrow transplant
B. blood transfusion
C. immunosuppression
D. splenectomy

MEDICAL RECORD ANALYSIS

MEDICAL RECORD 9-1

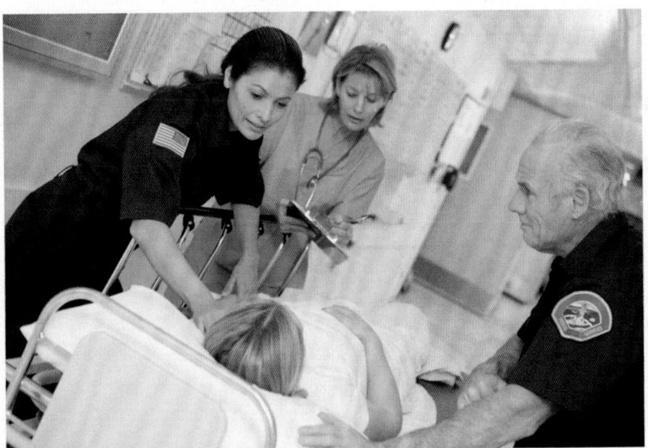

Emergency medical technicians are trained and certified to provide emergency medical services to the ill and injured.

Ms. Stinson sustained a snake bite while hiking in the desert. You are an emergency medical technician who transported her to the hospital and provided care en route. The documentation of her care at the hospital follows.

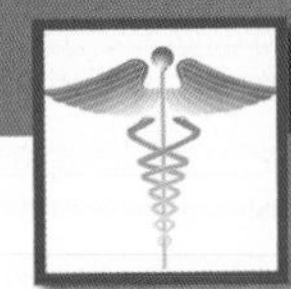

Medical Record

DISCHARGE SUMMARY

PATIENT: Carly Stinson **AGE:** 24-year-old female **DATE:** August 24, 20XX

FINAL DIAGNOSES:

1. Snake bite
2. Hemolysis
3. Thrombocytopenia
4. Nausea
5. Epistaxis
6. Hematuria
7. Tachycardia
8. Neurotoxicity
9. Hypotension

HOSPITAL COURSE: Patient reported to the emergency room within three hours of a presumed rattlesnake bite. She had been hiking in the desert when she was struck on the back of her right lower leg. She saw a large snake, over 6 ft long, with diamond-patterned skin. Her medical history is unremarkable for chronic illnesses. No known allergies (NKA). Medications are limited to birth control pills. She complained of anxiety, nausea, and tingling of her right lower extremity.

There were two visible entry wounds, with marked edema, ecchymosis, petechiae, and some early blisters. She complained of significant pain in the bite region. Her vital signs were consistent for hypotension at 98/60 with a tachycardic pulse at 136 BPM. Hemolytic effects from the snakebite venom started with epistaxis and slight hematuria.

TREATMENT: Administration of 20 vials of antivenin
Tetanus prophylaxis
Prophylactic antibiotic ordered because contact with a snake's mouth can cause a bacterial infection
Admitted to Intensive Care Unit
Cardiac monitoring with IV
Coagulation profile ordered q4–12h prn to monitor signs of hemolytic anemia, thrombocytopenia, or fibrinolysis

DISCHARGE INSTRUCTIONS: Patient was discharged after two days with symptoms subsiding. Will recheck patient at one week and four weeks postinjury.

DISCHARGE MEDICATIONS: Patient to complete the 10-day course of antibiotics.

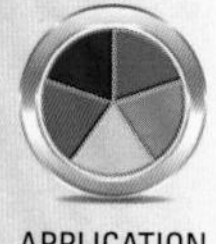
APPLICATION

Exercise 31

Write the appropriate medical terms used in this medical record on the blanks after their meanings. Note that not all the terms appear in the chapter, but you should be able to identify these terms based on word parts that are included in this chapter.

1. pertaining to the rupture or destruction of (red) blood (cells) __________

2. disorder involving low levels of platelets in blood __________

3. abbreviation for no known allergies __________

4. the abbreviation prn means __________

Bonus Question

5. Break the medical term *antibiotic* into its word parts, and define each part. Then define the medical term. (Hint: Refer to *Appendix A: Glossary of Combining Forms, Prefixes, and Suffixes* to recall the meaning of word parts learned earlier in the text.)

word parts: __________, __________, __________

meanings: __________, __________, __________

term meaning: __________

MEDICAL RECORD 9-2

Following is a clinic note in SOAP (subjective, objective, assessment, plan) format for a 42-year-old patient who was seen four weeks ago in an initial consultation by a rheumatologist. As an occupational therapist, you are reviewing her record before meeting with her to identify ways in which she can successfully perform her activities of daily living (ADLs) while managing her disease.

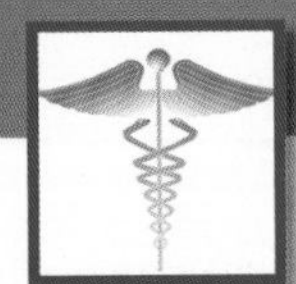

Medical Record

SOAP FOLLOW-UP FOR AUTOIMMUNE DISEASE

S: 42-year-old Debra Conner returns to the clinic for a one-month follow-up visit. She is married with two children and has a full-time career as a college instructor. She continues to complain of musculoskeletal aches, fatigue, and insomnia, which she admits has contributed to her stress level. She sometimes has trouble with activities of daily living because of her pain. She has had one episode of a urinary tract infection that was treated with a 10-day course of penicillin. She also takes an over-the-counter antiinflammatory drug to reduce her symptoms of muscle aches, which does provide some relief. She denies depressive episodes at this time.

O: Wt: 70 kg BP: 122/86 HR: 74 T: 98.8 R: 18
Laboratory Results: Positive ANA, ELISA method. Elevated rheumatoid factor, ESR, and complement levels. Negative EBV. CBC: WNL. Chemistry Profile: WNL

A: With the correlation of symptoms and laboratory data, my impressions are as follows:

1. Fibromyalgia
2. Sleep disorder
3. Fatigue
4. Systemic lupus erythematosus

P: Plan to decrease the inflammatory process with the following medications:
prednisone 10 mg daily
mycophenolate mofetil 500 mg b.i.d.

Patient may continue to take over-the-counter ibuprofen, on a prn basis, but not to exceed 1,600 mg/day. Patient instructed on stress reduction and was given written information on living with an autoimmune disease. Have ordered consultation with occupational therapy. Recommended she attend a SLE support group meeting.

Return to clinic in three months.

T. Gentry, MD
Rheumatology Associates

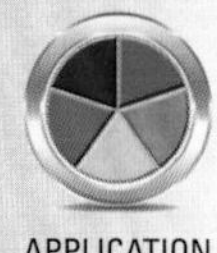

APPLICATION

Exercise 32

Read the medical report and circle the correct letter for each of the questions. Note: Although some of the medical terms in these questions do not appear in this chapter, you should understand them from their word parts.

1. What is the name of Mrs. Conner's autoimmune disease?

A. fibromyalgia
B. systemic lupus erythematosus
C. rheumatoid arthritis
D. fatigue

2. What does the abbreviation ANA stand for?

A. antinuclear antigen
B. antiinflammatory antigen
C. antinuclear antibody
D. autonomic nervous system

3. This patient is taking over-the-counter ibuprofen for

A. chemotherapy.
B. immunosuppression.
C. NSAID.
D. inflammation.

4. An elevated ESR level may indicate

A. inflammation.
B. infection.
C. immune disease.
D. clotting disorder.

5. What type of medical specialist should Mrs. Conner continue to see to monitor this disease on a regular basis?

A. rheumatologist
B. microbiologist
C. internist
D. allergologist

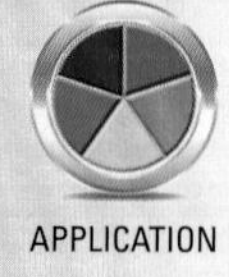

APPLICATION

Exercise 33

Write out the complete medical terms from the abbreviations used in the medical record above.

1. SLE ____________________

2. ESR ____________________

3. WBC ____________________

4. EBV test ____________________

5. ANA test ____________________

Bonus Question

6. SLE is an organ-threatening disease in which the kidneys can be a target, resulting in lupus nephritis. Therefore, many physicians will order routine urinalyses for SLE patients. Blood in the urine is an abnormal condition that needs immediate attention. Write in the correct

medical term for this condition: ____________________

Pronunciation and Spelling

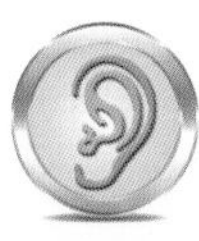

AUDITORY

Exercise 34

Review the Chapter 9 terms in the Dictionary/Audio Glossary in the Student Resources on thePoint, and practice pronouncing each term, referring to the pronunciation guide as needed.

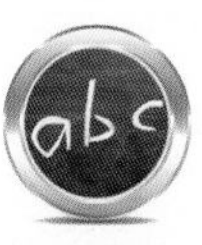

SPELLING

Exercise 35

Circle the correct spelling of each term.

1.	erithrocyte	erythrocyte	erythocyte
2.	granularcyte	granulacyte	granulocyte
3.	leukocyte	leukocite	luekocyte
4.	neutrophil	nuetrophyl	neutrophyll
5.	eaosinphil	eosinophil	eaosinphill
6.	agranulocyte	agranulcyte	agranulicyte
7.	erythropoetin	erythropoietin	erhythropoietin
8.	phagocitosis	phagocytosus	phagocytosis
9.	hemoglobin	hemeglobulin	hemoglobbin
10.	hemorrhagic	hemorhagic	hemmorrhagic
11.	virolent	virulent	virulant
12.	proliferation	proliforation	preliferation
13.	immunosuppressant	immunesupressant	imunosuppressant
14.	thalasemia	thalassemia	thallessemia
15.	thrombocytopenia	thrombecytopenia	trombocytopinia

Media Connection

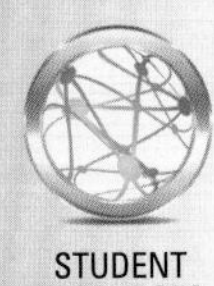

Exercise 36

Complete each of the following activities available with the Student Resources on thePoint. Check off each activity as you complete it, and record your score for the Chapter Quiz in the space provided.

Chapter Exercises

____ Flash Cards

____ Concentration

____ Abbreviation Match-Up

____ Roboterms

____ Word Anatomy

____ Fill the Gap

____ Break It Down

____ True/False Body Building

____ Quiz Show

____ Complete the Case

____ Medical Record Review

____ Look and Label

____ Image Matching

____ Spelling Bee

____ **Chapter Quiz** *Score:* _______%

Additional Resources

____ Animation: Wound Healing

____ Video: Venipuncture

____ Dictionary/Audio Glossary

____ Health Professions Careers: Emergency Medicine Technician

____ Health Professions Careers: Occupational Therapist

Cardiovascular and Lymphatic Systems

10

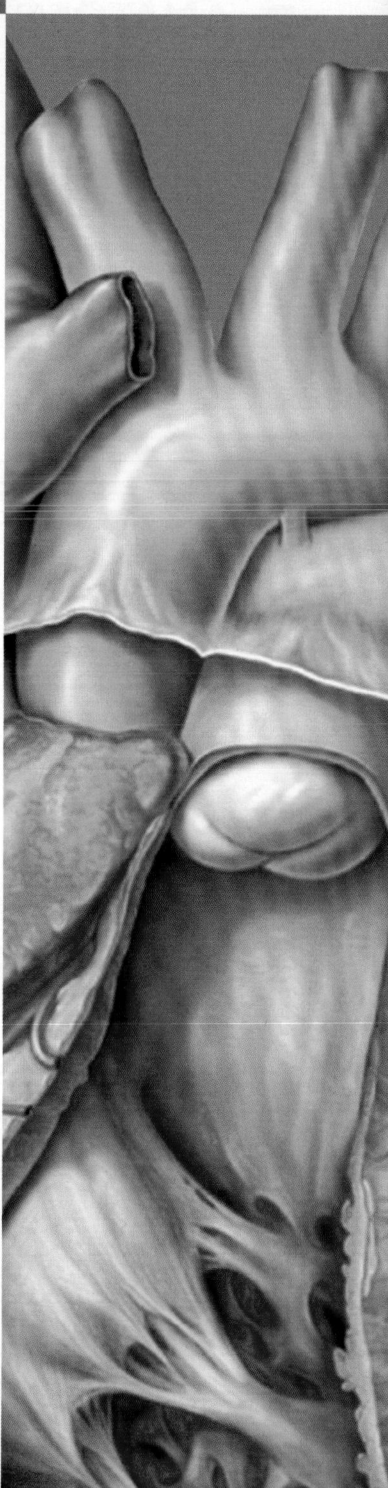

Chapter Outline

Introduction, 352

Anatomy and Physiology, 352
- Structures of the Cardiovascular System, 352
- Functions of the Cardiovascular System, 352
- Structures of the Lymphatic System, 352
- Functions of the Lymphatic System, 352
- Terms Related to the Cardiovascular and Lymphatic Systems, 353

Word Parts, 361
- Combining Forms, 361
- Prefixes, 362
- Suffixes, 362

Medical Terms, 365
- Adjectives and Other Related Terms, 365
- Medical Conditions, 367
- Tests and Procedures, 377
- Surgical Interventions and Therapeutic Procedures, 382
- Medications and Drug Therapies, 388
- Specialties and Specialists, 388
- Abbreviations, 389

Wrapping Up, 391

Chapter Review, 392

Learning Outcomes

After completing this chapter, you should be able to:

1. Describe the location of the main cardiovascular and lymphatic structures in the body.
2. Define terms related to the heart, blood vessels, and lymphatic system.
3. Define combining forms, prefixes, and suffixes related to the cardiovascular and lymphatic systems.
4. Define common medical terminology related to the cardiovascular and lymphatic systems, including adjectives and related terms; signs, symptoms, and medical conditions; tests and procedures; surgical interventions and therapeutic procedures; medications and drug therapies; and medical specialties and specialists.
5. Define common abbreviations related to the cardiovascular and lymphatic systems.
6. Successfully complete all chapter exercises.
7. Explain terms used in case studies and medical records involving the cardiovascular and lymphatic systems.
8. Successfully complete all exercises included with the companion Student Resources on thePoint.

INTRODUCTION

The heart and blood vessels make up the cardiovascular system, while the lymphatic system consists of the lymphatic vessels (lymphatics), lymph nodes, and lymphoid tissues. The cardiovascular and lymphatic systems are closely interrelated. Lymph is a fluid derived from the blood, and it contains white blood cells. Lymph is returned to the bloodstream at veins in the superior region of the chest. This chapter will focus on the integration of these two systems and will give the pertinent medical terminology associated with their structures, functions, and pathology.

ANATOMY AND PHYSIOLOGY

Structures of the Cardiovascular System

- The heart is a four-chambered organ consisting of two upper chambers called atria and two lower chambers called ventricles.
- The heart wall is made up of three tissue layers: the endocardium, myocardium, and pericardium.
- The heart's four chambers are aided by four valves to keep blood moving in one direction.
- The heart has specialized tissue that transmits electrical impulses.
- The heart muscle contracts in a rhythmic sequence, pushing blood through the chambers and vessels.
- Arteries carry blood away from the heart.
- Veins return blood back to the heart.
- Capillaries are fine branches of blood vessels that form a network between arteries and veins.

Functions of the Cardiovascular System

- Transporting blood throughout the body via blood vessels (**Figure 10-1**)
- Exchanging gases, nutrients, and wastes between the blood and body cells at capillaries
- Pumping blood through the systemic circuit, allowing blood to reach the whole body

Structures of the Lymphatic System

- Lymph is clear fluid consisting of white blood cells and a few red blood cells.
- Lymphatic vessels are structures that transport the lymph from the body tissues to the venous system.
- Lymphatic vessels have valves that promote one-way flow of lymph.
- Lymph nodes are small swellings along the length of lymphatic vessels that filter lymph.
- The lymph nodes are primarily concentrated in the neck, chest, armpits, and groin.
- Lymph capillaries are the beginning of the lymphatic system of vessels.

Functions of the Lymphatic System

- Returning lymph from body tissues to the blood (**Figure 10-1**)
- Protecting the body by filtering microorganisms and foreign particles from the lymph
- Maintaining the body's internal fluid level
- Absorbing fats from the small intestines through lymphatic structures called lacteals

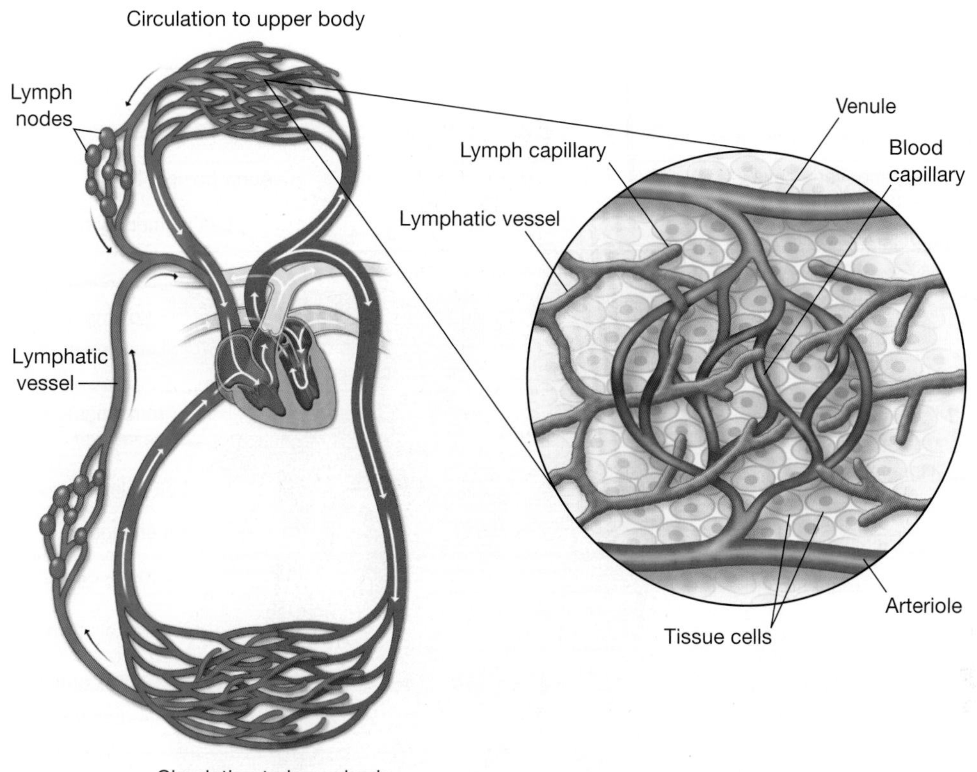

Figure 10-1 The relationship between the cardiovascular and lymphatic systems.

Terms Related to the Cardiovascular and Lymphatic Systems

Term	Pronunciation	Meaning
The Heart (Figures 10-2 and 10-3)		
cardiac cycle	kar′dē-ak sī′kl	one complete heartbeat that includes contraction (systole) and relaxation (diastole) of both atria (upper heart chambers) and both ventricles (lower heart chambers)
cardiovascular system	kar′dē-ō-vas′kyū-lăr sis′tĕm	composed of the heart and blood vessels that deliver oxygen and nutrients to the body cells and carry away cellular wastes (**Figure 10-4**)
heart	hart	hollow muscular organ that receives blood from the veins and propels blood through the arteries
apex	ā′peks	the lower pointed end of the heart formed by the left ventricle
coronary circulation	kōr′o-nār-ē ser′kyū-lā′shŭn	blood supply to the heart tissue (**Figure 10-5**)
septum	sep′tŭm	wall of heart tissue separating the right and left sides
atrium	ā′trē-ŭm	upper receiving chamber of the heart; right and left atria
ventricle	ven′tri-kĕl	lower pumping chamber of the heart; right and left ventricles
endocardium	en′dō-kar′dē-ŭm	inner lining of the heart
myocardium	mī′ō-kar′dē-ŭm	middle muscular layer of heart tissue
epicardium	ep′i-kar′dē-ŭm	outer lining of the heart

(continued)

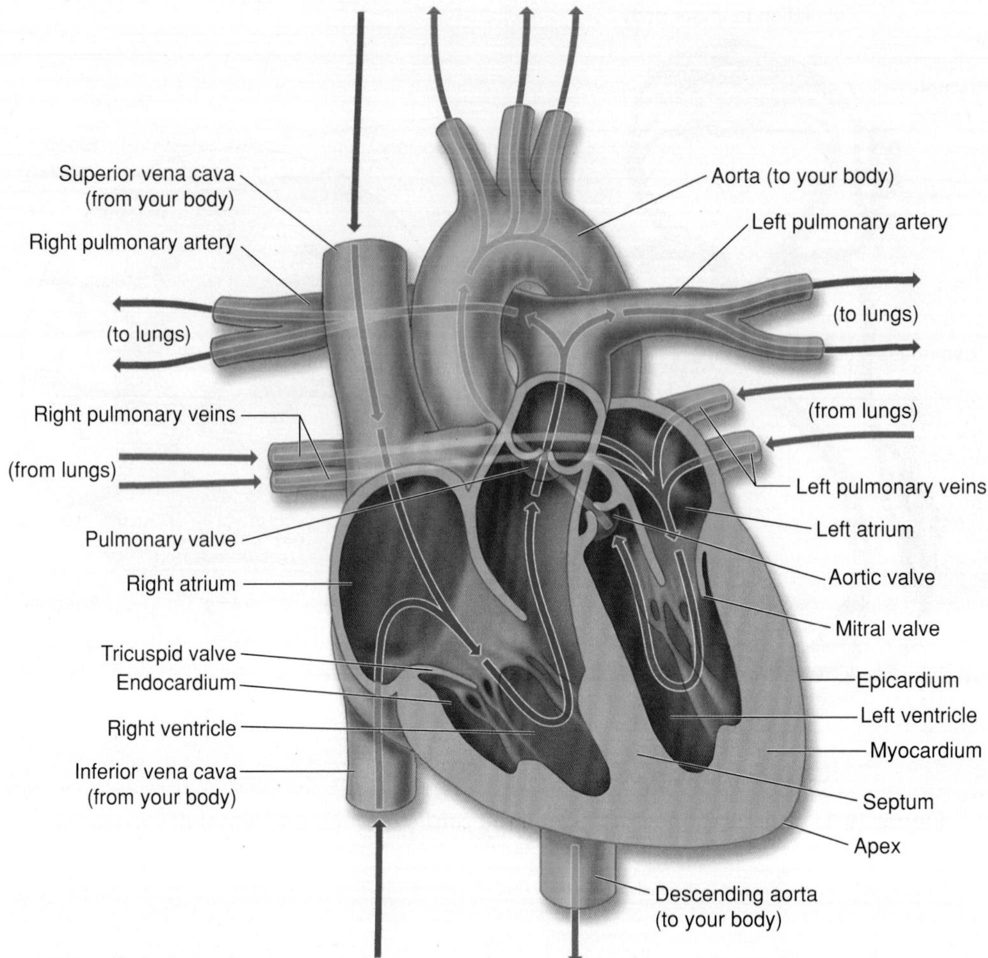

Figure 10-2 The heart and major blood vessels. Red blood vessels and arrows indicate oxygenated blood, and blue blood vessels and arrows indicate deoxygenated blood.

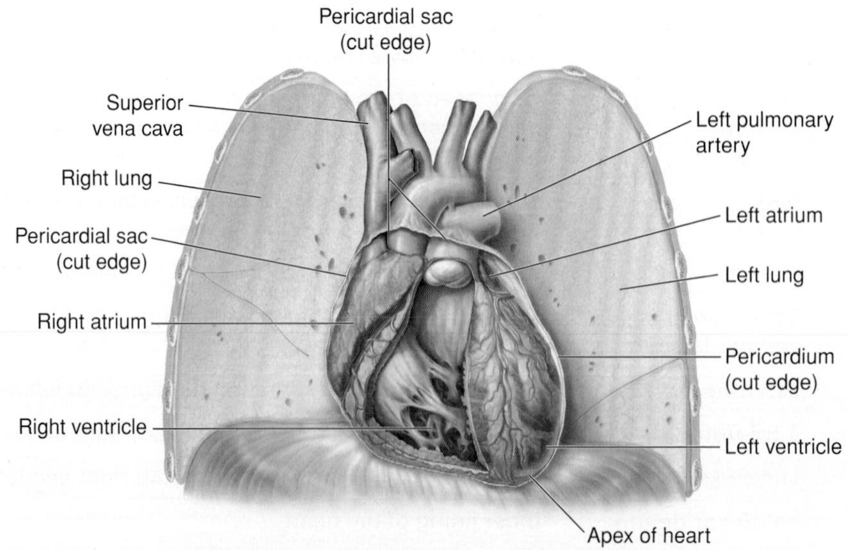

Figure 10-3 Cross-section of the heart and lungs showing the heart's relative position between the lungs.

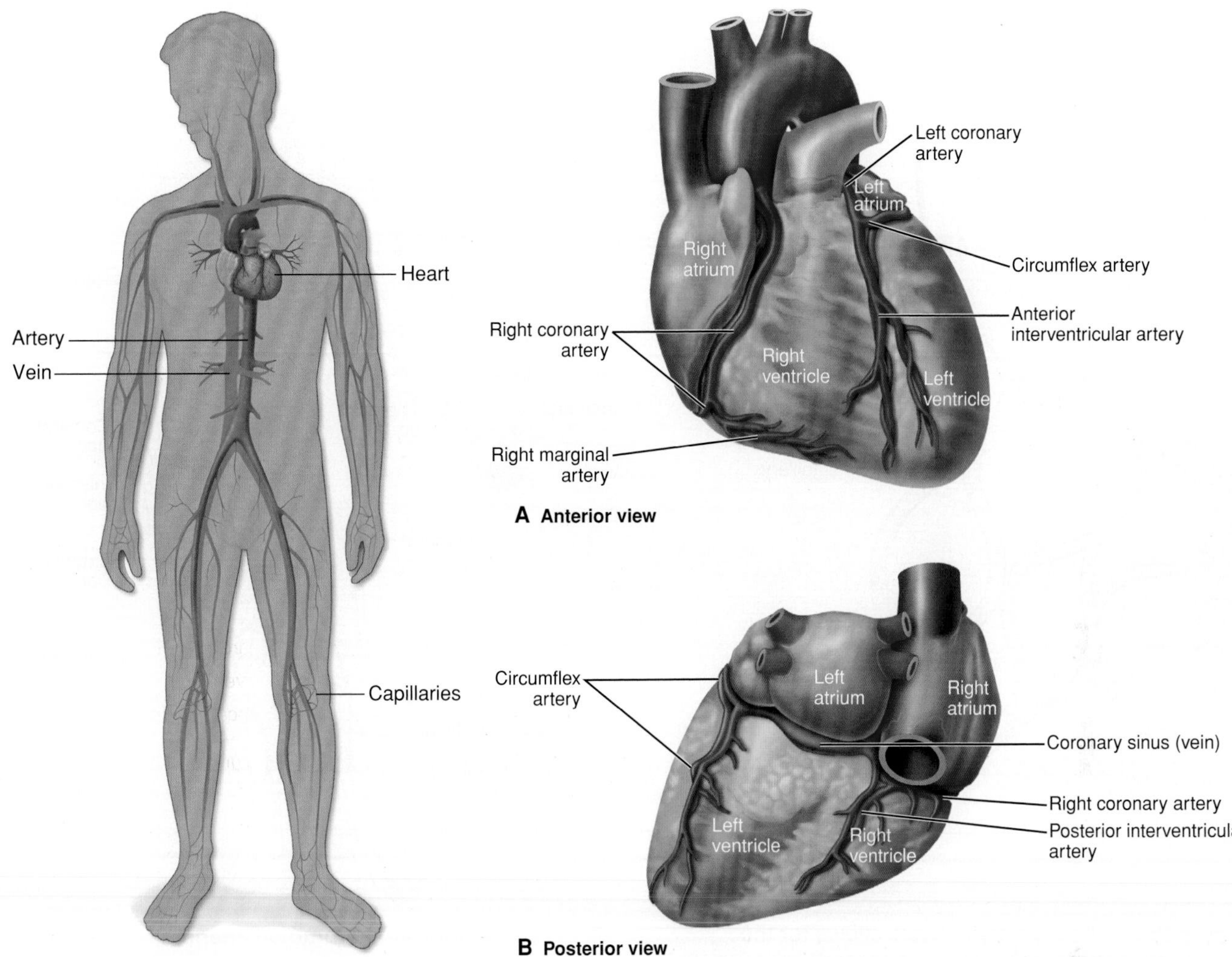

Figure 10-4 An overview of the cardiovascular system.

Figure 10-5 The coronary circulation, anterior **(A)** and posterior **(B)** views. Blood is supplied to the heart muscle via the coronary vessels. The major vessels of the coronary circulatory loop are shown here.

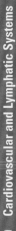

Terms Related to the Cardiovascular and Lymphatic Systems *(continued)*

Term	Pronunciation	Meaning
pericardium	per′i-kar′dē-ŭm	sac around the heart that facilitates movement of the heart as it beats
aortic valve	ā-ōr′tik valv	heart valve between the left ventricle and aorta (main artery of the heart)
mitral valve	mī′trăl valv	heart valve between the left atrium and left ventricle; also called a bicuspid valve
pulmonary valve	pul′mŏ-nār-ē valv	heart valve between the right ventricle and the pulmonary artery; also called a semilunar valve due to the half-moon shape of its three cusps
tricuspid valve	trī-kŭs′pid valv	heart valve between the right atrium and right ventricle

(continued)

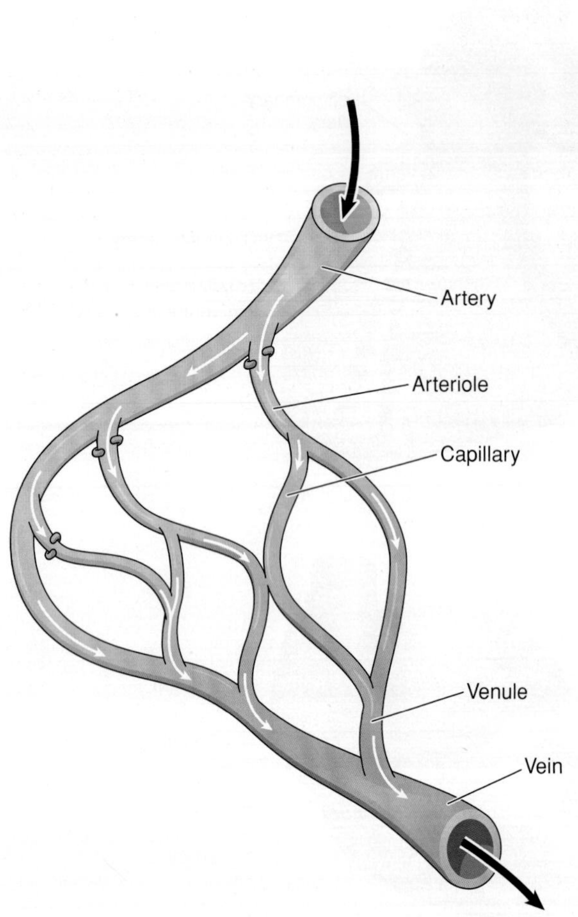

Figure 10-6 The capillary network allows for the exchange of gases, nutrients, and wastes between body cells and the blood.

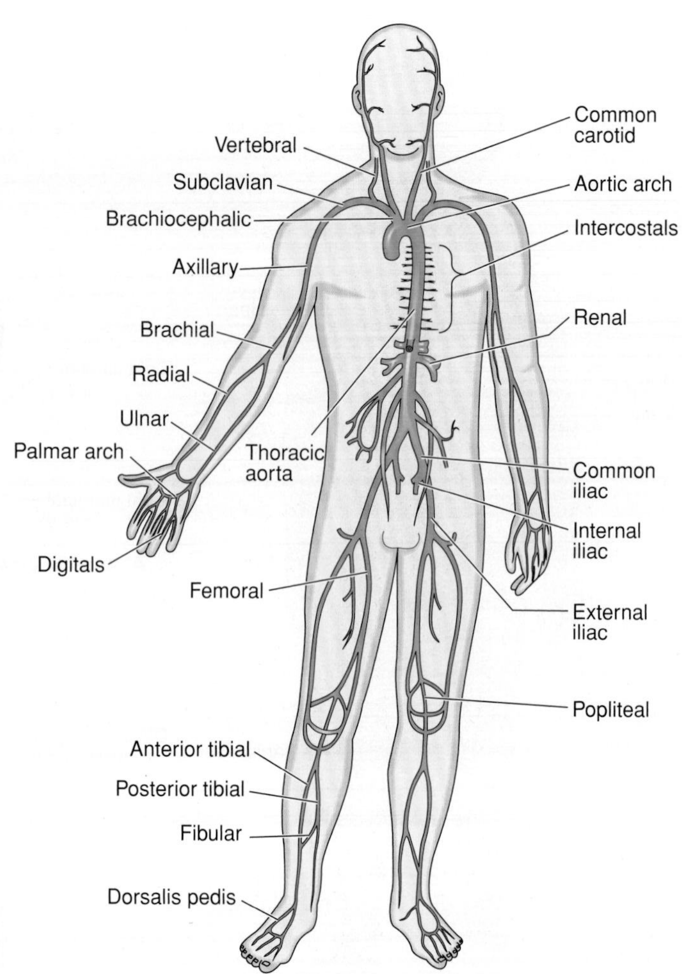

Figure 10-7 Common arteries.

Terms Related to the Cardiovascular and Lymphatic Systems *(continued)*

Term	Pronunciation	Meaning
		Blood Vessels (Figure 10-6)
blood vessels	blŭd ves'ĕlz	tubular structures that transport blood
capillary	kap'i-lār-ē	microscopic thin-walled vessel connecting arterioles and venules where gas, nutrient, and waste exchange take place between the blood and cells of the body
lumen	lū'mĕn	interior space of a vessel
		Arteries (Figure 10-7)
aorta	ā-ōr'tă	largest artery that begins as an arch from the left ventricle then branches and descends through the thoracic and abdominal cavities; carries oxygenated blood away from the heart
artery	ar'tĕr-ē	blood vessel that carries blood away from the heart
arteriole	ahr-tēr'ē-ōl	small artery that connects an artery to a capillary

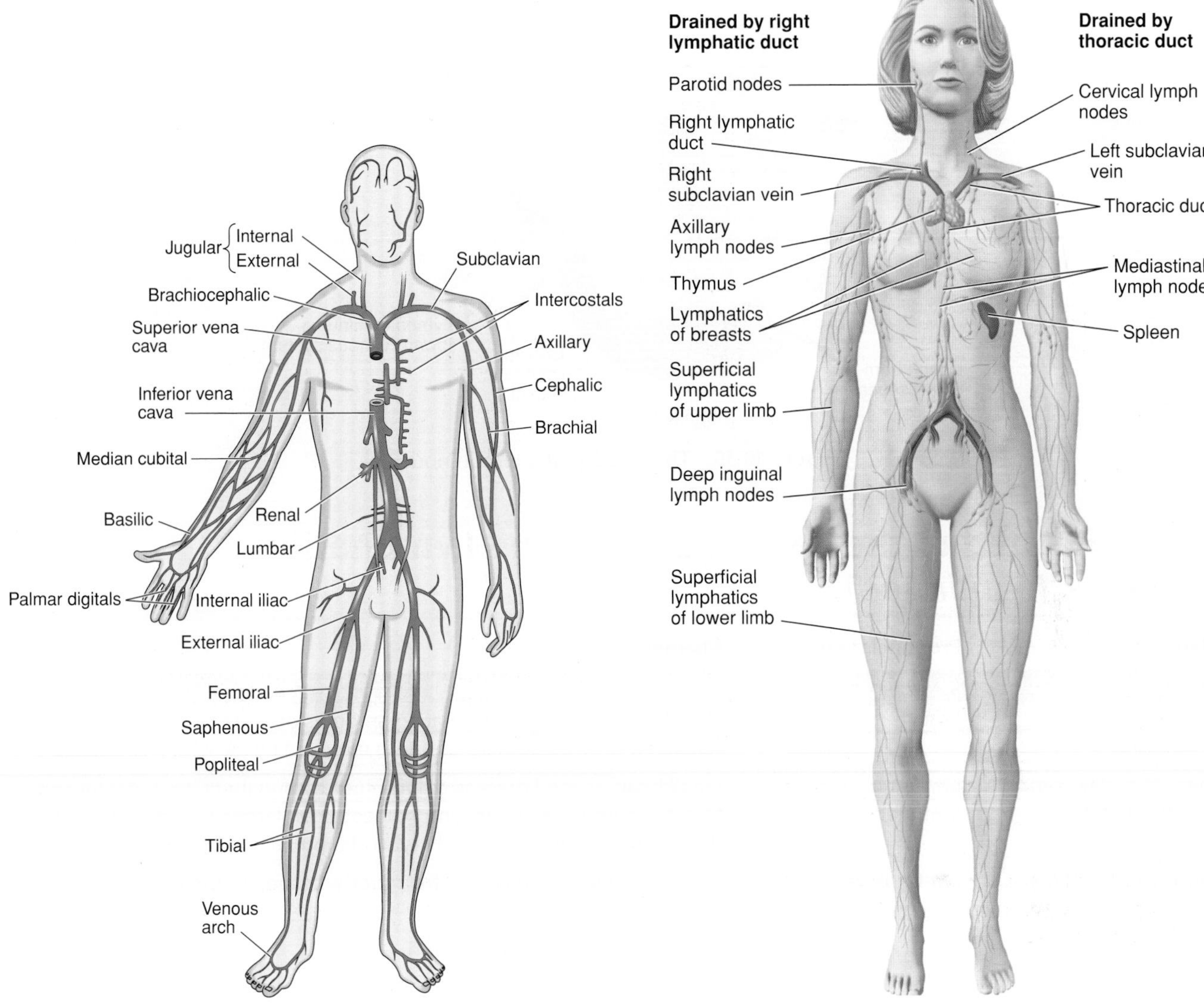

Figure 10-8 Common veins.

Figure 10-9 An overview of the lymphatic system.

Terms Related to the Cardiovascular and Lymphatic Systems

Term	Pronunciation	Meaning
		Veins (Figure 10-8)
inferior vena cava	in-fēr′ē-ŏr vē′nă kā′vă	large vein carrying blood to the heart from the lower part of the body (**Figure 10-2**)
superior vena cava	sŭ-pēr′ē-ŏr vē′nă kā′vă	large vein carrying blood to the heart from the upper part of the body (**Figure 10-2**)
venule	ven′yūl	small vein that connects a capillary to a vein
vein	vān	vessel carrying blood to the heart

(continued)

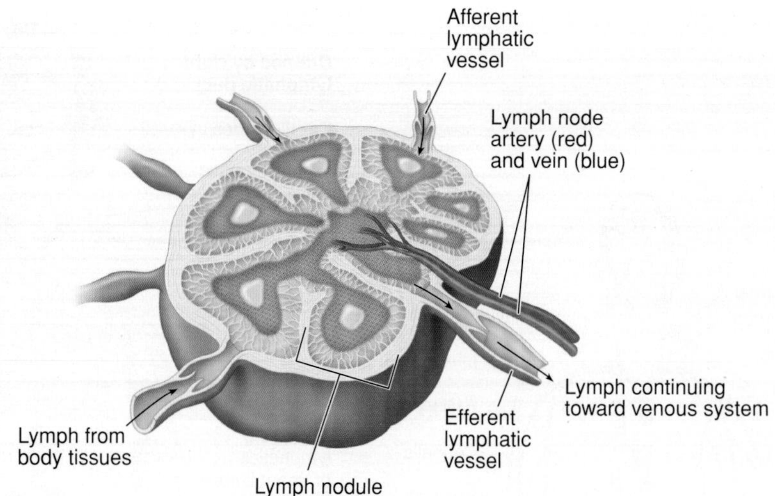

Figure 10-10 The interior of a lymph node.

Terms Related to the Cardiovascular and Lymphatic Systems *(continued)*

Term	Pronunciation	Meaning
The Lymphatic System (Figure 10-9)		
lymph	limf	clear fluid consisting of fluctuating amounts of white blood cells and a few red blood cells; bathes tissues and is removed by the lymph capillaries
lymph nodes; *syn.* lymph glands	limf nōdz; limf glandz	small bean-shaped masses of lymphatic tissue that filter bacteria and foreign material from the lymph; located on larger lymph vessels in the cervical, mediastinal, axillary, and inguinal regions (**Figure 10-10**)
lymphatic vessels	lim-fat′ik ves′ĕlz	vessels transporting lymph from body tissues to the venous system
lymph capillaries	limf kap′i-lar-ēz	microscopic thin-walled lymph vessels that pick up lymph, proteins, and waste from body tissues
lymph ducts	limf dŭkts	the largest lymphatic vessels that transport lymph to the venous system; right lymphatic duct and thoracic duct

ANIMATION

View the animation "Cardiac Cycle" on the Student Resources on thePoint to learn how blood flows through the heart.

Exercises: Anatomy and Physiology

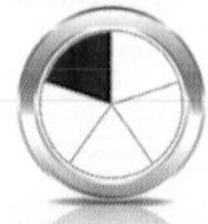
SIMPLE RECALL

Exercise 1

Write the correct anatomic structure for the meaning given.

1. upper chamber of the heart ____________

2. small vein ____________

3. middle muscular layer of heart ____________

4. valve between the left ventricle and aorta ______________________

5. wall of heart tissue separating right and left sides ______________________

6. small artery ______________________

7. large veins carrying blood to the heart ______________________

8. muscular pumping organ ______________________

9. inner lining of the heart ______________________

10. sac around the heart ______________________

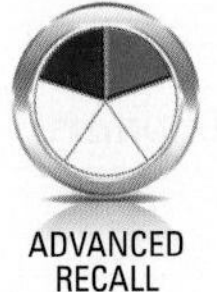

ADVANCED RECALL

Exercise 2

Write the meaning or function of the term given.

1. lymph ______________________

2. artery ______________________

3. vein ______________________

4. lymph capillaries ______________________

5. aorta ______________________

6. blood vessels ______________________

7. lymphatic vessels ______________________

8. lymph ducts ______________________

9. lymph nodes ______________________

10. tricuspid valve ______________________

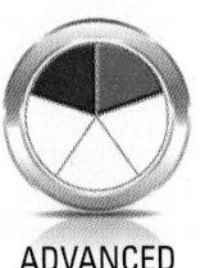

ADVANCED RECALL

Exercise 3

Circle the term that is most appropriate for the meaning of the sentence.

1. The two upper receiving chambers of the heart are called the right and left (*aortas, atria, ventricles*).

2. The epicardium is the (*inner, middle, outer*) lining of the heart.

3. The (*endocardium, myocardium, pericardium*) is the inner lining of the heart.

4. Another name for the mitral valve is the (*semilunar, bicuspid, tricuspid*) valve.

5. The largest artery in the body is the (*inferior vena cava, superior vena cava, aorta*).

6. The pulmonary valve is located between the right ventricle and the pulmonary (*vein, artery, vena cava*).

7. The lymph (*nodes, ducts, capillaries*) pick up lymph, proteins, and waste from the body tissues.
8. The inferior vena cava is a large (*artery, vein, capillary*).
9. The smallest blood vessel where gas and nutrients are exchanged is a(n) (*arteriole, capillary, venule*).
10. The (*aortic, mitral, tricuspid*) valve is also referred to as a semilunar valve.
11. The mitral valve has (*one, two, three*) cusps, or leaflets, that open and close.
12. The (*endocardium, myocardium, pericardium*) is the sac around the heart.
13. A small artery is called a(n) (*venule, arteriole, capillary*).
14. The muscular organ pumping blood through the body is the (*circulatory system, pulmonary system, heart*).

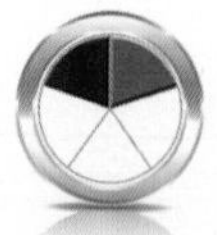

ADVANCED RECALL

Exercise 4

Match each medical term with its meaning.

myocardium	septum	lymph
pulmonary valve	lumen	apex

1. structure between the right ventricle and pulmonary artery ____________
2. middle muscular layer of heart tissue ____________
3. interior space of a vessel ____________
4. clear fluid that bathes tissues ____________
5. separating wall inside the heart ____________
6. the lower pointed end of the heart ____________

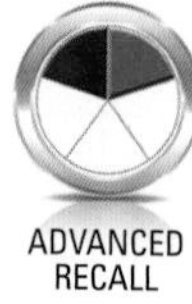

ADVANCED RECALL

Exercise 5

Complete each sentence by writing in the correct medical term.

1. Bacteria and foreign material are filtered out of the circulation by the ____________.
2. The bottom chambers of the heart responsible for forcing the blood through the body are the ____________.
3. The vessels that carry blood away from the heart are ____________.
4. The ____________ regulates the flow of blood between the left ventricle and the aorta.
5. The ____________ is a sac around the heart that facilitates movement as it beats.
6. The interior space of a vessel is called a(n) ____________.

7. A microscopic vessel that picks up fluid and proteins from the body tissues is a lymph

_______________________.

8. The lymph _______________________ are the largest lymphatic vessels.

9. The clear fluid that contains white blood cells and bathes body tissues is called

_______________________.

10. The _______________ vena cava carries blood to the heart from the lower part of the body.

WORD PARTS

The following tables list word parts related to the cardiovascular and lymphatic systems.

Combining Forms

Combining Form	Meaning
Related to the Cardiovascular System	
angi/o	vessel, vascular
aort/o	aorta
arteri/o	artery
ather/o	fatty, fatty deposit
atri/o	atrium
cardi/o	heart
coron/o	encircling, crown
electr/o	electric, electricity
my/o	muscle
phleb/o	vein
pulmon/o	lung
scler/o	hard
son/o	sound, sound waves
sphygm/o	pulse
steth/o	chest
thorac/o	chest, thorax
thromb/o	blood clot
valv/o, valvul/o	valve
vas/o, vascul/o	blood vessel
varic/o	swollen or twisted vein
ven/i, ven/o	veins
ventricul/o	normal cavity, ventricle
Related to the Lymphatic System	
aden/o	gland
lymph/o	lymph

Prefixes

Prefix	Meaning
Related to the Cardiovascular System	
brady-	slow
de-	away from, cessation, without
endo-	in, within
epi-	on, following
inter-	between
intra-	within
peri-	around, surrounding
tachy-	rapid, fast
tel-	end
trans-	across, through
tri-	three

Suffixes

Suffix	Meaning
Related to the Cardiovascular System	
-al, -ar, -ary, -ic	pertaining to
-ectasia	dilation, stretching
-gram	record, recording
-graph	instrument for recording
-graphy	recording, writing, description
-icle, -ole, -ule	small
-lytic	pertaining to destruction, breakdown, separation
-ium	tissue, structure
-stenosis	stricture, narrowing
-oid	resembling

Exercises: Word Parts

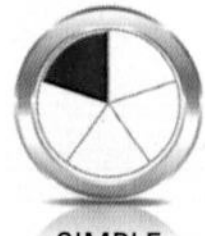

SIMPLE RECALL

Exercise 6

Write the meaning of the combining form given.

1. atri/o __________

2. my/o __________

3. vas/o __________

4. angi/o __________

5. ven/o ______

6. electr/o ______

7. arteri/o ______

8. cardi/o ______

9. ventricul/o ______

10. pulmon/o ______

11. coron/o ______

12. phleb/o ______

13. vascul/o ______

14. thorac/o ______

15. valvul/o ______

SIMPLE RECALL

Exercise 7

Write the correct combining form for the meaning given.

1. hard ______

2. pulse ______

3. swollen or twisted vein ______

4. lymph ______

5. valve ______

6. aorta ______

7. artery ______

8. atrium ______

9. heart ______

10. chest, thorax ______

SIMPLE RECALL

Exercise 8

Write the meaning of the prefix or suffix given.

1. -stenosis ______

2. -ule, -icle, -ole ______

3. tachy- ________________

4. trans- ________________

5. intra- ________________

6. inter- ________________

7. endo- ________________

8. -graph ________________

9. brady- ________________

10. epi- ________________

11. peri- ________________

12. -ium ________________

13. -al, -ar, -ary, -ic ________________

14. tri- ________________

15. de- ________________

16. -lytic ________________

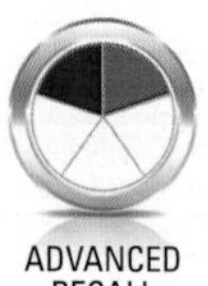

Exercise 9

Considering the meaning of the combining form from which the medical term is made, write the meaning of the medical term. (You have not yet learned many of these terms but can build their meanings from the word parts.)

Combining Form	Meaning	Medical Term	Meaning of Term
phleb/o	vein	phlebitis	1. ________
cardi/o	heart	cardiology	2. ________
my/o, cardi/o	muscle, heart	myocardium	3. ________
thromb/o	blood clot	thrombosis	4. ________
ven/o	vein	venogram	5. ________
ather/o	fatty, fatty deposit	atherectomy	6. ________
lymph/o	lymph	lymphoid	7. ________
aort/o	aorta	aortography	8. ________

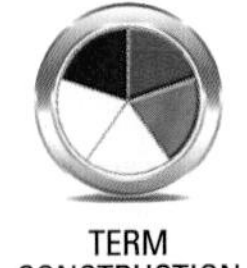

TERM CONSTRUCTION

Exercise 10

Using the given combining form, build a medical term for the meaning given.

Combining Form	Meaning of Medical Term	Medical Term
angi/o	surgical repair or reconstruction of a vessel	1. ________
thorac/o	pertaining to the chest	2. ________
arteri/o	small artery	3. ________
ven/o	small vein	4. ________
vascul/o	pertaining to blood vessels	5. ________
aden/o	resembling a gland	6. ________
lymph/o	disease of the lymphatic vessels or nodes	7. ________
son/o	process of recording using sound	8. ________

■ MEDICAL TERMS

The following table gives adjective forms and terms used in describing the cardiovascular and lymphatic systems.

Adjectives and Other Related Terms

Term	Pronunciation	Meaning
arteriovenous (AV)	ahr-tēr′ē-ō-vē′nŭs	relating to both an artery and a vein or both arteries and veins in general
atrioventricular (AV)	ā′trē-ō-ven-trik′yū-lăr	relating to both the atria and the ventricles of the heart
cardiovascular	kar′dē-ō-vas′kyū-lăr	pertaining to the heart and blood vessels
constriction	kŏn-strik′shŭn	contracted or narrowed portion of a structure
cyanotic	sī′ă-not′ik	pertaining to a blue or purple discoloration due to deoxygenated blood
deoxygenate	dē-ok′si-jĕ-nāt	to remove oxygen
diastole	dī-as′tŏ-lē	the relaxation phase of the heartbeat when the heart muscle relaxes and allows the chambers to fill with blood
ischemic	is-kē′mik	pertaining to a lack of blood flow
oxygenate	ok′si-jĕ-nāt′	to add oxygen
paroxysmal	par-ok-siz′măl	sudden
patent	pā′tĕnt	open or exposed
precordial	prē-kōr′dē-ăl	pertaining to the portion of body over the heart and the anterior lower chest

(continued)

Adjectives and Other Related Terms *(continued)*

Term	Pronunciation	Meaning
sphygmic	sfig′mik	pertaining to the pulse
stenotic	sten-ot′ik	pertaining to the condition of narrowing
supraventricular	sū′pră-ven-trik′yū-lăr	pertaining to above the ventricles
systole	sis′tŏ-lē	the contraction phase of the heartbeat when the heart muscle pumps blood from the chambers into the arteries and ventricles
thoracic	thōr-as′ik	pertaining to the chest
thrombotic	throm-bot′ik	pertaining to a thrombus or blood clot
varicose	var′i-kōs	pertaining to a swollen or twisted vein

Exercises: Adjectives and Other Related Terms

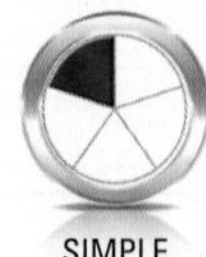

SIMPLE RECALL

Exercise 11

Circle the term that is most appropriate for the meaning of the sentence.

1. The term *supraventricular* refers to (*above, below, beside*) the ventricles.
2. A sudden arrhythmia, such as an atrial tachycardia, is described as (*stenotic, precordial, paroxysmal*).
3. An open coronary artery is referred to as (*patent, stenotic, varicose*).
4. A stenotic vessel is one that is (*widened, narrowed, stretched*).
5. The medical term used to describe a blue or purple discoloration is (*pathologic, varicose, cyanotic*).
6. (*Diastole, Systole, Stenosis*) refers to the contraction phase of the heartbeat.
7. The relaxation phase of the heartbeat is (*diastole, stenosis, systole*).

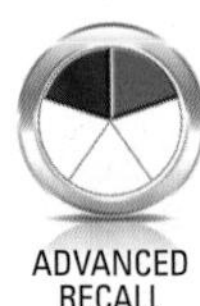

ADVANCED RECALL

Exercise 12

Match each medical term with its meaning.

precordial	constriction	cardiovascular	cyanotic	deoxygenate
varicose	oxygenate	atrioventricular	ischemic	thoracic

1. contracted or narrowed portion ____________
2. pertaining to the heart and blood vessels ____________
3. pertaining to a blue or purple discoloration ____________
4. pertaining to the anterior lower chest ____________
5. pertaining to twisted, swollen veins ____________

6. to add oxygen ______

7. pertaining to the chest ______

8. pertaining to lack of blood flow ______

9. pertaining to atria and ventricles ______

10. to remove oxygen ______

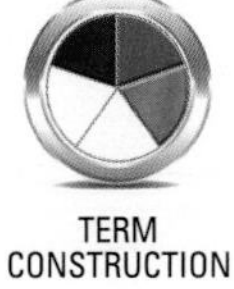

TERM CONSTRUCTION

Exercise 13

Write the combining form used in the medical term, followed by the meaning of the combining form.

Term	Combining Form	Combining Form Meaning
1. sphygmic	______	______
2. cardiovascular	______	______
3. varicose	______	______
4. arteriovenous	______	______
5. thrombosis	______	______

Medical Conditions

Term	Pronunciation	Meaning
Related to the Cardiovascular System		
Disorders of the Heart and Arteries		
acute coronary syndrome (ACS)	ă-kyūt′ kōr′ŏ-nār-ē sin′drōm	chest pain and other signs and symptoms associated with cardiac ischemia
aneurysm	an′yūr-izm	dilation of an artery; usually due to a weakness in the wall of the artery (**Figure 10-11**)
angina pectoris	an′ji-nă pek′tō′ris	chest pain or pressure resulting from lack of blood flow to the myocardium
angiostenosis	an′jē-ō-stĕ-nō′sis	narrowing of a blood vessel
aortic stenosis	ā-ōr′tik stĕ-nō′sis	narrowing of the aortic valve opening (**Figure 10-12**)
arteriosclerosis; *syn.* arteriosclerotic heart disease (ASHD)	ahr-tēr′ē-ō-skler-ō′sis; ahr-tēr′ē-ō-skler-ot′ik hart diz′ēz	hardening or loss of elasticity of the arteries (**Figure 10-13**)
atherosclerosis	ath′ĕr-ō-skler-ō′sis	buildup of plaque or fatty deposits on inner arterial walls (**Figure 10-13**)
cardiac arrest	kar′dē-ak ă-rest′	complete, sudden cessation of cardiac activity
cardiac tamponade	kar′dē-ak tam′pŏ-nahd′	compression of the heart due to an increase of fluid in the pericardium
cardiomegaly	kar′dē-ō-meg′ă-lē	enlargement of the heart

(continued)

Medical Conditions *(continued)*

Term	Pronunciation	Meaning
cardiomyopathy	kar′dē-ō-mī-op′ă-thē	disease of the heart muscle
cardiopathy	kar′dē-op′ă-thē	any disease of the heart

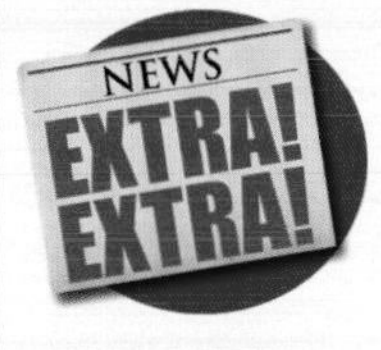

RISK FACTORS FOR CARDIOPATHY Risk factors for heart disease can be placed in two categories: those that are changeable and those that cannot be changed. Risk factors that are changeable include obesity, hypertension, smoking, lack of exercise, and poor diet. Diabetes and stress are also considered changeable risk factors because they can be controlled. Unchangeable risk factors include age, sex, ethnicity, and family history.

Term	Pronunciation	Meaning
cardiovalvulitis	kar′dē-ō-val-vyū-lī′tis	inflammation of the valves of the heart
coarctation of the aorta	kō′ahrk-tā′shŭn ā-ōr′tă	narrowing of the aorta causing hypertension, ventricular strain, and ischemia
congestive heart failure (CHF)	kŏn-jes′tiv hart fāl′yŭr	weakness of the heart causing an inability to circulate blood, leading to edema and fluid buildup in the lungs
coronary artery disease (CAD)	kōr′ŏ-nār-ē ahr′tĕr-ē di-zēz′	narrowing of coronary arteries causing a decrease of blood flow or ischemia to the myocardium
coronary occlusion	kōr′ŏ-nār-ē ŏ-klū′zhŭn	blockage of a coronary vessel often leading to a myocardial infarction
embolus	em′bō-lŭs	vascular blockage made up of a thrombus, bacteria, air, plaque, and/or other foreign material

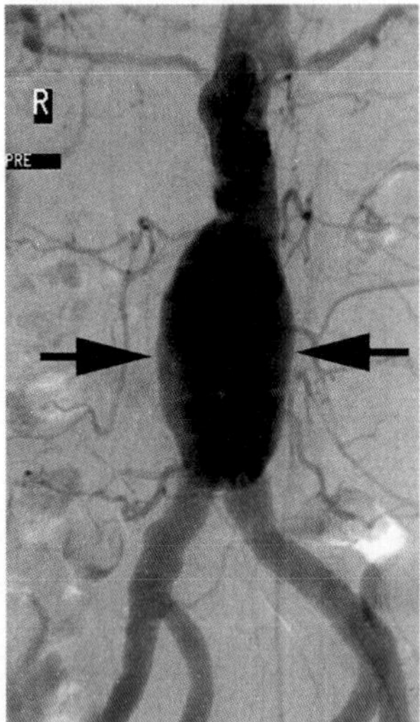

Figure 10-11 Aortic arteriogram in a 68-year-old man demonstrates an infrarenal abdominal aortic aneurysm (*arrows*).

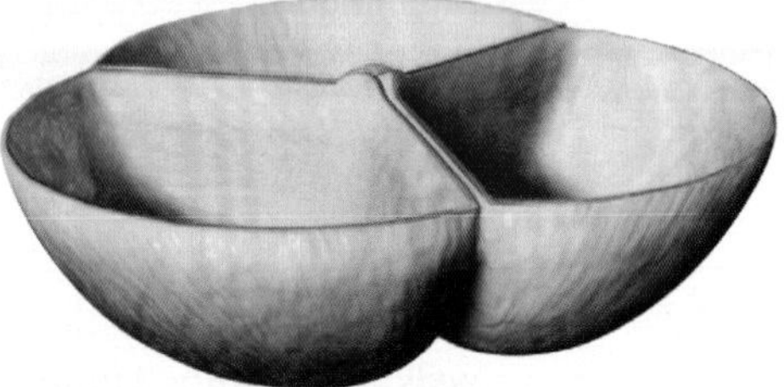
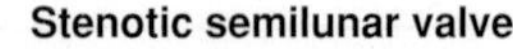

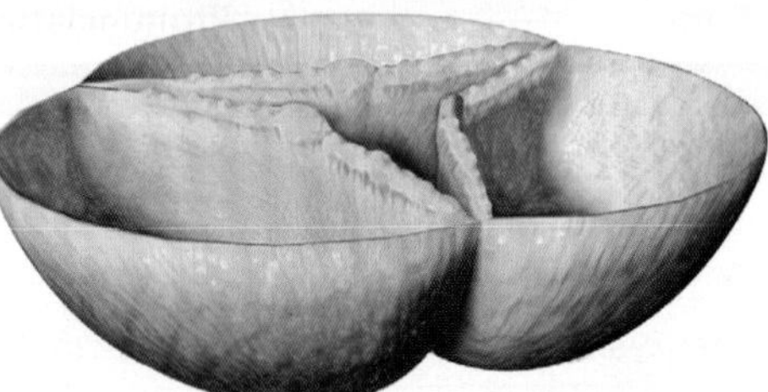

Figure 10-12 Stenosis of a semilunar valve. The aortic and pulmonary valves are semilunar valves.

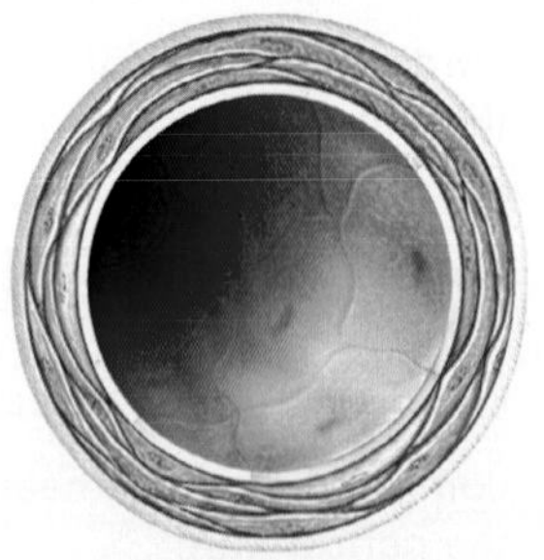
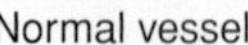

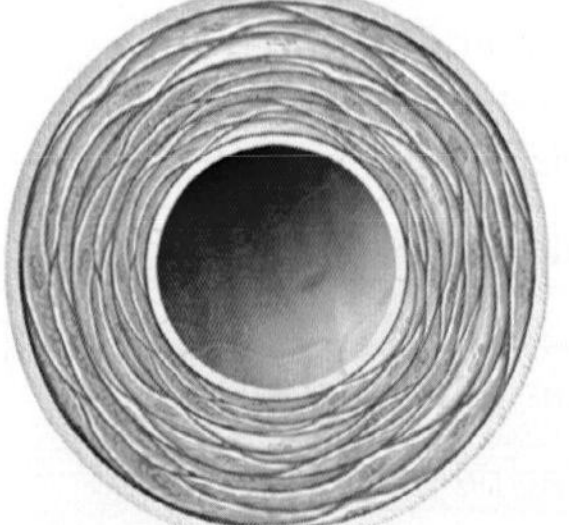

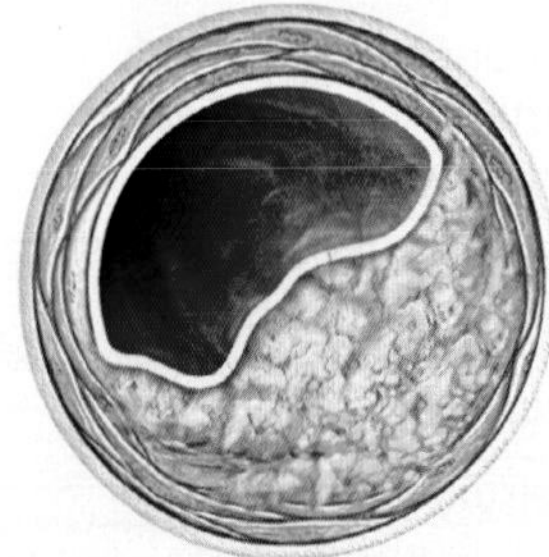

Figure 10-13 A comparison of arteriosclerosis with atherosclerosis.

Medical Conditions

Term	Pronunciation	Meaning
endocarditis	en′dō-kar-dī′tis	inflammation of the endocardium, usually caused by bacterial infection elsewhere in the body (**Figure 10-14**)
hypertension	hī′pĕr-ten′shŭn	persistently elevated (high) blood pressure
hypotension	hī′pō-ten′shŭn	blood pressure that is below normal
intermittent claudication	in′tĕr-mit′ĕnt klaw′di-kā′shŭn	cramping of the lower leg muscles, usually caused by lack of blood flow
ischemia	is-kē′mē-ă	inadequate supply of blood to the tissues
mitral valve prolapse	mī′trăl valv prō′laps	backward movement of the mitral valve cusps allowing regurgitation (backflow of blood)
mitral valve stenosis	mī′trăl valv stĕ-nō′sis	narrowing of the mitral valve opening, usually caused by scarring from rheumatic fever
murmur	mŭr′mŭr	abnormal heart sound
myocardial infarction (MI)	mī′ō-kar′dē-ăl in-fahrk′shŭn	death of heart tissue, usually due to coronary artery occlusion (**Figure 10-15**)
myocarditis	mī′ō-kar-dī′tis	inflammation of the heart muscle
occlusion	ŏ-klū′zhŭn	blockage or closure

(continued)

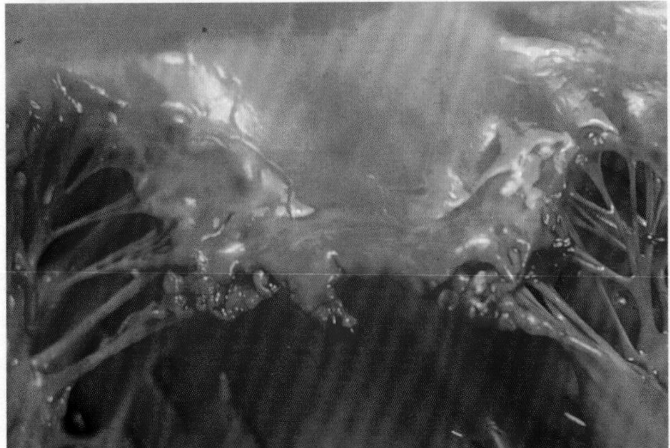

Figure 10-14 Bacterial endocarditis. The mitral valve shows destructive growths that have eroded through the valve.

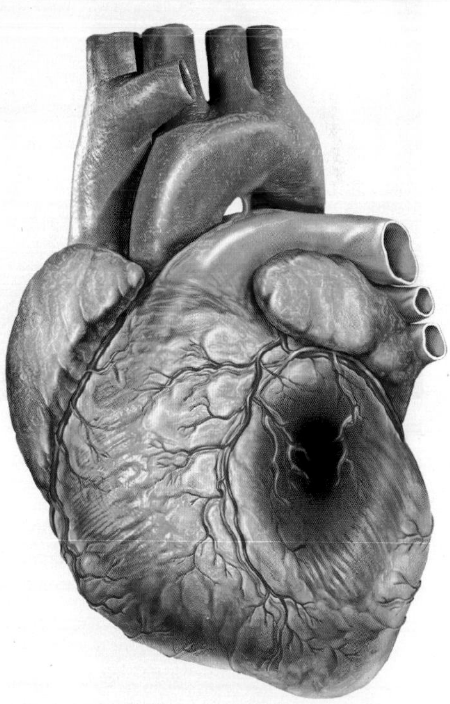

Figure 10-15 Myocardial infarction (MI) (*darkened area*).

Medical Conditions *(continued)*

Term	Pronunciation	Meaning
pericarditis	per′i-kar-dī′tis	inflammation of the pericardial sac around the heart (**Figure 10-16**)
peripheral arterial disease (PAD)	pĕr-if′ĕr-ăl ahr-tēr′ē-ăl di-zēz′	any disorder of the arteries outside, or peripheral to, the heart
plaque	plak	fat or lipid deposit on an arterial wall
polyarteritis	pol′ē-ahr-tĕr-ī′tis	inflammation of many arteries
Raynaud disease; *syn.* Raynaud syndrome	rā-nō′ diz′ēz; rā-nō′ sin′drōm	cyanosis of the fingers or toes due to vascular constriction, usually caused by cold temperatures or emotional stress (**Figure 10-17**)
rheumatic heart disease (RHD)	rū-mat′ik hart di-zēz′	valvular disease resulting from rheumatic fever, a syndrome that occurs after streptococcal bacterial infection (**Figure 10-18**)
stenosis	stĕ-nō′sis	abnormal narrowing of a vessel or body passage
thrombus	throm′bŭs	blood clot

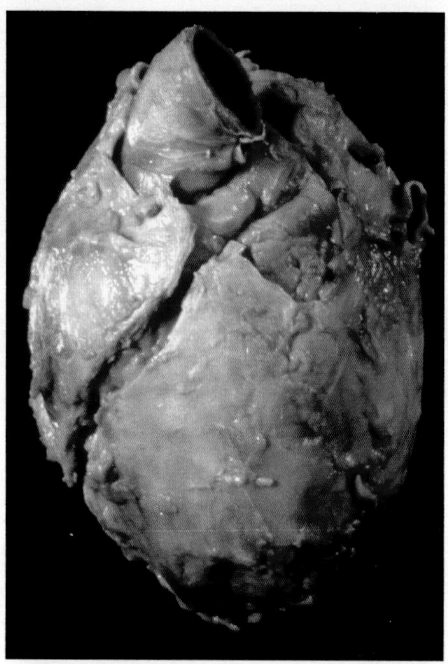

Figure 10-16 Pericarditis. The heart's pericardium is thickened and fibrotic.

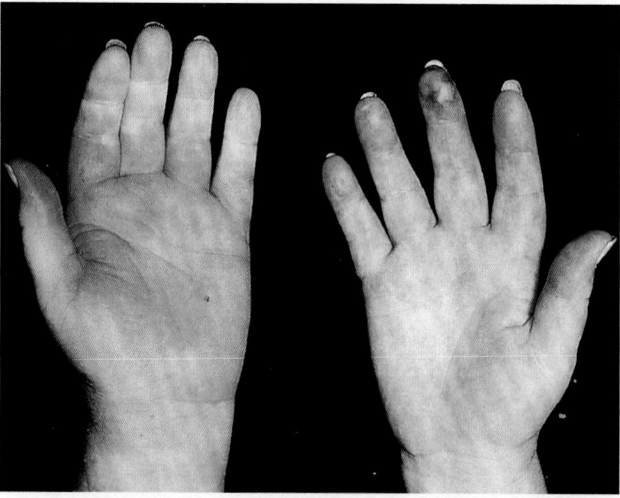

Figure 10-17 Raynaud disease is characterized by cyanosis (*bluish areas*) on the fingers.

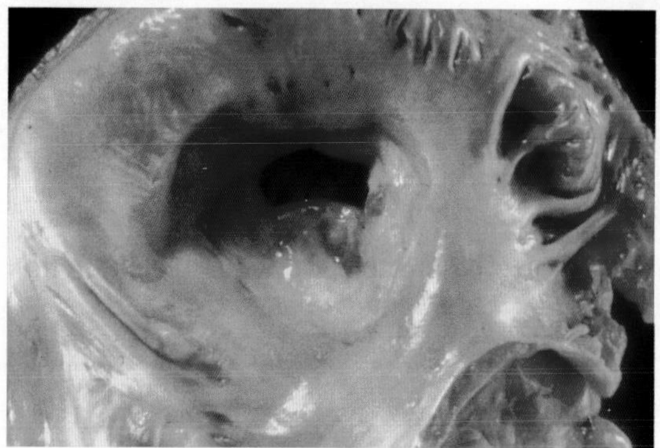

Figure 10-18 Rheumatic heart disease. A view of the mitral valve showing rigid, thickened and fused leaflets with a narrowing opening creating the characteristic "fish mouth" appearance.

Medical Conditions

Term	Pronunciation	Meaning
***Heart Rhythm and Conduction Disorders* (Figure 10-19)**		
arrhythmia	ā-rith′mē-ă	irregularity of the heartbeat resulting in abnormal rhythm
bradycardia	brad′ē-kar′dē-ă	slow heart rate (under 50 beats per minute)
dysrhythmia	dis-rith′mē-ă	defective heart rhythm
fibrillation	fib′ri-lā′shŭn	rapid irregular muscular contractions of the atria or ventricles
flutter	flŭt′ĕr	rapid regular muscular contractions of the atria or ventricles
palpitation	pal-pi-tā′shŭn	forceful or irregular heartbeat felt by the patient
premature ventricular contraction (PVC)	prē′mă-chŭr′ ven-trik′yū-lăr kŏn-trak′shŭn	early contraction of the ventricles
sinus rhythm	sī′nŭs rith′ŭm	normal cardiac rhythm proceeding from the sinoatrial node (the heart's pacemaker)
tachycardia	tak′i-kar′dē-ă	fast heart rate (over 90 beats per minute)
Disorders of the Veins		
deep vein thrombosis (DVT)	dēp vān throm-bō′sis	blood clot formation in a deep vein, usually in the legs or pelvic region
phlebitis	fle-bī′tis	inflammation of a vein
telangiectasia	tel-an′jē-ek-tā′zē-ă	dilation of capillaries
thrombophlebitis	throm′bō-flĕ-bī′tis	inflammation of a vein with formation of a blood clot
varicose vein	var′i-kōs vān	swollen and/or twisted veins, usually of the legs (**Figure 10-20**)
Related to the Lymphatic System		
edema	ĕ-dē′mă	accumulation of excess fluid in intercellular spaces; can be caused by blockage of lymphatic vessels
elephantiasis	el′ĕ-fan-tī′ă-sis	swelling in the lower extremities due to blockage of lymphatic vessels, commonly caused by filariae (parasitic worms) (**Figure 10-21**)
filariae	fi-lar′ē-ē	small parasitic worms that are transmitted by mosquitoes; the worms invade tissues as embryos and block lymphatic vessels as they grow
lymphadenitis	lim-fad′ĕ-nī′tis	inflammation of the lymph nodes
lymphadenopathy	lim-fad′ĕ-nop′ă-thē	disease of the lymph nodes; usually causes enlargement of the nodes
lymphangiitis	lim-fan′jē-ī′tis	inflammation of a lymphatic vessel
lymphedema	lim′fĕ-dē′mă	edema due to a blocked lymph node or lymphatic vessel
pitting edema	pit′ing ĕ-dē′mă	edema that retains an indentation of a finger that had been pressed firmly on the skin (**Figure 10-22**)

Normal sinus rhythm (NSR)

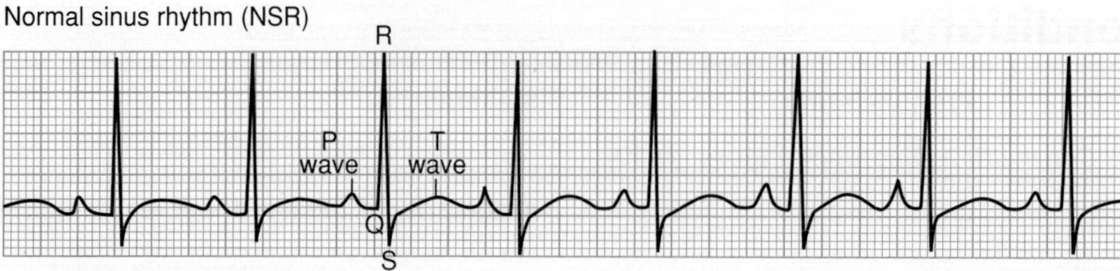

Bradycardia

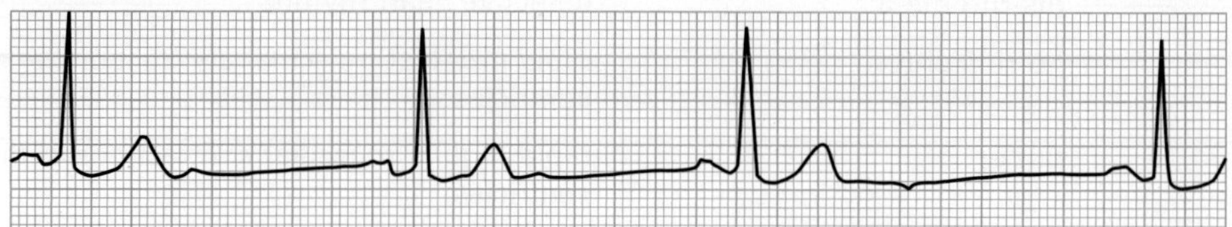

Fibrillation (ventricular)

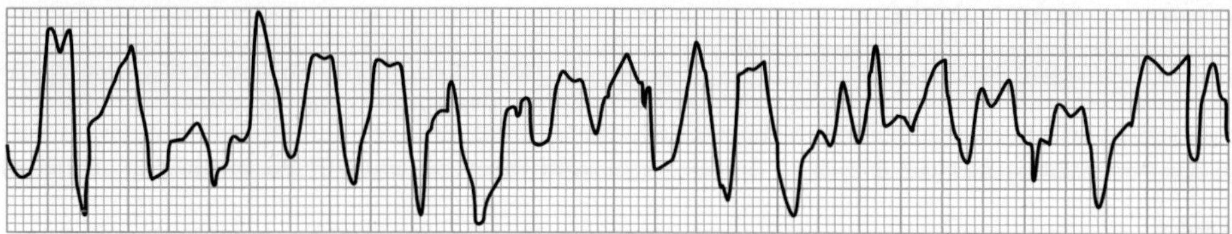

Flutter (atrial)

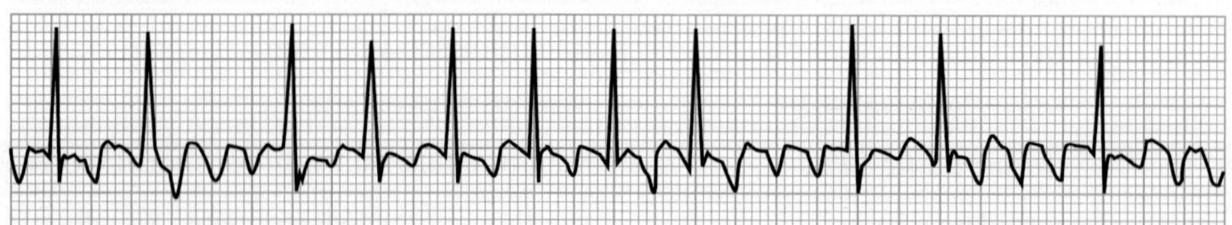

Premature ventricular contraction (PVC)

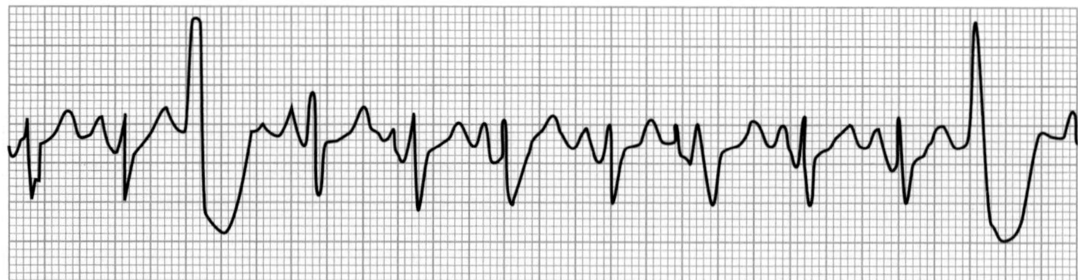

Tachycardia (sinus)

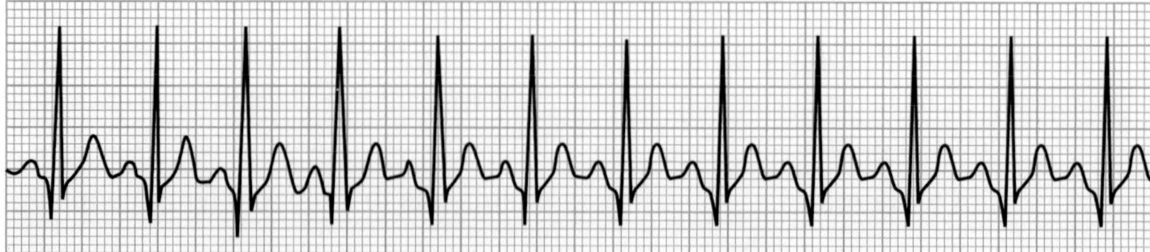

Figure 10-19 Common types of arrhythmias/dysrhythmias shown through electrocardiogram (ECG) tracings.

Learn how elevated blood pressure affects the heart and other organs of the body by viewing the animation "Hypertension" in the Student Resources on thePoint.

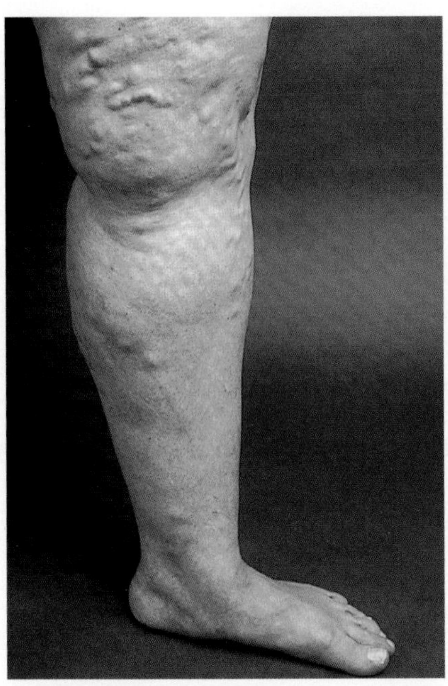

Figure 10-20 Varicose veins on a patient's leg.

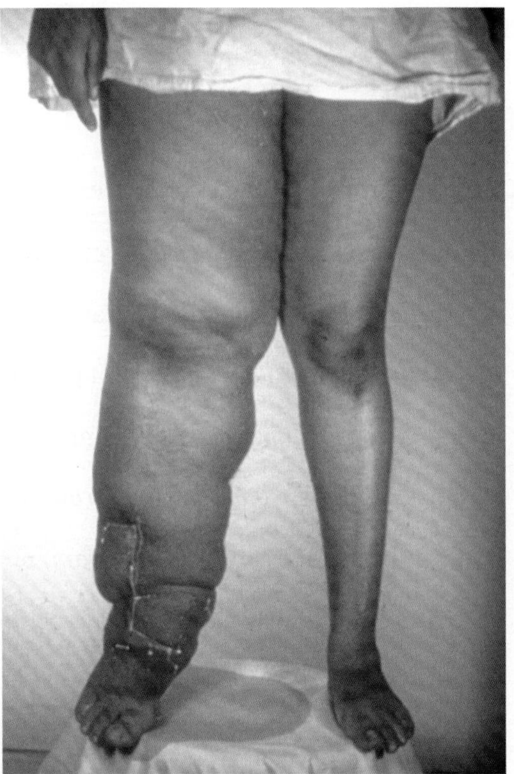

Figure 10-21 Edema of the right lower extremity in a patient with elephantiasis.

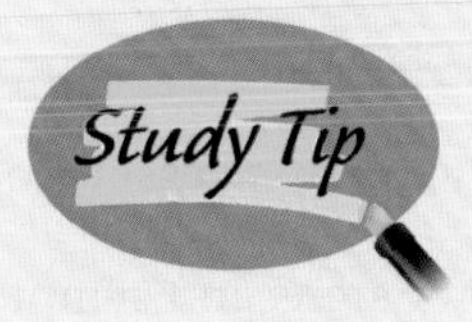

Arteriosclerosis Versus Atherosclerosis: To avoid confusing the meanings of the terms *arteriosclerosis* and *atherosclerosis,* focus on the word parts. Remember that *scler-* means hard and *-osis* means condition of. *Arterio-* means artery, so arteriosclerosis refers to hardening of the arteries. *Athero-* means fatty deposit, so atherosclerosis refers to buildup of a fatty deposit or plaque, which hardens the artery walls. Atherosclerosis is actually a type of arteriosclerosis.

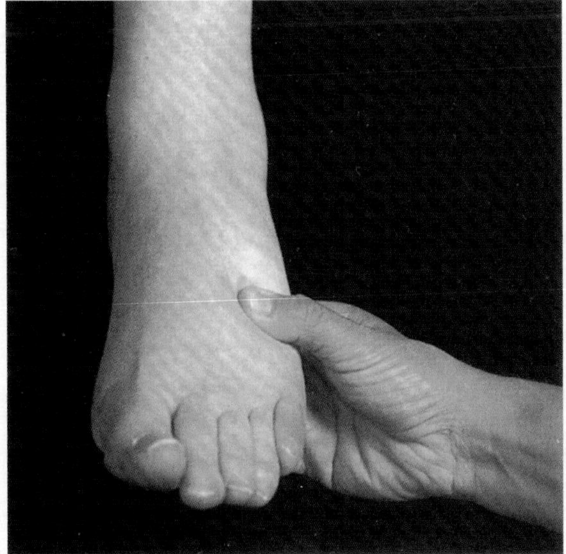

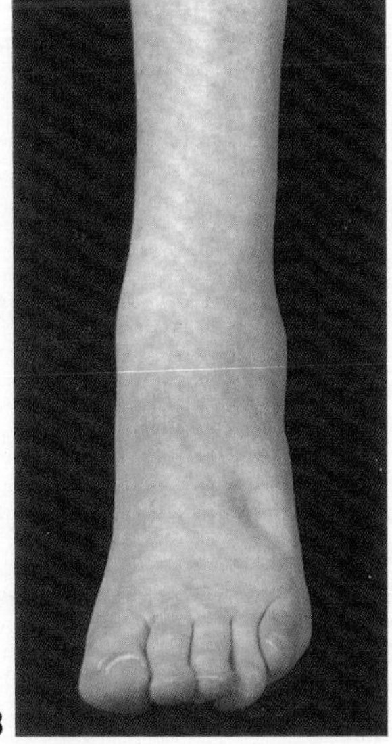

Figure 10-22 **A.** Palpation of the foot. **B.** Pitting edema.

Exercises: Medical Conditions

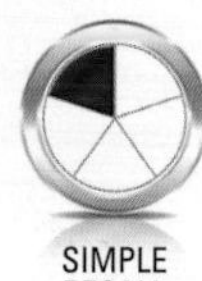
SIMPLE RECALL

Exercise 14

Circle the word that best completes the meaning given.

1. aneurysm = (*weakening, rupture*) of an arterial wall
2. atherosclerosis = condition of fatty buildup and (*enlarging, hardening*) of blood vessels
3. hypertension = (*low, high*) blood pressure
4. hypotension = (*low, high*) blood pressure
5. aortic stenosis = (*hardening, narrowing*) of the aortic valve opening
6. myocardial infarction = (*death, pain*) of the myocardium due to lack of blood supply
7. rheumatic heart disease = damage to the heart (*ventricle, valve*) due to rheumatic fever
8. ischemia = (*lack of, increase in*) blood flow
9. fibrillation = rapid (*irregular, regular*) heart contractions
10. flutter = rapid (*irregular, regular*) heart contractions
11. premature ventricular contraction = (*early, late*) contraction of the ventricles
12. murmur = (*normal, abnormal*) heart sounds
13. elephantiasis = (*anemia, edema*) of the lower extremities due to lymphatic vessel blockage
14. acute coronary syndrome = (*Raynaud disease, chest pain*) and other signs and symptoms associated with cardiac ischemia
15. intermittent claudication = (*cramping, edema*) of the lower leg muscles
16. peripheral artery disease = any disorder of the arteries (*inside, outside*) of, or peripheral to, the heart

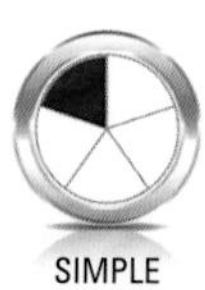
SIMPLE RECALL

Exercise 15

Circle the term that is most appropriate for the meaning of the sentence.

1. Mitral valve prolapse is when the blood flow moves (*backward, forward, circuitously*) through the valve.
2. Edema is the excess accumulation of intercellular (*blood, fluid, substances*).
3. In coarctation of the aorta, the aorta is (*widened, dilated, narrowed*).
4. Small parasitic worms that invade tissues and cause elephantiasis are called (*telangiectasia, filariae, ringworms*).
5. The death of heart tissue usually due to coronary artery occlusion is called (*cardiac arrest, myocardial infarction, angina pectoris*).

6. Chest pain or pressure resulting from lack of blood flow to the myocardium is called (*cardiac arrest, myocardial infarction, angina pectoris*).

7. The medical term for when the heart stops beating is (*cardiac arrest, myocardial infarction, angina pectoris*).

8. With Raynaud disease, the fingers and toes become (*cyanotic, diaphoretic, necrotic*) due to vascular constriction.

9. Congestive heart failure is inefficiency of cardiac (*circulation, valves, pressure*) causing edema and fluid buildup in the lungs.

10. A sudden onset of a fast heart rate is called (*tachycardia, palpitation, flutter*).

11. An inflammation of a vein is called (*phlebitis, telangiectasia, varicose vein*).

12. Coronary artery disease is a narrowing of the coronary arteries causing a(n) (*increase, decrease, leakage*) in blood flow to the myocardium.

13. A vascular blockage that is a combination of clotted blood and other foreign materials is a(n) (*regurgitation, embolus, thrombus*).

14. Deep vein thrombosis is (*plaque, fat, blood clot*) formation in a deep vein.

15. Swollen and/or twisted veins are called (*deep, varicose, phlebitis*) veins.

16. Blockage of a coronary vessel often leading to a myocardial infarction is called (*coronary stenosis, coronary occlusion, congestive heart failure*).

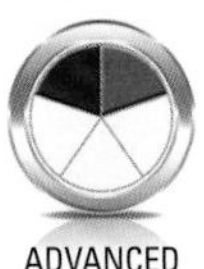

ADVANCED RECALL

Exercise 16

Match each medical term with its meaning.

palpitation	lymphedema	angiostenosis	dysrhythmia	cardiomegaly
lymphadenitis	occlusion	plaque	mitral valve stenosis	arrhythmia

1. narrowing of a blood vessel ____________________
2. forceful irregular heartbeat felt by the patient ____________________
3. abnormality or disturbance of heart rhythm ____________________
4. edema due to a blocked lymph node ____________________
5. blockage or closure ____________________
6. fat deposit on an arterial wall ____________________
7. narrowing of the mitral valve opening ____________________
8. inflammation of the lymph nodes ____________________
9. defective heart rhythm ____________________
10. enlargement of the heart ____________________

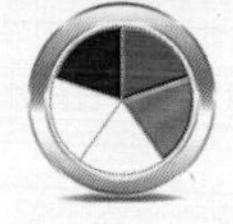

Exercise 17

Given their meanings, build a medical term from an appropriate prefix, combining form, and suffix.

Prefix	Combining Form	Suffix	Term
slow	heart	condition of	1. ________
around, surrounding	heart	inflammation	2. ________
in, within	heart	tissue, structure	3. ________
between	ventricles	pertaining to	4. ________
around, surrounding	heart	tissue, structure	5. ________
rapid, fast	heart	condition of	6. ________
many, much	artery	inflammation	7. ________

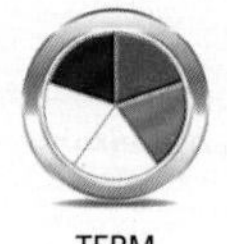

Exercise 18

Break the given medical term into its word parts and define each part. Then define the medical term.

For example:

pericarditis
word parts: peri-, cardi/o, -itis
meanings: around, surrounding; heart; inflammation
term meaning: inflammation of the pericardial sac around the heart

1. lymphangiitis
word parts: ________
meanings: ________
term meaning: ________

2. lymphadenopathy
word parts: ________
meanings: ________
term meaning: ________

3. thrombophlebitis
word parts: ________
meanings: ________
term meaning: ________

4. cardiomyopathy *word parts:* ______________________

meanings: ______________________

term meaning: ______________________

5. endocarditis *word parts:* ______________________

meanings: ______________________

term meaning: ______________________

6. cardiovalvulitis *word parts:* ______________________

meanings: ______________________

term meaning: ______________________

7. myocarditis *word parts:* ______________________

meanings: ______________________

term meaning: ______________________

8. telangiectasia *word parts:* ______________________

meanings: ______________________

term meaning: ______________________

Tests and Procedures

Term	Pronunciation	Meaning
Laboratory Tests Related to the Cardiovascular System		
cardiac enzyme tests	kar′dē-ak en′zīm tests	blood tests used to measure the levels of creatine kinase (CK), creatine phosphokinase (CPK), and lactate dehydrogenase (LDH); increases in such levels may indicate a myocardial infarction
cardiac troponin	kar′dē-ak trō′pō-nin	blood test used to measure the level of a protein that is released in the blood when myocardial (heart muscle) cells die
C-reactive protein (CRP)	sē-rē-ak′tiv prō′tēn	blood test used to measure the level of inflammation in the body; may indicate conditions that lead to cardiovascular disease
electrolyte panel	ĕ-lek′trō-līt pan′ĕl	blood test used to measure the levels of sodium (Na^+), potassium (K^+), chloride (Cl^-), and carbon dioxide (CO_2); used to diagnose an acid–base or pH imbalance that may cause arrhythmias, muscle damage, or death
lipid panel; *syn.* lipid profile	lip′id pan′ĕl; lip′id prō′fīl	blood test used to measure the levels of total cholesterol, high-density lipoprotein (HDL), low-density lipoprotein (LDL), and triglycerides, all of which may signal an increased risk of cardiovascular disease

(continued)

Tests and Procedures *(continued)*

Term	Pronunciation	Meaning
Diagnostic Procedures Related to the Cardiovascular System		
Imaging Studies		
angioscopy	an′jē-os′kŏ-pē	insertion of a catheter with an attached camera to visualize a structure or vessel
aortography	ā-ōr-tog′ră-fē	x-ray imaging of the aorta after injection of a dye
arteriography	ahr-ter′ē-og′ră-fē	x-ray imaging of an artery or arteries after injection of a dye
coronary angiography; *syn.* cardiac catheterization	kōr′ŏ-nār-ē an′jē-og′ră-fē; kar′dē-ak kath′ĕ-tĕr-ī-zā′shŭn	imaging of the circulation of the heart and major vessels after injection of a dye (**Figure 10-23**)
magnetic resonance imaging (MRI)	mag-net′ik rez′ŏ-năns im′ăj-ing	imaging technique that uses magnetic fields and radiofrequency waves to visualize anatomic structures
magnetic resonance angiography (MRA)	mag-net′ik rez′ŏ-năns an′jē-og′ră-fē	MRI of the heart and blood vessels with an injection of dye
multiple uptake gated acquisition (MUGA) scan	mŭl′ti-pĕl up′tāk gāt′ĕd ak-wi-zi′shŭn skan	nuclear medicine technique used to assess ventricular function by producing an image of a beating heart

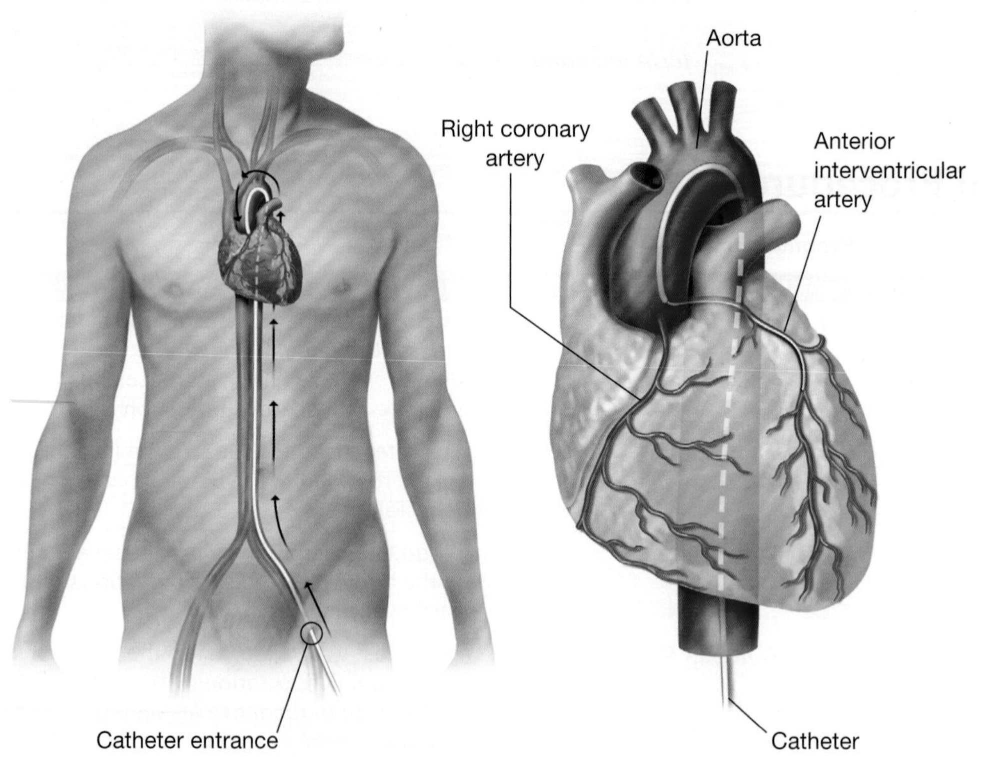

Figure 10-23 Coronary angiography.

Tests and Procedures

Term	Pronunciation	Meaning
sonography; *syn.* ultrasonography	sŏ-nog′ră-fē; ŭl′tră-sŏ-nog′ră-fē	use of ultrasonic sound waves to visualize internal organs
Doppler sonography (DS)	dop′lĕr sŏ-nog′ră-fē	technique used to record velocity of blood flow
echocardiography	ek′ō-kar-dē-og′ră-fē	the use of ultrasound to investigate heart function at rest and with exercise (**Figure 10-24**)
transesophageal echocardiography (TEE)	tranz-ē-sō-fā′jē-ăl ek′ō-kar-dē-og′ră-fē	placement of the ultrasonic transducer inside the patient's esophagus to assess cardiac function and examine cardiac structures
vascular sonography	vas′kyū-lăr sŏ-nog′ră-fē	placement of the ultrasound transducer at the tip of a catheter within a blood vessel to assess blood flow
single photon emission computed tomography (SPECT) scan	sing′gĕl fō′ton ē-mi′shŭn kŏm-pyūt′ĕd tŏ-mog′ră-fē skan	nuclear medicine technique used to assess ventricular function by producing a three-dimensional image of a beating heart
venography	vē-nog′ră-fē	x-ray imaging of a vein after injection of a dye
ventriculography	ven-trik′yū-log′ră-fē	imaging of the heart ventricles after injection of a dye or radioactive substance (radionuclide)
Other Procedures		
auscultation	aws′kŭl-tā′shŭn	listening to body sounds with a stethoscope
blood pressure (BP) monitoring	blŭd presh′ŭr mon′i-tŏr′ing	auscultation of the systolic and diastolic arterial pressure using a stethoscope and a sphygmomanometer (blood pressure cuff)
electrocardiography (ECG or EKG)	ĕ-lek′trō-kar-dē-og′ră-fē	graphic record of the heart's electrical activity; the waves are labeled with the letters P, Q, R, S, and T (**Figure 10-19**)

(continued)

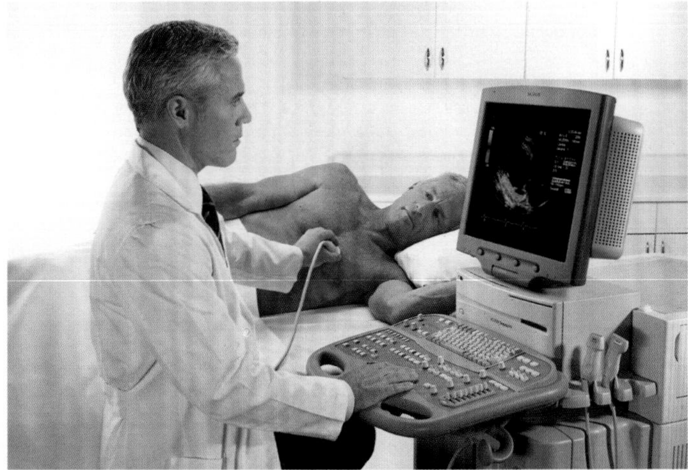

Figure 10-24 Echocardiography.

Tests and Procedures *(continued)*

Term	Pronunciation	Meaning
exercise stress test; *syn.* graded exercise test (GXT), stress electrocardiogram	eks'ĕr-sīz stres test; grād'ĕd eks'ĕr-sīz test, stres ĕ-lek'trō-kar'dē-ō-gram	electrocardiogram performed with controlled stress, usually with a treadmill or bicycle (**Figure 10-25**)
Holter monitor (HM)	hōl'tĕr mon'i-tŏr	portable electrocardiographic device usually worn for 24 hours
percussion	pĕr-kŭsh'ŭn	physical examination method of firmly tapping a part of the body to elicit vibrations and sounds to estimate the size, border, or fluid content of a cavity or organ
pulse	pŭls	palpable throbbing of an artery with each heartbeat, usually felt at the wrist or neck
sphygmomanometer	sfig'mō-mă-nom'ĕ-tĕr	device used for measuring blood pressure
stethoscope	steth'ō-skōp	instrument used to hear sounds within the body

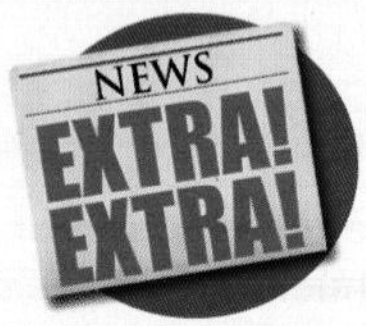

STETHOSCOPE Did you know that the first stethoscope was invented by a French physician who rolled paper into the shape of a cylinder to listen to heart sounds? Prior to this, physicians would listen to a patient's chest by placing their ear directly on the chest wall.

Diagnostic Procedures Related to the Lymphatic System		
lymphangiography	lim-fan'jē-og'ră-fē	imaging of the lymphatic vessels using an injected dye
scintigraphy	sin-tig'ră-fē	procedure using a scintillation (gamma) camera in which lymphatic absorption of a radioactive substance leads to a computer-generated image

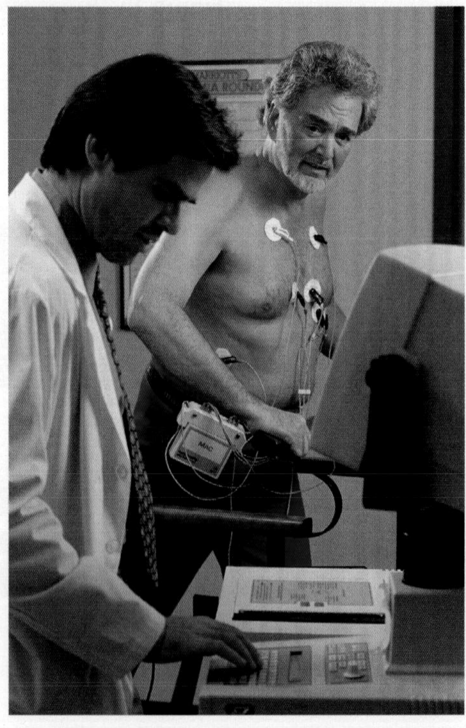

Figure 10-25 Exercise stress test.

Exercises: Tests and Procedures

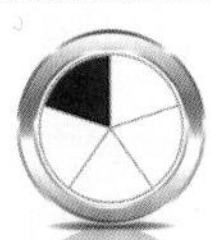

Exercise 19

Circle the term that is most appropriate for the meaning of the sentence.

1. A portable ECG monitoring device that can be worn for 24 hours is a(n) (*graded exercise test, Holter monitor, MUGA scan*).
2. X-ray imaging of an artery or arteries after injection of a dye is called (*arteriography, angiography, aortography*).
3. Imaging of the lymphatic vessels after injecting a dye is called (*angiography, vascular sonography, lymphangiography*).
4. Insertion of a catheter with a camera to visually assess a vessel is called (*angioscopy, fine-needle aspiration, cardiac catheterization*).
5. The process of listening to body sounds with a stethoscope is called (*echocardiography, ultrasound, auscultation*).
6. A graphic record of the heart's electrical activity is called (*echocardiography, electrocardiography, sonography*).
7. A(n) (*MUGA, MRI, SPECT*) scan produces a three-dimensional image of a beating heart.
8. Doppler (*electrocardiography, venography, sonography*) is used to record the velocity of blood flow.
9. The examination method of tapping a body part to elicit vibrations and sounds is called (*percussion, auscultation, blood pressure*).
10. An MRI of the heart and blood vessels with an injection of dye is called (*magnetic resonance imaging, MUGA, magnetic resonance angiography*).

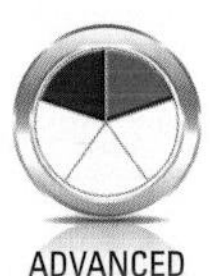

Exercise 20

Complete each sentence by writing in the correct medical term.

1. An ECG performed with controlled stress is a(n) ________________.
2. The use of ultrasound to investigate heart function at rest and with exercise called ________________.
3. To perform ________________, an ultrasound transducer is placed inside the patient's esophagus.
4. Two examples of nuclear medicine studies that assess ventricular function are

   ________________ and ________________.
5. Imaging of the circulation of the heart and major vessels after injection of a dye is called

   ________________ or ________________.
6. An echocardiogram assesses structure and function of the heart at rest and with

   ________________.

7. A ventriculography records the ______________________ after injection with dye.

8. Magnetic resonance imaging uses magnetic fields and ______________________ to visual anatomic structures.

9. Measurement of blood pressure requires a(n) ______________________.

10. Listening to body sounds is called ______________________ and requires one to use a ______________________ placed directly on the body.

Exercise 21

ADVANCED RECALL

Match each type of lab test with the description of the test.

cardiac troponin	electrolyte panel	C-reactive protein
lipid panel	cardiac enzyme tests	

1. evaluation of Na^+, K^+, Cl^-, and CO_2 ______________________
2. evaluation of CK, CPK, and LDH ______________________
3. evaluation of protein released when myocardial cells die ______________________
4. evaluation of cholesterol, HDL, LDL, and triglycerides ______________________
5. measurement of inflammation in the body ______________________

Exercise 22

TERM CONSTRUCTION

Using the given suffix, build a medical term for the meaning given.

Suffix	Meaning of Medical Term	Medical Term
-graphy	recording using sound waves	1. ______________________
-graphy	recording a vein	2. ______________________
-graphy	recording the ventricles	3. ______________________
-graphy	recording the aorta	4. ______________________
-graphy	recording a blood vessel	5. ______________________

Surgical Interventions and Therapeutic Procedures

Term	Pronunciation	Meaning
Related to the Cardiovascular System		
angioplasty	an′jē-ō-plas-tē	surgical repair of a vessel
aneurysmectomy	an′yūr-iz-mek′tō-mē	excision of an aneurysm
atherectomy	ath′er-ek′tō-mē	removal of fatty plaque from a vessel surgically or using catheterization

Surgical Interventions and Therapeutic Procedures

Term	Pronunciation	Meaning
cardiac pacemaker	kar′dē-ak pās′mā-kĕr	surgically placed mechanical device connected to stimulating leads (electrodes) on or within the heart, programmed to help maintain normal heart rate and rhythm (**Figure 10-26**)
cardioversion	kar′dē-ō-vĕr′zhŭn	use of defibrillation or drugs to restore the heart's normal rhythm
coronary artery bypass; *syn.* aortocoronary bypass (ACB)	kōr′ŏ-nār-ē ahr′tĕr-ē bī′pās; ā-ōr′tō-kōr′ō-nar-ē bī′pas	conduit, usually a vein graft or internal thoracic artery, surgically placed between the aorta and a coronary artery branch to shunt blood around an obstruction
coronary artery bypass graft (CABG)	kōr′ŏ-nār-ē ahr′tĕr-ē bī′pās graft	surgical procedure in which a damaged section of a coronary artery is replaced or bypassed with a graft vessel (**Figure 10-27**)

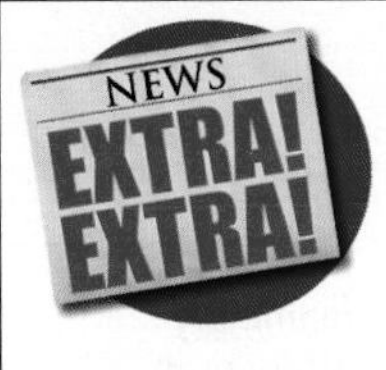

THE EVOLUTION OF CORONARY ARTERY BYPASS SURGERY Advances in technology have led to the development of several types of coronary artery bypass surgery. Traditionally, this procedure involved opening the chest via a large incision through the middle of the sternum; a heart–lung machine circulated the blood while the heart was stopped. A newer type of bypass surgery, called "off-pump," uses special agents to stabilize the heart while the surgery takes place. In addition, surgeons now perform minimally invasive bypass surgery, which uses small incisions in the side of the chest and special instruments for the operation.

Term	Pronunciation	Meaning
defibrillation	dē-fib′ri-lā′shŭn	use of an electric shock to stop fibrillation or cardiac arrest
embolectomy	em′bō-lek′tŏ-mē	surgical removal of an embolus or blood clot, usually with a catheter

(continued)

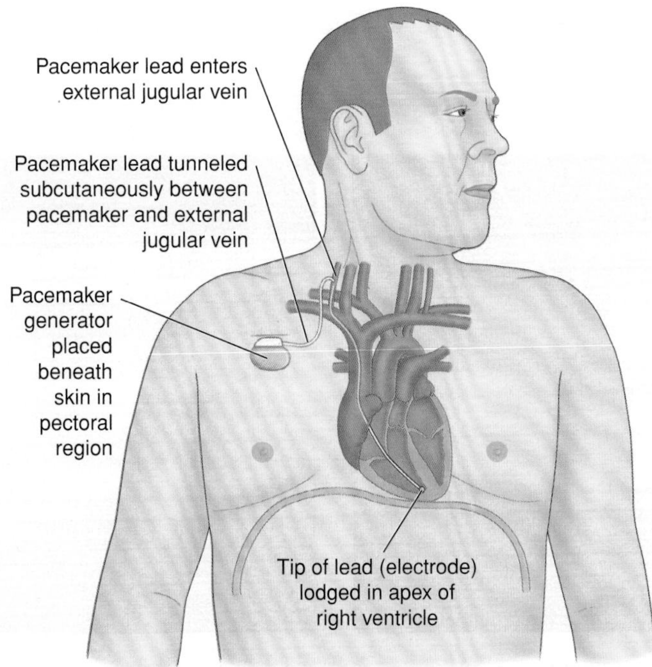

Figure 10-26 Insertion of a pacemaker.

Surgical Interventions and Therapeutic Procedures *(continued)*

Term	Pronunciation	Meaning
endarterectomy	end'ahr-tĕr-ek'tŏ-mē	surgical removal of fatty deposits in an artery
graft	graft	tissue, organ, or vessel used for transplantation
pericardiocentesis	per'i-kar'dē-ō-sen-tē'sis	surgical puncture to aspirate fluid from the pericardium
percutaneous transluminal coronary angioplasty (PTCA)	pĕr'kyū-tā'nē-ŭs trans-lū'mĕn-ăl kōr'ŏ-năr-ē an'jē-ō-plas-tē	procedure in which a balloon catheter is used to restore blood flow in a blocked vessel (**Figure 10-28**)

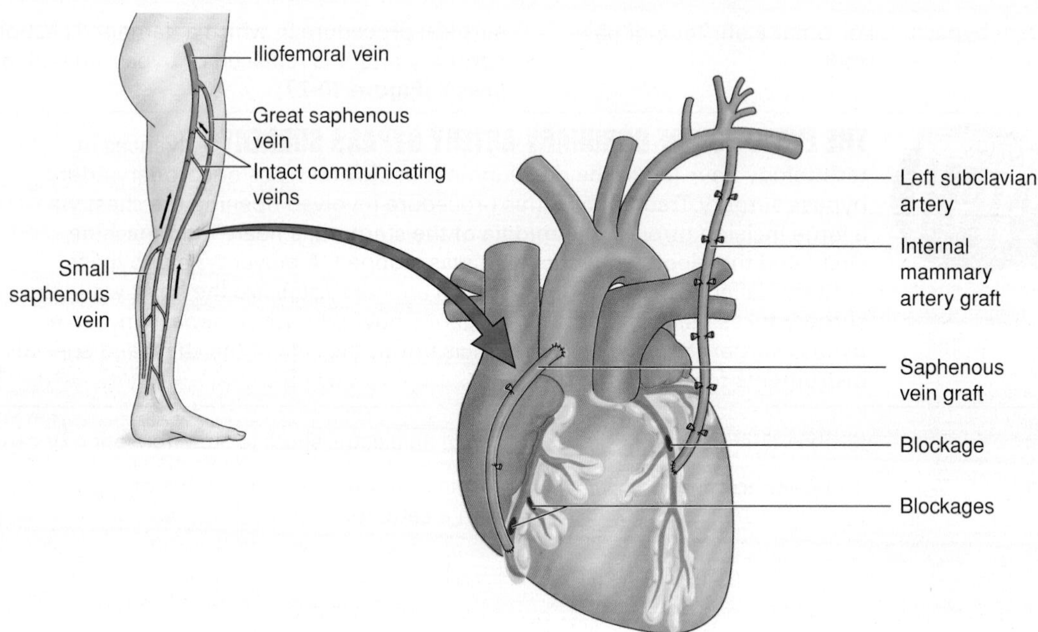

Figure 10-27 Coronary artery bypass graft (CABG).

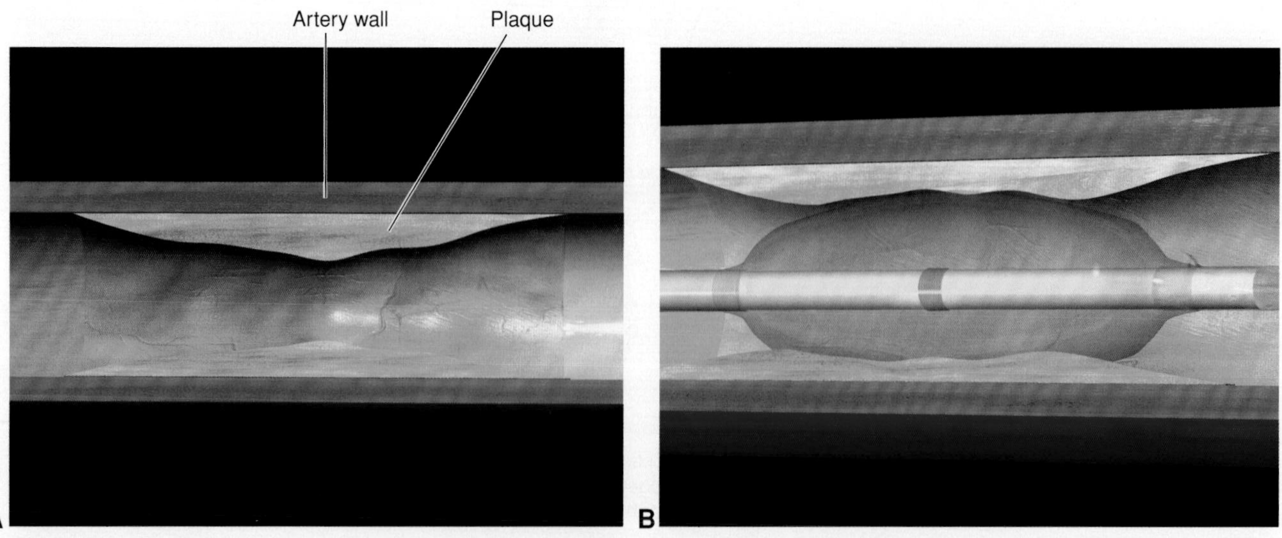

Figure 10-28 Coronary angioplasty (PTCA). **A.** Plaque buildup in an artery. **B.** Balloon inserted and inflated, thus enlarging the lumen.

Surgical Interventions and Therapeutic Procedures

Term	Pronunciation	Meaning
phlebectomy	fle-bek′tō-mē	excision of a segment of a vein, sometimes done to treat varicose veins
stent	stent	intravascular insertion of a hollow mesh tube designed to keep a vessel open or patent (**Figure 10-29**)
valve replacement	valv rē-plās′mĕnt	surgical replacement of a valve with a biologic or mechanical device (**Figure 10-30**)
valvotomy	val-vot′ŏ-mē	incision into a valve
valvuloplasty	val′vyū-lō-plas-tē	surgical repair of a valve
Related to the Lymphatic System		
adenectomy	ad′ĕ-nek′tŏ-mē	excision of a gland
lymphadenectomy	lim-fad′ĕ-nek′tŏ-mē	excision of a lymph node
lymphadenotomy	lim-fad′ĕ-not′ŏ-mē	incision into a lymph node

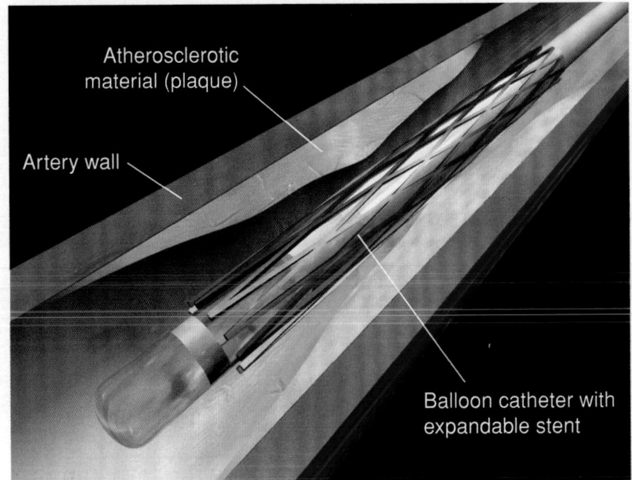

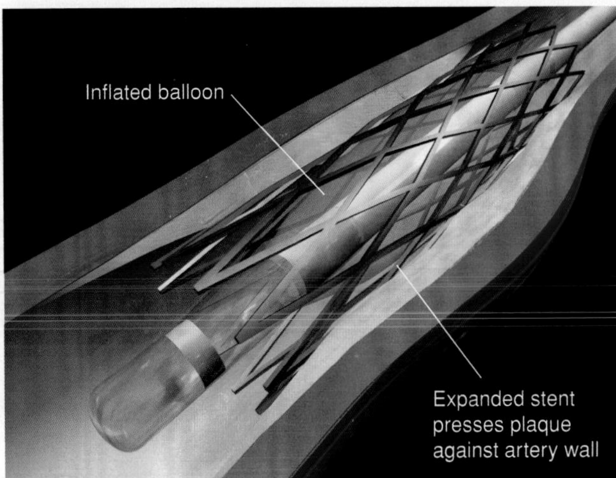

Figure 10-29 Arterial stent.

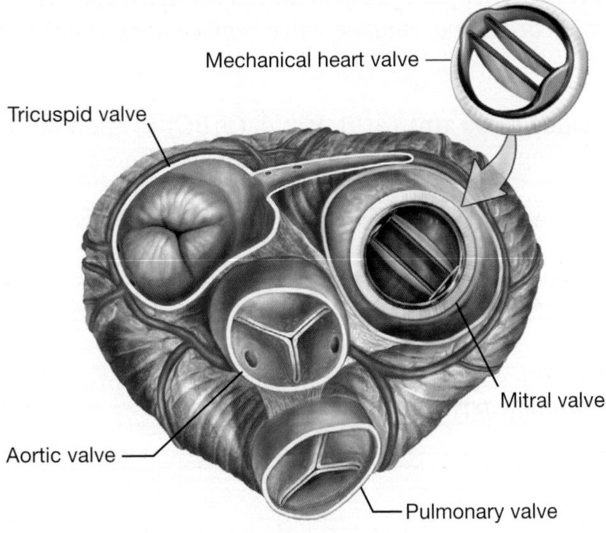

Figure 10-30 Mitral valve replacement.

Exercises: Surgical Interventions and Therapeutic Procedures

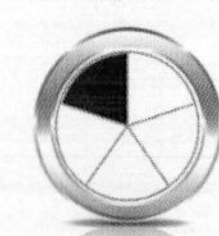

SIMPLE RECALL

Exercise 23

Write the correct medical term for the meaning given.

1. excision of a gland ____________
2. inflation of a balloon catheter in a coronary artery ____________
3. surgical removal of an embolus or blood clot ____________
4. surgical repair of a valve ____________
5. surgical removal of fatty plaque ____________
6. excision of a lymph node ____________
7. incision into a lymph node ____________

ADVANCED RECALL

Exercise 24

Circle the correct term that is appropriate for the meaning of the sentence.

1. Dr. Johansson explained to Mr. Curren that his (*valvuloplasty, valve replacement, atherectomy*) would be with a biologic or mechanical device.
2. A(n) (*angioplasty, cardioversion, valve replacement*) was performed on Mrs. Campbell to correct her irregular and fast heart rate.
3. Mr. Torres had a(n) (*endarterectomy, embolectomy, stent*) to surgically remove the fatty buildup in his carotid artery.
4. After having several syncopal episodes due to bradycardia, Mr. DeHaan was scheduled for implantation of a (*cardiac pacemaker, valve replacement, stent*) to help maintain normal heart rate and rhythm.
5. Dr. LaPenna decided to do a(n) (*ACB, PTCA, CABG*) to open Mr. Thompson's narrowed coronary artery using a catheter with a balloon attachment.
6. A (*pacemaker, PTCA, stent*) was inserted in Ms. Andretti's coronary artery to help keep it open.
7. After documenting the restenosis of his coronary arteries by angiography, Dr. Ayerdi advised Mr. Johnson to have a(n) (*CABG, cardioversion, adenectomy*).
8. Dr. Nowak grafted the saphenous vein to the aorta in a procedure called a(n) (*aortocoronary bypass, endarterectomy, PTCA*).

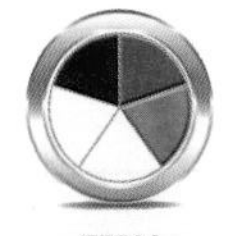
TERM CONSTRUCTION

Exercise 25

Using the given suffix, build a medical term for the meaning given.

Suffix	Meaning of Medical Term	Medical Term
-plasty	surgical repair of a blood vessel	**1.** ________
-ectomy	excision of an aneurysm	**2.** ________
-centesis	puncture to aspirate fluid from the pericardium	**3.** ________
-ectomy	excision of a gland	**4.** ________
-tomy	incision into a valve	**5.** ________

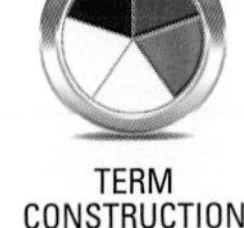
TERM CONSTRUCTION

Exercise 26

Break the given medical term into its word parts, and define each part. Then define the medical term.

For example:

carditis
word parts: cardi/o, -itis
meanings: heart, inflammation
term meaning: inflammation of the heart

1. valvuloplasty
word parts: ________
meanings: ________
term meaning: ________

2. angioplasty
word parts: ________
meanings: ________
term meaning: ________

3. atherectomy
word parts: ________
meanings: ________
term meaning: ________

4. phlebectomy
word parts: ________
meanings: ________
term meaning: ________

5. valvotomy
word parts: ________
meanings: ________
term meaning: ________

Medications and Drug Therapies

Term	Pronunciation	Meaning
anticoagulant	an′tē-kō-ag′yŭ-lănt	drug used to prevent or inhibit blood clotting
antiarrhythmic agent	an′tē-ā-rith′mik ā′jĕnt	drug used to suppress fast or irregular heart rhythms
hemostatic agent	hē′mō-stat′ik ā′jĕnt	drug that stops the flow of blood within vessels
hypolipidemic agent	hī′pō-lip′id-ē-mĭc a′jĕnt	drug used to lower blood cholesterol levels
nitroglycerin	nī′trŏ-glis-er-in	vasodilator used for angina pectoris
thrombolytic therapy	throm′bō-lit′ik thār′ă-pē	administration of an intravenous (IV) drug to dissolve a blood clot
vasoconstrictor	vā′sō-kŏn-strik′tŏr	drug that narrows (constricts) blood vessel diameter, which increases blood pressure
vasodilator	vā′sō-dī′lā-tŏr	drug that increases (dilates) blood vessel diameter, which decreases blood pressure

Exercise: Medications and Drug Therapies

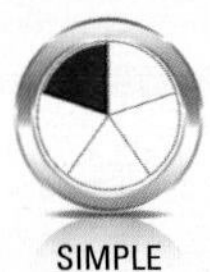

SIMPLE RECALL

Exercise 27

Write the correct medication or drug therapy term for the meaning given.

1. drug that decreases blood vessel diameter ____________
2. drug that prevents or inhibits blood clotting ____________
3. administration of an IV drug to dissolve a clot ____________
4. drug that increases the diameter of blood vessels ____________
5. drug that stops the flow of blood ____________
6. drug that suppresses fast or irregular heart rhythms ____________
7. drug used for angina pectoris ____________
8. drug used to lower blood cholesterol ____________

Specialties and Specialists

Term	Pronunciation	Meaning
cardiology	kar′dē-ol′ŏ-jē	medical specialty concerned with diagnosis and treatment of heart disease
cardiologist	kar′dē-ol′ŏ-jist	physician who specializes in cardiology
cardiac electrophysiology	kar′dē-ak ĕ-lek′trō-fiz′ē-ol′ŏ-jē	medical specialty concerned with the electrical activities of the heart
cardiac electrophysiologist	kar′dē-ak ĕ-lek′trō-fiz′ē-ol′ŏ-jist	physician who specializes in cardiac electrophysiology
lymphedema therapy	lim′fĕ-dē′mă thār′ă-pē	medical specialty concerned with the treatment of lymphedema
lymphedema therapist	lim′fĕ-dē′mă thār′ă-pist	one who specializes in lymphedema therapy

Exercise: Specialties and Specialists

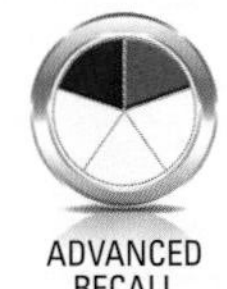
ADVANCED RECALL

Exercise 28

Match each medical specialty or specialist with its description.

cardiac electrophysiology | cardiologist | cardiology
lymphedema therapy | lymphedema therapist | cardiac electrophysiologist

1. study of heart disease __________
2. specialty related to the treatment of lymphedema __________
3. physician who specializes in heart disease __________
4. specialty related to the heart's electrical activities __________
5. one who specializes in lymphedema therapy __________
6. physician specialized in the heart's electrical activities __________

Abbreviations

Abbreviation	Meaning
Related to the Cardiovascular System	
ACB	aortocoronary bypass
ACS	acute coronary syndrome
ASHD	arteriosclerotic heart disease
AV	arteriovenous, atrioventricular
BP	blood pressure
CABG	coronary artery bypass graft
CAD	coronary artery disease
CHF	congestive heart failure
DS	Doppler sonography
DVT	deep vein thrombosis
ECG or EKG	electrocardiography
GXT	graded exercise test
HM	Holter monitor
HTN	hypertension
MI	myocardial infarction
MRA	magnetic resonance angiography
MRI	magnetic resonance imaging
MUGA	multiple uptake gated acquisition
PAD	peripheral arterial disease

(continued)

Abbreviations *(continued)*

Abbreviation	Meaning
PTCA	percutaneous transluminal coronary angioplasty
PVC	premature ventricular contraction
RHD	rheumatic heart disease
SPECT	single photon emission computed tomography
TEE	transesophageal echocardiography

Exercises: Abbreviations

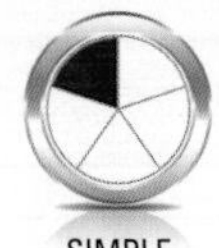
SIMPLE RECALL

Exercise 29

Write the meaning of each abbreviation.

1. CHF ______
2. ACB ______
3. SPECT ______
4. ASHD ______
5. DVT ______
6. PVC ______
7. BP ______
8. ACS ______
9. HTN ______
10. CABG ______

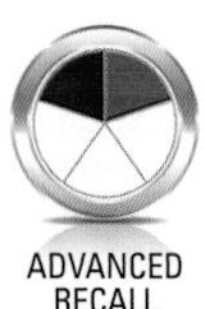
ADVANCED RECALL

Exercise 30

Write the meaning of each abbreviation used in these sentences.

1. Dr. Erickson ordered an **HM** for Mr. Hadley to investigate his complaints of irregular heartbeats.

______

2. Mrs. Cuthbert underwent a **PTCA** to enlarge the lumen of her stenotic artery.

______

3. The cardiologist ordered an **MRA** of the brain to locate the blocked vessel.

______

4. Dr. Anderson's specialty is repair of **AV** defects.

____

5. Dr. Macken had difficulty visualizing the heart structures on the echocardiogram, so he ordered a **TEE,** a procedure in which the patient swallows the transducer, to obtain a different perspective.

____

6. Angie Smith was diagnosed with **CAD** because of her ischemia.

____

7. Mr. Javovich's heart valve was damaged after having **RHD** as a child.

____

8. Mr. John's **GXT** was performed using a treadmill.

____

9. Dr. Francis diagnosed Ms. Snyder with an **MI** caused by coronary artery occlusion.

____

10. Mrs. Adkins was diagnosed with **PAD** through the use of Doppler sonography.

____

ADVANCED RECALL

Exercise 31

Match each abbreviation with the appropriate description.

DS	MUGA	MRA
MRI	ECG	

1. recording of the heart's electrical activity _______________
2. imaging technique using magnetic fields and radiofrequency waves _______________
3. MRI of the heart and blood vessels with an injection of dye _______________
4. technique used to record velocity of blood flow _______________
5. nuclear medicine technique used to assess ventricular function _______________

WRAPPING UP

- The cardiovascular and lymphatic systems are closely related. Their purpose is to circulate blood and lymph throughout the body using blood vessels (arteries and veins) and lymphatic vessels.
- In this chapter, you learned medical terminology including word parts, prefixes, suffixes, adjectives, conditions, tests, procedures, medications, specialties, and abbreviations related to both the cardiovascular and lymphatic systems.

Chapter Review

Review of Terms for Anatomy and Physiology

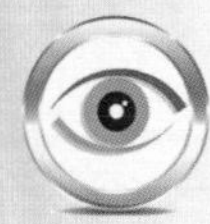

Exercise 32

Write the correct terms on the blanks for the anatomic structures indicated.

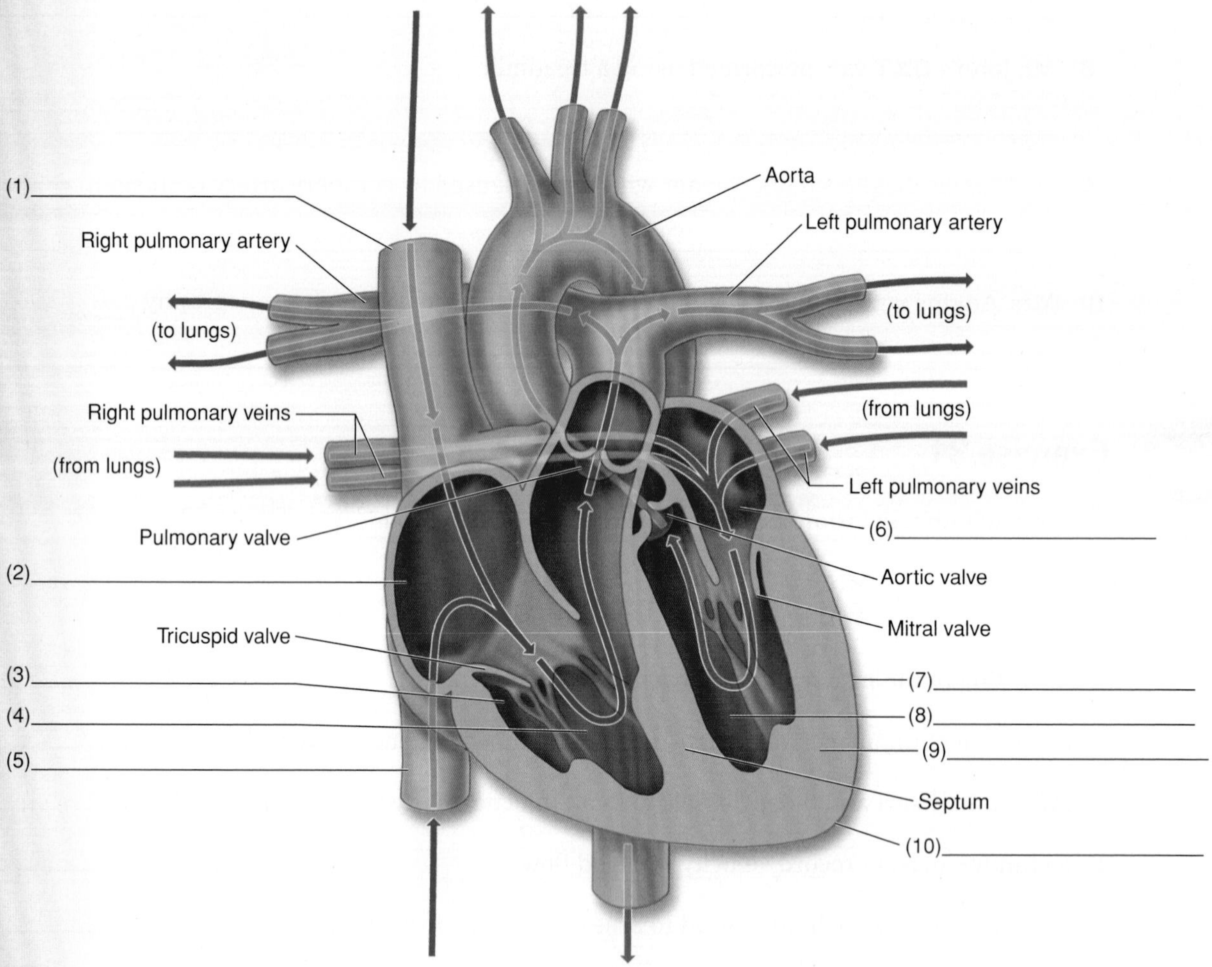

(1)________________
Aorta
Right pulmonary artery
Left pulmonary artery
(to lungs)
(to lungs)
Right pulmonary veins
(from lungs)
(from lungs)
Left pulmonary veins
Pulmonary valve
(6)________________
(2)________________
Aortic valve
Mitral valve
Tricuspid valve
(3)________________
(7)________________
(4)________________
(8)________________
(5)________________
(9)________________
Septum
(10)________________

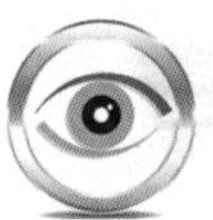

Exercise 33

Write the correct terms on the blanks for the anatomic structures indicated.

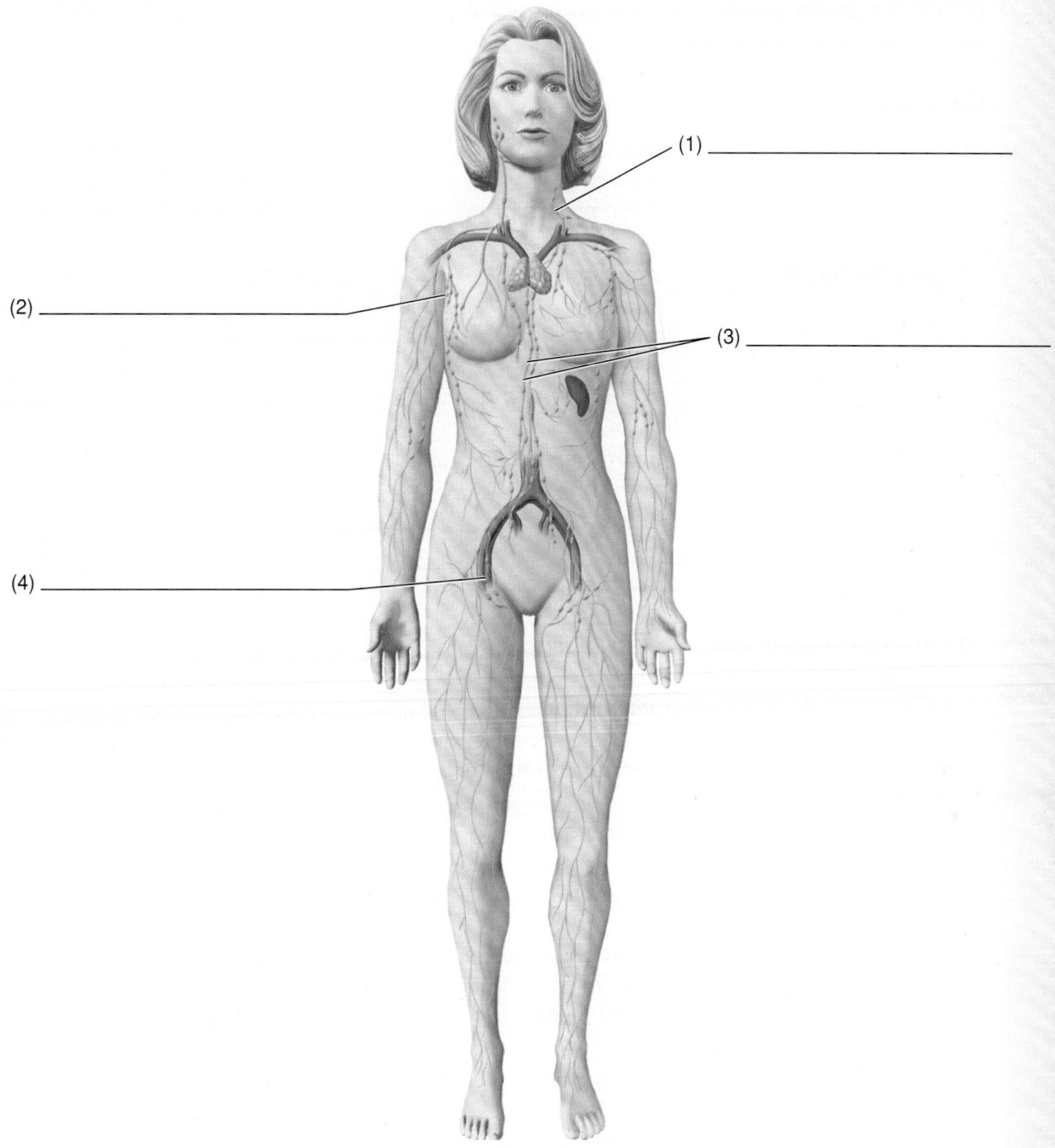

(1) ______________________

(2) ______________________

(3) ______________________

(4) ______________________

Understanding Term Structure

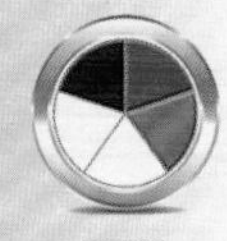

Exercise 34

Break the given medical term into its word parts and define each part. Then define the medical term.

For example:

carditis	*word parts:*	cardi/o, -itis
	meanings:	heart, inflammation
	term meaning:	inflammation of the heart

1. angiostenosis	*word parts:*	______
	meanings:	______
	term meaning:	______
2. phlebitis	*word parts:*	______
	meanings:	______
	term meaning:	______
3. electrocardiography	*word parts:*	______
	meanings:	______
	term meaning:	______
4. atrioventricular	*word parts:*	______
	meanings:	______
	term meaning:	______
5. tachycardia	*word parts:*	______
	meanings:	______
	term meaning:	______
6. interventricular	*word parts:*	______
	meanings:	______
	term meaning:	______
7. thrombosis	*word parts:*	______
	meanings:	______
	term meaning:	______

8. polyarteritis
word parts: ______
meanings: ______
term meaning: ______

9. thrombophlebitis
word parts: ______
meanings: ______
term meaning: ______

10. cardiomyopathy
word parts: ______
meanings: ______
term meaning: ______

11. arteriosclerosis
word parts: ______
meanings: ______
term meaning: ______

12. sphygmic
word parts: ______
meanings: ______
term meaning: ______

13. venography
word parts: ______
meanings: ______
term meaning: ______

14. bradycardia
word parts: ______
meanings: ______
term meaning: ______

15. atherosclerosis
word parts: ______
meanings: ______
term meaning: ______

16. myocardium
word parts: ______
meanings: ______
term meaning: ______

17. valvulotomy *word parts:* ______

meanings: ______

term meaning: ______

18. lymphadenopathy *word parts:* ______

meanings: ______

term meaning: ______

19. lymphangiitis *word parts:* ______

meanings: ______

term meaning: ______

20. thrombolytic *word parts:* ______

meanings: ______

term meaning: ______

Comprehension Exercises

COMPREHENSION

Exercise 35

Fill in the blank with the correct term.

1. The ______ is located between the endocardium and epicardium.
2. The wall that separates the right and left sides of the heart is called the ______.
3. A(n) ______ is one who specializes in the study of the heart.
4. The heart valve between the right ventricle and the pulmonary artery is called the ______ valve.
5. The ______ carries oxygenated blood away from the heart.
6. When the ventricles are in the relaxation phase of the heartbeat, it is referred to as ______.
7. Dilation of small terminal vessels is a condition called ______.
8. Swollen or twisted veins are referred to as ______ veins.
9. A rhythm of rapid regular contractions of the atria is called atrial ______.
10. A rhythm of rapid irregular contractions of the ventricles is called ventricular ______.

11. ______________________ is the enlargement of the lower extremities due to worms blocking the lymph vessels.

12. Cramping of the legs due to lack of blood flow is called ______________________.

13. Lack of blood flow is a condition called ______________________.

14. When the heart muscle is deprived of oxygen or blood flow for a significant amount of time, tissue death may occur. Death of heart muscle is called ______________________.

15. Cardiac arrest is complete, sudden cessation of ______________________ activity.

16. Prolonged immobility during air travel can increase the risk of blood clot formation in the large veins, causing a condition called ______________________.

17. An early contraction of the ventricles is referred to as a(n) ______________________.

18. Abnormal heart sounds are also referred to as ______________________.

19. Patent means ______________________, such as in a patent ductus arteriosus in which the fetal circulatory vessels fail to close.

20. C-reactive protein is a blood test used to measure the level of ______________ in the body.

Exercise 36

COMPREHENSION

Write a short answer for each question.

1. Which type of drug stops the flow of blood within vessels? ______________________
2. The pulse is usually felt at which two points on the body? ______________________
3. During vascular sonography, where is the catheter placed? ______________________
4. What four substances are measured in a lipid panel? ______________________
5. What is the difference between hypotension and hypertension? ______________________
6. Blood pressure monitoring involves the use of what two instruments? ______________________
7. The drug nitroglycerin is used to treat what condition? ______________________

8. What procedure might be used to treat fluid around the pericardium? ____________

9. What physical activity does a physician perform during percussion? ____________

10. Why might a SPECT scan be performed to diagnose arrhythmias? ____________

____

11. What two types of treatment might be done in cardioversion? ____________

____

12. What is the opposite of tachycardia? ____________

13. In what two situations might a defibrillation be performed? ____________

____

14. Which two procedures are done to bypass damaged coronary arteries? ____________

____

15. How does the balloon attachment function in a PTCA? ____________

____

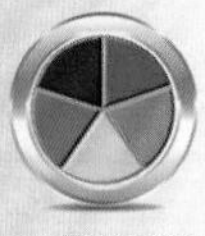

APPLICATION

Exercise 37

Circle the letter of the best answer in the following questions.

1. Which of the following would not be used to describe an abnormal heartbeat?

   A. aneurysm
   B. dysrhythmia
   C. tachycardia
   D. palpitation

2. Using the plural form of the term, the two upper receiving chambers of the heart are called the

   A. aorta.
   B. atria.
   C. arterioles.
   D. atrium.

3. Inflammation of the lymphatic vessels is referred to as

   A. lymphangiitis.
   B. lymphadenitis.
   C. lymphedema.
   D. lymphadenopathy.

4. Edema that retains an indentation of a pressed finger is called

   A. dissecting.
   B. pitting.
   C. ischemic.
   D. stenotic.

5. Cardiac tamponade is compression of the heart. Which procedure might be used to treat this condition?

   A. angioplasty
   B. cardioversion
   C. myocentesis
   D. pericardiocentesis

6. A patient with mitral valve stenosis might have previously had which condition?

   A. rheumatic fever
   B. Raynaud syndrome
   C. murmur
   D. peripheral arterial disease

7. Which of the following is not a diagnostic test designed to record arrhythmias?

A. lipid profile
B. graded exercise test
C. electrocardiogram
D. Holter monitor

8. ECG electrodes are usually placed at the precordial region, or the

A. abdomen.
B. anterior lower chest.
C. anterior right chest.
D. shoulders.

9. CABG stands for

A. coronary artery bypass graft.
B. cardiac artery bypass graft.
C. cerebrovascular accident bypass graft.
D. aortocoronary bypass.

10. During a PTCA, a catheter is advanced *through a vessel.* Which term pertains to the italicized phrase?

A. percutaneous
B. transluminal
C. coronary
D. angiogram

11. Which of the following is a hollow mesh tube used to keep a vessel patent?

A. pacemaker
B. valvotomy
C. defibrillation
D. stent

12. What substance is injected during a cardiac catheterization?

A. fluid
B. dye
C. blood
D. lymph

13. Which blood test diagnoses an acid–base or pH imbalance?

A. cardiac enzyme test
B. C-reactive protein
C. cardiac troponin
D. electrolyte panel

14. Filariae cause elephantiasis by blocking which type of vessels?

A. arteries
B. veins
C. lymphatic
D. capillaries

15. A patient who states that she can "feel her heartbeat" is experiencing

A. palpitations.
B. tachycardia.
C. bradycardia.
D. percussion.

16. Vessels carrying blood *to* the heart might be tested using which diagnostic procedure?

A. arteriography
B. aortography
C. transesophageal echocardiography
D. venography

17. Which condition is not a heart rhythm or conduction disorder?

A. bradycardia
B. tachycardia
C. phlebitis
D. dysrhythmia

18. Lack of blood flow to the lower limbs causes

A. phlebitis.
B. lymphangiitis.
C. intermittent claudication.
D. thrombus.

19. Which procedure treats the buildup of plaque or fatty deposits inside arterial walls?

A. pericardiocentesis
B. atherectomy
C. valve replacement
D. aneurysmectomy

20. An ECG produces a recording of the heart's electrical activity in what type of format?

A. x-ray
B. three-dimensional image
C. sonogram
D. graph

Application and Analysis

CASE STUDIES

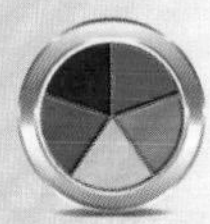
APPLICATION

Exercise 38

Read the case studies, and circle the correct letter for each of the questions.

CASE 10-1

Mr. Terrigo reported to the emergency room with complaints of chest pressure and palpitations. He has a history of a triple CABG done in March 20XX with a history of atrial fibrillation prior to surgery. He was doing well until this morning when he started feeling chest pressure and palpitations. Dr. Francis ordered an ECG that showed evidence of premature ventricular contractions and ST-segment depression. A cardiac catheterization and subsequent PTCA were performed on the stenotic right coronary artery.

1. What of the following best describes a CABG?

A. noninvasive procedure to open a clogged artery
B. surgical replacement or bypass of a damaged coronary artery
C. removal of a clot using catheterization
D. intravascular insertion of a hollow mesh tube

2. Atrial fibrillation is best described as

A. rapid irregular rhythm of the lower heart chambers.
B. rapid regular rhythm of the upper heart chambers.
C. rapid irregular rhythm of the upper heart chambers.
D. rapid regular rhythm of the lower heart chambers.

3. Mr. Terrigo's signs and symptoms could best be described as

A. acute coronary syndrome.
B. cardiac arrest.
C. intermittent claudication.
D. Raynaud disease.

4. Which of the following are waves found on an ECG?

A. QRS waves
B. TUV waves
C. ultrasound waves
D. Doppler waves

5. Which of the following would typically not be true of stenotic coronary arteries?

A. caused by CAD
B. caused by a thrombus
C. caused by atherosclerosis
D. caused by lymphedema

6. Which of the following would not be true for a PTCA?

A. attempts to enlarge the vessel lumen
B. involves a cardiac catheter
C. involves the use of electric shock
D. uses a balloon catheter attachment

CASE 10-2

Mr. Peterson had signs and symptoms of fatigue, cough, and a fever over the past few days. Last night he began experiencing chest pain radiating to his back, which was worse lying down and relieved by sitting up. During the precordial examination, Dr. Macken detected by auscultation a "squeaky leather" sound characteristic of a pericardial rub. An ECG and echocardiogram were performed. Mr. Peterson was diagnosed with pericarditis (**Figure 10-31**) and placed on antiinflammatory drugs.

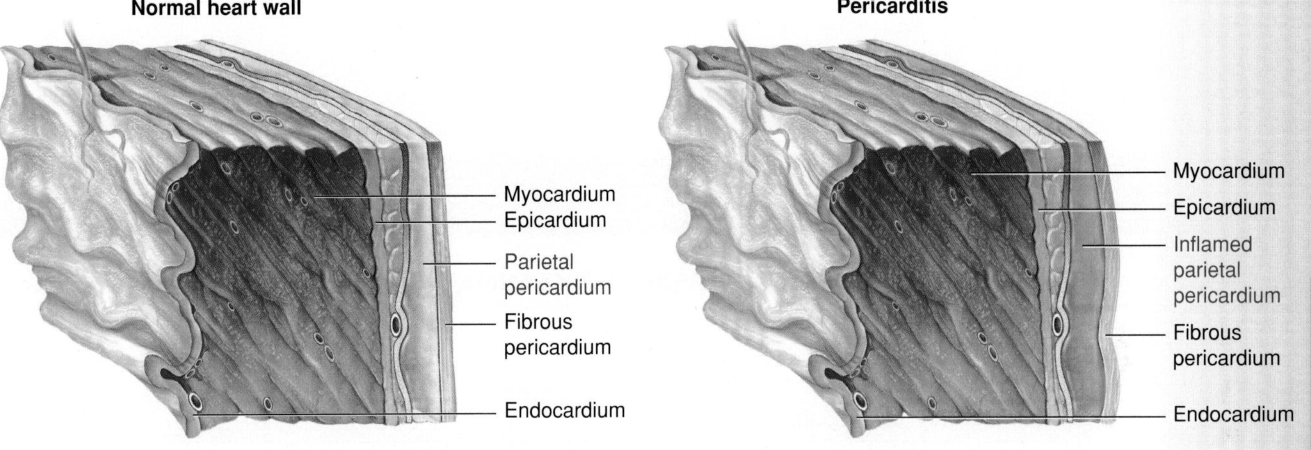

Figure 10-31 Tissue changes in pericarditis.

7. The pericardium is

A. a membrane that protects the heart valves.
B. the heart muscle.
C. inside the heart.
D. the sac surrounding the heart.

8. Cardiac tamponade can occur if which condition progresses?

A. occlusion
B. chest pain
C. fatigue
D. pericarditis

9. Auscultation is an examination by

A. microscope.
B. viewing through a scope or tube.
C. palpation.
D. listening.

10. The term *precordial* refers to the

A. anterior right chest.
B. anterior left chest.
C. heart.
D. lungs.

11. An echocardiogram uses _______ to assess heart structure and function.

A. radiographic rays
B. electrical waves
C. ultrasound waves
D. nuclear imaging

MEDICAL RECORD ANALYSIS

MEDICAL RECORD 10-1

As a clinical medical assistant working in a cardiac clinic, you work directly with patients, measuring vital signs, assisting with examinations, and performing other procedures as directed by the physician. Last week one of the clinic's patients, Mr. Johnson, was admitted to the hospital for chest pain. He has now been discharged and is returning to the clinic. You are reviewing the history and physical examination from his hospital admission.

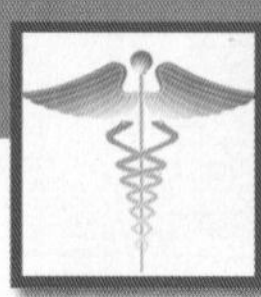

Medical Record

HISTORY AND PHYSICAL EXAMINATION

HISTORY

CHIEF COMPLAINT: Chest pain.

HISTORY OF PRESENT ILLNESS: Mr. Johnson presents here today with complaints of chest pressure with pain radiating to left arm and jaw. Onset four days ago. These symptoms usually begin when he has been jogging for 1 to 2 miles and get worse when he runs uphill. The pain subsides if he slows down or rests. He has admitted to diaphoresis and shortness of breath during these episodes. He exercises five to seven times per week, usually running or jogging 3 to 5 miles per day. He is not on any medications at this time other than an over-the-counter daily vitamin.

MEDICAL HISTORY: His family history is positive for heart disease because his father died at the age of 61 from a myocardial infarction.

SOCIAL HISTORY: Nondrinker, nonsmoker.

OCCUPATIONAL HISTORY: Has been working at the executive level for a land development company for 27 years.

REVIEW OF SYSTEMS: On review of systems, his medical history is unremarkable. He denies any cognitive, visual, auditory, musculoskeletal, digestive, or urinary problems.

PHYSICAL EXAMINATION

GENERAL APPEARANCE: On examination this patient is a well-developed, well-nourished 57-year-old man in no acute distress.

VITAL SIGNS: BP 122/78; P 59 reg; R 12; T 98.8; Wt. 85 kg; Ht. 6′1″

HEENT: Pupils are equal, round, and reactive to light and accommodation.

NECK: The neck is supple. Carotid pulses are strong. No masses or tenderness.

LUNGS: Clear to percussion and auscultation. Breath sounds are easily heard and normal.

HEART: The heart rate and rhythm are regular. Pulse is 59. No murmurs, gallops, or rubs.

EXTREMITIES: No clubbing, cyanosis, or edema.

DIAGNOSTICS: Chest x-ray: suggestive of slight left ventricular enlargement, ECG: positive for ST-segment depression, occasional PVC.

ASSESSMENT

IMPRESSION: Rule out ischemia, rule out cardiovascular disease.

PLAN: CBC, chemistry profile, echocardiogram, and GXT today. If positive, schedule cardiac catheterization within a week. Instructions were given to patient to discontinue jogging until further notice. Patient was given a sample of sublingual nitroglycerin and instructed on its use.

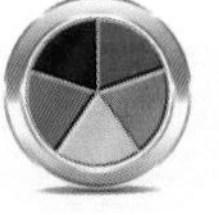
APPLICATION

Exercise 39

Write the appropriate medical terms used in this medical record on the blanks after their meanings. Note that not all the terms appear in the chapter, but you should be able to identify these terms based on word parts that are included in this chapter.

1. pertaining to the heart and vessels ____________________
2. ultrasound recording of heart structure ____________________
3. GXT is an abbreviation for ____________________
4. death of heart tissue ____________________
5. pertaining to a ventricle ____________________
6. abnormal condition characterized by purple or blue discoloration ____________________

Bonus Questions

Atherosclerosis is a form of arteriosclerosis. These two medical terms sound similar but have two different meanings. Write in the correct term after each meaning.

7. hardening of the arteries ____________________
8. hardening of vessels due to plaque buildup ____________________

MEDICAL RECORD 10-2

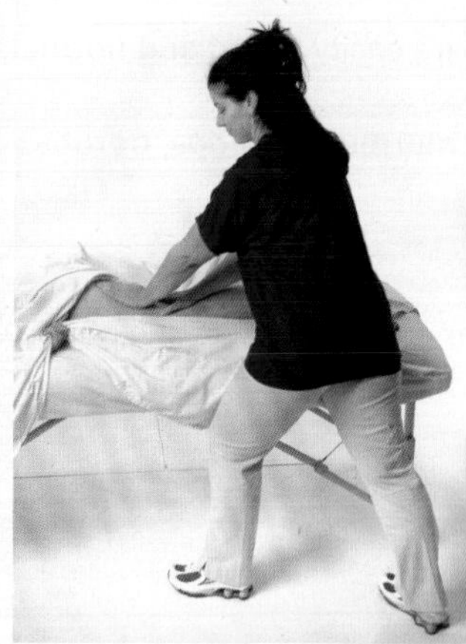

A massage therapist uses touch to assist patients with various conditions.

You are a massage therapist seeing Mr. Van den Berg for the first time for treatment of his lymphedema. He and his wife were missionaries for the past 10 years in Ethiopia, Africa, where he contracted filarial elephantiasis. He has brought his medical record from his last physician visit.

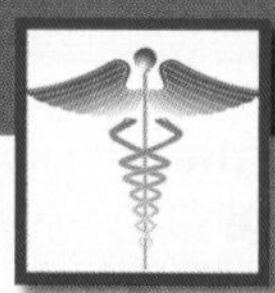

Medical Record

FOLLOW-UP FOR FILARIAL ELEPHANTIASIS

SUBJECTIVE: Patient returns for follow-up after starting chemotherapy for his condition. He complains of continued edema in both of his lower extremities. This is probably due to lymphangiitis and the interrupted flow of lymph and fluid buildup. He has signs and symptoms of chills, fever, and general malaise, which are all to be expected for this stage of his illness.

OBJECTIVE: Lab results confirm the presence of a bacterial infection from adult filarial worms. His temperature is 100.5°F today. His weight has stayed around 210 lb, which is up 2 lb from last visit. On palpation of lower extremities, there is pitting edema, and the right lower leg is erythematic.

ASSESSMENT

1. Filarial elephantiasis
2. Lymphedema
3. Lymphangiitis
4. Fever
5. General malaise

PLAN

1. Review appropriate hygiene plan.
2. Continue with chemotherapy as prescribed.
3. Begin massage therapy as tolerated for lymphedema.
4. Follow up in one month to monitor signs of lymphadenitis or lymphadenopathy.

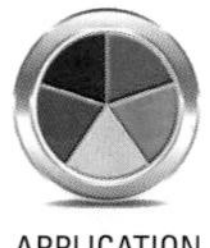

APPLICATION

Exercise 40

Read the medical report and circle the correct letter for each of the following questions. Note: Although some of the medical terms in these questions do not appear in this chapter, you should understand them from their word parts.

1. What is causing Mr. Van den Berg's elephantiasis?

A. red clay soil
B. filariae
C. food poisoning
D. heat

2. What is lymphedema?

A. infection of a lymph node
B. inflammation of a lymph node
C. swelling due to blocked blood vessels
D. swelling due to blocked lymphatic vessels and fluid buildup

3. What are filariae?

A. worms
B. bacteria
C. germs
D. fleas

4. What is lymphangiitis?

A. infection of a lymphatic vessel
B. inflammation of a lymph node
C. inflammation of a lymphatic vessel
D. malignant tumor of lymph tissue

5. Which of the following statements about elephantiasis is *not* true?

A. It occurs most commonly in South America.
B. Filariae get into a body via mosquito bites.
C. Filariae block lymphatic vessels.
D. Lymphedema and lymphangiitis are common signs.

Bonus Question

6. Although this chapter does not describe this term, what does the word *erythema* mean?

Pronunciation and Spelling

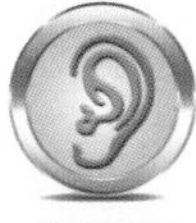

AUDITORY

Exercise 41

Review the Chapter 10 terms in the Dictionary/Audio Glossary in the Student Resources on thePoint and practice pronouncing each term, referring to the pronunciation guide as needed.

SPELLING

Exercise 42

Circle the correct spelling of each term.

1. aneurism	anyerism	aneurysm
2. lymphangeitis	lymphangiitis	lymphanitis
3. valvoplasty	valvuplasty	valvuloplasty

4.	telangietasia	telengiectasia	telangiectasia
5.	Dopplier	Dopler	Doppler
6.	sphygmomanometer	sphymonometer	sphymomenometer
7.	vasoconstrictor	vasoconstricter	vasoconstitor
8.	diastoli	diestole	diastole
9.	ascultation	ausultation	auscultation
10.	elephantiasis	elephanitis	elephantiosis
11.	paroxismal	paroxysmal	paroximal
12.	ischimic	iskemic	ischemic
13.	dysrhythmia	dysrrythmia	dysrythmia
14.	arrhythmia	arrythmia	arythmia
15.	claudication	claudacation	claudocation

Media Connection

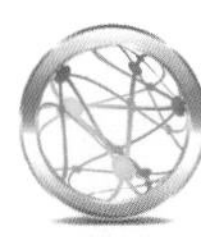
STUDENT RESOURCES

Exercise 43

Complete each of the following activities available with the Student Resources on thePoint. Check off each activity as you complete it, and record your score for the Chapter Quiz in the space provided.

Chapter Exercises

____ Flash Cards

____ Concentration

____ Abbreviation Match-Up

____ Roboterms

____ Word Anatomy

____ Fill the Gap

____ Break It Down

____ True/False Body Building

____ Quiz Show

____ Complete the Case

____ Medical Record Review

____ Look and Label

____ Image Matching

____ Spelling Bee

____ **Chapter Quiz** *Score:*________%

Additional Resources

____ Animation: *Cardiac Cycle*

____ Animation: *Hypertension*

____ Dictionary/Audio Glossary

____ Health Professions Careers: Clinical Medical Assistant

____ Health Professions Careers: Massage Therapist

Respiratory System 11

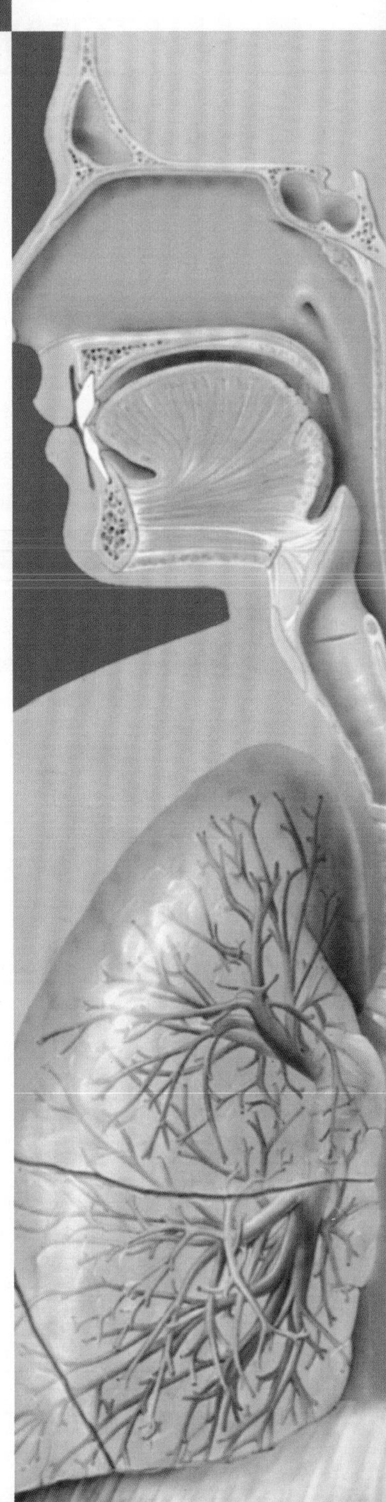

Chapter Outline

Introduction, 410

Anatomy and Physiology, 410
- Structures, 410
- Functions, 411
- Terms Related to the Respiratory System, 411

Word Parts, 416
- Combining Forms, 416
- Prefixes, 417
- Suffixes, 418

Medical Terms, 422
- Adjectives and Other Related Terms, 422
- Medical Conditions, 424
- Tests and Procedures, 434
- Surgical Interventions and Therapeutic Procedures, 440
- Medications and Drug Therapies, 445
- Specialties and Specialists, 446
- Abbreviations, 447

Wrapping Up, 448

Chapter Review, 449

Learning Outcomes

After completing this chapter, you should be able to:

1. List the structures and functions of the respiratory system.
2. Define terms related to the upper and lower respiratory tracts and to respiration.
3. Define combining forms, prefixes, and suffixes related to the respiratory system.
4. Define common medical terminology related to the respiratory system, including adjectives and related terms; signs, symptoms, and medical conditions; tests and procedures; surgical interventions and therapeutic procedures; medications and drug therapies; and medical specialties and specialists.
5. Define common abbreviations related to the respiratory system.
6. Successfully complete all chapter exercises.
7. Explain terms used in case studies and medical records involving the respiratory system.
8. Successfully complete all exercises included with the companion Student Resources on thePoint.

INTRODUCTION

Body cells need oxygen, and the job of the respiratory system is to ensure that cells' oxygen requirements are met. In previous chapters, you learned the roles of the red blood cells and the circulatory system in delivering oxygen to the cells. Carbon dioxide, a byproduct of cellular metabolism, is also exchanged for oxygen at the cellular level and then transported back to the lungs to be "blown off." This chapter focuses on the basic anatomy and physiology of the respiratory system and gives terms related to normal and abnormal functioning.

ANATOMY AND PHYSIOLOGY

Structures

- The respiratory system consists of an upper respiratory tract and a lower respiratory tract.
- The upper and lower respiratory tracts work together to supply oxygen to the lungs and to eliminate carbon dioxide from the lungs **(Figure 11-1)**.

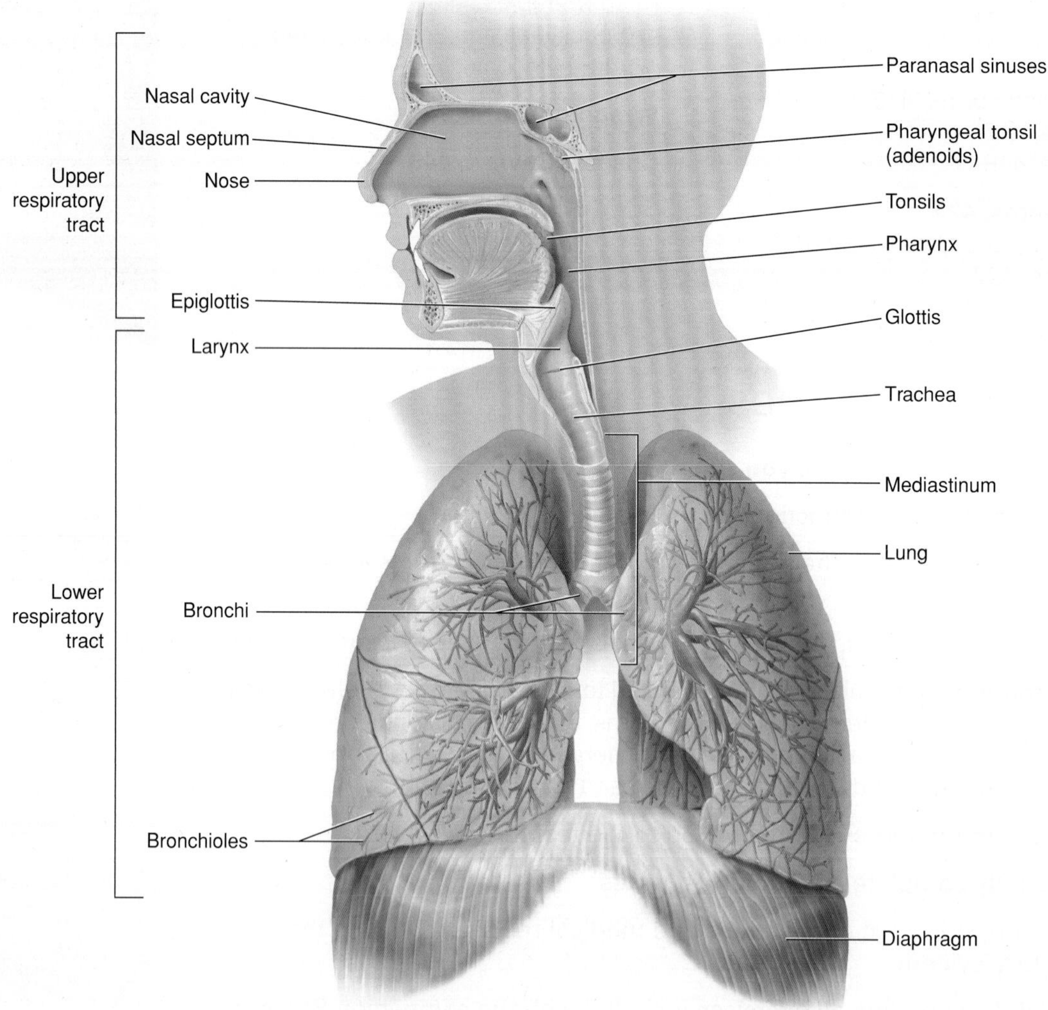

Figure 11-1 The structures of the respiratory system.

Functions

- Supplying oxygen to body cells and tissues via the bloodstream
- Eliminating carbon dioxide from the body
- Providing airflow between the upper and lower respiratory tracts through the larynx and vocal cords, making human vocal sounds possible

Terms Related to the Respiratory System

Term	Pronunciation	Meaning
The Upper Respiratory Tract (Figure 11-2)		
nose	nōz	anatomic structure at the entrance to the respiratory system that conducts, warms, humidifies, and cleans inhaled air
nasal cavity	nā′zăl kav′i-tē	the space on either side of the nasal septum extending from the nares (nostrils) to the pharynx
nasal septum	nā′zăl sep′tŭm	dividing wall between the right and left nasal cavities
paranasal sinuses	par′ă-nă′zăl sīnŭ-sez′	paired air-filled cavities in the bones of the face that are connected to the nasal cavity; these include the frontal, sphenoidal, maxillary, and ethmoidal sinuses **(Figure 11-3)**
pharynx; *syn.* throat	far′ingks; thrōt	space behind the mouth that serves as a passage for food from the mouth to the esophagus and for air from the nose and mouth to the larynx; made up of the nasopharynx, oropharynx, and laryngopharynx
adenoids	ad′ĕ-noydz	pharyngeal tonsil located on the posterior wall of the nasopharynx that enlarges during childhood and shrinks during puberty
tonsils	ton′silz	lymphatic structures including the pharyngeal tonsil (adenoids), palatine tonsil, and lingual tonsil **(Figure 11-4)**

(continued)

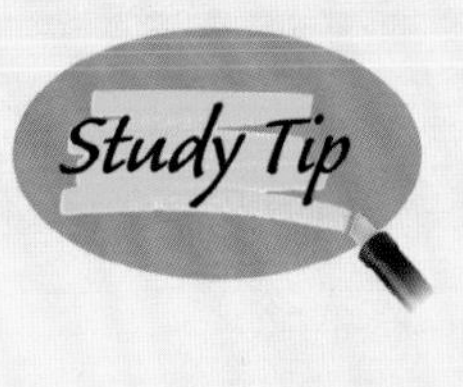

Adenoids and Pharyngeal Tonsil: *Adenoids* are a normal collection of folded unencapsulated lymphatic tissue in the nasopharynx that are also known as the *pharyngeal tonsil.* A single fold of this lymphatic tissue is called an *adenoid.* The tissue forms a mass in the roof and posterior wall of the nasopharynx, undergoes enlargement during childhood, and then regresses during puberty. When this tissue is inflamed, it can lead to otitis media (inflammation of the middle ear), nasal obstruction, sinusitis, and obstructive sleep apnea (recurrent interruptions of breathing during sleep).

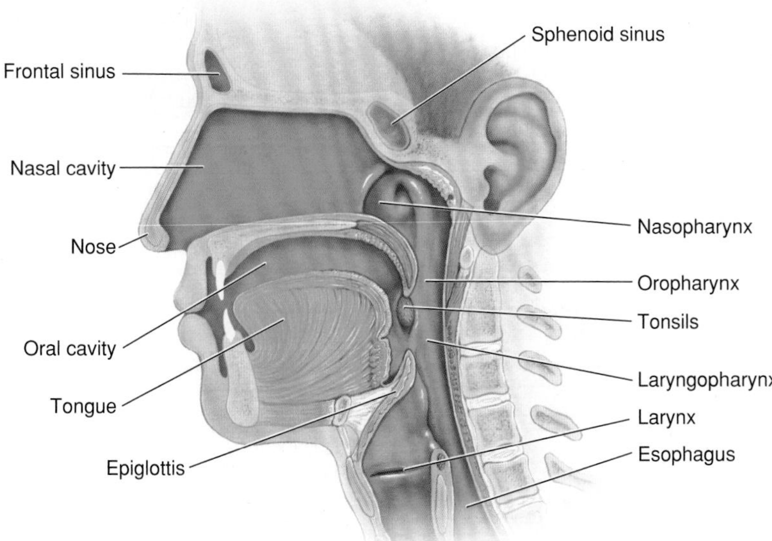

Figure 11-2 The structures of the upper respiratory tract.

Terms Related to the Respiratory System *(continued)*

Term	Pronunciation	Meaning
The Lower Respiratory Tract (Figure 11-5)		
cilia	sil'ē-ă	fine hair-like projections lining the mucous membranes
larynx	lar'ingks	air passageway located between the pharynx and the trachea that holds the vocal cords; commonly called the voice box
epiglottis	ep'i-glot'is	flap of cartilage that covers the upper region of the larynx during swallowing to prevent food or other matter from entering the lungs
glottis	glot'is	part of the larynx consisting of the vocal folds (vocal cords) and the slit-like opening between the folds
trachea; *syn.* windpipe	tră'kē-ă; wind'pīp	air passage extending from the larynx into the thorax; also called the windpipe

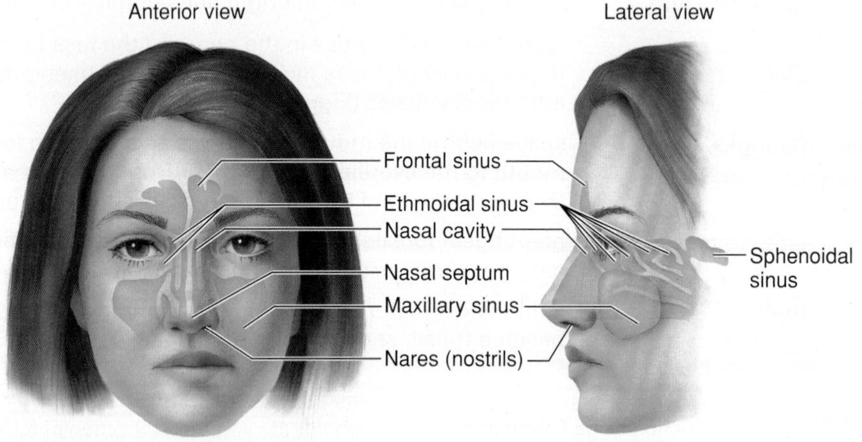

Figure 11-3 The nasal cavity and paranasal sinuses.

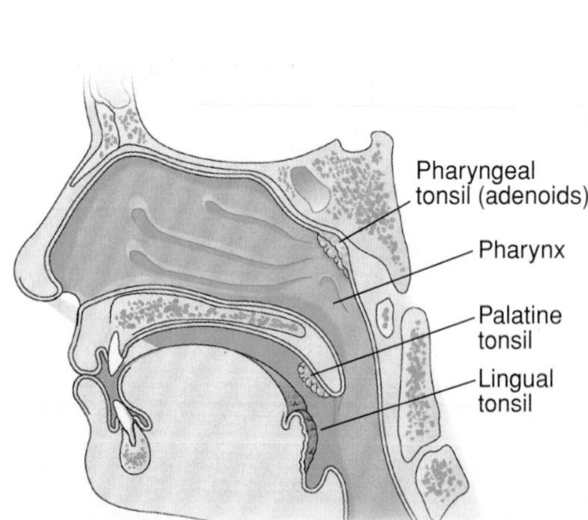

Figure 11-4 The pharynx and tonsils. The pharyngeal tonsil, or adenoids, are located in the nasopharynx (upper portion of the throat). The palatine tonsils are located in the oropharynx (back of the mouth). The lingual tonsils are located at the base of the tongue.

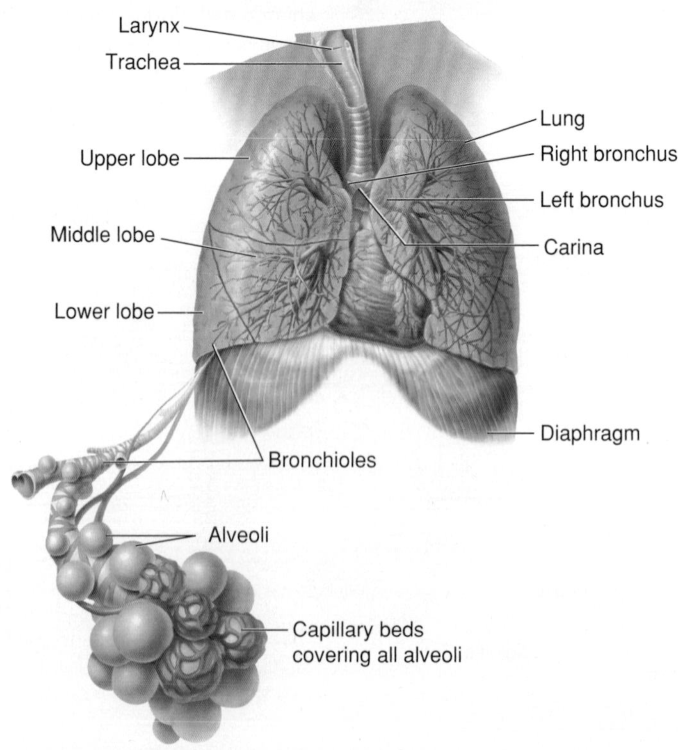

Figure 11-5 The structures of the lower respiratory tract.

Terms Related to the Respiratory System

Term	Pronunciation	Meaning
bronchi	brong′kī	two main branches (left bronchus and right bronchus) off the trachea that convey air to and from the lungs
carina; *syn.* carina of trachea	kă-rī′nă; kă-rī′nă ov tră′kē-ă	cartilaginous ridge at the point where the trachea divides into the two (right and left) bronchi
alveoli	al-vē′ō-lī	tiny air sacs in the lungs where the exchange of oxygen and carbon dioxide occurs between the lungs and blood
bronchioles	brong′kē-ōlz	finer subdivisions of the bronchi located in the lungs
lungs	lŭngz	paired organs of breathing in which blood is aerated
lobes	lōbz	subdivisions of the lungs: there are three on the right (upper, middle, and lower) and two on the left (upper and lower)
pleura	plūr′ă	serous membrane surrounding the lungs and lining the walls of the pulmonary (lung) cavities
parietal layer	pă-rī′ĕ-tăl lā′ĕr	outer layer of the pleura that attaches to the chest wall; also called parietal pleura
pleural cavity	plūr′ăl kav′i-tē	space between the layers of the pleura
visceral layer	vis′ĕr-ăl lā′ĕr	inner layer of the pleura that attaches to the lungs; also called visceral pleura
thorax; *syn.* chest	thō′raks; chest	upper part of the trunk between the neck and the abdomen; formed by the sternum, the thoracic vertebrae, and the ribs, extending to the diaphragm
diaphragm	dī′ă-fram	muscular partition between the abdominal and thoracic cavities; the contraction and relaxation of the diaphragm causes inspiration and expiration

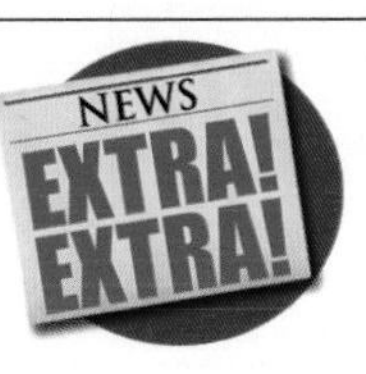

THE DIAPHRAGM The diaphragm assists in breathing. When air is taken into the lungs (inspiration), the diaphragm contracts, or is pushed down (inferiorly). As the muscle relaxes, it forces air back out of the lungs (expiration). When people experience a "stitch" while exercising, they are actually experiencing a spasm of the diaphragm. Physicians agree that the best way to prevent a stitch is to breathe deeply while exercising. This puts less stress on the diaphragm.

Term	Pronunciation	Meaning
mediastinum	me′dē-as-tī′nūm	area of the thoracic cavity between the lungs that contains the heart, aorta, esophagus, trachea, and thymus
Respiration (Breathing)		
airway	ār′wā	any part of the respiratory tract through which air passes during breathing
eupnea	yūp-nē′ă	normal breathing
expiration; *syn.* exhalation	eks′pi-rā′shŭn; eks′hă-lā′shŭn	the process of breathing out **(Figure 11-6)**

(continued)

ANIMATION

Learn more about the structures and functions of the respiratory system by viewing the animation "The Respiratory System" included in the Student Resources on thePoint.

11 Respiratory System

Terms Related to the Respiratory System *(continued)*

Term	Pronunciation	Meaning
external respiration; *syn.* breathing	eks-tĕr′năl res′pi-rā′shŭn; brēth′ing	the exchange of respiratory gases (oxygen and carbon dioxide) in the lungs
inspiration; *syn.* inhalation	in-spi-rā′shŭn; in′hă-lā′shŭn	the process of breathing in **(Figure 11-6)**
internal respiration	in-ter′năl res′pi-rā′shŭn	the exchange of gases between the blood and the tissues; also called tissue respiration
patent	pā′tĕnt	open or unobstructed
respiration	res′pi-rā′shŭn	the process involving the exchange of oxygen and carbon dioxide between the environment and body cells; also called breathing or pulmonary ventilation
sputum	spyū′tŭm	mixture of saliva and mucus coughed up (expectorated) from the respiratory tract; also called phlegm
ventilation	ven-ti-lā′shŭn	movement of gases into and out of the lungs; also called respiration

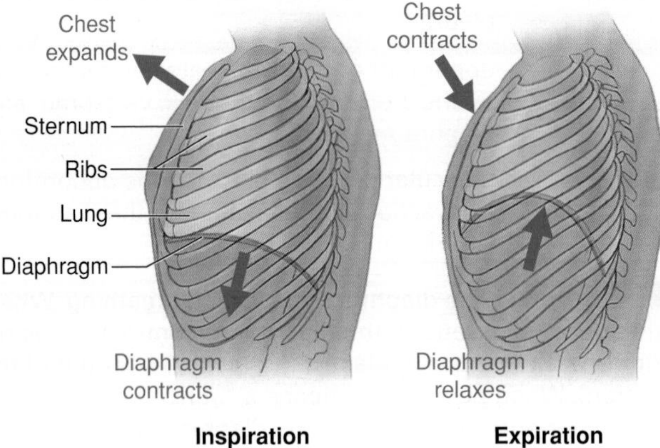

Figure 11-6 The process of breathing.

To see a visual representation of the ventilation process, view the animation "Pulmonary Ventilation" in the Student Resources on thePoint.

Exercises: Anatomy and Physiology

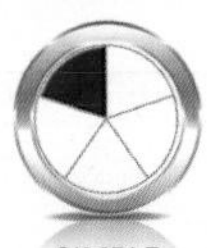

Exercise 1

Write the correct anatomic term for the definition given.

1. subdivisions of the left and right lungs ________________

2. the process of breathing out ________________

3. prevents food or other materials from entering the lungs during swallowing __________

4. normal breathing __________

5. air passageway located between the pharynx and the trachea __________

6. space behind the mouth where food and air pass __________

7. process of breathing in __________

8. muscular partition between the thoracic and abdominal cavities __________

9. anatomic structure at entrance to the respiratory system that conducts, warms, humidifies, and cleans inhaled air __________

10. the exchange of respiratory gases (oxygen and carbon dioxide) in the lungs __________

11. dividing wall between the nasal cavities __________

12. the two main branches off the trachea __________

13. tiny air sacs in the lungs where the exchange of oxygen and carbon dioxide occurs between the lungs and blood __________

14. inner layer of pleura that attaches to the lungs __________

15. mixture of saliva and mucus coughed up (expectorated) from the respiratory tract __________

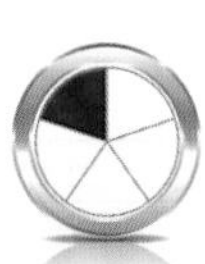
SIMPLE RECALL

Exercise 2

Circle the term that is most appropriate for the meaning of the sentence.

1. The major structures of the upper respiratory system are the (*nose and pharynx, pharynx and lungs, larynx and diaphragm*).

2. The (*paranasal sinuses, cilia*) are fine hair-like projections lining the (*serous membranes, mucous membranes*).

3. When the (*sputum, trachea, ventilation*) is blocked, air cannot pass through the respiratory tract.

4. Human speech is made possible when air enters the (*pharynx, larynx, pleura*).

5. The (*laryngopharynx, epiglottis, sputum*) prevents food from entering the lower respiratory tract.

6. The (*bronchus, glottis, pharynx*) is a branch off the trachea.

7. The bronchi further divide into finer subdivisions in the lungs called (*bronchioles, alveoli, cilia*).

8. The (*mediastinum, diaphragm, thorax*) separates the thoracic cavity from the abdominal cavity.

9. The air-filled cavities in the bones of the face are called (*alveoli, adenoids, paranasal sinuses*).

10. The (*carina, alveolus, diaphragm*) divides into the left and right bronchi.

11. The outer layer of the pleura that attaches to the chest wall is called the (*visceral layer, pleural cavity, parietal layer*).

12. The (*mediastinum, pleural cavity, thorax*) is the space between the layers of the pleura.

13. The process involving the exchange of oxygen and carbon dioxide between the environment and body cells is called (*ventilation, expiration, respiration*).

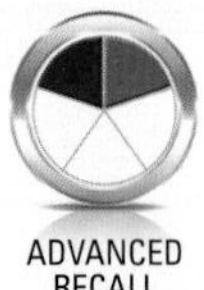
ADVANCED RECALL

Exercise 3

Match each medical term with its meaning.

glottis	patent	pleura	mediastinum
lungs	thorax	adenoid	internal respiration

1. the exchange of gases between the blood and the tissues ____________
2. part of the larynx consisting of the vocal folds (vocal cords) and the slit-like opening between the folds ____________
3. lymphatic structures located on the wall of the nasopharynx ____________
4. part of the thoracic cavity between the lungs ____________
5. paired organs of breathing in which blood is aerated ____________
6. the membrane surrounding the lungs ____________
7. open or unobstructed ____________
8. region of the body formed by the sternum, thoracic vertebrae, and ribs ____________

WORD PARTS

The following tables list word parts related to the respiratory system.

Combining Forms

Combining Form	Meaning
adenoid/o	adenoid
alveol/o	alveolus
aspir/o	to breathe in or suck in
atel/o	incomplete

Combining Forms

Combining Form	Meaning
ausculat/o	listening
bronchi/o, bronch/o	bronchus (windpipe)
capn/o, capn/i	carbon dioxide
cost/o	rib
diaphragmat/o	diaphragm
epiglott/o	epiglottis
laryng/o	larynx
lob/o	lobe
mediastin/o	mediastinum (middle septum)
muc/o	mucus
nas/o	nose
ox/o, ox/a	oxygen
pector/o	chest
pharyng/o	pharynx (throat)
phon/o	sound, voice
phren/o	diaphragm
pleur/o	rib, side, pleura (lung)
pneum/o, pneumat/o, pneumon/o	lung, air
pulmon/o	lung
rhin/o	nose
sept/o	septum, thin wall
sinus/o	sinus, hollow space
spir/o	breathe
thorac/o	thorax, chest
tonsill/o	tonsil
trache/o	trachea

Prefixes

Prefix	Meaning
a-, an-	without, not
dys-	painful, difficult, abnormal
em-	in
eu-	good, normal
hypo-	below, deficient
in-	not
pan-	all, entire
per-	through
tachy-	rapid, fast

Suffixes

Suffix	Meaning
-algia	pain
-al, -ar, -ary, -ic	pertaining to
-cele	herniation, protrusion
-centesis	puncture to aspirate
-ectasis	dilation, stretching
-ectomy	excision, surgical removal
-emia	blood (condition of)
-graphy	a writing, description
-itis	inflammation
-metry	measurement of
-phonia	condition of the voice
-plasty	surgical repair, reconstruction
-plegia	paralysis
-pnea	breathing
-rrhagia	flowing forth
-rrhea	flow, discharge
-scopy	process of examining, examination
-spasm	involuntary movement
-stomy	artificial or surgical opening
-tomy	incision (a cutting operation)

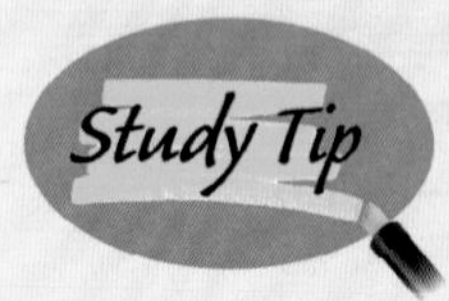

Tonsil and Tonsill/o: The word tonsil just has one "L" but the combining form for tonsil contains two L's. Any word built from this combining form will have two L's.

Exercises: Word Parts

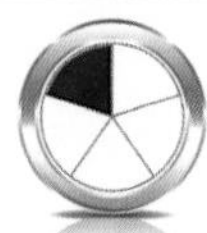

SIMPLE RECALL

Exercise 4

Write the meaning of the combining form given.

1. capn/o ______________________
2. trache/o ______________________
3. epiglott/o ______________________
4. thorac/o ______________________

5. aspir/o ______________________________

6. sept/o ______________________________

7. pleur/o ______________________________

8. mediastin/o ______________________________

9. bronchi/o ______________________________

10. muc/o ______________________________

11. tonsill/o ______________________________

12. auscultat/o ______________________________

13. pneumat/o ______________________________

14. pulmon/o ______________________________

15. atel/o ______________________________

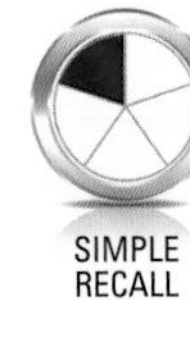
SIMPLE RECALL

Exercise 5

Write the correct combining form for the meaning given.

1. chest ______________________________

2. tonsils ______________________________

3. sound, voice ______________________________

4. thorax, chest ______________________________

5. pharynx ______________________________

6. larynx ______________________________

7. pleura ______________________________

8. breathe ______________________________

9. lobe ______________________________

10. bronchus ______________________________

11. sinus ______________________________

12. nose ______________________________

13. diaphragm ______________________________

14. oxygen ______________________________

15. carbon dioxide ______________________________

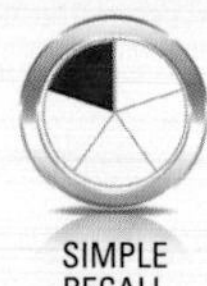

Exercise 6

Write the meaning of the suffix or prefix given.

1. per- __________
2. hypo- __________
3. em- __________
4. -pnea __________
5. tachy- __________
6. -rrhagia __________
7. pan- __________
8. -spasm __________
9. -plegia __________
10. -cele __________
11. -ectomy __________
12. -emia __________
13. -scopy __________
14. a-, an- __________
15. -graphy __________

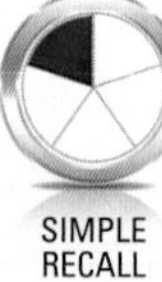

Exercise 7

Write the correct suffix or prefix for the meaning given.

1. measurement of __________
2. pertaining to __________
3. flow, discharge __________
4. condition of the voice __________
5. blood (condition of) __________
6. puncture to aspirate __________
7. dilation, stretching __________
8. painful, difficult, abnormal __________

9. artificial or surgical opening ______
10. through ______
11. good, normal ______
12. surgical repair ______
13. inflammation ______
14. protrusion ______
15. incision (a cutting operation) ______

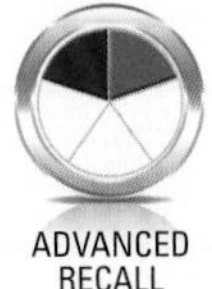

Exercise 8

Considering the meaning of the combining form from which the medical term is made, write the meaning of the medical term. (You have not yet learned many of these terms but can build their meaning from the word parts.)

Combining Form	Meaning	Medical Term	Meaning of Term
adenoid/o	adenoid	adenoidectomy	1. ______
alveol/o	alveolus	alveolitis	2. ______
bronch/o	bronchus	bronchoscope	3. ______
diaphragmat/o	diaphragm	diaphragmatocele	4. ______
epiglott/o	epiglottis	epiglottitis	5. ______
laryng/o	larynx	laryngoscope	6. ______
lob/o	lobe	lobar	7. ______
nas/o	nose	nasal	8. ______
pharyng/o	pharynx	pharyngospasm	9. ______
pleur/o	pleura	pleuritis	10. ______

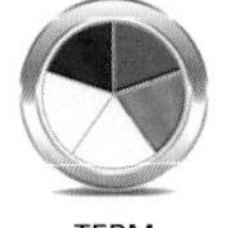

Exercise 9

Using the given combining form and a word part learned previously, build a medical term for the meaning given.

Combining Form	Meaning of Medical Term	Medical Term
pneum/o	inflammation of the lung	1. ______
sept/o	surgical repair of the septum	2. ______
trache/o	incision of the trachea	3. ______

thorac/o	surgical opening into the chest	**4.** ____________
tonsill/o	inflammation of the tonsils	**5.** ____________
sinus/o	inflammation of sinus	**6.** ____________
laryng/o	inflammation of larynx	**7.** ____________
lob/o	pertaining to the lobes (of the lungs)	**8.** ____________
alveol/o	pertaining to the alveolus	**9.** ____________
pharyng/o	inflammation of pharynx	**10.** ____________

MEDICAL TERMS

The following table gives adjective forms and terms used in describing the respiratory system and its conditions.

Adjectives and Other Related Terms

Term	Pronunciation	Meaning
alveolar	al-vē′ŏ-lăr	pertaining to the alveoli
anoxic	an-ok′sik	pertaining to the absence of oxygen
apneic	ap′nē-ik	pertaining to or suffering from apnea
bronchial	brong′kē-ăl	pertaining to the bronchus
diaphragmatic	dī′ă-frag-mat′ik	pertaining to the diaphragm
endotracheal	en′dō-trā′kē-ăl	pertaining to within the trachea
hypoxic	hī-pok′sik	pertaining to a low level of oxygen
intercostal	in′tĕr-kos′tăl	pertaining to the area between the ribs
laryngeal	lă-rin′jē-ăl	pertaining to the larynx
lobar	lō′bahr	pertaining to any lobe of the lungs
mediastinal	mē′dē-as-tī′năl	pertaining to the mediastinum
mucous	myū′kŭs	pertaining to mucus or a mucous membrane
nasal	nā′zăl	pertaining to the nose
pectoral	pek′tō-răl	pertaining to the chest
pharyngeal	făr-in′jē-ăl	pertaining to the pharynx
phrenic	fren′ik	pertaining to the diaphragm
pleural	plūr′ăl	pertaining to the pleura
pleuritic	plūr-it′ik	pertaining to pleurisy
pulmonary	pul′mŏ-năr-ē	pertaining to the lungs
respiratory	res′pi-ră-tōr′ē	pertaining to respiration
thoracic	thō-ras′ik	pertaining to the thorax (chest)
tonsillar	ton-sil′lăr	pertaining to the tonsil
tracheal	trā′kē-ăl	pertaining to the trachea

Exercises: Adjectives and Other Related Terms

Exercise 10

SIMPLE RECALL

Write the meaning of the term given.

1. apneic ______________________
2. tracheal ______________________
3. phrenic ______________________
4. hypoxic ______________________
5. pleuritic ______________________
6. respiratory ______________________
7. tonsillar ______________________
8. endotracheal ______________________
9. mediastinal ______________________
10. mucous ______________________

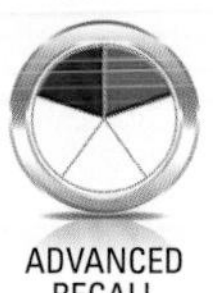

Exercise 11

ADVANCED RECALL

Match each medical term with its meaning.

alveolar	thoracic	pharyngeal	bronchial	intercostal
diaphragmatic	anoxic	pleural	pectoral	lobar

1. pertaining to the thorax ______________________
2. pertaining to the bronchus ______________________
3. pertaining to the pleura ______________________
4. pertaining to the alveoli ______________________
5. pertaining to the diaphragm ______________________
6. pertaining to any lobe ______________________
7. pertaining to the absence of oxygen ______________________
8. pertaining to the pharynx ______________________
9. pertaining to the area between the ribs ______________________
10. pertaining to the chest ______________________

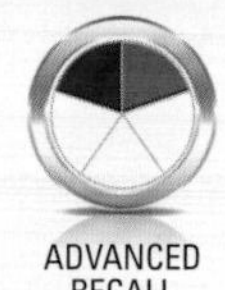

Exercise 12

ADVANCED RECALL

Circle the term that is most appropriate for the meaning of the sentence.

1. Mr. Mullins was treated in the emergency department for a (*pleuritic, pulmonary*) infection within the lower right (*lobar, thoracic*) portion of his lung.
2. Ms. Lane was diagnosed with a fractured rib based on her report of pain and the results of the x-ray of the (*thoracic, pharyngeal, nasal*) cavity.
3. When the physician asked Gabriel where he felt pain, the child pointed at his throat. The physician noted that the reported pain was in the (*pharyngeal, alveolar, pectoral*) area.
4. Mr. Bolling's left lung biopsy involved surgery within the (*laryngeal, tracheal, mediastinal*) cavity.
5. Diagnosing Ms. Hatfield's respiratory condition required an examination of each of the (*lobar, thoracic, pleural*) areas within the lung.

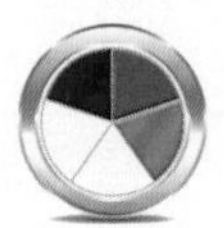

Exercise 13

TERM CONSTRUCTION

Write the combining form used in the medical term, followed by the meaning of the combining form.

Term	Combining Form	Meaning of Combining Form
1. lobar	________	________
2. phrenic	________	________
3. pleural	________	________
4. nasal	________	________
5. pulmonary	________	________

Medical Conditions

Term	Pronunciation	Meaning
acute respiratory distress syndrome (ARDS)	ă-kyūt′ res′pi-ră-tōr′ē dis-tres′ sin′drōm	respiratory failure that can occur with underlying illnesses or injury
aphonia	ă-fō′nē-ă	loss of the voice as a result of disease or injury to the larynx
apnea	ap′nē-ă	absence of breathing
asthma	az′mă	chronic severe breathing disorder characterized by attacks of wheezing due to inflammation and narrowing of the airways **(Figure 11-7)**
atelectasis	at-ĕ-lek′tă-sis	decrease or loss of air in the lung, causing loss of lung volume and possible lung collapse
bronchiectasis	brong′kē-ek′tă-sis	an irreversible widening of portions of the bronchi resulting from damage to the airway wall

Medical Conditions

Term	Pronunciation	Meaning
bronchitis	brong-kī′tis	inflammation of the bronchi
bronchiolitis obliterans with organizing pneumonia (BOOP)	brong′kē-ō-lī′tis ob-lit′ĕr-ā′nz with ōr′gă-ni-zing nūmō′nē-ă	non-infectious pneumonia characterized by inflammation of the bronchioles and surrounding lung tissue
chronic obstructive pulmonary disease (COPD)	kron′ik ob-strŭk′tiv pul′mō-nār′ē di-zēz′	general term used for those disorders with permanent or temporary narrowing of small bronchi, in which forced expiratory flow is slowed
Cheyne–Stokes respiration	chān-stōks res′pi-rā′shŭn	respiratory pattern that involves alternating periods of apnea and deep, rapid breathing
croup	krūp	acute obstruction of the upper airway in infants and children characterized by a barking cough with difficult and noisy respiration
cystic fibrosis (CF)	sis′tik fī-brō′sis	inherited disorder characterized by the production of thick mucus that blocks the internal passages, including the bronchi and lungs, often resulting in respiratory infection
diaphragmatocele	dī′ă-frag-mat′ō-sēl	hernia (abnormal protrusion) of the diaphragm
dysphonia	dis-fō′nē-ă	altered voice production; difficulty speaking due to vocal cord disorder
dyspnea	disp-nē′ă	difficulty breathing
emphysema	em′fi-sē′mă	chronic lung disorder characterized by enlarged alveoli (air sacs) **(Figure 11-8)**
empyema	em′pī-ē′mă	localized collection of pus in the thoracic cavity resulting from an infection in the lungs
epistaxis	ep′i-stak′sis	bleeding from the nose
hemothorax	hē′mō-thōr′aks	blood in the pleural cavity
hypoxemia	hī′pok-sē′mē-ă	decreased level of oxygen in the blood
hypoxia	hī-pok′sē-ă	decreased level of oxygen in the tissues
influenza; *syn.* flu	in-flū-en′ză; flū	an acute contagious respiratory illness caused by influenza viruses

(continued)

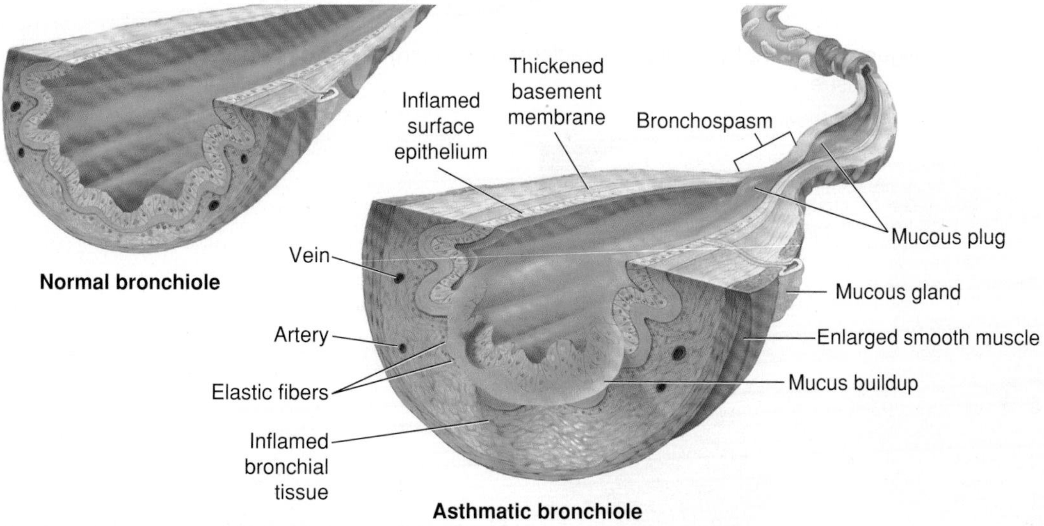

Figure 11-7 Asthma as characterized by obstructed airways.

Medical Conditions *(continued)*

Term	Pronunciation	Meaning
interstitial lung disease (ILD); *syn.* pulmonary fibrosis	in′tĕr-stish′ăl lŭng di-zēz; pul′mŏ-nār-ē fī-brō′sis	a group of chronic lung disorders affecting the tissue between the air sacs of the lungs causing irreversible inflammation and fibrosis (scarring) **(Figure 11-9)**
laryngitis	lar′in-jī′tis	inflammation of the larynx
laryngospasm	lă-ring′gō-spazm	involuntary movement of the larynx
nasopharyngitis	nā-so-fă-rin-jī′tis	inflammation of the nasal cavity and pharynx
orthopnea	ōr′thop-nē′ă	discomfort in breathing that is brought on or aggravated by lying flat
pansinusitis	pan-sī-nŭ-sī′tis	inflammation of all sinuses

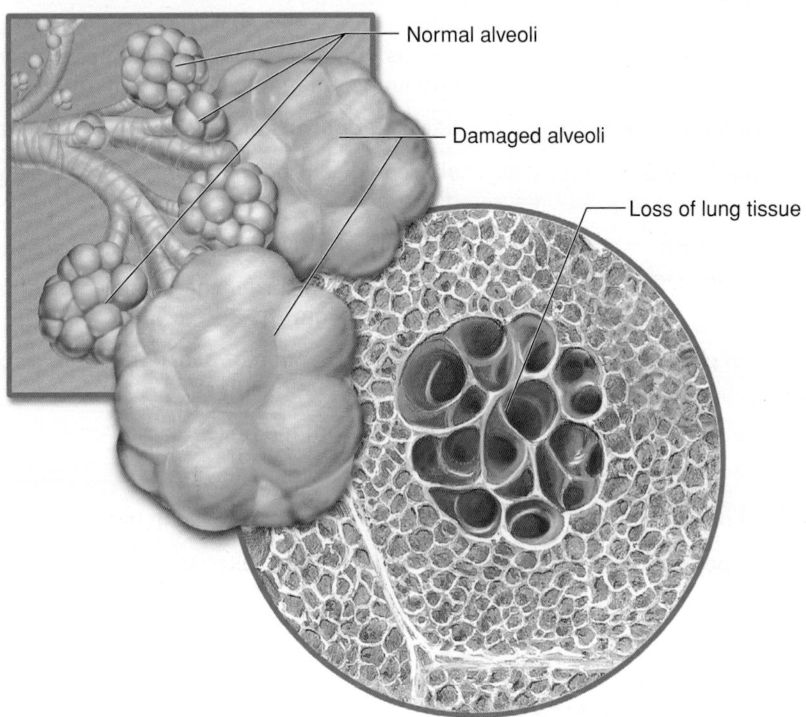

Figure 11-8 Emphysema as characterized by enlarged alveoli and loss of lung tissue.

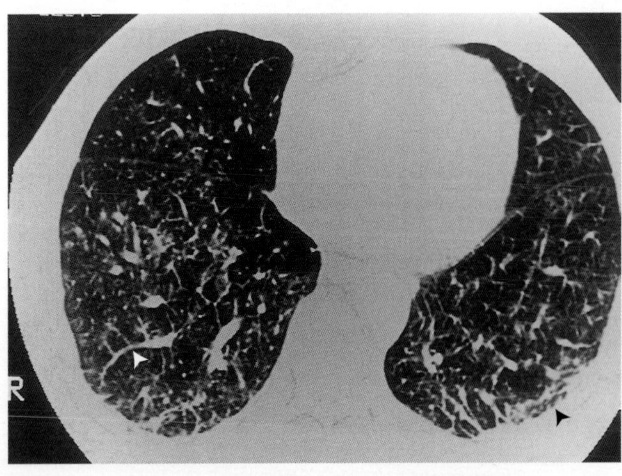

Figure 11-9 Cross-section computed tomography (CT) scan of the chest revealing markings in the lungs consistent with interstitial lung disease (*arrowheads*).

Medical Conditions

Term	Pronunciation	Meaning
pertussis; *syn.* whooping cough	per-tŭs′is; hūp′ing kawf	an acute infectious inflammation of the larynx, trachea, and bronchi caused by the bacterium *Bordetella pertussis*
pharyngitis	fă-rin-jī′tis	inflammation of the pharynx
pleural effusion	plūr′ăl e-fyū′zhŭn	collection of fluid or blood in the pleural space around the lung
pleuritis	plū-rī′tis	inflammation of the pleura
pneumonia	nū-mō′nē-ă	bacterial infection and inflammation within the lobes of the lungs **(Figure 11-10)**
bacterial pneumonia	bak-tēr′ē-ăl nū-mō′nē-ă	pneumonia caused by a bacterial infection
bronchopneumonia	brong′ko-nū-mō′nē-ă	infection of the smaller bronchial tubes of the lungs
lobar pneumonia	lō′bar nū-mō′nē-ă	pneumonia affecting one or more lobes of the lung, often due to bacterial infection, such as infection by *Streptococcus pneumoniae*
pneumococcal pneumonia	nū′mō-kok′ăl nū-mō′nē-ă	form of pneumonia caused by the bacterial species *Streptococcus pneumoniae*
pneumonitis	nū′mō-nī′tis	inflammation of the lungs
pneumothorax	nŭ′mō-thōr′aks	the presence of air or gas in the pleural cavity causing collapse of the lung **(Figure 11-11)**
pulmonary edema	pul′mō-nār′ē e-dē′mă	buildup of fluid in the lungs

(continued)

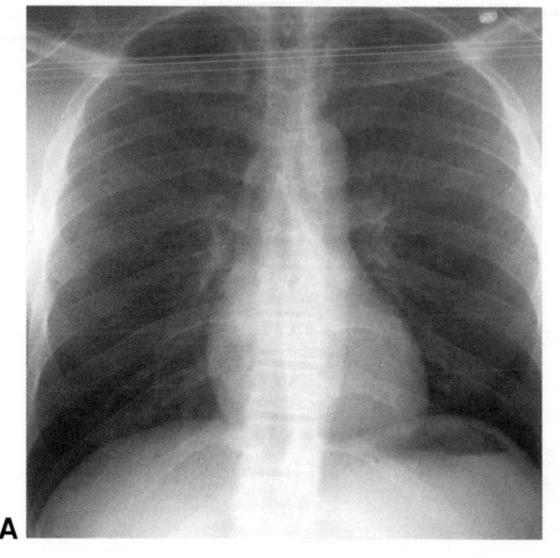

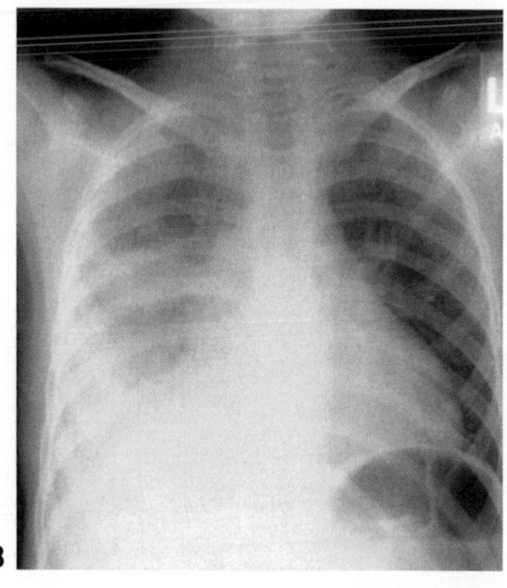

Figure 11-10 **A.** X-ray of a normal lung. **B.** X-ray of the lungs of a child with bacterial pneumonia. The white area of the right lung demonstrates pneumonia.

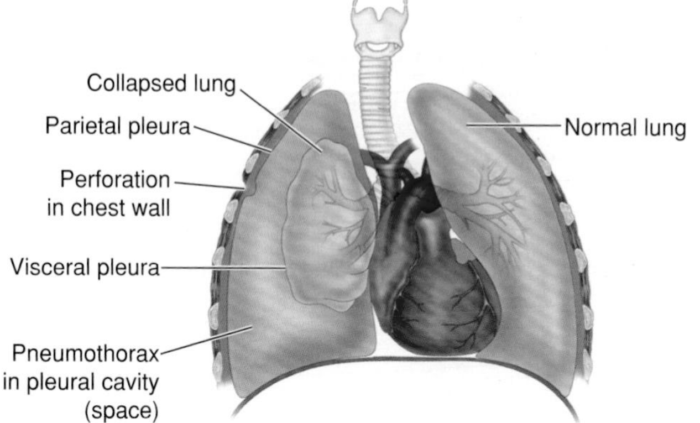

Figure 11-11 A pneumothorax can be caused by many factors, including lung disease or a perforation in the chest wall.

Medical Conditions *(continued)*

Term	Pronunciation	Meaning
pulmonary embolism	pul′mō-năr′ē em′bō-lizm	obstruction of the pulmonary circulation by a blood clot **(Figure 11-12)**
rales; *syn.* crackles	rahlz; krak′ĕlz	crackling or bubbling lung noises heard on inspiration that indicate fibrosis or fluid in the alveoli
reactive airway disease (RAD)	rē-ak′ti-v ār′wā di-zēz′	respiratory condition characterized by wheezing, shortness of breath (SOB), and coughing after exposure to an irritant
respiratory failure (RF)	res′pi-ră-tōr′ē fāl′yūr	condition in which the level of oxygen in the blood becomes dangerously low and/or the level of carbon dioxide becomes dangerously high
rhinitis	rī-nī′tis	inflammation of the mucous membranes within the nasal cavity
rhonchi	rong′kī	abnormal whistling, humming, or snoring sounds heard during inspiration or expiration
rubs	rŭbz	friction sounds in the lungs caused by inflammation of the pleura
sinusitis	sī′nŭ-sī′tis	inflammation of the sinus
stridor	strī′dōr	a whistling sound heard on inspiration that indicates partial obstruction of the trachea or larynx
tachypnea	tak-ip-nē′ă	abnormally rapid breathing

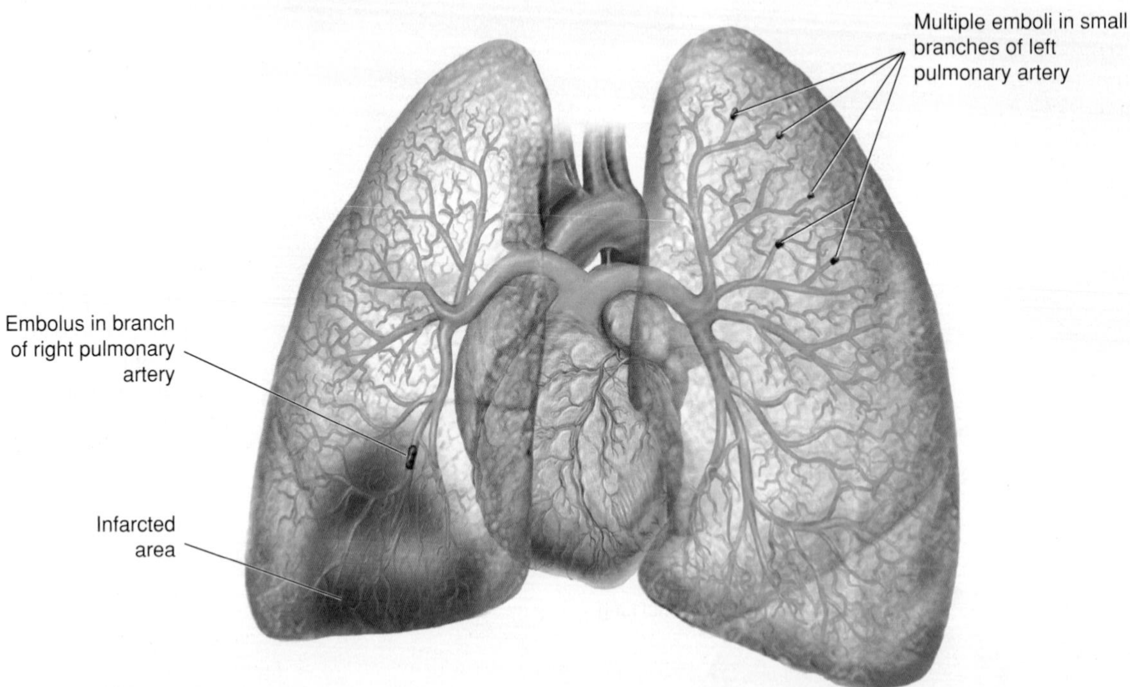

Figure 11-12 Pulmonary embolism. Pulmonary emboli (clots) obstruct pulmonary blood flow and impede oxygen delivery, which leads to infarction (tissue death).

Medical Conditions

Term	Pronunciation	Meaning
tonsillitis	ton′si-lī′tis	inflammation of one or both tonsils
tracheitis	trā-kē-ī′tis	inflammation of the trachea
tracheorrhagia	trā′kē-ō-rā′jē-ă	bleeding from the lining of the trachea
tuberculosis (TB)	tū-ber′kyū-lō′sis	infection caused by *Mycobacterium tuberculosis,* a bacterium that attacks the lungs and is spread through the air from one person to another **(Figure 11-13)**
upper respiratory infection (URI)	ŭp′r res′pi-ră-tōr′ē in-fek′shŭn	acute infection involving the nose, sinuses, or pharynx; commonly called a cold
wheeze	wēz	whistling or squeaking breath sound made as a result of airway obstruction

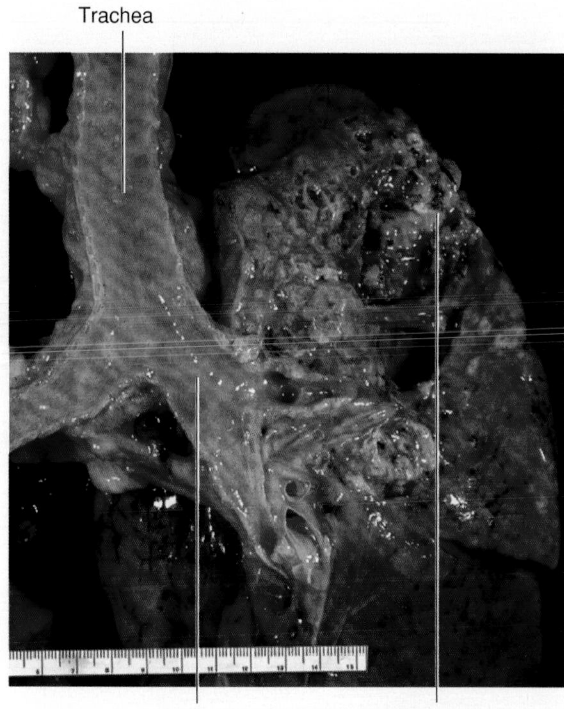

Figure 11-13 Tuberculosis is an infectious disease that causes rounded swellings called tubercles to appear in the lungs.

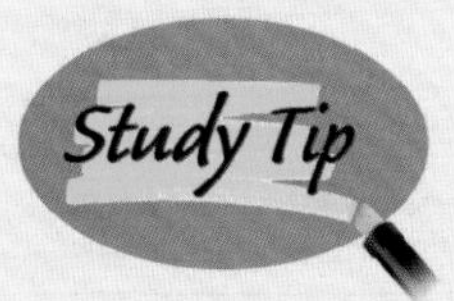

Pulmonary Embolism: A pulmonary embolism is a traveling clot (thrombus) from an injured or inflamed blood vessel anywhere in the body, or a clot that has formed and broken loose from the right side of the heart. The clot travels into the pulmonary artery, where it lodges in the vessel. Smaller pulmonary emboli can form in the branches of the pulmonary arteries.

Exercises: Medical Conditions

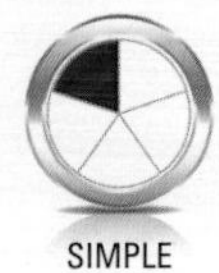

Exercise 14

Write the correct medical term for the meaning given.

1. decreased level of oxygen in the blood ______
2. inflammation of the tonsils ______
3. an acute infection involving the nose, sinus, or pharynx ______
4. chronic enlargement of the bronchi ______
5. inflammation within the bronchi of the lung ______
6. buildup of fluid in the space around the lungs ______
7. inflammation of the mucous membranes in the nasal cavity ______
8. bleeding from the lining of the trachea ______
9. bleeding from the nose ______
10. pneumonia affecting one or more lobes of the lung, often due to bacterial infection ______
11. inflammation of the pharynx ______
12. inflammation of all sinuses ______
13. decrease or loss of air in the lung, resulting in loss of lung volume ______
14. inflammation of the lungs ______
15. abnormal whistling, humming, or snoring sounds ______
16. difficulty breathing ______
17. friction sounds caused by inflammation of the pleura ______
18. airy, whistling type of sound made while breathing ______
19. group of disorders involving narrowing of small bronchi ______

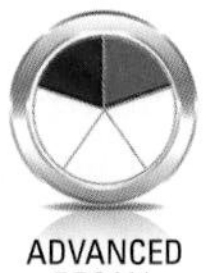
ADVANCED RECALL

Exercise 15

Match each medical term with its meaning.

pertussis	bronchopneumonia	adult respiratory distress syndrome	hemothorax
pansinusitis	influenza	pulmonary embolism	pulmonary edema
empyema	tuberculosis	pleuritis	

1. buildup of fluid in the lungs ______________
2. an infection of the smaller bronchial tubes of the lungs ______________
3. acute highly contagious viral infection, also known as flu ______________
4. blood located in the pleural cavity ______________
5. a localized collection of pus in the thoracic cavity ______________
6. an acute infectious inflammation of the larynx, trachea, and bronchi caused by the bacterium *Bordetella pertussis* ______________
7. inflammation of all sinuses ______________
8. respiratory failure that can occur with underlying illnesses or injury ______________
9. inflammation of the pleura ______________
10. an infection caused by *Mycobacterium tuberculosis* ______________
11. an obstruction of the pulmonary circulation by a blood clot ______________

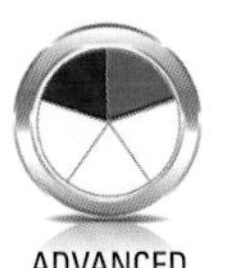
ADVANCED RECALL

Exercise 16

Circle the term that is most appropriate for the meaning of the sentence.

1. When Timmy Smith presented with a barking cough and difficult and noisy respirations, his physician diagnosed (*asthma, croup, dysphonia*).
2. Mr. Hannah was seen in follow-up for (*asthma, emphysema, empyema*), a chronic severe breathing disorder that includes attacks of wheezing.
3. Dr. Thomas informed Mr. Jenkins that severe (*stridor, hypoxia, pulmonary embolism*) can occur in respiratory failure.
4. Mrs. Lin was diagnosed with (*tuberculosis, emphysema, pneumococcal pneumonia*) when the lab discovered *Streptococcus pneumoniae* in her sputum.
5. On auscultation of the child's chest, Dr. Daughtry heard these two types of breath sounds: rhonchi and (*rales, rhinitis, dyspnea*).
6. Dr. Bazel explained to the patient that (*bacterial pneumonia, interstitial lung disease, chronic obstructive pulmonary disease*) is a group of chronic lung disorders affecting the tissue between the air sacs of the lungs.
7. After his x-ray report showed an obstruction of pulmonary circulation due to a blood clot, the patient was told that he had a (*pneumothorax, pulmonary embolism, pneumonitis*).

8. Mrs. Green had (*chronic obstructive pulmonary disease, interstitial lung disease, bronchiolitis obliterans with organizing pneumonia*), a condition in which her bronchioles were filled with granulated tissue plugs.

9. The physician diagnosed Ms. Thatcher with (*emphysema, empyema, dyspnea*) after testing showed permanent destruction of very fine airways and alveoli.

10. Mr. McGrath was diagnosed with (*respiratory failure, reactive airway disease, rales*) after he inhaled a toxic substance and began wheezing, coughing, and experiencing shortness of breath.

11. Jon Burns suffered from alternating periods of apnea and deep, rapid breathing known as (*respiratory failure, dyspnea, Cheyne–Stokes respiration*).

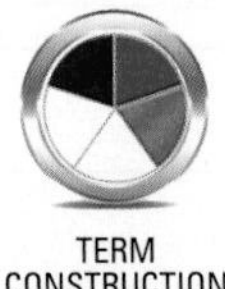

TERM CONSTRUCTION

Exercise 17

Break the given medical term into its word parts, and define each part. Then define the medical term.

For example:

bronchoplasty	*word parts:*	bronch/o, -plasty
	meanings:	bronchus; surgical repair, reconstruction
	term meaning:	surgical repair of the bronchus

1. pneumonia — *word parts:* ____ *meanings:* ____ *term meaning:* ____

2. aphonia — *word parts:* ____ *meanings:* ____ *term meaning:* ____

3. bronchiectasis — *word parts:* ____ *meanings:* ____ *term meaning:* ____

4. bronchopneumonia — *word parts:* ____ *meanings:* ____ *term meaning:* ____

5. laryngospasm — *word parts:* ____ *meanings:* ____ *term meaning:* ____

6. pleuritic — *word parts:* ____ *meanings:* ____ *term meaning:* ____

7. apnea
word parts: ______________________
meanings: ______________________
term meaning: ______________________

8. laryngitis
word parts: ______________________
meanings: ______________________
term meaning: ______________________

9. pneumonitis
word parts: ______________________
meanings: ______________________
term meaning: ______________________

10. sinusitis
word parts: ______________________
meanings: ______________________
term meaning: ______________________

11. tracheitis
word parts: ______________________
meanings: ______________________
term meaning: ______________________

12. diaphragmatocele
word parts: ______________________
meanings: ______________________
term meaning: ______________________

13. nasopharyngitis
word parts: ______________________
meanings: ______________________
term meaning: ______________________

14. dysphonia
word parts: ______________________
meanings: ______________________
term meaning: ______________________

15. pharyngitis
word parts: ______________________
meanings: ______________________
term meaning: ______________________

Tests and Procedures

Term	Pronunciation	Meaning
Laboratory Tests		
acid-fast bacilli (AFB) smear	as'id-fast bă-sil'ī smēr	clinical test performed on sputum to determine the presence of acid-fast bacilli, the bacteria that cause tuberculosis **(Figure 11-14)**
arterial blood gases (ABGs)	ahr-tēr'ē-ăl blŭd gas'ĕz	test performed on arterial blood to determine levels of oxygen, carbon dioxide, and other gases present
purified protein derivative (PPD) skin test	pyū'ri-fied prō'tēn dĕ-riv'ă-tiv skin test	skin test used to determine whether the patient has developed an immune response to the bacteria that cause tuberculosis
Diagnostic Procedures		
Imaging Studies		
chest radiograph (CXR)	chest rā'dē-ō-graf	radiographic image (x-ray) of chest used to evaluate the lungs and the heart
computed tomography (CT) scan	kŏm-pyū'tĕd tŏ-mog'ră-fē skan	x-ray technique producing computer-generated cross-sectional images
magnetic resonance imaging (MRI)	mag-net'ik rez'ŏ-năns im'ăj-ing	imaging technique that uses magnetic fields and radiofrequency waves to visualize anatomic structures; often used to diagnose lung disorders
radiography	rā'dē-og'ră-fē	examination of any part of the body for diagnostic purposes by means of x-rays, with the record of the findings exposed onto photographic film
ventilation–perfusion (V/Q) scan	ven'ti-lā'shŭn-pĕr-fyū'zhŭn skan	test used to assess distribution of blood flow and ventilation through both lungs **(Figure 11-15)**; V = ventilation: the air that reaches the alveoli, and Q = perfusion: the blood that reaches the alveoli

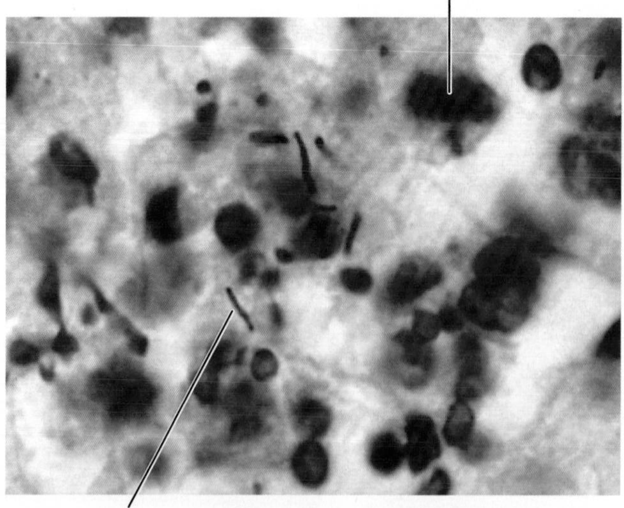

Figure 11-14 Acid-fast bacilli smear showing *Mycobacterium tuberculosis,* the bacterium that causes tuberculosis, as seen under a microscope.

Tests and Procedures

Term	Pronunciation	Meaning
Other Diagnostic Procedures		
auscultation	aws′kŭl-tā′shŭn	physical examination method of listening to body sounds using a stethoscope **(Figure 11-16)**
bronchoalveolar lavage (BAL)	brong′kō-al-vē′ō-lăr lă-vahzh′	procedure performed during bronchoscopy to collect cells of the alveoli; saline solution is instilled into distal bronchi, that solution is then withdrawn along with the alveolar cells
bronchoscopy	brong-kos′kŏ-pē	examination of the trachea and bronchial tree through a bronchoscope **(Figure 11-17)**
endoscopy	en-dos′kŏ-pē	examination of the interior of the body by means of a special instrument called an endoscope
laryngoscopy	lar′ing-gos′kŏ-pē	endoscopic examination of the larynx
nasopharyngoscopy	nā′zō-far-in-gos′kŏ-pē	endoscopic examination of the nasal passages and the pharynx

(continued)

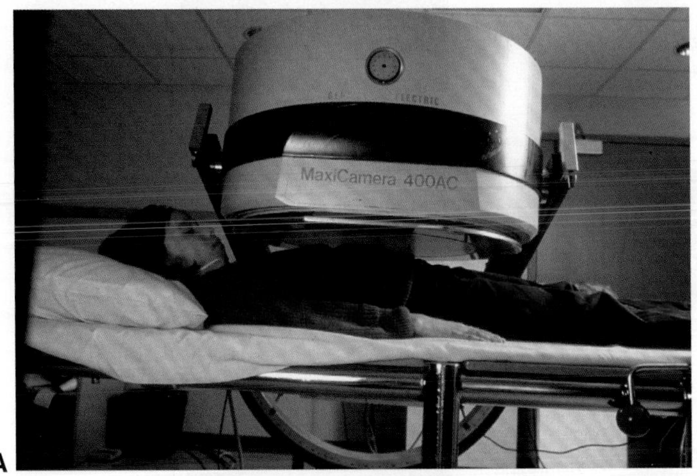

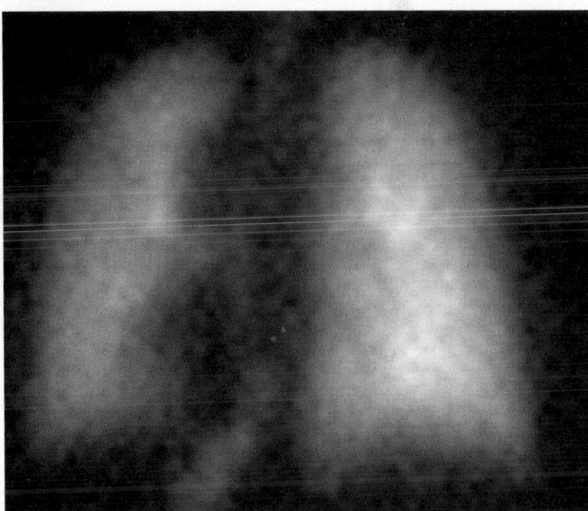

Figure 11-15 Ventilation–perfusion scanning. **A.** Nuclear medicine scanner. **B.** Ventilation–perfusion scan showing posterior view of the lungs.

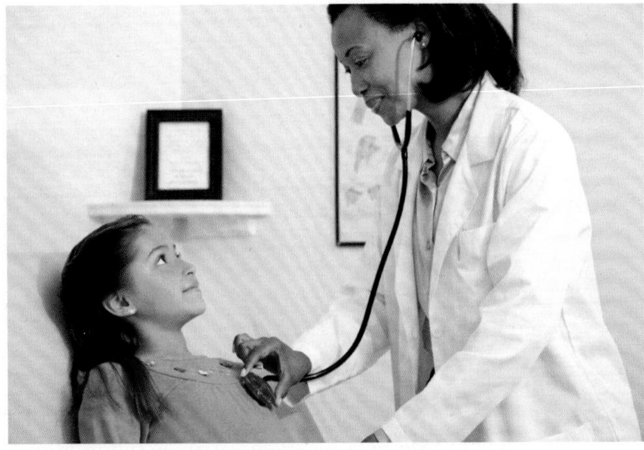

Figure 11-16 Auscultation.

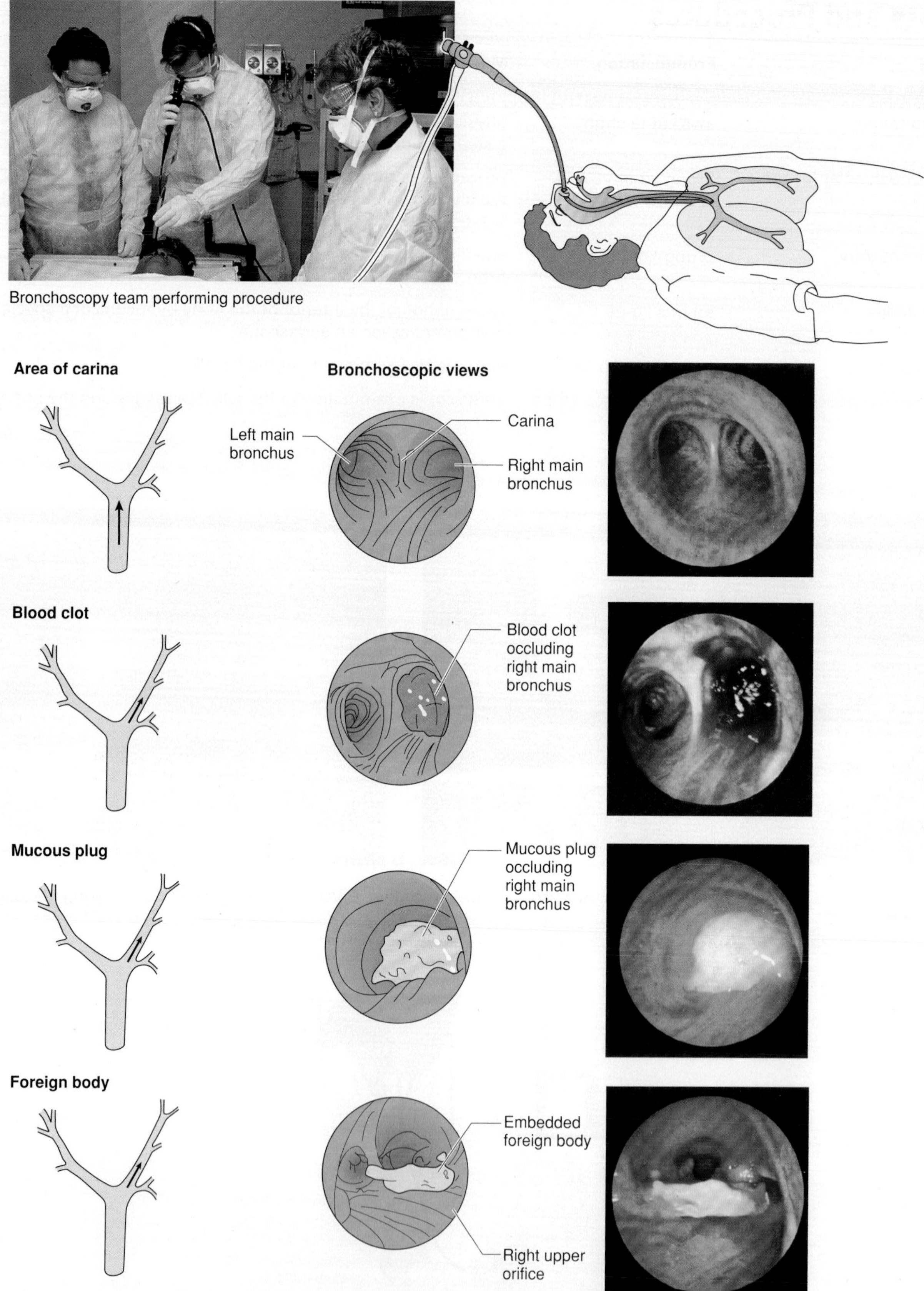

Figure 11-17 Bronchoscopy done through a fiberoptic scope can show many different problems occurring in the bronchi.

Tests and Procedures *(continued)*

Term	Pronunciation	Meaning
peak flow monitoring	pēk flō mon′i-tŏr′ing	test that measures the rate of air flow, or how fast air is able to pass through the airways
percussion	pĕr-kŭsh′ŭn	physical examination method of tapping over the body to elicit vibrations and sounds to estimate the size, border, or fluid content of a cavity, such as the chest
pharyngoscopy	far′ing-gos′kō-pē	endoscopic examination of the pharynx
polysomnography	pol′ē-som-nog′ră-fē	monitoring and recording normal and abnormal activity during sleep, including neural and respiratory functions
pulmonary function tests (PFTs)	pul′mŏ-nār-ē fŭngk′shŭn tests	group of tests performed to measure breathing; used to determine respiratory function or abnormalities; useful in distinguishing chronic obstructive pulmonary diseases from asthma
pulse oximetry	pŭls ok-sim′ĕ-trē	measurement of oxygen saturation in the blood **(Figure 11-18)**

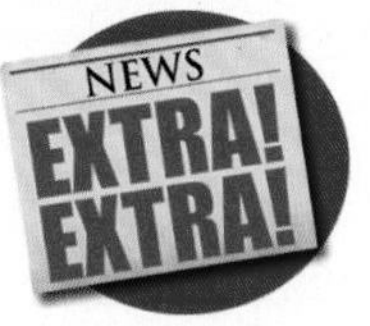

PULSE OXIMETRY MEASUREMENTS Pulse oximetry is measured via a probe placed on either the finger or the ear of the patient. If placed on the patient's finger, it is important to note that a patient should not have fingernail polish on the digit used for monitoring. Readings between 95% and 100% are acceptable ranges for pulse oximetry. When measurements are documented, it is noted if the reading was obtained on room air or on supplemental oxygen. If a patient is receiving oxygen, then the amount of oxygen the patient is receiving is also documented.

Term	Pronunciation	Meaning
rhinoscopy	rī-nos′kŏ-pē	endoscopic examination of the nasal cavity
spirometry	spī-rom′ĕ-trē	procedure for measuring air flow and volume of air inspired and expired by the lungs using a device called a spirometer
thoracoscopy	thōr-ă-kos′kŏ-pē	endoscopic examination of the thorax done through a small opening in the chest wall
video-assisted thoracoscopic surgery (VATS)	vid′ē-o-ă-sis′ted thō′ră-kŏ-skop′ik sŭr′jĕr-ē	thoracic surgery performed using endoscopic cameras, optical systems, and display screens, as well as specially designed surgical instruments, which enables surgeons to view the inside of the chest cavity and remove tissue to test for disease **(Figure 11-19)**

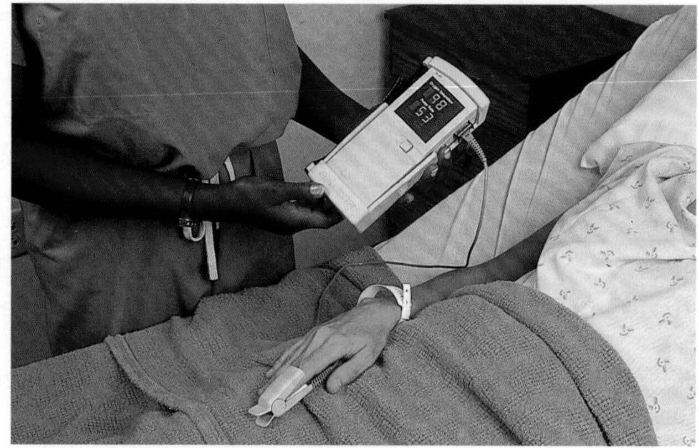

Figure 11-18 Pulse oximetry taken via the finger.

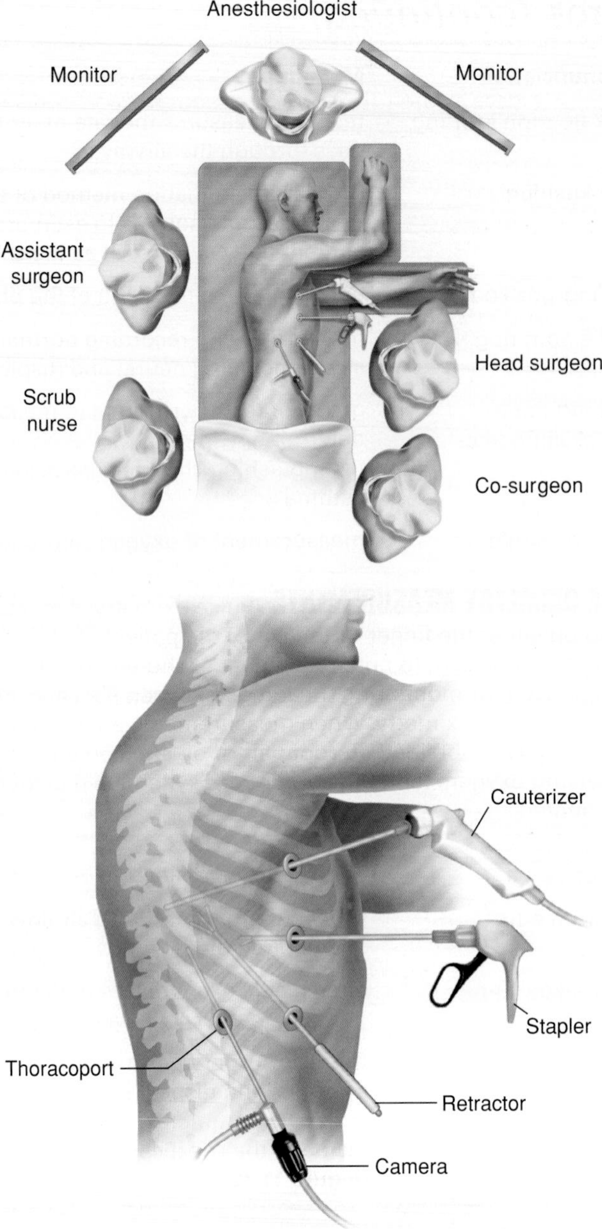

Figure 11-19 VATS procedure.

ANIMATION

For a visual and audio tour of some of the sounds heard on auscultation, view the animation "Change in Breathing Sounds" on the Student Resources on thePoint.

Exercises: Tests and Procedures

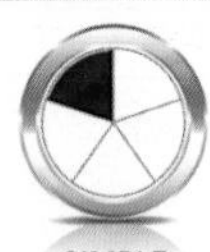
SIMPLE RECALL

Exercise 18

Circle the term that is most appropriate for the meaning of the sentence.

1. (*Computed tomography, Thoracoscopy, Bronchoscopy*) is an x-ray technique producing computer-generated cross-sectional images.

2. An x-ray procedure used to evaluate the lungs and the heart is called a(n) (*arthrogram, chest radiograph, bronchoscopy*).

3. (*Magnetic resonance imaging, Computed tomography, V/Q scan*) is a test used to assess distribution of blood flow and ventilation through both lungs.

4. The skin test used to determine the immune response to the bacteria that cause tuberculosis is called (*AFB smear, PPD test, ABGs*).

5. (*Thoracoscopy, Computed tomography, Bronchoalveolar lavage*) is performed during bronchoscopy to collect cells of the alveoli.

6. The imaging technique that uses magnetic fields and radiofrequency waves is called (*magnetic resonance imaging, computed tomography, chest radiography*).

7. (*CT, VATS, MRI*) allows surgeons to view the inside of the chest cavity and remove tissue for testing.

8. A procedure for measuring air flow and volume of air inspired and expired by the lungs is called (*spirometry, radiography, pulse oximetry*).

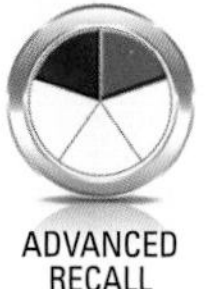

ADVANCED RECALL

Exercise 19

Complete each sentence by writing in the correct medical term.

1. The measurement of oxygen saturation in the blood is called ____________.

2. A test performed on arterial blood to determine levels of oxygen, carbon dioxide, and other gases present is called ____________.

3. A method of physical examination that uses a tapping motion over the body to elicit vibrations and sounds to estimate the size, border, or fluid content of a cavity is called ____________.

4. The test performed on sputum to determine the presence of acid-fast bacilli, the bacteria that causes tuberculosis, is called ____________.

5. Examination of any part of the body for diagnostic purposes by means of x-rays with the record of the findings exposed onto photographic film is called ____________.

6. An endoscopic examination of the larynx is called a(n) ____________.

7. A group of tests used to determine respiratory function or abnormalities that is useful in distinguishing chronic obstructive pulmonary diseases from asthma is called ____________.

8. The monitoring and recording of normal and abnormal activity during sleep, including neural and respiratory function, is called ____________.

9. A physical examination method of listening to the sounds of the respiratory system with the aid of a stethoscope is called ____________.

10. A test that measures the rate of air flow, or how fast air is able to pass through the airways, is called ____________.

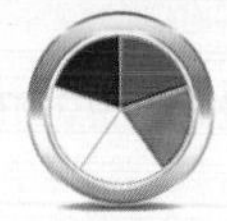

TERM CONSTRUCTION

Exercise 20

Using the given combining form, build a medical term for the meaning given.

Combining Form	Meaning of Medical Term	Medical Term
thorac/o	endoscopic examination of the thorax	**1.** ______________
rhin/o	endoscopic examination of the nasal cavity	**2.** ______________
pharyng/o	endoscopic examination of the pharynx	**3.** ______________
bronch/o	endoscopic examination of the trachea and bronchial tree	**4.** ______________
laryng/o	endoscopic examination of the larynx	**5.** ______________

Surgical Interventions and Therapeutic Procedures

Term	Pronunciation	Meaning
adenoidectomy	ad′ĕ-noyd-ek′tŏ-mē	operation to remove adenoid tissue from the nasopharynx
aspiration	as′pi-rā′shŭn	removal of accumulated fluid by suction
bronchoplasty	brong′kō-plas-tē	surgical repair of the bronchus
cardiopulmonary resuscitation (CPR)	kar′dē-ō-pŭl′mo-nār-ē rē-sŭs′i-tā′shŭn	medical procedure to ventilate the lungs and artificially circulate the blood if a patient has stopped breathing and the heart has stopped
continuous positive airway pressure (CPAP) therapy	kon-tin′yū-us poz′i-tiv ār′wā presh′ŭr thār′ă-pē	breathing apparatus that pumps constant pressurized air through the nasal passages via a mask to keep the airway patent (open) **(Figure 11-20)**
endotracheal intubation	en′dō-trā′kē-ăl in′tū-bā′shŭn	medical procedure in which a tube is passed through the mouth into the trachea to maintain the airway during anesthesia or to establish an airway for breathing purposes **(Figure 11-21)**

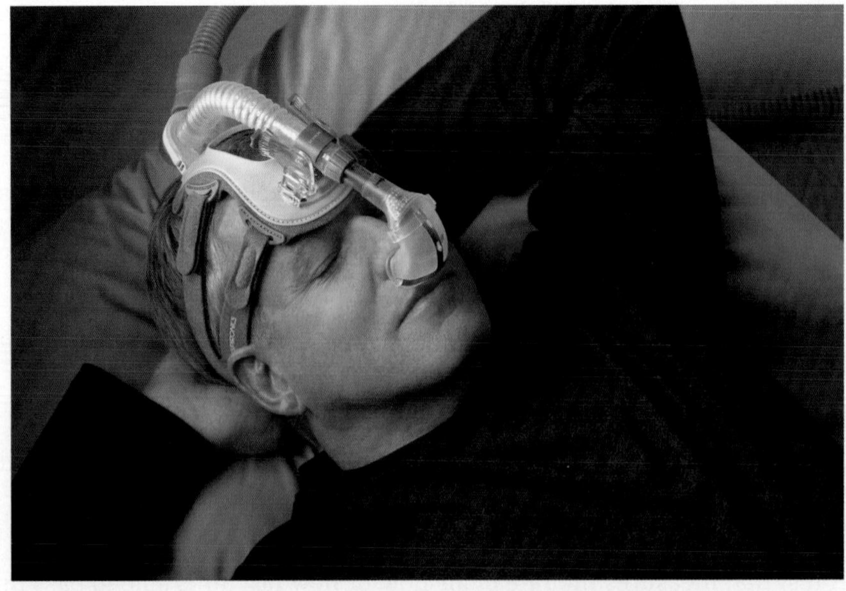

Figure 11-20 Continuous positive airway pressure (CPAP) therapy.

Surgical Interventions and Therapeutic Procedures

Term	Pronunciation	Meaning
hyperbaric medicine	hī′pĕr-băr′ik med′i-sin	medicinal use of high barometric pressure, usually in specially constructed chambers, to increase oxygen content of blood and tissues
incentive spirometry	in-sen′tiv spī-rom′ĕ-trē	medical procedure to encourage patients to breathe deeply by using a portable plastic device called a spirometer that gives visual feedback as the patient inhales forcefully **(Figure 11-22)**
laryngectomy	lar′in-jek′tŏ-mē	excision of the larynx
laryngotracheotomy	lă-ring′gō-trā-kē-ot′ŏ-mē	incision into the larynx and trachea
lobectomy	lō-bek′tŏ-mē	excision of a lobe (of the lung)
mechanical ventilation	mĕ-kan′i-kăl ven-ti-lā′shŭn	use of an automatic mechanical device to perform all or part of the work of breathing **(Figure 11-23)**

(continued)

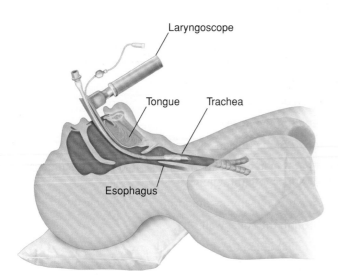

Figure 11-21 Endotracheal intubation.

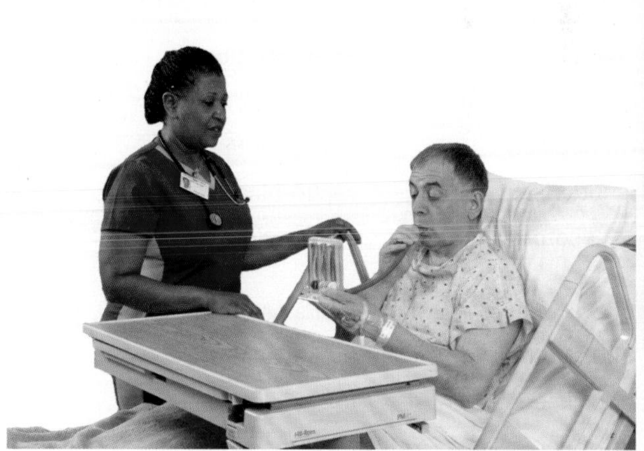

Figure 11-22 Incentive spirometry.

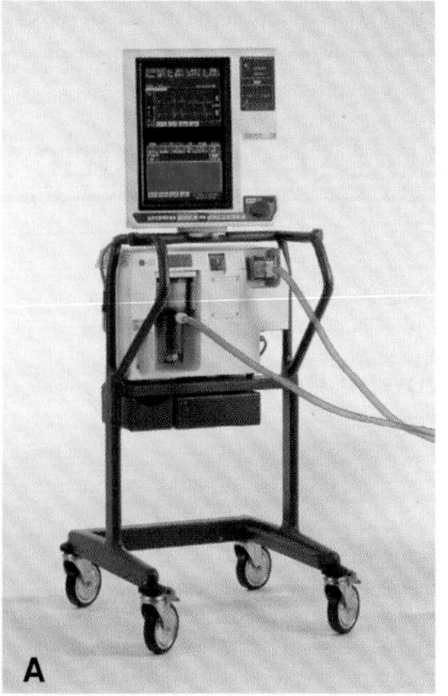

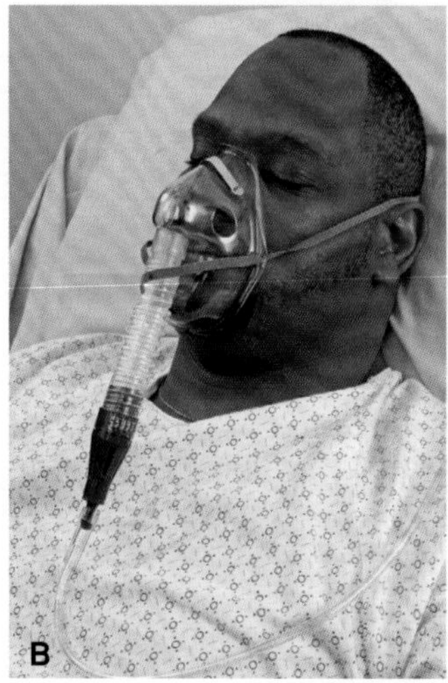

Figure 11-23 **A.** Mechanical ventilation system. **B.** Patient on mechanical ventilation via mask attached to system.

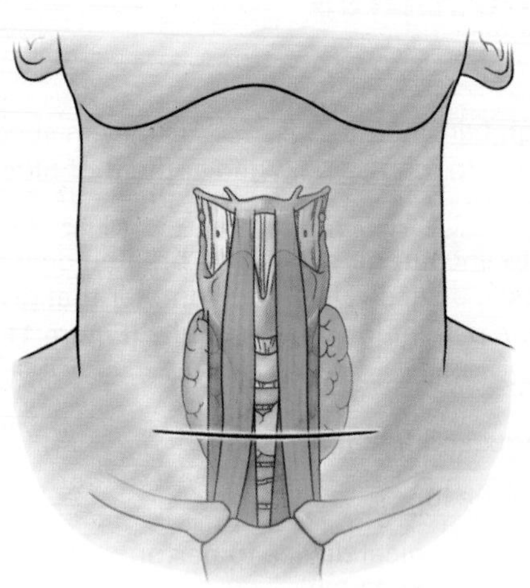
Skin incision for tracheostomy

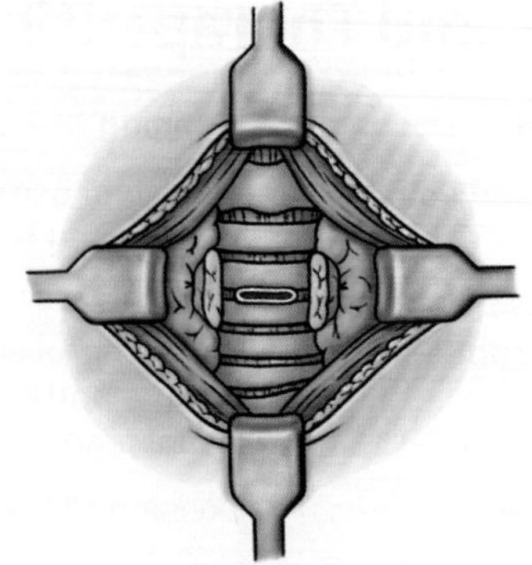
Incision in trachea after retracting infrahyoid muscles and incising isthmus of thyroid gland

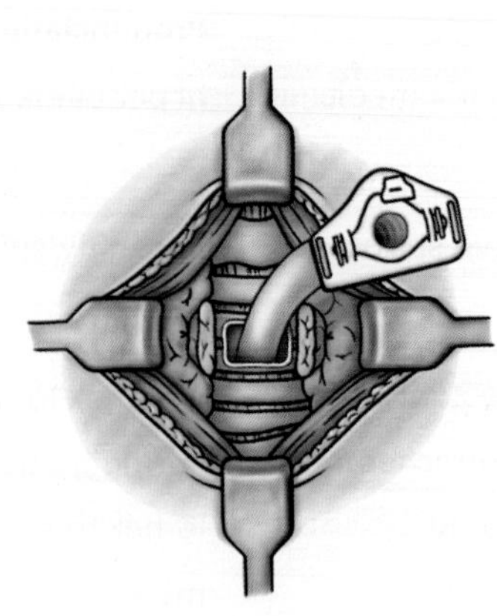
Tracheostomy tube inserted in tracheal opening

Figure 11-24 Tracheostomy.

Surgical Interventions and Therapeutic Procedures *(continued)*

Term	Pronunciation	Meaning
pneumonectomy	nū′mō-nek′tŏ-mē	removal of an entire lung
rhinoplasty	rī′nō-plas-tē	surgical repair of the nose
septoplasty	sep′tō-plas-tē	surgical repair of the (nasal) septum
sinusotomy	sī′nŭ-sot′ŏ-mē	surgical operation in which an incision is made into a sinus to prevent or reduce inflammation
thoracentesis	thōr′ă-sen-tē′sis	surgical puncture to aspirate fluid from the chest cavity
thoracotomy	thōr′ă-kot′ŏ-mē	incision through the chest wall
tonsillectomy	ton′si-lek′tŏ-mē	surgical removal of the tonsil(s)
tracheoplasty	trā′kē-ō-plas-tē	surgical repair of the trachea
tracheostomy; *syn.* tracheotomy	trā′kē-os′tŏ-mē; trā′kē-ot′ŏ-mē	an operation to make an opening into the trachea **(Figure 11-24)**
tracheostomy tube	trā′kē-os′tŏ-mē tūb	breathing tube inserted into a tracheotomy **(Figure 11-24)**

■ Exercises: Surgical Interventions and Therapeutic Procedures

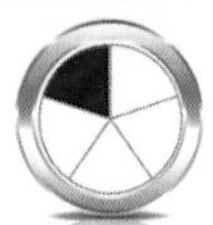
SIMPLE RECALL

Exercise 21

Write the correct medical term for the meaning given.

1. incision through the chest wall ____________
2. operation to remove adenoid tissue ____________
3. surgical repair of the trachea ____________
4. use of high barometric pressure to increase oxygen content of blood and tissues ____________

5. use of an automatic mechanical device to perform all or part of the work of breathing ________________

6. removal of accumulated fluid by suction ________________

7. breathing apparatus that pumps air through the nasal passages to keep the airway patent (open) ________________

8. incision into the trachea ________________

9. incision into the larynx and trachea ________________

10. breathing tube inserted into a tracheotomy ________________

11. surgical repair of the bronchus ________________

12. procedure in which a tube is passed through the mouth into the trachea to maintain the airway ________________

13. removal of an entire lung ________________

14. medical procedure to encourage patients to breathe deeply ________________

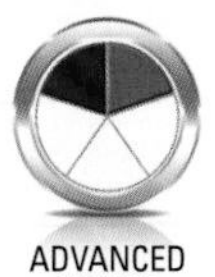
ADVANCED RECALL

Exercise 22

Circle the term that is most appropriate for the meaning of the sentence.

1. Mr. Martinez required a (*laryngectomy, tracheoplasty, tracheotomy*) to create an opening to ensure normal breathing processes could occur.

2. Mr. Browder had a very sore throat and inflamed left tonsil for a long time but was nonetheless reluctant to undergo (*lobectomy, tonsillectomy, laryngectomy*) to remove it.

3. The boxer's nose was injured during the ninth round of the match, which required (*rhinoplasty, tracheoplasty, bronchoplasty*) surgery to fix his nasal injury.

4. Following surgical removal of a tumor in the right lung, Mr. Hunnicutt required extensive (*thoracentesis, thoracoscopy, thoracotomy*) to remove the buildup of fluid in the thoracic cavity.

5. The patient's heart stopped, causing the medical team to begin (*BOOP, CPAP, CPR*) immediately.

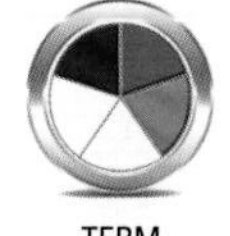
TERM CONSTRUCTION

Exercise 23

Using the given suffix, build a medical term for the meaning given.

Suffix	Meaning of Medical Term	Medical Term
-plasty	surgical repair of the nasal septum	1. ____________
-ectomy	excision of the larynx	2. ____________
-centesis	surgical puncture of the chest cavity	3. ____________
-scopy	process of examining the bronchus	4. ____________
-tomy	surgical opening of the thorax	5. ____________

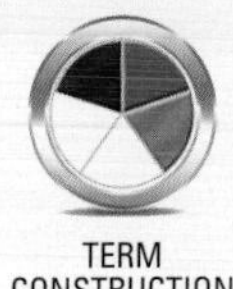
TERM CONSTRUCTION

Exercise 24

Break the given medical term into its word parts, and define each part. Then define the medical term.

For example:

pleuritis
word parts: pleur/o, -itis
meanings: pleura, inflammation
term meaning: inflammation of the pleura

1. laryngoscope
word parts: ____________
meanings: ____________
term meaning: ____________

2. rhinoplasty
word parts: ____________
meanings: ____________
term meaning: ____________

3. laryngostomy
word parts: ____________
meanings: ____________
term meaning: ____________

4. pneumonectomy
word parts: ____________
meanings: ____________
term meaning: ____________

5. sinusotomy
word parts: ____________
meanings: ____________
term meaning: ____________

6. bronchoplasty
word parts: ____________
meanings: ____________
term meaning: ____________

7. thoracentesis
word parts: ____________
meanings: ____________
term meaning: ____________

8. tracheotomy
word parts: ____________
meanings: ____________
term meaning: ____________

9. adenoidectomy *word parts:* ______________________

meanings: ______________________

term meaning: ______________________

10. tracheostomy *word parts:* ______________________

meanings: ______________________

term meaning: ______________________

Medications and Drug Therapies

Term	Pronunciation	Meaning
antibiotic	an′tē-bī-ot′ik	drug that kills or inhibits the growth of microorganisms
antihistamine	an′tē-his′tă-mēn	drug used to stop the effects of histamine in the respiratory tract
antitubercular drug	an′tē-tū-ber′kyū-lăr drŭg	antibiotic used in the prevention and treatment of tuberculosis; used to lower the risk of getting tuberculosis in people who may be exposed to the disease
antitussive	an′tē-tŭs′iv	drug used to prevent or relive a cough
bronchodilator	brong′kō-dī-lā′ter	drug that dilates the bronchial tube, allowing air to pass through and relieving breathing difficulties
corticosteroid	kōr′ti-kō-stĕr′oyd	drug that reduces bronchial inflammation and airway obstruction and thereby improves lung function
decongestant	dē′kon-jes′tant	drug that relieves congestion by reducing tissue swelling in the nasal passages and blood vessels
expectorant	ek-spek′tō-rănt	drug that helps bring up mucus and other material from the lungs, bronchi, and trachea to be coughed up and out; also helps to lubricate the irritated respiratory tract
nebulizer; *syn.* atomizer	neb′yū-līz′ĕr; at′ŏm-ī-zĕr	device for administering a drug by spraying a fine mist into the nose **(Figure 11-25)**

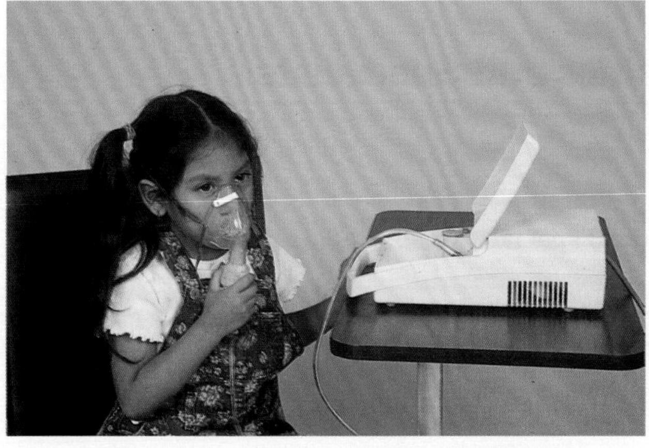

Figure 11-25 Child using a portable nebulizer.

Exercise: Medications and Drug Therapies

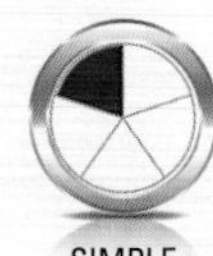

SIMPLE RECALL

Exercise 25

Write the correct medication or drug therapy term for the meaning given.

1. device for administering a medication by spraying a fine mist into the nose __________
2. drug that helps bring up mucus and other material from the lungs, bronchi, and trachea __________
3. drug that reduces bronchial inflammation and airway obstruction __________
4. drug used to prevent or relieve a cough __________
5. drug used to stop the effects of histamine __________
6. drug that dilates the bronchial tube __________
7. drug that kills or inhibits the growth of microorganisms __________
8. drug that relieves congestion by reducing tissue swelling in the nasal passages and blood vessels __________
9. antibiotic used in the prevention and treatment of tuberculosis __________

Specialties and Specialists

Term	Pronunciation	Meaning
otorhinolaryngology	ō′tō-rī′nō-lar-in-gol′ŏ-jē	medical specialty concerned with diagnosis and treatment of diseases of the ear, nose, and throat (pharynx and larynx)
otorhinolaryngologist	ō′tō-rī′nō-lar-in-gol′ŏ-jist	physician who specializes in otorhinolaryngology
pulmonology	pul′mō-nol′ŏ-jē	medical specialty concerned with diseases of the lungs and the respiratory tract
pulmonologist	pul′mō-nol′ŏ-jist	physician who specializes in pulmonology

Exercise: Specialties and Specialists

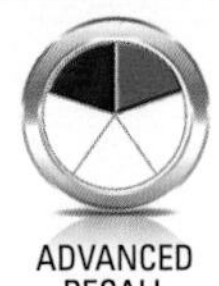

ADVANCED RECALL

Exercise 26

Match each medical specialty or specialists with its description.

otorhinolaryngology
otorhinolaryngologist
pulmonology
pulmonologist

1. physician who specializes in otorhinolaryngology __________
2. physician who specializes in pulmonology __________

3. medical specialty concerned with diseases of the ear, nose, and throat ______

4. medical specialty concerned with diseases of the lungs and the respiratory tract ______

Abbreviations

Abbreviation	Meaning
ABG	arterial blood gas
AFB	acid-fast bacilli
ARDS	acute respiratory distress syndrome
BAL	bronchoalveolar lavage
BOOP	bronchiolitis obliterans with organizing pneumonia
CF	cystic fibrosis
COPD	chronic obstructive pulmonary disease
CPAP	continuous positive airway pressure
CPR	cardiopulmonary resuscitation
CT	computed tomography (scan)
CXR	chest x-ray
ILD	interstitial lung disease
INH	isoniazid; isonicotinic acid hydrazide
MRI	magnetic resonance imaging
PFTs	pulmonary function tests
PPD	purified protein derivative
RAD	reactive airway disease
RF	respiratory failure
SOB	shortness of breath
TB	tuberculosis
URI	upper respiratory infection
V/Q	ventilation–perfusion (scan)
VATS	video-assisted thoracoscopic surgery

Exercises: Abbreviations

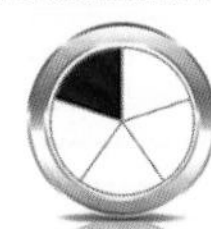

SIMPLE RECALL

Exercise 27

Write the meaning of each abbreviation.

1. RAD ______
2. CT ______
3. URI ______
4. V/Q ______

5. TB ____________________

6. CPR ____________________

7. MRI ____________________

8. PPD ____________________

9. VATS ____________________

10. ABG ____________________

11. CPAP ____________________

12. BAL ____________________

SIMPLE RECALL

Exercise 28

Write the meaning of each abbreviation used in these sentences.

1. After completing the examination, Dr. Gaskill diagnosed Mr. Stewart with **COPD** complicated with **ILD.**

   ____________________ ____________________

2. A college student underwent **PFTs** when she noticed shortness of breath related to her **CF.**

   ____________________ ____________________

3. The physician concluded the patient suffered from **ARDS** and was admitted to the hospital for treatment.

   ____

4. The physician ordered an **AFB** test to help determine if the patient had tuberculosis or **BOOP.**

   ____________________ ____________________

5. The patient's **CXR** showed a small nodule in the left upper lobe.

   ____

WRAPPING UP

- The respiratory system is divided into the upper respiratory tract and lower respiratory tract, which work together to supply oxygen to the lungs and eliminate carbon dioxide from the lungs.
- The cardiovascular system then carries oxygen from the lungs to the rest of the body.
- In this chapter, you learned medical terminology including word parts, prefixes, suffixes, adjectives, conditions, tests, procedures, medications, specialties, and abbreviations related to the respiratory system.

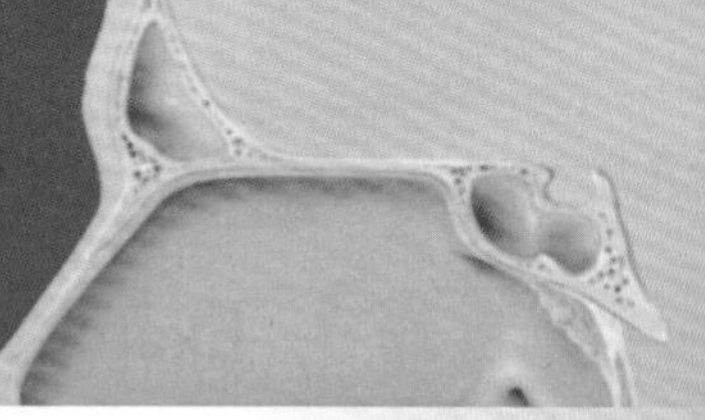

Chapter Review

Review of Terms for Anatomy and Physiology

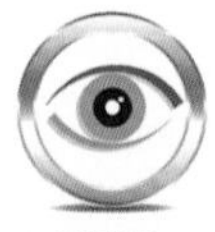

Exercise 29

Write the correct terms on the blanks for the anatomic structures indicated.

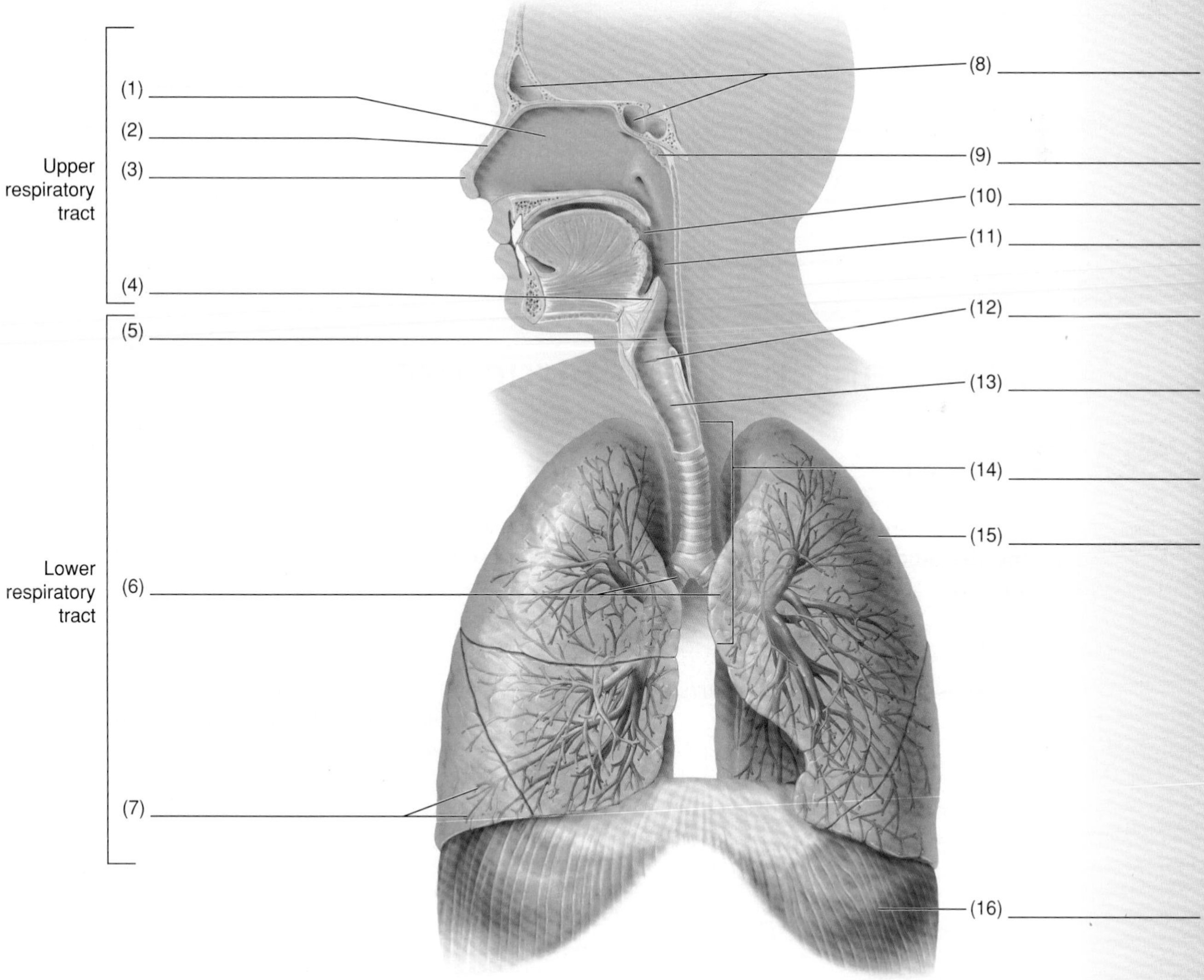

Upper respiratory tract

(1) ______________________

(2) ______________________

(3) ______________________

(4) ______________________

Lower respiratory tract

(5) ______________________

(6) ______________________

(7) ______________________

(8) ______________________

(9) ______________________

(10) ______________________

(11) ______________________

(12) ______________________

(13) ______________________

(14) ______________________

(15) ______________________

(16) ______________________

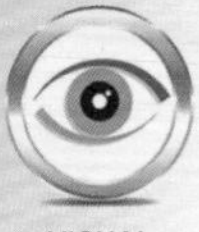

VISUAL

Exercise 30

Write the correct terms on the blanks for the anatomic structures indicated.

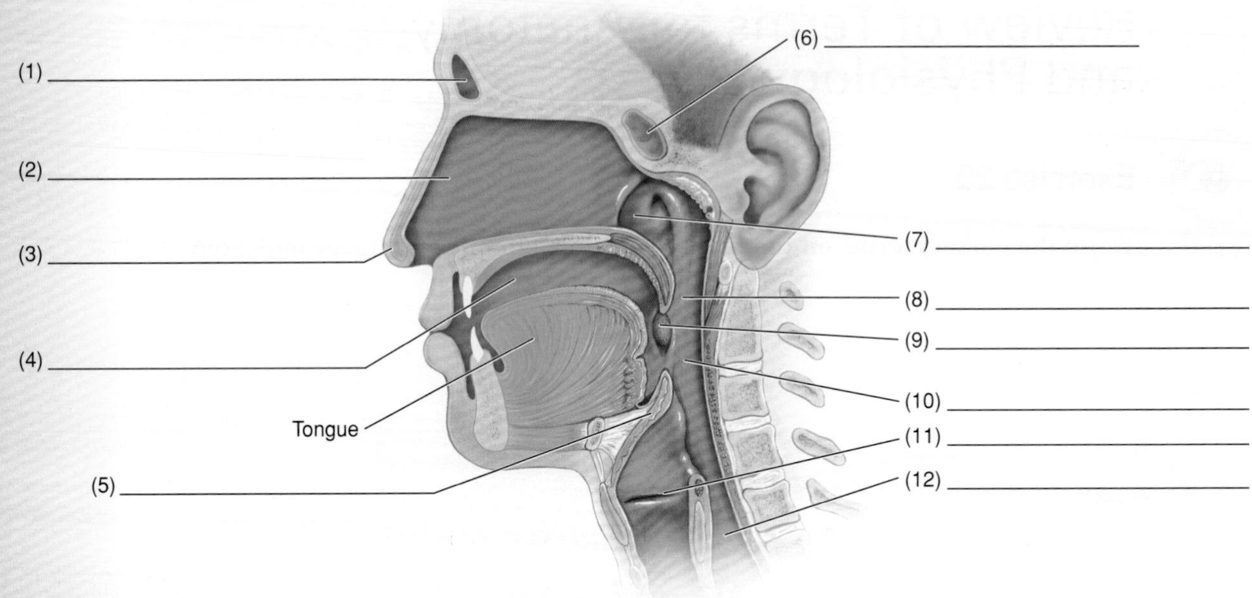

Understanding Term Structure

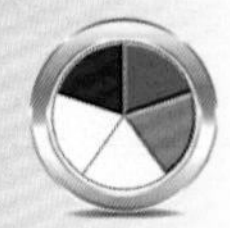

TERM CONSTRUCTION

Exercise 31

Break the given medical term into its word parts, and define each part. Then define the medical term. (Note: You may need to use word parts from other chapters.)

For example:

laryngospasm	*word parts:*	laryng/o, -spasm
	meanings:	larynx, involuntary movement
	term meaning:	involuntary movement of the larynx
1. laryngeal	*word parts:*	______
	meanings:	______
	term meaning:	______
2. rhinorrhea	*word parts:*	______
	meanings:	______
	term meaning:	______

3. pulmonary
   word parts: __________
   meanings: __________
   term meaning: __________

4. phrenospasm
   word parts: __________
   meanings: __________
   term meaning: __________

5. thoracotomy
   word parts: __________
   meanings: __________
   term meaning: __________

6. tachypnea
   word parts: __________
   meanings: __________
   term meaning: __________

7. thoracic
   word parts: __________
   meanings: __________
   term meaning: __________

8. bronchospasm
   word parts: __________
   meanings: __________
   term meaning: __________

9. pulmonology
   word parts: __________
   meanings: __________
   term meaning: __________

10. bronchoscopy
   word parts: __________
   meanings: __________
   term meaning: __________

Comprehension Exercises

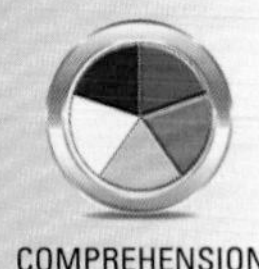
COMPREHENSION

Exercise 32

Fill in the blank with the correct term.

1. The layer of the pleura that is closest to the lung is known as the ______.
2. Tiny air sacs in the lungs where gas exchange occurs are the ______.
3. The ______ acts as a cover over the entrance to the esophagus.
4. Abnormally fast breathing is termed ______.
5. ______ is a term used to describe blood located in the pleural cavity.
6. During a(n) ______ attack, a person has attacks of wheezing due to inflammation and obstruction of the airways.
7. A sudden involuntary movement of the larynx is a(n) ______.
8. The ______ tract is composed of the nose and pharynx.
9. ______ is a sound indicating obstruction of the airway.
10. Inflammation of the ______ is commonly known as a sore throat.

COMPREHENSION

Exercise 33

Write a short answer for each question.

1. What body structures make up the lower respiratory tract? ______
2. Name the structure that allows humans to form sounds. ______
3. Describe the thoracic region. ______
4. How many lobes are present within each lung? ______
5. What is the term for a procedure that requires the creation of an artificial opening in the trachea? ______
6. What is another name for interstitial lung disease? ______
7. Why would a thoracentesis be performed? ______

8. How does a CPAP work? ______________________________

____

9. What does a spirometer measure? ______________________________

10. What is another common name for the trachea? ______________________________

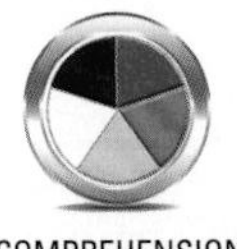
COMPREHENSION

Exercise 34

Circle the letter of the best answer in the following questions.

1. The term that most specifically applies to inflammation of the structure between the pharynx and trachea is
   A. epiglottitis.
   B. laryngitis.
   C. pharyngitis.
   D. pleuritis.

2. Which procedure would be performed when a patient's heart and breathing stop?
   A. CPR
   B. VATS
   C. CXR
   D. CPAP

3. What is the condition that causes a progressive loss of lung function?
   A. asthma
   B. diphtheria
   C. pneumonia
   D. emphysema

4. Which term describes the condition commonly known as whooping cough?
   A. pyothorax
   B. pertussis
   C. pleuritis
   D. pneumonitis

5. Which of the following tests sputum for tuberculosis?
   A. arterial blood gases
   B. peak flow monitoring
   C. purified protein derivative test
   D. acid-fast bacilli smear

6. Every year, a highly contagious viral infection causes many adults and children to seek medical treatment for a disease, commonly known as the flu. The medical term for this infection is
   A. emphysema.
   B. influenza.
   C. croup.
   D. asthma.

7. What is the name of the test used to examine the nasal passages and the pharynx to diagnose structural abnormalities?
   A. auscultation
   B. nasopharyngoscopy
   C. laryngopharyngoscopy
   D. laryngoscopy

8. Which of these tests is used to measure breathing?
   A. PPD
   B. PFT
   C. PEFR
   D. PF

9. Even if you had never heard of this condition, you might assume that sinusitis refers to
   A. surgical repair of the sinus.
   B. incision of the sinus.
   C. inflammation of the sinus.
   D. excision of the sinus.

10. Which combining form refers to the structure that takes in air?
   A. sinus/o
   B. sept/o
   C. adenoid/o
   D. rhin/o

Application and Analysis

CASE STUDIES

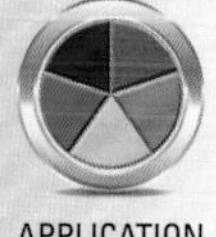

Exercise 35

APPLICATION

Read the case studies and circle the correct letter for each of the questions.

CASE 11-1

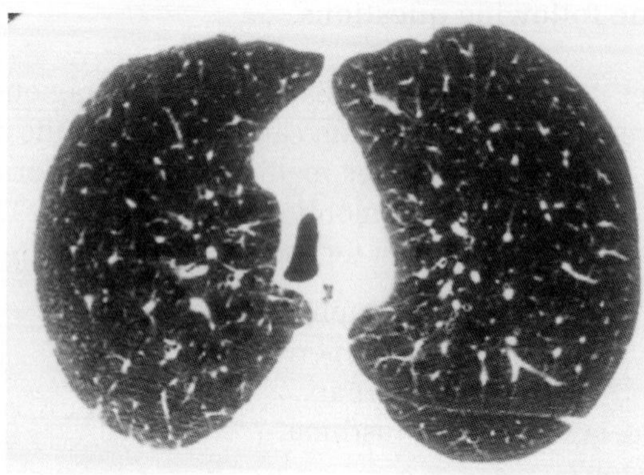

Figure 11-26 CT scan of the chest of a patient diagnosed with COPD.

After working 25 years in the coal-mining industry, Mr. Orbin Davis, age 65, is undergoing a series of pulmonary function tests to investigate issues related to his progressive loss of lung function and inability to breathe normally. During the procedures, an instrument was used to measure Mr. Davis's breathing rate by estimating the amount of air exhaled after normal inspiration. Ms. Whalen, a nurse practitioner, also performed a test that measured the amount of air exhaled after a maximal inspiration. This group of tests will assist in determining whether Mr. Davis suffers from COPD or from asthma. Depending on the test results, a CT scan may also be ordered to confirm COPD (**Figure 11-26**).

1. The term for an instrument used to measure breathing is

A. spirometry.
B. spirometer.
C. percussion.
D. capnometer.

2. The abbreviation COPD stands for

A. chronic obstructive pneumonia dyspnea.
B. chronic olfactory pharyngitis disease.
C. caustic other pneumonic disease.
D. chronic obstructive pulmonary disease.

3. What group of tests will assist in determining whether the patient has COPD or asthma?

A. PFT
B. RR
C. AFB
D. ABG

4. A sign or symptom related to asthma is

A. a progressive loss of lung function.
B. lack of expansion of a lung.
C. wheezing.
D. severe headaches.

5. Mr. Davis's pulmonary function test revealed an abnormal amount of fluid inside various lobes within the lungs. This condition is known as

A. pleurodesis.
B. pleural effusion.
C. pulmonary edema.
D. pneumothorax.

CASE 11-2

Ms. Beverly Bonner, age 58, requested an office appointment. Ms. Bonner stated she suffered from a sore throat, fever, chills, and depression. Dr. Wallace physically examined her, took a chest x-ray, and measured her breathing. Using a stethoscope, she established the presence of fluid in Ms. Bonner's lungs via auscultation and palpable vibrations within her pleural cavity. After reviewing the results of the tests and examination, Dr. Wallace diagnosed Ms. Bonner with pneumococcal pneumonia.

6. What bacterial species is the cause of pneumococcal pneumonia?

A. *Pneumococcus aureus*
B. *Streptococcus pneumoniae*
C. *Mycopneumonia streptococcus*
D. *Pneumococcus pneumoniae*

7. The throat is the common name for which structure?

A. pharynx
B. larynx
C. nasopharynx
D. glottis

8. An instrument that measures breathing is called a(n)

A. oximeter.
B. peak flow meter.
C. spirometer.
D. tidal volume meter.

9. What is the name of the physical examination involving listening inside the pleural cavity that relies on the use of a stethoscope?

A. percussion
B. auscultation
C. polysomnography
D. spirometry

10. What is the name of the physical examination of the pleural cavity that relies on the use of tapping over the body to elicit vibrations and sounds?

A. percussion
B. auscultation
C. polysomnography
D. spirometry

MEDICAL RECORD ANALYSIS

MEDICAL RECORD 11-1

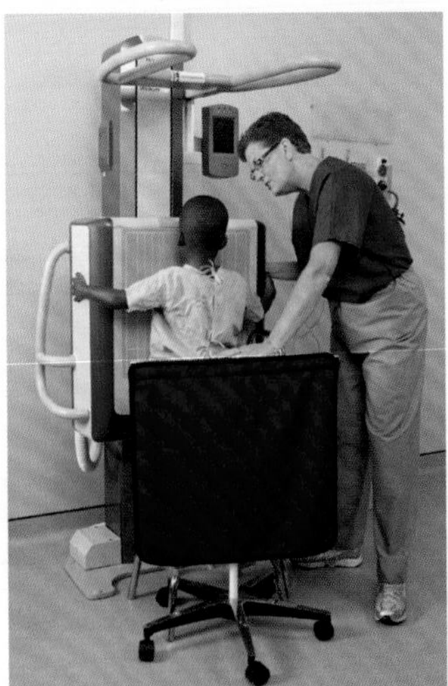

A radiologic technician prepares patients for and performs radiologic examinations.

Travis Reynolds is a patient who is returning to the office with his mother after a routine tuberculosis skin test was performed a couple of days ago. As the radiologic technologist, you are reviewing the record in preparation for performing his chest x-ray.

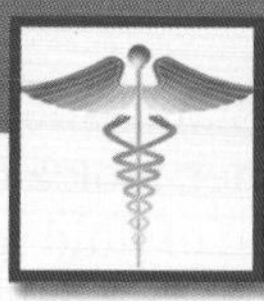

Medical Record

POSITIVE TUBERCULIN SKIN TEST

SUBJECTIVE: This 4-year-old boy is a patient of our clinic who came here today for a tuberculosis test reading. The patient had a TB test placed previously and today, 48 hours later, shows a positive reaction. TB test was present in the left forearm, and there is an area of erythema and induration corresponding to about 20 mm. This was measured by the nurse and verified to me.

Mom denies child being exposed to anyone with tuberculosis. He had been tested a couple of times during the past year, but mom had never come in for the reading. She said there was no reaction to it on either occasion except this one time. She also says that he is only around the family and the kids in school. She is not aware of anyone being diagnosed with tuberculosis and child has been completely fine, alert, active, and feeding well with no problems.

OBJECTIVE: Temperature 98.8, blood pressure 80/60, weight 14.5 kg, heart rate 80. General: Alert, active, well nourished. Neck: Supple, no lymphadenopathy. Heart: Regular rate and rhythm, no heart murmurs. Lungs: Clear to auscultation bilaterally. No rhonchi, rales, crackles, or wheezing.

ASSESSMENT AND PLAN: Patient is a 4-year-old boy with positive tuberculin skin test result, recent converter. I ordered chest x-rays to rule out active tuberculosis. The patient very likely has latent TB and mom was told that her son would be a good candidate for INH prophylaxis. The patient is to return to clinic in the next couple of weeks. Mom voiced understanding and agrees to follow up accordingly.

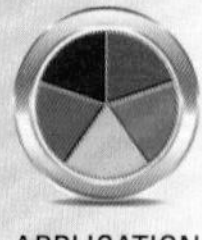

APPLICATION

Exercise 36

Write the appropriate medical terms used in this medical record on the blanks after their definitions. Note that not all the terms appear in the chapter, but you should be able to identify these terms based on word parts that are included in this chapter.

1. redness ______________________
2. infection by a bacterium that attacks the lungs ______________________
3. abnormal whistling, humming, or snoring sounds during breathing ______________________
4. listening with aid of a stethoscope ______________________
5. an airy, whistling type sound ______________________
6. pertaining to both sides ______________________

Bonus Question

7. Why were chest x-rays ordered? ______________________

MEDICAL RECORD 11-2

You are a respiratory therapist working at a private hospital and will be treating Mr. Samuel Burnett, who suffers from chronic obstructive pulmonary disease. Prior to his appointment, you reviewed the medical record from his recent hospitalization.

The numbered blanks in this medical record are part of Exercise 37.

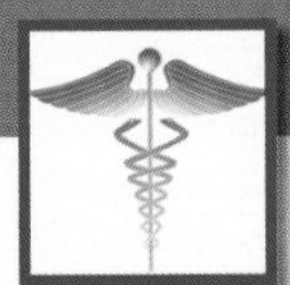

Medical Record

BRONCHITIS WITH COPD

DIAGNOSES

1. (1) ____________________
2. Chronic obstructive pulmonary disease.
3. Coronary artery disease.

PROCEDURES: Chest x-ray that had the following result: The patient had increased markings in left lower lung, possibly early left lower lobe pneumonia versus chronic fibrosis, minimal hyperinflation with flattened diaphragms, decreased lung markings in both upper lungs, and increased AP diameter. Chest compatible with emphysema. Moderate diffuse osteoporosis. Wedging one midthoracic vertebral body.

HISTORY AND HOSPITAL COURSE: The patient was admitted with a chief complaint of cough with white (2) ________________ with shortness of breath and (3) ________________ on exertion, worse for three days.

This is an 83-year-old male with COPD and diagnosed with a non–ST-elevation MI 1 and 1/2 months ago. Patient underwent cardiac catheterization at that time and was discharged on Plavix. The patient reports ongoing dyspnea on exertion and shortness of breath since then. Most recently, the patient complained of very severe cough with white sputum. The patient denies chest pain. He does have nocturia and paroxysmal nocturnal dyspnea, subjective hot and cold flashes, but denies night sweats or weight loss.

I believe the patient has severe COPD, but the patient does not want to have PFTs done because he does not want to pay the expense since he can get them done for free at the VA. The patient also does not want to have a CT to make sure he does not have a (4) ________________, although my previous assessment of probability for a PE was low. The patient also refuses to be transferred to the VA where he can receive these studies for free. The patient decided he would rather be discharged.

The patient was treated for bronchitis with doxycycline with improvement in his symptoms. He was discharged to home in stable condition. He will be discharged on Atrovent MDI two puffs every six hours and doxycycline 100 mg by mouth two times per day for 10 days. The patient was told to go to the VA to set up home physical therapy and (5) ________________ rehab. No activity restrictions, but he should walk with assistance. He should continue to be active. He will call the VA to set up home physical therapy and pulmonary rehabilitation.

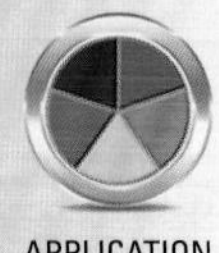
APPLICATION

Exercise 37

Fill in the blanks in the medical record above with the correct medical terms. The definitions of the missing terms are listed below.

1. inflammation of the bronchi
2. expectorated matter
3. difficulty breathing
4. blockage of the pulmonary artery by a blood clot
5. pertaining to the lungs

Bonus Question

6. Which type of physician specialist would most likely have treated this patient?

____

Pronunciation and Spelling

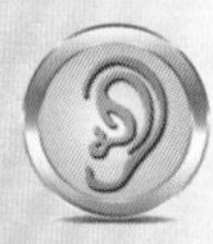
AUDITORY

Exercise 38

Review the Chapter 11 terms in the Dictionary/Audio Glossary in the Student Resources on thePoint, and practice pronouncing each term, referring to the pronunciation guide as needed.

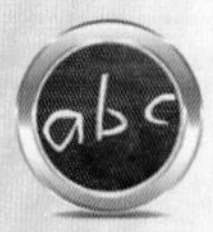

SPELLING

Exercise 39

Check the spelling of each term. If it is correct, check off the correct box. If incorrect, write the correct spelling on the line.

1. alveolor ☐ _______________
2. pulomonary ☐ _______________
3. bronchiolitis ☐ _______________
4. diaphragm ☐ _______________
5. pneumopluritis ☐ _______________
6. pleuraglia ☐ _______________
7. rhinorrhea ☐ _______________
8. bronchography ☐ _______________
9. tonsilar ☐ _______________
10. dispena ☐ _______________

Media Connection

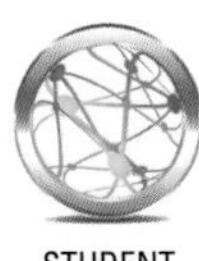
STUDENT RESOURCES

Exercise 40

Complete each of the following activities available with the Student Resources on thePoint. Check off each activity as you complete it, and record your score for the Chapter Quiz in the space provided.

Chapter Exercises

____ Flash Cards

____ Concentration

____ Abbreviation Match-Up

____ Roboterms

____ Word Anatomy

____ Fill the Gap

____ Break It Down

____ True/False Body Building

____ Quiz Show

____ Complete the Case

____ Medical Record Review

____ Look and Label

____ Image Matching

____ Spelling Bee

____ **Chapter Quiz** *Score:*________%

Additional Resources

____ Animation: The Respiratory System

____ Animation: Pulmonary Ventilation

____ Animation: Change in Breathing Sounds

____ Dictionary/Audio Glossary

____ Health Professions Careers: Radiologic Technician

____ Health Professions Careers: Respiratory Therapist

Digestive System

12

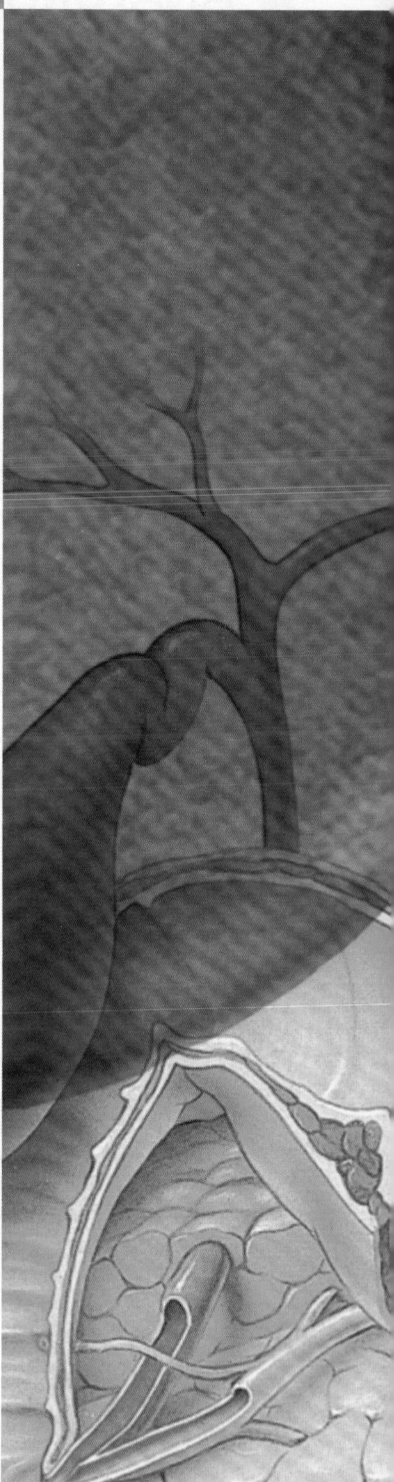

Chapter Outline

Introduction, 462

Anatomy and Physiology, 462
- Structures, 462
- Functions, 462
- Terms Related to the Digestive System, 462

Word Parts, 467
- Combining Forms, 467
- Prefixes, 468
- Suffixes, 469

Medical Terms, 475
- Adjectives and Other Related Terms, 475
- Medical Conditions, 477
- Tests and Procedures, 484
- Surgical Interventions and Therapeutic Procedures, 487
- Medications and Drug Therapies, 492
- Specialties and Specialists, 493
- Abbreviations, 493

Wrapping Up, 494

Chapter Review, 495

Learning Outcomes

After completing this chapter, you should be able to:

1. List the structures and functions of the digestive system.
2. Define terms related to the digestive system.
3. Define combining forms, prefixes, and suffixes related to the digestive system.
4. Define common medical terminology related to the digestive system, including adjectives and related terms; signs, symptoms and medical conditions; tests and procedures; surgical interventions and therapeutic procedures; medications and drug therapies; and medical specialties and specialists.
5. Define abbreviations related to the digestive system.
6. Successfully complete all chapter exercises.
7. Explain terms used in case studies and medical records involving the digestive system.
8. Successfully complete all exercises included with the companion Student Resources on thePoint.

INTRODUCTION

The digestive system, also known as the gastrointestinal (GI) system, begins with the mouth and ends with the anus. Its purpose is to break down food into smaller, usable forms that can be used by the body. Anything the body cannot use is then excreted as waste. This chapter discusses the anatomy, physiology, and pathology of digestion and provides important medical terms associated with the digestive system.

ANATOMY AND PHYSIOLOGY

Structures

- The digestive system is made up of the digestive tract and its associated glands and organs.
- The digestive tract leads from the mouth through the pharynx, esophagus, stomach, and intestines to the anus.
- The digestive tract is also known as the gastrointestinal tract or the alimentary canal.
- The small and large intestines are also called the bowels or guts.

Functions

- Bringing in food to provide nutrients to the body
- Breaking down food into usable nutrients
- Absorbing nutrients from the breakdown of food
- Eliminating the solid wastes not used by the body

Terms Related to the Digestive System

Term	Pronunciation	Meaning
Primary Digestive Structures (Figure 12-1)		
mouth; *syn.* oral cavity	mowth; ōr'ăl kav'i-tē	opening where food enters the body and undergoes the first process of digestion
palate	pal'ăt	the roof of the mouth; separates the oral cavity from the nasal cavity
uvula; *syn.* uvula of soft palate	yū'vyū-lă; yū'vyū-lă ov sôft pal'ăt	small piece of tissue that hangs in the posterior portion of the oral cavity
tongue	tŭng	muscular organ at the floor of the mouth; assists in swallowing and speaking (**Figure 12-2**)
teeth	tēth	structures that provide the hard surfaces needed for chewing (mastication)
salivary glands	sal'i-var-ē glandz	saliva-secreting glands in the oral cavity; include the parotid, sublingual, and submandibular glands (**Figure 12-2**)
saliva	să-lī'vă	clear, tasteless, slightly acidic (pH 6.8) fluid that helps to lubricate food in the mouth

Terms Related to the Digestive System

Term	Pronunciation	Meaning
pharynx; *syn.* throat	far′ingks; thrōt	space behind the mouth that serves as a passage for food from the mouth to the esophagus and for air from the nose and mouth to the larynx
esophagus	ĕ-sof′ă-gŭs	muscular tube that moves food from the pharynx to the stomach
stomach	stŏm′ăk	sac-like organ in which chemical and mechanical digestion take place (**Figure 12-3**)
cardia	kahr′dē-ă	region where the esophagus connects to the stomach
fundus	fŭn′dŭs	superior dome-shaped region of the stomach
body	bod′ē	largest region of the stomach, between the fundus and pylorus
lower esophageal sphincter (LES)	lō′wĕr ĕ-sof′ă-jē′ăl sfingk′tĕr	ring of muscle between the esophagus and the stomach
pyloric sphincter	pī-lōr′ik sfingk′tĕr	ring of muscle between the stomach and the first segment of the small intestine (duodenum)
pylorus	pī-lōr′ŭs	lower region of the stomach that connects to the small intestine
rugae	rū′gē	folds in the stomach lining that increase the surface area for absorption of nutrients

(continued)

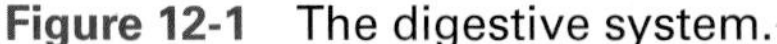

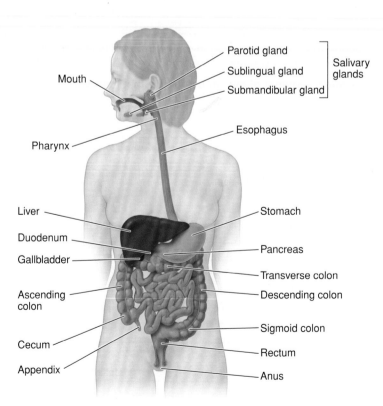

Figure 12-1 The digestive system.

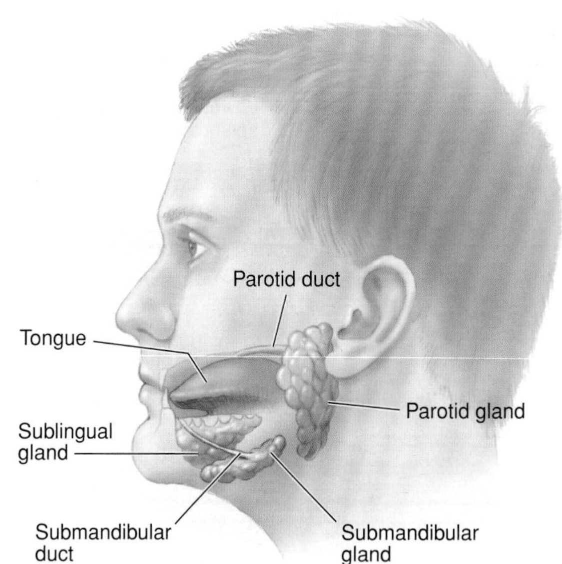

Figure 12-2 The salivary glands secrete enzymes that break down food.

Terms Related to the Digestive System *(continued)*

Term	Pronunciation	Meaning
small intestine	smôl in-tes′tin	section of digestive tube between the stomach and cecum where most absorption of nutrients occurs (**Figure 12-4**)
duodenum	dū′ō-dē′nŭm	first segment of the small intestine
jejunum	je-jū′nŭm	the middle segment of the small intestine
ileum	il′ē-ŭm	the last segment of the small intestine that connects to the large intestine
large intestine	larj in-tes′tin	distal section of digestive tube, extending from the small intestine to the anus, where water and electrolytes are absorbed and wastes are formed (**Figure 12-4**)
cecum	sē′kŭm	first segment of the large intestine
appendix; *syn.* vermiform appendix	ă-pen′diks; vĕr′mi-fōrm ă-pen′diks	finger-like projection off the cecum of the large intestine
colon	kō′lŏn	segment of the large intestine that extends from the cecum to the rectum and is divided into four parts
ascending colon	ă-send′ing kō′lŏn	segment of the large intestine on the right side between the cecum and the right colic flexure
right colic flexure; *syn.* hepatic flexure	rīt kol′ik flek′shŭr; he-pat′ik flek′shŭr	the bend of the colon between the ascending and transverse sections
transverse colon	trans-vĕrs′ kō′lŏn	segment of the large intestine between the ascending colon and descending colon
left colic flexure; *syn.* left splenic flexure	left kol′ik flek′shŭr; left splen′ik flek′shŭr	the bend of the colon between the transverse and descending sections
descending colon	dĕ-send′ing kō′lŏn	segment of the large intestine on the left side between the left colic flexure and the sigmoid colon
sigmoid colon	sig′moyd kō′lŏn	terminal segment of the large intestine that joins with the rectum

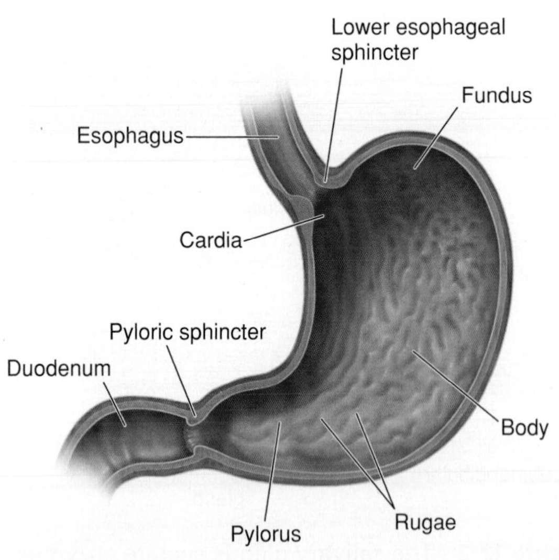

Figure 12-3 The stomach and its sections.

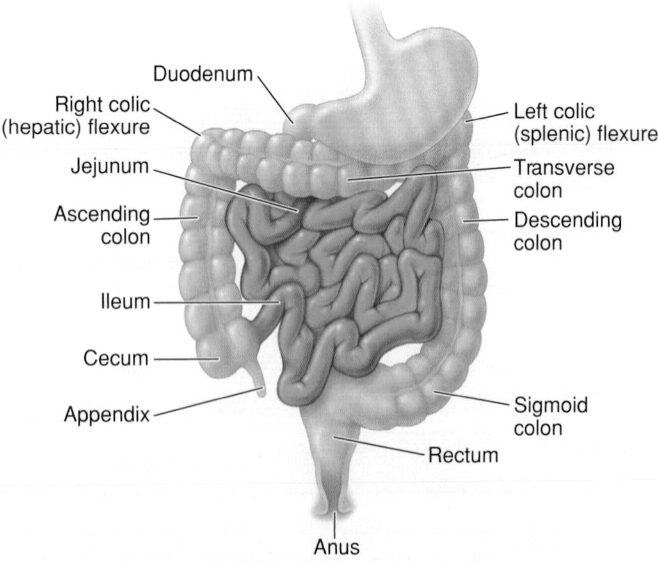

Figure 12-4 The small and large intestines.

Terms Related to the Digestive System

Term	Pronunciation	Meaning
rectum	rek'tŭm	extension of the large intestine; a pouch that holds solid waste before elimination from the body
anus	ā'nŭs	opening at the end of the digestive tract through which solid waste exits the body
Accessory Digestive Organs (Figure 12-5)		
liver	liv'ĕr	large glandular organ that produces and secretes bile into the gallbladder
bile	bīl	fluid that is secreted by the liver into the duodenum and aids in the digestion of fats
gallbladder	gawl'blad-ĕr	sac-shaped organ beneath the liver that stores bile secreted by the liver and releases it into the small intestine
pancreas	pan'krē-ăs	organ that secretes pancreatic juice (digestive enzymes) into the small intestine; its endocrine part secretes insulin and glucagon into the bloodstream

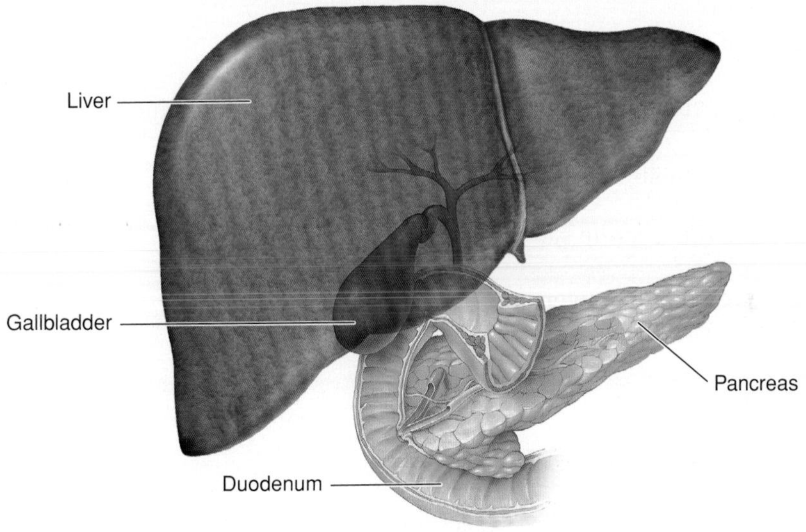

Figure 12-5 Accessory organs of the digestive system.

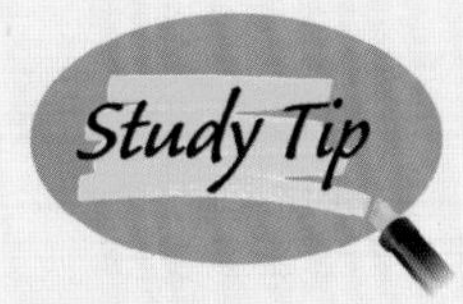

Segments of the Small Intestine: To remember the segments of the small intestine from proximal to distal, think "**D**on't **J**ump **I**n" for **d**uodenum, **j**ejunum, and **i**leum.

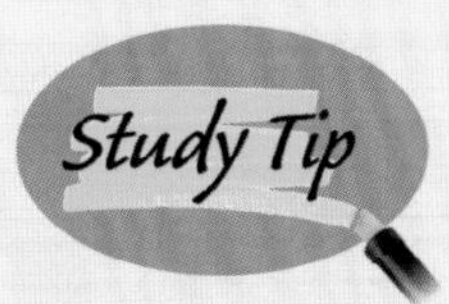

Spelling Homonyms—Ilium and Ileum: Ilium and ileum are homonyms; that is, they are spelled differently but sound alike. Here is an easy way to remember the difference in meaning and spelling. Ilium is the upper section of the hip bone, and both hip and ilium contain the letter "i." For ileum, remember that it is part of the small intestine and that both intestine and its combining form enter/o contain the letter "e."

Learn more about digestion and the organs involved in the digestion process by viewing the animation "General Digestion" on the Student Resources on thePoint.

Exercises: Anatomy and Physiology

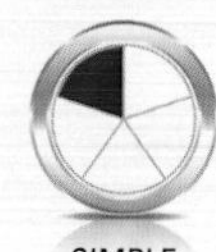
SIMPLE RECALL

Exercise 1

Write the correct anatomic structure for the meaning given.

1. middle segment of the small intestine ______________________
2. finger-like projection located on the large intestine ______________________
3. organ that stores bile ______________________
4. site where food enters the body ______________________
5. the roof of the mouth ______________________
6. medical term for throat ______________________
7. superior dome-shaped region of stomach ______________________
8. organ that secretes bile ______________________
9. segment of small intestine that connects with large intestine ______________________
10. structure through which solid wastes pass to exit the body ______________________
11. structures that secrete saliva ______________________
12. fluid secreted by the liver ______________________

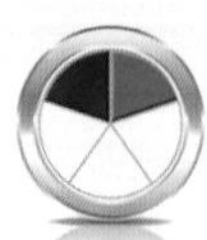
ADVANCED RECALL

Exercise 2

Match each medical term with its meaning.

rugae	esophagus	rectum	cecum	sigmoid colon
duodenum	pancreas	descending colon	uvula	pylorus

1. first segment of the small intestine ______________________
2. organ that secretes juices that aid in digestion ______________________
3. muscular tube that moves food to the stomach ______________________
4. segment of colon between the descending colon and rectum ______________________
5. region of stomach that connects to the small intestine ______________________
6. area where solid waste is temporarily stored ______________________
7. first segment of the large intestine ______________________
8. segment of the large intestine between the left colic flexure and the sigmoid colon ______________________

9. structure that hangs in the posterior oral cavity ______________

10. folds in the stomach lining ______________

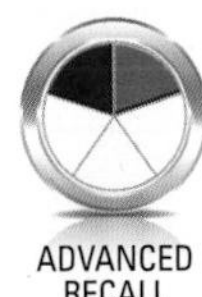

Exercise 3

Circle the term that is most appropriate for the meaning of the sentence.

1. The (*duodenum, stomach, large intestine*) is where chemical digestion begins.
2. Located in the mouth, the (*salivary glands, rugae, teeth*) provide the hard surfaces for mastication.
3. The (*transverse, ascending, sigmoid*) colon is the second segment of the colon.
4. The muscular organ on the floor of the mouth is called the (*palate, tongue, uvula*).
5. The large intestine reabsorbs (*food, waste, water*) and produces solid wastes.
6. The region of the stomach where the esophagus connects is called the (*fundus, cardia, body*).
7. The small intestine is made up of (*two, three, four*) segments.
8. The fluid that helps lubricate food in the mouth is called (*bile, saliva, rugae*).
9. The largest region of the stomach is called the (*body, fundus, pylorus*).
10. The (*ascending, descending, sigmoid*) colon arises from the cecum and joins the transverse colon.

WORD PARTS

The following tables list word parts related to the digestive system.

Combining Forms

Combining Form	Meaning
abdomin/o	abdomen
aliment/o	nourishment, nutrition
an/o	anus
appendic/o	appendix
bil/o	bile
bucc/o	cheek
cec/o	cecum
cheil/o	lip
chol/e	bile
cholecyst/o	gallbladder

(continued)

Combining Forms *(continued)*

Combining Form	Meaning
col/o, colon/o	colon
dent/o	tooth
duoden/o	duodenum
enter/o	small intestine
esophag/o	esophagus
diverticul/o	diverticulum (pouch opening from a tubular organ)
gastr/o	stomach
hemat/o, hem/o	blood
hepat/o	liver
herni/o	hernia (protrusion)
ile/o	ileum
jejun/o	jejunum
labi/o	lip
lapar/o	abdomen
lingu/o	tongue
lith/o	stone, calculus
odont/o	tooth
or/o	mouth
palat/o	palate
pancreat/o	pancreas
peps/o	digestion
phag/o	eat, swallow
pharyng/o	pharynx
polyp/o	polyp
proct/o	rectum, anus
pylor/o	pylorus
rect/o	rectum
sial/o	saliva
sigmoid/o	sigmoid colon
stomat/o	mouth

Prefixes

Prefix	Meaning
endo-	in, within
hyper-	above, excessive
peri-	around, surrounding
post-	after, behind
retro-	backward, behind

Suffixes

Suffix	Meaning
-algia	pain
-ase	enzyme
-cele	herniation, protrusion
-centesis	puncture to aspirate
-dynia	pain
-emesis	vomiting
-gen	origin, production
-gram	record, recording
-graphy	technique of producing images
-iasis	condition of
-logist	one who specializes in
-logy	study of
-malacia	softening
-megaly	enlargement
-prandial	meal
-ptosis	prolapse, drooping, sagging
-rrhaphy	suture
-scope	instrument for examination
-scopy	viewing or examining with an instrument
-stenosis	stricture, narrowing
-stomy	surgical opening
-tomy	incision
-tripsy	crushing

Exercises: Word Parts

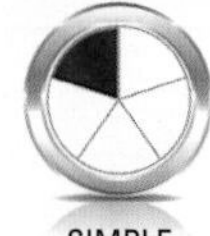

SIMPLE RECALL

Exercise 4

Write the meaning of the combining form given.

1. duoden/o ____________________
2. stomat/o ____________________
3. pancreat/o ____________________
4. enter/o ____________________
5. cheil/o ____________________
6. sial/o ____________________

7. hepat/o ______________________

8. bucc/o ______________________

9. an/o ______________________

10. peps/o ______________________

11. pharyng/o ______________________

12. proct/o ______________________

13. pylor/o ______________________

14. col/o ______________________

15. sigmoid/o ______________________

16. odont/o ______________________

17. lapar/o ______________________

Exercise 5

SIMPLE RECALL

Write the correct combining form for the meaning given.

1. jejunum ______________________

2. appendix ______________________

3. eat, swallow ______________________

4. blood ______________________

5. stomach ______________________

6. esophagus ______________________

7. cheek ______________________

8. rectum ______________________

9. polyp ______________________

10. gallbladder ______________________

11. cecum ______________________

12. tongue ______________________

13. ileum ______________________

14. tooth ______________________

15. colon ______

16. stone, calculus ______

17. palate ______

18. bile ______

19. hernia ______

20. abdomen ______

21. nourishment ______

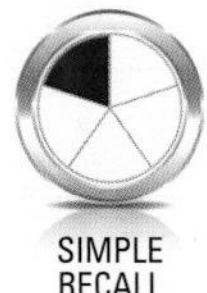

Exercise 6

Write the meaning of the prefix or suffix given.

1. endo- ______
2. -tripsy ______
3. -ase ______
4. peri- ______
5. -stomy ______
6. -iasis ______
7. -logist ______
8. -cele ______
9. -gen ______
10. -megaly ______
11. retro- ______
12. -ptosis ______
13. -scopy ______
14. -prandial ______
15. post- ______
16. hyper- ______
17. -dynia ______
18. -malacia ______

19. -graphy ______________________________

20. -emesis ______________________________

21. -scope ______________________________

22. -centesis ______________________________

23. -stenosis ______________________________

24. -gram ______________________________

25. -rrhaphy ______________________________

26. -algia ______________________________

27. -tomy ______________________________

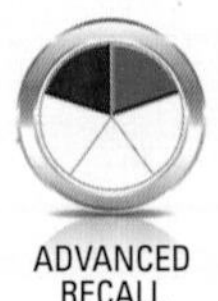

ADVANCED RECALL

Exercise 7

Considering the meaning of the combining form from which the medical term is made, write the meaning of the medical term. (You have not yet learned many of these terms but can build their meanings from the word parts.)

Combining Form	Meaning	Medical Term	Meaning of Term
pancreat/o	pancreas	pancreatitis	1. ______________
sigmoid/o	sigmoid colon	sigmoidoscope	2. ______________
aliment/o	nutrition	alimentary	3. ______________
col/o	colon	colostomy	4. ______________
cholecyst/o	gallbladder	cholecystectomy	5. ______________
diverticul/o	diverticulum	diverticulitis	6. ______________

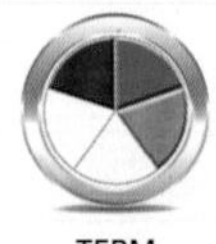

TERM CONSTRUCTION

Exercise 8

Build a medical term for each meaning using one of the listed combining forms and one of the listed suffixes.

Combining Forms		Suffixes	
gastr/o	lith/o	-logist	-al
abdomin/o	hepat/o	-itis	-centesis
an/o	proct/o	-scopy	-ectomy
bucc/o	colon/o	-tripsy	-plasty

1. one who specializes in disorders of the rectum and anus ______________

2. inflammation of the liver ______________

3. pertaining to the cheek ______________________

4. crushing of stones ______________________

5. puncture to aspirate (fluid) from the abdomen ______________________

6. surgical repair of the anus ______________________

7. surgical removal of the stomach ______________________

8. visual examination of the colon ______________________

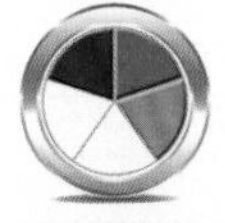
TERM CONSTRUCTION

Exercise 9

Build a medical term for each meaning using one of the listed combining forms and one of the listed suffixes.

Use Combining Form for	Use Suffix for	Term
esophagus	inflammation	1. ______________
appendix	surgical removal	2. ______________
stomach	examination	3. ______________
colon	surgical opening	4. ______________
lip	suture	5. ______________
abdomen	incision	6. ______________
gallbladder	record, recording	7. ______________
mouth	pertaining to	8. ______________
nourishment	pertaining to	9. ______________
liver	inflammation	10. ______________
pancreas	disease	11. ______________

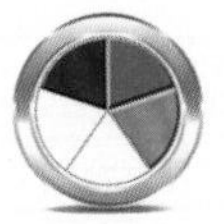
TERM CONSTRUCTION

Exercise 10

Break the given medical term into its word parts, and define each part. Then define the medical term.

For example:

appendicitis	*word parts:*	appendic/o, -itis
	meanings:	appendix, inflammation of
	term meaning:	inflammation of the appendix

1. gastroenterologist *word parts:* ______________________

meanings: ______________________

term meaning: ______________________

2. dyspepsia *word parts:* ____________________

meanings: ____________________

term meaning: ____________________

3. hyperemesis *word parts:* ____________________

meanings: ____________________

term meaning: ____________________

4. colectomy *word parts:* ____________________

meanings: ____________________

term meaning: ____________________

5. herniorrhaphy *word parts:* ____________________

meanings: ____________________

term meaning: ____________________

6. dysphagia *word parts:* ____________________

meanings: ____________________

term meaning: ____________________

7. cholelithiasis *word parts:* ____________________

meanings: ____________________

term meaning: ____________________

8. hematemesis *word parts:* ____________________

meanings: ____________________

term meaning: ____________________

9. rectocele *word parts:* ____________________

meanings: ____________________

term meaning: ____________________

10. palatoplasty *word parts:* ____________________

meanings: ____________________

term meaning: ____________________

11. ileostomy *word parts:* ____________

meanings: ____________

term meaning: ____________

12. sublingual *word parts:* ____________

meanings: ____________

term meaning: ____________

■ MEDICAL TERMS

The following table gives adjective forms and terms used in describing the digestive system and its conditions.

Adjectives and Other Related Terms

Term	Pronunciation	Meaning
anorexia	an′ŏ-rek′sē-ă	decrease in or loss of appetite
bolus	bō′lŭs	ball of chewed food that is ready to be swallowed
chyme	kīm	partially digested food that passes from the stomach into the duodenum
defecation; *syn.* bowel movement (BM)	def-ĕ-kā′shun; bow′ĕl mūv′mĕnt	passage of solid wastes (feces) from the body
deglutition	dē-glū-tish′ŭn	the act of swallowing
digestion	di-jes′chŭn	the mechanical, chemical, and enzymatic process of breaking down food into substances the body can use
eructation	ē-rŭk-tā′shŭn	the voiding of gas or acidic fluid from the stomach through the mouth; commonly called a burp or belch
feces	fē′sēz	waste matter discharged from the bowels
flatus	flā′tŭs	gas that passes through the anus
halitosis	hal-i-tō′sis	bad breath
hematochezia	hē′mă-tō-kē′zē-ă	the passage of bloody stools
inguinal	ing′gwi-năl	relating to the groin
mastication	mas′ti-kā′shŭn	chewing
melena	mĕ-lē′nă	black, tarry stools due to the presence of blood altered by intestinal juices
nausea	naw′zē-ă	the urge to vomit
occult blood	ŏ-kŭlt′ blŭd	blood in the feces in amounts that are too small to be seen by the naked eye but detectable by chemical tests

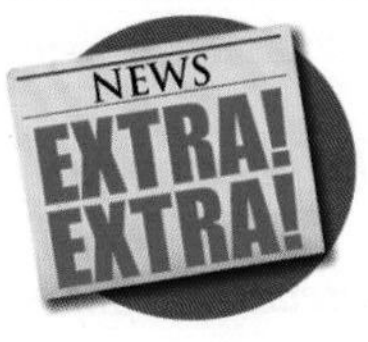

FECAL OCCULT BLOOD TEST The easiest and first screening test done to check for colon cancer involves checking the feces for hidden blood. This test, called the fecal occult blood test (FOBT) can also be used to check for bleeding in the digestive tract, which can be a cause of anemia. The patient can do the FOBT at home, or a physician can perform the test in the office during a routine physical examination.

(continued)

Adjectives and Other Related Terms *(continued)*

Term	Pronunciation	Meaning
peristalsis	per'i-stal'sis	involuntary contraction and relaxation of smooth muscles of the GI tract creating wave-like movements that push substances along its length (**Figure 12-6**)
postprandial	pōst-pran'dē-ăl	after a meal
vomit; *syn.* regurgitate	vom'it; rē-gŭr'ji-tāt	to eject matter from the stomach through the mouth

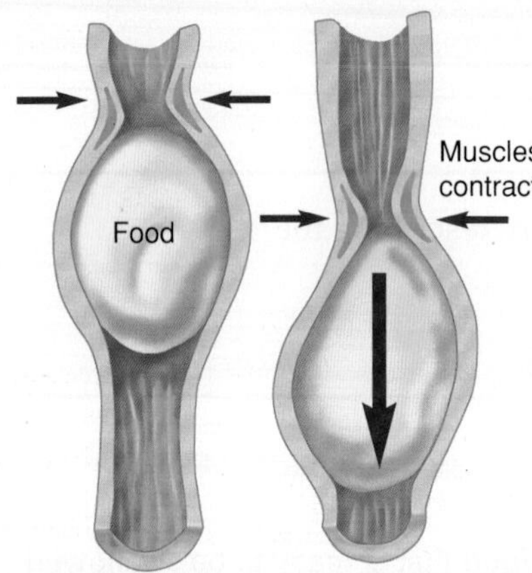

Figure 12-6 Peristalsis. The muscles in the esophagus contract to move food toward the stomach.

Exercises: Adjectives and Other Related Terms

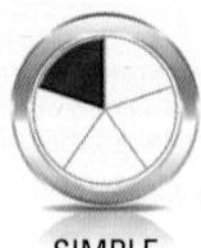
SIMPLE RECALL

Exercise 11

Circle the term that is most appropriate for the meaning of the sentence.

1. To remove gas from the body through the mouth is called (*flatus, vomit, eructation*).
2. Blood that is hidden in the stools is known as (*halitosis, occult, chyme*).
3. The solid wastes that are removed from the body are known as (*vomitus, melena, feces*).
4. Moving food through the digestive system using wave-like motions is known as (*peristalsis, regurgitation, retroflexed*).
5. The first step in the digestion of food is called (*regurgitation, mastication, eructation*).
6. Someone who has forgotten to brush his teeth may have a condition known as (*eructation, halitosis, flatus*).
7. The mechanical, chemical, and enzymatic process of breaking down food into usable substances is (*peristalsis, digestion, mastication*).
8. A ball of chewed food that is ready for swallowing is called a (*bolus, chyme, melena*).
9. Another term that means having a bowel movement is (*mastication, defecation, peristalsis*).
10. The term hematochezia means the passing of (*vomit, bloody stools, chyme*).

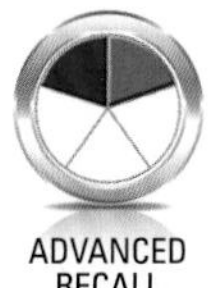
ADVANCED RECALL

Exercise 12

Match each medical term with its meaning.

melena	nausea	deglutition	flatus
inguinal	chyme	vomit	anorexia

1. swallowing ______
2. black, tarry stools ______
3. relating to the groin ______
4. the urge to vomit ______
5. gas that passes through the anus ______
6. partially digested food ______
7. to eject matter from the stomach ______
8. decreased or loss of appetite ______

Medical Conditions

Term	Pronunciation	Meaning
anorexia nervosa	an-ō-rek′sē-ă nĕr-vō′să	eating disorder characterized by an extreme fear of becoming obese and by an aversion to eating
ascites	ă-sī′tēz	accumulation of fluid in the abdominal/peritoneal cavity (**Figure 12-7**)
cholecystitis	kō′lĕ-sis-tī′tis	inflammation of the gallbladder
cholelithiasis	kō′le-li-thī′ă-sis	presence of stones in the gallbladder or bile ducts; formation of gallstones (**Figure 12-8**)
cirrhosis	sir-ō′sis	chronic liver disease characterized by gradual failure of liver cells and loss of blood flow in the liver
constipation	kon′sti-pā′shŭn	decreased number of bowel movements often associated with hard stools
Crohn disease; *syn.* regional enteritis	krōn di-zēz′; rē′jŭn-ăl en′tĕr-ī′tis	chronic intestinal inflammation of unknown cause that is characterized by deep ulcers and thickening of the intestine
diarrhea	dī′ă-rē′ă	abnormally frequent discharge of semisolid or liquid feces
diverticulitis	dī′vĕr-tik′yū-lī′tis	inflammation of a diverticulum
diverticulum	dī′vĕr-tik′yū-lŭm	an abnormal pouch on the wall of a hollow organ that protrudes outward (**Figure 12-9**)
dysentery	dis′ĕn-tar′ē	infection of the intestines resulting in severe diarrhea containing blood and mucus
dyspepsia	dis-pep′sē-ă	indigestion or upset stomach
dysphagia	dis-fā′jē-ă	difficulty swallowing

(continued)

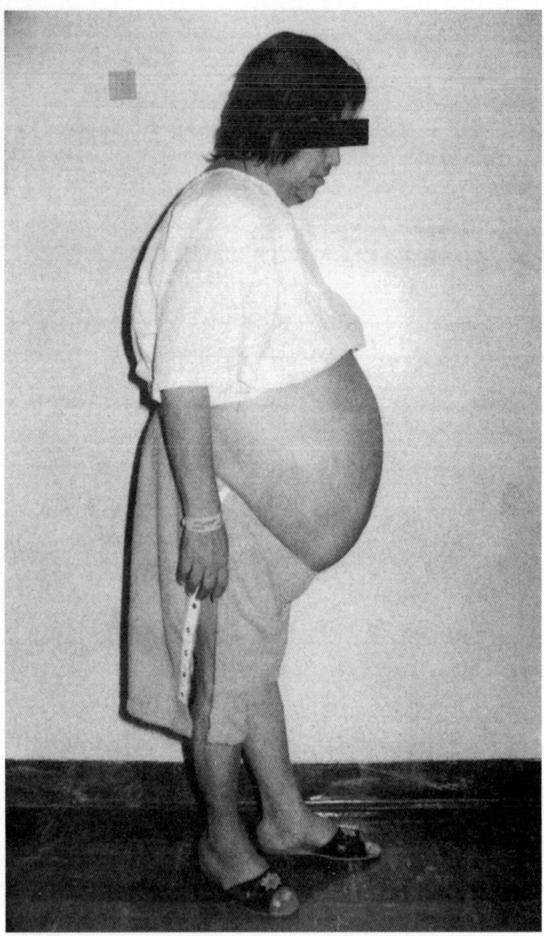

Figure 12-7 Patient with ascites as indicated by the protruding abdomen.

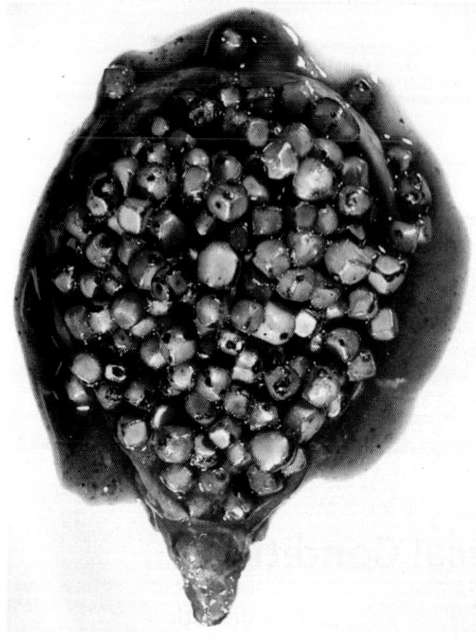

Figure 12-8 Cholelithiasis. The gallbladder has been opened to reveal numerous yellow gallstones made up of cholesterol.

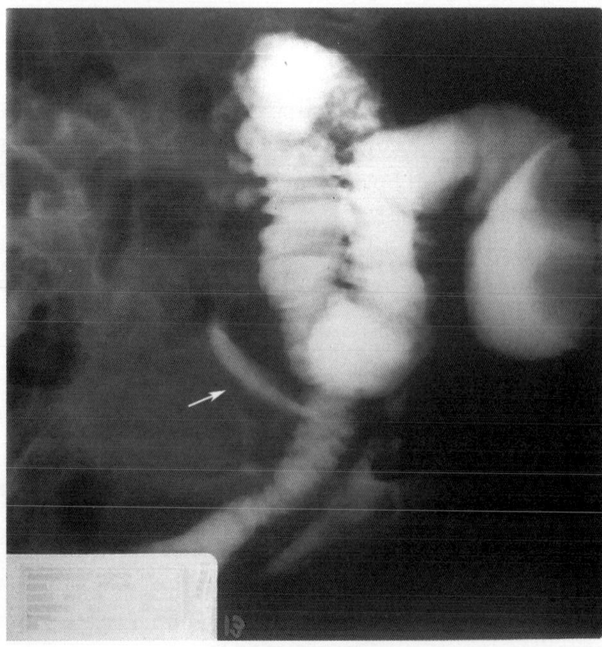

Figure 12-9 Barium enema showing a ruptured diverticulum, which is the elongated extension off the intestine.

Medical Conditions *(continued)*

Term	Pronunciation	Meaning
gastric ulcer	gas'trik ŭl'sĕr	sore on the stomach lining with inflammation (**Figure 12-10**)
gastroenteritis	gas'trō-en-tĕr-ī'tis	inflammation of the stomach and intestines
gastroesophageal reflux disease (GERD)	gas'trō-ĕ-sŏ-fā'jē-ăl rē'flŭks di-zēz'	backward flow of stomach acid into the esophagus
hemorrhoids	hem'ŏr-oydz	swollen (varicose) veins in the anal region; may be internal or external (**Figure 12-11**)
hepatomegaly	hep'ă-tō-meg'ă-lē	enlargement of the liver

(continued)

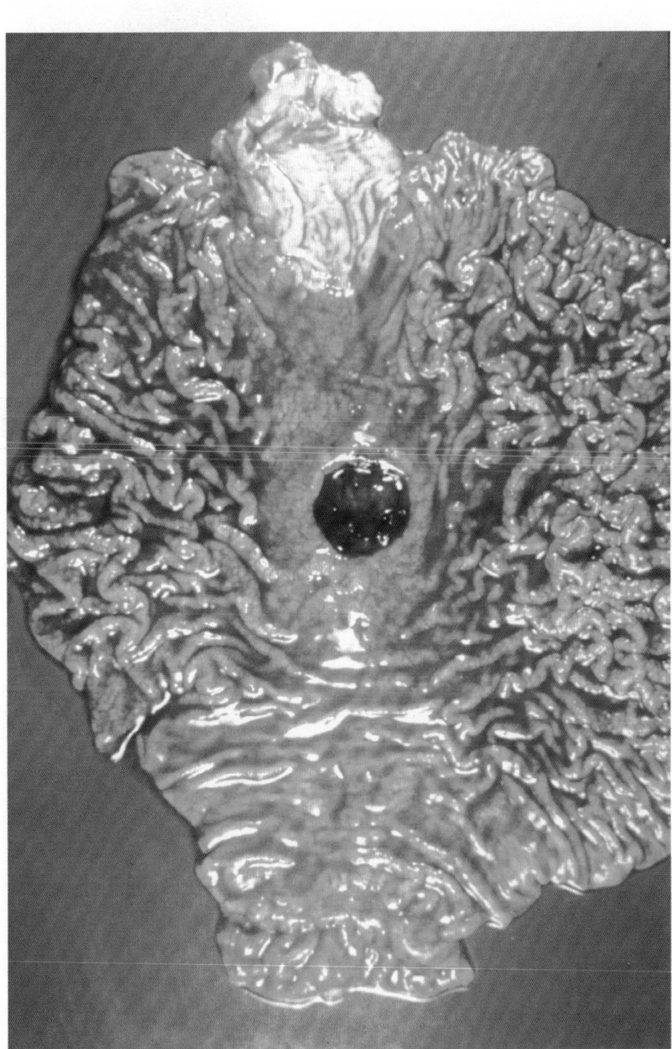

Figure 12-10 The stomach has been opened to reveal a deep gastric ulcer.

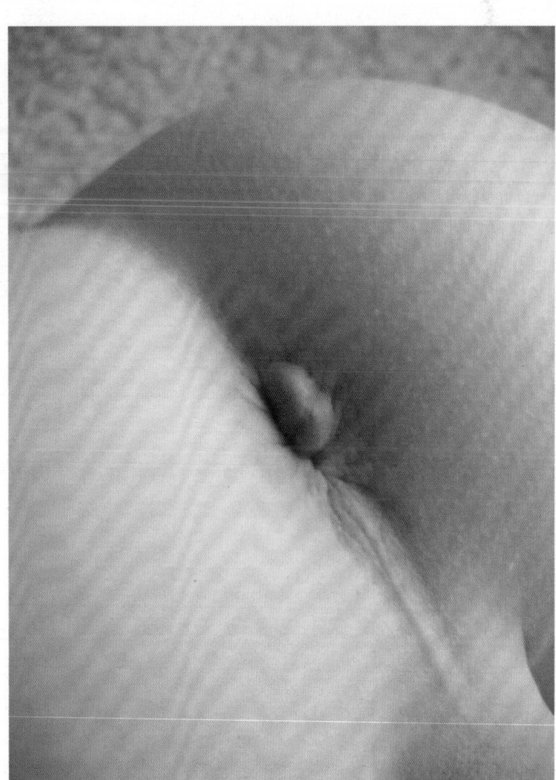

Figure 12-11 External hemorrhoid in a 2-year-old boy who with recurrent straining due to chronic constipation.

Medical Conditions *(continued)*

Term	Pronunciation	Meaning
hiatal hernia	hī-ā'tăl hĕr'nē-ă	protrusion of a part of the stomach through the esophageal hiatus (opening) in the diaphragm (**Figure 12-12**)
ileus	il'ē-ŭs	an obstruction of the intestine
incontinence	in-kon'ti-nĕns	inability to prevent the discharge of feces or urine
intussusception	in'tŭs-sŭs-sep'shŭn	the sliding (enfolding) of one section of the intestine into an adjacent section, much like the parts of a collapsible telescope (**Figure 12-13**)
irritable bowel syndrome (IBS); *syn.* spastic colon	ir'i-tă-bĕl bow'ĕl sin'drōm; spas'tik kō'lŏn	painful intestinal disease characterized by constipation alternating with diarrhea
pancreatitis	pan'krē-ă-tī'tis	inflammation of the pancreas

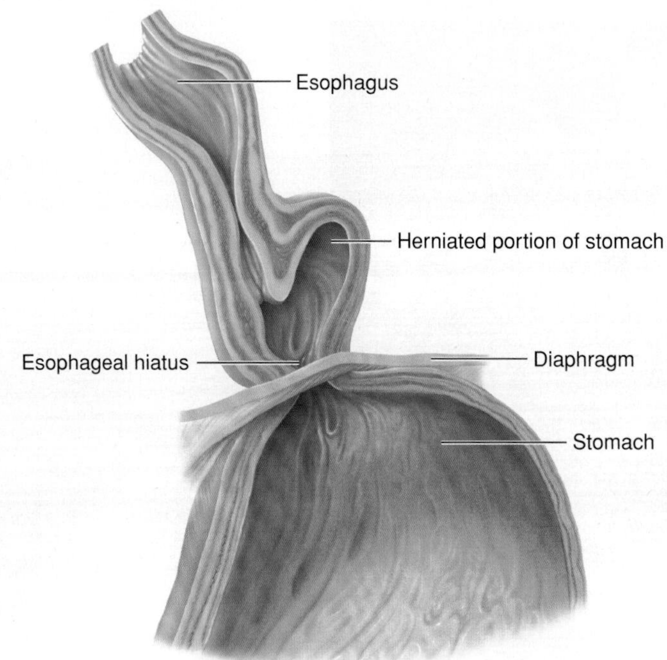

Figure 12-12 Hiatal hernia.

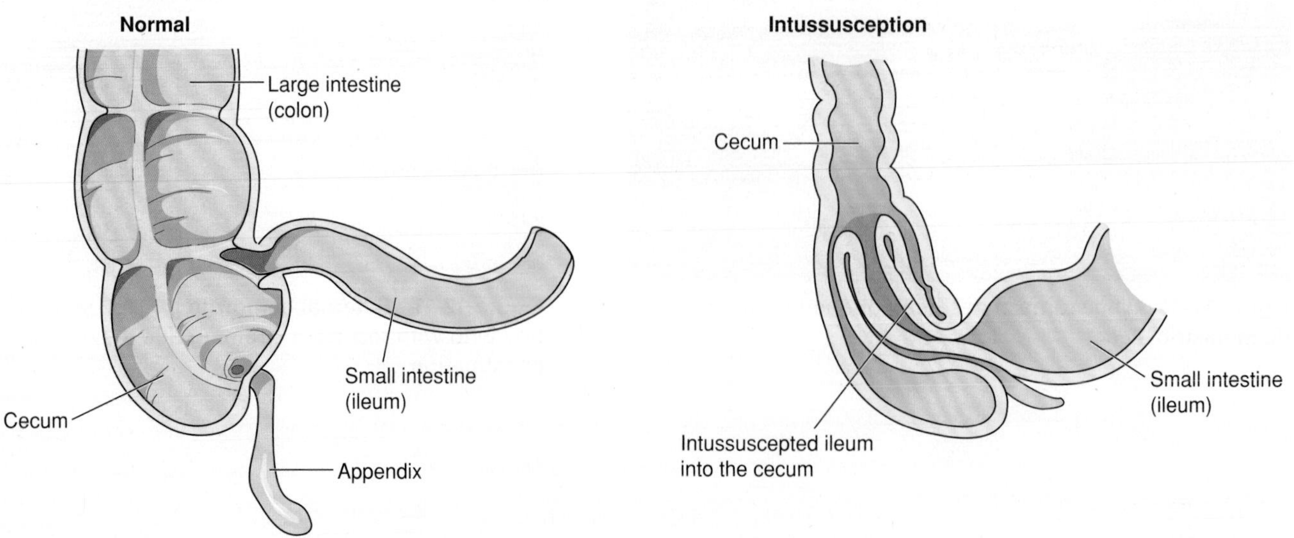

Figure 12-13 Intussusception of the ileum.

Medical Conditions

Term	Pronunciation	Meaning
peptic ulcer; *syn.* peptic ulcer disease (PUD)	pep′tik ŭl′ser; pep′tik ŭl′ser di-zēz′	ulcer of the stomach or duodenum that is caused by gastric acid
peritonitis	per′i-tō-nī′tis	inflammation of the peritoneal cavity
polyp	pol′ip	section of tissue that grows abnormally and protrudes from a surface (**Figure 12-14**)
polyposis	pol′i-pō′sis	condition characterized by the presence of several polyps
pruritus ani	prūr-ī′tŭs ā′nī	itching around the opening of the anus
ulcerative colitis	ŭl′sĕr-ă-tiv kō-lī′tis	painful condition in which ulcers form in the colon and rectum (**Figure 12-15**)
volvulus	vol′vyū-lŭs	a twisting of the intestine that can cause obstruction

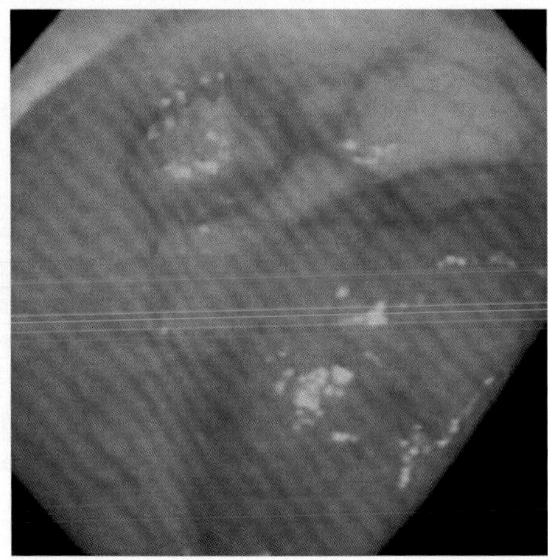

Figure 12-14 Polyp as seen through an endoscope.

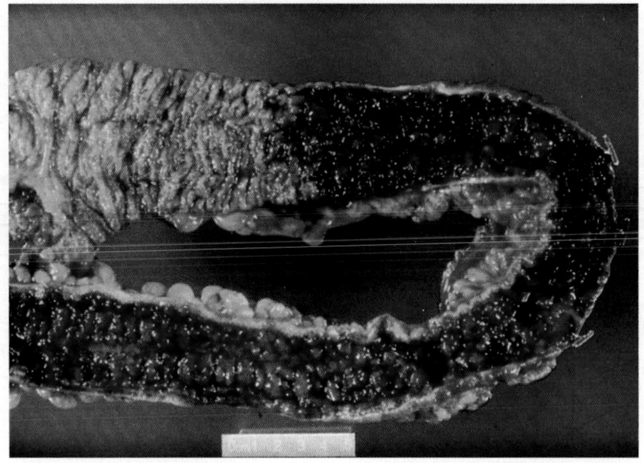

Figure 12-15 Ulcerative colitis of the ascending colon and rectosigmoid area.

Exercises: Medical Conditions

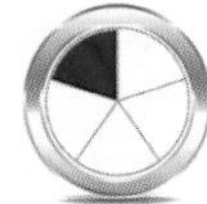

SIMPLE RECALL

Exercise 13

Write the correct medical term for the meaning given.

1. fluid in the abdominal cavity ______________________
2. eating disorder involving an aversion to eating ______________________
3. a twisting of the intestine ______________________

4. backward flow of stomach acids into the esophagus __________

5. chronic enteritis __________

6. an obstruction of the intestine __________

7. inability to prevent the discharge of feces or urine __________

8. anal itching __________

9. sore on the stomach lining __________

10. protrusion of the stomach through the diaphragm __________

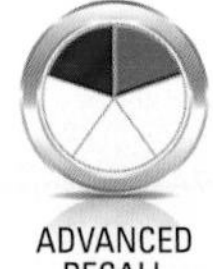

ADVANCED RECALL

Exercise 14

Circle the term that is most appropriate for the meaning of the sentence.

1. During the sigmoidoscopy, Ms. Heller was found to have in her colon several abnormal pouches known as (*volvulus, intussusception, diverticula*).

2. After three treatments of peritoneal dialysis inflamed her peritoneum, Mrs. Jonas developed an infection that was diagnosed as (*cholecystitis, gastritis, peritonitis*).

3. Ms. Amity was constantly straining with bowel movements and subsequently began to have irregular bowel movements with hard and small stools. This is known as (*pancreatitis, constipation, polyposis*).

4. The medical assistant noticed that Ms. LaRocca had lost weight during her last four visits and asked Ms. LaRocca about her appetite. The patient stated she had lost interest in food and was not eating a normal amount each day. The physician is concerned that Ms. LaRocca has (*pruritus ani, ulcerative colitis, anorexia nervosa*).

5. Mr. Hernandez has a disease with frequent watery, bloody diarrhea; this disease is called (*Crohn disease, gastroenteritis, dysentery*).

6. When the patient complained of extreme pain in the stomach, the physician ran tests for (*incontinence, peptic ulcer disease, hemorrhoids*).

7. The physician diagnosed Mr. Smith with the chronic liver disease called (*cholelithiasis, cholecystitis, cirrhosis*).

8. Mr. Hansen complained of abdominal pain, constipation, and diarrhea and was found to have (*intussusception, irritable bowel syndrome, ulcerative colitis*).

9. During an endoscopic examination, Mrs. Reyes was found to have a (*pruritus ani, spastic colon, polyp*), which is a section of tissue that grows abnormally and protrudes from a surface.

10. After surgery, Ms. Adams was told that part of her intestine had folded inside itself, a condition known as (*intussusception, ileus, incontinence*).

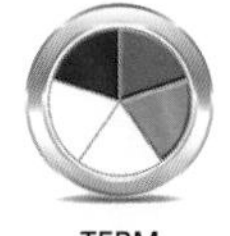

TERM CONSTRUCTION

Exercise 15

Using the given suffix, build a medical term for the meaning given.

Suffix	Meaning of Medical Term	Medical Term
-itis	inflammation of the pancreas	1. ______
-algia	pain in the stomach	2. ______
-osis	abnormal condition of polyps	3. ______
-itis	inflammation of the stomach and small intestine	4. ______
-megaly	enlargement of the liver	5. ______
-iasis	condition of gallstones	6. ______
-itis	inflammation of the gallbladder	7. ______

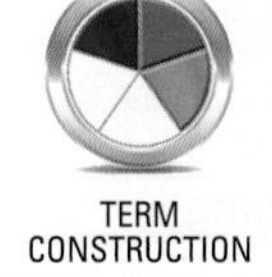

TERM CONSTRUCTION

Exercise 16

Write the combining form used in the medical term, followed by the meaning of the combining form.

Term	Combining Form	Combining Form Meaning
1. polyposis	______	______
2. hepatomegaly	______	______
3. diverticulitis	______	______
4. esophageal	______	______
5. cholecystitis	______	______
6. stomatitis	______	______
7. hematemesis	______	______
8. appendicitis	______	______
9. dysphagia	______	______
10. cheilosis	______	______

Tests and Procedures

Term	Pronunciation	Meaning
Laboratory Tests		
occult blood test; *syn.* hemoccult test	ŏ-kŭlt′ blŭd test; hēm′ō-kŭlt′ test	screening test that detects hidden blood in feces; the amount of blood is too small to be seen, but is detectable by chemical tests
stool culture	stūl kŭl′chŭr	microscopic examination of feces for identification of possible pathogens
Diagnostic Procedures		
abdominal ultrasound	ab-dom′ĭ-năl ŭl′tră-sownd	use of sound waves to view digestive system organs/structures (**Figure 12-16**)
abdominocentesis; *syn.* paracentesis	ab-dom′i-nō-sen-tē′sis; par′ă-sen-tē′sis	puncture into the abdomen to obtain fluid for culture or to relieve pressure
barium enema (BE)	bar′ē-ŭm en′ĕ-mă	use of contrast dye to view the lower gastrointestinal tract (**Figure 12-17**)
cholecystogram	kō′lĕ-sis′tŏ-gram	x-ray record of the gallbladder
colonoscopy	kō′lŏn-os′kŏ-pē	visual examination of the colon using an endoscope
endoscopy	en-dos′kŏ-pē	visual examination of organ interior using an endoscope (**Figure 12-18**)
esophagogastroduodenoscopy (EGD)	ĕ-sof′ă-gō-gas′trō-dū′ō-den-os′kŏ-pē	visual examination of the esophagus, stomach, and duodenum, usually using a fiberoptic endoscope
flexible sigmoidoscopy	fleks′i-bĕl sig′moy-dos′kŏ-pē	visual examination of the interior of the sigmoid colon using a fiberoptic endoscope (**Figure 12-19**)
laparoscopy	lap′ă-ros′kŏ-pē	visual examination of the abdominopelvic cavity with a type of endoscope called a laparoscope (**Figure 12-20**)
proctoscopy	prok-tos′kŏ-pē	visual examination of the rectum and anus with an endoscope
upper gastrointestinal series (UGI); *syn.* barium swallow	ŭp′ĕr gas′trō-in-tes′ti-năl sēr′ēz; bar′ē-ŭm swahl′ō	radiographic contrast (x-ray with contrast dye) study of the esophagus, stomach, and duodenum

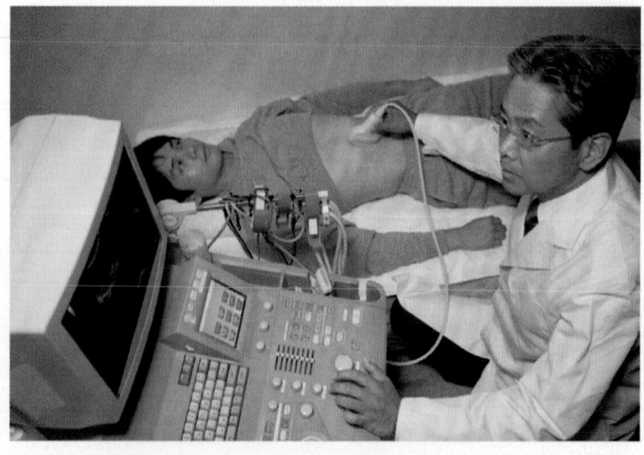

Figure 12-16 Abdominal ultrasound.

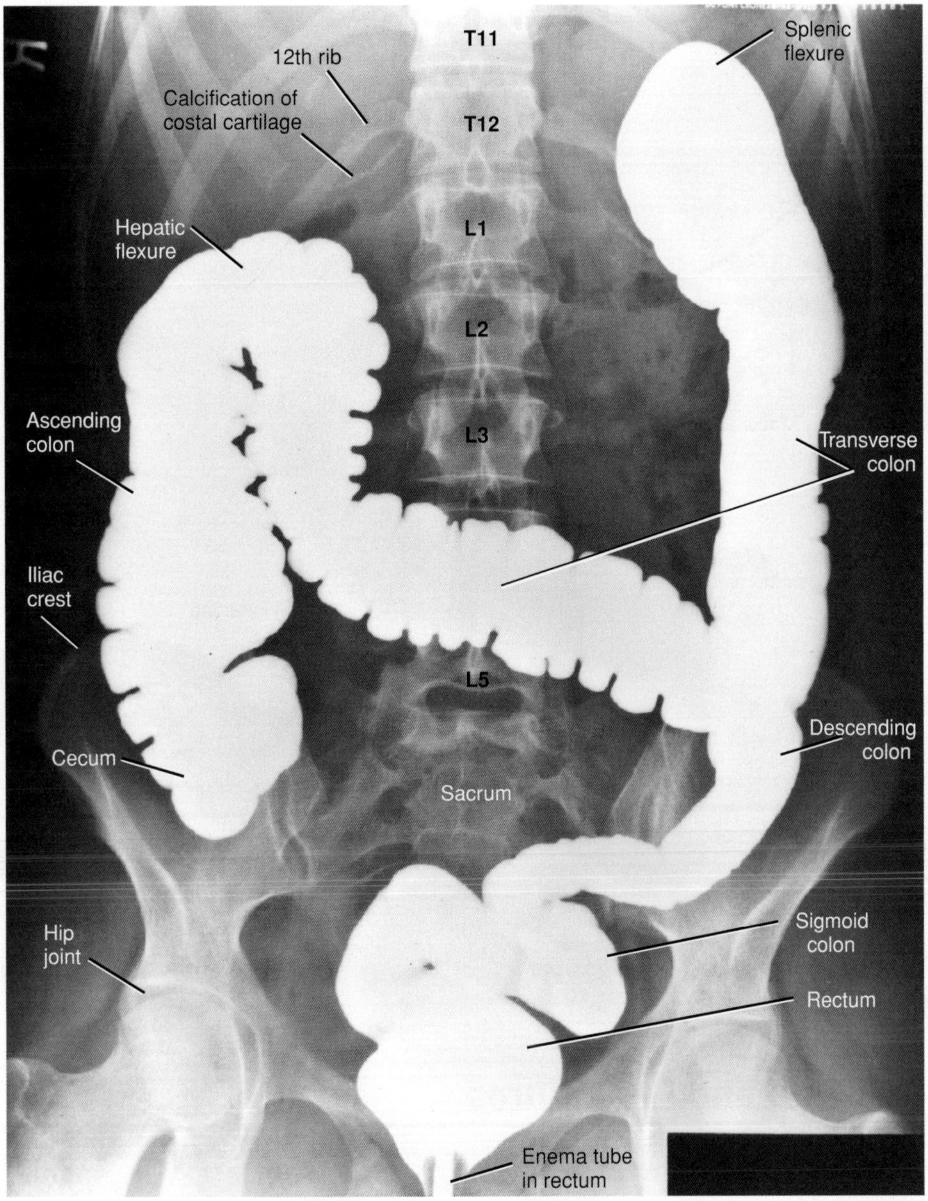

Figure 12-17 Barium enema.

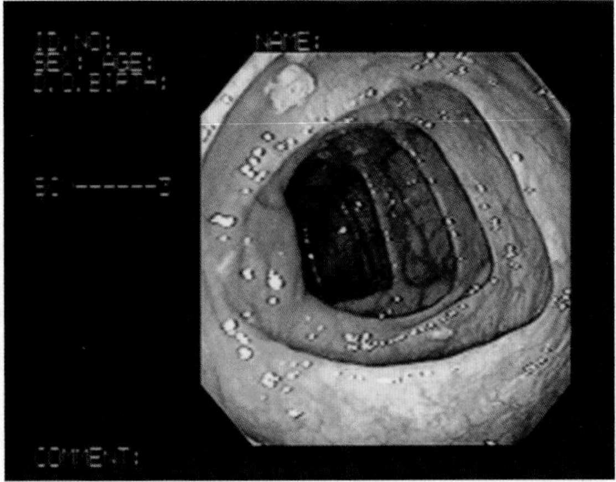

Figure 12-18 Endoscopic view of cecum.

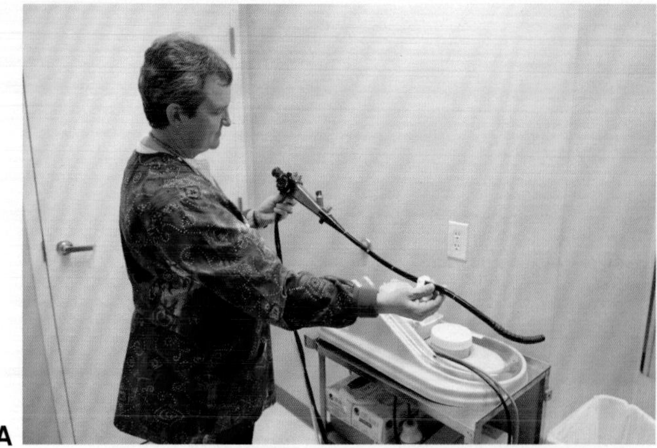

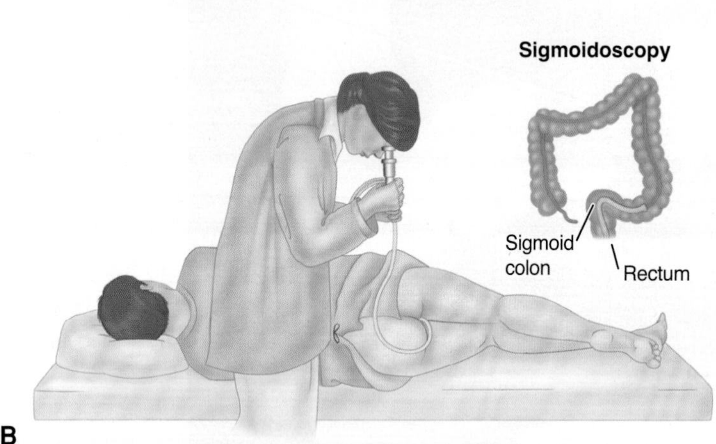

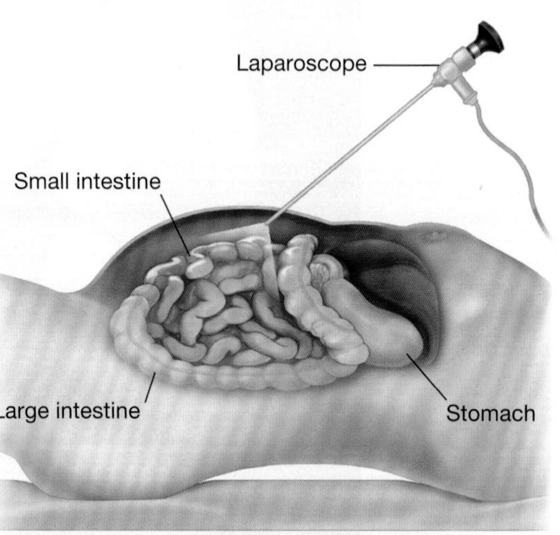

Figure 12-19 **A.** Medical assistant prepares a flexible sigmoidoscope. **B.** Flexible sigmoidoscopy.

Figure 12-20 Laparoscopy.

Exercises: Tests and Procedures

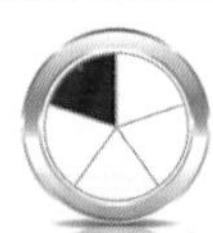

Exercise 17

Circle the term that is most appropriate for the meaning of the sentence.

1. A microscopic examination of feces for identification of possible pathogens is called a(n) (*occult blood test, proctoscopy, stool culture*).

2. A (*barium enema, barium swallow, colonoscopy*) is the viewing of the esophagus, stomach, and the duodenum with the use of contrast dye.

3. The use of an endoscope to examine the inside of organs is called (*endoscopy, colonoscopy, proctoscopy*).

4. Another name for abdominocentesis is (*barium enema, barium swallow, paracentesis*).

5. A (*hemoccult test, stool culture, proctoscopy*) is a type of test used to locate hidden blood in the feces.

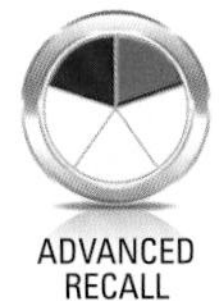
ADVANCED RECALL

Exercise 18

Complete each sentence by writing in the correct medical term.

1. Visual examination of the rectum and anus with an endoscope is called ____.
2. Visual examination of the interior of the sigmoid colon using a fiberoptic endoscope is called a(n) ____________________.
3. Visual examination of the colon using an endoscope is called a(n) ____.
4. The use of sound waves to view the digestive system is called ____________________.
5. The use of contrast dye to view the lower gastrointestinal tract is called a(n) ____________________.
6. An x-ray record of the gallbladder is called a(n) ____________________.
7. Visual examination of the esophagus, stomach, and duodenum, usually using a fiberoptic endoscope, is called ____________________.

TERM CONSTRUCTION

Exercise 19

Write the combining form used in the medical term, followed by the meaning of the combining form.

Term	Combining Form	Combining Form Meaning
1. abdominocentesis	________	________
2. cholecystogram	________	________
3. laparoscopy	________	________
4. sigmoidoscopy	________	________
5. colonoscopy	________	________
6. proctoscopy	________	________

Surgical Interventions and Therapeutic Procedures

Term	Pronunciation	Meaning
abdominoperineal resection (APR)	ab-dom′i-nō-per-i-nē′ăl rē-sek′shŭn	surgical removal of the colon and rectum by both abdominal and perineal approaches; includes a colostomy and is performed to treat severe lower intestinal diseases including cancer
abdominoplasty	ab-dom′i-nō-plas-tē	surgical repair of the abdominal area
anastomosis	ă-nas′tŏ-mō′sis	a connection made surgically between two structures, such as adjacent parts of the intestine
appendectomy	ap′pĕn-dek′tŏ-mē	surgical removal of the appendix

(continued)

Surgical Interventions and Therapeutic Procedures *(continued)*

Term	Pronunciation	Meaning
bariatric surgery	bar'ē-at'rik sŭr'jĕr-ē	surgical removal of parts of the stomach and/or intestines to induce weight loss

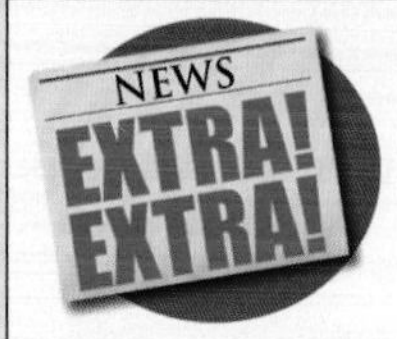

OBESITY Bariatric surgery is used for treatment of obesity. Obesity is defined as a body mass index of greater than 30 kg/m^2. Normal body mass index is between 18 and 24 kg/m^2.

Term	Pronunciation	Meaning
gastric bypass surgery	gas'trik bī'pas sŭr'jĕr-ē	surgical procedure in which the stomach is divided into a small upper pouch and a larger lower pouch and then the small intestine is rearranged and connected to both pouches (**Figure 12-21**)
cholecystectomy	kō'lĕ-sis-tek'tŏ-mē	removal of the gallbladder
cholelithotripsy	kō'lĕ-lith'ō-trip-sē	crushing of gallstones
colostomy	kō-los'tŏ-mē	surgical construction of an artificial opening between the colon and the body exterior; done to bypass a damaged part of the colon, so the sites vary (**Figure 12-22**)
gastrectomy	gas-trek'tŏ-mē	removal of the stomach

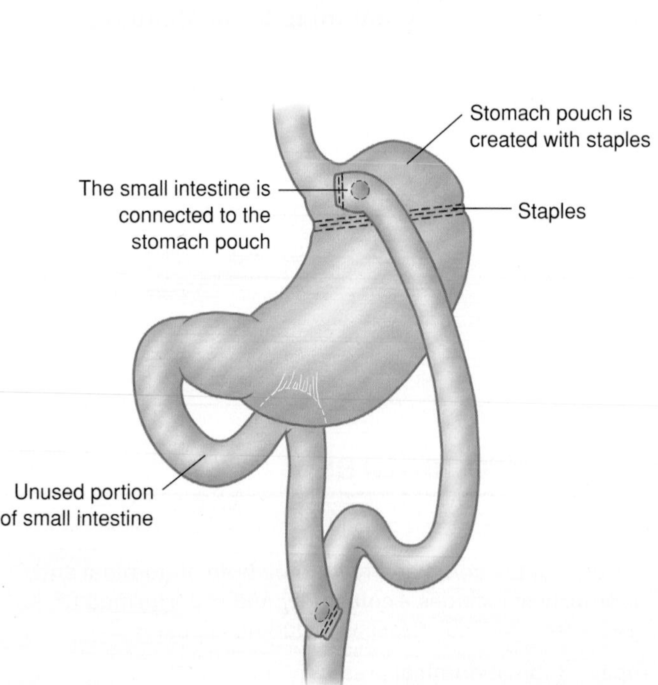

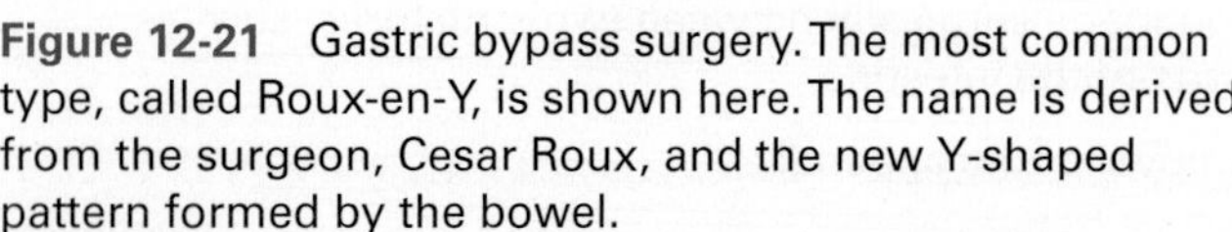
Figure 12-21 Gastric bypass surgery. The most common type, called Roux-en-Y, is shown here. The name is derived from the surgeon, Cesar Roux, and the new Y-shaped pattern formed by the bowel.

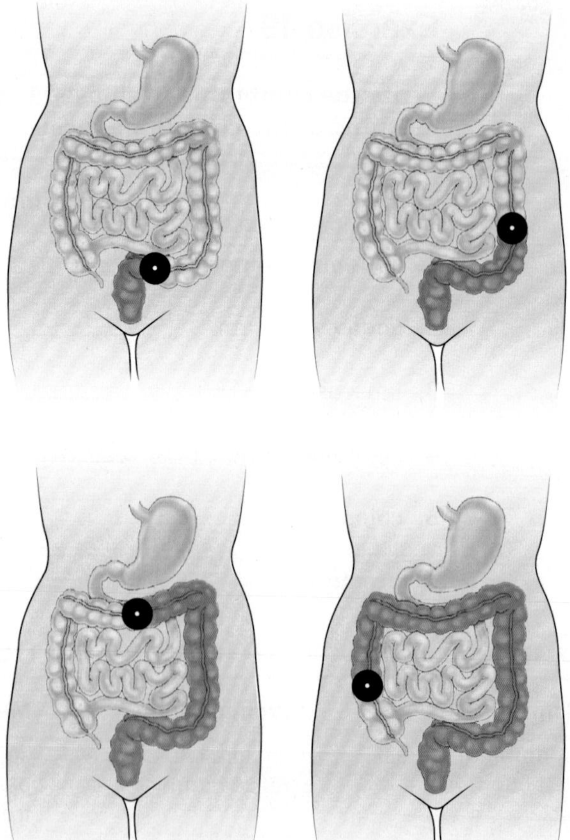
Figure 12-22 Various sites for a colostomy.

Surgical Interventions and Therapeutic Procedures

Term	Pronunciation	Meaning
gastric lavage	gas'trik lă-vahzh'	insertion of a tube from the mouth into the stomach to wash and suction out its contents for examination and treatment; usually done to remove blood clots or monitor bleeding
gastric resection	gas'trik rē-sek'shŭn	removal of a section of the stomach
gavage	gă-vahzh'	process of feeding a patient through nasogastric intubation
glossorrhaphy	glos-ōr'ă-fē	suturing of the tongue
herniorrhaphy	hĕr'nē-ōr'ă-fē	suturing of a hernia
ileostomy	il'ē-os'tŏ-mē	surgical construction of an artificial opening between the ileum and the body exterior; done to bypass a damaged part of the ileum
laparotomy	lap'ă-rot'ŏ-mē	surgical incision into the abdominal cavity
nasogastric (NG) intubation	nā'zō-gas'trik in'tū-bā'shŭn	insertion of a tube from the nose into the stomach for feeding or suctioning stomach contents
palatoplasty	pal'ă-tō-plas-tē	surgical repair of the roof of the mouth
polypectomy	pol'i-pek'tŏ-mē	surgical removal of polyps (**Figure 12-23**)
total parenteral nutrition (TPN)	tō'tăl pă-ren'tĕr-ăl nū-trish'ŭn	feeding a person intravenously or by a nasogastric tube

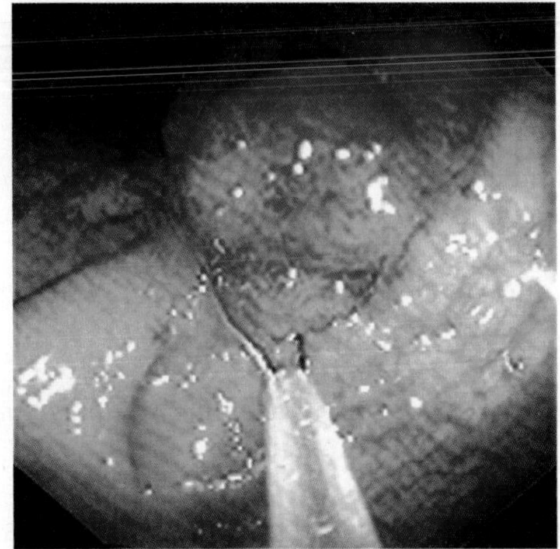

Figure 12-23 Endoscopic colon polypectomy.

Exercises: Surgical Interventions and Therapeutic Procedures

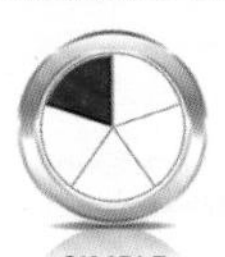

Exercise 20

Write the meaning of the term given.

1. laparotomy ______________________
2. glossorrhaphy ______________________

3. gastrectomy ______________________

4. gavage ______________________

5. palatoplasty ______________________

6. gastric resection ______________________

7. anastomosis ______________________

8. cholelithotripsy ______________________

9. appendectomy ______________________

10. ileostomy ______________________

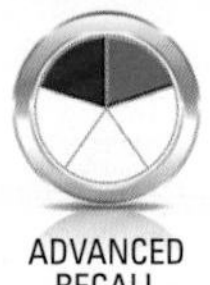

Exercise 21

Circle the term that is most appropriate for the meaning of the sentence.

1. Mr. Juno was morbidly obese, so his physician suggested (*abdominoperineal resection, bariatric surgery, gastric lavage*) to manage his condition.

2. Due to severe intestinal disease, Mrs. Wainwright underwent a(n) (*gavage, gastrectomy, abdominoperineal resection*), which included a colostomy.

3. After the car accident, the patient was unable to eat due to his comatose state and had to be fed by a process known as (*anoscopy, gavage, laparotomy*).

4. To correct the condition of cleft palate, the patient underwent a (*glossorrhaphy, lingulectomy, palatoplasty*).

5. Mr. Ruiz underwent an ileocolostomy, which is an (*anastomosis, oligodontia, effusion*) between the large intestine and the ileum.

6. Because Mr. Taylor had been diagnosed with multiple gallstones, the physician suggested that he have a(n) (*colotomy, appendectomy, cholecystectomy*) to treat the condition.

7. Mr. Gray had a large amount of blood in his stomach, so the physician ordered (*gastric lavage, total parenteral nutrition, gastric bypass*).

8. A patient who has a tube inserted through the nose and into the stomach has had (*herniorrhaphy, gastric lavage, nasogastric intubation*).

9. The physician ordered (*TPN, NG, GL*), which is feeding a person intravenously or by a nasogastric tube.

10. Mrs. Anderson had a(n) (*gastric lavage, gastric bypass, abdominoperineal resection*), which included a stomach stapling and anastomosis to the jejunum.

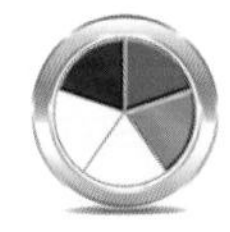

Exercise 22

TERM CONSTRUCTION

Build the correct medical term for the meaning given. Write the term in the blank and then indicate the word parts (P = prefix, CF = combining form, S = suffix).

1. surgical opening into the colon ______/______
   CF S
2. producing images of the pancreas ______/______
   CF S
3. pertaining to surrounding the tooth ______/______/______
   P CF S
4. suture of the lip ______/______
   CF S
5. surgical incision into the ileum ______/______
   CF S
6. crushing of stones in the gallbladder ______/______/______
   CF CF S
7. surgical removal of polyps ______/______
   CF S
8. surgical removal of half the colon ______/______/______
   P CF S
9. surgical repair of the abdomen ______/______
   CF S

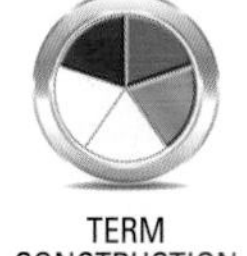

Exercise 23

TERM CONSTRUCTION

For each term, first write the meaning of the term. Then write the meanings of the word parts in that term.

1. palatoplasty ______
   palat/o ______
   -plasty ______
2. colostomy ______
   colon/o ______
   -stomy ______
3. herniorrhaphy ______
   herni/o ______
   -rrhaphy ______

4. ileostomy ______________________

ile/o ______________________

-tomy ______________________

5. appendectomy ______________________

appendic/o ______________________

-ectomy ______________________

6. glossorrhaphy ______________________

gloss/o ______________________

-rrhaphy ______________________

Medications and Drug Therapies

Term	Pronunciation	Meaning
antacid	ant-as′id	drug used to reduce stomach acid or neutralize acidity
antidiarrheal	an′tē-dī-ă-rē′ăl	drug used to treat or prevent diarrhea
antiemetic	an′tē-ĕ-met′ik	drug used to treat or prevent nausea and vomiting
emetic	ĕ-met′ik	drug used to induce vomiting
laxative; *syn.* cathartic	lak′să-tiv; kă-thahr′tik	drug used to promote the expulsion of feces

■ Exercise: Medications and Drug Therapies

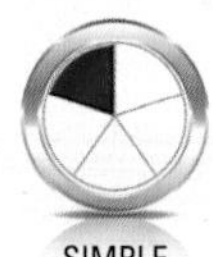
SIMPLE RECALL

Exercise 24

Write the correct medication or drug therapy term for the meaning given.

1. used to stop diarrhea ______________________

2. used to relieve constipation ______________________

3. used to decrease stomach acid or neutralize acidity ______________________

4. used to induce vomiting ______________________

5. used to stop vomiting ______________________

Specialties and Specialists

Term	Pronunciation	Meaning
bariatrics	bar′ē-at′riks	branch of medicine concerned with the prevention and control of obesity and allied diseases
gastroenterology	gas′trō-en-tĕr-ol′ŏ-jē	medical specialty concerned with diagnosis and treatment of disorders of the gastrointestinal tract
gastroenterologist	gas′trō-en-tĕr-ol′ŏ-jist	physician who specializes in gastroenterology
proctology	prok-tol′ŏ-jē	medical specialty concerned with diagnosis and treatment of disorders of the rectum and anus
proctologist	prok-tol′ŏ-jist	physician who specializes in proctology

■ Exercise: Specialties and Specialists

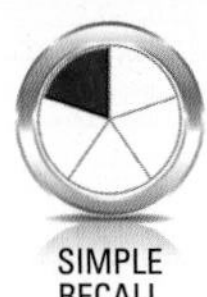

Exercise 25

Write the meaning of the term given.

1. gastroenterology ______________________
2. proctologist ______________________
3. proctology ______________________
4. gastroenterologist ______________________
5. bariatrics ______________________

Abbreviations

Abbreviation	Meaning
APR	abdominoperineal resection
BE	barium enema
BM	bowel movement
EGD	esophagogastroduodenoscopy
GERD	gastroesophageal reflux disease
GI	gastrointestinal
IBS	irritable bowel syndrome
LES	lower esophageal sphincter
NG	nasogastric
PUD	peptic ulcer disease
TPN	total parenteral nutrition
UGI	upper gastrointestinal

Exercises: Abbreviations

Exercise 26

SIMPLE RECALL

Write the meaning of each abbreviation.

1. GI ________________
2. BE ________________
3. TPN ________________
4. EGD ________________
5. NG ________________
6. UGI ________________
7. GERD ________________

Exercise 27

ADVANCED RECALL

Match each abbreviation with the appropriate description.

BE	PUD	IBS
BM	APR	

1. intestinal condition with symptoms of gas, bloating, diarrhea, constipation, and pain ________________
2. passage of feces ________________
3. condition that affects the stomach ________________
4. surgical removal of the colon and rectum ________________
5. use of contrast dye to view the lower gastrointestinal tract ________________

WRAPPING UP

- The gastrointestinal tract is a continuous tube that runs from the mouth to the anus.
- Rhythmic contractions (peristalsis) move material all the way through the body.
- The function of the digestive system (also called the gastrointestinal system) is to break down food into components that the body can use. If the body cannot use something, it is stored or excreted as feces.
- In this chapter, you learned medical terminology including word parts, prefixes, suffixes, adjectives, conditions, tests, procedures, medications, specialties, and abbreviations related to the digestive system.

Chapter Review

Review of Terms for Anatomy and Physiology

Exercise 28

Write the correct terms on the blanks for the anatomic structures indicated.

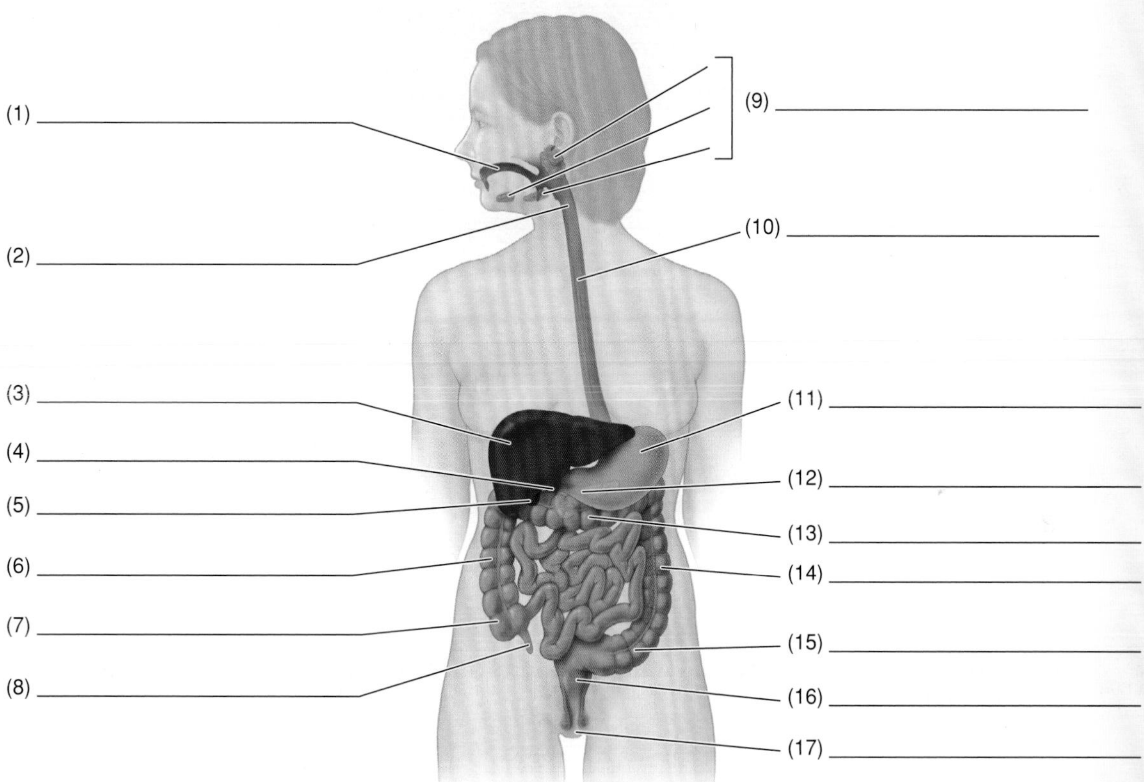

12 Digestive System

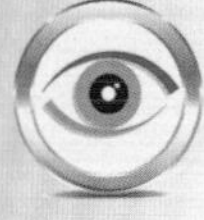

Exercise 29

Write the correct terms on the blanks for the anatomic structures indicated.

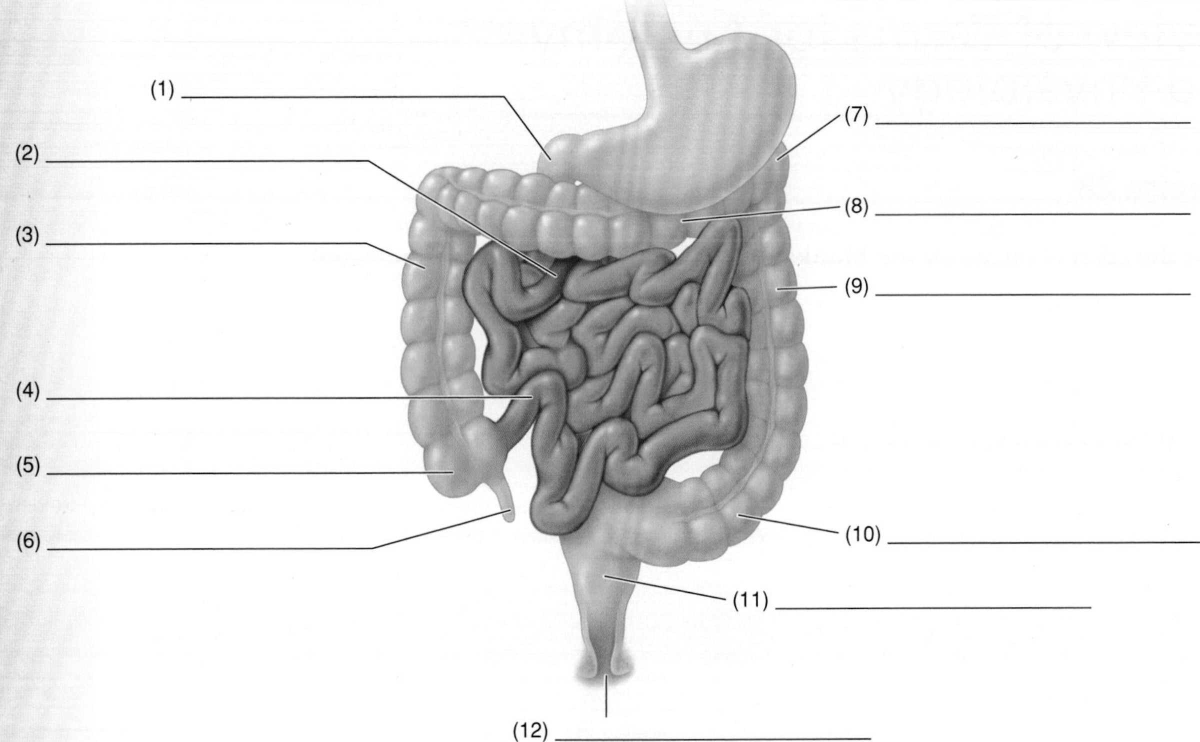

Understanding Term Structure

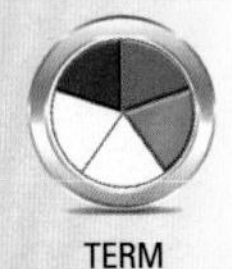

Exercise 30

For each term, first write the meaning of the term. Then write the meanings of the word parts in that term.

1. pyloroplasty ______________________

pylor/o ______________________

-plasty ______________________

2. esophagocele ______________________

esophag/o ______________________

-cele ______________________

3. gastrodynia ______________________

gastr/o ______________________

-dynia ______________________

4. stomatomalacia __________

stomat/o __________

-malacia __________

5. hepatomegaly __________

hepat/o __________

-megaly __________

6. laparogastroscopy __________

lapar/o __________

gastr/o __________

-scopy __________

7. anoscope __________

an/o __________

-scope __________

8. cheilophagia __________

cheil/o __________

-phagia __________

9. sigmoidoproctostomy __________

sigmoid/o __________

proct/o __________

-stomy __________

10. enterocolitis __________

enter/o __________

col/o __________

-itis __________

11. rectostenosis __________

rect/o __________

-stenosis __________

12. cheilorrhaphy ______________________

cheil/o ______________________

-rrhaphy ______________________

13. odontalgia ______________________

odont/o ______________________

-algia ______________________

14. appendicopathy ______________________

appendic/o ______________________

-pathy ______________________

15. cholelithotomy ______________________

chol/e ______________________

lith/o ______________________

-tomy ______________________

16. jejunostomy ______________________

jejun/o ______________________

-stomy ______________________

17. esophagogastrectomy ______________________

esophag/o ______________________

gastr/o ______________________

-ectomy ______________________

18. proctoptosis ______________________

proct/o ______________________

-ptosis ______________________

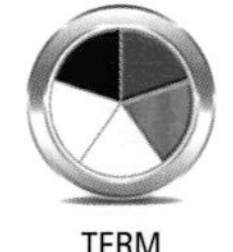
TERM CONSTRUCTION

Exercise 31

Write the combining form used in the medical term, followed by the meaning of the combining form.

Term	Combining Form	Combining Form Meaning
1. sialocele	__________	__________
2. alimentary	__________	__________
3. pylorostenosis	__________	__________
4. pharyngospasm	__________	__________
5. duodenorrhaphy	__________	__________
6. gastroenteropathy	__________	__________
7. hepatectomy	__________	__________
8. palatoplasty	__________	__________
9. buccopharyngeal	__________	__________
10. dentofacial	__________	__________
11. cecostomy	__________	__________
12. proctologist	__________	__________
13. polyposis	__________	__________

Comprehension Exercises

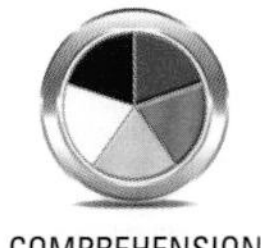
COMPREHENSION

Exercise 32

Fill in the blank with the correct term.

1. Puncture into the abdomen to remove fluid and relieve abdominal pressure is called ____________________.
2. A specialist whose focus is on disorders of the rectum and anus is called a(n) ____________________.
3. The test used to identify the presence of occult blood is called a(n) ____________________.
4. When stomach acid begins to flow backward into the esophagus, this disease is called ____________________.
5. Excessive vomiting is called ____________________.

6. To remove stones from the pancreas, a patient would have a surgery known as
_______________.

7. An anastomosis between the stomach and the small intestine is called a(n) _______________
_______________.

Exercise 33

COMPREHENSION

Circle the letter of the best answer in the following questions.

1. A patient diagnosed with _______________ experiences problems during mastication.
   A. esophagitis
   B. odontitis
   C. hepatitis
   D. laryngitis

2. Which of the following is not a primary organ of the digestive system?
   A. liver
   B. stomach
   C. large intestine
   D. pharynx

3. The substance that helps to form a bolus in the mouth is called
   A. chyme.
   B. stoma.
   C. saliva.
   D. uvula.

4. The correct order of the segments of the small intestine is
   A. duodenum, jejunum, ileum.
   B. duodenum, ileum, jejunum.
   C. ileum, duodenum, jejunum.
   D. jejunum, duodenum, ileum.

5. Surgical repair of the rectum is called
   A. anoplasty.
   B. sigmoidoplasty.
   C. rectoplasty.
   D. hepatoplasty.

6. Which condition does not involve the passing of hard stools?
   A. spastic colon
   B. dysentery
   C. constipation
   D. irritable bowel syndrome

7. A gastric lavage is performed for blood clots in the
   A. stomach.
   B. palate.
   C. mouth.
   D. anus.

8. A dangerous twisting of the colon is called
   A. ileus.
   B. ilius.
   C. volvulus.
   D. intussusception.

9. Black, tarry stools contain what substance?
   A. diarrhea
   B. melena
   C. blood
   D. flatus

10. Increased fluid in the abdominal area that is not a normal finding is called
    A. ascites.
    B. eructation.
    C. cirrhosis.
    D. cholestasis.

11. Difficulty in the act of deglutition is called
    A. dyspepsia.
    B. dysentery.
    C. dysodontiasis.
    D. dysphagia.

12. Which condition involves the large organ that produces and secretes bile into the gallbladder?
    A. cirrhosis
    B. dysentery
    C. dysodontiasis
    D. pancreatitis

13. The procedure used to treat stones in the gallbladder without removing the gallbladder is called

    A. cholecystectomy.
    B. cholecystostomy.
    C. cholelithotripsy.
    D. cholelithiasis.

14. An incision into the duodenum is called a

    A. duodenoscopy.
    B. duodenostomy.
    C. duodenotomy.
    D. duodenorrhaphy.

15. The condition known as halitosis occurs in the

    A. stomach.
    B. rectum.
    C. anus.
    D. mouth.

Application and Analysis

CASE STUDIES

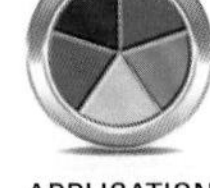

APPLICATION

Exercise 34

Read the case studies, and circle the correct letter for each of the questions.

CASE 12-1

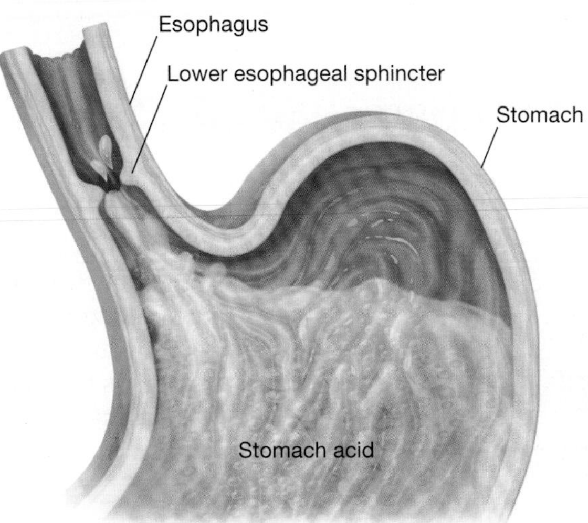

Figure 12-24 Stomach acid flowing back into the esophagus in gastroesophageal reflux disease (GERD).

Mr. Patel complained of dysphagia and dyspepsia. He stated these problems had been occurring for the past six months and were increasing in frequency. His physician diagnosed him with GERD (**Figure 12-24**) and encouraged him to stay away from chocolate and to decrease his caffeine intake.

1. The patient has been diagnosed with

    A. gastric regurgitation disease.
    B. gastroesophageal rectal disease.
    C. gastroesophageal reflux disease.
    D. gastric reflux disease.

2. Because of his dyspepsia, the patient has

    A. trouble with pepsin production.
    B. painful digestion.
    C. enlarged liver.
    D. decreased stomach acid production.

3. Backward flow of stomach acid into the esophagus is known as

A. dyspepsia.
B. gastric reflux.
C. dysphagia.
D. esophagitis.

CASE 12-2

Mr. Desalvo had been experiencing abdominal pain and anorexia for the past day, but when it became unbearable he went to the ER. This evening, the ER physician determined that Mr. Desalvo had peritonitis resulting from a ruptured appendix.

4. Peritonitis is defined as

A. inflammation of the palate.
B. inflammation of the pharynx.
C. inflammation of the peritoneum.
D. inflammation of the polyps.

5. To treat the ruptured appendix, the patient would have to undergo emergency

A. appendicolith.
B. appendectomy.
C. appendicostomy.
D. appendicopathy.

6. Anorexia is a condition characterized by

A. decreased flatus.
B. decreased bowel movements.
C. decreased appetite.
D. decreased digestion.

MEDICAL RECORD ANALYSIS

MEDICAL RECORD 12-1

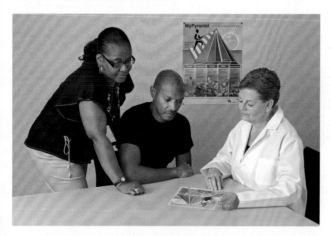

A nutritionist meets with a patient and his family to discuss his diet.

Mr. Riggins was recently seen by his family physician after finding blood in his stool. After Mr. Riggins's clinic visit, he was referred to you, a nutritionist, to answer any questions he and his family might have concerning the addition of fiber to his diet.

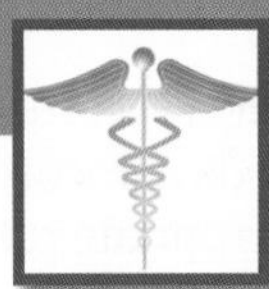

Medical Record

ANAL FISSURE

PATIENT: David Riggins
CHART NUMBER: 00675

PHYSICIAN: Dr. Henry Preston
DATE: March 21, 20XX

Patient presented to the clinic today with having had a BM this morning in which he noticed a large amount of bright red blood in the toilet. He denied any pain with the BM. This was the first time this has happened. No associated nausea and vomiting or diarrhea. He did mention that he has been constipated for the past week or so. He stated he had small, hard stools that he had to strain to pass a couple of times during the last week. The patient has no history of peptic ulcers or gastrointestinal cancer.

OBJECTIVE: Wt. 90 kg, BP 160/88, P 88. The patient is a well-developed, well-nourished male in no acute distress. Examination of the rectal area reveals a small tear in the rectal mucosa.

MEDICATIONS: Ibuprofen p.r.n.; metoprolol 50 mg b.i.d.

ASSESSMENT: The patient has a small anal fissure. This is most likely caused from several incidences of constipation with associated straining.

PLAN: The patient was instructed to increase the amount of fiber in his diet as well as to use an OTC laxative to increase the frequency of his BM and to soften the stool. He was advised to not strain, as this would increase the likelihood that any hard stools that are passed will worsen the tear. This should resolve on its own. The patient is instructed to call the clinic should he continue to have issues.

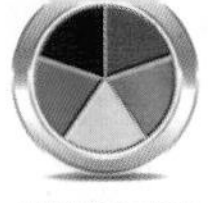

APPLICATION

Exercise 35

Write the appropriate medical terms used in this medical record on the blanks after their meanings. Note that not all the terms appear in the chapter, but you should be able to identify these terms based on word parts that are included in this chapter.

1. pertaining to the stomach and intestines ____________________
2. abnormally frequent discharge of semisolid or liquid feces ____________________
3. decreased number of bowel movements with passage of hard stools ____________________
4. passage of solid wastes (abbreviation) ____________________
5. the urge to vomit ____________________
6. pertaining to the anus ____________________
7. condition of the stomach or duodenum caused by gastric acid ____________________

Bonus Question

8. Recalling the meaning of the term fissure in Chapter 4, what is the definition of an anal fissure? ____________________

MEDICAL RECORD 12-2

As a medical coding specialist, you are responsible for evaluating patient medical records and documenting to accurately bill for services provided. You are reviewing the medical record that follows to determine the codes needed for submission to the insurance company for appropriate reimbursement.

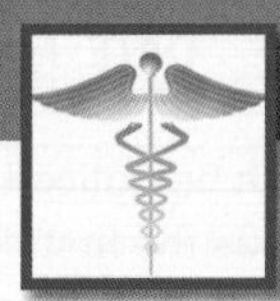

Medical Record

GERD

PATIENT: Adrian Edwards **PHYSICIAN:** Dr. Carter Price
CHART NUMBER: 03151 **DATE:** March 21, 20XX

Mr. Edwards came to the clinic today with complaints of heartburn and postprandial regurgitation. He states that these symptoms increase in severity soon after he lies down in his recliner after eating to watch TV. He is on no regular medications, except that he does take occasional Maalox when his symptoms are "too much to handle." These symptoms have only started to bother him recently, within the past month or so. He also complains of some flatus.

OBJECTIVE: This is an obese, well-developed male. Currently, he is in no distress. Weight today is 134 kg. This is an increase since his last visit six months ago when he weighed 116 kg. He has just recently lost his job and has stopped going to the gym because he let his membership lapse.

ASSESSMENT: GERD with increase in weight and decreased activity.

PLAN: Starting proton pump inhibitor b.i.d. Encouraged patient to try to get back into routine of exercise. Discussed dietary guidelines to decrease fatty food intake. Discussed the need to abstain from coffee, tea, chocolate, and activities such as lying down or reclining immediately or soon after eating. The patient was encouraged to raise the head of his bed about 2 in. If symptoms persist, Mr. Edwards is to return to clinic. More aggressive evaluation with endoscopy will then be scheduled.

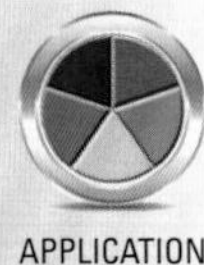

APPLICATION

Exercise 36

Read the medical report, and circle the letter of your answer choice for the following questions.

1. In GERD, the backward flow of acid into the esophagus comes from the

A. small intestine.
B. pharynx.
C. stomach.
D. mouth.

2. If the patient is scheduled for an endoscopy, the physician will

A. use an endoscope to examine the inside of the upper gastrointestinal tract.
B. obtain an x-ray examination of the esophagus.
C. view the condition of the mouth.
D. obtain a recording of the large intestine.

3. When does the patient experience regurgitation?

A. after meals
B. after defecating
C. after waking
D. before leaving for work

4. Flatus is

A. bile.
B. feces.
C. gas.
D. urine.

Bonus Question

5. Why is the patient encouraged to raise the head of his bed?______________________

____

Pronunciation and Spelling

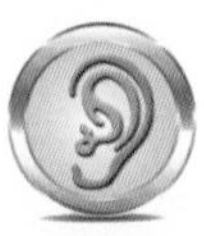
AUDITORY

Exercise 37

Review the Chapter 12 terms in the Dictionary/Audio Glossary in the Student Resources on thePoint, and practice pronouncing each term, referring to the pronunciation guide as needed.

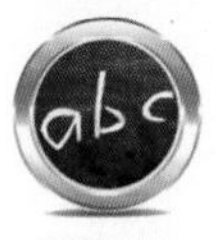
SPELLING

Exercise 38

Circle the correct spelling of each term.

1.	ruggae	rugay	rugae
2.	cecum	cecome	secum
3.	tonge	tunge	tongue
4.	regurgitation	regergatation	regergitashun
5.	illeus	ileus	eelius
6.	feeces	feces	fesees
7.	acult	ocult	occult
8.	pieloris	pilorus	pylorus
9.	youvyoula	uvule	uvula
10.	gavage	gabage	gavach
11.	nawsea	nausea	nalsea
12.	mastication	mastikashun	mustication
13.	polyposias	poliposis	polyposis
14.	pilate	palate	palit
15.	incontinence	incontinance	incontinense

Media Connection

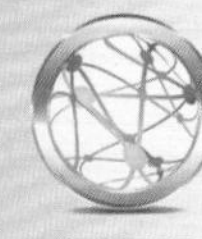
STUDENT RESOURCES

Exercise 39

Complete each of the following activities available with the Student Resources on thePoint. Check off each activity as you complete it, and record your score for the Chapter Quiz in the space provided.

Chapter Exercises

____ Flash Cards

____ Concentration

____ Abbreviation Match-Up

____ Roboterms

____ Word Anatomy

____ Fill the Gap

____ Break It Down

____ True/False Body Building

____ Quiz Show

____ Complete the Case

____ Medical Record Review

____ Look and Label

____ Image Matching

____ Spelling Bee

____ **Chapter Quiz** *Score:*________%

Additional Resources

____ Animation: *General Digestion*

____ Dictionary/Audio Glossary

____ Health Professions Careers: Nutritionist

____ Health Professions Careers: Medical Coding Specialist

Urinary System

13

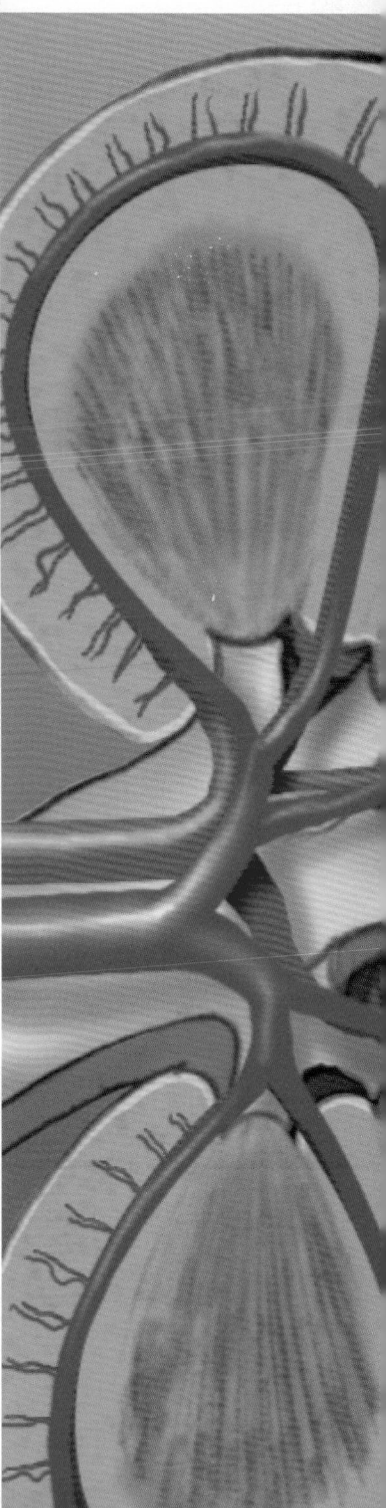

Chapter Outline

Introduction, 508

Anatomy and Physiology, 508
- Structures, 508
- Functions, 508
- Terms Related to the Urinary System, 509

Word Parts, 512
- Combining Forms, 512
- Prefixes, 512
- Suffixes, 512

Medical Terms, 516
- Adjectives and Other Related Terms, 516
- Medical Conditions, 518
- Tests and Procedures, 525
- Surgical Interventions and Therapeutic Procedures, 529
- Medications and Drug Therapies, 534
- Specialties and Specialists, 534
- Abbreviations, 535

Wrapping Up, 536

Chapter Review, 437

Learning Outcomes

After completing this chapter, you should be able to:

1. Describe the structures and functions of the urinary system.
2. Define terms related to the urinary system.
3. Define combining forms, prefixes, and suffixes related to the urinary system.
4. Define common medical terminology related to the urinary system, including adjectives and related terms; signs, symptoms, and medical conditions; tests and procedures; surgical interventions and therapeutic procedures; medications and drug therapies; and medical specialties and specialists.
5. Define abbreviations related to the urinary system.
6. Successfully complete all chapter exercises.
7. Explain terms used in case studies and medical records involving the urinary system.
8. Successfully complete all exercises included with the companion Student Resources on thePoint.

INTRODUCTION

The urinary system plays important roles in maintaining fluid and electrolyte (mineral) balance. It also rids the body of wastes, toxins, and drugs. The formation of urine begins with blood. As the blood is filtered through the kidneys, substances the body can use are retained, and those it cannot use are excreted as urine. This chapter gives an overview of the basic anatomy, physiology, and pathology of the urinary system while providing medical terms related to normal and abnormal functions.

ANATOMY AND PHYSIOLOGY

Structures (Figure 13-1)

- The kidneys remove wastes from the blood in the form of urine.
- The ureters carry urine from the kidneys to the bladder.
- The bladder stores urine prior to urination.
- The urethra carries urine from the bladder to the outside of the body.

Functions

- Filtering wastes from the body
- Regulating fluid levels and electrolytes and reclaiming important electrolytes and water
- Contributing to blood pressure control
- Playing a role in red blood cell production via the hormone erythropoietin, which is produced in the kidneys
- Carrying urine through the system until it is excreted during the process of urination

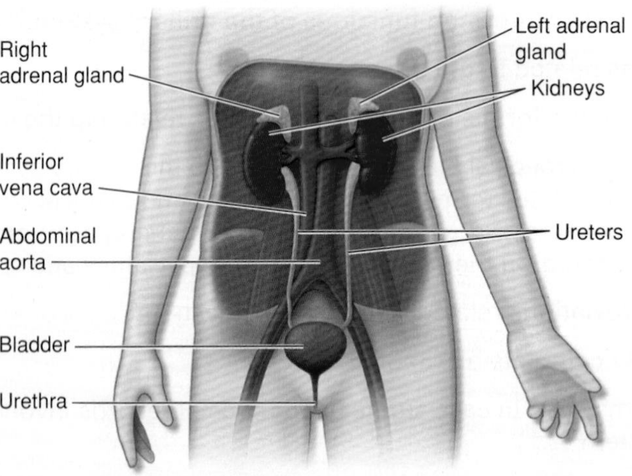

Figure 13-1 The urinary system.

Terms Related to the Urinary System

Term	Pronunciation	Meaning
kidney	kid′nē	one of two bean-shaped organs that remove wastes from the blood and help maintain fluid and electrolyte balance in the body **(Figure 13-2)**
calyx	kā′liks	cup-like structure that drains into the renal pelvis
renal artery	rē′năl ar′ter-ē	one of two vessels that branch off the abdominal aorta and supply the kidney with blood; left renal artery and right renal artery
renal cortex	rē′năl kōr′teks	outer part of the kidney
renal medulla	rē′năl me-dūl′ă	inner part of the kidney
renal pelvis	rē′năl pel′vis	a reservoir in each kidney that collects urine
renal vein	rē′năl vān	one of two blood vessels that drain the kidney and connect to the inferior vena cava; left renal vein and right renal vein
nephron	nef′ron	microscopic functional unit of the kidney that forms urine; found in the cortex and medulla, it consists of a renal corpuscle and its associated tubule; each kidney contains about 1 million nephrons **(Figure 13-3)**
renal corpuscle	rē′năl kōr′pŭs-ĕl	structure composed of the glomerulus and the glomerular capsule
glomerulus	glō-mer′yū-lŭs	one of several capillary clusters at the entrance of each nephron that initiate the process of filtering of the blood

(continued)

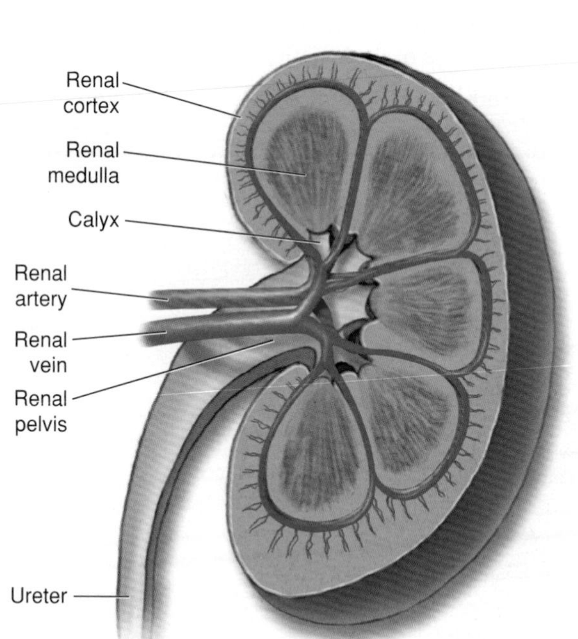

Figure 13-2 Cross-section of the left kidney.

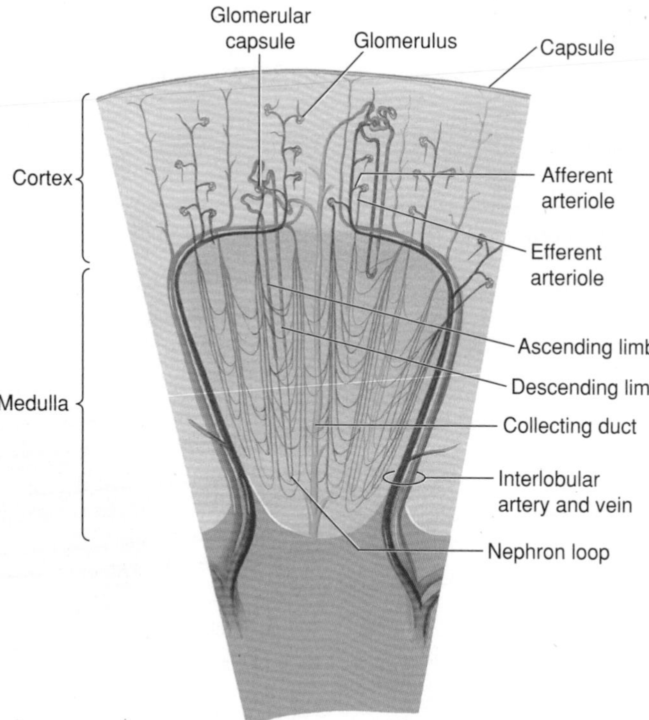

Figure 13-3 A representative nephron.

Terms Related to the Urinary System *(continued)*

Term	Pronunciation	Meaning
glomerular capsule; *syn.* Bowman capsule	glō-mer′yū-lăr kap′sūl; bō′măn kap′sūl	sac that surrounds the glomerulus (tuft of capillaries) and marks the beginning of the nephron
afferent arteriole	af′ĕr-ĕnt ar-tēr′ē-ōl	blood vessel that supplies the nephron
collecting duct	kə′lekt-ing dŭkt	tubule that connects the nephrons to the renal pelvis
distal convoluted tubule (DCT)	dis′tăl kon′vō-lūt′ed tū′byūl	segment of the nephron between the nephron loop and the collecting duct
efferent arteriole	ef′ĕr-ent ar-tēr′ē-ōl	blood vessel that forms from the convergence of the glomerular capillaries; takes blood to capillaries of proximal convoluted tubule
nephron loop	nef′ron lūp	U-shaped segment of the nephron between the proximal convoluted tubule and the distal convoluted tubule
peritubular capillaries	per′ē-tū′byū-lăr kap′i-lār-ēz	tiny blood vessels alongside the nephrons where reabsorption and secretion between the blood and the nephron takes place
proximal convoluted tubule (PCT)	prok′si-măl kon′vō-lūt′ed tū′byūl	segment of the nephron between the glomerular capsule and the nephron loop
ureter	yū′re-tur	one of two narrow tubes that carry urine from the kidneys to the bladder
urethra	yū-rē′thră	tubular structure through which urine passes from the urinary bladder to the outside of the body
urinary bladder[a]	yūr′i-nār′ē blad′er	muscular organ that holds the urine until it is released **(Figure 13-4)**
detrusor muscle	dē-trū′sŏr mŭs′ĕl	muscle that forms the urinary bladder
external urethral orifice	eks-ter′năl yū-rē′thrăl or′i-fis	opening that carries urine from the urethra to the outside of the body; external urethral meatus (opening) (see also **Figure 13-6A**)
trigone of bladder	trī′gōn ov blad′er	triangular region at the base of the urinary bladder between the openings of the two ureters and the urethra
urine	yūr′in	water, waste products, and other substances excreted by the kidneys

[a]The term *bladder* will refer to the urinary bladder in this chapter.

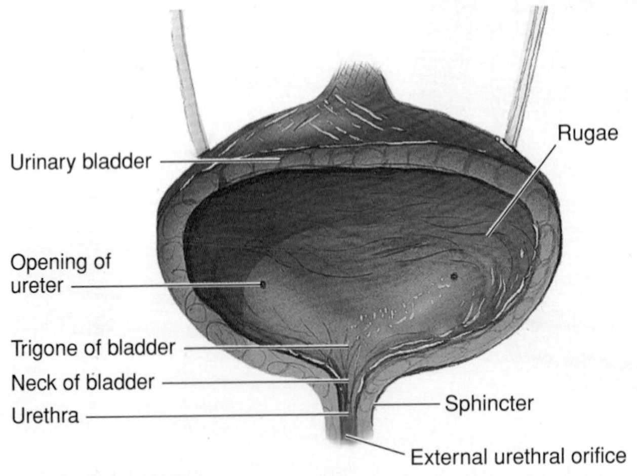

Figure 13-4 The urinary bladder.

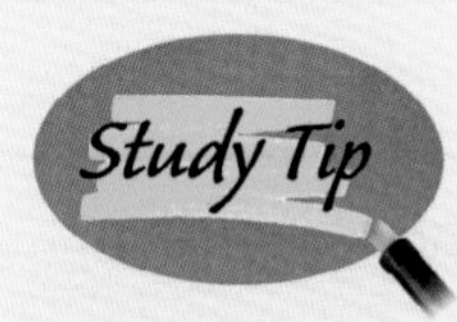

Ureters Versus Urethra: Here is an easy way to remember the difference between the ureters and the urethra: There are two ureters in the body, and the word *ureter* has two Es. There is only one urethra in the body, and the word *urethra* has only one "E."

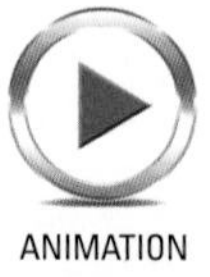
ANIMATION

To learn more about the function of the kidneys, view the animation "Renal Function" on the Student Resources on thePoint.

Exercises: Anatomy and Physiology

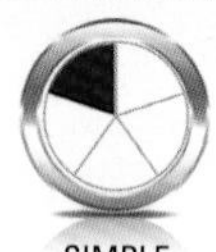
SIMPLE RECALL

Exercise 1

Write the meaning of the anatomic structure given.

1. external urethral orifice ______________________________
2. ureter ______________________________
3. kidney ______________________________
4. nephron ______________________________
5. renal pelvis ______________________________

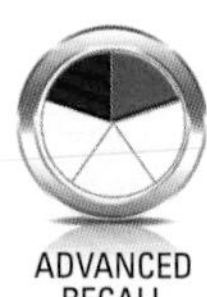
ADVANCED RECALL

Exercise 2

Match each medical term with its meaning.

renal cortex	glomerular capsule	glomerulus	urine
trigone of bladder	urethra	urinary bladder	

1. capillary cluster at entrance to nephrons ______________________________
2. outer part of kidney ______________________________
3. sac that surrounds the glomerulus ______________________________
4. tube carrying urine from bladder to outside of body ______________________________
5. muscular organ that holds urine until it is released ______________________________
6. triangular region at the base of the urinary bladder ______________________________
7. fluid excreted by the kidneys ______________________________

WORD PARTS

The following tables list word parts related to the urinary system.

Combining Forms

Combining Form	Meaning
albumin/o	albumin
bacteri/o	bacteria
cyst/o[a]	fluid-filled sac (urinary bladder)
enur/o	to urinate in
glomerul/o	glomerulus
glyc/o, glycos/o	glucose, sugar
hemat/o	blood
hydr/o	water, fluid
lith/o	stone, calculus
meat/o	meatus (opening)
nephr/o	kidney
noct/i	night
olig/o	scanty, few
py/o	pus
pyel/o	renal pelvis
ren/o	kidney
son/o	sound, sound waves
ureter/o	ureter
urethr/o	urethra
ur/o, urin/o	urine, urinary system/tract
vesicul/o, vesic/o	fluid-filled sac (urinary bladder)

[a]The combining form *cyst/o* may also refer to a cyst but will refer to the urinary bladder in this chapter unless otherwise noted.

Prefixes

Prefix	Meaning
dys-	painful, difficult, abnormal
gluco-	glucose (sugar)
poly-	many, much
ure-	urea, urine

Suffixes

Suffix	Meaning
-cele	herniation, protrusion
-emia	blood (condition of)
-iasis	condition of
-esis	condition of

Suffixes

Suffix	Meaning
-lith	stone, calculus
-lysis	destruction, breakdown, separation
-ptosis	prolapse, drooping, sagging
-scopy	viewing or examining with an instrument
-stenosis	stricture, narrowing
-stomy	surgical opening
-tripsy	crushing
-uria	urine, urination

Exercises: Word Parts

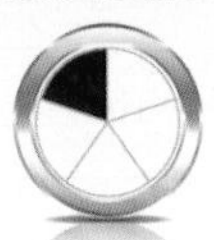

SIMPLE RECALL

Exercise 3

Write the correct combining form for the meaning given.

1. meatus ______________________________
2. scanty ______________________________
3. urine ______________________________
4. kidney ______________________________
5. water, fluid ______________________________
6. renal pelvis ______________________________
7. night ______________________________
8. stone ______________________________
9. to urinate in ______________________________

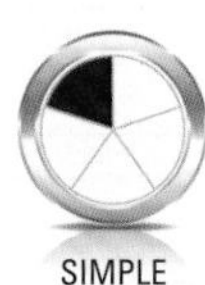

SIMPLE RECALL

Exercise 4

Write the correct suffix for the meaning given.

1. surgical opening ______________________________
2. stone ______________________________
3. herniation ______________________________
4. process of examining ______________________________
5. drooping, sagging ______________________________
6. blood (condition of) ______________________________
7. condition of ______________________________
8. stricture, narrowing ______________________________

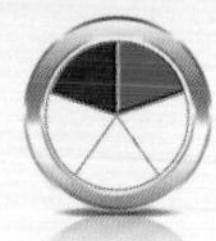

Exercise 5

Match each combining form with its meaning.

py/o	hydr/o	son/o	nephr/o
urethr/o	ureter/o	vesic/o	

1. kidney ____________________
2. pus ____________________
3. urethra ____________________
4. sound, sound waves ____________________
5. urinary bladder ____________________
6. ureter ____________________
7. water, fluid ____________________

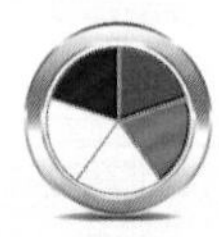

Exercise 6

Given their meanings, build a medical term from the appropriate combining form and suffix.

Use Combining Form for	Use Suffix for	Term
blood	urine, urination	**1.** __________
ureter	stricture, narrowing	**2.** __________
stone, calculus	crushing	**3.** __________
urine	blood (condition of)	**4.** __________
glomerulus	inflammation	**5.** __________
ureter	stone, calculus	**6.** __________
sound, sound waves	record	**7.** __________
bladder	viewing with an instrument	**8.** __________

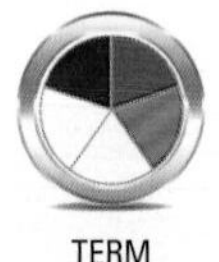

Exercise 7

Using the given suffix, build a medical term for the meaning given.

Suffix	Meaning of Medical Term	Medical Term
-uria	pus in the urine	**1.** __________
-uria	blood in the urine	**2.** __________

-uria	albumin in the urine	**3.** ______________________
-uria	glucose in the urine	**4.** ______________________
-uria	scanty amounts of urine	**5.** ______________________
-uria	bacteria in the urine	**6.** ______________________
-uria	much urination	**7.** ______________________
-uria	painful urination	**8.** ______________________

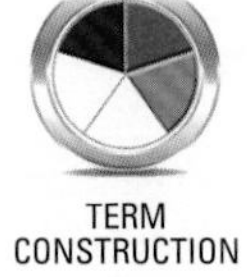

TERM CONSTRUCTION

Exercise 8

Break the given medical term into its word parts, and define each part. Then define the medical term.

For example:

urethritis	*word parts:*	urethr/o, -itis
	meanings:	urethra, inflammation
	term meaning:	inflammation of the urethra
1. nephromegaly	*word parts:*	______________________
	meanings:	______________________
	term meaning:	______________________
2. cystoscope	*word parts:*	______________________
	meanings:	______________________
	term meaning:	______________________
3. nocturia	*word parts:*	______________________
	meanings:	______________________
	term meaning:	______________________
4. ureterostomy	*word parts:*	______________________
	meanings:	______________________
	term meaning:	______________________
5. renogram	*word parts:*	______________________
	meanings:	______________________
	term meaning:	______________________

6. nephrolysis — *word parts:* ______________
meanings: ______________
term meaning: ______________

7. vesicular — *word parts:* ______________
meanings: ______________
term meaning: ______________

8. nephrorrhaphy — *word parts:* ______________
meanings: ______________
term meaning: ______________

MEDICAL TERMS

The following table gives adjective forms and terms used in describing the urinary system and its conditions.

Adjectives and Other Related Terms

Term	Pronunciation	Meaning
cystic; *syn.* vesical	sis′tik; ves′i-kăl	pertaining to the urinary bladder
genitourinary (GU)	jen′i-tō-yūr′i-nar-ē	pertaining to the organs of reproduction and urination
meatal	mē-ā′tăl	pertaining to the meatus
micturate	mik′chū-rāt	to urinate
micturition	mik′chū-rish′ŭn	urination
nephric; *syn.* renal	nef′rik; rē′năl	pertaining to the kidney
ureteral	yū-rē′tĕr-ăl	pertaining to the ureter
urethral	yū-rē′thrăl	pertaining to the urethra
urinary	yūr′i-năr′ē	pertaining to urine
urinate; *syn.* void	yūr′i-nāt; voyd	to pass urine

Exercises: Adjectives and Other Related Terms

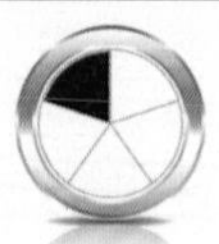

SIMPLE RECALL

Exercise 9

Write the meaning of the term given.

1. void ______________

2. renal ______________

3. cystic ______

4. micturate ______

5. urethral ______

6. urinary ______

ADVANCED RECALL

Exercise 10

Match each medical term with its meaning.

urinate	vesical	nephric	genitourinary
meatal	ureteral	micturition	

1. urination ______
2. pertaining to the bladder ______
3. pertaining to the meatus ______
4. pertaining to the organs of reproduction and urination ______
5. pertaining to the kidney ______
6. to pass urine ______
7. pertaining to a ureter ______

TERM CONSTRUCTION

Exercise 11

Break the given medical term into its word parts, and define each part. Then define the medical term.

For example:

meatal	*word parts:*	meat/o, -al
	meanings:	urethra, inflammation
	term meaning:	pertaining to the meatus
1. urinary	*word parts:*	______
	meanings:	______
	term meaning:	______
2. renal	*word parts:*	______
	meanings:	______
	term meaning:	______

3. cystic *word parts:* ______

meanings: ______

term meaning: ______

4. urethral *word parts:* ______

meanings: ______

term meaning: ______

5. ureteral *word parts:* ______

meanings: ______

term meaning: ______

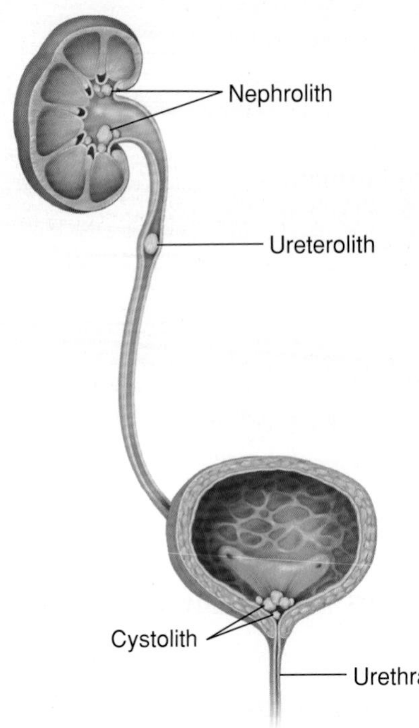

Figure 13-5 Calculi throughout the urinary system.

Medical Conditions

Term	Pronunciation	Meaning
albuminuria	al-bū-min-yū′rē-ă	presence of albumin (a blood protein) in the urine; usually a sign of disease
anuria	an-yū′rē-ă	absence of urine formation; failure of the kidneys to produce urine
bacteriuria	bak-tēr′ē-yū′rē-ă	bacteria in the urine
cystitis	sis-tī′tis	inflammation of the bladder
cystocele	sis′tō-sēl	protrusion of the bladder
cystolith	sis′tō-lith	stone in the bladder **(Figure 13-5)**

Medical Conditions

Term	Pronunciation	Meaning
diuresis	dī'yū-rē'sis	increased or excessive production of urine
dysuria	dis-yū'rē-ă	difficulty urinating; painful urination
end-stage renal disease (ESRD); *syn.* renal failure	end-stāj rē'năl diz-ēz'; rē'năl fāl'yūr	loss of kidney function; the final phase of chronic kidney disease
enuresis	en'yū-rē'sis	involuntary urination
epispadias	ep'i-spā'dē-ăs	congenital defect in which the urethral opening (orifice) is located on the upper surface of a nonerect penis **(Figure 13-6B)**
glomerulonephritis	glō-mer'yū-lō-ne-frī'tis	inflammation of the glomeruli of the kidney
glucosuria; *syn.* glycosuria	glū'kō-syū'rē-ă; glī'kō-syū'rē-ă	glucose in the urine
hematuria	hē'mă-tyū'rē-ă	blood in the urine
hydronephrosis	hī'drō-ne-frō'sis	dilation of the renal pelvis and calyces of one or both kidneys caused by obstruction of urine flow (urine builds up) usually due to a stone or stricture; literally "water inside the kidney" **(Figure 13-7)**
hydroureter	hī'drō-yūr'ē- tĕr	dilation of a ureter caused by obstruction of urine flow usually due to a stone or stricture; literally "water inside the ureter" **(Figure 13-7)**
hypospadias	hī'pō-spā'dē-ăs	congenital defect in which the urethral opening (orifice) is located on the underside of a nonerect penis **(Figure 13-6C)**
nephritis	ne-frī'tis	inflammation of the kidney
nephrolith; *syn.* renal calculus	nef'rō-lith; rē'năl kal'kyū-lŭs	kidney stone **(Figure 13-5)**
nephrolithiasis	nef'rō-li-thī'ă-sis	presence of kidney stones
nephromegaly	nef'rō-meg'ă-lē	enlargement of the kidney
nephroptosis	nef'rop-tō'sis	drooping of the kidney

(continued)

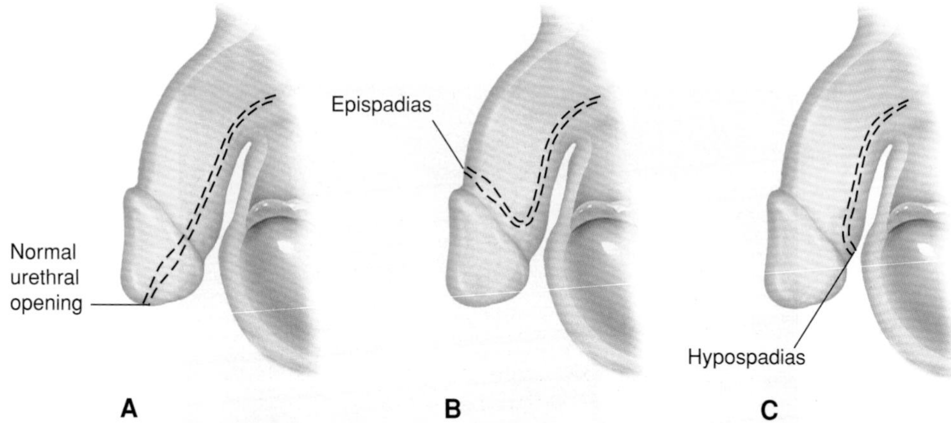

Figure 13-6 **A.** Normal urethral opening. **B.** Epispadias. **C.** Hypospadias.

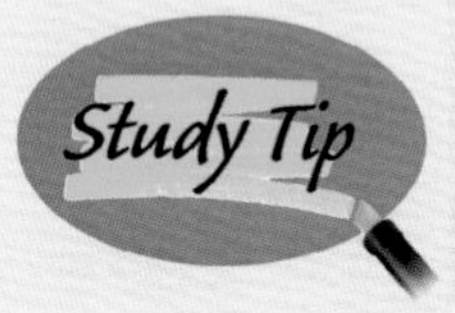

Epispadias and Hypospadias: To avoid confusing the terms epispadias and hypospadias, focus on the prefixes. *Epi-* means on or upon, so epispadias is the urinary opening on the *upper* side of a nonerect penis. *Hypo-* means less than or below, so hypospadias is the urinary opening on the *under-* side of a nonerect penis.

Medical Conditions *(continued)*

Term	Pronunciation	Meaning
nocturia	nokt-yū′rē-ă	excessive urination at night
nocturnal enuresis	nok-ter′năl en′yū-rē′sis	involuntary urination at night; bed-wetting
oliguria	ol′i-gyū′rē-ă	scanty amount of urine
polycystic kidney disease	pol′ē-sis′tik kid′nē diz-ēz′	condition in which many cysts occur within and upon the kidneys, resulting in the loss of functional renal tissue **(Figure 13-8)**

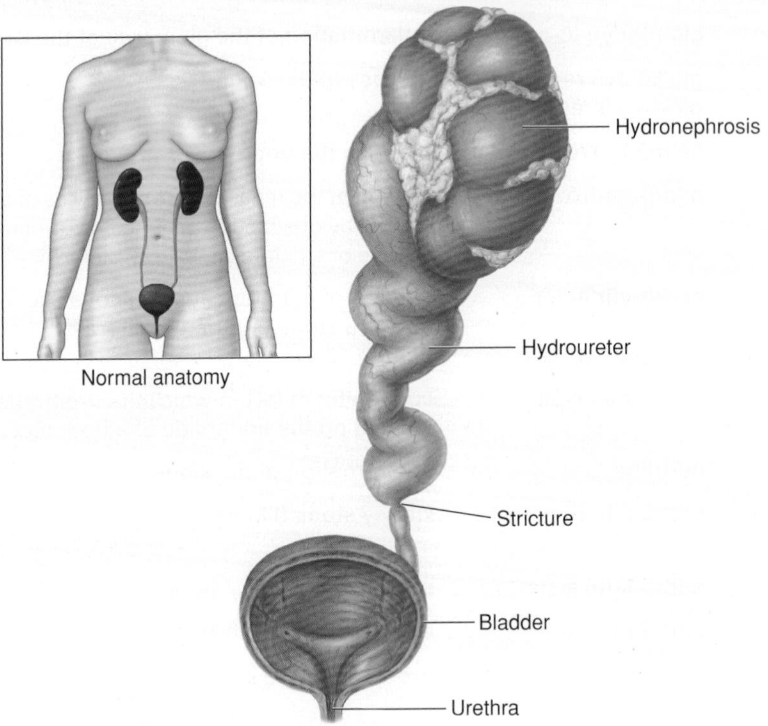

Figure 13-7 Hydronephrosis and hydroureter from a stricture.

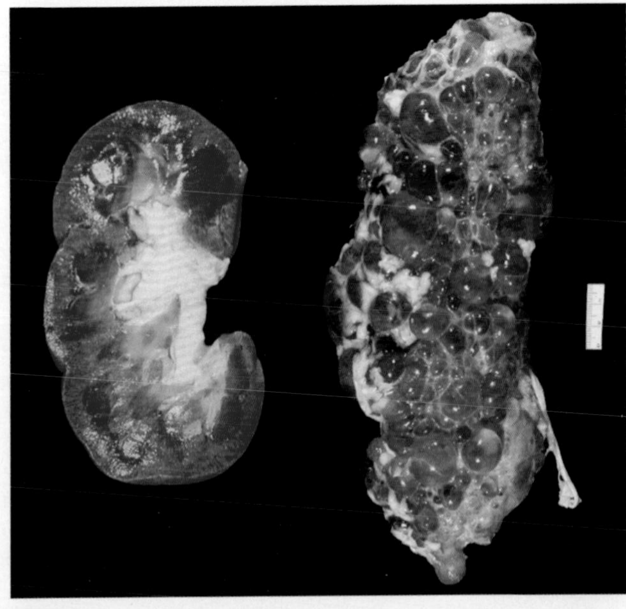

Figure 13-8 Normal kidney (**left**). Polycystic kidney (**right**).

Medical Conditions

Term	Pronunciation	Meaning
polyuria	pol′ē-yū′rē-ă	excessive and frequent urination
proteinuria	prō′tē-nūr′ē-ă	protein in the urine
pyelitis	pī′ĕ-lī′tis	inflammation of the renal pelvis
pyelonephritis	pī′ĕ-lō-ne-frī′tis	inflammation of the renal pelvis and kidney
pyuria	pī-yūr′ē-ă	pus in the urine
renal failure	rē′năl fāl′yŭr	significant decline in kidney function resulting in uremia (excess urea in the blood); two forms are acute renal failure (ARF) and chronic renal failure (CRF)
renal hypertension	rē′năl hī′pĕr-ten′shŭn	elevated blood pressure resulting from kidney disease
stress urinary incontinence (SUI)	stres yūr′i-nār′ē in-kon′ti-nens	involuntary urinating during coughing, straining, or sudden movements due to loss of sphincter strength
stricture	strik′chūr	narrowing of an organ
uremia	yū-rē′mē-ă	excess blood level of urea and other nitrogenous wastes that are normally eliminated by the kidneys
ureteritis	yū′rē-tĕr-ī′tis	inflammation of the ureter
ureterocele	yū-rē′tĕr-ō-sēl′	protrusion of the ureter into the bladder forming a sac-like pouch
ureterolith	yū-rē′tĕr-ō-lith	stone in the ureter **(Figure 13-5)**
ureterostenosis	yū-rē′tĕr-ō-ste-nō′sis	narrowing of the ureter
urethral stenosis	yū-rē′thrăl ste-nō′sis	narrowing of the urethra
urethritis	yū′rĕ-thrī′tis	inflammation of the urethra
urinary retention	yūr′i-nār′ē rē-ten′shŭn	abnormal accumulation of urine in the bladder due to inability to empty the bladder
urinary suppression	yūr′i-nār′ē sŭ-presh′ŭn	stoppage or reduction of urine formation
urinary tract infection (UTI)	yūr′i-nār′ē trakt in-fek′shŭn	infection in one or more organs of the urinary system
urge incontinence	ŭrj in-kon′ti-nens	involuntary leakage of urine with a strong, sudden desire to urinate

Exercises: Medical Conditions

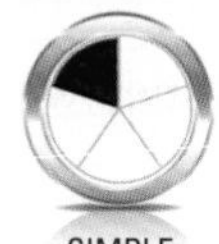

SIMPLE RECALL

Exercise 12

Write the correct medical term for the definition given.

1. narrowing of an organ ____________________
2. involuntary urination ____________________
3. kidney stone ____________________
4. presence of stones in the kidney ____________________

5. significant decline in kidney function ____________________

6. narrowing of the urethra ____________________

7. infection in urinary system organ(s) ____________________

8. excess blood level of urea ____________________

9. urinary opening on underside of penis ____________________

10. absence of urine formation ____________________

11. dilation of the renal pelvis and calyces with urine buildup ____________________

12. excessive urination ____________________

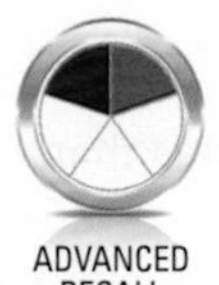

ADVANCED RECALL

Exercise 13

Circle the term that is most appropriate for the meaning of the sentence.

1. Mrs. Canter's urine leakage when she coughs is due to (*hypospadias, glycosuria, stress urinary incontinence*).

2. The medication caused (*epispadias, diuresis, pyuria*), so Mr. Samuels had to urinate frequently.

3. A stone in the patient's ureter caused a backup of urine, a condition that the physician called (*hydroureter, hematuria, ureterocele*).

4. Mr. Gill complained of fatigue from having to get up so many times at night because of his (*hypospadias, nocturia, nephroma*).

5. Laboratory testing showed that the patient was not urinating enough due to (*nocturnal enuresis, uremia, urinary suppression*).

6. Mr. Horvath was diagnosed with (*ureteritis, polycystic kidney disease, anuria*) because his right kidney contained cysts.

7. The patient's prostate enlargement had caused him to develop (*diuresis, urinary retention, nephroptosis*) because he was having trouble emptying his bladder.

8. The physician explained to Mrs. Marianas that the medical term for her drooping kidney was (*nephroptosis, oliguria, urethral stenosis*).

9. A urinalysis revealed (*ureterocele, cystolith, hematuria*) because it was positive for the presence of blood in the urine sample.

10. Mrs. Katz had difficulty traveling because she had leaking of urine with a strong desire to urinate, which the physician called (*urethritis, anuria, urge incontinence*).

11. The newborn's examination revealed (*hypospadias, epispadias, enuresis*) when the physician noticed that the urinary opening was on the upper surface of the penis.

12. Dr. Delgado told Mr. Peterson that his dysuria was due to (*proteinuria, urethritis, urethral stenosis*), which caused the urine to flow through a narrow urethra.

13. Mr. Berger's kidney disease led to elevated blood pressure called (*renal hypertension, hydroureter, enuresis*).

14. The parents expressed concern to Dr. Dodge about their son's (*oliguria, nephritis, nocturnal enuresis*), because the bed-wetting was affecting him socially.

15. Mr. Segel had (*chronic renal failure, end-stage renal disease, acute renal failure*), which is the final phase of chronic renal disease.

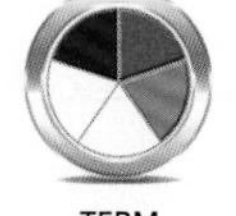

TERM CONSTRUCTION

Exercise 14

Build the correct medical term for the meaning given. Write the term in the blank, and then indicate the word parts (CF = combining form, S = suffix).

1. stone in the ureter ____________/____________
   CF S

2. protein in the urine ____________/____________
   CF S

3. albumin in the urine ____________/____________
   CF S

4. urea in the blood ____________/____________
   CF S

5. inflammation of the urethra ____________/____________
   CF S

6. glucose in the urine ____________/____________
   CF S

7. inflammation of the ureter ____________/____________
   CF S

8. inflammation of the renal pelvis and kidney ____________/____________
   CF S

9. condition of stones in the kidney ____________/____________
   CF S

10. inflammation of the glomeruli of the kidney ____________/____________
   CF S

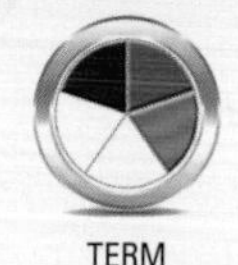

TERM CONSTRUCTION

Exercise 15

Write the remainder of the term for the meaning given.

1. stone in the ureter — uretero ________________
2. pus in the urine — ________________ uria
3. inflammation of the bladder — cyst ________________
4. drooping of the kidney — nephro ________________
5. protrusion of the bladder — ________________ cele
6. difficulty urinating — ________________ uria
7. excessive amounts of urine — poly ________________
8. inflammation of the renal pelvis — ________________ itis
9. scanty amounts of urine — ________________ uria
10. protrusion of the ureter — uretero ________________
11. inflammation of the kidney — ________________ itis
12. stone in the bladder — cysto ________________
13. bacteria in the urine — ________________ uria
14. enlargement of the kidney — nephro ________________
15. narrowing of the ureter — uretero ________________

Tests and Procedures

Term	Pronunciation	Meaning
Laboratory Tests		
blood urea nitrogen (BUN)	blŭd yū-rē′ă nī′trō-jen	blood test that measures the amount of urea in the blood; used to evaluate kidney function
creatinine clearance test	krē-at′i-nēn klēr′ăns test	test done to measure the total amount of creatinine (product of protein metabolism) excreted in the urine, usually in a 24-hour period, to assess kidney function
specific gravity (SG)	spĕ-sif′ik grav′i-tē	test to measure the concentration (density) of urine; used to evaluate the ability of the kidneys to concentrate or dilute urine
urinalysis (UA)	yūr′i-nal′i-sis	series of tests done to analyze a sample of urine

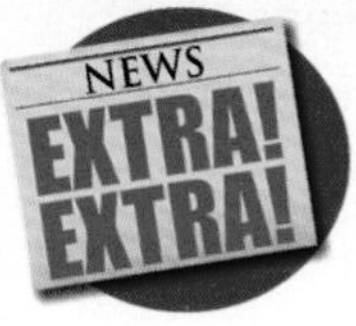

DIPSTICK URINALYSIS A dipstick urinalysis involves dipping a type of chemical analysis strip into a sample of urine and reading the colors of the squares. The test measures the specific gravity, acidity (pH), glucose, ketones (compound produced during fat metabolism), blood, leukocytes (type of white blood cell), nitrites (a salt), bilirubin (pigment formed by hemoglobin breakdown), and urobilinogen (byproduct of bilirubin) levels in the sample. Abnormal findings in the assessment can indicate urinary system diseases and the progression of diseases such as hypertension or diabetes.

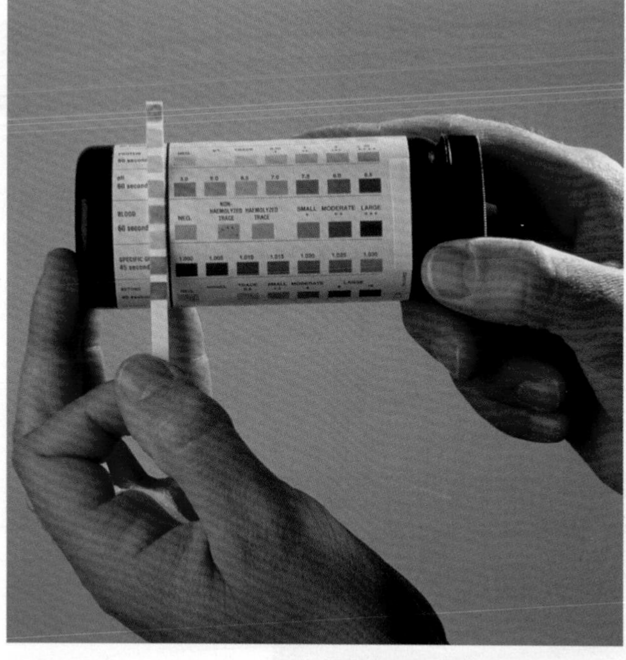

Term	Pronunciation	Meaning
urinometer	yūr′i-nom′ĕ-tĕr	instrument for measuring the specific gravity of urine

(continued)

Tests and Procedures *(continued)*

Term	Pronunciation	Meaning
Diagnostic Procedures		
cystogram	sis′tō-gram	radiographic (x-ray) image of the bladder filled with contrast dye **(Figure 13-9)**
cystography	sis-tog′ră-fē	radiography of the bladder after injection of a radiopaque dye
cystometrogram (CMG)	sis′tō-met′rō-gram	graphic recording of urinary bladder pressure at various volumes to evaluate bladder function
cystoscope	sis′tō-skōp	instrument for examining the bladder interior
cystoscopy	sis-tos′kŏ-pē	examination of the bladder using a cystoscope **(Figure 13-10)**
intravenous pyelography (IVP); *syn.* intravenous urography (IVU)	in′tră-vē′nŭs pī′ĕ-log′ră-fē; in′tră-vē′nŭs yūr-og′ră-fē	radiologic (x-ray or CT scan) examination of the kidneys, ureters, and bladder after intravenous injection of a contrast dye **(Figure 13-11)**
kidneys, ureters, and bladder (KUB) x-ray	kid′nēz, yūr′ĕ-tĕrz, and blad′ĕr	radiograph (x-ray) of the kidneys, ureters, and bladder

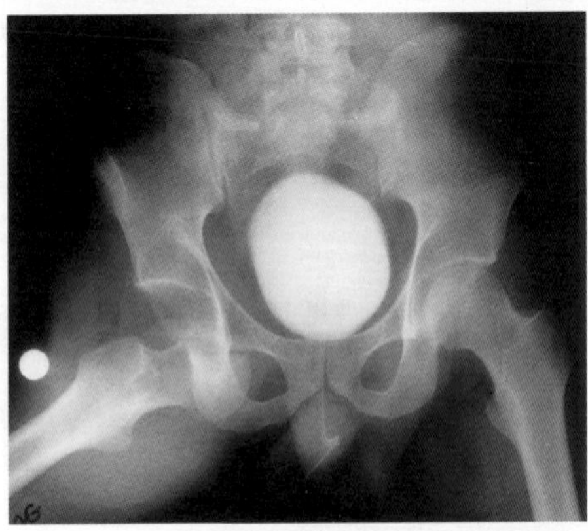

Figure 13-9 Normal cystogram showing contrast-filled bladder for a patient with a dislocated hip.

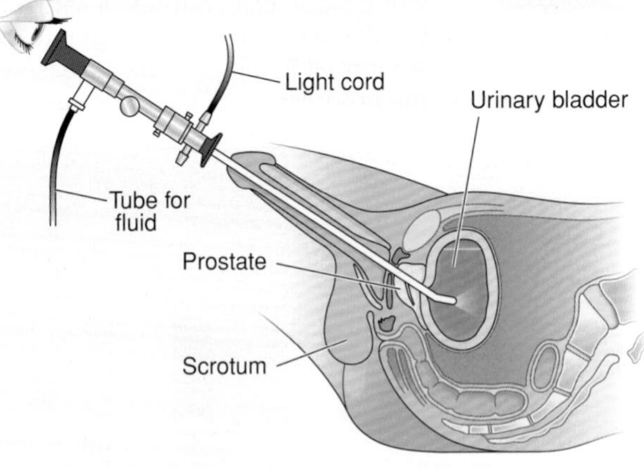

Figure 13-10 Cystoscopy. A lighted cystoscope is inserted into the bladder of a male. Sterile fluid is used to inflate the bladder.

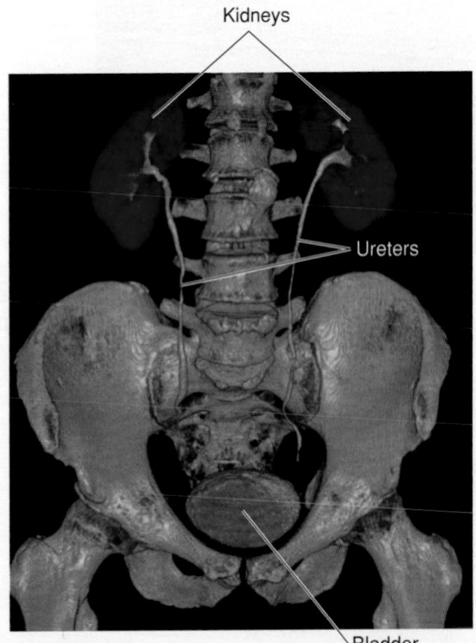

Figure 13-11 Computerized tomography (CT) intravenous pyelogram (IVP).

Tests and Procedures

Term	Pronunciation	Meaning
nephrogram	nef′rō-gram	radiographic (x-ray) examination of the kidney after intravenous injection of a contrast dye
nephrography	ne-frog′ră-fē	radiography (x-ray) of the kidney
nephroscope	nef′rō-skōp	endoscope passed into the renal pelvis
nephroscopy	nef-ros′kŏ-pē	examination of the kidney(s) using a nephroscope
nephrosonography	nef′rō-sŏ-nog′ră-fē	examination of the kidneys using sound waves (ultrasound)
nephrotomogram	nef′rō-tō′mō-gram	computed tomographic (CT) examination of the kidneys after intravenous injection of contrast dye; used to visualize renal parenchymal (connective tissue framework) abnormalities
renogram	rē′nō-gram	assessment of kidney function by external radiation detectors after intravenous injection of a radioactive dye; note that this is not an x-ray view
retrograde pyelogram	ret′rō-grād pī′el-ō-gram′	radiologic study of the kidneys, ureters, and bladder after injection of a contrast dye into the ureters; retrograde means to move backward (opposite to normal flow)
urethroscope	yū-rē′thrō-skōp	instrument used for examining the urethra
urethroscopy	yū′rē-thros′kŏ-pē	examination of the urethra using a urethroscope
urodynamics	yūr′ō-dī-nam′iks	diagnostic study of urine storage, bladder pressure, and urine flow throughout the urinary tract
voiding cystourethrogram (VCUG)	voy′ding sis′tō-yū-rēth′rō-gram	radiologic study of the bladder and urethra during urination after filling the bladder with a contrast dye

Exercises: Tests and Procedures

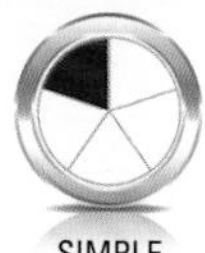
SIMPLE RECALL

Exercise 16

Write the correct medical term for the meaning given.

1. test for measuring creatinine in urine ______________
2. instrument for examining the bladder ______________
3. x-ray of kidneys, ureters, and bladder ______________
4. assessment of kidney function by external radiation detectors after intravenous injection of a radioactive dye ______________
5. tests that analyze a urine sample ______________
6. test of the concentration of urine ______________
7. examination of the urethra ______________

8. radiologic examination of the urinary tract after injecting dye ____________

9. x-ray of kidney after injection of a contrast dye ____________

10. blood test for measuring urea in the blood ____________

ADVANCED RECALL

Exercise 17

Match each medical term with its meaning.

urinometer	retrograde pyelogram	voiding cystourethrogram
urodynamics	cystometrogram	nephrosonography
nephrotomogram	urinalysis	

1. recording of pressure measurements in the bladder ____________
2. radiologic study of renal pelvis and kidneys after dye injection ____________
3. diagnostic study of the force and flow of urine ____________
4. examination of the kidneys using sound waves ____________
5. radiologic study of the bladder and urethra during urination after filling the bladder with a contrast dye ____________
6. computed tomographic (CT) examination of the kidneys after intravenous injection of contrast dye ____________
7. instrument for measuring the specific gravity of urine ____________
8. series of tests that analyze a sample of urine ____________

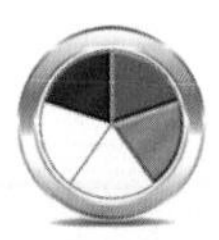

TERM CONSTRUCTION

Exercise 18

Using the given suffix, build a medical term for the meaning given.

Suffix	Meaning of Medical Term	Medical Term
-scopy	examination of the kidney	1. ____________
-gram	x-ray of the bladder	2. ____________
-graphy	process of x-raying the kidney	3. ____________
-scope	instrument for examining the urethra	4. ____________
-scopy	examination of the bladder	5. ____________
-gram	recording of kidney function	6. ____________
-graphy	process of x-raying the bladder	7. ____________
-scope	instrument for examining the kidney	8. ____________

Surgical Interventions and Therapeutic Procedures

Term	Pronunciation	Meaning
catheterization (cath)	kath′ĕ-ter-ī-zā′shŭn	procedure of inserting a tube through the urethra into the bladder to drain it of urine; a Foley catheter is an indwelling catheter with a retaining balloon to prevent it from slipping out **(Figure 13-12)**
cystectomy	sis-tek′tō-mē	surgical removal of the bladder
cystolithotomy	sis′tō-li-thot′ō-mē	incision into the bladder to remove a stone
cystoplasty	sis′tō-plas′tē	repair of the bladder
cystorrhaphy	sis-tōr′ă-fē	suturing of the bladder
cystostomy	sis-tos′tō-mē	creating a surgical opening into the bladder
extracorporeal shock wave lithotripsy (ESWL)	eks′tră-kōr-pōr′ē-ăl shok wāv lith′ō-trip′sē	breaking up of renal or ureteral calculi by focused ultrasound energy **(Figure 13-13)**

(continued)

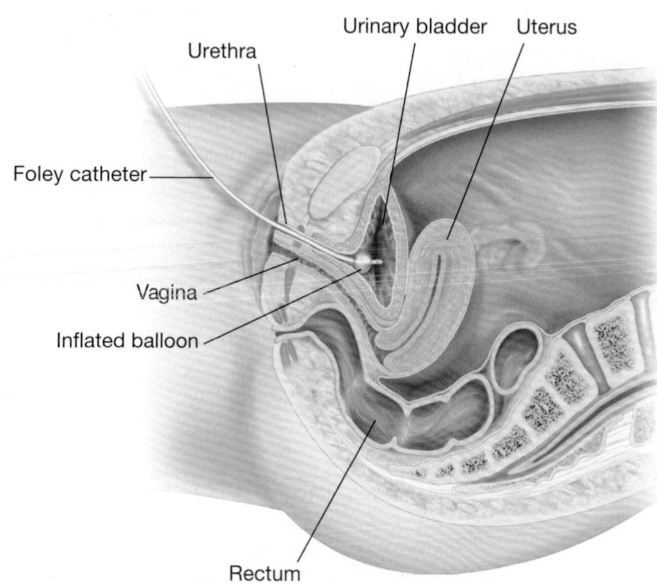

Figure 13-12 Foley catheterization.

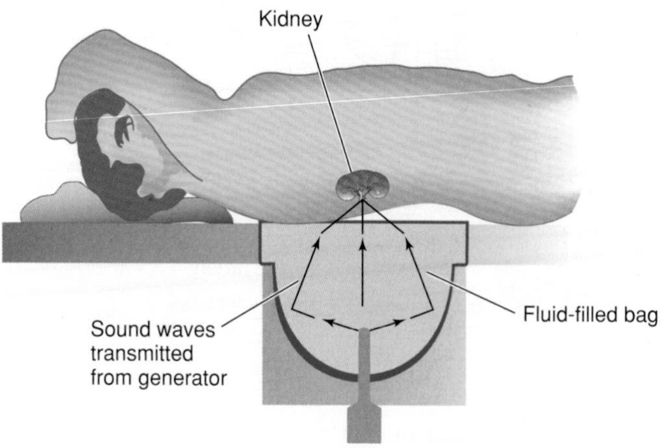

Figure 13-13 Extracorporeal shock wave lithotripsy (ESWL). (Note that the kidney is not drawn anatomically correct but is for visualization purposes only.)

Surgical Interventions and Therapeutic Procedures *(continued)*

Term	Pronunciation	Meaning
hemodialysis	hē′mō-dī-al′i-sis	removal of wastes from the blood by pumping the blood through a machine that works as an artificial kidney **(Figure 13-14)**
kidney transplant; *syn.* renal transplant	kid′nē trans′plant; rē′năl trans′plant	operation in which a donor kidney is placed into a recipient **(Figure 13-15)**

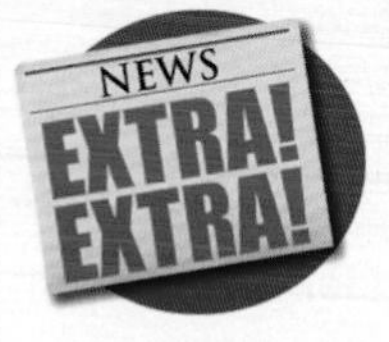

KIDNEY TRANSPLANT In most kidney transplant cases, the diseased or damaged kidney is not removed, and the right donor kidney is placed on the left side and the left donor kidney is placed on the right side of the recipient. This reversal is done to allow easier access to the renal artery.

Term	Pronunciation	Meaning
lithotomy	li-thot′ŏ-mē	incision made to remove a stone surgically

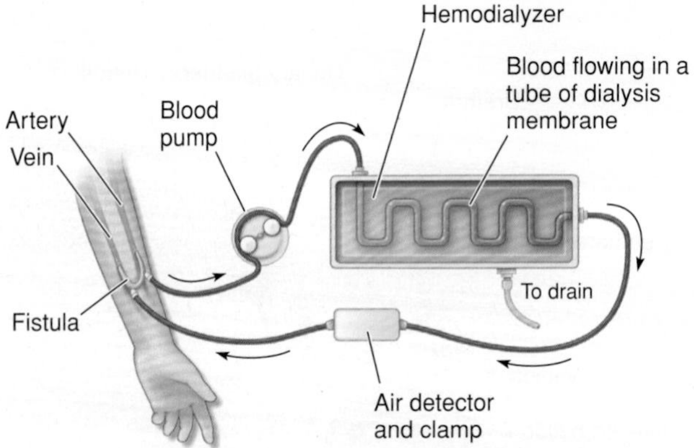

Figure 13-14 Hemodialysis.

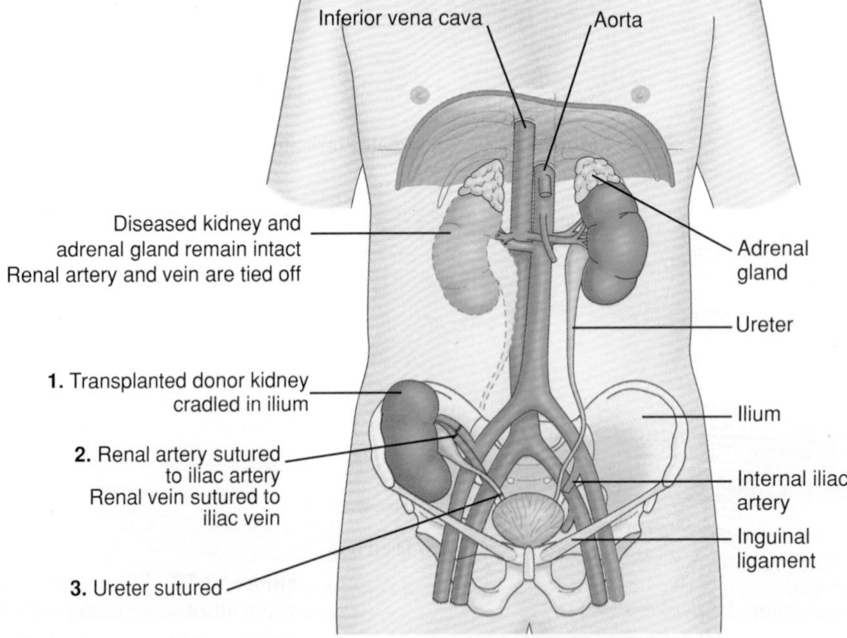

Figure 13-15 Kidney transplant.

Surgical Interventions and Therapeutic Procedures

Term	Pronunciation	Meaning
lithotripsy	lith′ō-trip′sē	crushing of a stone
meatotomy	mē′ă-tot′ŏ-mē	incision into a meatus
nephrectomy	ne-frek′tō-mē	surgical removal of a kidney
nephrolithotomy	nef′rō-li-thot′ŏ-mē	incision into a kidney to remove a stone
nephrolysis	ne-frol′i-sis	separation of the kidney from adhesions
nephropexy	nef′rō-pek′sē	surgical fixation of a drooping kidney
nephrotomy	ne-frot′ŏ-mē	incision into a kidney
peritoneal dialysis	per′i-tō-nē′ăl dī-al′i-sis	removal of wastes from the blood or impurities from the body by using the peritoneum of the abdominal cavity as a filter **(Figure 13-16)**
pyelolithotomy	pī′ĕ-lō-li-thot′ŏ-mē	incision into the renal pelvis to remove a stone
pyeloplasty	pī′ĕ-lō-plas′tē	repair of a renal pelvis
ureterectomy	yū′rē-tĕr-ek′tŏ-mē	excision of a ureter
ureterostomy	yū-rē′tĕr-os′tŏ-mē	creation of a surgical opening into a ureter
ureterotomy	yū-rē′tĕr-ot′ō-mē	incision into a ureter
urethroplasty	yū-rē′thrō-plas′tē	repair of the urethra
urethrotomy	yū′rĕ-throt′ŏ-mē	incision into the urethra
vesicourethral suspension	ves′i-kō-yū-rē′thrăl sŭs-pen′shŭn	surgical elevation and support of the bladder and urethra to control stress urinary incontinence (SUI)

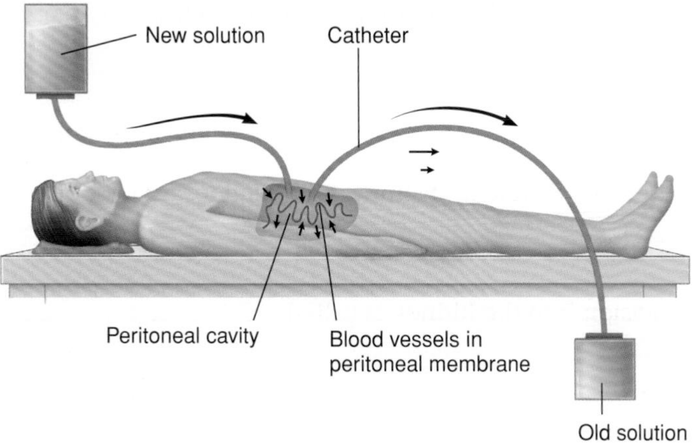

Figure 13-16 Peritoneal dialysis.

Exercises: Surgical Interventions and Therapeutic Procedures

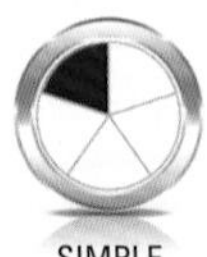
SIMPLE RECALL

Exercise 19

Write the meaning of the term given.

1. catheterization ____________________

2. cystolithotomy ____________________

3. nephropexy ______________________
4. cystostomy ______________________
5. pyelolithotomy ______________________
6. ureterectomy ______________________
7. urethroplasty ______________________
8. cystectomy ______________________
9. extracorporeal shock wave lithotripsy ______________________

Exercise 20

ADVANCED RECALL

Complete each sentence by writing in the correct medical term.

1. The removal of wastes from the blood by pumping the blood through a machine that works as an artificial kidney is called ______________________.
2. An operation in which a donor kidney is placed into a recipient is called a(n) ______________________.
3. ______________________ is an incision made into a kidney to remove a stone.
4. ______________________ means to create a surgical opening into a ureter.
5. Removing wastes from the blood or impurities from the body using the peritoneum as a filter is called ______________________.
6. ______________________ means to repair the bladder.
7. A procedure done to elevate and support the bladder and urethra to correct SUI is called a(n) ______________________.
8. To make an incision into the kidney is called ______________________.

Exercise 21

TERM CONSTRUCTION

Break the given medical term into its word parts, and define each part. Then define the medical term.

For example:

cystectomy	*word parts:*	cyst/o, -ectomy
	meanings:	urinary bladder, excision, surgical removal
	term meaning:	excision of the bladder

1. lithotomy *word parts:* ______________________
meanings: ______________________
term meaning: ______________________

2. cystorrhaphy *word parts:* ______

meanings: ______

term meaning: ______

3. ureterotomy *word parts:* ______

meanings: ______

term meaning: ______

4. nephrectomy *word parts:* ______

meanings: ______

term meaning: ______

5. pyeloplasty *word parts:* ______

meanings: ______

term meaning: ______

6. meatotomy *word parts:* ______

meanings: ______

term meaning: ______

7. lithotripsy *word parts:* ______

meanings: ______

term meaning: ______

8. nephrolysis *word parts:* ______

meanings: ______

term meaning: ______

9. urethrotomy *word parts:* ______

meanings: ______

term meaning: ______

Medications and Drug Therapies

Term	Pronunciation	Meaning
antibacterial	an'tē-bak-tēr'ē-ăl	drug used to destroy or prevent the growth of bacteria
antibiotic	an'tē-bī-ot'ik	drug that kills or inhibits the growth of microorganisms
diuretic	dī-yūr-et'ik	drug that increases the amount of urine secreted
urinary analgesic	yūr'i-nār-ē an'ăl-jē'zik	drug used to relieve pain within the urinary system

Exercise: Medications and Drug Therapies

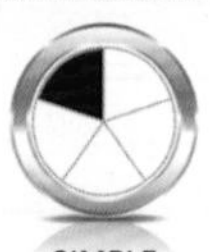

SIMPLE RECALL

Exercise 22

Write the correct medication or drug therapy term for the definition given.

1. relieves pain within the urinary system __________
2. acts on susceptible microorganisms __________
3. increases the amount of urine secreted __________
4. destroys or prevents the growth of bacteria __________

Specialties and Specialists

Term	Pronunciation	Meaning
nephrology	ne-frol'ŏ-jē	medical specialty focusing on the study and treatment of kidney conditions
nephrologist	nef'rol'ŏ-jist	physician who specializes in nephrology
urology	yū-rol'ŏ-jē	medical specialty focusing on the study and treatment of conditions of the urinary system
urologist	yū-rol'ŏ-jist	physician who specializes in urology

Exercise: Specialties and Specialists

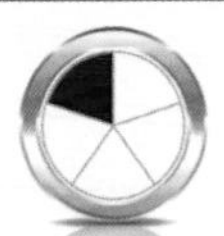

SIMPLE RECALL

Exercise 23

Write the correct medical term for the definition given.

1. physician who specializes in the study and treatment of kidney conditions __________
2. specialty focusing on the study and treatment of urinary system conditions __________
3. physician who specializes in the study and treatment of urinary system conditions __________
4. specialty focusing on the study and treatment of kidney conditions __________

Abbreviations

Term	Meaning
ARF	acute renal failure
BUN	blood urea nitrogen
cath	catheter; catheterize; catheterization
CMG	cystometrogram
CRF	chronic renal failure
DCT	distal convoluted tubule
ESRD	end-stage renal disease
ESWL	extracorporeal shock wave lithotripsy
GU	genitourinary
IVP	intravenous pyelogram; intravenous pyelography
IVU	intravenous urogram; intravenous urography
KUB	kidneys, ureters, and bladder (x-ray)
PCT	proximal convoluted tubule
SG	specific gravity
SUI	stress urinary incontinence
UA	urinalysis
UTI	urinary tract infection
VCUG	voiding cystourethrogram; voiding cystourethrography

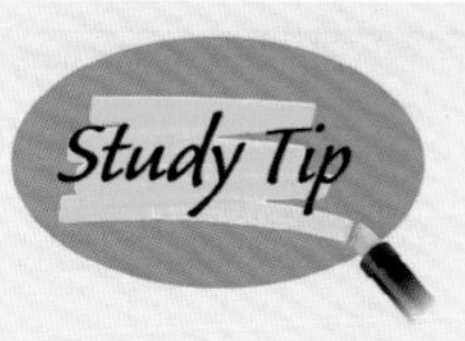

Same Abbreviation, Different Meanings: Some abbreviations can stand for two (or even more) medical terms, depending on the context in which they are used. For example, the abbreviation *cath* (see Abbreviations table) can stand for three variations of the word *catheter.* Also, words that have the same prefix and combining form but a different suffix (most commonly *-gram* or *-graphy*) can have the same abbreviation (see IVP, IVU, and VCUG in the Abbreviations table).

Exercises: Abbreviations

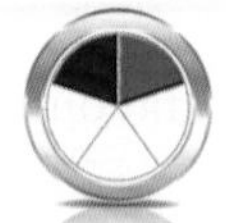

ADVANCED RECALL

Exercise 24

Write the meaning for each abbreviation.

1. UTI ____________________
2. IVP ____________________
3. ESRD ____________________
4. SG ____________________
5. cath ____________________

6. VCUG ______________________

7. BUN ______________________

8. ARF ______________________

9. GU ______________________

10. IVU ______________________

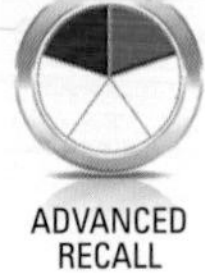

ADVANCED RECALL

Exercise 25

Write the meaning of each abbreviation used in these sentences.

1. The physician told Mrs. Cooper that a **KUB** was needed to look for stones in her urinary system.

____

2. Dr. Shapiro ordered **ESWL** to try to break up the stones found in the patient's bladder.

____

3. Mr. Kent's **CRF** was probably due to diabetic nephropathy.

____

4. A **UA** was ordered to help diagnose the cause of the patient's dysuria.

____

5. Ms. Stefano's physician told her that her urinary leakage when she coughs is a condition known as **SUI.**

____

WRAPPING UP

- The urinary system consists of two kidneys, two ureters, one bladder, and one urethra.
- The function of the urinary system is to eliminate waste from the blood, to regulate blood volume and blood pressure, and to maintain fluid and electrolyte balance.
- In this chapter, you learned medical terminology including word parts, prefixes, suffixes, adjectives, conditions, tests, procedures, medications, specialties, and abbreviations related to the urinary system.

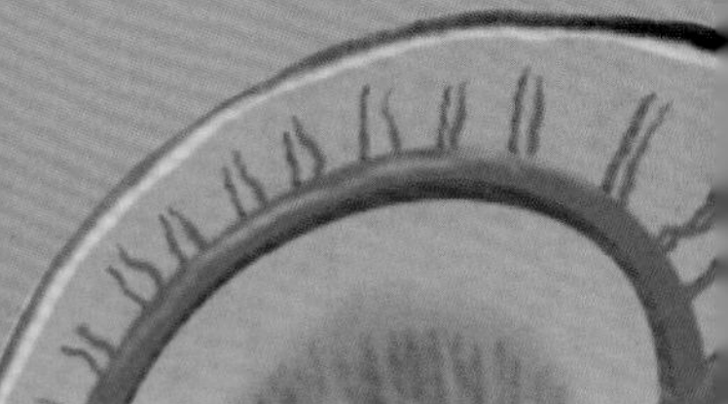

Chapter Review

Review of Terms for Anatomy and Physiology

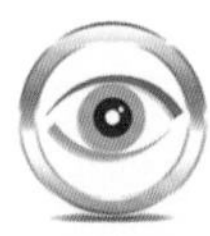

VISUAL

Exercise 26

Write the correct terms on the blanks for the anatomic structures indicated.

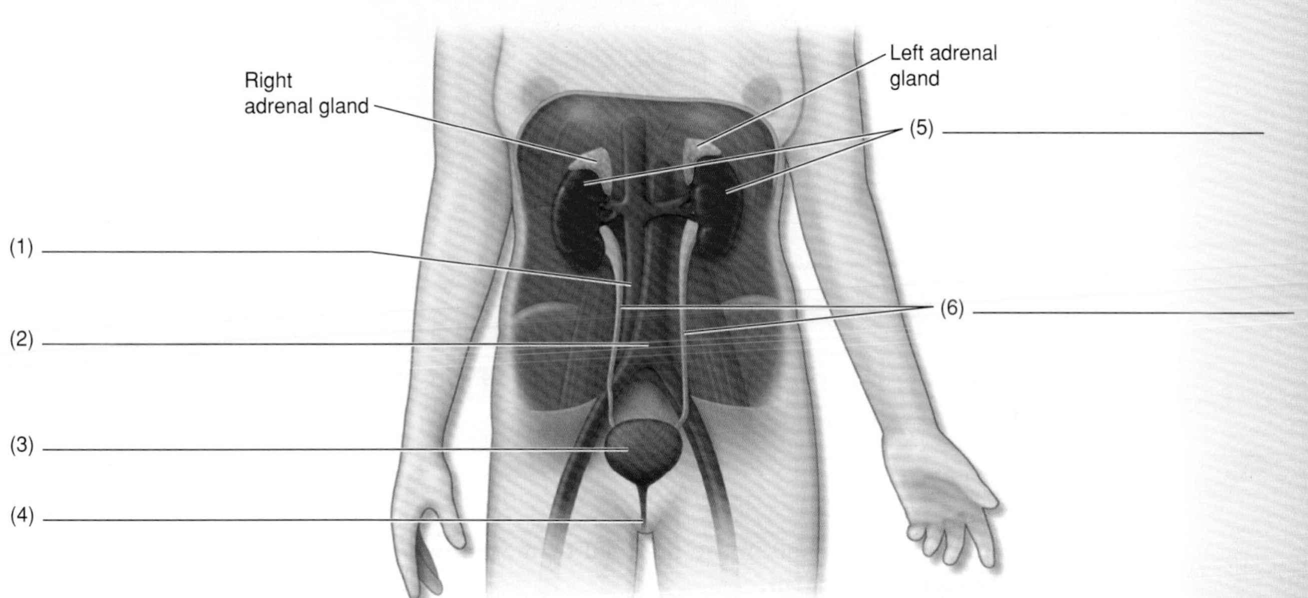

13 Urinary System

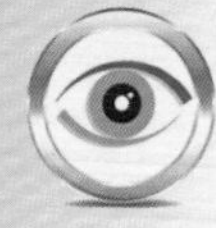
VISUAL

Exercise 27

Write the correct terms on the blanks for the anatomic structures indicated.

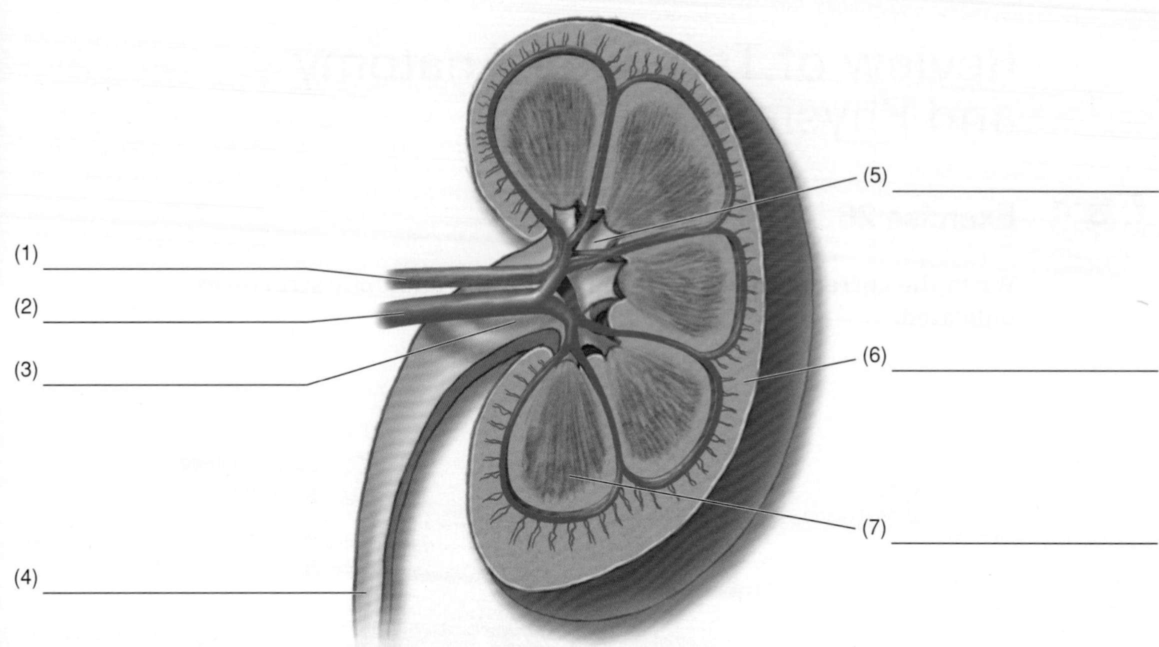

Understanding Term Structure

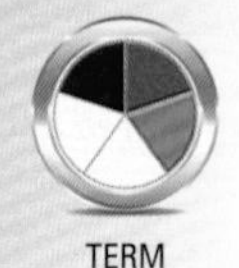
TERM CONSTRUCTION

Exercise 28

Write the combining form used in the medical term, followed by the meaning of the combining form.

Term	Combining Form	Combining Form Definition
1. cystorrhaphy	____________	____________
2. meatal	____________	____________
3. urethritis	____________	____________
4. hematuria	____________	____________
5. cystitis	____________	____________
6. renal	____________	____________
7. ureterostenosis	____________	____________
8. pyuria	____________	____________
9. pyelitis	____________	____________

10. urethroscope ______________ ______________

11. glycosuria ______________ ______________

12. nephrectomy ______________ ______________

13. vesical ______________ ______________

14. nocturia ______________ ______________

15. uremia ______________ ______________

16. cystoscopy ______________ ______________

17. nephrogram ______________ ______________

18. urethroplasty ______________ ______________

19. oliguria ______________ ______________

20. ureterolith ______________ ______________

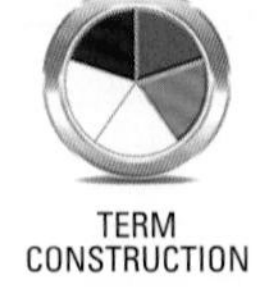

TERM CONSTRUCTION

Exercise 29

Break the given medical term into its word parts, and define each part. Then define the medical term.

For example:

cystectomy
word parts: cyst/o, -ectomy
meanings: urinary bladder; excision, surgical removal
term meaning: excision of the bladder

1. ureterolith
word parts: ______________
meanings: ______________
term meaning: ______________

2. glycosuria
word parts: ______________
meanings: ______________
term meaning: ______________

3. nephroptosis
word parts: ______________
meanings: ______________
term meaning: ______________

4. ureterostenosis
word parts: ______________
meanings: ______________
term meaning: ______________

5. nephrotomy *word parts:* ____________________

meanings: ____________________

term meaning: ____________________

6. uremia *word parts:* ____________________

meanings: ____________________

term meaning: ____________________

7. pyelitis *word parts:* ____________________

meanings: ____________________

term meaning: ____________________

8. glomerulonephritis *word parts:* ____________________

meanings: ____________________

term meaning: ____________________

Comprehension Exercises

Exercise 30

COMPREHENSION

Fill in the blank with the correct term.

1. ____________________ is a test that measures the concentration (density) of urine.

2. An x-ray of the kidneys, ureters, and bladder is commonly referred to by its abbreviation ____________________.

3. When a stone causes urine to back up in the ureter, the condition is called ____________________.

4. The process of inserting a tube into the bladder to drain it is termed ____________________.

5. A condition involving protein in the urine is known as ____________________.

6. Removing wastes from the blood by pumping the blood through an artificial kidney is called ____________________.

7. Involuntary release of urine when coughing or sneezing is called ____________________.

8. High blood pressure caused by kidney disease is known as ____________________.

9. The procedure for elevating and supporting the bladder and urethra to hold them in the proper position is called ____________________.

10. A prolapsed or "drooping" kidney is called ____________________.

11. A(n) ______________________ is a recording of pressure measurements in the bladder.

12. A(n) ______________________ is a series of tests done to analyze a urine sample.

13. A buildup of urine in the bladder due to the inability to release it is called ______________.

14. The term for involuntary release of urine during the night is ______________________.

15. ______________________ is a congenital defect in which the urinary opening is located on the underside of the penis.

Exercise 31

COMPREHENSION

Write a short answer for each question.

1. What does a BUN test for? ______________________

2. What organ is implanted in a renal transplant? ______________________

3. What kind of a sample is obtained for a specific gravity test? ______________________

4. Why might a patient with a renal calculus also have hydronephrosis? ______________________

____

5. Why is voiding an important function of the body? ______________________

____

6. Why would a patient with a cystolith require a lithotripsy? ______________________

____

7. What organ is examined using a nephroscope? ______________________

8. What type of physician would treat polycystic kidney disease? ______________________

9. What type of drug would be prescribed to relieve a patient of dysuria? ______________________

____

10. What substance cannot flow properly if a patient has a ureteral stricture? ______________________

11. What anatomic structures are suspended in the surgical treatment of stress urinary incontinence? ______________________

12. What procedure might be used to treat urinary retention? ______________________

13. What specialty might involve studying new treatment options for cystitis? ______________________

14. What does a lithotomy enable a physician to do? ______________________

____

15. What is fixated in a nephropexy? ________________

16. What is protruding in a ureterocele? ________________

17. What x-ray of a single organ would be used to diagnose a cystolith? ________________

18. What instrument is used to measure specific gravity? ________________

19. What two types of drugs might be used to treat bacteriuria? ________________

____

20. What organ is examined in a nephrotomogram? ________________

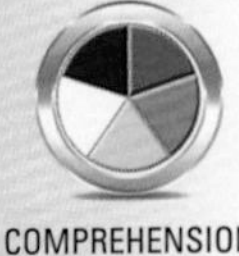

COMPREHENSION

Exercise 32

Circle the letter of the best answer in the following questions.

1. In the condition hypospadias, what structure is displaced?
   A. glomerulus
   B. renal pelvis
   C. urethra
   D. opening (orifice)

2. A condition that results from nonfunctioning nephrons is
   A. dysuria.
   B. anuria.
   C. urinary retention.
   D. nephromegaly.

3. Which pair of terms indicates the same condition?
   A. cystocele and ureterolith
   B. nephritis and cystitis
   C. epispadias and hypospadias
   D. nephrolith and renal calculus

4. The procedure that produces an ultrasound recording of the kidney is called
   A. nephrosonography.
   B. nephrography.
   C. nephrotomography.
   D. cystometrography.

5. Which of these conditions is a congenital defect?
   A. hydromegaly
   B. epispadias
   C. diuresis
   D. cystitis

6. Which term indicates that the nephrons are not functioning properly?
   A. urinary suppression
   B. dysuria
   C. renal hypertension
   D. micturition

7. Which test does not involve the testing of urine?
   A. specific gravity
   B. BUN
   C. urinalysis
   D. creatinine clearance

8. The procedure that involves making an incision into the reservoir of the kidney to remove a stone is called
   A. nephrolithotomy.
   B. cystolithotomy.
   C. lithotripsy.
   D. pyelolithotomy.

9. Which condition does not indicate an abnormal substance in the urine?
   A. pyuria
   B. hematuria
   C. dysuria
   D. proteinuria

10. Which procedure involves the use of the patient's own body for the removal of wastes from the blood?

A. peritoneal dialysis
B. hemodialysis
C. nephrosonography
D. urodynamics

11. Which procedure records the backward flow of dye through the urinary tract?

A. intravenous pyelogram
B. cystometrogram
C. retrograde pyelogram
D. renogram

12. A patient who is excreting increased amounts of urine has

A. diuresis.
B. urge incontinence.
C. stress urinary incontinence.
D. hydronephrosis.

13. The procedure that is done during micturition is called a

A. nephrogram
B. cystometrogram
C. voiding cystourethrogram
D. retrograde pyelogram

14. Which procedure does not involve fixation or repair?

A. nephrolysis
B. nephropexy
C. cystoplasty
D. pyeloplasty

15. Narrowing of the structure that carries urine to the body exterior is known as

A. urethritis.
B. ureteritis.
C. ureterostenosis.
D. urethrostenosis.

Application and Analysis

CASE STUDY

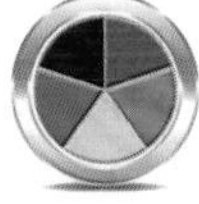

APPLICATION

Exercise 33

Read the case study and circle the correct letter for each of the questions.

CASE 13-1

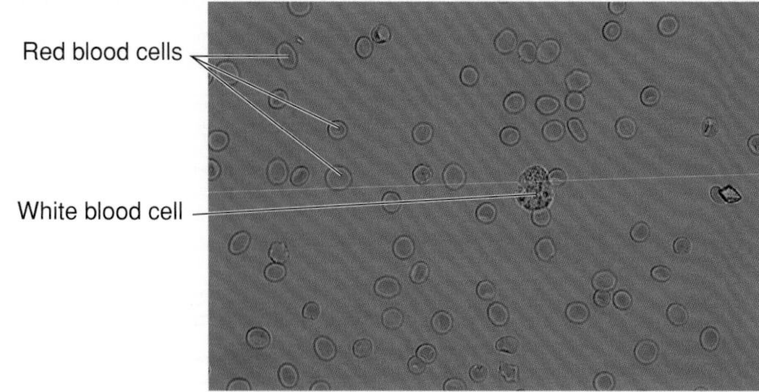

Figure 13-17 Hematuria. Microscopic view of a urine sample shows a large number of red blood cells (RBCs) accompanied by a single while blood cell near the center.

Mrs. Kendall was seen in the office today for complaints of dysuria, polyuria, and hematuria **(Figure 13-17)**. She has a history of urge incontinence and polycystic kidneys. A urinalysis was performed, which revealed elevated leukocytes and the presence of some blood. The diagnosis was a urinary tract infection; she was started on antibiotic therapy for this condition.

1. Which term indicates that the patient had excessive urination?

   A. hematuria
   B. polyuria
   C. urge incontinence
   D. dysuria

2. The patient's history indicates that she sometimes has leakage accompanied by a sudden and strong urge to urinate. What is the term used in the case for this condition?

   A. urge incontinence
   B. urinary tract infection
   C. hematuria
   D. polycystic kidney disease

3. The term for the presence of blood in the urine is

   A. dysuria.
   B. pyuria.
   C. hematuria.
   D. proteinuria.

4. Which is a test that analyzes a urine sample?

   A. cystogram
   B. nephrogram
   C. renogram
   D. urinalysis

5. Which is the term for an infection in one or more organs of the urinary system?

   A. urge incontinence
   B. hematuria
   C. urinary tract infection
   D. polycystic kidneys

MEDICAL RECORD ANALYSIS

MEDICAL RECORD 13-1

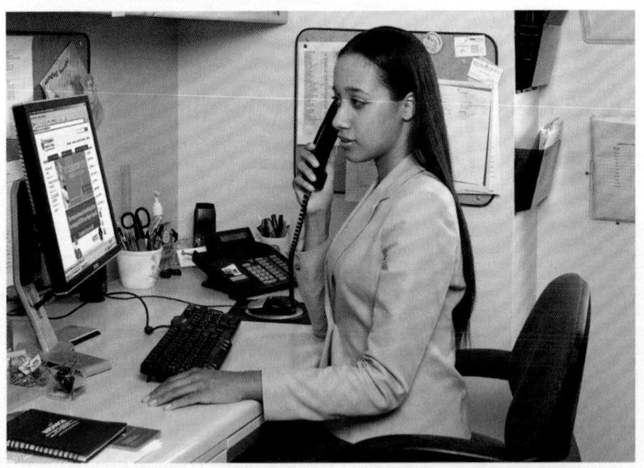

An administrative medical assistant performs critical medical office duties.

As the administrative medical assistant working in a physician's office, you have been asked to abstract information from the patient's medical record to obtain a rush authorization from his insurance company for a procedure. The patient's progress note from today's visit is as follows.

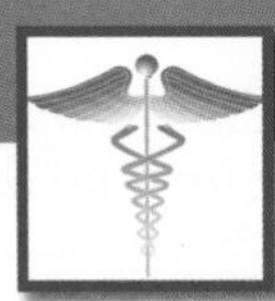

Medical Record

PROBLEM WITH URINATION

SUBJECTIVE: The patient presented in the office today with complaints of a feeling of fullness in his pelvic area as well as oliguria for the past three days. He feels the need to urinate and "not much comes out." He states that he also had some nocturnal enuresis off and on over the past week. He has a history of pyelonephritis one year ago.

OBJECTIVE: The patient is a 52-year-old underweight male in obvious discomfort. Examination of the abdomen and pelvis was notable for pain on palpation of the pelvic area over the bladder. Percussion of this area revealed a distended bladder. A digital rectal examination was performed and revealed no enlargement of the prostate.

A urinalysis was ordered, but the patient was unable to void, so in-and-out catheterization was performed and the bladder was drained. Urinalysis was performed on a sample of the urine and revealed dark color and a high SG.

ASSESSMENT: Diagnosis is urinary retention due to a probable stone in the urinary tract causing hydroureter or hydronephrosis.

PLAN: A stat KUB was ordered. I will call the patient as soon as I have the results of the KUB. Treatment will be determined based on the results of the x-ray.

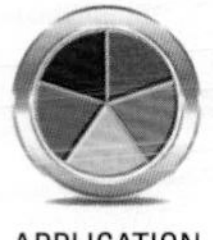

APPLICATION

Exercise 34

Write the appropriate medical terms or abbreviations used in this medical record on the blanks after their definitions.

1. scanty amounts of urine ______
2. involuntary release of urine at night ______
3. inflammation of the renal pelvis and kidneys ______
4. condition of fluid in the kidney(s) ______
5. series of tests done to analyze a urine sample ______
6. inserting a tube into the bladder to drain it of urine ______
7. specific gravity (abbreviation) ______
8. abnormal accumulation of urine in the bladder ______
9. backing up of urine in the ureter ______
10. x-ray of the kidney, ureters, and bladder (abbreviation) ______

Bonus Question

11. According to the Assessment section of the report, what does the physician expect the KUB to reveal? ______

MEDICAL RECORD 13-2

You are a medical laboratory technologist working in a physician's office. Mrs. Talbot, a patient in your office, was referred to a urologist one month ago and is returning for a preoperative clearance. You are to perform the urinalysis in the office laboratory.

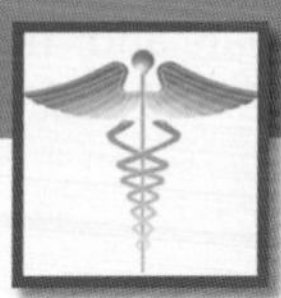

Medical Record

UROLOGY CONSULTATION REPORT

I saw Mrs. Talbot today on referral by your office. She presented as a pleasant 45-year-old woman with a history of stress urinary incontinence for the past year. She states that the symptoms have been increasing in severity over the past two months and that you referred her for possible surgical correction of the problem.

Medical history reveals a right nephrectomy due to polycystic kidneys. She has no history of frequent urinary tract infections. The patient is multigravida. She had four vaginal deliveries without complications. She is also an asthmatic and finds the symptoms worse when an asthma exacerbation causes increased coughing.

Examination revealed an overweight female in no acute distress. Pelvic examination revealed a cystocele. Urinalysis done in the office today was normal.

The patient was scheduled for cystoscopy, urodynamics, a pelvic ultrasound, and a voiding cystourethrogram. I informed the patient that her SUI is likely caused by weakness of the pelvic floor muscles due to multiple childbirths that have left her with a prolapsed bladder. She may be an excellent candidate for a transvaginal tape procedure. We will discuss this further following her workup, and I will keep you updated as to the results.

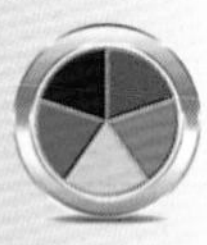

APPLICATION

Exercise 35

Read the medical report and circle the correct letter for each of the questions.

1. The urologist indicated that the patient's SUI is likely due to weakness of the pelvic floor muscles. What does the abbreviation SUI mean?

   A. strong urinary infection
   B. stressing urinary infection
   C. stress urinary incontinence
   D. stress urethral incontinence

2. The pelvic examination revealed a cystocele. What is a cystocele?

   A. protrusion of the rectum
   B. protrusion of the bladder
   C. inflammation of the bladder
   D. stone in the bladder

3. The term that means an x-ray of the bladder and urethra made during urination is

   A. nephrogram.
   B. intravenous pyelogram.
   C. retrograde pyelogram.
   D. voiding cystourethrogram.

4. What procedure was previously performed because of the patient's polycystic kidney?

   A. nephrectomy
   B. renography
   C. nephrolysis
   D. nephrostomy

5. The diagnostic test that will record the force and flow of urine is a(n)

   A. urethroscopy.
   B. cystometrogram.
   C. urodynamics.
   D. intravenous pyelogram.

6. Which test ordered by the urologist will involve examination of the bladder using a scope?

   A. nephroscopy
   B. cystoscopy
   C. urethroscopy
   D. cystography

7. Which of the patient's conditions would result in loss of functioning kidney tissue?

   A. SUI
   B. polycystic kidneys
   C. prolapsed bladder
   D. cystocele

Bonus Question

8. If the term *vaginal* means "pertaining to the vagina," what does the term *transvaginal* mean?

____

Pronunciation and Spelling

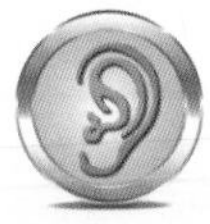

AUDITORY

Exercise 36

Review the Chapter 13 terms in the Dictionary/Audio Glossary in the Student Resources on thePoint, and practice pronouncing each term, referring to the pronunciation guide as needed.

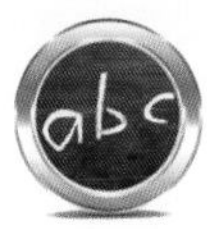

SPELLING

Exercise 37

Check the spelling of each term. If it is correct, check off the correct box. If incorrect, write the correct spelling on the line.

1. glomarulus ☐ ______________
2. meatis ☐ ______________
3. cistic ☐ ______________
4. vesical ☐ ______________
5. micturate ☐ ______________
6. nefromegaly ☐ ______________
7. oliguria ☐ ______________
8. cystosele ☐ ______________
9. dieuresis ☐ ______________
10. glycosuria ☐ ______________
11. hydrourether ☐ ______________
12. incontinence ☐ ______________

13. creatinine ☐ ____________________

14. urinanalysis ☐ ____________________

15. cistoscopy ☐ ____________________

Media Connection

STUDENT RESOURCES

Exercise 38

Complete each of the following activities available with the Student Resources on thePoint. Check off each activity as you complete it, and record your score for the Chapter Quiz in the space provided.

Chapter Exercises

____ Flash Cards

____ Concentration

____ Abbreviation Match-Up

____ Roboterms

____ Word Anatomy

____ Fill the Gap

____ Break It Down

____ True/False Body Building

____ Quiz Show

____ Complete the Case

____ Medical Record Review

____ Look and Label

____ Image Matching

____ Spelling Bee

____ **Chapter Quiz** *Score:*________%

Additional Resources

____ Animation: Renal Function

____ Dictionary/Audio Glossary

____ Health Professions Careers: Administrative Medical Assistant

____ Health Professions Careers: Medical Laboratory Technologist

Male Reproductive System

14

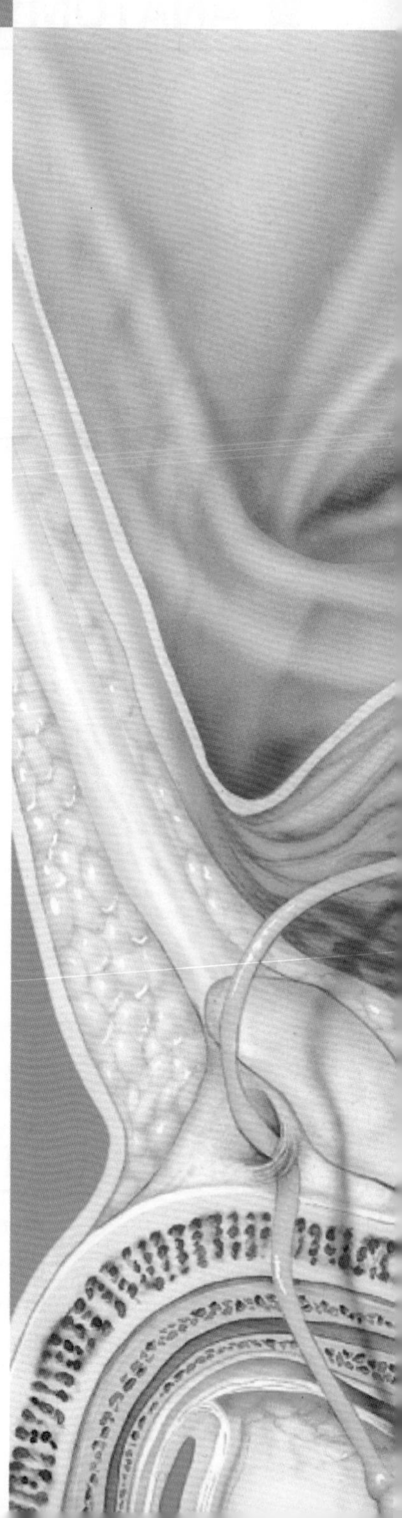

Chapter Outline

Introduction, 550

Anatomy and Physiology, 550
- Structures, 550
- Functions, 550
- Terms Related to the Male Reproductive System, 550

Word Parts, 553
- Combining Forms, 553
- Prefixes, 553
- Suffixes, 554

Medical Terms, 556
- Adjectives and Other Related Terms, 556
- Medical Conditions, 557
- Tests and Procedures, 564
- Surgical Interventions and Therapeutic Procedures, 565
- Medications and Drug Therapies, 569
- Specialties and Specialists, 569
- Abbreviations, 570

Wrapping Up, 571

Chapter Review, 572

Learning Outcomes

After completing this chapter, you should be able to:

1. List the structures and functions of the male reproductive system.
2. Define terms related to the male reproductive system.
3. Define combining forms, prefixes, and suffixes related to the male reproductive system.
4. Define common medical terminology related to the male reproductive system, including adjectives and related terms; signs, symptoms, and medical conditions; tests and procedures; surgical interventions and therapeutic procedures; medications and drug therapies; and medical specialties and specialists.
5. Define common abbreviations related to the male reproductive system.
6. Successfully complete all chapter exercises.
7. Explain terms used in case studies and medical records involving the male reproductive system.
8. Successfully complete all exercises included with the companion Student Resources on thePoint.

INTRODUCTION

The male reproductive system is made up of organs and hormones with the purpose of producing offspring. Biologists may call this sexual reproduction or procreation. The major organs include external genitalia (penis and testes) and internal genitalia (glands, ducts, and other structures). Hormones will play important roles in the proper functioning of this system.

ANATOMY AND PHYSIOLOGY

Structures

- The penis is the external organ of urination and sexual intercourse.
- Testes (testicles) are paired structures found in the cavity of the scrotum. They produce sperm (spermatozoa) and testosterone.
- Sperm (spermatozoa) are the male reproductive (sex) cells.
- The scrotum is a muscular sac formed of skin that encloses the testes.
- The bulbourethral (Cowper) glands are two pea-sized glands at the base of the penis that secrete an alkaline fluid, which lubricates the tip of the penis. Bulbourethral glands are homologous (have the same evolutionary origin) to the greater vestibular (Bartholin) glands in females.
- The prostate gland, commonly called the prostate, is a chestnut-shaped structure that surrounds the beginning of the urethra. It secretes a milky fluid into the prostatic urethra.
- The seminal vesicles, also known as the seminal glands, produce fluids that help sperm motility.
- Semen is the fluid produced by the glands in the male reproductive system.
- Fluids from the bulbourethral glands, prostate gland, and seminal vesicles make up about 35% of the total volume of semen. Semen is ejaculated fluid that contains a mixture of secretions and sperm. Alkaline fluid from the prostate gland and paired seminal vesicles helps neutralize the acidity of the female vagina to prolong the life of ejaculated sperm.
- The epididymis and the ductus deferens (vas deferens) transport sperm and semen.
- Testosterone is the male sex hormone.

Functions

- Producing the hormone testosterone
- Producing and storing the male reproductive cells called spermatozoa (sperm)
- Producing, transporting, and releasing semen

Terms Related to the Male Reproductive System (Figure 14-1)

Term	Pronunciation	Meaning
bulbourethral glands	bŭl′bō-yū-rē′thrăl glandz	the two glands inferior to (below) the prostate gland that secrete a sticky fluid that becomes a component of semen
ejaculation	ē-jak′yū-lā′shŭn	action of ejecting semen from the genital ducts to the exterior

Terms Related to the Male Reproductive System

Term	Pronunciation	Meaning
epididymis	ep′i-did′i-mis	long coiled duct located on the posterior surface (behind) each testis that stores, matures, and transports sperm between the testis and the ductus deferens
gamete	gam′ēt	any sex cell; male sperm cell or female oocyte
gonad	gō′nad	organ that produces gametes; a male testis or female ovary
penis	pē′nis	external male organ used in urination and sexual intercourse
glans penis	glanz pē′nis	rounded tip at the end of the penis
prepuce; *syn.* foreskin	prē′pūs; fōr′skin	fold of skin that covers the glans penis in uncircumcised males
prostate gland; *syn.* prostate	pros′tāt gland; pros′tāt	gland that surrounds the beginning of the urethra (immediately inferior to the bladder) that secretes a fluid that becomes part of semen
scrotum	skrō′tŭm	sac (pouch) that is suspended on either side of and behind the penis that encloses the testes and epididymis
semen	sē′mĕn	viscous fluid containing sperm and secretions of the testes and seminal vesicles, prostate gland, and bulbourethral glands
seminal vesicles; *syn.* seminal glands	sem′i-năl ves′i-kălz; sem′i-năl glandz	two glands posterior to the urinary bladder that produce seminal fluid, which becomes a component of semen

(continued)

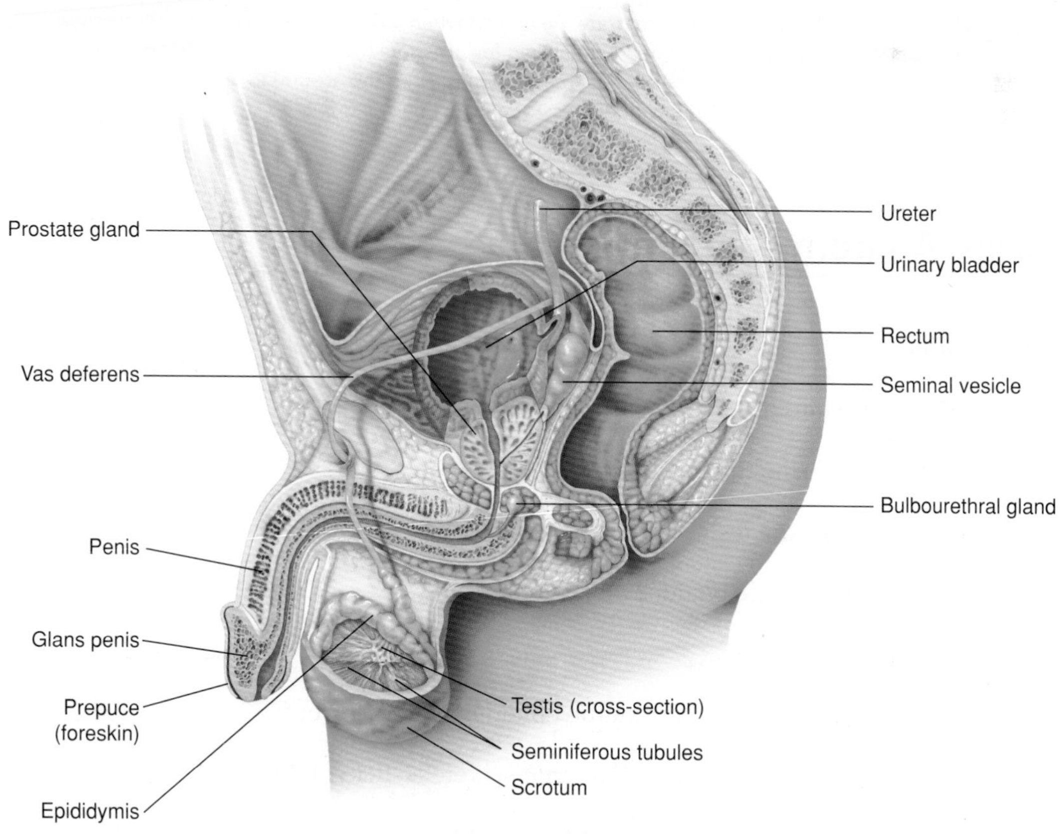

Figure 14-1 The male reproductive system.

Terms Related to the Male Reproductive System *(continued)*

Term	Pronunciation	Meaning
seminiferous tubules	sem′i-nif′ĕr-ŭs tū′byūlz	coiled tubes in the testes where spermatozoa are formed
sperm; *syn.* spermatozoon	sperm; sper′mă-tō-zō′on	male sex cell produced by the testes that can fertilize an oocyte in a female to produce offspring
spermatic cord	sper-mat′ik kōrd	cord-like structure consisting of a bundle of nerves, ducts, and blood vessels extending from the deep inguinal ring through the inguinal canal into the scrotum
testis; *syn.* testicle	tes′tis; tes′ti-kĕl	one of two oval male gonads (reproductive organs) located in the scrotum that produce sperm and testosterone
testosterone	tes-tos′tĕ-rōn	male hormone produced by the testes
vas deferens; *syn.* ductus deferens	vas def′ĕr-enz; dŭk′tŭs def′ĕr-enz	duct that carries spermatozoa from the epididymis to the urethra

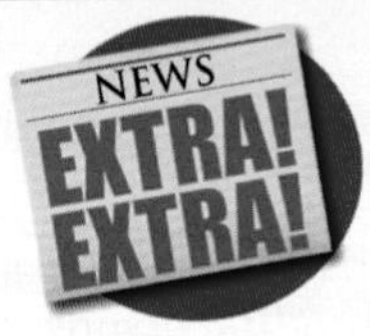

MALE URETHRA The male urethra has two separate functions. It carries urine from the urination, and it transports semen from the vas deferens during ejaculation. During sexual intercourse, bladder neck muscles connecting the urinary bladder to the urethra contract and prevent urine from escaping with the ejaculate. This same muscle group keeps urine in the bladder until the muscles relax for urination. Retrograde ejaculation is a condition in which these bladder neck muscles do not tighten and semen enters the bladder during ejaculation. Retrograde ejaculation can occur with neurologic disease, in cases of diabetes, and sometimes after prostate gland surgery.

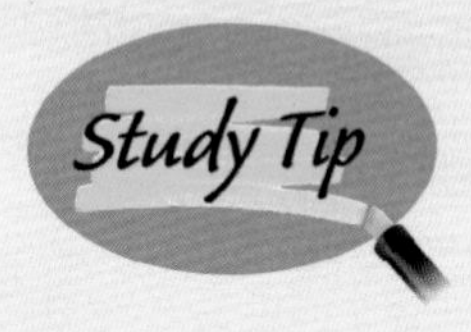

Prostate Versus Prostrate: Be careful when writing or saying the word *prostate* (one *R*). It is frequently mistaken for *prostrate* (two *Rs*). *Prostate* refers to the gland, whereas *prostrate* means lying flat on the ground in face-down position or to be overcome with distress or exhaustion.

Exercises: Anatomy and Physiology

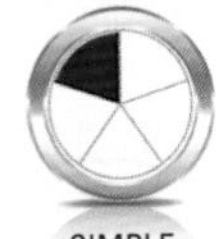

SIMPLE RECALL

Exercise 1

Write the correct anatomic structure for the definition given.

1. fold of skin covering the glans penis __________
2. sac that contains the testes and epididymis __________
3. glands posterior to the bladder that produce fluid __________
4. male sex cell __________
5. ducts carrying spermatozoa from the epididymis to the urethra __________
6. glands inferior to the prostate gland that secrete a sticky fluid __________
7. external male organ of urination and intercourse __________
8. coiled tubes in the testes where spermatozoa are formed __________

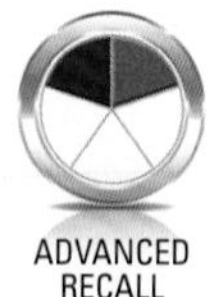
ADVANCED RECALL

Exercise 2

Match each medical term with its meaning.

epididymis	semen	testis
testosterone	glans penis	prostate gland

1. male hormone produced by the testes ____________

2. rounded tip of the penis ____________

3. coiled duct behind the testes that transports sperm ____________

4. fluid containing sperm and fluids from other glands ____________

5. gland that surrounds the beginning of the urethra ____________

6. male reproductive organ that produces sperm and testosterone ____________

WORD PARTS

The following tables list word parts related to the male reproductive system.

Combining Forms

Combining Form	Meaning
andr/o	male
balan/o	glans penis
epididym/o	epididymis
orch/o, orchi/o, orchid/o	testis, testicle
prostat/o	prostate
sperm/o, spermat/o	sperm, spermatozoon
test/o, testicul/o	testis, testicle
vas/o	duct, vessel, vas deferens[a]
vesicul/o	fluid-filled sac (seminal vesicle)[a]

[a]In this chapter, the combining form vas/o will refer specifically to the vas deferens, and the combining form vesicul/o will refer to the seminal vesicle.

Prefixes

Prefix	Meaning
an-	without, not
andro-	masculine, male
crypt-	hidden

Suffixes

Suffix	Meaning
-cele	herniation, protrusion
-genesis	originating, producing
-ism	condition of
-lith	stone, calculus
-lysis	destruction, breakdown, separation
-pathy	disease
-pexy	surgical fixation
-plasty	surgical repair, reconstruction
-rrhea	flow, discharge
-stomy	surgical opening
-tomy	incision

Exercises: Word Parts

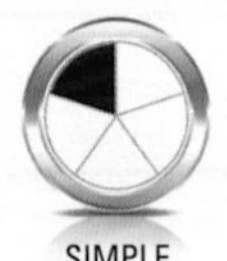

SIMPLE RECALL

Exercise 3

Write the meaning of the combining form given.

1. prostat/o ____________
2. sperm/o ____________
3. andr/o ____________
4. vesicul/o ____________
5. orchid/o ____________
6. balan/o ____________
7. epididym/o ____________
8. spermat/o ____________
9. vas/o ____________
10. test/o ____________

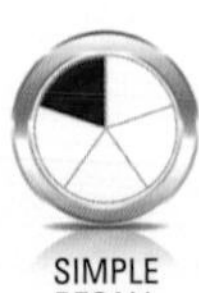
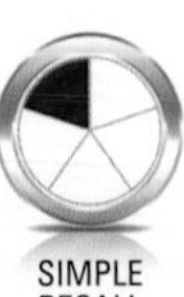

SIMPLE RECALL

Exercise 4

Write the correct prefix or suffix for the meaning given.

1. hidden ____________
2. destruction, breakdown ____________
3. condition of ____________
4. herniation ____________

5. incision ______
6. without ______
7. surgical fixation ______
8. surgical repair ______
9. surgical opening ______
10. originating, producing ______

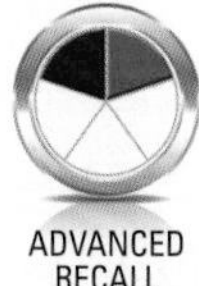

ADVANCED RECALL

Exercise 5

Match each combining form with its meaning.

orchi/o balan/o prostat/o
vas/o vesicul/o

1. male reproductive gland that produces spermatozoa and testosterone ______
2. rounded tip of the penis ______
3. fluid-filled sac (seminal vesicle) ______
4. a duct or a vessel ______
5. gland that surrounds the beginning of the urethra ______

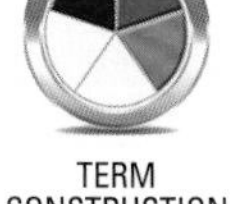

TERM CONSTRUCTION

Exercise 6

Build a medical term for each definition, using one of the listed combining forms and one of the listed suffixes.

Combining Forms	Suffixes
orchi/o	-genesis
andr/o	-rrhea
vas/o	-ectomy
spermat/o	-lith
balan/o	-pathy
prostat/o	-itis
vesicul/o	-pexy

1. excision of the vas deferens ______
2. disease found only in males ______
3. stone in the prostate gland ______
4. inflammation of a seminal vesicle ______
5. formation of spermatozoa ______
6. discharge from the glans penis ______
7. surgical fixation of a testicle ______

MEDICAL TERMS

The following table gives adjective forms and terms used in describing the male reproductive system.

Adjectives and Other Related Terms

Term	Pronunciation	Meaning
balanic	ba-lan′ik	pertaining to the glans penis
coitus	kō′i-tŭs	sexual intercourse
condom	kŏn′dom	sheath for the penis worn during intercourse to prevent conception (fertilization of oocyte by a sperm) or infection
ejaculation	ē-jak′yū-lā′shŭn	expulsion of semen from the male urethra
epididymal	ep′i-did′i-măl	pertaining to the epididymis
prostatic	pros-tat′ik	pertaining to the prostate
puberty	pyū′bĕr-tē	period of development when secondary sex characteristics (physical characteristic typical to a male or female such as men's beards and women's breasts) develop and the ability to reproduce begins
spermatic	spĕr-mat′ik	pertaining to sperm
spermicide	spĕr′mi-sīd	substance that kills spermatozoa
testicular	tes-tik′yū-lăr	pertaining to a testicle

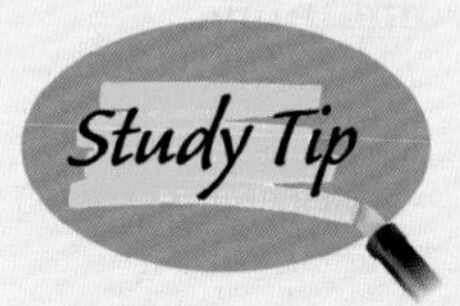

Prostatic Versus Prosthetic: Avoid confusing these sound-alike terms. Prostatic means relating to the prostate. A prosthetic relates to an artificial body part.

Exercises: Adjectives and Other Related Terms

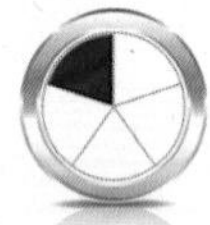

SIMPLE RECALL

Exercise 7

Write the correct medical term for the definition given.

1. pertaining to the prostate ________________

2. pertaining to a testicle ________________

3. sheath for the penis worn during intercourse ________________

4. expulsion of semen from a male urethra ________________

5. pertaining to the epididymis ____________

6. pertaining to sperm ____________

7. pertaining to the glans penis ____________

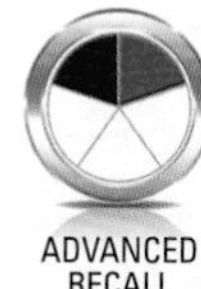

Exercise 8

ADVANCED RECALL

Circle the term that is most appropriate for the meaning of the sentence.

1. Mrs. Perez's preferred form of birth control is a(n) (*coitus, spermicide, ejaculation*).
2. Dr. Smyth suspected that Mr. Lee had a problem with his testes, so he performed a (*prostatic, balanic, testicular*) examination.
3. The patient reported fluid coming from his penis; this is known as a(n) (*balanic, testicular, epididymal*) discharge.
4. Dr. Jovan explained that the patient's prostate had increased in size, a condition also referred to as (*testicular, prostatic, spermatic*) enlargement.
5. Because of his developmental changes, 13-year-old Jimmy Petit was thought to be going through (*ejaculation, puberty, spermatic*).
6. Mr. Cuomo was diagnosed with a(n) (*epididymal, balanic, spermatic*) infection, which is located in the coiled duct on the posterior surface of the testes.
7. The physician asked Mr. Ackerman if he knew the correct way to use a (*coitus, puberty, condom*).

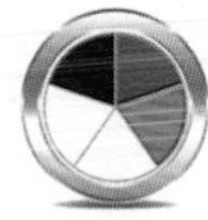

Exercise 9

TERM CONSTRUCTION

Write the combining form used in the medical term, followed by the meaning of the combining form.

Term	Combining Form	Combining Form Definition
1. testicular	____________	____________
2. prostatic	____________	____________
3. balanic	____________	____________
4. epididymal	____________	____________
5. spermicide	____________	____________

Medical Conditions

Term	Pronunciation	Meaning
andropathy	an-drop′ă-thē	disease found only in males
anorchism	an-ōr′kizm	absence of the testes; may be congenital or acquired
aspermia	ā-spĕr′mē-ă	absence of sperm; inability to produce sperm
balanitis	bal′ă-nī′tis	inflammation of the glans penis

(continued)

Medical Conditions *(continued)*

Term	Pronunciation	Meaning
balanorrhea	bal′ă-nō-rē′ă	abnormal discharge from the glans penis
benign prostatic hyperplasia (BPH); *syn.* benign prostatic hypertrophy (BPH)	bē-nīn′ pros-tat′ik hī-pĕr-plā′zhē-ă; hī-pĕr′trō-fē	enlargement of the prostate gland (**Figure 14-2**)
cryptorchidism	krip-tōr′ki-dizm	condition of hidden testis (or testes); failure of the testes to descend into the scrotum before birth (**Figure 14-3**)
epididymitis	ep′i-did-i-mī′tis	inflammation of the epididymis
erectile dysfunction (ED)	ē-rek′tīl dis-fŭnk′shŭn	inability of a man to attain or maintain an erection
hydrocele	hī′drō-sēl	accumulation of fluid in the scrotum (**Figure 14-4**)
oligospermia	ol′i-gō-spĕr′mē-ă	deficiency of sperm in the semen
orchitis; *syn.* testitis	ōr-kī′tis; tes-tī′tis	inflammation of a testis or testicle

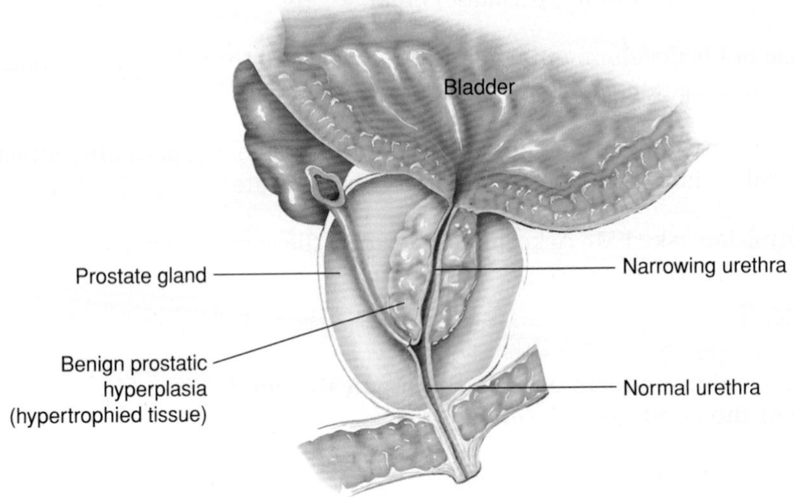

Figure 14-2 Benign prostatic hyperplasia.

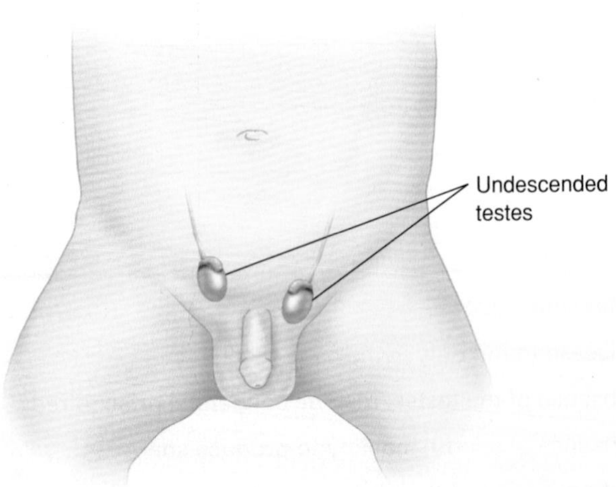

Figure 14-3 Cryptorchidism.

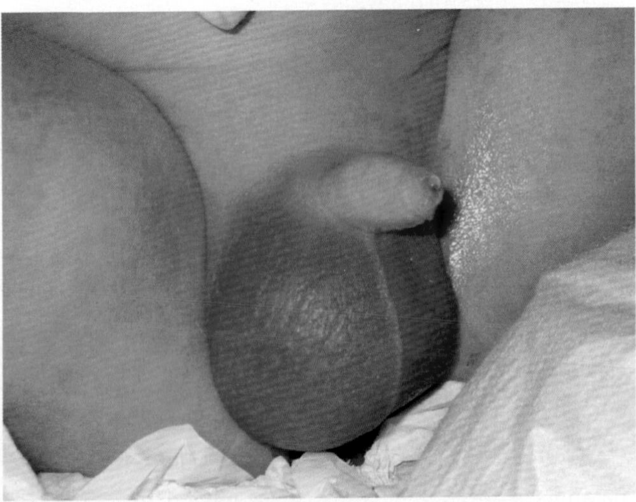

Figure 14-4 Infant with hydrocele.

Medical Conditions

Term	Pronunciation	Meaning
Peyronie disease	pā-rō-nē′ di-zēz′	condition of abnormal fibrous tissue in the erectile tissues of the penis, causing penile bending and pain during erection (**Figure 14-5**)
phimosis	fī-mō′sis	narrowing of the penis foreskin opening that prevents it from being retracted over the glans penis (**Figure 14-6**)
priapism	prī′ă-pizm	abnormal persistent and painful erection of the penis
prostatic calculus; *syn.* prostatolith	pros-tat′ik kal′kyū-lŭs; pros-tat′-ō-lith	stone formed in the prostate gland
prostatitis	pros′tă-tī′tis	inflammation of the prostate gland
prostatorrhea	pros′tă-tō-rē′ă	discharge from the prostate gland
spermatocele	spĕr′mă-tō-sēl′	sperm-containing cyst in the epididymis (**Figure 14-7**)
testicular torsion	tes-tik′yū-lăr tōr′shŭn	twisting of the spermatic cord, causing a decrease in blood flow to the penis (**Figure 14-8**)
varicocele	var′i-kō-sēl′	enlargement of veins in the spermatic cord (**Figure 14-9**)

(continued)

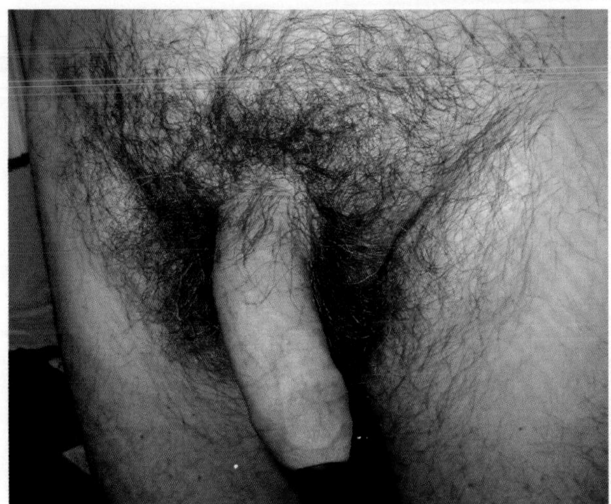

Figure 14-5 Peyronie disease causing bending of the penis.

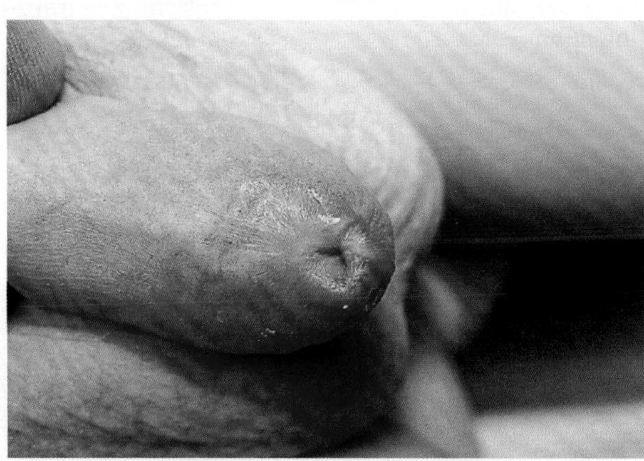

Figure 14-6 With phimosis, the foreskin cannot be retracted over the penis tip.

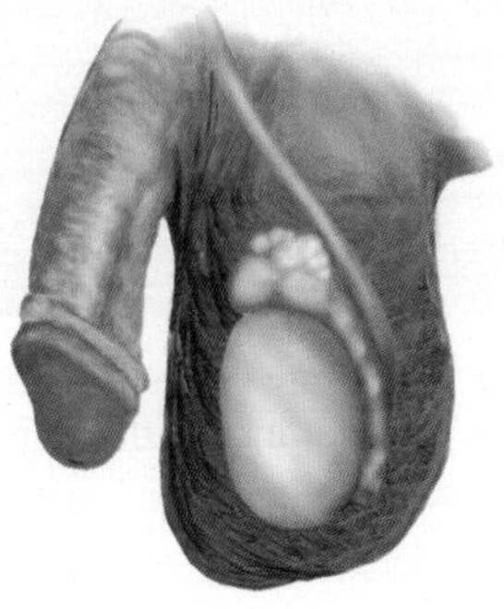

Figure 14-7 Spermatocele. Mass located just above the testis indicates a spermatocele that contains sperm.

Medical Conditions *(continued)*

Term	Pronunciation	Meaning
	Sexually Transmitted Diseases (STDs)	
acquired immunodeficiency syndrome (AIDS)	ă-kwīrd′ im′yū-nō-dē-fish′en-sē sin′drōm	disease of the immune system caused by infection with human immunodeficiency virus (HIV)
chlamydia	klă-mid′ē-ă	bacterial sexually transmitted disease that can occur with no symptoms (sometimes referred to as the silent sexually transmitted disease) until it progresses to where it damages organs; the most common STD in the United States
condyloma	kon′di-lō′mă	a wart-like lesion on the genitals
genital herpes	jen′i-tăl hĕr′pēz	inflammatory sexually transmitted disease caused by the herpes simplex virus; symptoms include blisters or ulcerative lesions on the genitals
gonorrhea	gon′ō-rē′ă	contagious, inflammatory, sexually transmitted disease affecting mucous membranes of the genitals and urinary system
human immunodeficiency virus (HIV)	hyū′măn im′yū-nō-dē-fish′en-sē vī′rŭs	a virus that weakens the body's immune system and can cause AIDS
human papillomavirus (HPV)	hyū′măn pap′i-lō′mă-vī′rŭs	viral sexually transmitted disease that causes genital warts and other symptoms (**Figure 14-10**)
sexually transmitted disease (STD); *syn.* venereal disease (VD), sexually transmitted infection	sek′shū-ă-lē tranz-mit′ĕd di-zēz′; vĕ-nēr′ē-ăl di-zēz′, sek′shū-ă-lē tranz-mit′ĕd in-fek′shŭn	any contagious disease acquired during sexual contact
syphilis	sif′i-lis	bacterial sexually transmitted disease that causes sores called chancres (shan′kerz); can spread to other parts of the body (**Figure 14-11**)

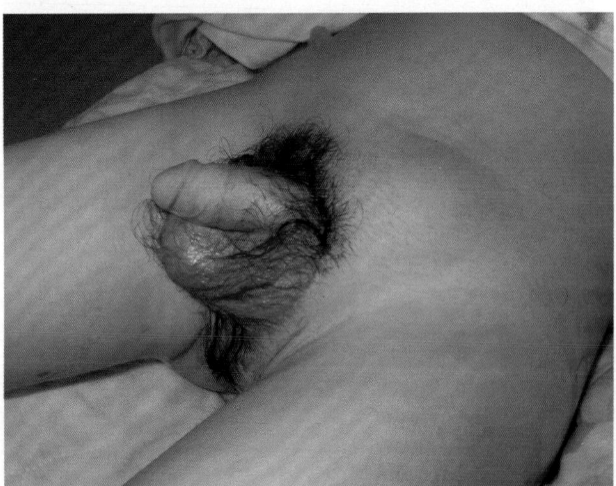

Figure 14-8 Adolescent with testicular torsion.

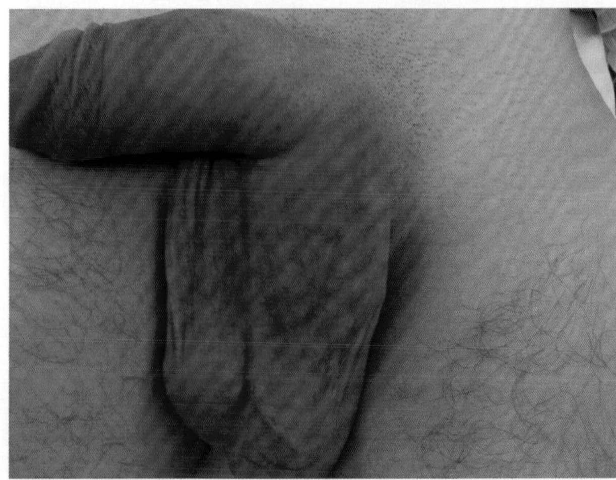

Figure 14-9 Varicocele with characteristic "bag of worms" appearance within the testicle.

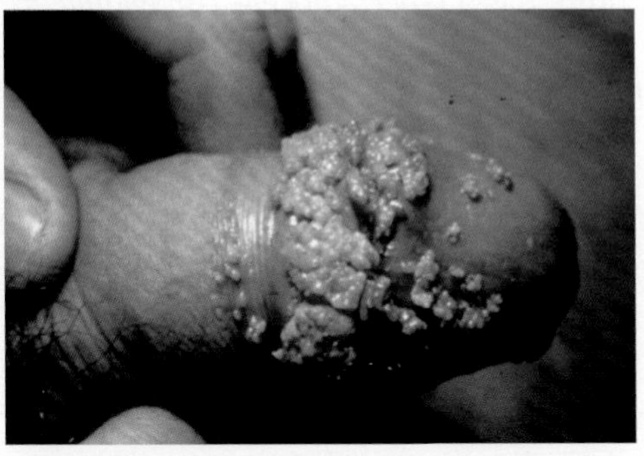
Figure 14-10 Genital warts caused by human papillomavirus (HPV).

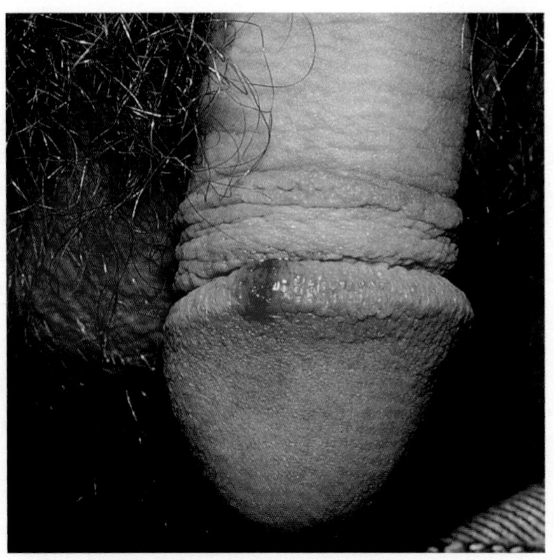
Figure 14-11 Syphilitic chancres.

Exercises: Medical Conditions

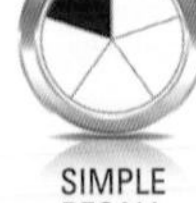
SIMPLE RECALL

Exercise 10

Write the meaning of the term given.

1. prostatitis ______________________
2. priapism ______________________
3. aspermia ______________________
4. balanorrhea ______________________
5. epididymitis ______________________
6. phimosis ______________________
7. condyloma ______________________

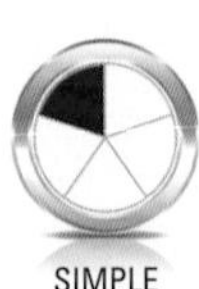
SIMPLE RECALL

Exercise 11

Circle the term that is most appropriate for the meaning of the sentence.

1. The bacterial sexually transmitted disease that can occur with no symptoms until it reaches a serious stage is called (*syphilis, chlamydia, gonorrhea*).
2. (*Gonorrhea, Human papillomavirus, Genital herpes*) is a sexually transmitted disease that causes blisters or ulcerative lesions on the genitals.
3. When veins in the spermatic cord enlarge, it is called a (*phimosis, varicocele, prostatolith*).

4. (*Gonorrhea, Condyloma, Genital herpes*) is a sexually transmitted disease that affects the mucous membranes of the genitals and urinary system.

5. A disease of the immune system caused by infection with HIV is called (*human papillomavirus, syphilis, acquired immunodeficiency syndrome*).

6. A patient with an accumulation of fluid in the scrotum has a (*spermatocele, condyloma, hydrocele*).

7. (*Erectile dysfunction, Benign prostatic hypertrophy, Priapism*) is a condition in which the prostate gland is enlarged.

8. When a patient cannot attain or maintain an erection, he has a condition called (*chlamydia, phimosis, erectile dysfunction*).

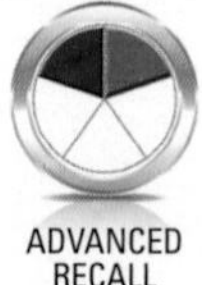
ADVANCED RECALL

Exercise 12

Complete each sentence by writing in the correct medical term.

1. A sexually transmitted disease that causes genital warts is ______________________.

2. Enlargement of the prostate gland is called ______________________.

3. The virus that weakens the body's immune system and causes AIDS is known as ______________________.

4. Any disease transmitted through sexual contact is known as a(n) ______________________.

5. An epididymal cyst containing sperm is a(n) ______________________.

6. A condition in which there is twisting of the spermatic cord is a(n) ______________________.

7. A sexually transmitted disease that causes chancres is ______________________.

8. Development of abnormal fibrous tissue in erectile tissues inside the penis is called ______________________.

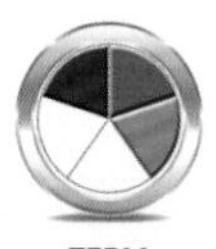
TERM CONSTRUCTION

Exercise 13

Build the correct medical term for the meaning given. Write the term in the blank and then indicate the word parts (P = prefix, CF = combining form, S = suffix).

1. cyst in the epididymis containing spermatozoa ____________ / ____________
   CF S

2. inflammation of the prostate ____________ / ____________
   CF S

3. abnormal discharge from the glans penis ____________ / ____________
   CF S

4. absence of sperm ________ / ________ / ________
   P CF S

5. inflammation of a testis ________ / ________ (CF / S)

6. inflammation of the glans penis ________ / ________ (CF / S)

7. condition of hidden testes ________ / ________ / ________ (P / CF / S)

8. inflammation of the epididymis ________ / ________ (CF / S)

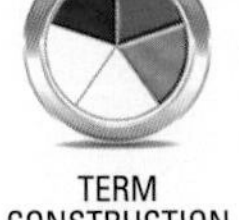
TERM CONSTRUCTION

Exercise 14

Break the given medical term into its word parts, and define each part. Then define the medical term.

For example:

orchitis
word parts: orchi/o, -itis
meanings: testicle, inflammation of
term meaning: inflammation of the testicles

1. andropathy
word parts: ________
meanings: ________
term meaning: ________

2. prostatolith
word parts: ________
meanings: ________
term meaning: ________

3. balanitis
word parts: ________
meanings: ________
term meaning: ________

4. oligospermia
word parts: ________
meanings: ________
term meaning: ________

5. anorchism
word parts: ________
meanings: ________
term meaning: ________

6. prostatorrhea *word parts:* ______

meanings: ______

term meaning: ______

7. cryptorchidism *word parts:* ______

meanings: ______

term meaning: ______

Tests and Procedures

Term	Pronunciation	Meaning
Laboratory Test		
prostate-specific antigen (PSA) test	pros′tāt-spĕ-sif′ik an′ti-jen test	blood test that measures the amount of an enzyme released by the prostate gland known as prostate-specific antigen; increased levels indicate benign prostatic hyperplasia (BPH) or prostate cancer
Diagnostic Procedures		
digital rectal examination (DRE)	dij′i-tăl rek′tăl ek-zam′i-nā′shŭn	assessment done by inserting a finger into the male rectum to determine the size and shape of the prostate gland through the rectal wall (**Figure 14-12**)
transrectal ultrasound (TRUS)	trans-rek′tăl ŭl′tră-sownd	ultrasound imaging of the prostate gland done through the rectum

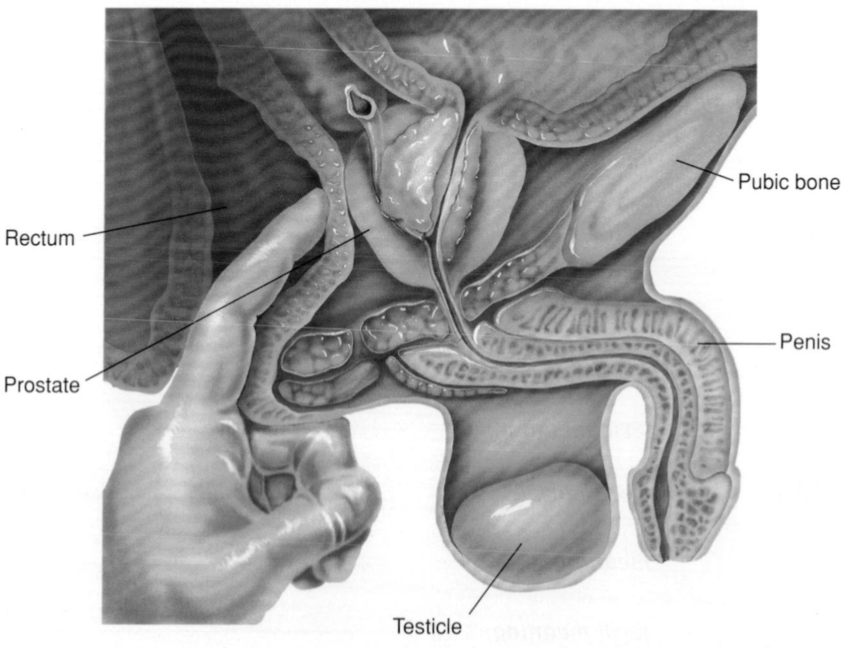

Figure 14-12 Digital rectal examination (DRE).

Exercise: Tests and Procedures

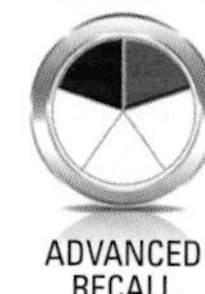

ADVANCED RECALL

Exercise 15

Match each medical term with its meaning.

digital rectal examination prostate-specific antigen transrectal ultrasound

1. ultrasound imaging of the prostate through the rectum ______________________
2. examination of the prostate by inserting a finger into the rectum ______________________
3. blood test that screens for BPH or prostate cancer ______________________

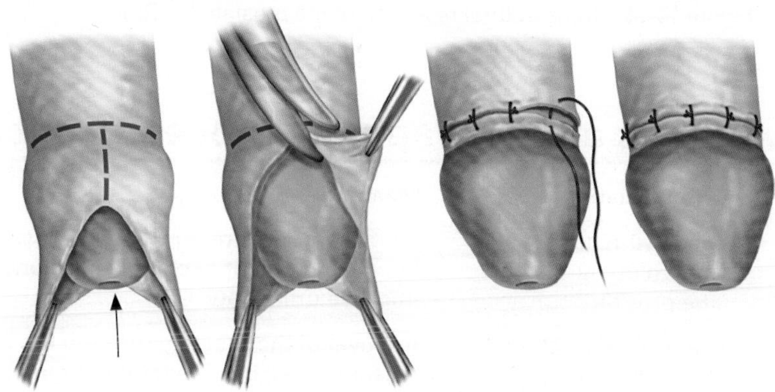

Figure 14-13 Circumcision.

Surgical Interventions and Therapeutic Procedures

Term	Pronunciation	Meaning
balanoplasty	bal′ăn-ō-plas′tē	surgical repair or reconstruction of the glans penis
circumcision	ser′kŭm-sizh′ŭn	operation to remove the prepuce (foreskin) from the penis (**Figure 14-13**)
epididymectomy	ep′i-did-i-mek′tŏ-mē	operation to remove the epididymis
orchiectomy; *syn.* orchidectomy	ōr′kē-ek′tŏ-mē; ōr′ki-dek′tŏ-mē	removal of one or both testes
orchiopexy; *syn.* orchidopexy	ōr′kē-ō-pek′sē; ōr-kid′ō-peks′ē	surgical treatment of an undescended testicle by freeing it and implanting it into the scrotum
orchiotomy; *syn.* orchotomy	ōr′kē-ot′ŏ-mē; ōr-kot′ŏ-mē	incision into a testis
orchioplasty	ōr′kē-ō-plas′tē	surgical repair or reconstruction of a testis
penile implant	pē′nīl im′plant	device that is surgically placed in the penis to produce an erection; used to treat erectile dysfunction (ED)
prostatectomy	pros′tă-tek′tŏ-mē	surgical procedure to remove all or part of the prostate
prostatolithotomy	pros′tă-tō-li-thot′ŏ-mē	incision into the prostate to remove a stone

(continued)

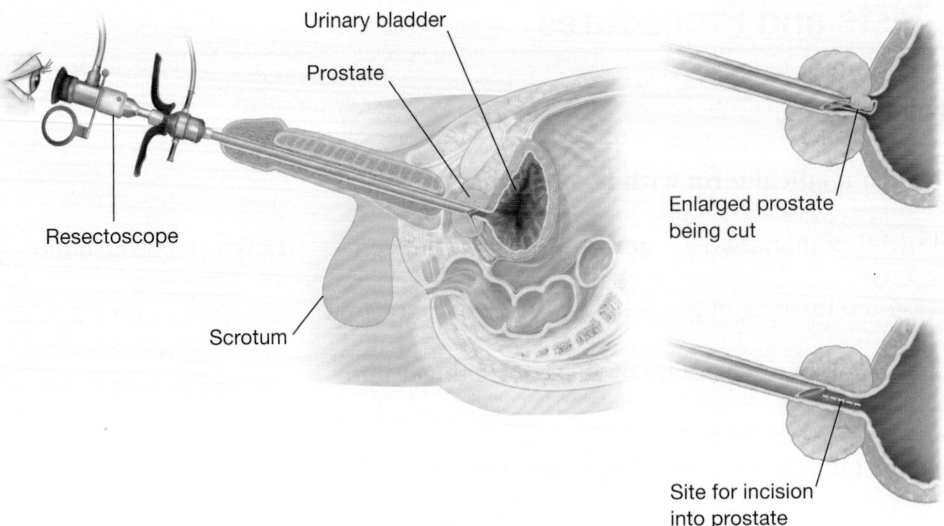

Figure 14-14 Transurethral resection of the prostate (TURP).

Surgical Interventions and Therapeutic Procedures *(continued)*

Term	Pronunciation	Meaning
transurethral incision of the prostate (TUIP or TIP)	trans′yū-rē′thrăl in-sizh′ŭn ov the pros′tāt	surgical procedure for treating prostate gland enlargement by making one or two small incisions in the prostate to improve urine flow
transurethral resection of the prostate (TURP)	trans′yū-rē′thrăl rē-sek′shŭn ov the pros′tāt	removal of the prostate through the urethra using a resectoscope; used to treat benign prostatic hyperplasia (**Figure 14-14**)
vasectomy	va-sek′tŏ-mē	surgical excising and closing off (ligating) of a segment of each vas deferens (ductus deferens) to cause male sterility (**Figure 14-15**)
vasovasostomy	vā′sō-vă-sos′tŏ-mē	surgical reconnecting of the vasa deferentia in a male with a vasectomy to restore fertility; vasectomy reversal operation

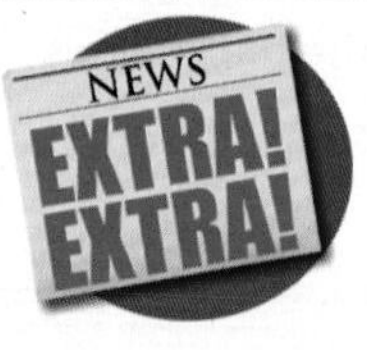

VASECTOMY AND VASOVASOSTOMY In order to understand how a vasectomy works, you have to know the pathway a sperm travels to reach the body's exterior. The seminiferous tubules within the testes produce sperm, which are then matured and stored in the epididymis. From there, sperm travel from the tail of the epididymis into the ductus (vas) deferens → seminal vesicle → ejaculatory duct → through prostate gland → out urethra. During ejaculation, rhythmic muscle contractions propel the sperm forward and out of the body. A vasectomy cuts off the pathway at the vas deferens so no live sperm can complete the transit. The sperm are instead absorbed by the body and do not become part of seminal fluid. It is important to note that a vasectomy is a bilateral procedure, because there are two vasa deferentia, one on the right and one on the left. To reverse the procedure an operation called vasovasostomy is performed. During a vasovasostomy, the tubes that were cut during a vasectomy are reconnected. Think *vaso vaso* means "duct duct" and *ostomy* refers to a surgical opening. So this surgery recreates the opening between the two cut ducts. If a vasovasostomy is done within three years of a vasectomy, pregnancy results about 50% of the time. As time goes on, the pregnancy success rate decreases and the incidence of abnormal sperm production increases.

vesiculectomy	vě-sik′ū-lek′tŏ-mē	surgical removal of a part or all of a seminal vesicle

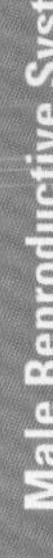

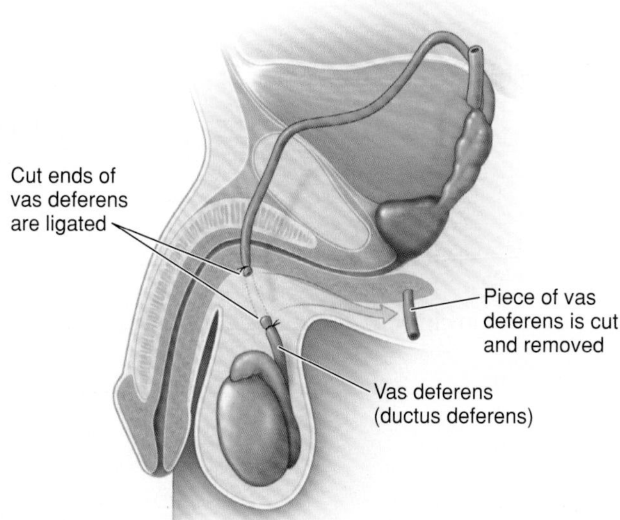

Figure 14-15 In a vasectomy, a piece of the vas deferens is cut and removed, and the loose ends are ligated (tied).

Exercises: Surgical Interventions and Therapeutic Procedures

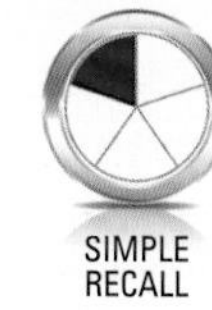
SIMPLE RECALL

Exercise 16

Write the meaning of the term given.

1. vasovasostomy __________
2. circumcision __________
3. orchiectomy __________
4. prostatolithotomy __________
5. transurethral resection of the prostate __________
6. penile implant __________

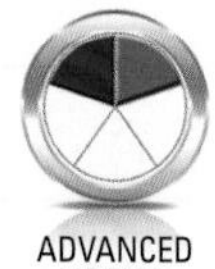
ADVANCED RECALL

Exercise 17

Match each medical term with its meaning.

prostatolithotomy	orchiectomy	epididymectomy
vasectomy	prostatectomy	orchioplasty

1. surgical repair of a testicle __________
2. operation to remove an epididymis __________
3. incision to remove a stone from the prostate __________
4. removal of a testicle __________
5. male sterilization procedure __________
6. removal of the prostate __________

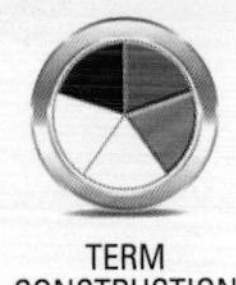

Exercise 18

TERM CONSTRUCTION

Write the remainder of the term for the meaning given.

1. removal of the epididymis ______________ ectomy
2. surgical repair or reconstruction of a testis orchio ______________
3. removal of a seminal vesicle vesicul ______________
4. incision into a testis orchido ______________
5. excision of the vas deferens ______________ ectomy

Exercise 19

TERM CONSTRUCTION

Break the given medical term into its word parts, and define each part. Then define the medical term.

For example:

orchitis	*word parts:*	orchi/o, -itis
	meanings:	testes, inflammation of
	term meaning:	inflammation of the testicles

1. orchiotomy
   word parts: ______________
   meanings: ______________
   term meaning: ______________
2. balanoplasty
   word parts: ______________
   meanings: ______________
   term meaning: ______________
3. prostatectomy
   word parts: ______________
   meanings: ______________
   term meaning: ______________
4. orchiopexy
   word parts: ______________
   meanings: ______________
   term meaning: ______________
5. vasectomy
   word parts: ______________
   meanings: ______________
   term meaning: ______________

Medications and Drug Therapies

Term	Pronunciation	Meaning
antiretroviral	an′tē-ret′rō-vī′răl	drug used for the treatment of infection by a retrovirus, primarily human immunodeficiency virus (HIV)
antiviral	an′tē-vī′răl	drug used specifically for treating viral infections
impotence agent	im′pŏ-tĕns ā′jĕnt	drug used to treat erectile dysfunction (ED)
vasodilator	vā′sō-dī′lā-tŏr	drug used to open blood vessels; may be used to treat benign prostatic hypertrophy and erectile dysfunction

■ Exercise: Medications and Drug Therapies

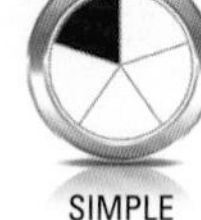
SIMPLE RECALL

Exercise 20

Write the correct medication or drug therapy term for the definition given.

1. drug used to treat erectile dysfunction ______________________
2. drug used to treat infection caused by a retrovirus ______________________
3. drug used to open blood vessels ______________________
4. drug used specifically to treat viral infections ______________________

Specialties and Specialists

Term	Pronunciation	Meaning
urology	yū-rol′ŏ-jē	medical specialty focusing on the study and treatment of conditions of the urinary system and male reproductive system
urologist	yū-rol′ŏ-jist	physician who specializes in urology

■ Exercise: Specialties and Specialists

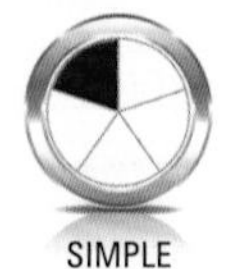
SIMPLE RECALL

Exercise 21

Write the correct medical term for the definition given.

1. specialty concerned with conditions of the urinary system ______________________
2. physician who specializes in urology ______________________

Abbreviations

Abbreviation	Meaning
AIDS	acquired immunodeficiency syndrome
BPH	benign prostatic hyperplasia; benign prostatic hypertrophy
DRE	digital rectal examination
ED	erectile dysfunction
HIV	human immunodeficiency virus
HPV	human papillomavirus
PSA	prostate-specific antigen
STD	sexually transmitted disease
STI	sexually transmitted infection
TIP	transurethral incision of the prostate
TRUS	transrectal ultrasound
TUIP	transurethral incision of the prostate
TURP	transurethral resection of the prostate
VD	venereal disease

Exercises: Abbreviations

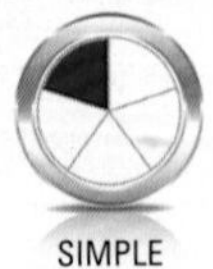

SIMPLE RECALL

Exercise 22

Write the meaning of each abbreviation.

1. BPH ______________________________
2. TUIP ______________________________
3. ED ______________________________
4. HIV ______________________________
5. PSA ______________________________
6. STI ______________________________
7. TRUS ______________________________
8. TIP ______________________________

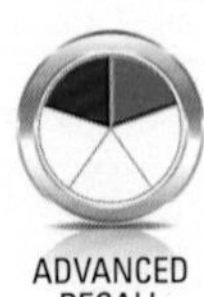

ADVANCED RECALL

Exercise 23

Write the meaning of each abbreviation used in these sentences.

1. The patient had an enlarged prostate, so the physician scheduled him for a **TURP.**

____

2. The physician counseled the patient about the risks of getting an **STD.**

____

3. At the patient's annual physical, the physician performed a **DRE.**

____

4. The patient's genital warts were caused by an **HPV** infection.

____

5. The human immunodeficiency virus caused the patient to develop **AIDS.**

____

6. The patient's oliguria was caused by **BPH.**

____

WRAPPING UP

- The main male reproductive organs (the penis and testicles) are located outside the body.
- The main function of the male reproductive system is to produce semen and sperm.
- In this chapter, you learned medical terminology including word parts, prefixes, suffixes, adjectives, conditions, tests, procedures, medications, specialties, and abbreviations related to the reproductive system.

Chapter Review

Review of Terms for Anatomy and Physiology

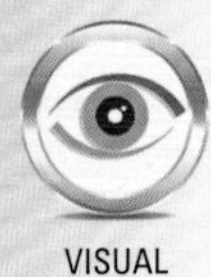

VISUAL

Exercise 24

Write the correct terms on the blanks for the anatomic structures indicated.

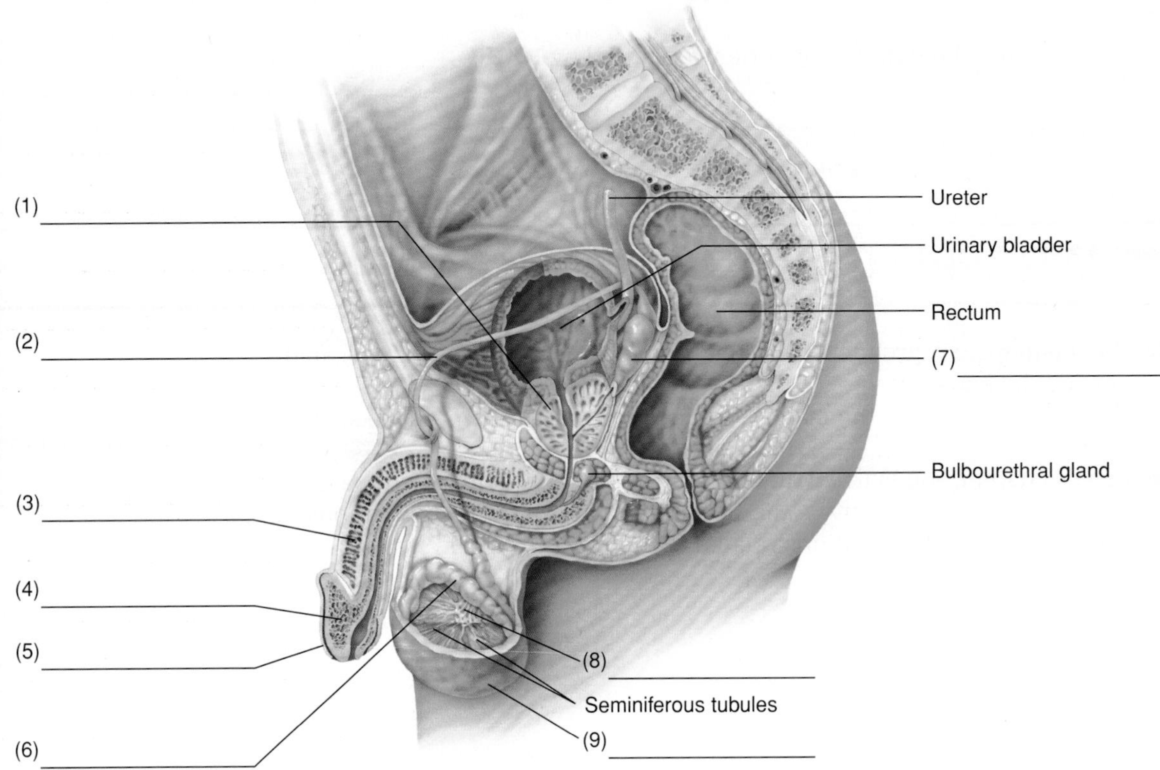

Understanding Term Structure

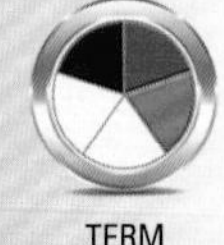

TERM CONSTRUCTION

Exercise 25

Write the combining form used in the medical term followed by the meaning of the combining form.

Term	Combining Form	Combining Form Definition
1. testicular		
2. prostatitis		
3. balanorrhea		

4. anorchism ______ ______

5. epididymectomy ______ ______

6. spermatic ______ ______

7. vesiculectomy ______ ______

8. andropathy ______ ______

Exercise 26

TERM CONSTRUCTION

For each term, first write the meaning of the term. Then write the meanings of the word parts in that term.

1. vasectomy ______
   vas/o ______
   -ectomy ______
2. prostatorrhea ______
   prostat/o ______
   -rrhea ______
3. balanitis ______
   balan/o ______
   -itis ______
4. epididymal ______
   epididym/o ______
   -al ______
5. orchidopexy ______
   orchid/o ______
   -pexy ______
6. prostatolith ______
   prostat/o ______
   -lith ______
7. orchioplasty ______
   orchid/o ______
   -plasty ______
8. vesiculectomy ______
   vesicul/o ______
   -ectomy ______

Comprehension Exercises

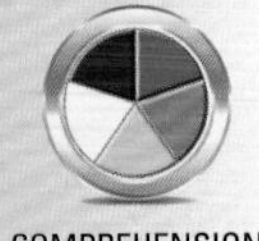

Exercise 27

Write a short answer for each question.

1. How is gonorrhea transmitted? ____________
2. Why would a patient undergo a vasovasostomy? ____________
3. What is the name of the hormone produced by the testes? ____________
4. In addition to sperm, what other substances make up semen? ____________
5. What is a cyst in the epididymis that contains sperm called? ____________
6. Genital warts are a sign of what sexually transmitted disease? ____________
7. What structure is assessed during a digital rectal examination? ____________
8. What fold of skin is left intact on an uncircumcised male penis? ____________
9. Which medical condition involves the testes and occurs before birth? ____________
10. Males who no longer want to produce offspring often have which procedure? ____________
11. Where does abnormal fibrous tissue form in a patient with Peyronie disease? ____________

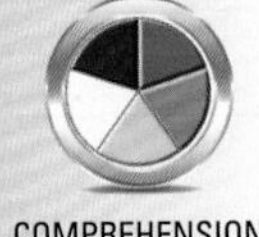

Exercise 28

Circle the letter of the best answer in the following questions.

1. Which procedure involves the removal of prostatic tissue with a resectoscope?
   A. vasovasostomy
   B. transurethral resection of the prostate
   C. orchiectomy
   D. circumcision

2. An examination of the prostate gland might reveal which condition?
   A. phimosis
   B. condyloma
   C. varicocele
   D. benign prostatic hyperplasia

3. Reproduction is not possible until a male goes through what period of development?
   A. prepuce
   B. puberty
   C. balanorrhea
   D. epididymis

4. Which test is performed to screen for BPH?
   A. transrectal ultrasound
   B. transurethral resection of the prostate
   C. prostate-specific antigen test
   D. balanoplasty

5. Another term for sexual intercourse is
   A. coitus.
   B. prepuce.
   C. priapism.
   D. puberty.

6. When there is an abnormal persistent erection of the penis, the condition is called
   A. benign prostatic hypertrophy.
   B. erectile dysfunction.
   C. priapism.
   D. syphilis.

7. Which of the following conditions is an STD?
   A. condyloma
   B. hydrocele
   C. varicocele
   D. anorchism

8. What is the name of the male sex cell needed to fertilize an oocyte?
   A. testosterone
   B. bulbourethral glands
   C. glans penis
   D. spermatozoon

9. A patient with chancres would likely be diagnosed with which condition?
   A. AIDS
   B. gonorrhea
   C. syphilis
   D. chlamydia

10. Twisting of the spermatic cord is known as
    A. anorchism.
    B. testicular torsion.
    C. testicular cancer.
    D. spermatocele.

11. The procedure that involves an ultrasound of the prostate done through the rectum is called a
    A. digital rectal examination.
    B. prostatolithotomy.
    C. circumcision.
    D. transrectal ultrasound.

12. A sheath for the penis worn during intercourse to prevent conception or infection is a
    A. condyloma.
    B. semen.
    C. condom.
    D. coitus.

13. A patient wanting to reverse his vasectomy needs to undergo a(n)
    A. orchioplasty.
    B. vasovasostomy.
    C. transurethral resection of the prostate.
    D. vesiculectomy.

14. When semen is expelled from the male urethra, it is called
    A. ejaculation.
    B. orchiotomy.
    C. erectile dysfunction.
    D. priapism.

15. The sexually transmitted disease that can occur with no signs or symptoms until it becomes severe is
    A. chlamydia.
    B. syphilis.
    C. gonorrhea.
    D. human papillomavirus.

16. An agent that is used to prevent pregnancy by killing the male sex cell is called
    A. prostate-specific antigen.
    B. testosterone.
    C. ejaculation.
    D. spermicide.

17. Which condition might be resolved as a result of circumcision?
    A. varicocele
    B. phimosis
    C. priapism
    D. testicular torsion

18. The male hormone produced by the testes is
    A. semen.
    B. testosterone.
    C. prostatorrhea.
    D. balanorrhea.

Application and Analysis

CASE STUDIES

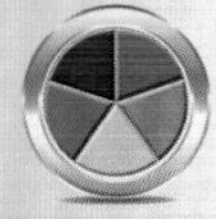
APPLICATION

Exercise 29

Read the case studies, and circle the correct letter for each of the questions.

CASE 14-1

Mr. Kendall was seen in the office because of a lump he discovered in his testes when he performed a testicular self-examination. He was concerned about the possibility of having testicular cancer. He denied having any balanorrhea. Examination revealed a circumcised male with an enlargement in the scrotum consistent with a varicocele.

1. The term that means abnormal discharge from the glans penis is

A. semen.
B. testosterone.
C. prostatorrhea.
D. balanorrhea.

2. The term that means enlargement of veins in the spermatic cord is

A. spermatocele.
B. varicocele.
C. hydrocele.
D. cystocele.

3. The term that refers to the sac that contains the testes is

A. testicular.
B. varicocele.
C. scrotum.
D. circumcised.

CASE 14-2

Mr. Glower was seen in the office today for consideration of a vasovasostomy. He underwent a vasectomy five years ago. He had a history of an STD. Findings of genital examination today were significant for a single condylomatous lesion on the penis as well as for phimosis. After discussion of the risks and benefits of surgery, he has decided to go ahead with it. The procedure has been scheduled for next week.

4. The term that involves creating a new opening between two severed pieces of vas deferens is

A. vasectomy.
B. vasovasostomy.
C. phimosis.
D. balanoplasty.

5. The condyloma on the patient's penis could be described as a(n)

A. blister or ulcerative lesion.
B. enlargement of the veins.
C. agent that kills sperm.
D. wart-like lesion.

6. The term *phimosis* means there is a(n)

A. narrowing of the prepuce.
B. enlargement of the penis.
C. enlargement of the veins in the spermatic cord.
D. accumulation of fluid in the scrotum.

MEDICAL RECORD ANALYSIS

MEDICAL RECORD 14-1

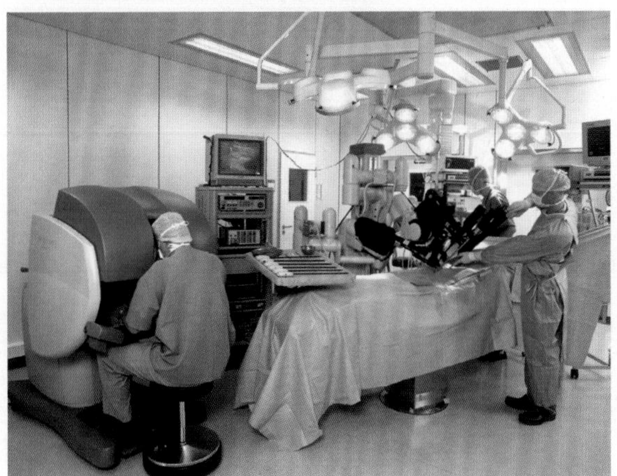

Figure 14-16 Robotic-assisted laparoscopic prostatectomy.

The patient in the Medical Record that follows, was previously diagnosed with prostate cancer and is being admitted to County General Hospital for a robotic-assisted laparoscopic prostatectomy **(Figure 14-16)**. As a diagnostic medical sonographer, you performed the transrectal ultrasound that helped to confirm the presence of this patient's tumor.

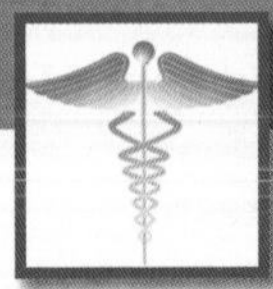

Medical Record

HISTORY AND PHYSICAL

HPI: The patient was seen in the office one month ago for symptoms of dysuria, oliguria, and nocturia, which had been worsening over the preceding three weeks. He was concerned about possible recurrence of BPH.

PMH: Medical history was remarkable for benign prostatic hyperplasia, which was treated medically three years ago with good results. He also reported having a hydrocele about five years ago and an orchiopexy as a child for cryptorchidism. He also has hypertension, which is under good control with medication and diet.

PE: Physical examination revealed no tenderness to palpation of the pubic area. A digital rectal examination was performed and revealed enlargement of the prostate gland. The gland was notably firm and nodular. Examination was otherwise unremarkable.

Laboratory and radiologic testing was ordered. A PSA was highly elevated at 25 ng/mL. A prostatic acid phosphatase test revealed elevated enzyme levels. Transrectal ultrasound was also performed and confirmed the presence of a tumor. Using ultrasound guidance, a needle biopsy of the prostate was also performed and revealed the presence of malignant cells.

Dx: Diagnosis was prostate cancer.

PLAN: Patient is admitted at this time for a robotic-assisted laparoscopic wprostatectomy **(Figure 14-16)** for minimally invasive removal of his tumor.

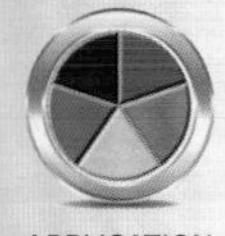

APPLICATION

Exercise 30

Write the appropriate medical terms used in this medical record on the blanks after their definitions. Note that not all the terms appear in the chapter, but you should be able to identify these terms based on word parts that are included in this chapter.

1. examination by feeling the prostate through the rectal wall ____________

2. painful urination ____________

3. accumulation of fluid in the scrotum ____________

4. surgical treatment of an undescended testicle ____________

5. imaging of the prostate done through the rectum ____________

APPLICATION

Exercise 31

Read the medical report, and circle the correct letter for each of the questions.

1. The medical record indicates that the patient's PSA level was highly elevated. The abbreviation PSA stands for

A. prostatic acid phosphatase.
B. prostate-specific alkaline.
C. prostate symptom analysis.
D. prostate-specific antigen.

2. Which of the patient's signs indicates he is urinating frequently at night?

A. oliguria
B. nocturia
C. dysuria
D. hematuria

3. As a child, the patient underwent surgery to correct

A. an undescended testicle.
B. enlargement of veins in the spermatic cord.
C. condition of being without testes or a testis.
D. abnormal persistent erection of the penis.

4. The patient is admitted for a prostatectomy, or

A. excision of a segment of the vas deferens.
B. incision into a testis.
C. surgical fixation of a testis.
D. removal of the prostate.

5. The abbreviation for enlargement of the prostate gland is

A. DRE.
B. PSA.
C. UTI.
D. BPH.

Bonus Question

6. In what two procedures was ultrasound imaging used? ____________

____

MEDICAL RECORD 14-2

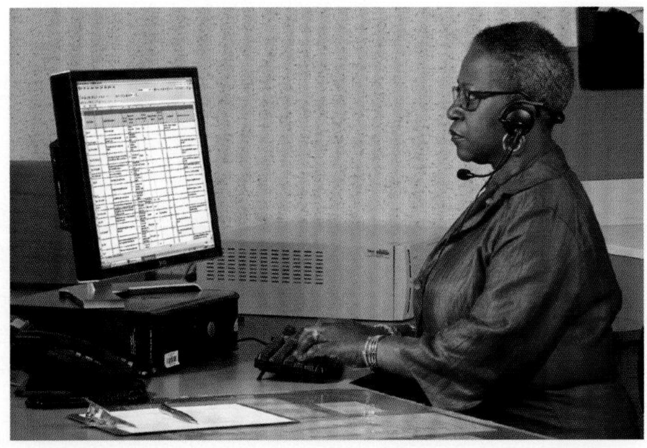

A medical transcriptionist transcribes the physician's dictated report.

Mr. Roberts was recently seen by his physician, who dictated his findings on completion of the examination. You, as a medical transcriptionist, transcribed the physician's dictated report to become a permanent part of the patient's medical record. The final transcribed record follows.

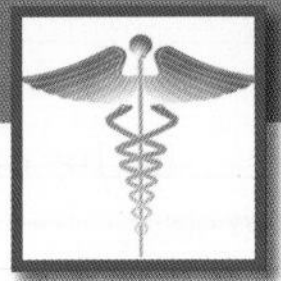

Medical Record

PROGRESS NOTE

SUBJECTIVE: The patient presents today with complaints of burning during urination, orchialgia, and balanorrhea for the past week. He denies having any condylomata, chancres, or other sores in the genital area or elsewhere on his body. He had one episode of syphilis many years ago, which was successfully treated with antibiotics. He admits to having unprotected coitus in the past few weeks. Contraceptive method is spermicide. The patient denies any other previous history of STDs.

OBJECTIVE: Examination is within normal limits with the exception of scant yellow discharge from the glans penis, urethritis, and testicular edema. A culture was taken from the discharge and Gram stain was performed revealing gonorrhea bacterium. A urine sample was obtained and will be sent to the lab for STD screening to rule out concurrent chlamydial infection.

ASSESSMENT: Gonorrhea. Rule out chlamydia.

PLAN: Rocephin 1 g injection as administered for treatment of gonorrhea. Should the lab testing prove positive for chlamydia, oral antibiotics will be prescribed. The patient was also counseled regarding the transmission of STDs and safe sex measures, including the use of condoms. He was advised to notify his sexual partners about his diagnosis so they can be tested too. He was further advised to return should his signs and symptoms return or not resolve following antibiotic therapy.

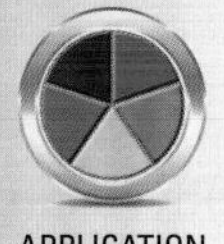

Exercise 32

APPLICATION

Write the appropriate medical terms used in this medical record on the blanks after their definitions. Note that not all these terms appear in the chapter, but you should be able to identify these terms based on word parts that are included in this chapter.

1. testicular pain ______________________
2. discharge from the glans penis ______________________
3. agent that kills sperm ______________________
4. genital warts ______________________
5. inflammation of the urethra ______________________

Exercise 33

APPLICATION

Read the medical report, and circle the correct letter for each of the questions.

1. The STD that affects the mucous membranes of the genitals and urinary system is
   A. genital herpes.
   B. chlamydia.
   C. syphilis.
   D. gonorrhea.

2. The term for a sore caused by syphilis is
   A. chancre.
   B. genital herpes.
   C. condyloma.
   D. chlamydia.

3. The term for the silent STD is
   A. human papillomavirus.
   B. chlamydia.
   C. syphilis.
   D. genital herpes.

4. ______________ is the medical term for sexual intercourse.
   A. Prepuce
   B. Edema
   C. Coitus
   D. Priapism

5. ______________ is the STD that causes chancres and can spread to other parts of the body.
   A. Gonorrhea
   B. Syphilis
   C. Genital herpes
   D. Chlamydia

Bonus Question

6. Using your medical dictionary, look up the word *edema,* and write the definition.

____

Pronunciation and Spelling

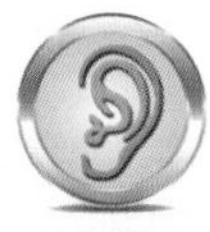

Exercise 34

Review the Chapter 14 terms in the Dictionary/Audio Glossary in the Student Resources on thePoint, and practice pronouncing each term, referring to the pronunciation guide as needed.

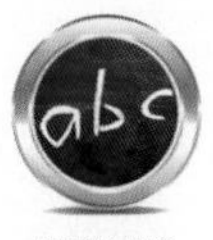

Exercise 35

Circle the correct spelling of each term.

1. skrotum	scrotum	scrotim
2. spermatozoen	spermtozoon	spermatozoon
3. semin	semun	semen
4. prostate gland	prostrate gland	prostat gland
5. coytus	coitis	coitus
6. epididimis	epididymus	epididymis
7. balanorrhea	balanorhea	balanorrhia
8. aspermea	aspermia	aspirmea
9. fimosis	phimosis	phemosis
10. hydroceel	hydrocele	hydroseal
11. prostatitis	prostratitis	prostatittis
12. vericocel	varicoseal	varicocele
13. chlamydia	clamydia	chlamidia
14. condiloma	condyloma	condylloma
15. sifilus	syphilis	syphilus

Media Connection

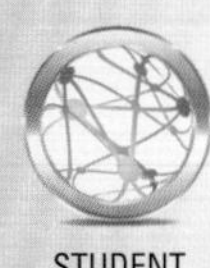

Exercise 36

Complete each of the following activities available with the Student Resources on thePoint. Check off each activity as you complete it, and record your score for the Chapter Quiz in the space provided.

Chapter Exercises

____ Flash Cards

____ Concentration

____ Abbreviation Match-Up

____ Roboterms

____ Word Anatomy

____ Fill the Gap

____ Break It Down

____ True/False Body Building

____ Quiz Show

____ Complete the Case

____ Medical Record Review

____ Look and Label

____ Image Matching

____ Spelling Bee

____ **Chapter Quiz** *Score:* ______%

Additional Resources

____ Dictionary/Audio Glossary

____ Health Professions Careers: Diagnostic Medical Sonographer

____ Health Professions Careers: Medical Transcriptionist

Female Reproductive System, Obstetrics, and Neonatology

15

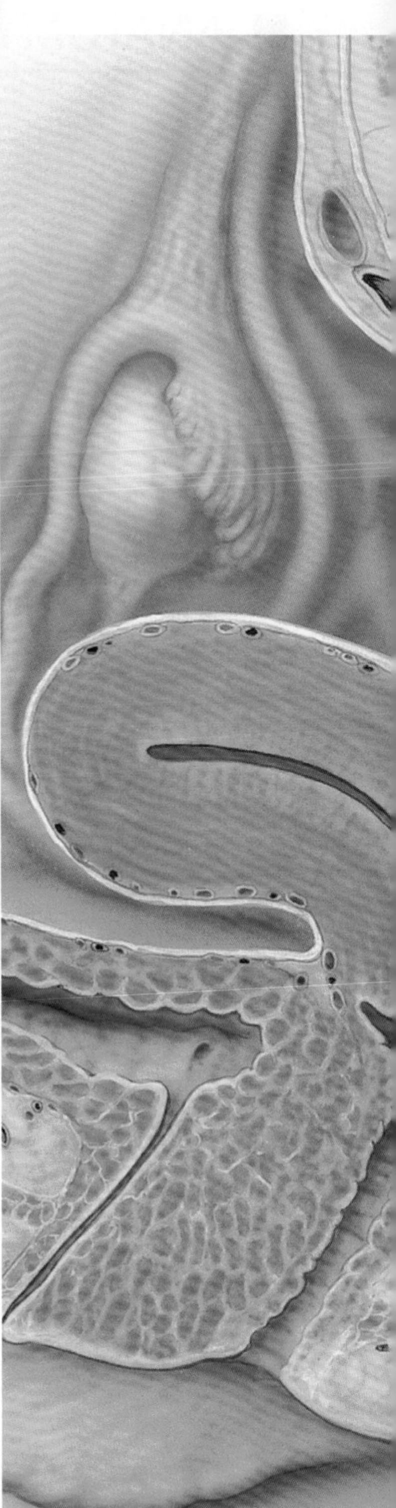

Chapter Outline

Introduction, 584

Anatomy and Physiology, 584
- Structures, 584
- Functions, 584
- Terms Related to the Female Reproductive System, 585
- Terms Related to Obstetrics and Neonatology, 588

Word Parts, 593
- Combining Forms, 593
- Prefixes, 594
- Suffixes, 595

Medical Terms, 598
- Adjectives and Other Related Terms, 598
- Medical Conditions, 602
- Tests and Procedures, 610
- Surgical Interventions and Therapeutic Procedures, 614
- Medications and Drug Therapies, 619
- Specialties and Specialists, 620
- Abbreviations, 622

Wrapping Up, 624

Chapter Review, 625

Learning Outcomes

After completion of this chapter, you should be able to:

1. List the structures and functions of the female reproductive system.
2. Describe terms related to the menstrual cycle and obstetrics.
3. Define combing forms, prefixes, and suffixes related to the female reproductive system, obstetrics, and neonatology.
4. Define common medical terminology related to the female reproductive system, obstetrics, and neonatology, including adjectives and related terms; signs, symptoms and conditions; tests and procedures; surgical interventions and therapeutic procedures; medications and drug therapies; and medical specialties and specialists.
5. Define abbreviations related to the female reproductive system, obstetrics, and neonatology.
6. Successfully complete all chapter exercises.
7. Explain terms used in case studies and medical records involving the female reproductive system and obstetrics.
8. Successfully complete all exercises included with the companion Student Resources on thePoint.

INTRODUCTION

This chapter focuses on the female reproductive system, obstetrics, and neonatology. The main purpose of the female reproductive system is to produce the female sex cells known as oocytes, to nourish a developing embryo and fetus, and to nurse an infant. Obstetrics is the field of medicine concerned chiefly with childbirth and the care of women throughout their pregnancy. Neonatology, also known as neonatal medicine, deals with the care of a newborn and includes the study of disorders of the newborn.

ANATOMY AND PHYSIOLOGY

Structures

- The external genitalia, commonly known as the genitals or vulva, include the mons pubis, labia majora (*sing.,* majus) and labia minora (*sing.,* minus), clitoris, the vestibule (surrounding area) of the vagina and its glands, and the openings of the urethra and vagina. These organs enable spermatozoa to enter the body, protect the internal genital organs from infectious organisms, and provide sexual pleasure (**Figure 15-1**).
- The internal genitalia are the passages involved in human reproduction. These structures form a pathway called the genital tract.
- The breasts are functionally a part of the female reproductive system because they contain the milk-producing structures that nourish an infant.

Functions

- Producing female sex hormones
- Propagating life by producing oocytes, the female sex cells

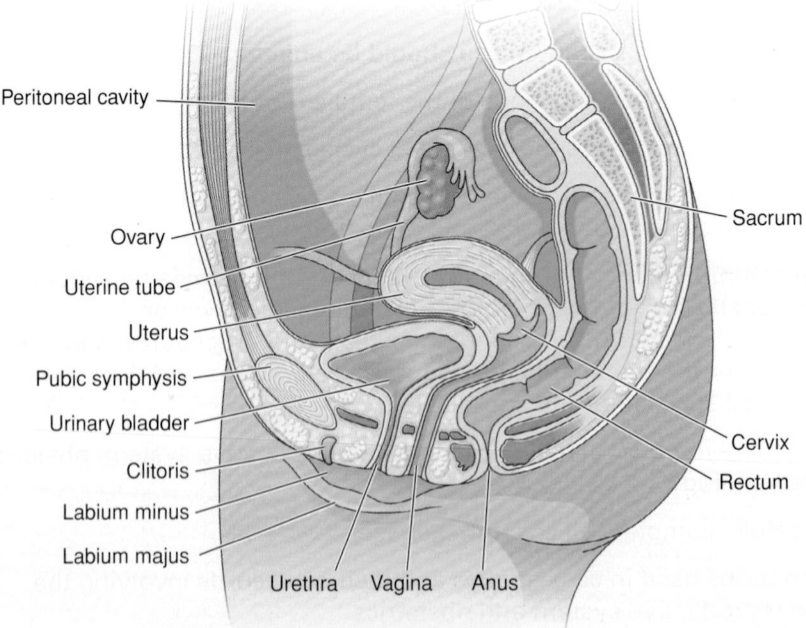

Figure 15-1 The female reproductive system.

- Transporting oocytes to a site where they may be fertilized by spermatozoa to form ova
- Supporting and nurturing a developing embryo and fetus in a favorable environment until birth
- Providing an infant's first source of nutrition and protective antibodies after birth through breast milk

Terms Related to the Female Reproductive System

Term	Pronunciation	Meaning
breasts; *syn.* mammary glands	brests'; mam'ă-rē glandz	modified sweat glands that produce milk (**Figure 15-2**)
areola	ă-rē'ō-lă	pigmented area around the breast nipple
lactiferous ducts	lak-tif'ĕr-ŭs dŭkts	channels that carry breast milk to the nipple
lactiferous sinuses	lak-tif'ĕr-ŭs sī'nŭs-ĕz	expanded chambers that converge on the nipple surface
lobes of mammary gland	lōbz uv mam'ă-rē gland	15–20 separate portions of the mammary gland that radiate from the central area deep to the nipple-like wheel spokes and comprise the body of the mammary gland; each is drained by a single lactiferous duct
lobules of mammary gland	lob'yūlz uv mam'ă-rē gland	subdivisions of the lobes of the mammary gland that make breast milk; also called lactiferous lobules

(continued)

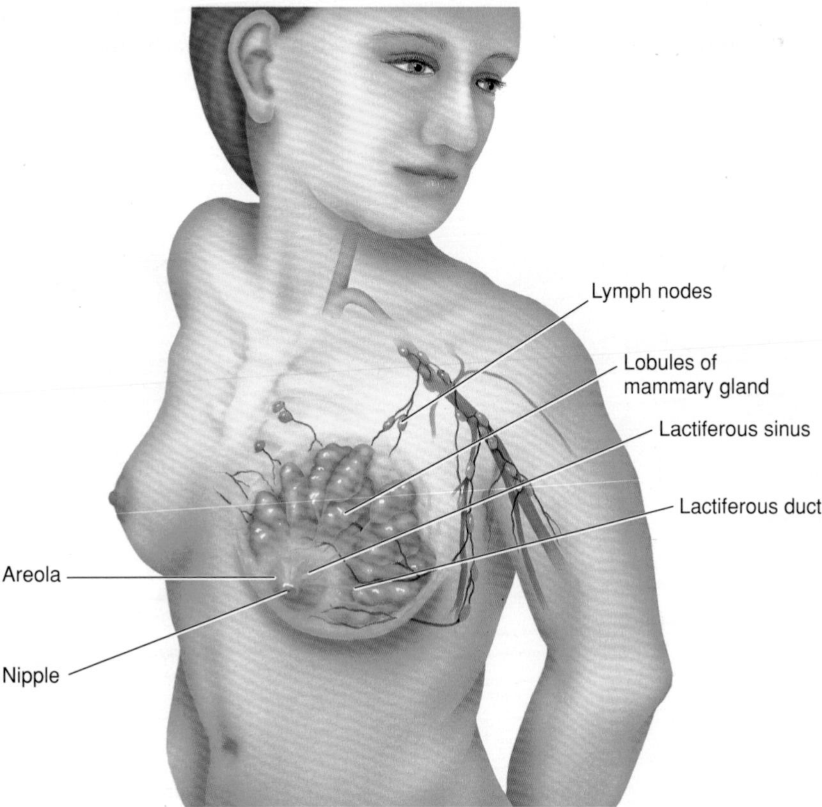

Figure 15-2 Frontal view of the breasts.

Terms Related to the Female Reproductive System *(continued)*

Term	Pronunciation	Meaning
nipple	nip'ĕl	projection on the breast surface through which milk can be secreted
genitalia	jen'i-tā'lē-ă	external and internal organs of reproduction
ovaries	ō'vă-rēz	pair of oval reproductive glands that produce hormones and release oocytes (**Figure 15-3**)
oocyte	ō'ō-sīt	female gamete or sex cell; when fertilized by a sperm, it develops into an ovum and is capable of developing into a new individual
corpus luteum	kōr'pŭs lū'tē-ŭm	temporary endocrine gland formed in the ovary that secretes the hormone progesterone during the second half of the menstrual cycle
menstrual cycle	men'strū-ăl sī'kl	period of time in which an oocyte matures, is ovulated, and enters the uterus through the uterine tubes; during this time, ovarian hormonal secretions effect endometrial changes; if fertilization does not occur, the endometrium is shed and menstrual flow begins; the cycle lasts about 28 days
vesicular ovarian follicles; *syn.* graafian follicles	vĕ-sik'yū-lăr ō-var'ē-ăn fol'i-kĕlz; grah'fē-ăn fol'i-kĕlz	fluid-filled sacs in the ovaries in which the primary oocyte matures
ovum, *pl.* ova	ō'vŭm, ō'vă	oocyte that has been fertilized by a spermatozoon; an egg cell
uterine tubes; *syn.* salpinges, fallopian tubes	yū'tĕr-in tūbz; sal-pin'jēz, fă-lō'pē-ăn tūbz	tubular structures that carry the oocyte from the ovary to the uterus (**Figure 15-3**)
fimbriae	fim'brē-ē	finger-like extensions of each uterine tube that drape over each ovary

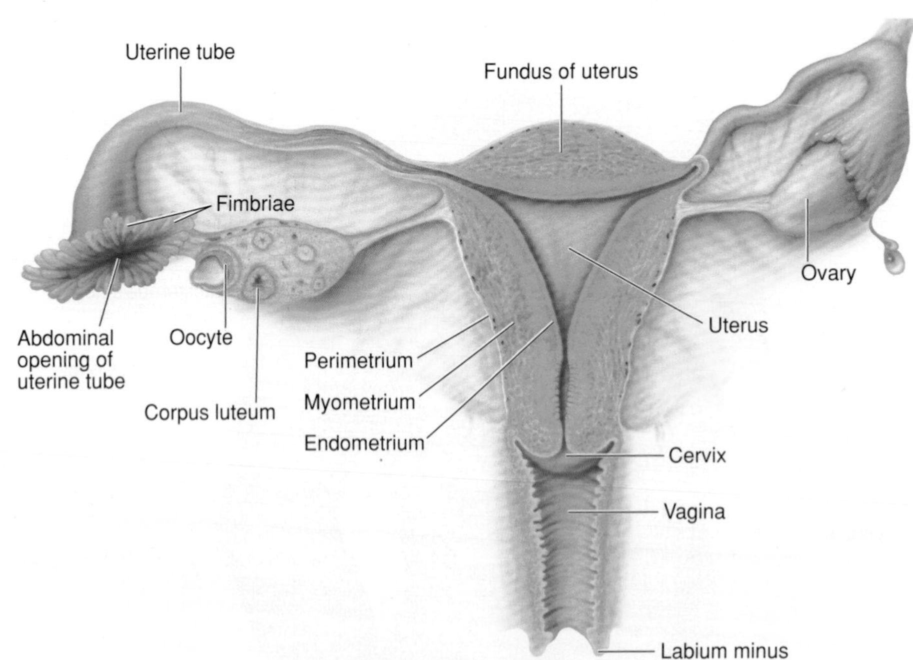

Figure 15-3 The ovaries, uterine tubes, uterus, and vagina.

Terms Related to the Female Reproductive System

Term	Pronunciation	Meaning
uterus; *syn.* womb	yū'tĕr-ŭs; wūm	pear-shaped organ located in the middle of the pelvis that supports a growing embryo and fetus and is the site of menstruation (**Figure 15-3**)
adnexa	ad-nek'să	appendages or adjunct parts; the adnexa of the uterus consist of the uterine tubes, the ovaries, and the ligaments that hold them together
endometrium	en'dō-mē'trē-ŭm	inner layer that lines the uterus; this layer is shed during menstruation
myometrium	mī'ō-mē'trē-ŭm	thick, muscular middle layer of the uterus
perimetrium	per'i-mē'trē-ŭm	outer layer of the uterus that covers the body of the uterus and part of the cervix
cervix	sĕr'viks	tubular, lower portion of the uterus that opens into the vagina
cervical os	ser'vĭ-kăl oz	vaginal opening of the uterus; also called external os of uterus
fundus	fŭn'dŭs	dome-shaped top portion of the uterus that lies above the entrance of the uterine tubes
vagina; *syn.* birth canal	vă-jī'nă; bĭrth kă-nal'	muscular tube projecting inside a female that connects the uterus to the outside of the body (**Figure 15-3**)
vulva	vŭl'vă	the female external genital organs (**Figure 15-4**)

(continued)

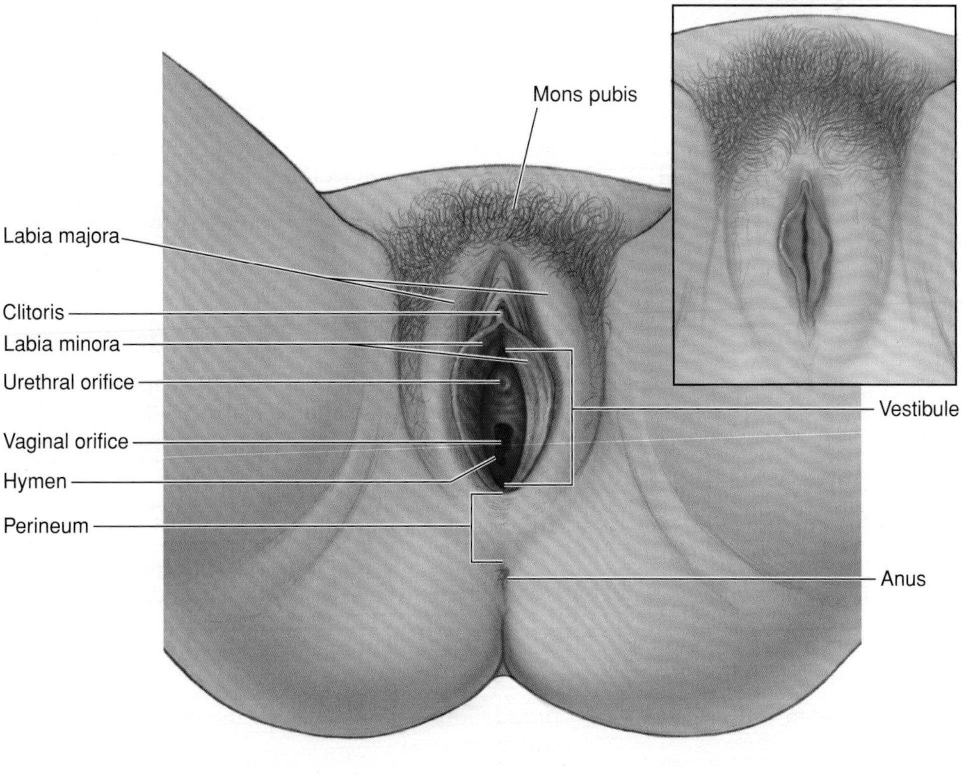

Figure 15-4 Structures of the vulva.

Terms Related to the Female Reproductive System *(continued)*

Term	Pronunciation	Meaning
clitoris	klit'ŏr-is	small (less than 2 cm) mass of erectile tissue in females that responds to sexual stimulation
hymen	hī'men	thin fold of mucous membrane covering the entrance to the vagina
greater vestibular glands; *syn.* Bartholin glands	grā'tĕr ves-tib'yū-lăr glandz; bahr'tō-lin glandz	glands that keep the vagina moist and provide a lubricant for the vagina during sexual intercourse
labia	lā'bē-ă	two sets of skin folds that cover the female external genital organs and tissues
labia majora; *syn.* labium majus	lā'bē-ă mă-jōr'ă; lā'bē-ŭm mā'jŭs	part of the labia that covers and protects the female external genital organs
labia minora; *syn.* labium minus	lā'bē-ă mi-nō'ră; lā'bē-ŭm mi'nus	inner folds of the labia that surround the openings to the vagina and urethra
mons pubis	monz pyū'bis	rounded mound of fatty tissue that covers the pubic bone
perineum	per'i-nē'ŭm	surface area between the thighs extending from the coccyx to the pubis that includes the anus posteriorly and the external genitalia anteriorly
vaginal orifice; *syn.* introitus	vaj'i-năl or'i-fis; in-trō'i-tŭs	opening of the vagina
vestibule	ves'ti-byūl	central space between the labia minora

Terms Related to Obstetrics and Neonatology

Term	Pronunciation	Meaning
amnion	am'nē-on	inner layer of membrane surrounding the fetus and containing the amniotic fluid (**Figure 15-5**)
amnionic fluid; *syn.* amniotic fluid	am'nē-on'ik flū'id; am'nē-ot'ik flū'id	fluid that encases the fetus and provides a cushion for the fetus as the mother moves (**Figure 15-5**)
chorion	kōr'ē-on	outermost membrane surrounding the fetus (**Figure 15-5**)
conception; *syn.* fertilization	kŏn-sep'shŭn; fĕr'til-ī-zā'shŭn	fertilization of an oocyte by a sperm
effacement	ē-fās'mĕnt	thinning of the cervix in preparation for delivery
embryo	em'brē-ō	the developing organism from conception until the end of the eighth week of gestation (**Figure 15-6**)
fetus	fē'tŭs	developing embryo from the end of the eighth week of gestation until delivery (**Figure 15-6**)
gamete	gam'ēt	an organism's reproductive cell, such as sperm or oocytes
gestation; *syn.* pregnancy	jes-tā'shŭn; preg'năn-sē	period of development from fertilization until birth
human chorionic gonadotropin (hCG)	hyū'măn kōr'ē-on'ik gō-nad'ō-trō'pin	hormone secreted by the fertilized ovum soon after conception
lactation	lak-tā'shŭn	production of breast milk by the mammary glands after childbirth
lochia	lō'kē-ă	normal vaginal discharge consisting of mucus, blood, and tissue debris following childbirth

(continued)

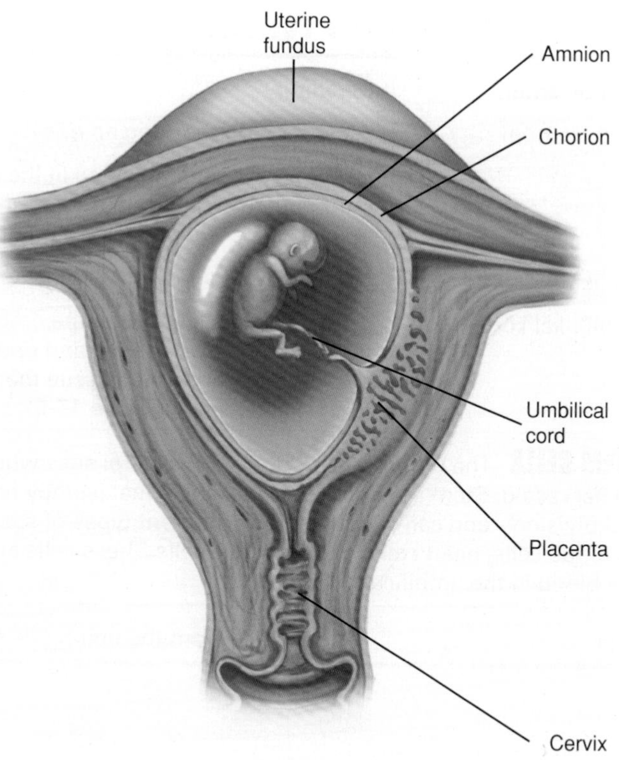

Figure 15-5 The embryo is floating in amniotic fluid surrounded by the protective fetal membranes (amnion and chorion).

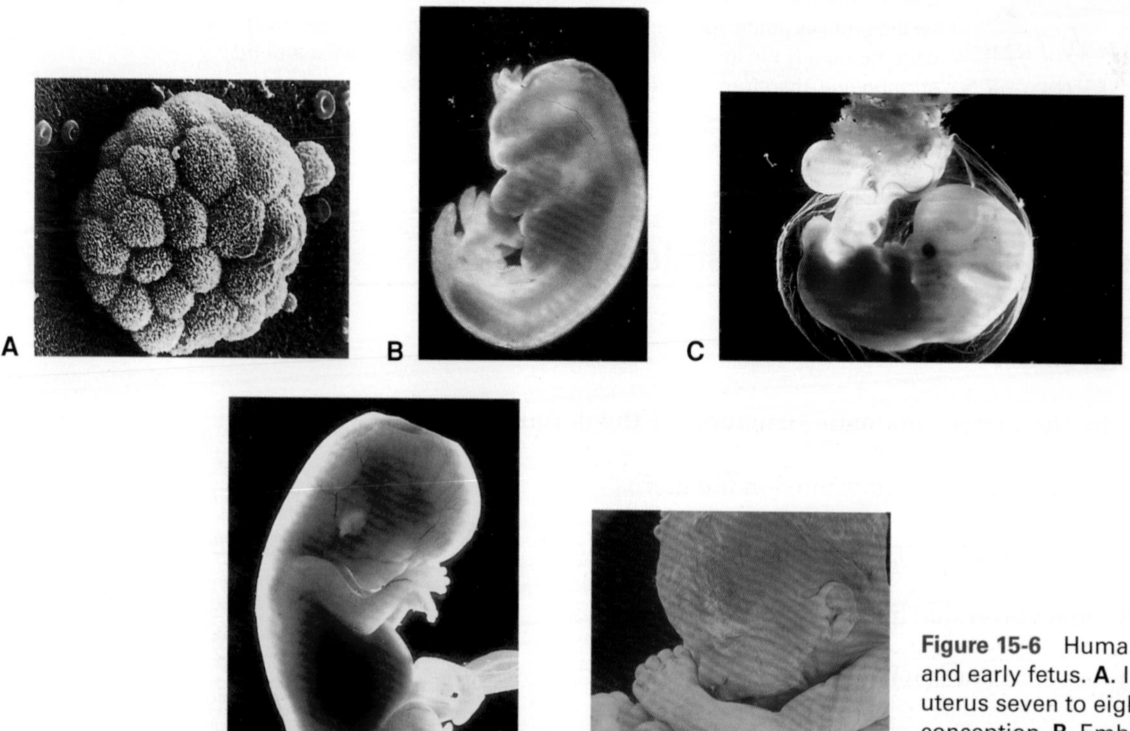

Figure 15-6 Human embryos and early fetus. **A.** Implantation in uterus seven to eight days after conception. **B.** Embryo at 32 days. **C.** Embryo at 37 days. **D.** Embryo at 41 days. **E.** Fetus between 12 and 15 weeks.

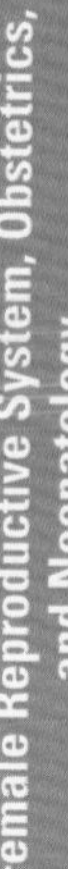

Terms Related to Obstetrics and Neonatology *(continued)*

Term	Pronunciation	Meaning
ovulation	ov'yū-lā'shŭn	process of discharging an oocyte from an ovary
placenta	plă-sen'tă	temporary organ implanted in the uterus through which the embryo/fetus receives nutrients and oxygen from the mother's blood and passes waste through the umbilical cord (**Figure 15-5**)
prolactin	prō-lak'tin	hormone that stimulates breast growth and milk secretion
umbilical cord	ŭm-bil'i-kăl kōrd	connecting stalk between the embryo/fetus and the placenta that contains two arteries and one vein cord composed of blood vessels and connective tissue that is connected to the fetus from the placenta (**Figure 15-5**)

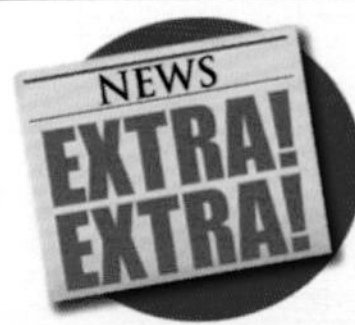

STEM CELLS The umbilical cord is one of several sites where stem cells can be harvested. Stem cells are self-renewing—that is, they reproduce through cell division—and can produce many different types of specialized cells, such as blood cells, heart cells, or pancreatic cells. These cells are retrieved from the blood in the umbilical cord.

Term	Pronunciation	Meaning
zygote	zī'gōt	cell resulting from the union of a sperm and oocyte

ANIMATION

View the animation "Ovulation and Fertilization" included with the Student Resources on thePoint for an illustration of the process of ovulation.

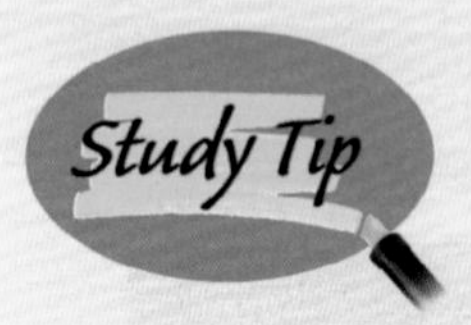

Endometrium and Perimetrium: When memorizing these layers of the uterus, let the prefixes guide you. Remember that *endo-* means *in, within;* thus, the endometrium is the inner layer that lines the uterus. *Peri-* means *around, surrounding;* therefore, the perimetrium is the outer layer that covers (surrounds) the body of the uterus.

Exercises: Anatomy and Physiology

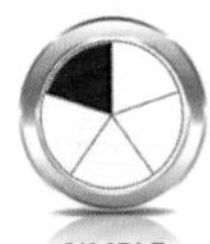
SIMPLE RECALL

Exercise 1

Write the correct anatomic structure for the definition given.

1. temporary organ implanted in the uterus ____________________
2. channels that carry breast milk to the nipple ____________________
3. inner layer that lines the uterus ____________________
4. modified sweat glands that produce milk ____________________
5. external and internal organs of reproduction ____________________

6. a fertilized oocyte ______

7. inner layer of membrane that surrounds the fetus ______

8. connecting stalk between the fetus and the placenta ______

9. projection on the breast surface through which milk can be secreted ______

10. dome-shaped top portion of the uterus ______

11. pigmented area around the nipple ______

12. temporary endocrine gland formed in the ovary ______

13. fluid-filled sacs in the ovaries in which the primary oocyte mature ______

14. glands that keep the vagina moist ______

15. cell resulting from union of sperm and oocyte ______

SIMPLE RECALL

Exercise 2

Write the meaning of the term given.

1. perimetrium ______

2. amniotic fluid ______

3. cervix ______

4. human chorionic gonadotropin (hCG) ______

5. oocyte ______

6. chorion ______

7. uterine tubes ______

8. gestation ______

9. lobules of mammary gland ______

10. prolactin ______

11. uterus ______

12. labia majora ______

13. embryo ______

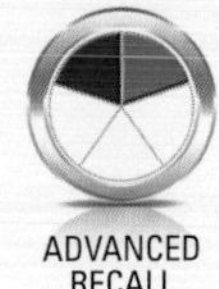

Exercise 3

Circle the term that is most appropriate for the meaning of the sentence.

1. The (*corpus luteum, clitoris, mammary gland*) secretes progesterone.
2. The (*labia, ovaries, adnexa*) cover the female external genital organs.
3. (*Oocytes, Fimbriae, Lobules*) are like fingers that extend over the ovaries.
4. The fatty tissue that covers the pubic bone is called the (*mons pubis, perineum, vulva*).
5. An oocyte is discharged from the ovary in a process called (*pregnancy, fertilization, ovulation*).
6. Another name for the vaginal opening is the (*uterus, introitus, vulva*).
7. The (*labia minora, labia majora, mons pubis*) surround the opening of the vagina.
8. One purpose of the (*salpinges, uterus, ovaries*) is to release oocytes.
9. Another name for the (*uterus, cervix, vagina*) is the "birth canal."
10. A(n) (*fetus, zygote, oocyte*) is an early embryo.

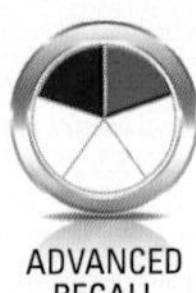

Exercise 4

Match each medical term with its meaning.

lobules of mammary gland	gamete	ovaries	lochia
effacement	vulva	vagina	lactation
fetus	cervical os		

1. area containing the external genital organs ____________________
2. embryo from the end of the eighth week until delivery ____________________
3. vaginal opening of the uterus ____________________
4. the production of breast milk ____________________
5. thinning of the cervix for delivery ____________________
6. an organism's reproductive cell ____________________
7. vaginal discharges following childbirth ____________________
8. the birth canal ____________________
9. glands in the breasts that make milk ____________________
10. produce hormones and release oocytes ____________________

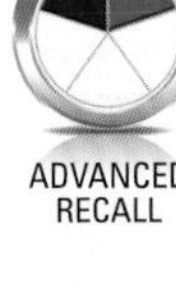

Exercise 5

Complete each sentence by writing in the correct medical term.

1. The inner lining of the uterus is called the ____________________.
2. The ________________ is a structure that responds to sexual stimulation.
3. The __________________ are the two sets of skin folds that cover the external genital organs and tissues.
4. The surface area between the thighs from the coccyx to the mons pubis is called the

   __________________________.
5. The ______________________ prepare for milk production for a newborn.
6. The organs of reproduction are generally referred to as ____________________.
7. A general term for appendages or adjunct parts is ________________.
8. The ______________________ is the thick, muscular middle layer of the uterus.

WORD PARTS

The following tables list word parts related to the reproductive system, obstetrics, and neonatology.

Combining Forms

Combining Form	Meaning
Related to the Female Reproductive System	
cervic/o	neck, cervix (neck of uterus)
colp/o	vagina
episi/o	vulva (external genitalia; wrapper)
gyn/o, gynec/o	woman
hyster/o	uterus (womb)
men/o, menstru/o	menstruation
metr/o, metri/o	uterus
my/o	muscle (uterus)
oophor/o	ovary
ovari/o	ovary
pelv/i	pelvis, pelvic cavity
perine/o	perineum (area between the anus and vulva)
salping/o	salpinx, uterine tube, fallopian tube

(continued)

Combining Forms *(continued)*

Combining Form	Meaning
uter/o	uterus
vagin/o	vagina
vulv/o	vulva (external genitalia; wrapper)
Related to Obstetrics and Neonatology	
amni/o, amnion/o	amnion
cephal/o	head
chori/o	chorion (membrane)
embry/o, embryon/o	embryo, immature form
fet/o	fetus
fund/o	fundus (part farthest from opening or exit)
galact/o	milk
gestat/o	from conception to birth
gravid/o	pregnancy
hydr/o	water, fluid
lact/o	milk
mamm/o	breast, mammary gland
mast/o	breast, mammary gland
nat/o	birth
olig/o	scanty, few
omphal/o	umbilicus, navel
pub/o	pubis
toc/o	labor, birth

Prefixes

Prefix	Meaning
ante-	before
dys-	painful, difficult, abnormal
ecto-	outer, outside
endo-	in, within
micro-	small
multi-	many
neo-	new
nulli-	none
poly-	many, much
post-	after, behind
pre-	before
supra-	above

Suffixes

Suffix	Meaning
-arche	beginning
-asthenia	weakness
-cele	herniation, protrusion
-centesis	puncture to aspirate
-ia	condition of
-ism	condition of
-metry	measurement of
-partum	childbirth, labor
-pexy	surgical fixation
-plasia	formation, growth
-plasty	surgical repair, reconstruction
-rrhage, -rrhagia	flowing forth
-rrhaphy	suture
-rrhea	flow, discharge
-scopy	process of examining, examination
-tomy	incision

Exercises: Word Parts

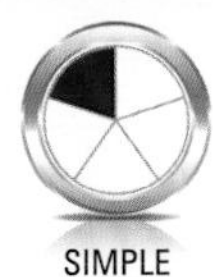
SIMPLE RECALL

Exercise 6

Write the meaning of the combining form given.

1. fund/o ______
2. pelv/i ______
3. cervic/o ______
4. mast/o ______
5. gestat/o ______
6. pub/o ______
7. salping/o ______
8. colp/o ______
9. gravid/o ______
10. olig/o ______

11. uter/o ______
12. galact/o ______
13. nat/o ______
14. chori/o ______
15. perine/o ______

Exercise 7

SIMPLE RECALL

Write the correct combining form or forms for the meaning given.

1. vagina ______
2. woman ______
3. muscle (uterus) ______
4. salpinx ______
5. breast, mammary gland ______
6. head ______
7. pregnancy ______
8. perineum ______
9. water, fluid ______
10. labor, birth ______
11. menstruation ______
12. cervix ______
13. milk ______
14. vulva ______
15. pubis ______

Exercise 8

SIMPLE RECALL

Write the meaning of the prefix or suffix given.

1. supra- ______
2. -plasty ______
3. -tomy ______

4. nulli- ____________________

5. -cele ____________________

6. -metry ____________________

7. -rrhea ____________________

8. -ia ____________________

9. neo- ____________________

10. -arche ____________________

11. -rrhaphy ____________________

12. -centesis ____________________

13. ante- ____________________

14. endo- ____________________

15. -partum ____________________

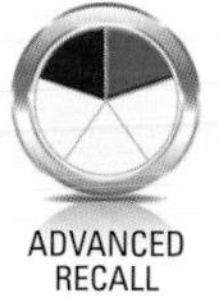

ADVANCED RECALL

Exercise 9

Considering the meaning of the combining form from which the medical term is made, write the meaning of the medical term. (You have not yet learned many of these terms but can build their meaning from the word parts.)

Combining Form	Meaning	Medical Term	Meaning of Term
metr/o	uterus	metrorrhagia	1. ____________
gynec/o	woman	gynecology	2. ____________
hyster/o	uterus	hysterectomy	3. ____________
mamm/o	breast	mammogram	4. ____________
episi/o	vulva	episiotomy	5. ____________
colp/o	vagina	colporrhaphy	6. ____________
oophor/o	ovary	oophorectomy	7. ____________
cervic/o	cervix	cervicitis	8. ____________
vagin/o	vagina	vaginoplasty	9. ____________
salping/o	salpinx	salpingectomy	10. ____________

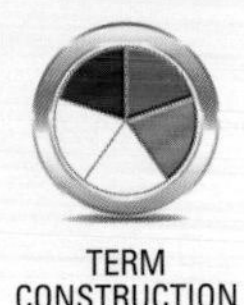
TERM CONSTRUCTION

Exercise 10

Using the given combining form and word part from the earlier tables, build a medical term for the meaning given.

Combining Form	Meaning of Medical Term	Medical Term
gynec/o	one who specializes in the study of women	**1.** ________
hyster/o	process of examining the uterus	**2.** ________
colp/o	suturing of the vagina	**3.** ________
omphal/o	herniation of the umbilical cord	**4.** ________
vagin/o	inflammation of the vagina	**5.** ________
mamm/o	recording (making an image of) the breast	**6.** ________
amni/o	incision of the amnion (to induce labor)	**7.** ________
fet/o	pertaining to a fetus	**8.** ________
embry/o	study of an embryo	**9.** ________
mast/o	excision or surgical removal of a breast	**10.** ________

MEDICAL TERMS

The following table gives adjective forms and terms used in describing the digestive system and its conditions.

Adjectives and Other Related Terms

Term	Pronunciation	Meaning
abdominopelvic	ab-dom′i-nō-pel′vik	pertaining to the abdomen and pelvis
amnionic; *syn.* amniotic	am′nē-on′ik; am′nē-ot′ik	relating to the amnion
chorionic	kōr′ē-on′ik	pertaining to the chorion (surrounding membrane)
congenital	kŏn-jen′i-tăl	existing at birth
cystic	sis′tik	pertaining to or containing cysts
date of birth (DOB)	dāt uv bĭrth	the day of birth of a patient
embryonic	em′brē-on′ik	pertaining to an embryo
endometrial	en′dō-mē′trē-ăl	pertaining to or composed of endometrium

Adjectives and Other Related Terms

Term	Pronunciation	Meaning
estimated date of confinement (EDC); *syn.* estimated date of delivery (EDD)	es'ti-mā'ted dāt uv kŏn-fīn'mĕnt; es'ti-mā'ted dāt uv dē-liv'ĕr-ē	the date an infant is expected to be born, calculated by counting forward 280 days (40 weeks) from the first day of the mother's last menstrual period (LMP); also called the due date

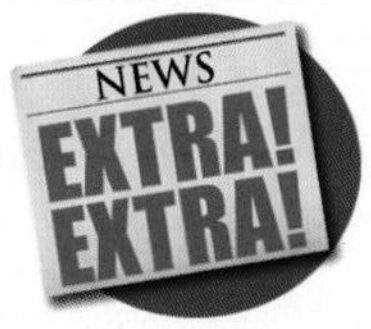

CALCULATING THE EDC A pregnant woman's "due date" is usually determined by the 280-day rule, which is based on a regular 28-day menstrual cycle. Assuming that the patient has regular periods every 28 days, the estimated date of confinement is calculated by counting 40 weeks, or 280 days, from the first day of her last cycle. If the patient's cycles are not right on target, then the resulting date is only a very good estimate of the actual due date.

Term	Pronunciation	Meaning
fetal	fē'tăl	pertaining to a fetus
gestational	jes-tā'shŭn-ăl	pertaining to pregnancy
gravida	grav'i-dă	a pregnant woman
in vitro	in vē'trō	in an artificial environment
intrauterine	in'tră-yū'tĕr-in	within the uterus
last menstrual period (LMP)	last men'strū-ăl pēr'ē-ŏd	the date indicating the first day of a patient's last menstruation (menstrual period)
meconium	mē-kō'nē-ŭm	greenish-black first feces of a newborn
menarche	men'ahr'kē	a girl's first menstrual period
menstruation; *syn.* menses	men'strū-ā'shŭn; men'sēz	cyclic shedding of endometrial lining and discharge of bloody fluid from the uterus; occurs approximately every 28 days
neonatal	nē'ō-nā'tăl	pertaining to the period immediately after an infant's birth and continuing through the first 28 days of life
neonate; *syn.* newborn	nē'ō-nāt; nū'bōrn	a newborn infant
nulligravida	nŭl-i-grav'i-dă	a woman who has never conceived a child
nullipara	nŭ-lip'ă-ră	a woman who has never given birth to a child
ovarian	ō-var'ē-ăn	pertaining to an ovary
para	par'ă	a woman who has given birth
pelvic	pel'vik	pertaining to the pelvis
perineal	per'i-nē'ăl	pertaining to the perineum
postpartum	pōst-pahr'tŭm	the period of time after birth
prenatal	prē-nā'tăl	the period of time preceding birth
primigravida	prī'mi-grav'i-dă	a woman who has had one pregnancy
suprapubic	sū'pră-pyū'bik	above the pubic bone
transabdominal	tranz'ab-dom'ĭ-năl	across or through the abdomen
transvaginal	trans-vaj'i-năl	across or through the vagina
stillbirth	stil'bĭrth	the birth of an infant who has died before delivery
uterine	yū'tĕr-in	pertaining to the uterus

Exercises: Adjectives and Other Related Terms

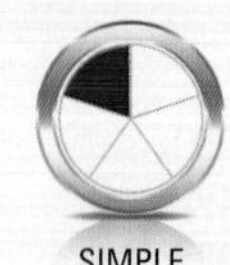
SIMPLE RECALL

Exercise 11

Circle the term that is most appropriate for the meaning of the sentence.

1. The area above the pubic bone is referred to as the (*transvaginal, intrauterine, suprapubic*) area.
2. Birth control products implanted in the uterus are typically called (*ovarian, intrauterine, perineal*) devices.
3. The word that describes a female's first menstrual period is (*nulligravida, menarche, meconium*).
4. A patient's due date is also called the (*last menstrual period, date of birth, estimated date of confinement*).
5. The birth of an infant who has died before delivery is called a (*stillbirth, gravida, neonate*).
6. The word that describes a woman who has given birth is (*gravida, para, congenital*).
7. The period of time preceding birth is known as the (*postnatal, perinatal, prenatal*) period.
8. A newborn's first feces is called (*menstruation, meconium, menarche*).
9. The term (*nulligravida, gravida, primigravida*) refers to a woman who has had one pregnancy.

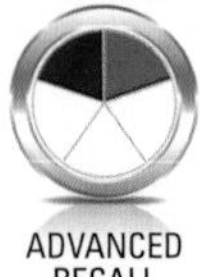
ADVANCED RECALL

Exercise 12

Match each medical term with its meaning.

congenital	cystic	chorionic	gravida
nullipara	transabdominal	neonate	gestational

1. relating to the chorion ________________
2. woman who has never given birth ________________
3. across or through the abdomen ________________
4. a newborn infant ________________
5. existing at birth ________________
6. containing cysts ________________
7. relating to pregnancy ________________
8. a pregnant woman ________________

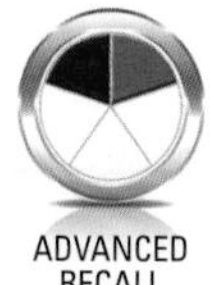
ADVANCED RECALL

Exercise 13

Circle the term that is most appropriate for the meaning of the sentence.

1. After having failed at conception several times, Mr. and Mrs. Timmeney decided to undergo fertilization in an artificial environment, also known as (*in vitro, congenital, transvaginal*) fertilization.
2. The physician diagnosed a(n) (*ovarian, chorionic, suprapubic*) cyst, which is a very painful cyst on an ovary.
3. On pelvic examination, Mrs. Veras displayed no (*uterine, nulligravida, in vitro*) tenderness.
4. Ms. Smith will return six weeks after the delivery of her child for (*postpartum, prenatal, perineal*) care.
5. Our practice provides (*neonatal, gestational, congenital*) care for the infant for the first 28 days of life.
6. Mrs. Wu came in complaining of a rash involving the surface area between her thighs, also known as the (*perineal, peritoneal, endometrial*) area.
7. An adolescent girl typically begins her (*neonatal, para, menses*), or cyclic shedding of the endometrial lining, around the age of 12.
8. Ms. Patton was born on September 20, 1978; that day is called her (*estimated date of confinement, due date, date of birth*).
9. Mrs. Lau indicated that her most recent menses had started on July 12; this date was noted in her medical record as her (*estimated date of confinement, date of birth, last menstrual period*).
10. Mrs. Johnson has not been able to conceive; her medical record would note that she is (*gravida, nullipara, nulligravida*).

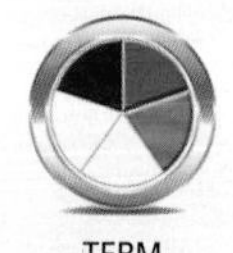
TERM CONSTRUCTION

Exercise 14

Write the combining form used in the medical term followed by the meaning of the combining form.

Term	Combining Form	Combining Form Definition
1. fetal	________	________
2. transvaginal	________	________
3. pelvic	________	________
4. endometrial	________	________
5. abdominopelvic	________	________
6. embryonic	________	________
7. transabdominal	________	________
8. ovarian	________	________

Medical Conditions

Term	Pronunciation	Meaning
Related to the Female Reproductive System		
adenomyosis	ad'ĕ-nō-mī-ō'sis	the presence of endometrial tissue growing through the myometrium
amenorrhea	ā-men-ŏr-ē'ă	abnormal absence of menstrual bleeding
atrophic vaginitis	ā-trō'fik vaj'i-nī'tis	inflammation of the vagina due to the thinning and shrinking of the tissues, as well as decreased lubrication
bacterial vaginosis	bak-tēr'ē-ăl vaj'i-nō'sis	infection of the vagina caused by the disruption of the normal balance of bacteria, in which "good" bacteria is replaced by "harmful" bacteria
cervical dysplasia	sĕr'vi-kăl dis-plā'zē-ă	development of abnormal cells in the lining of the cervix
cervicitis	sĕr'vi-sī'tis	inflammation of the cervix (**Figure 15-7**)
dysmenorrhea	dis-men'ōr-ē'ă	difficult or painful menstruation
dyspareunia	dis'păr-ū'nē-ă	condition of experiencing pain during sexual intercourse
endometriosis	en'dō-mē-trē-ō'sis	the presence of functional endometrial tissue somewhere other than in the lining of the uterus (**Figure 15-8**)
endometritis	en'dō-mē-trī'tis	inflammation of the endometrium
mastitis	mas-tī'tis	inflammation of the breast(s)
mastodynia	mas'tō-din'ē-ă	pain in the breast(s)
menopause	men'ō-pawz	permanent ceasing of menses
menorrhagia	men'ō-rā'jē-ă	abnormally heavy or prolonged bleeding during menstruation
metrorrhagia	mē'trō-rā'jē-ă	irregular bleeding from the uterus between menstrual periods

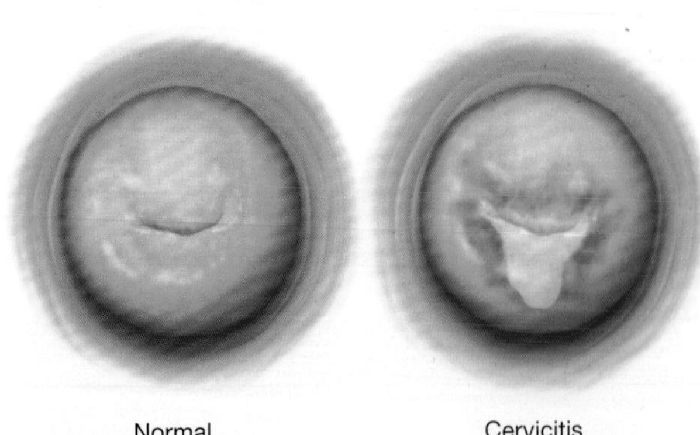

Figure 15-7 Inflammation and discharge are signs of cervicitis.

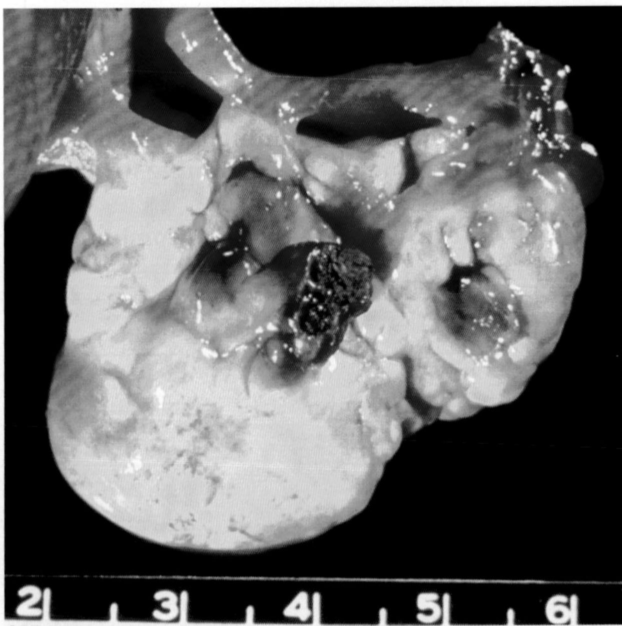

Figure 15-8 Endometriosis. Implants of endometriosis on the ovary appear as red-blue nodules.

Medical Conditions

Term	Pronunciation	Meaning
uterine fibroid; *syn.* leiomyoma, fibromyoma, myoma	yū'tĕr-in fī'broyd; lī'ō-mī-ō'mă, fī'brō-mī-ō'mă, mī-ō'mă	benign growth that develops from the smooth muscular tissue of the uterus (**Figure 15-9**)
pelvic inflammatory disease (PID)	pel'vik in-flam'ă-tōr-ē di-zēz'	inflammation of the female pelvic organs (ovaries, uterine tubes, and uterus) caused by infection by any of several microorganisms, such as *Neisseria gonorrhoeae* and *Chlamydia trachomatis*
polycystic ovary syndrome	pol'ē-sis'tik ō'văr-ē sin'drōm	condition characterized by irregular menstrual periods, excess hair growth, obesity, and enlarged ovaries due to hormone imbalance (**Figure 15-10**)
salpingitis	sal'pin-jī'tis	inflammation of the uterine tube (salpinx)
sexually transmitted disease (STD)[a]	sek'shū-ă-lē tranz-mit'ĕd di-zēz'	any contagious disease acquired during sexual contact; also called sexually transmitted infection
uterine prolapse	yū'tĕr-in prō'laps	protrusion of the uterus into or through the vagina
vulvodynia	vŭl'vō-din'ē-ă	chronic vulvar discomfort with complaints of burning and superficial irritation

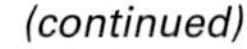
(continued)

[a]See Chapter 14: Male Reproductive System for coverage of specific sexually transmitted diseases.

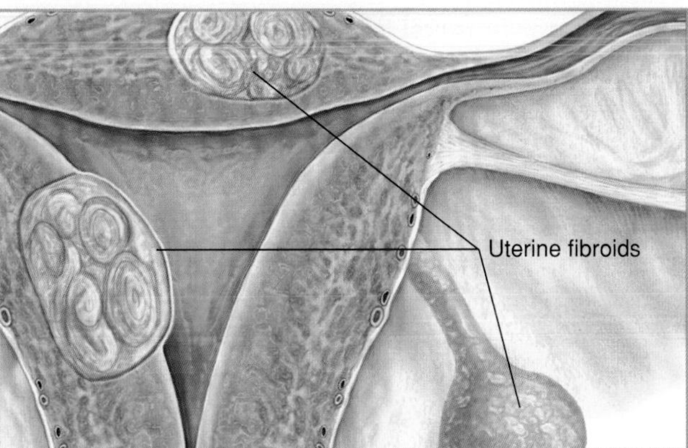

Figure 15-9 Uterine fibroids.

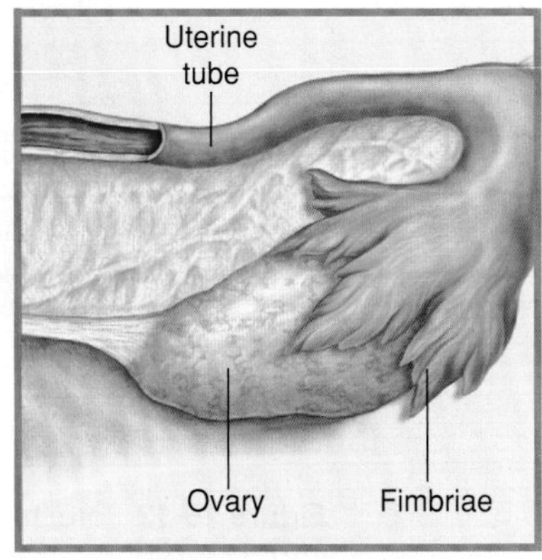

Normal ovary

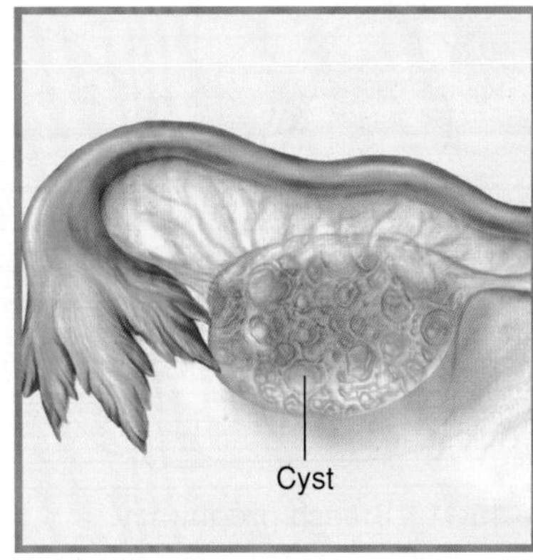

Polycystic ovary

Figure 15-10 Polycystic ovary syndrome.

Medical Conditions *(continued)*

Term	Pronunciation	Meaning
Related to Obstetrics		
abortion (AB); *syn.* spontaneous abortion (SAB)	ă-bōr′shŭn; spon-tā′nē-ŭs ă-bōr′shŭn	expulsion of an embryo or fetus (products of conception) from the uterus before viability; also called a miscarriage
incomplete abortion	in′kŏm-plēt′ ă-bōr′shŭn	abortion in which part of the products of conception have passed but part (usually the placenta) remains in the uterus
abruptio placentae	ăb-rŭp′shē-ō plă-sen′tē	premature detachment of a normally situated placenta
Braxton Hicks contractions; *syn.* false labor	braks′tŏn-hiks kŏn-trak′shŭns; fawls lā′bŏr	irregular weak uterine contractions that occur during pregnancy that usually cause little or no pain
breech pregnancy	brēch preg′năn-sē	pregnancy in which the buttocks of the baby present at the bottom of the uterus, while the head remains in the upper part of the uterus (**Figure 15-11**)
dystocia	dis-tō′sē-ă	difficult childbirth
eclampsia	ek-lamp′sē-ă	seizures or coma in a patient with pregnancy-induced hypertension
ectopic pregnancy	ek-top′ik preg′năn-sē	a pregnancy that occurs when the zygote implants itself outside the uterus
gestational diabetes	jes-tā′shŭn-ăl dī-ă-bē′tēz	diabetes that develops or first occurs during pregnancy
infertility	in′fĕr-til′i-tē	inability of a couple to conceive, regardless of the cause
lithotomy position	li-thot′ŏ-mē pŏ-zish′ŭn	supine position with buttocks at the end of the operating table, hips and knees are fully flexed, and the feet are strapped in position; common position for childbirth
nuchal cord	nū′kăl kōrd	loop(s) of umbilical cord wrapped around the neck of the fetus, posing risk of intrauterine hypoxia, fetal distress, or death (**Figure 15-12**)

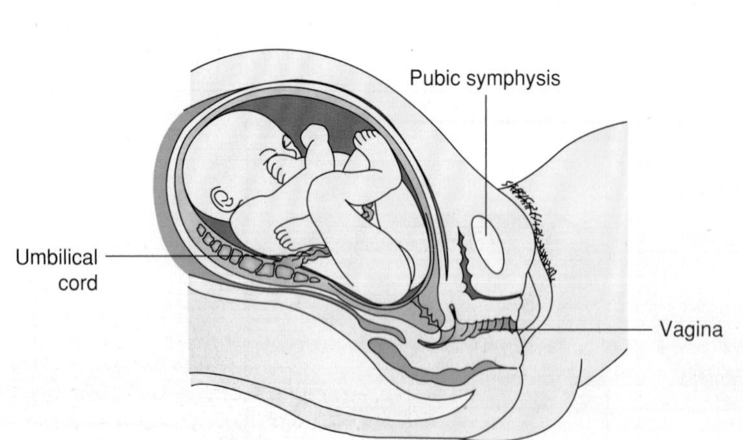

Figure 15-11 Breech pregnancy.

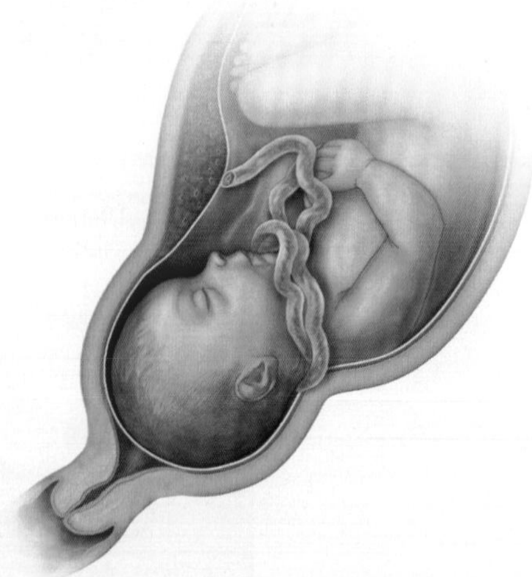

Figure 15-12 Nuchal cord. The umbilical cord is wrapped around the neck of the fetus.

Medical Conditions

Term	Pronunciation	Meaning
oligohydramnios	ol′i-gō-hī-dram′nē-os	an insufficient amount of amniotic fluid
placenta previa	plă-sen′tă prē′vē-ă	condition in which the placenta is implanted in the lower segment of the uterus instead of the upper part (**Figure 15-13**)
postpartum depression	pōst-pahr′tŭm dĕ- presh′ŭn	form of clinical depression suffered by the mother that occurs soon after giving birth
preeclampsia	prē′ē-klamp′sē-ă	development of hypertension with proteinuria, edema, or both, due to pregnancy
prolapsed cord	prō-lapst kōrd	slipping of the umbilical cord into the vagina before delivery
rupture of membranes	rŭp′chŭr uv membrānz	spontaneous rupture of the amniotic sac with release of fluid preceding childbirth
toxoplasmosis	tok′sō-plaz-mō′sis	infection caused by the protozoan parasite *Toxoplasma gondii* transmitted to humans through cat feces; if contracted by a pregnant woman, the infection can affect the fetus in many ways, including profound physical abnormalities
vertex	ver′teks	normal birth position of the fetus so that the crown of the head presents first in the cervix and vaginal canal
Related to Neonatology		
atresia	ă-trē′zē-ă′	congenital absence of a normal opening, such as the esophagus or anus
atrial septal defect (ASD)	ā′trē-ăl sep′tăl dē′fekt	failure of an opening or foramen to close between the atria after birth
cleft lip	kleft lip	congenital split in the upper lip associated with a cleft palate (**Figure 15-14**)
cleft palate	kleft pal′ăt	congenital split in the roof of the mouth caused by failure of the embryonic facial bones to fuse; often associated with cleft lip (**Figure 15-14**)

(continued)

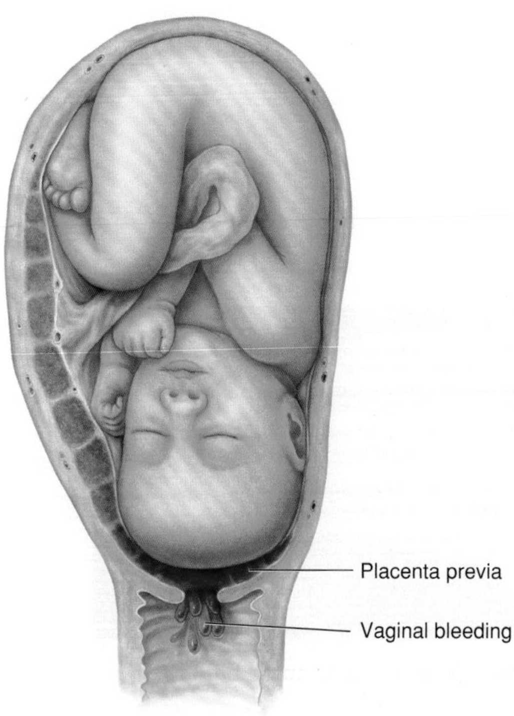

Figure 15-13 Placenta previa.

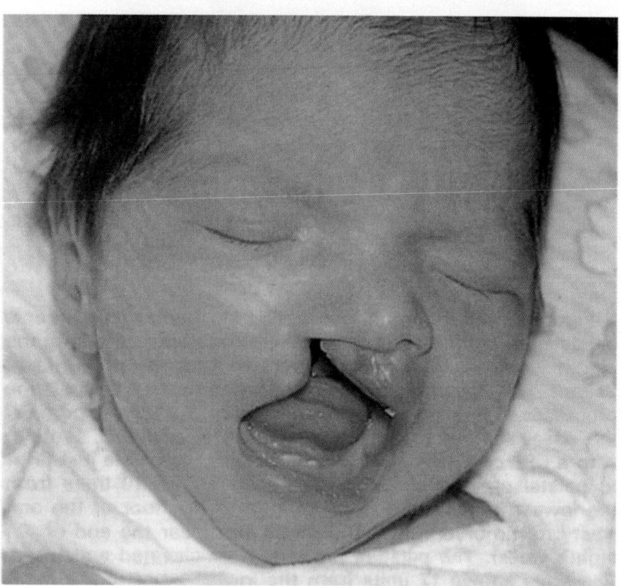

Figure 15-14 Cleft lip and cleft palate in an infant.

Medical Conditions *(continued)*

Term	Pronunciation	Meaning
Down syndrome	down sin′drōm	congenital disorder characterized by intellectual impairment and physical abnormalities caused by a tripling of chromosome 21; also called trisomy 21 (**Figure 15-15**)
gastroschisis	gas-tros′ki-sis	congenital defect in the anterior abdominal wall, usually accompanied by protrusion of the intestines
jaundice of newborn	jawn′dis uv nū′bōrn	inability of an infant's liver to metabolize bilirubin; usually disappears within 48–72 hours after birth
microcephaly	mī′krō-sef′ă-lē	congenital condition characterized by an abnormally small head; usually associated with intellectual impairment
omphalocele	om-fal′ŏ-sēl	congenital herniation in which abdominal organs protrude into a baby's umbilical cord
patent ductus arteriosus (PDA)	pā′tent dŭk′tŭs ahr-tē-rē-ō′sus	congenital disorder in which a fetal blood vessel connecting the left pulmonary artery with the descending aorta fails to close after birth
spina bifida	spī′nă bif′i-dă	congenital defect of incomplete vertebral closure that allows the spinal cord or meninges to protrude through a gap in the backbone (**Figure 15-16**)
tetralogy of Fallot	te-tral′ŏ-jē uv fahl-ō′	set of four congenital heart defects: ventricular septal defect, pulmonic valve stenosis, malposition of the aorta, and right ventricular hypertrophy
Turner syndrome	tŭr′nĕr sin′drōm	congenital disorder in which affected women have only one X chromosome instead of two, causing developmental abnormalities and infertility
ventricular septal defect (VSD)	ven-trik′yū-lăr sep′tăl dē-fekt′	failure of an opening or foramen to close between the heart ventricles after birth

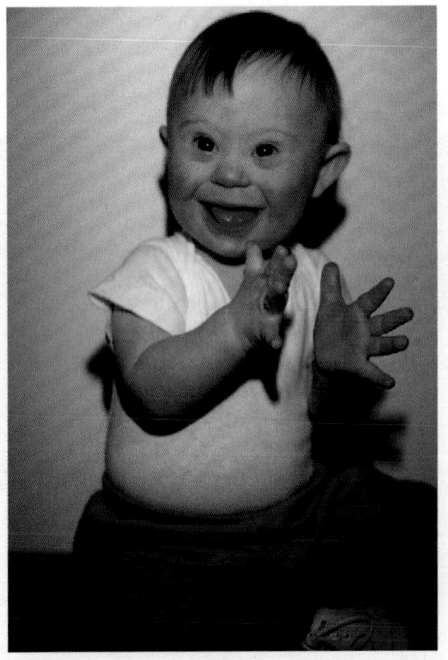

Figure 15-15 Physical traits characteristic of Down syndrome.

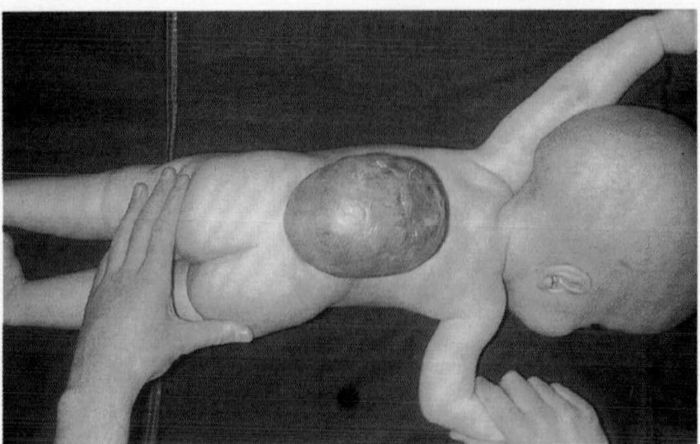

Figure 15-16 An infant with spina bifida.

Exercises: Medical Conditions

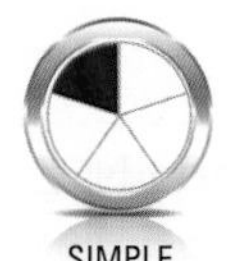
SIMPLE RECALL

Exercise 15

Write the correct medical term for the definition given.

1. contagious disease spread through sexual contact ____________
2. an insufficient amount of amniotic fluid ____________
3. congenital defect in the abdominal wall ____________
4. abnormal cells in the lining of the cervix ____________
5. congenital disorder in which a woman has only one X chromosome ____________
6. a pregnancy that develops outside the uterus ____________
7. ceasing of menses ____________
8. failure of the foramen of the atria to close after birth ____________
9. congenital split in the upper lip ____________
10. loops of umbilical cord wrapped around the neck of the fetus ____________
11. expulsion of an embryo or fetus before viability ____________
12. an infection caused by a parasite transmitted by cats ____________
13. loss of fluid from the amniotic sac preceding childbirth ____________
14. failure of a fetal blood vessel to close after birth ____________
15. premature detachment of the placenta ____________
16. set of four congenital heart defects ____________
17. disruption of the normal balance of bacteria in the vagina ____________
18. inflammation of the female pelvic organs ____________
19. congenital absence of a normal opening ____________
20. pregnancy in which the buttocks of the baby present first ____________

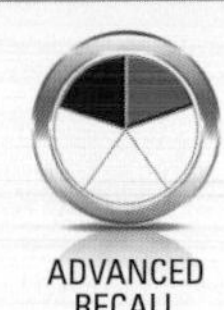

ADVANCED RECALL

Exercise 16

Circle the term that is most appropriate for the meaning of the sentence.

1. Mrs. Murphy experienced irregular bleeding from the uterus between menstrual periods, which is referred to as (*menorrhagia, metrorrhagia, vulvodynia*).

2. After hearing the patient's symptom of painful intercourse, the physician diagnosed her with (*bacterial vaginosis, oophoritis, dyspareunia*).

3. The couple was suffering from (*endometriosis, eclampsia, infertility*), which means they could not conceive a child.

4. Dr. Jones noticed excess hair growth in Ms. Allen, which is a characteristic of a hormonal disorder known as (*salpingitis, menopause, polycystic ovary syndrome*).

5. The baby suffered from a(n) (*atrial septal defect, tetralogy of Fallot, ventricular septal defect*) characterized by the failure of the foramen to close between the heart ventricles after birth.

6. My sister suffered from (*Braxton Hicks, eclampsia, syphilis*) contractions, or false labor, during all three of her pregnancies.

7. Mrs. Tobias was diagnosed with (*preeclampsia, erythroblastosis fetalis, gestational diabetes*), which is a type of diabetes that develops during pregnancy.

8. The patient's preeclampsia developed into (*ectopic pregnancy, abruption placentae, eclampsia*), which caused her to have a seizure.

9. Some women suffer from a mental disorder called (*postpartum depression, oligohydramnios, nuchal cord*) after the birth of their babies.

10. The physician explained to Mrs. Lane that her (*atrophic vaginitis, bacterial vaginosis, dyspareunia*) was due to thinning and shrinking of vaginal tissues.

11. The baby was diagnosed with (*spina bifida, cleft palate, microcephaly*), a congenital condition in which the vertebra surrounding the spinal cord does not close properly.

12. The woman developed a protrusion of the uterus through the vagina, which is known as (*vaginitis, uterine prolapse, pelvic inflammatory disease*).

13. The infant had difficulty feeding because of a (*cleft chin, cleft palate, cleft mouth*), a congenital split (fissure) that is often associated with a cleft lip.

14. The pregnancy was complicated by (*menopause, infertility, placenta previa*).

15. Mrs. Brown experienced a slipping of the umbilical cord into the vagina before delivery, which is called (*premature cord, prolapsed cord, presenting cord*).

16. Mr. Marfin's daughter was born with Down syndrome, a (*contracted, contraindicated, congenital*) chromosomal condition.

17. The baby suffered from (*Down syndrome, Turner syndrome, jaundice of newborn*), which cleared within 48 hours of birth.

18. Ms. Lloyd experienced a(n) (*spontaneous abortion, rupture of membranes, incomplete abortion*) when all the products of conception were not expelled.

19. The patient was diagnosed with (*endometriosis, endometritis, adenomyosis*) after endometrial tissue was found growing through the muscular lining of her uterus.

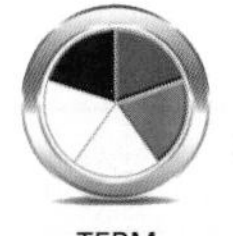

Exercise 17

Break the given medical term into its word parts, and define each part. Then define the medical term.

For example:

urethritis	*word parts:*	urethr/o, -itis
	meanings:	urethra, inflammation of
	term meaning:	inflammation of the urethra

1. amenorrhea
   word parts: ____________
   meanings: ____________
   term meaning: ____________
2. salpingitis
   word parts: ____________
   meanings: ____________
   term meaning: ____________
3. mastitis
   word parts: ____________
   meanings: ____________
   term meaning: ____________
4. endometriosis
   word parts: ____________
   meanings: ____________
   term meaning: ____________
5. vulvodynia
   word parts: ____________
   meanings: ____________
   term meaning: ____________
6. microcephaly
   word parts: ____________
   meanings: ____________
   term meaning: ____________
7. myoma
   word parts: ____________
   meanings: ____________
   term meaning: ____________

8. omphalocele *word parts:* ____________

meanings: ____________

term meaning: ____________

9. mastodynia *word parts:* ____________

meanings: ____________

term meaning: ____________

10. dysmenorrhea *word parts:* ____________

meanings: ____________

term meaning: ____________

Tests and Procedures

Term	Pronunciation	Meaning
Laboratory Tests Related to the Female Reproductive System and Obstetrics		
group B streptococcus	grūp B strep'tō-kok'ŭs	test for bacterium that, if transmitted from the mother, can cause life-threatening infections in newborns
Papanicolaou (Pap) test	pa-pă-ni'kō-lō (pap) test	microscopic examination of cells collected from the vagina and cervix to detect abnormal changes (e.g., cancer)
pregnancy test	preg'năn-sē test	blood test to determine the presence of the hormone human chorionic gonadotropin (hCG) secreted by the placenta
quad marker screen	kwahd mark'ĕr skrēn	blood test that measures the levels of four substances (alpha-fetoprotein, human chorionic gonadotropin, estriol, and inhibin A) to determine the risk of having a baby with a birth defect

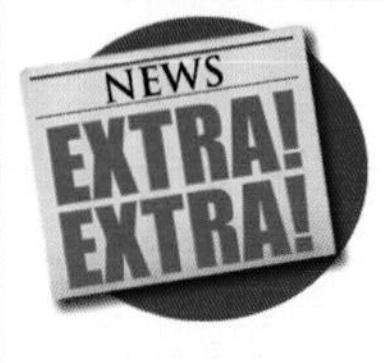

QUAD SCREEN is the shortened name for the quadruple marker test. This test is typically done during the second trimester of pregnancy, and its results indicate a mother's likelihood of carrying a baby with birth defects. The test measures four substances (one protein and three hormones) found in the blood of a pregnant woman. Alpha-fetoprotein (AFP) is a protein that is made by the baby's liver, and levels can help detect spina bifida. Human chorionic gonadotropin (hCG) and inhibin A are hormones made by the placenta, and estriol is a hormone made by the placenta and baby's liver.

Term	Pronunciation	Meaning
TORCH panel	tōrch pan'ĕl	group of tests that screen for antibodies to common infections that can be transmitted from mother to fetus; it is an acronym for toxoplasmosis, other infections, rubella, cytomegalovirus, and herpes simplex (**Figure 15-17**)

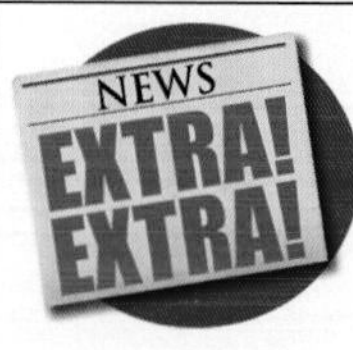

CHEAP TORCHES is an expansion of the original TORCH acronym and includes the following conditions: C = Chickenpox, H = Hepatitis, E = Enteroviruses, A = AIDS (HIV infection), P = Parvovirus B19, T = Toxoplasmosis, O = Other (group B streptococcus, listeria, candida, Lyme disease), R = Rubella, C = Cytomegalovirus, H = Herpes simplex, E = Everything else sexually transmitted, and S = Syphilis.

Tests and Procedures

Term	Pronunciation	Meaning
Diagnostic Procedures Related to the Female Reproductive System, Obstetrics, and Neonatology		
amniocentesis	am′nē-ō-sen-tē′sis	transabdominal aspiration of fluid from the amniotic sac to test for fetal lung immaturity or certain fetal problems, such as genetic defects or infections (**Figure 15-18**)
Apgar score	ap′gahr skōr	numeric result of a test conducted on an infant immediately after delivery to evaluate quickly the newborn's physical condition

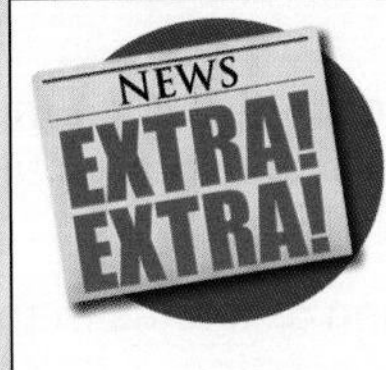

APGAR SCORE Part of a pediatrician's examination of an infant immediately after birth includes assigning an Apgar score. Developed in 1952 by anesthesiologist Virginia Apgar, the test is designed to quickly evaluate a newborn's physical condition after delivery and to determine any immediate need for extra medical or emergency care. The score evaluates heart rate, breathing, skin color, muscle tone, and response to stimulation, which are rated 0, 1, or 2 at 1 and 5 minutes after birth. Each set of ratings is totaled, and both totals are reported.

(continued)

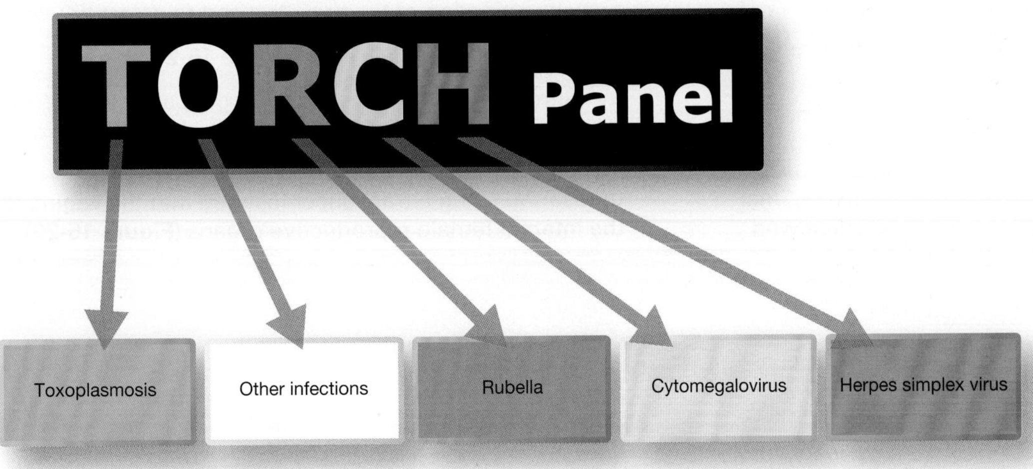

Figure 15-17 TORCH panel.

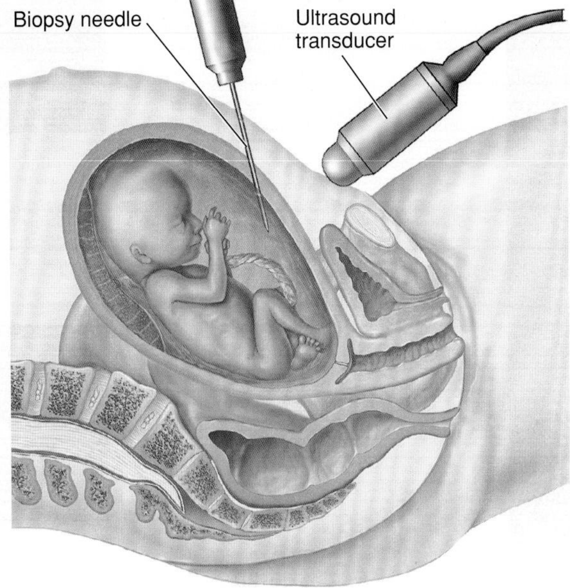

Figure 15-18 Amniocentesis.

Tests and Procedures *(continued)*

Term	Pronunciation	Meaning
chorionic villus sampling (CVS)	kōr′ē-on′ik vil′ŭs samp′ling	removal of a small piece of placental tissues (the villi of the chorion, which forms part of the placenta) during early pregnancy to test for fetal abnormalities
colposcope	kol′pō-skōp	a thin lighted endoscope inserted into the vagina to allow for direct visualization of the vagina and cervix
colposcopy	kol-pos′kŏ-pē	visual examination of the tissues of the cervix and vagina (**Figure 15-19**)
fetal ultrasound; *syn.* obstetric ultrasound	fē′tăl ŭl′tră-sownd; ob-stet′rik ŭl′tră-sownd	ultrasound done during pregnancy that uses reflected sound waves to produce a picture of a fetus, the placenta that nourishes it, and the amniotic fluid that surrounds it
fetoscope	fē′tō-skōp	special type of stethoscope used for listening to a fetus in the womb, usually used after about 18 weeks' gestation
hysterosalpingography (HSG)	his′tĕr-ō-sal-ping-gog′ră-fē	x-ray examination of the uterus and uterine tubes after injection of contrast dye
mammography	mă-mog′ră-fē	x-ray examination of the breasts; used to detect breast tumors
pelvic ultrasound	pel′vik ŭl′tră-sownd	ultrasound of the pelvic area (**Figure 15-20**)
pelvimetry	pel-vim′ĕ-trē	measurement of the dimensions of the pelvis to determine whether a woman can give birth through the vagina or if a cesarean section (C-section) will be required
transvaginal ultrasound	trans-vaj′i-năl ŭl′tră-sownd	ultrasound using a transducer inserted into the vagina to view the internal female reproductive organs (**Figure 15-20**)

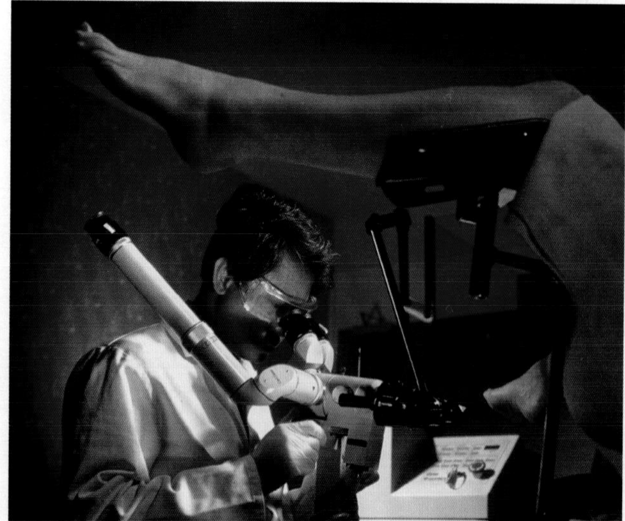

Figure 15-19 Colposcopy. Patient is in the lithotomy position.

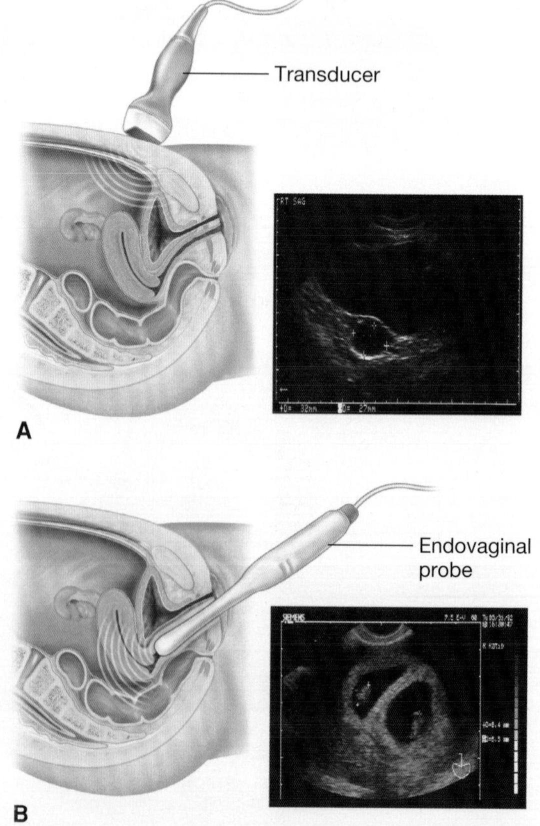

Figure 15-20 Ultrasound. **A.** Pelvic ultrasound. **B.** Transvaginal ultrasound.

Exercises: Tests and Procedures

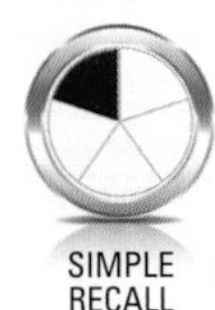
SIMPLE RECALL

Exercise 18

Circle the term that is most appropriate for the meaning of the sentence.

1. The physician listened to the fetus in the womb by using a (*hysteroscope, stethoscope, fetoscope*).
2. An ultrasound using a transducer inserted into the vagina to view the internal female reproductive organs is called a (*fetal ultrasound, transvaginal ultrasound, pelvic ultrasound*).
3. An x-ray examination of the uterus and uterine tubes is called a (*colposcopy, pelvimetry, hysterosalpingography*).
4. The (*pelvimetry, CVS, Apgar*) is a numeric score that indicates an infant's condition immediately after birth.
5. A test for antibodies against infectious agents that can be transmitted from the mother to the fetus is called a (*TORCH panel, group B streptococcus, pregnancy test*).
6. A (*quad marker screen, chorionic villus sampling, pelvic ultrasound*) is a blood test to determine the risk of carrying a baby with a birth defect.
7. The (*pregnancy test, quad marker screen, Papanicolaou test*) is the microscopic examination of cells collected from the vagina and cervix to detect abnormal changes.

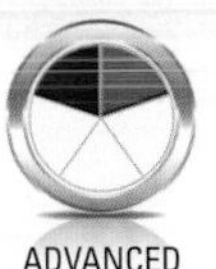
ADVANCED RECALL

Exercise 19

Complete each sentence by writing in the correct medical term.

1. An ultrasound of the pelvic area that can be used to reproduce images of a fetus is called ________________.
2. A visual examination of the cervix and vagina is called a(n) ________________.
3. A blood test to determine the presence of the hormone human chorionic gonadotropin secreted by the placenta is called a(n) ________________.
4. An x-ray examination of the breasts used to detect breast tumors is called ________________.
5. A procedure whereby a sample of placental tissue is removed from the uterus to detect fetal abnormalities is called ________________.
6. Transabdominal aspiration of fluid from the amniotic sac to test for certain problems in the fetus is called a(n) ________________.
7. A group of tests for antibodies to infectious organisms that cause congenital infections transmitted from mother to fetus is called a(n) ________________.

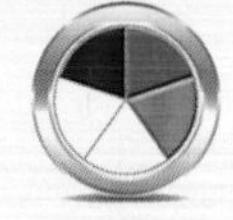

TERM CONSTRUCTION

Exercise 20

Considering the meaning of the combining form from which the medical term is made, write the meaning of the medical term.

Combining Form	Meaning	Medical Term	Meaning of Term
amni/o	amnion	amniocentesis	**1.** ______________
colp/o	vagina	colposcope	**2.** ______________
hyster/o, salping/o	uterus, salpinges (uterine tubes)	hysterosalpingography	**3.** ______________
mamm/o	breast	mammography	**4.** ______________
fet/o	fetus	fetoscope	**5.** ______________
colp/o	vagina	colposcopy	**6.** ______________

Surgical Interventions and Therapeutic Procedures

Term	Pronunciation	Meaning
Related to the Female Reproductive System		
colporrhaphy; *syn.* anterior/posterior repair	kol-pōr′ă-fē; an-tēr′ē-ōr/pos-tēr′ē-ŏr rē-pār′	surgical procedure that repairs a defect in the wall of the vagina
cryosurgery	krī′ō-sŭr′jĕr-ē	in gynecology, a procedure that uses liquid nitrogen to freeze a section of the cervix to destroy abnormal or precancerous cervical cells
dilatation and curettage (D&C); *syn.* dilation and curettage (D&C)	dī′lă-tā-shŭn and kūr′ĕ-tahzh′; dī-lā′shŭn and kūr′ĕ-tahzh′	surgical procedure in which the cervix is dilated and the endometrial lining of the uterus is scraped with a curette (**Figure 15-21**)

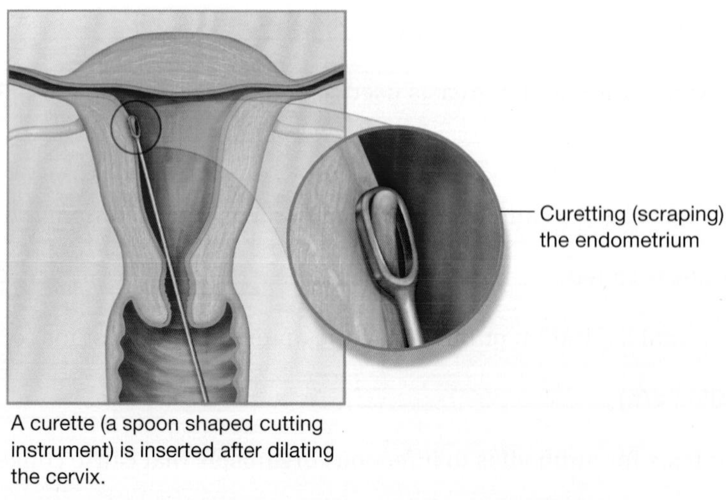

Curetting (scraping) the endometrium
A curette (a spoon shaped cutting instrument) is inserted after dilating the cervix.

Figure 15-21 Dilatation and curettage (D&C).

Surgical Interventions and Therapeutic Procedures

Term	Pronunciation	Meaning
hysterectomy	his′tĕr-ek′tŏ-mē	surgical removal of the uterus and cervix (**Figure 15-22**)
total abdominal hysterectomy (TAH)	tō′tăl ab-dom′i-năl his′tĕr-ek′tŏ-mē	surgical removal of the uterus and cervix (with or without removal of the ovaries and uterine tubes) through an incision in the abdomen
vaginal hysterectomy	vaj′i-năl his′tĕr-ek′tŏ-mē	surgical removal of the uterus and cervix through an incision deep inside the vagina
laparotomy	lap′ă-rot′ō-mē	surgical incision into the abdominal cavity
loop electrosurgical excision procedure (LEEP); *syn.* loop excision	lūp ē-lek′trō-sĭr′jik-ăl ek-sizh′ŭn prŏ-sē′jŭr; lūp ek-sizh′ŭn	gynecologic procedure that uses a thin, low-voltage electrified wire loop to cut out abnormal tissue in the cervix
mammoplasty	mam′ō-plas-tē	surgical repair of the breast
mastopexy	mas′tō-pek-sē	plastic surgery (fixation) to elevate and reshape a breast by removing excess skin and tightening the surrounding tissue
myomectomy	mī′ō-mek′tŏ-mē	surgical removal of a uterine myoma
oophorectomy	ō′of-ōr-ek′tŏ-mē	surgical removal of an ovary
pessary	pes′ă-rē	an elastic or rigid device inserted into the vagina to support the uterus or to correct any displacement
salpingectomy; *syn.* tubectomy	sal′pin-jek′tŏ-mē; tū-bek′tŏ-mē	surgical removal of a uterine tube
salpingo-oophorectomy	sal-ping′gō-ō-of′ŏr-ek′tŏ-mē	surgical removal of the ovary and its uterine tube (salpinx)
uterotomy; *syn.* hysterotomy	yū′tĕr-ot′ŏ-mē; his′tĕr-ot′ŏ-mē	incision of the uterus
vulvectomy	vŭl-vek′tŏ-mē	surgical removal of all or part of the vulva

(continued)

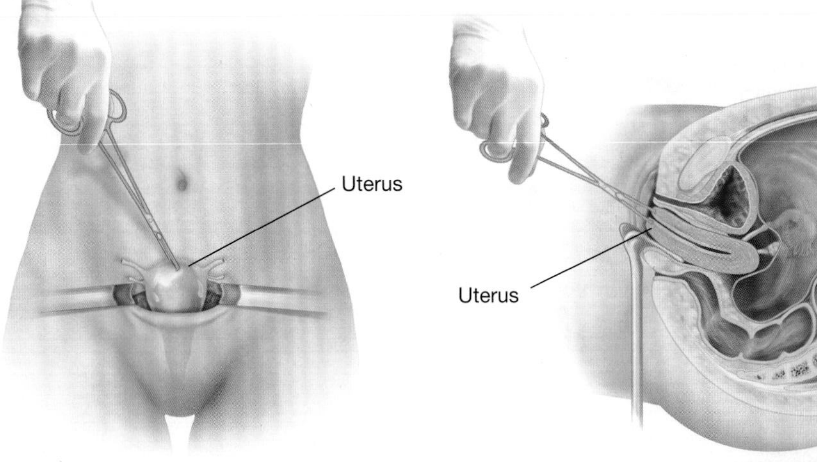

Figure 15-22 Hysterectomy.

Surgical Interventions and Therapeutic Procedures *(continued)*

Term	Pronunciation	Meaning
Related to Obstetrics		
amniotomy; *syn.* artificial rupture of membranes	am′nē-ot′ŏ-mē; ahr′ti-fish′ăl rup′shŭr mem′brānz	artificial (purposeful) tearing of the amniotic sac to induce or accelerate labor
cerclage	ser-klazh′	placement of a nonabsorbable suture, ring, or loop around a malfunctioning (incompetent) cervical opening
cesarean section (C-section)	se-zā′rē-ăn sek′shŭn	surgical operation for delivering a baby by cutting through the mother's abdominal wall and uterus
episiotomy	e-piz′ē-ot′ŏ-mē	surgical incision through the perineum to enlarge the vagina and assist childbirth
induction of labor	in-duk′shŭn uv lā′bŏr	attempt to start the childbirth process artificially by administering a drug to start labor or by puncturing the amniotic sac
in vitro fertilization (IVF)	in vē′trō fĕr′til-ī-zā′shŭn	process whereby oocytes are placed in a medium to which spermatozoa are added for fertilization, which produces a zygote; the zygote is then introduced into the uterus to establish a successful pregnancy
sterilization	ster′ĭl-i-zā′shŭn	rendering a person incapable of reproducing
therapeutic abortion (TAB)	thār-ă-pyū′tik ă-bōr′shŭn	abortion performed for medical reasons (such as when the mother's life is threatened by the pregnancy)
tubal ligation	tū′băl lī-gā′shŭn	sterilization technique in which a woman's uterine tubes are surgically blocked by tying (ligating), cutting, cauterizing, or a device to prevent oocytes from reaching the uterus; also known as having one's "tubes tied" (**Figure 15-23**)

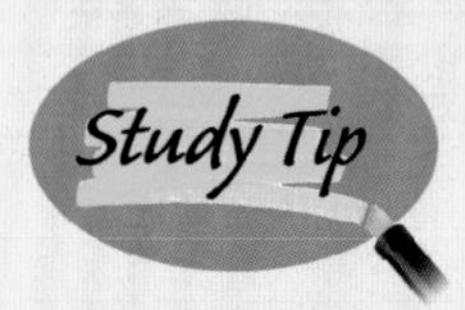

Salpingo-oophorectomy: The spelling of salpingo-oophorectomy (surgical removal of the ovary and salpinx) includes a hyphen because of the presence of three like vowels in a row. Always include the hyphen whether the term is handwritten or typed.

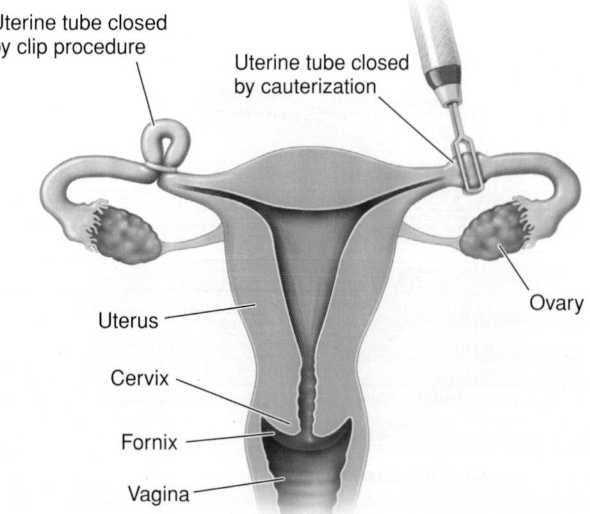

Figure 15-23 Two different procedures for tubal ligation.

Exercises: Surgical Interventions and Therapeutic Procedures

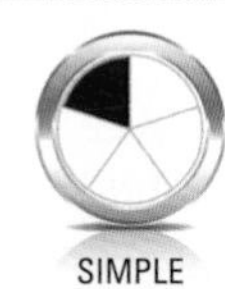

Exercise 21

Write the correct medical term for the definition given.

1. procedure whereby the cervix is dilated and the uterus is scraped ____________
2. surgical removal of a uterine myoma ____________
3. device inserted into the vagina to support the uterus ____________
4. surgical removal of the uterus and cervix through the abdomen ____________
5. placement of a nonabsorbable suture around an incompetent cervical opening ____________
6. surgical removal of the uterus and cervix through a vaginal incision ____________
7. inducing childbirth artificially with drugs or by puncturing the amniotic sac ____________
8. process whereby oocytes and spermatozoa are placed in a medium to produce a zygote ____________
9. procedure using an electrified wire loop to cut out abnormal tissue in the cervix ____________
10. artificial rupture of the amniotic sac to induce or accelerate labor ____________

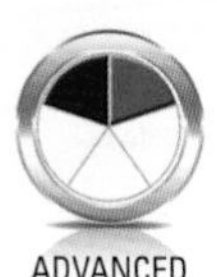

Exercise 22

Circle the term that is most appropriate for the meaning of the sentence.

1. After having four children, Ms. Thompson decided on a(n) (*vulvectomy, episiotomy, tubal ligation*) as a permanent contraceptive measure.
2. Dr. Adams used (*LEEP, cryosurgery, colporrhaphy*) to freeze abnormal cells from the patient's cervix.
3. Mrs. Kumar's surgeon performed a bilateral (*salpingo-oophorectomy, oophorectomy, salpingectomy*), a procedure whereby both the ovaries and uterine tubes are removed.
4. Mrs. Grace underwent a (*vulvectomy, lumpectomy, salpingectomy*) to remove a diseased portion of her uterine tube.
5. After her car accident, Mrs. Nabors had a (*therapeutic abortion, missed abortion, spontaneous abortion*) to save her life.
6. As a vaginal birth was not possible, Mrs. Nguyen delivered the child by means of (*cesarean section, hysterectomy, myomectomy*).

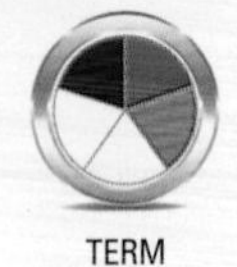
TERM CONSTRUCTION

Exercise 23

Using the given suffix, build a medical term for the meaning given.

Suffix	Meaning of Medical Term	Medical Term
-plasty	surgical repair of the breast	**1.** ____________
-tomy	incision into the amniotic sac	**2.** ____________
-pexy	surgical fixation of the breast	**3.** ____________
-plasty	surgical repair of the uterus	**4.** ____________
-tomy	surgical incision of the vulva to assist in childbirth	**5.** ____________

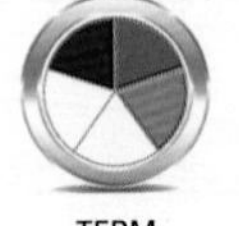
TERM CONSTRUCTION

Exercise 24

Break the given medical term into its word parts, and define each part. Then define the medical term.

For example:

mastitis	*word parts:*	mast /o, -itis
	meanings:	breast, inflammation of
	term meaning:	inflammation of the breast

1. salpingo-oophorectomy
word parts: ____________
meanings: ____________
term meaning: ____________

2. colporrhaphy
word parts: ____________
meanings: ____________
term meaning: ____________

3. uterotomy
word parts: ____________
meanings: ____________
term meaning: ____________

4. mammoplasty
word parts: ____________
meanings: ____________
term meaning: ____________

5. hysterectomy
word parts: ____________
meanings: ____________
term meaning: ____________

6. episiotomy *word parts:* ______

meanings: ______

term meaning: ______

7. salpingectomy *word parts:* ______

meanings: ______

term meaning: ______

8. oophorectomy *word parts:* ______

meanings: ______

term meaning: ______

9. mastopexy *word parts:* ______

meanings: ______

term meaning: ______

10. vulvectomy *word parts:* ______

meanings: ______

term meaning: ______

Medications and Drug Therapies

Term	Pronunciation	Meaning
Related to the Female Reproductive System		
contraceptive	kon'tră-sep'tiv	device or drug that prevents conception (pregnancy)
hormone replacement therapy (HRT)	hōr'mōn rĕ-plās'mĕnt thār'ă-pē	administration of hormones (e.g., estrogen, progesterone) to women after menopause or oophorectomy
Related to Obstetrics		
abortifacient	ă-bōr'ti-fā'shĕnt	drug that produces abortion
ovulation induction	ov'yū-lā'shŭn in-dŭk'shŭn	use of hormone therapy to stimulate ovulation (release of mature oocytes)
oxytocin	ok'sē-tō'sin	hormone that causes contractions and promotes milk release during lactation; also used to induce or stimulate labor
tocolytic	tō'kō-lit'ik	drug used to suppress uterine contractions, often used in an attempt to arrest premature birth

Exercise: Medications and Drug Therapies

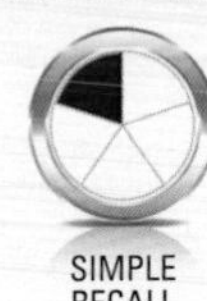
SIMPLE RECALL

Exercise 25

Write the correct medication or drug therapy term for the definition given.

1. a hormone that causes uterine contractions and promotes milk release ______________
2. drug that produces abortion ______________
3. device or drug that prevents conception ______________
4. hormone therapy to stimulate the development of mature oocytes ______________
5. drug used to suppress uterine contractions ______________
6. administration of hormones to women after menopause ______________

Specialties and Specialists

Term	Pronunciation	Meaning
gynecology (GYN)	gī'nĕ-kol'ŏ-jē	medical specialty concerned with the functions and diseases of the female genital tract, as well as endocrinology and reproductive physiology of the female
gynecologist (GYN)	gī'nĕ-kol'ŏ-jist	physician who specializes in gynecology
midwifery	mid-wif'ĕ-rē	practice of providing holistic health care to the childbearing woman and newborn
midwife	mid'wīf	health professional who practices midwifery
neonatal intensive care unit (NICU)	nē'ō-nā'tăl in-ten'siv kār yū'nit	hospital department designed for care of critically ill premature and full-term infants
neonatology	nē'ō-nā-tol'ŏ-jē	medical subspecialty of pediatrics concerned with the medical needs of newborn babies through the 28th day of life
neonatologist	nē'ō-nā-tol'ŏ-jist	pediatrician specializing in neonatology
obstetrics (OB)	ob-stet'riks	medical specialty concerned with childbirth and care of the mother
obstetrician (OB)	ob-stĕ-trish'ŭn	physician who specializes in obstetrics
pediatrics	pē-dē-at'riks	medical specialty concerned with the study and treatment of children in health and disease during development from birth through adolescence
pediatrician	pē'dē-ă-trish'ăn	physician who specializes in pediatrics
reproductive endocrinology	rē'prō-dŭk'tiv en'dō-kri-nol'ŏ-jē	medical subspecialty within gynecology and obstetrics that addresses hormonal functioning as it pertains to reproduction as well as the issue of infertility
reproductive endocrinologist	rē'prō-dŭk'tiv en'dō-kri-nol'ŏ-jist	physician who practices reproductive endocrinology

Exercise: Specialties and Specialists

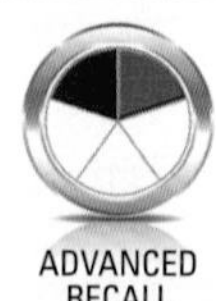
ADVANCED RECALL

Exercise 26

Match each medical specialty or specialist with its description.

gynecology	neonatology	obstetrics	reproductive endocrinologist
midwifery	pediatrics	gynecologist	neonatal intensive care unit
pediatrician	midwife	obstetrician	neonatologist
reproductive endocrinology			

1. provider of holistic health care to the childbearing woman ____________
2. hospital department caring for critically ill infants ____________
3. addresses hormonal functioning as it relates to pregnancy and infertility ____________
4. medical subspecialty that focuses on care and treatment of newborns up to 28 days ____________
5. branch of medicine dealing with childbirth and care of the mother ____________
6. the study and treatment of children from birth through adolescence ____________
7. pediatrician who specializes in caring and treating newborns up to 28 days ____________
8. practice that focuses on providing holistic health care to the childbearing woman and newborn ____________
9. physician who specializes in hormonal functioning as it relates to pregnancy and infertility ____________
10. the study and treatment of diseases of the female genital tract ____________
11. physician who specializes in childbirth and care of the mother ____________
12. physician who studies and treats children from birth through adolescence ____________
13. physician who specializes in diseases of the female genital tract ____________

Abbreviations

Abbreviation	Meaning
AB	abortion
AFP	alpha-fetoprotein
C-section	cesarean section
CVS	chorionic villus sampling
D&C	dilatation and curettage; dilation and curettage
DOB	date of birth
EDC	estimated date of confinement
EDD	estimated date of delivery
GBS	group B streptococcus
GYN	gynecology; gynecologist
hCG	human chorionic gonadotropin
HRT	hormone replacement therapy
HSG	hysterosalpingogram
IVF	in vitro fertilization
LEEP	loop electrosurgical excision procedure
LMP	last menstrual period
NICU	neonatal intensive care unit
OB	obstetrics; obstetrician
PID	pelvic inflammatory disease
SAB	spontaneous abortion
STD	sexually transmitted disease
TAB	therapeutic abortion
TAH	total abdominal hysterectomy

Exercises: Abbreviations

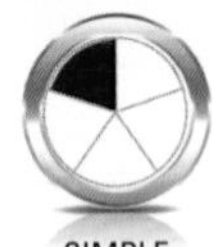

SIMPLE RECALL

Exercise 27

Write the meaning of each abbreviation.

1. TAH ______________________________
2. SAB ______________________________
3. AB ______________________________
4. PID ______________________________
5. STD ______________________________

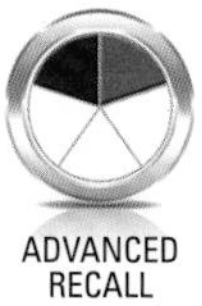

Exercise 28

Write the meaning of each abbreviation used in these sentences.

1. The infant was born six weeks prematurely and was sent to the **NICU** for further care.

____

2. Ms. McNeal saw her **OB** regularly until the birth of her baby last year.

____

3. Mrs. Hajdu's gynecologist started her on **HRT** to help minimize the symptoms of menopause.

____

4. A **TAH** is a common type of surgery performed on women who require removal of the uterus and cervix.

____

5. A **TAB** may be performed when the mother's life is threatened by the pregnancy.

____

6. Given the date of conception, the obstetrician placed Ms. Ellys's **EDD** at December 25.

____

7. Part of Mrs. Winn's gynecologic record includes the date of her **LMP**, which was sometime in March.

____

8. Ms. Hernandez underwent **IVF** because she could not conceive a child normally.

____

9. The patient underwent a **D&C** following her therapeutic abortion to remove any remaining products of conception.

____

10. Theresa underwent an **LEEP** to remove abnormal tissue in her cervix.

____

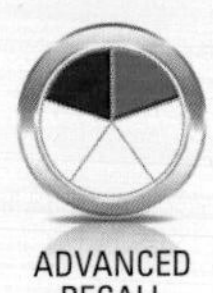

Exercise 29

Match each abbreviation with the appropriate description.

GYN	DOB	CVS
hCG	D&C	HSG

1. removal of endocervical tissue using a curette ____________
2. examination of placental tissue ____________
3. x-ray examination of the uterus and salpinges ____________
4. one who practices gynecology ____________
5. date of birth of a patient ____________
6. hormone produced in pregnancy ____________

WRAPPING UP

- Female reproductive system: main functions are to produce female sex cells (oocytes), nourish a developing embryo and fetus, and nurse an infant.
- Obstetrics: field of medicine concerned with childbirth and the care of women during pregnancy.
- Neonatology: pediatric subspecialty that deals with the care of a newborn and disorders of the newborn.
- In this chapter, you learned medical terminology including word parts, prefixes, suffixes, adjectives, conditions, tests, procedures, medications, specialties, and abbreviations related to the female reproductive system, obstetrics, and neonatology.

Chapter Review

Review of Terms for Anatomy and Physiology

Exercise 30

Write the correct terms on the blanks for the anatomic structures indicated.

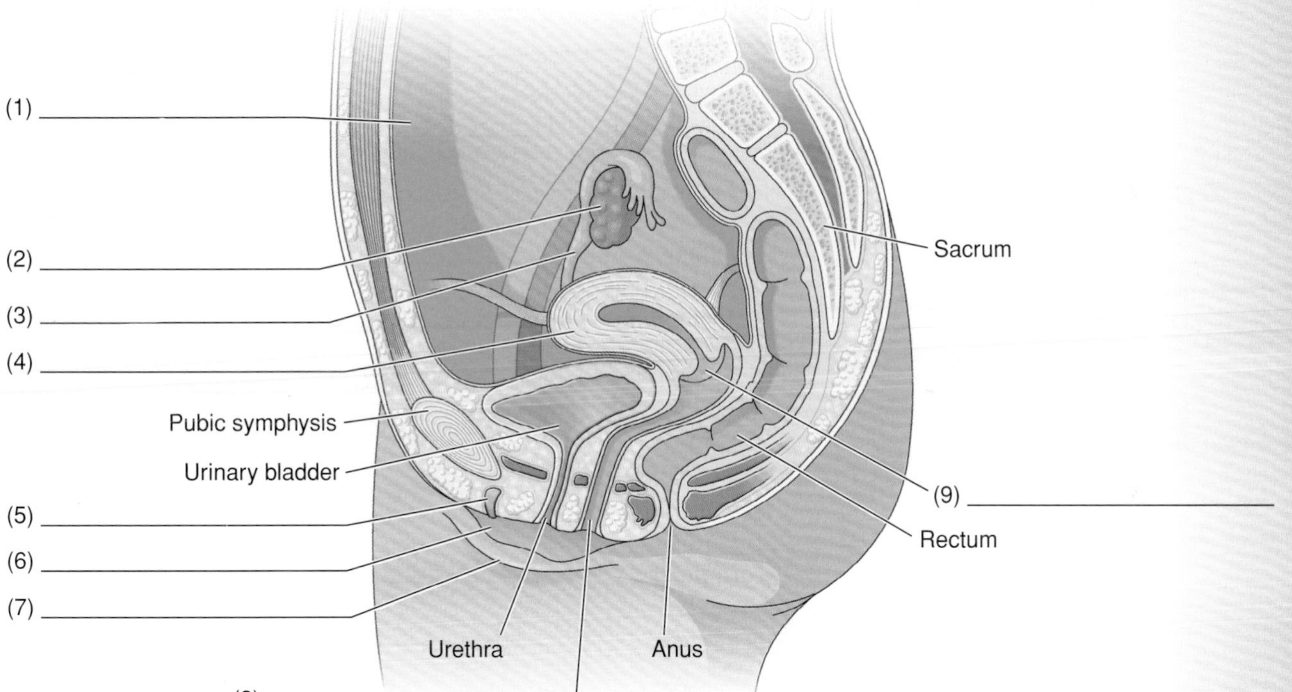

Understanding Term Structure

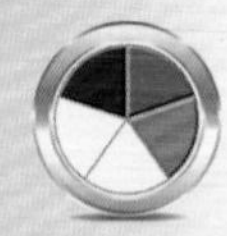
TERM CONSTRUCTION

Exercise 31

Break the given medical term into its word parts, and define each part. Then define the medical term. (Note: You may need to use word parts from other chapters.)

For example:

mastitis	*word parts:*	mast/o, -itis
	meanings:	breast, inflammation of
	term meaning:	inflammation of the breast

1. hysterosalpingography	*word parts:*	______________________
	meanings:	______________________
	term meaning:	______________________
2. episiotomy	*word parts:*	______________________
	meanings:	______________________
	term meaning:	______________________
3. colporrhaphy	*word parts:*	______________________
	meanings:	______________________
	term meaning:	______________________
4. endocervical	*word parts:*	______________________
	meanings:	______________________
	term meaning:	______________________
5. pelvimetry	*word parts:*	______________________
	meanings:	______________________
	term meaning:	______________________
6. oophorectomy	*word parts:*	______________________
	meanings:	______________________
	term meaning:	______________________
7. mammography	*word parts:*	______________________
	meanings:	______________________
	term meaning:	______________________

8. metrorrhagia *word parts:* ______
meanings: ______
term meaning: ______

9. oligomenorrhea *word parts:* ______
meanings: ______
term meaning: ______

10. mammoplasty *word parts:* ______
meanings: ______
term meaning: ______

11. salpingectomy *word parts:* ______
meanings: ______
term meaning: ______

12. colposcopy *word parts:* ______
meanings: ______
term meaning: ______

13. vaginitis *word parts:* ______
meanings: ______
term meaning: ______

14. cervicitis *word parts:* ______
meanings: ______
term meaning: ______

Comprehension Exercises

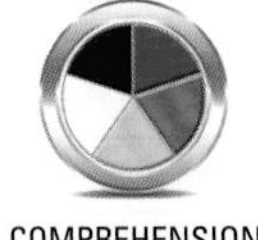
COMPREHENSION

Exercise 32

Fill in the blank with the correct term.

1. A(n) ______ pregnancy occurs when a fertilized ovum implants itself outside the uterus.

2. The term ______ means no pregnancies.

3. ______________________ is the inability of a couple to achieve fertilization.

4. ______________________ is a method of conception that takes place outside of the uterus.

5. ______________________ is a method to extract the fetus other than through the birth canal.

6. A(n) ______________________ poses the risk of intrauterine hypoxia, fetal distress, and death because the structure wraps around the fetal neck.

Exercise 33

COMPREHENSION

Write a short answer for each question.

1. In what surgical procedure is the adnexa of the uterus removed? ______________________

____

2. What is the name given to a developing infant between the zygote and fetus stages? ______________________

____

3. What structure enables an oocyte to travel from the ovary to the uterus? ______________________

____

4. How do the meanings of the terms *nulligravida, primigravida,* and *gravida* differ? ______________________

____

5. Name the three layers making up the wall of the uterus. ______________________

____

6. What is the difference between gynecology and obstetrics? ______________________

____

7. Where can endometriosis occur? ______________________

____

8. What is the difference between rupture of membranes and an amniotomy? ______________________

____

9. For what reason would a physician perform amniocentesis? ______________________

____

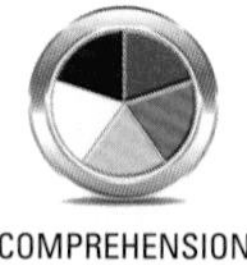

COMPREHENSION

Exercise 34

Circle the letter of the best answer in the following questions.

1. Which of the following structures might be involved if a woman has PID?

A. ovaries
B. uterus
C. salpinges
D. all of the above

2. The cervix is a part of which structure?

A. uterus
B. vagina
C. It is a separate structure.
D. none of the above

3. The structures that store oocytes and produce hormones are the

A. salpinges.
B. ovaries.
C. labia.
D. fimbriae.

4. A girl's first menses is referred to as

A. menarche.
B. menopause.
C. date of last menstrual period.
D. menstruation.

5. A ______________ can be performed either transvaginally or through the abdomen.

A. mastectomy
B. laparotomy
C. hysterectomy
D. myomectomy

6. The estimated date of confinement is calculated from the patient's

A. EDC.
B. LMP.
C. DOB.
D. EDD.

7. Which test is done to examine tissues inside the placenta?

A. Apgar score
B. chorionic villus sampling
C. quad marker screen
D. pregnancy test

8. The term that indicates a patient's obstetric history in which there have been no deliveries of viable offspring is

A. gravida.
B. nulligravida.
C. primigravida.
D. nullipara.

Application and Analysis

CASE STUDIES

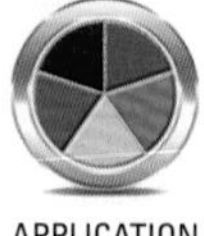

APPLICATION

Exercise 35

Read the case studies, and circle the correct letter for each of the questions.

CASE 15-1

Mrs. Andresson, who had been seen in the emergency room for vaginal bleeding last week, came into the medical office for follow-up. She had a positive pregnancy test result more than 11 weeks ago and had recently begun passing several clots. A specimen was sent for testing. It was explained to her that this was a spontaneous abortion because her hCG levels have decreased, and the specimen showed products of conception. She was provided emotional support and given instructions to take a multivitamin as needed.

1. What is hCG?

A. a hormone produced in the pancreas
B. a growth hormone
C. a hormone produced in pregnancy that is made by the developing embryo and placenta soon after conception
D. a hormone that causes pregnancy

2. What was the patient's diagnosis?

A. a therapeutic abortion
B. a spontaneous abortion
C. a missed abortion
D. a D&C

3. Decreasing levels of hCG probably indicate

A. a spontaneous abortion.
B. a growing baby.
C. a conflict in blood types between mother and baby.
D. a twin gestation.

4. What was the initial sign or symptom that brought the patient to the emergency room?

A. headaches
B. decreasing hCG levels
C. vaginal bleeding
D. a positive pregnancy test

5. The specimen showed products of conception; this also indicated a

A. spontaneous abortion.
B. rupture of membranes.
C. congenital defect.
D. placenta previa.

CASE 15-2

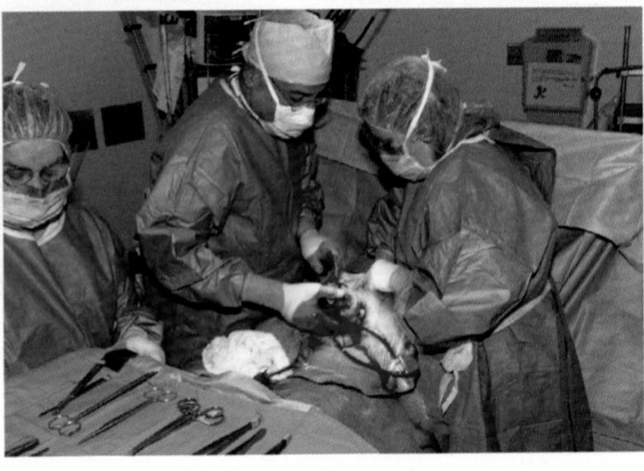

Cesarean section.

Ms. Jamesly is seen in the office for follow-up. She was admitted to the hospital last week to deliver her baby. On examination, the baby was found to be in a breech presentation. Ms. Jamesly was taken to the operating room, where a cesarean section was performed. She also had a tubal ligation. Her incision appears normal and she says that her breast milk is coming in. She states that baby is being treated for jaundice but is feeding well.

6. In a breech presentation, the infant's buttocks

A. appear last.
B. appear first.
C. do not appear at all.
D. none of the above

7. What is the medical term for production of breast milk?

A. lactation
B. lochia
C. prolactin
D. milk production

8. A cesarean section involves removing the fetus via an incision in the abdominal wall and the

A. perineum.
B. vagina.
C. uterus.
D. peritoneum.

9. A tubal ligation is a(n) ________________ procedure for women.

A. sterilization
B. uterine
C. conception
D. in vitro fertilization

10. Jaundice is the inability of the infant's liver to metabolize

A. prolactin.
B. fat.
C. breast milk.
D. bilirubin.

MEDICAL RECORD ANALYSIS

MEDICAL RECORD 15-1

Ms. Brown is a patient who is being observed for suspicious-looking lesions on a Pap test with subsequent evaluation of those lesions, as detailed in the medical record that follows. She is now returning for a follow-up Pap test. You are the cytotechnologist who will be analyzing the specimen from the test.

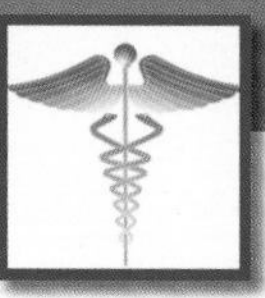

Medical Record

CLINIC NOTE

SUBJECTIVE: This patient is a 36-year-old gravida 3, para 3–0–0–3 with a history of conization in September 20xx, which showed precancerous cells and a negative endocervical curettage. Prior to that, the patient had had a colposcopy revealing precancerous cells in August 20xx. The patient has had follow-up after her colposcopy with a Pap test.

Later the patient had another Pap test that was negative and a colposcopy performed that was negative. No lesions or metastases were seen at that time and no biopsies were taken, as such. The Pap test again returned as normal. Today the patient comes back for a Pap test. She has no changes in her interval history. She denies any sexually transmitted diseases.

OBJECTIVE: On examination, the external genitalia appeared to be within normal limits and without any obvious lesions. The speculum was inserted into the vaginal canal, and the vaginal mucosa appeared to be pink and healthy. The cervix was visualized and noted to be free of lesions, although at the 9 o'clock position, a suture was seen. A Pap test was performed. There was some stenosis of the cervical os. The patient tolerated the procedure well.

ASSESSMENT AND PLAN: The test results and plan for follow-up will be mailed to patient when available.

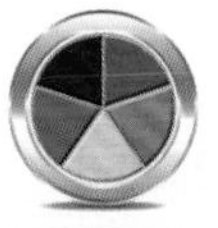

APPLICATION

Exercise 36

Write the appropriate medical terms used in this medical record on the blanks after their definitions. Note that not all the terms appear in the chapter, but you should be able to identify these terms based on word parts that are included in this chapter.

1. infectious disease spread through sexual contact ________________
2. scraping within the cervix with a curette ________________
3. process of examining the vagina and cervix ________________
4. narrowing of a structure ________________

Bonus Questions

5. What is meant by the phrase *gravida 3*? ________________
6. What is the full term for *Pap test*? ________________

MEDICAL RECORD 15-2

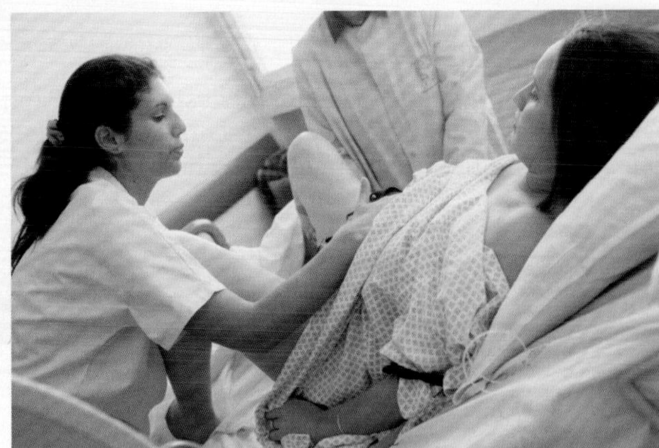

Nurse midwife assisting a patient in labor.

As a nurse midwife, you have cared for the patient in the following medical record throughout her pregnancy and delivery. You are now documenting the delivery through this medical record.

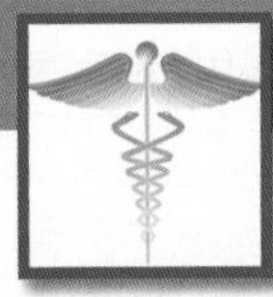

Medical Record

DELIVERY NOTE

PROCEDURES

1. Controlled vaginal delivery.
2. Repair of episiotomy.

PROCEDURE IN DETAIL: The patient is a primigravida 27-year-old white female who received (1) ____________________ care throughout her pregnancy. She has remained normotensive throughout her pregnancy, and dipsticks remained negative. Maternal blood type is O-negative, so RhoGAM was administered postdelivery.

The patient arrived in active labor with a good mechanism at 0430 hours. She was 80% effaced with the (2) ____________________ dilated to 4 cm. The fetus was noted to be in a vertex presentation at a –2 station. She progressed rapidly in labor, and by 1045 hours, she was 100% effaced and dilated to 5 cm. An epidural was started by anesthesia at the patient's request. The fetus remained in the vertex presentation and had normal fetal monitoring strips throughout labor, with a heart rate ranging from 120 to 152.

At 1205 hours, the patient was moved to delivery. The epidural was continued. The patient's vagina and perineum were prepped, and drapes were applied after the patient was placed in Allen stirrups in the lithotomy position. It was felt that is was necessary to do a midline (3) ____________________. The infant's head was delivered, and the nose and oropharynx were suctioned with a bulb. The shoulders were gently rotated, and the infant was delivered and placed on the mother's abdomen. The infant cried spontaneously and vigorously. The mouth and nose were once again suctioned. The cord was clamped and cut. Cord blood was obtained from a three-vessel cord. The infant was handed off the field to the (4) ____________________ in attendance. The infant's blood type will be determined, and the infant will be closely monitored for any signs of Rh incompatibility, but none was apparent at birth.

The patient delivered a viable male infant weighing 7 lb 9 oz with an (5) ____________________ of 8 at one minute and 10 at five minutes. RhoGAM will be administered. The midline episiotomy was repaired without complications. The infant was sent to the newborn nursery, and the mother will be closely observed prior to returning to her room for recovery.

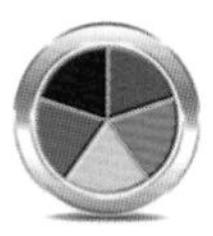
APPLICATION

Exercise 37

Fill in the blanks in the medical record above with the correct medical terms. The definitions of the missing terms are listed below.

1. period of time preceding birth
2. tubular, lower portion of the uterus
3. surgical incision of the perineum to assist childbirth
4. pediatrician specializing in neonatology
5. numeric result of a test to evaluate a newborn's physical condition quickly

Bonus Question

6. Why was an episiotomy performed? ______________________________

____

Pronunciation and Spelling

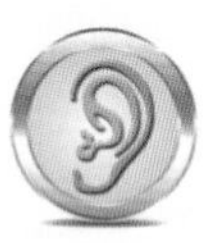
AUDITORY

Exercise 38

Review the Chapter 15 terms in the Dictionary/Audio Glossary in the Student Resources on thePoint, and practice pronouncing each term, referring to the pronunciation guide as needed.

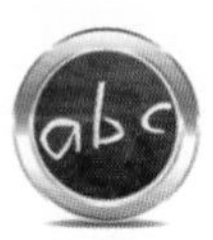
SPELLING

Exercise 39

Circle the correct spelling of each term.

1. histerectomy	hysterectomy	hystirectomy
2. suprapubic	suprepubic	suprepublic
3. cervicitis	cervisitis	servicitis
4. cystic	cystik	cistic
5. laparotomy	laprotome	laperotomy
6. mastectomy	mastectome	mestectomy
7. indometrial	endometrial	endometreal
8. ovvulation	ovulation	oveulation
9. perimetrum	perimetrium	parimetrium

10. mammographe	mammography	mamography
11. placenta	plasenta	plecenta
12. clytoris	clitoris	cleitoris
13. ariola	areolla	areola
14. colposcopy	culposcopy	colposcopey
15. zygote	zygoote	zygotte

Media Connection

Exercise 40

Complete each of the following activities available with the Student Resources on thePoint. Check off each activity as you complete it, and record your score for the Chapter Quiz in the space provided.

Chapter Exercises

_____ Flash Cards

_____ Concentration

_____ Abbreviation Match-Up

_____ Roboterms

_____ Word Anatomy

_____ Fill the Gap

_____ Break It Down

_____ True/False Body Building

_____ Quiz Show

_____ Complete the Case

_____ Medical Record Review

_____ Look and Label

_____ Image Matching

_____ Spelling Bee

_____ **Chapter Quiz** *Score:*________%

Additional Resources

_____ Animation: Ovulation and Fertilization

_____ Dictionary/Audio Glossary

_____ Health Professions Careers: Cytotechnologist

_____ Health Professions Careers: Nurse-Midwife

Oncology

16

Chapter Outline

Introduction, 638

Word Parts, 638
- Combining Forms, 638
- Prefixes, 639
- Suffixes, 639

Medical Terms, 642
- General Terms Related to Oncology, 642
- Selected Types of Cancer by Body System, 647
- Laboratory Tests, 655
- Diagnostic Procedures, 656
- Surgical Interventions, 661
- Therapeutic Procedures, 663
- Medications and Drug Therapies, 666
- Specialties and Specialists, 668
- Abbreviations, 670

Wrapping Up, 672

Chapter Review, 673

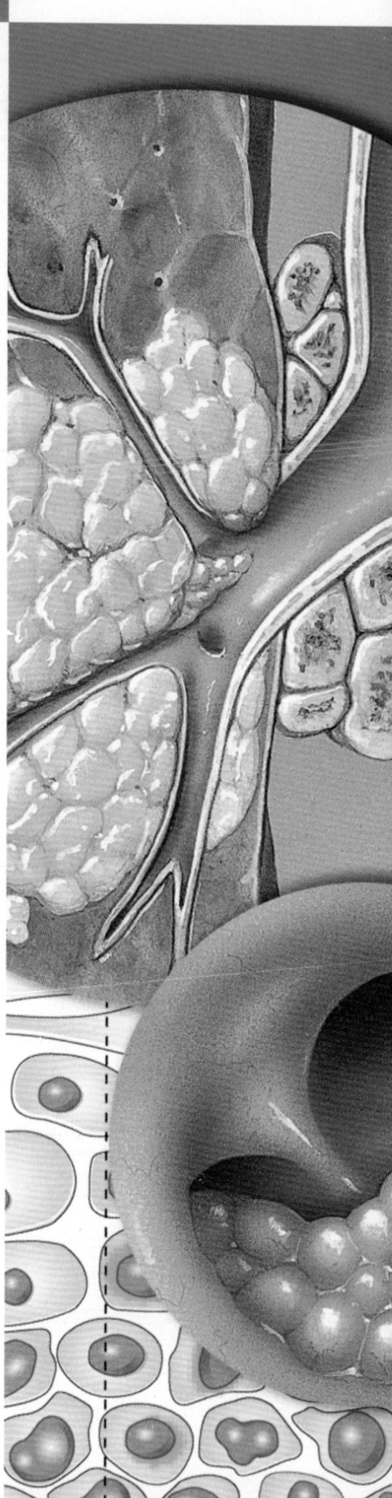

Learning Outcomes

After completing this chapter, you should be able to:

1. Define combing forms, prefixes, and suffixes related to oncology.
2. Define general terms related to oncology.
3. Define terms related to cancers of different body systems.
4. Define common medical terminology related to oncology, including tests and procedures; surgical interventions and therapeutic procedures; medications and drug therapies; and medical specialties and specialists used to evaluate and identify cancer and cancer progression.
5. Define abbreviations for terms related to oncology and cancers of various body systems.
6. Successfully complete all chapter exercises.
7. Explain terms used in case studies and medical records involving cancers of the various body systems.
8. Successfully complete all exercises included with the companion Student Resources on thePoint.

INTRODUCTION

Oncology is the study and treatment of new, abnormal tissue known as neoplasms. Typically, it refers to cancer, the disease characterized by uncontrolled cell division that leads to abnormal cells. Cancer is a leading public health issue worldwide. Among men, the most common type of cancer is prostate (26%); among women, the most common cancer is breast (29%). This chapter focuses on word parts and medical terms related to oncology.

WORD PARTS

The following tables list word parts related to oncology. Note that some word parts introduced earlier in the book may not be repeated here.

Combining Forms

Combining Form	Meaning
ablat/o	to take away
bi/o	life
cancer/o	cancer
carcin/o	cancer
chem/o	chemical, drug
cry/o	cold
cyt/o	cell
kary/o	nucleus
lapar/o	abdomen
leuk/o	white
melan/o	black, dark
onc/o	tumor
path/o	disease
plas/o	growth, formation
radi/o	x-rays, radiation
rhabd/o	striated muscle
sarc/o	muscle, flesh
squam/o	scale-like structure

Prefixes

Prefix	Meaning
chondro-	cartilage
dys-	painful, difficult, abnormal
intra-	within
leio-	smooth
mal-	bad, poor
meta-	change, beyond
neo-	new
para-	beside
trans-	across, through

Suffixes

Suffix	Meaning
-gen	origin, production
-genic	originating, producing
-oma	tumor or neoplasm
-scopy	viewing, examining, or observing with an instrument

Exercises: Word Parts

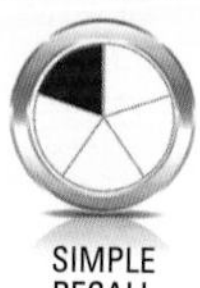

SIMPLE RECALL

Exercise 1

Write the meaning of the combining form given.

1. path/o ______________________
2. carcin/o ______________________
3. onc/o ______________________
4. cancer/o ______________________
5. cry/o ______________________
6. melan/o ______________________
7. leuk/o ______________________
8. sarc/o ______________________
9. radi/o ______________________
10. lapar/o ______________________

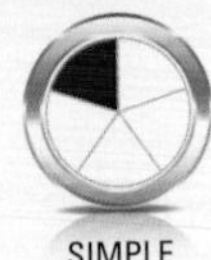

Exercise 2

Write the correct combining form for the meaning given.

1. cell _______________
2. nucleus _______________
3. chemical, drug _______________
4. cancer _______________
5. striated muscle _______________
6. scale-like structure _______________
7. growth, formation _______________
8. life _______________
9. to take away _______________
10. muscle, flesh _______________

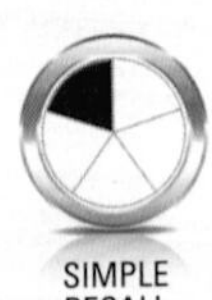

Exercise 3

Write the meaning of the prefix or suffix given.

1. meta- _______________
2. -scopy _______________
3. -oma _______________
4. -gen _______________
5. intra- _______________
6. mal- _______________
7. leio- _______________
8. neo- _______________
9. dys- _______________
10. -genic _______________
11. para- _______________
12. trans- _______________

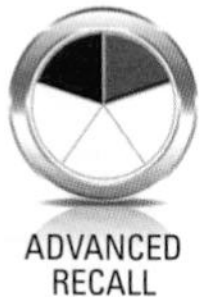
ADVANCED RECALL

Exercise 4

Considering the meaning of the combining form from which the medical term is made, write the meaning of the medical term. (You have not yet learned many of these terms but can build their meanings from the word parts).

Combining Form	Meaning	Medical Term	Meaning of Term
oste/o	bone	osteoma	1. ____________
chondr/o	cartilage	chondroma	2. ____________
lei/o, my/o	smooth, muscle	leiomyoma	3. ____________
carcin/o	cancer	carcinoma	4. ____________
leuk/o	white	leukemia	5. ____________
my/o	muscle	myoma	6. ____________
duct/o	duct	ductal	7. ____________

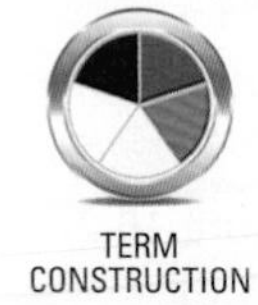
TERM CONSTRUCTION

Exercise 5

Using the given combining form and a word part from the earlier tables, build a medical term for the meaning given.

Combining Form	Meaning of Medical Term	Medical Term
cyt/o	study of cells	1. ____________
squam/o	pertaining to a scale-like structure	2. ____________
lei/o, my/o	tumor of smooth muscle	3. ____________
melan/o	tumor of melanin-forming cells	4. ____________
aden/o	tumor of glandular tissue	5. ____________
lymph/o	tumor of lymphoid tissue	6. ____________
myel/o	tumor of the bone marrow	7. ____________
nephr/o	tumor of the kidney	8. ____________
angi/o	tumor consisting of a mass of blood vessels	9. ____________
neur/o	tumor of nervous tissue	10. ____________

MEDICAL TERMS

General Terms Related to Oncology

Term	Pronunciation	Meaning
General Terms		
benign	bĕ-nīn′	nonmalignant form of a neoplasm
cancer (CA)	kan′sĕr	general term for a group of diseases characterized by an abnormal, uncontrolled growth of cells
cancerous	kan′sĕr-ŭs	pertaining to cancer
carcinogen	kar-sin′ŏ-jen	any cancer-causing substance or organism
differentiation	dif′ĕr-en′shē-ā′shŭn	acquiring characteristics or functions different from that of the original cell
dysplasia	dis-plā′zē-ă	abnormal growth of tissue (**Figure 16-1**)
in situ	in sī′tū	in the original place or site without any expansion or spread (**Figure 16-1**)
invasion	in-vā′zhŭn	the direct migration and penetration of cancerous cells into neighboring tissues
lesion	lē′zhŭn	a pathologic change in tissue resulting from disease or injury
malignant	mă-lig′nănt	tumor that invades surrounding tissue and may spread to other body parts; cancerous (**Figure 16-1**)
metastasis	mĕ-tas′tă-sis	spread of disease from one part of the body to another (**Figure 16-2**)
oncogenes	ong′kō-jenz	mutated forms of genes that cause normal cells to grow out of control and become cancer cells
oncogenic	ong′kō-jen′ik	causing or being suitable for the development of a tumor

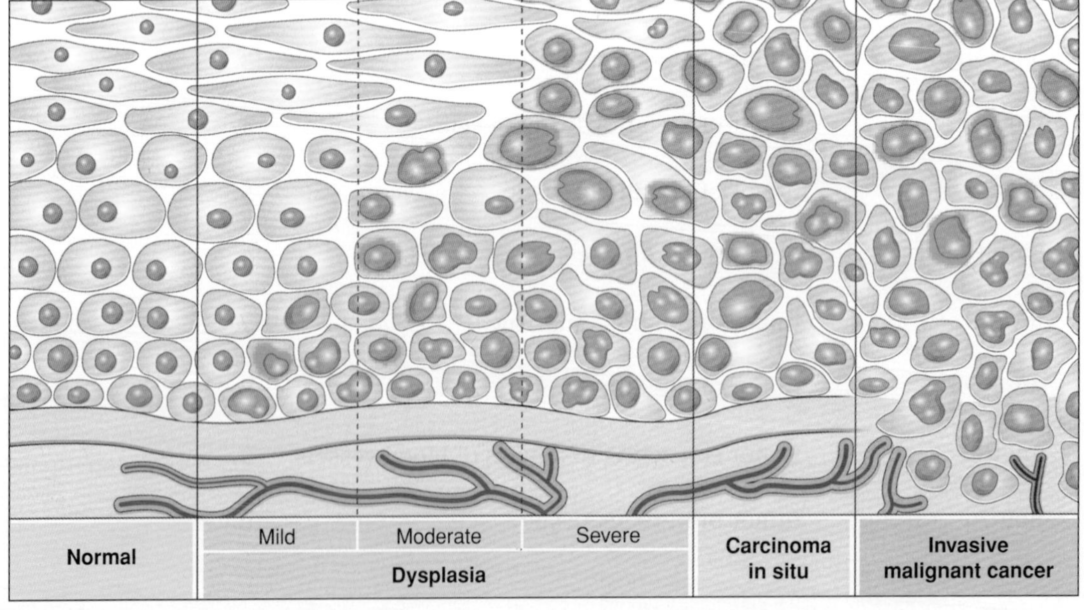

Figure 16-1 Examples of tissue showing cell changes related to cancer.

General Terms Related to Oncology

Term	Pronunciation	Meaning
recurrence	rē-kŭr′ĕns	the return of cancer or disease
remission	rē-mish′ŭn	lessening in severity of disease symptoms; the period of time when a cancer is responding to treatment or is under control
TNM staging	tē en em stāj′ing	abbreviation for cancer classification based on characteristics of the tumors, nodal involvement, and extent of metastasis (**Figure 16-3**)
tumor staging	tū′mŏr stāj′ing	the extent of spread of a cancer from its original site

(continued)

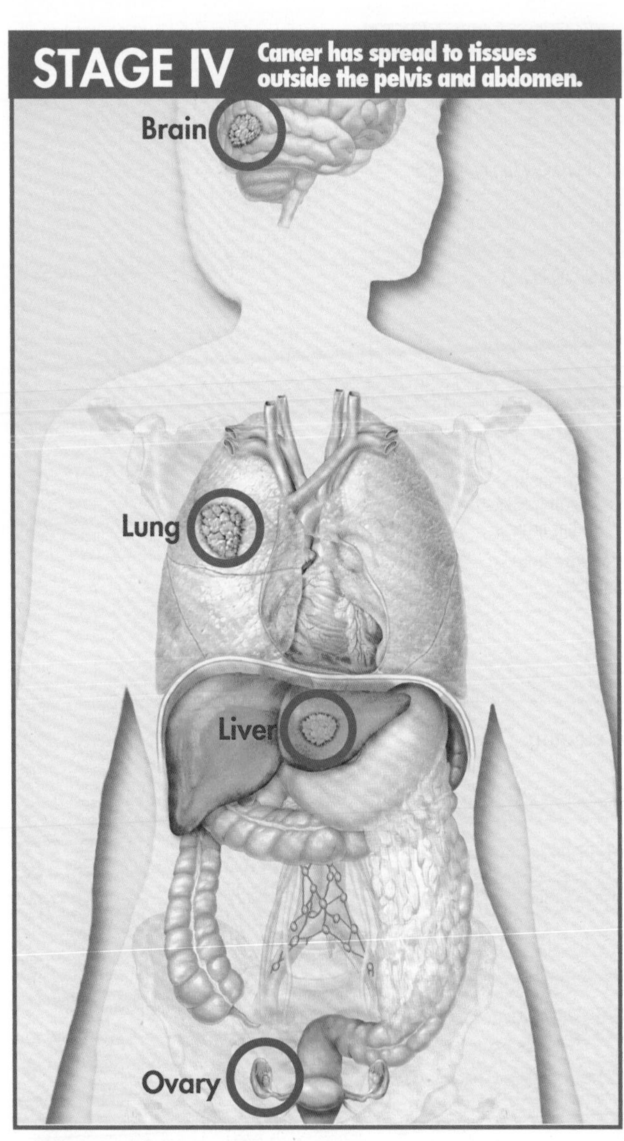

Figure 16-2 Metastatic ovarian cancer. The original cancer site was located in the ovary, and it has spread to the brain, lung, and liver.

General Terms Related to Oncology *(continued)*

Term	Pronunciation	Meaning
Types of Tumors		
adenocarcinoma	ad′ĕ-nō-kar′si-nō′mă	malignant neoplasm composed of glandular tissue (**Figures 16-4** and **16-5**)

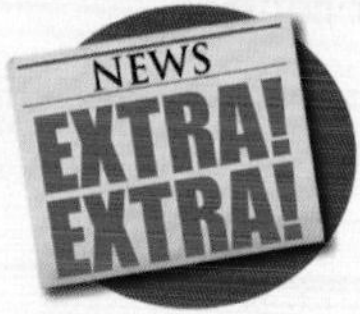

UNDERSTANDING TUMORS Many cancers involve the formation of malignant tumors derived from glandular structures in epithelial tissue, meaning that they are adenocarcinomas. For example, approximately 95% of prostate cancer is classified as adenocarcinoma of the prostate, and many breast cancers are determined to be adenocarcinoma of the breast.

TNM staging

T — primary tumor	
TX	primary tumor cannot be judged
T0	no basis for primary tumor
Tis	carcinoma/tumor in situ
T1, T2, T3, T4	increasing sizes and/or extent of primary tumor invasion
N — regional lymph nodes	
NX	regional lymph nodes cannot be judged
N0	no regional lymph node metastases
N1, N2, N3	increasing invasion of regional lymph nodes
M — metastasis	
MX	existence of metastases cannot be judged
M0	no metastases
M1	metastases present

the category M1 can be subdivided as follows:

lung	PUL	marrow	MAR
bone	OSS	rib	PLE
liver	HEP	peritoneum	PER
brain	BRA	skin	SKI
lymph nodes	LYM	other organs	OTH

G — histopathologic differentiation grade (grading)	
GX	differentiation grade cannot be determined
G1	well-differentiated
G2	moderately differentiated
G3	poorly differentiated
G4	undifferentiated

Figure 16-3 TNM staging.

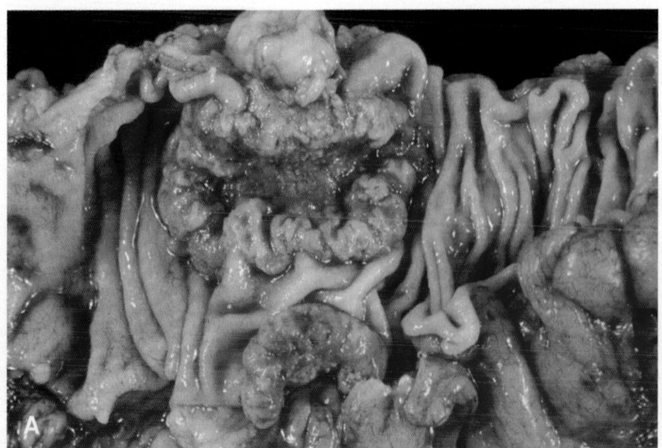

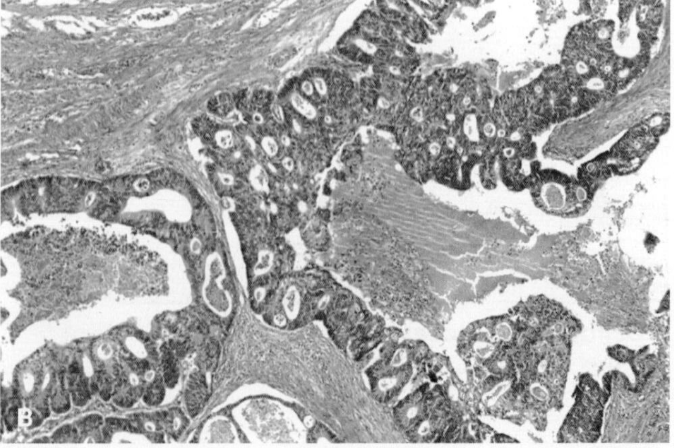

Figure 16-4 Adenocarcinoma of the colon. **A.** A resected colon shows an ulcerated mass with enlarged, firm, rolled borders. **B.** Microscopically, this adenocarcinoma consists of moderately differentiated glands.

General Terms Related to Oncology

Term	Pronunciation	Meaning
adenoma	ad′ĕ-nō′mă	benign neoplasm composed of glandular tissue
carcinoma (CA)	kar′si-nō′mă	malignant neoplasm derived from epithelial tissue, chiefly glandular (adenocarcinoma) or squamous (squamous cell carcinoma)
fibroma	fī-brō′mă	benign neoplasm of fibrous connective tissue
fibrosarcoma	fī′brō-sar-kō′mă	malignant neoplasm of deep fibrous tissue (**Figure 16-5**)
lipoma	li-pō′mă	benign neoplasm of adipose (fat) tissue
liposarcoma	lip′ō-sar-kō′mă	malignant neoplasm of adipose (fat) tissue (**Figure 16-5**)
malignant neoplasm	mă-lig′nănt nē′ō-plazm	tumor that invades surrounding tissue and is usually capable of metastasizing; can be located in any organ or tissue in the body
melanoma	mel′ă-nō′mă	tumor characterized by a dark appearance; most commonly occurs in the skin or in the eye (**Figure 16-5**)

(continued)

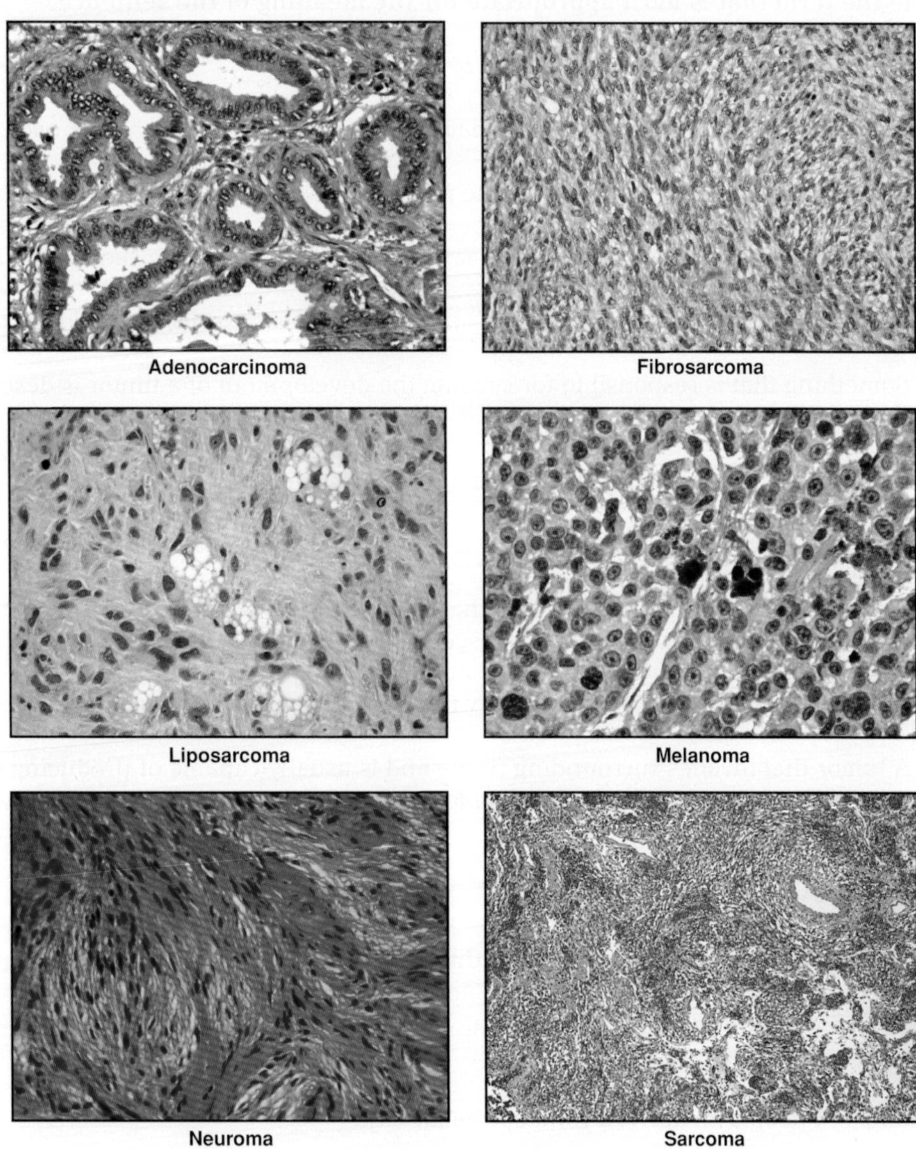

Figure 16-5 Types of tumors seen under the microscope.

General Terms Related to Oncology *(continued)*

Term	Pronunciation	Meaning
neoplasm; *syn.* tumor	nē′ō-plazm; tū′mŏr	abnormal growth of new tissue into a mass; can be benign or malignant
neuroma	nūr-ō′mă	tumor derived from nervous tissue (**Figure 16-5**)
myeloma	mī′ĕ-lō′mă	tumor composed of cells derived from bone marrow (**Figure 16-5**)
sarcoma	sar-kō′mă	malignant neoplasm of connective tissue or nonepithelial tissue

Exercises: General Terms Related to Oncology

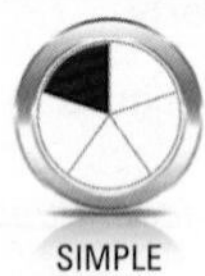

Exercise 6

Circle the term that is most appropriate for the meaning of the sentence.

1. A nonmalignant tumor is (*oncogenic, benign, invasive*).
2. A liposarcoma is different from a lipoma in that it is a(n) (*malignant, benign, oncogenic*) neoplasm.
3. Tumors derived from cells in the bone marrow are called (*lipomas, sarcomas, myelomas*).
4. A tumor characterized by a dark appearance is called a (*sarcoma, melanoma, myeloma*).
5. An adenocarcinoma is composed of (*squamous cells, nerve cells, glandular tissue*).
6. Something that is responsible for causing the development of a tumor is described as (*malignant, oncogenic, recurrent*).
7. Cancer that has returned is known as a (*promotion, progression, recurrence*).
8. A tumor derived from nervous tissue is called a (*nucleus, recurrence, neuroma*).
9. A tumor that is locally invasive and characterized by destructive growth and metastasis is referred to as (*benign, malignant, oncogenic*).
10. A benign neoplasm derived from fatty tissue is referred to as a (*neuroma, lipoma, fibroma*).
11. A tumor that invades surrounding tissue and is usually capable of producing metastasis is known as a(n) (*malignant neoplasm, adenoma, carcinoma*).

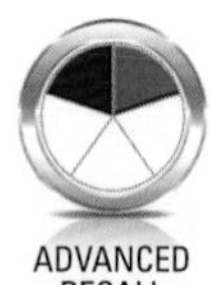

Exercise 7

Match each medical term with its meaning.

dysplasia	lesion	in situ	invasion	benign
cancer	metastasis	tumor	carcinoma	

1. malignant neoplasm derived from epithelial tissue ____________
2. nonmalignant form of a neoplasm ____________

3. pathologic change in tissue ______________________

4. abnormal growth of tissue ______________________

5. abnormal growth of new tissue into a mass ______________________

6. general term for a group of diseases characterized by an abnormal, uncontrolled growth of cells ______________________

7. in the original place or site ______________________

8. direct migration of cancerous cells to neighboring tissues ______________________

9. spread of disease from one part of the body to another ______________________

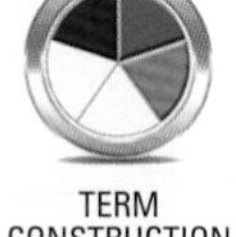

TERM CONSTRUCTION

Exercise 8

Build a medical term from the appropriate combining form and suffix, given their meanings.

Use Combining Form for	Use Suffix for	Term
gland	tumor	1. ______________
fiber	tumor	2. ______________
disease	originating, producing	3. ______________
fatty tissue	tumor	4. ______________
muscle, flesh	tumor	5. ______________
bone marrow	tumor	6. ______________
cancer	pertaining to	7. ______________
fiber; connective tissue	tumor	8. ______________

Selected Types of Cancer by Body System

This table lists common cancers by body system. Adenocarcinomas, such as prostate cancer and breast cancer, are not listed.

Term	Pronunciation	Meaning
Related to the Integumentary System		
basal cell carcinoma (BCC)	bā′săl sel kar′si-nō′mă	a cancer that begins in the lowest layer of the epidermis of the skin (**Figure 16-6**)
Kaposi sarcoma	kap-ŏ′zē sar-kō′mă	cancer of the skin and sometimes lymph codes that causes purplish-red patches on the skin; most commonly seen in patients with acquired immunodeficiency syndrome (AIDS) (**Figure 16-7**)

(continued)

Selected Types of Cancer by Body System *(continued)*

Term	Pronunciation	Meaning
melanoma	mel′ă-nō′mă	a malignant skin cancer that arises from the melanocytes in the epidermis, usually caused by exposure to ultraviolet (UV) radiation

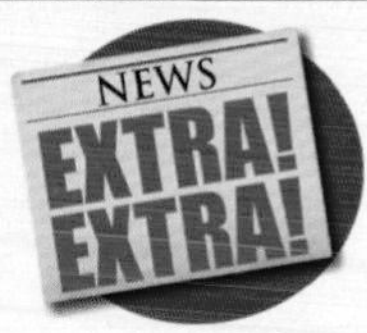

ABCD SIGNS OF MELANOMA UVA and UVB rays are the two types of ultraviolet rays from the sun that cause our skin to age prematurely and make us more susceptible to melanoma. The American Cancer Society encourages people to check their skin at least once a month to look for signs of melanoma. These signs can be remembered with the acronym ABCD:

- A is for *asymmetry.* Look for any areas of skin, pigmentation, or moles that are not the same all around.
- B stands for border. Check to be sure that any suspicious areas do not have a ragged border.
- C is for color. If an area is changing in color or is not the same color throughout, this is a clear sign that the area needs to be checked by a health care professional.
- D is for the diameter. Check for spots that are the size of a pencil eraser or larger.

The American Academy of Dermatology adds a fifth sign, *E,* that stands for *evolving.* A dermatologist should examine an area of skin, a mole, or any pigmentation that changes in any way from one skin check to the next (**Figure 16-8**).

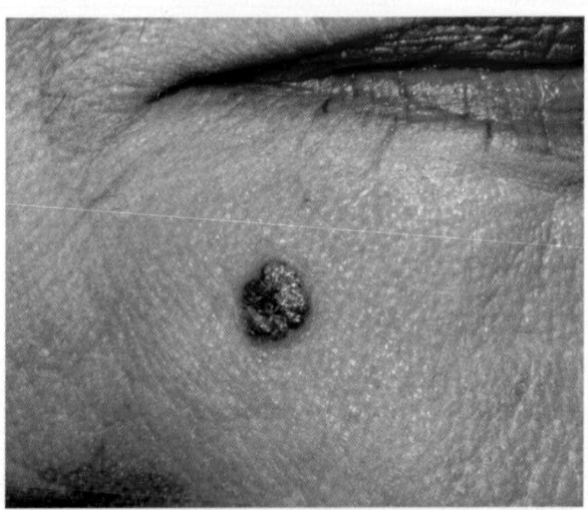

Figure 16-6 Basal cell carcinoma. Note the irregular surface.

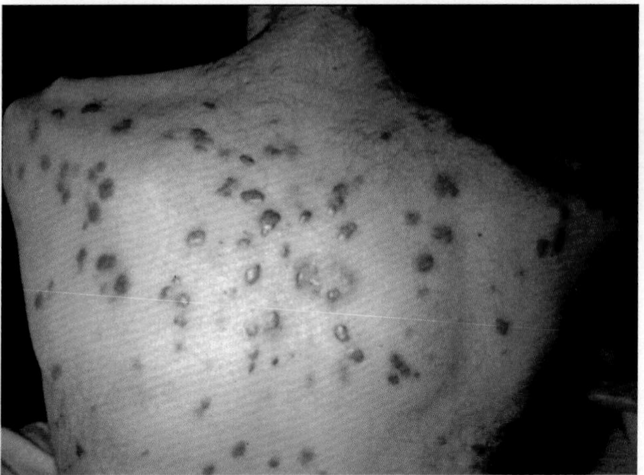

Figure 16-7 Kaposi sarcoma.

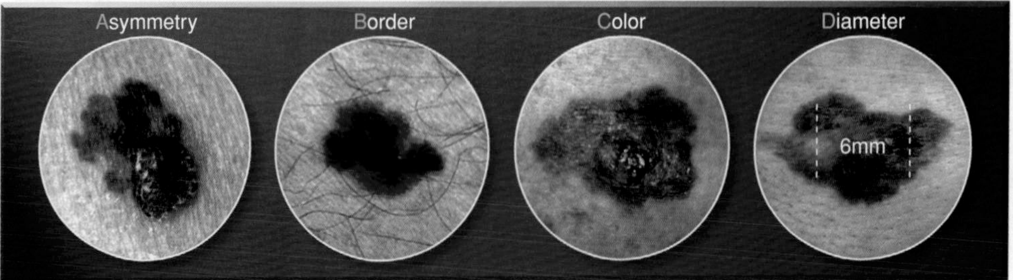

Figure 16-8 The ABCD signs of melanoma.

Selected Types of Cancer by Body System

Term	Pronunciation	Meaning
squamous cell carcinoma (SCC)	skwā′mŭs sel kar′si-nō′mă	a cancer that begins in the squamous cells located in the upper levels of the epidermis of the skin (**Figure 16-9**)
Related to the Musculoskeletal System		
chondroma	kon-drō′mă	a common benign tumor arising from cartilage cells
chondrosarcoma	kon′drō-sar-kō′mă	a large malignant tumor arising from cartilage cells
Ewing tumor; *syn.* Ewing sarcoma	ū′ing tū′mŏr; ū′ing sar-kō′mă	a malignant tumor found in bone or soft tissue
giant cell tumor	jī′ănt sel tū′mŏr	a tumor of the tendon sheath that can be either benign or malignant
leiomyoma	lī′ō-mī-ō′mă	benign tumor of smooth (nonstriated) muscle
leiomyosarcoma	lī′ō-mī′ō-sar-kō′mă	malignant tumor of smooth (nonstriated) muscle
liposarcoma	lip′ō-sar-kō′mă	a malignant tumor of adipose (fat) tissue in deep soft tissue; occurs in the retroperitoneal tissues and the thigh
osteofibroma	os′tē-ō-fī-brō′mă	benign lesion of bone consisting mainly of fairly dense, moderately cellular, fibrous connective tissue
osteosarcoma	os′tē-ō-sar-kō′mă	fast-growing malignant type of bone cancer that develops in the bone-forming cells (osteoblasts); most common and most malignant of bone sarcomas (**Figure 16-10**)
rhabdomyoma	rab′dō-mī-ō′mă	benign tumor of striated (skeletal) muscle
rhabdomyosarcoma	rab′dō-mī′ō-sar-kō′mă	a highly malignant tumor of striated (skeletal) muscle

(continued)

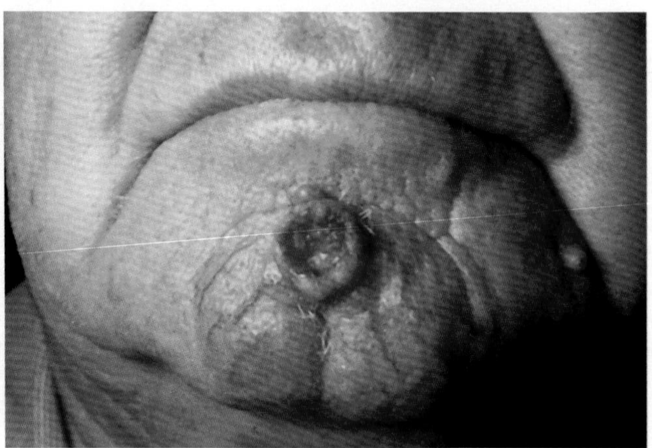

Figure 16-9 Squamous cell carcinoma on the chin.

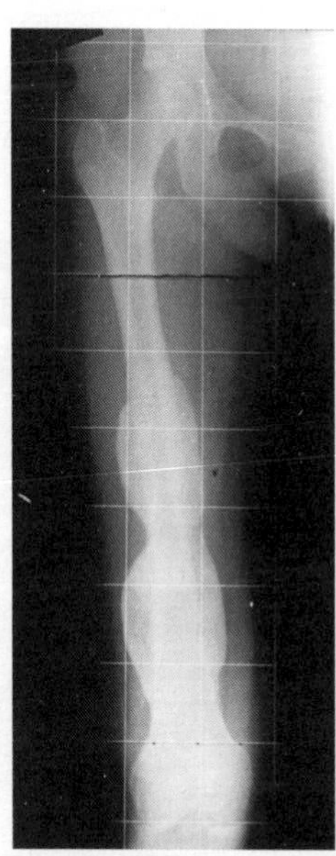

Figure 16-10 X-ray of 29-year-old woman showing femur with osteosarcoma. The multiple expansions demonstrate bone cancer.

Selected Types of Cancer by Body System *(continued)*

Term	Pronunciation	Meaning
Related to the Nervous System		
astrocytoma	as'trō-sī-tō'mă	a tumor that arises from small, star-shaped cells (astrocytes) in the brain and spinal cord
glioma	glī-ō'mă	cancer that arises from the glial cells of the nervous system
medulloblastoma	mĕ-dŭl'ō-blas-tō'mă	cancer that develops from the primitive nerve cells in the medullary tube and is usually located in the cerebellum
meningioma	mĕ-nin'jē-ō'mă	benign and slow-growing tumor of the meninges
neuroblastoma	nūr'ō-blas-tō'mă	malignant tumor of embryonic nerve cells (neuroblasts); neuroblastomas frequently occur in infants and children, and 30% are associated with the adrenal glands
Related to Special Senses		
intraocular melanoma	in'tră-ok'yū-lăr mel'ă-nō'mă	a malignant cancer that forms in the tissues of the eye
retinoblastoma	ret'i-nō-blas-tō'mă	a malignant ocular tumor of the retina that affects young children
Related to the Endocrine System		
multiple endocrine neoplasia (MEN)	mŭl'ti-pĕl en'dō-krin nē-ōplā'zē-ă	a group of disorders characterized by functioning tumors in more than one endocrine gland
pheochromocytoma	fē'ō-krō'mō-sī-tō'mă	a vascular tumor of the adrenal gland (**Figure 16-11**)
pituitary adenoma	pi-tū'i-tar-ē ad'ĕ-nō'mă	a benign tumor arising in the pituitary gland
Related to Blood and the Immune System		
Hodgkin disease	hoj'kin di-zēz'	cancer of the immune system marked by the presence of Reed–Sternberg cells (large, transformed pathogenic cells derived from B lymphocytes) (**Figure 16-12**)
leukemia	lū-kē'mē-ă	cancer of the blood indicated by malignant increase in the number of white blood cells
lymphangioma	lim-fan'jē-ō'mă	mass or tumor of lymphatic vessels

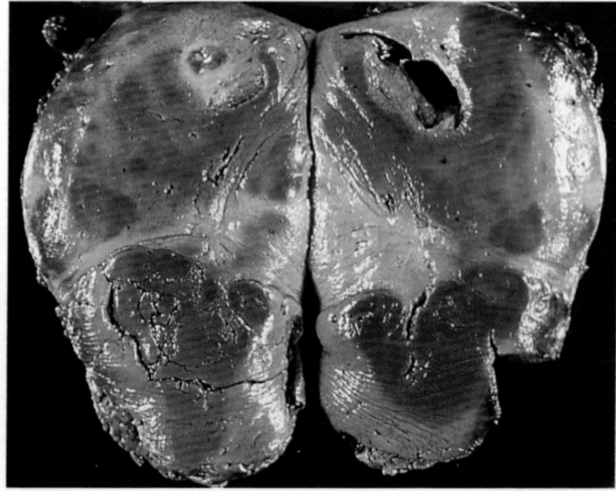

Figure 16-11 Pheochromocytoma. Adrenal gland with dark brown coloration demonstrating the tumor.

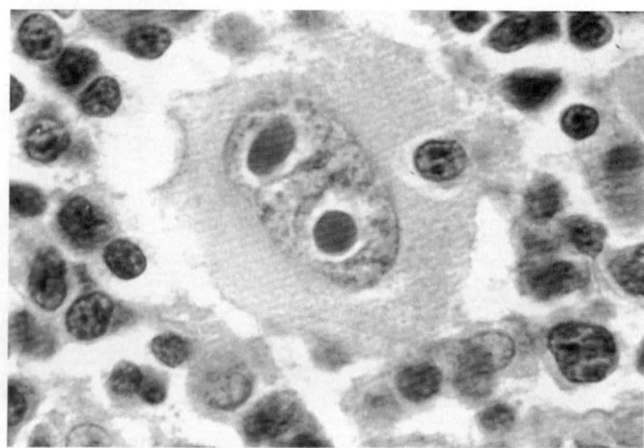

Figure 16-12 Reed–Sternberg cells as seen in Hodgkin disease. A typical Reed–Sternberg cell has two nuclei with large, dark-staining nucleoli.

Selected Types of Cancer by Body System

Term	Pronunciation	Meaning
lymphoma	lim-fō′mă	cancer that begins in immune system cells
non-Hodgkin lymphoma (NHL)	non-hoj′kin lim-fō′mă	any of a large group of cancers of lymphocytes; lymphoma other than Hodgkin disease
Related to the Respiratory System		
bronchogenic carcinoma; *syn.* non-small cell carcinoma	brong′kō-jen′ik kar′si-nō′mă; non smôl sel kar′si-nō′mă	lung cancer; cancer that arises from the lung or bronchial tract

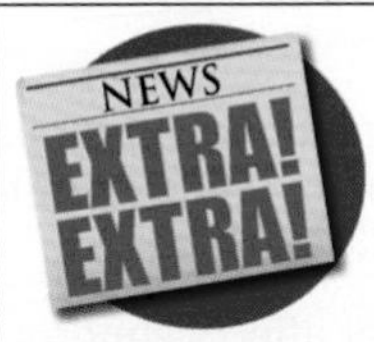

TOBACCO USE AND CANCERS Tobacco use, which is the most preventable cause of cancer, can be linked to at least 15 different types of cancers. These include bronchogenic carcinoma and other cancers of the lung, as well as pancreatic, uterine, mouth, nose, throat, larynx, stomach, kidney, and bladder cancers.

Term	Pronunciation	Meaning
mesothelioma	mez′ō-thē-lē-ō′mă	cancer of the epithelium lining the lungs (pleura) or the epithelium lining the heart (pericardium), usually associated with exposure to asbestos dust
oat cell carcinoma; *syn.* small cell carcinoma	ōt sel kar′si-nō′mă; smôl sel kar′si-nō′mă	highly malignant form of lung or bronchogenic cancer in which cells appear small and rounded under a microscope (**Figure 16-13**)

(continued)

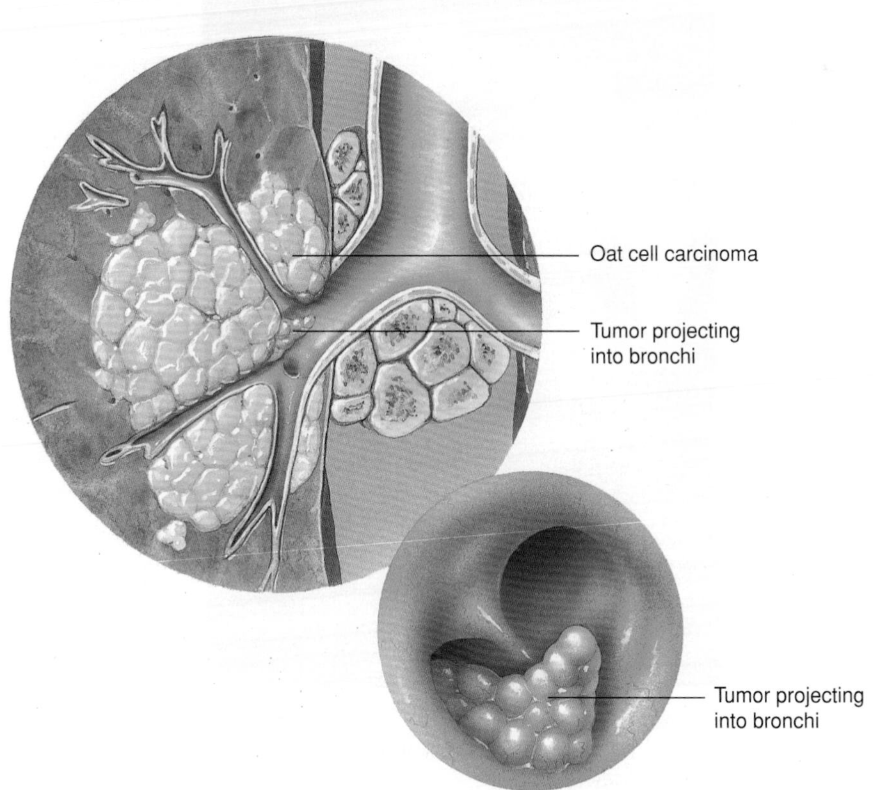

Figure 16-13 Oat cell carcinoma.

Selected Types of Cancer by Body System *(continued)*

Term	Pronunciation	Meaning
Related to the Digestive System		
colon cancer	kō′lon kan′ser	cancer that forms in the tissues of the colon
gastrointestinal stromal tumor (GIST)	gas′trō-in-tes′ti-năl strō′măl tū′mŏr	benign or malignant tumor of the gastrointestinal tract, with most occurring in the stomach
Related to the Urinary System		
bladder cancer	blad′ĕr kan′ser	cancer that forms in the tissues of the urinary bladder
nephroma	ne-frō′mă	tumor of the kidney
urothelial carcinoma; *syn.* transitional cell carcinoma	yūr′ō-thē′lē-ăl kar′si-nō′mă; tran-zish′ŭn-ăl sel kar′sinō′mă	cancer derived from the transitional epithelium, occurring mainly in the urinary bladder, ureters, or renal pelves
Wilms tumor	vilmz tū′mŏr	malignant kidney cancer that affects children (**Figure 16-14**)
Related to the Female Reproductive System		
ductal carcinoma in situ (DCIS); *syn.* intraductal carcinoma	dŭk′tăl kar′si-nō′mă in sī′tū; in′tră-dŭk′tăl kar′si-nō′mă	form of cancer derived from the epithelial lining of ducts in the breast; in most cases, it is confined to the ducts (in situ means "in place") and does not spread into the surrounding breast tissue (**Figure 16-15**)
germ cell tumor (GCT)	jĕrm sel tū′mŏr	cancerous or noncancerous neoplasm derived from the germ cells (sex cells) of the ovaries

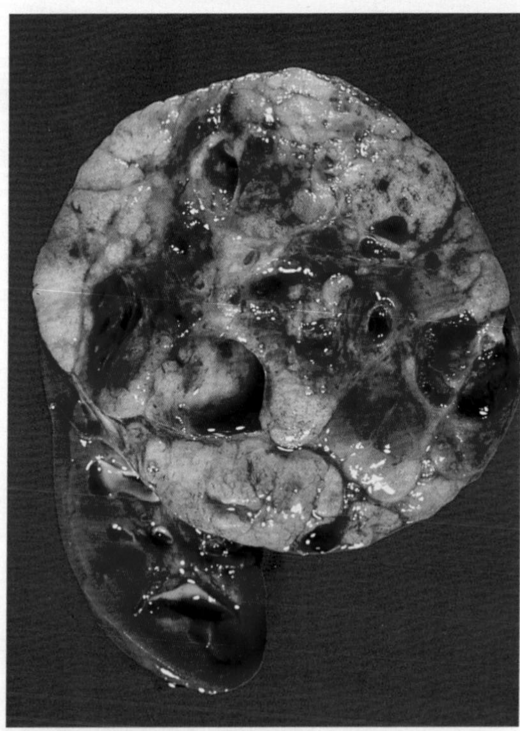

Figure 16-14 Wilms tumor. A cross-section of a whitish, pale tan neoplasm is attached to a portion of the kidney.

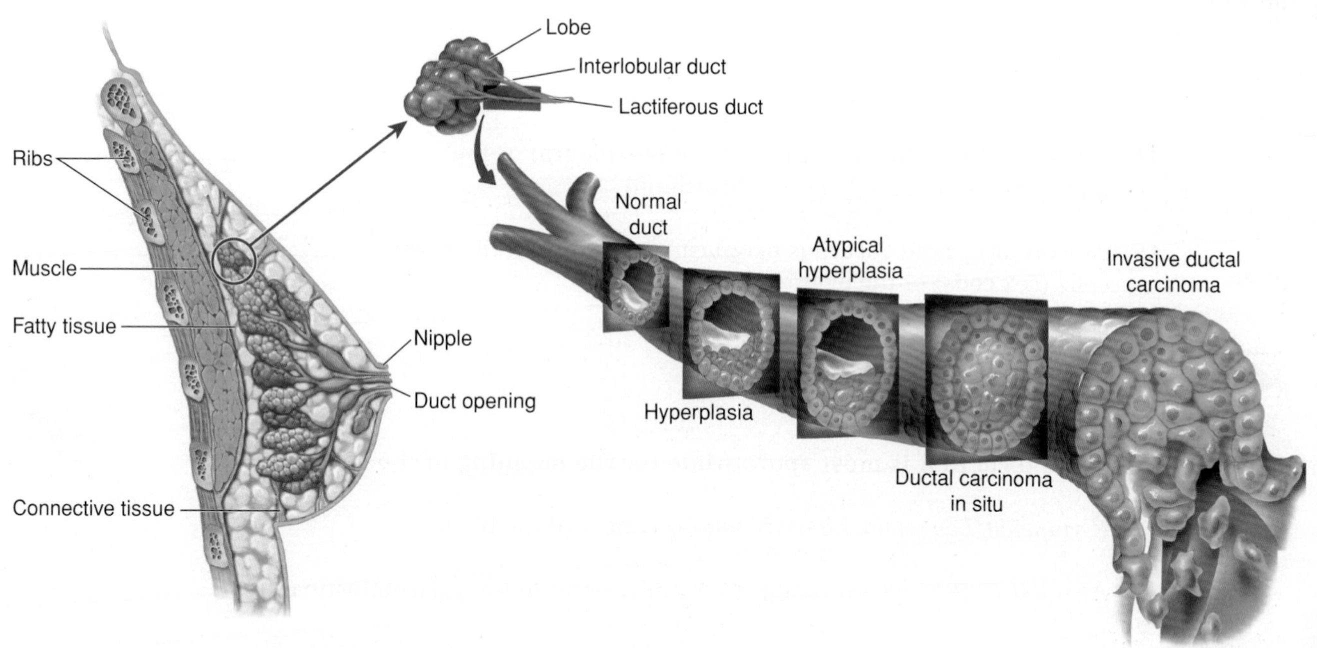

Figure 16-15 Progression to ductal carcinoma in situ and invasive ductal carcinoma of the breast.

Exercises: Selected Types of Cancer by Body System

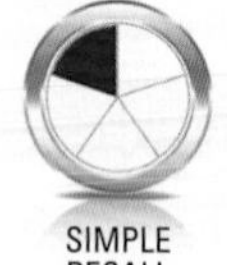
SIMPLE RECALL

Exercise 9

Write the correct medical term for the meaning given.

1. cancer that begins in immune system cells ____________
2. lung cancer; cancer that arises from the lung or bronchial tract ____________
3. benign tumor of smooth (nonstriated) muscle ____________
4. benign tumor of cartilage cells ____________
5. malignant tumor arising from bone-forming cells ____________
6. malignant tumor of fat cells ____________
7. tumor of lymphatic vessels ____________
8. malignant kidney cancer that affects children ____________
9. skin cancer usually caused by UV radiation ____________
10. tumor of the glial cells ____________
11. benign, fibrous tumor of bone ____________

12. tumor of the tendon sheath ________________

13. benign tumor of striated muscle ________________

14. cancer of the epithelium lining the lungs (pleura) or the epithelium lining the heart (pericardium) ________________

15. cancerous or noncancerous neoplasm derived from the germ cells (sex cells) of the ovaries ________________

Exercise 10

SIMPLE RECALL

Circle the term that is most appropriate for the meaning of the sentence.

1. (*Cytopenia, Leukemia, Liposarcoma*) is cancer of the blood.
2. A(n) (*GIST, SCC, DCIS*) tumor is typically found in the gastrointestinal tract.
3. A type of kidney cancer that affects children is known as a(n) (*Ewing, Kaposi, Wilms*) tumor.
4. The presence of Reed–Sternberg cells signifies (*non-Hodgkin, Hodgkin, Ewing*) disease.
5. A vascular tumor of the adrenal gland is known as a(n) (*adrenal adenoma, pheochromocytoma, vascular adenoma*).
6. Ewing sarcoma is a malignant tumor found in (*skin, bone, cartilage*) or soft tissue.
7. A(n) (*osteofibroma, leiomyoma, chondrosarcoma*) is a malignant tumor arising from cartilage cells.
8. A (*giant cell tumor, GIST, sarcoma*) involves the tendon sheaths.
9. A(n) (*adenoma, leiomyosarcoma, retinoblastoma*) could eventually lead to blindness.
10. A (*myoma, squamous cell carcinoma, meningioma*) grows from the meninges.

Exercise 11

ADVANCED RECALL

Match each medical term with its meaning.

neuroblastoma	ductal carcinoma in situ	basal cell carcinoma	Kaposi sarcoma
medulloblastoma	oat cell carcinoma	squamous cell carcinoma	

1. cancer that develops from the primitive nerve cells in the medullary tube and is usually located in the cerebellum ________________
2. cancer confined to the ducts of the breast ________________
3. highly malignant form of lung cancer ________________

4. a cancer in the upper layer of the epidermis ______________

5. a cancer in the lowest (deepest) layer of the epidermis ______________

6. a cancer of the nervous system ______________

7. cancer most commonly seen in patients with AIDS ______________

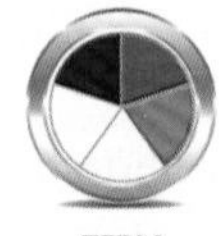

TERM CONSTRUCTION

Exercise 12

Build a medical term for each meaning, using one or more of the listed combining forms and prefixes and one of the listed suffixes. (Note: Combining forms, prefixes, and suffixes may be used more than once.)

Combining Forms and Prefixes		Suffixes
my/o	gli/o	-oma
leio-	sarc/o	-emia
aden/o	astr/o	
cyt/o	carcin/o	
rhabd/o	lymph/o	
nephr/o	leuk/o	

1. tumor of the kidney ______________

2. tumor of lymphatic tissue ______________

3. cancer of the blood ______________

4. tumor of glial cells ______________

5. tumor of a gland ______________

6. benign tumor of smooth (nonstriated) muscle ______________

7. malignant tumor of smooth (nonstriated) muscle ______________

8. tumor arising from star-like cells ______________

9. malignant neoplasm of epithelial tissue ______________

10. malignant tumor of nonsmooth (striated) muscle ______________

Laboratory Tests

Term	Pronunciation	Meaning
alpha fetoprotein (AFP) test	al′fă fē′tō-prō′tēn test	blood test for substance produced by tumor cells in the body; found in elevated levels in patients with ovarian cancer
estrogen receptor test	es′trŏ-jen rĕ-sep′tŏr test	blood test for a type of protein present on some breast cancer cells to which estrogen attaches; if cells have estrogen receptors, they need estrogen to grow, and knowing this determines treatment type

(continued)

Laboratory Tests *(continued)*

Term	Pronunciation	Meaning
human chorionic gonadotropin (hCG) test	hyū'măn kōr'ē-on'ik gō-nad'ō-trō'pin test	blood test for the substance that, in elevated levels, may indicate cancer in the testis, ovary, liver, stomach, pancreas, or lung
Papanicolaou (Pap) test	pa-pă-ni'kō-lō (pap) test	microscopic examination of cells collected from the vagina and cervix to detect abnormal changes (e.g., cancer)
prostate-specific antigen (PSA) test	pros'tāt-spĕ-sif'ik an'ti-jen test	blood test for substance produced only by the prostate; elevated levels may indicate prostate cancer in its early stages
tumor marker test	tū'mŏr mark'ĕr test	various blood tests for specific substances produced by certain types of tumors

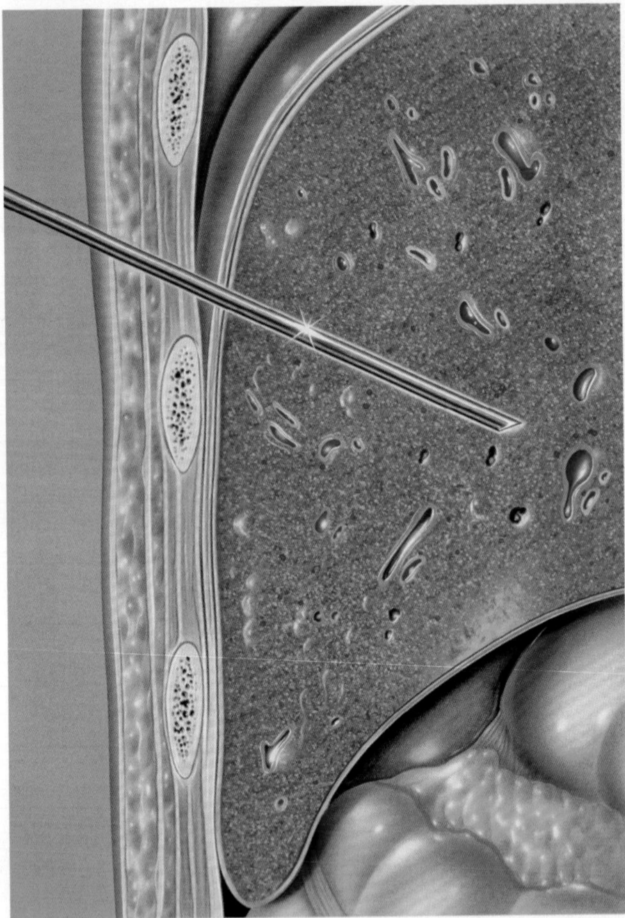

Figure 16-16 Fine-needle aspiration of the liver.

Diagnostic Procedures

Term	Pronunciation	Meaning
General Diagnostic Procedures		
biopsy	bī'op-sē	the process of removing tissue from living patients for diagnostic examination
fine-needle aspiration (FNA)	fīn-nē'dĕl as-pir-ā'shŭn	procedure of withdrawing cells from a lesion for examination with a fine needle on a syringe (**Figure 16-16**)

Diagnostic Procedures

Term	Pronunciation	Meaning
radionuclide scan	rā′dē-ō-nū′klīd skan	imaging scan in which a small amount of radioactive substance is injected into the vein; a machine measures levels of radioactivity in certain organs, which may indicate abnormal areas or tumors
sentinel lymph node biopsy	sen′ti-nĕl limf nōd bī′op-sē	removal and examination of the sentinel nodes, which are the first lymph nodes to which cancer cells are likely to spread from a primary tumor
single photon emission computed tomography (SPECT) scan	sing′gĕl fō′ton ē-mi′shŭn kŏm-pyūt′ĕd tŏ-mog′ră-fē skan	type of nuclear imaging test that shows how blood flows to tissues and organs; can help identify certain types of tumors
Related to the Integumentary System		
punch biopsy	pŭnch bī′op-sē	removal of a small oval core of skin for laboratory analysis using a sharp, hollow instrument (**Figure 16-17**)
shave biopsy	shāv bī′op-sē	removal of a sample of skin for laboratory analysis using a scalpel to slice the specimen from the site
Related to the Musculoskeletal System		
bone scan	bōn skan	technique used to create images of bone by injecting the patient with radioactive dye that is taken up by bone tissue (**Figure 16-18**)
bone marrow aspiration and biopsy	bōn ma′rō as-pir-ā′shŭn and bī′op-sē	procedure in which a small sample of bone marrow and bone is removed for evaluation using a special needle that is pushed into the bone (**Figure 16-19**)
Related to the Nervous System		
stereotactic biopsy	ster′ē-ō-tak′tik bī′op-sē	precise procedure that uses a computer and three-dimensional scanner to find a tumor and remove it
Related to the Blood and Immune System		
bone marrow aspiration	bōn mar′ō as-pirā′shŭn	removal of a small amount of fluid and cells from inside the bone with a needle and syringe

(continued)

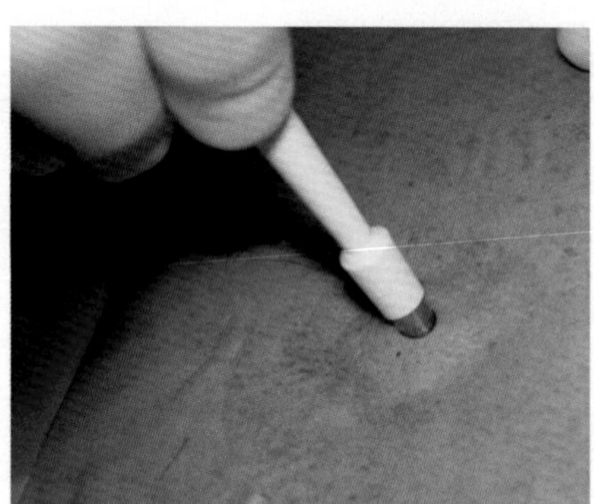

Figure 16-17 Punch biopsy.

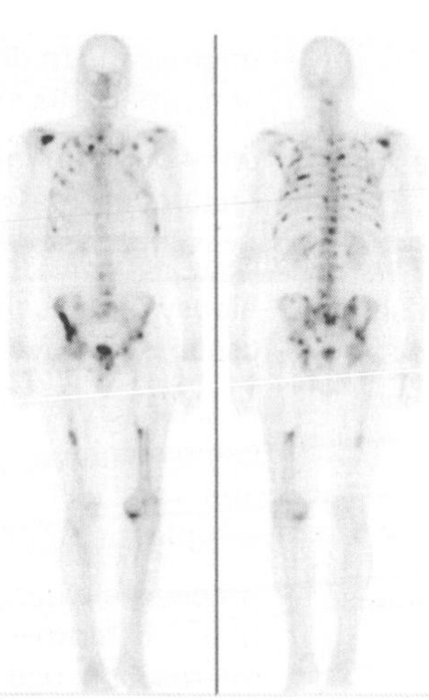

Figure 16-18 Bone scan of a 68-year-old male with lung cancer showing extensive metastases to the bones.

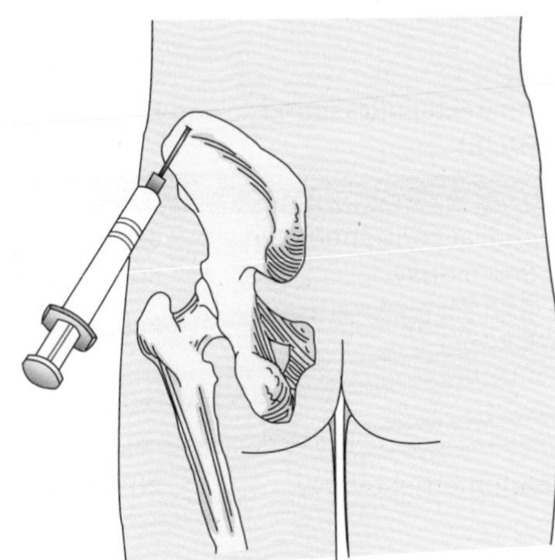

Figure 16-19 Bone marrow aspiration. Posterior view of pelvic region showing a common site for bone marrow aspiration and biopsy.

Diagnostic Procedures *(continued)*

Term	Pronunciation	Meaning
bone marrow biopsy	bōn mar′ō bī′op-sē	removal and evaluation of a small amount of bone along with fluid and cells from inside the bone
lumbar puncture (LP)	lŭm′bar pŭnk′chūr	the process of inserting a needle into the subarachnoid space of the lumbar spine to obtain cerebrospinal fluid for analysis; used to determine if leukemic cells are present
Related to the Lymphatic System		
lymph node biopsy	limf nōd bī′op-sē	removal of lymph node tissue for pathologic evaluation
Related to the Respiratory System		
thoracoscopy; *syn.* pleuroscopy	thōr-ă-kos′kŏ-pē; plūr-os′kŏ-pē	endoscopic examination of the pleural cavity made through a small opening in the chest wall
Related to the Digestive System		
cholescintigraphy; *syn.* hepatobiliary iminodiacetic acid (HIDA) scan	kō′lē-sin-tig′ră-fē; hĕ-pat′ō-bil′ē-ar-ē i′mĕ-nō-dī-ă-sē′tik as′id skan	imaging test used to examine the function of the liver, gallbladder, and bile ducts
endoscopic retrograde cholangiopancreatography (ERCP)	en′dō-skop′ik ret′rōgrād kō-lan′jē-ō-pan′krē-ă-tog′ră-fē	procedure using x-ray and injectable dye to examine disorders in the bile ducts, gallbladder, and pancreas
endoscopic ultrasound (EUS)	en′dō-skop′ik ŭl′tră-sownd	procedure using an ultrasound imaging device on the tip of an endoscope for evaluation of the bowel wall and adjacent structures
magnetic resonance cholangiopancreatography (MRCP)	mag-net′ik rez′ŏ-nănskō-lan′jē-ō-pan′krē-ătog′ră-fē	procedure using magnetic resonance imaging and an injectable dye to examine problems in the bile ducts, gallbladder, and pancreas
Related to the Male Reproductive System		
digital rectal examination (DRE)	dij′i-tăl rek′tăl ek-zam′	examination in which the clinician inserts a lubricated, gloved finger into the rectum to check anatomic structures for abnormalities (see **Figure 14-12**)
prostate biopsy	pros′tāt bī′op-sē	a procedure in which prostate gland tissue samples are removed from the body for examination under a microscope to determine whether cancerous or other abnormal cells are present
transrectal ultrasound (TRUS)	trans-rek′tăl ŭl′trăsownd	ultrasound imaging of the prostate done through the rectum; used to diagnose prostate cancer
Related to the Female Reproductive System		
cervical conization; *syn.* cone biopsy	sĕr′vi-kăl kon′i-zā′shŭn; kōn bī′op-sē	biopsy of the cervix in which a cone-shaped sample of tissue is removed from the cervix
colposcopy	kol-pos′kŏ-pē	visual examination of the tissues of the cervix and vagina using a lighted microscope (colposcope) to identify abnormal cell growth and if necessary, remove a tissue sample for biopsy
endometrial biopsy	en′dō-mē′trē-ăl bīop-sē	procedure whereby a sample of the endometrium of the uterus is removed from the body and examined under a microscope; used to check for uterine cancer
mammography	mă-mog′ră-fē	an x-ray examination of the breasts; used to detect breast tumors (**Figure 16-20**)

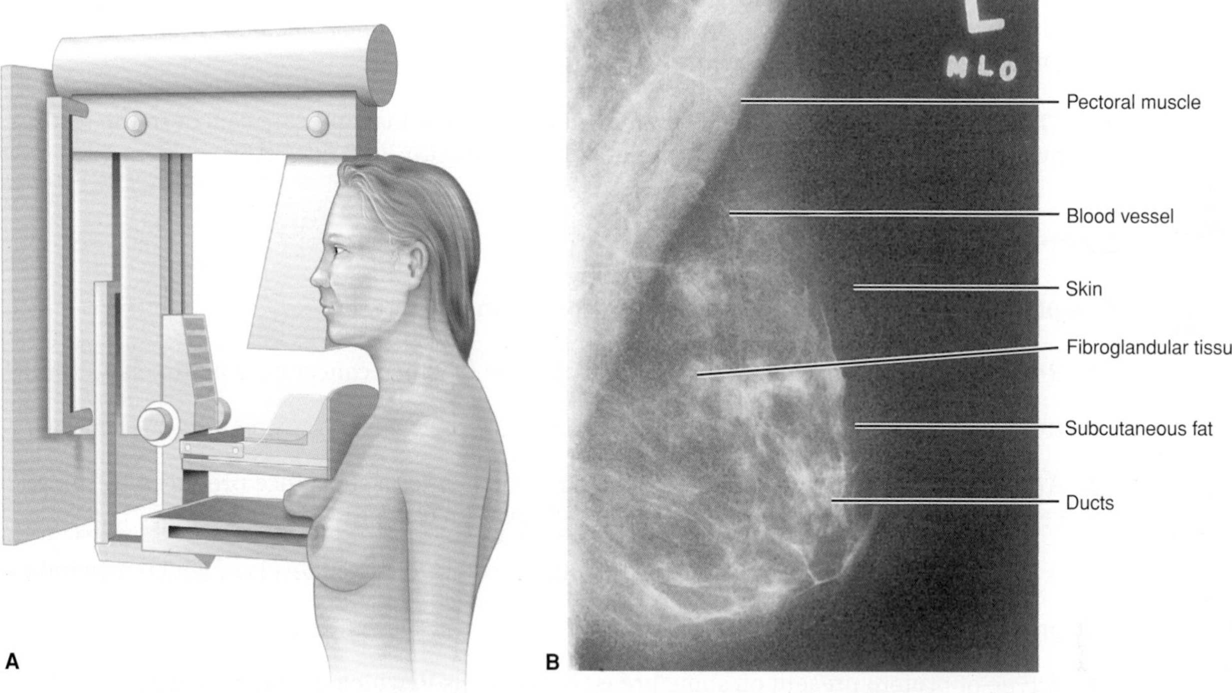

Figure 16-20 Mammography. **A.** Mammography is the radiologic examination of the breast. **B.** Image displayed from a mammogram.

Exercises: Laboratory Tests and Diagnostic Procedures

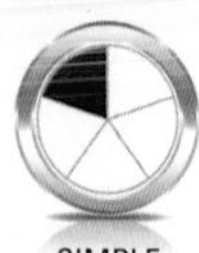

Exercise 13

Circle the term that is most appropriate for the meaning of the sentence.

1. A scan that measures levels of radioactivity in certain organs is called a (*single photon emission computed tomography scan, radionuclide scan, cholescintigraphy*).
2. (*Endoscopic retrograde cholangiopancreatography, Magnetic resonance imaging, Magnetic resonance cholangiopancreatography*) is a procedure using x-ray and injectable dye.
3. A gallbladder function problem may be diagnosed by a(n) (*endometrial biopsy, pleuroscopy, cholescintigraphy*).
4. A (*transrectal ultrasound, lumbar puncture, fine-needle aspiration*) withdraws cells from a lesion for examination with a fine needle on a syringe.
5. To help determine if leukemic cells are present in the cerebrospinal fluid, a patient may undergo a (*lumbar puncture, bronchoscopy, colonoscopy*).
6. An examination of cells obtained from the cervix is called a (*prostate biopsy, prostate-specific antigen, Pap test*).
7. Various blood tests for specific substances produced by certain types of tumors are called (*tumor marker, progesterone receptor, estrogen receptor*) tests.
8. To investigate carcinoma of the lung, a surgeon may make a small opening in the chest wall to perform a (*bone marrow biopsy, hepatobiliary iminodiacetic acid scan, thoracoscopy*).

9. To help identify certain types of tumors, a physician may order a test that shows an image of blood flow to tissues and organs, called a (*mammography, single photon emission computed tomography scan, computed tomography scan*).

10. The blood test for the substance that, in elevated levels, may indicate cancer in the testis, ovary, liver, stomach, pancreas, or lung is abbreviated (*SPECT, hCG, AFP.*)

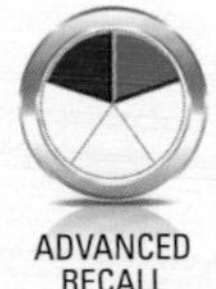

ADVANCED RECALL

Exercise 14

Complete each sentence by writing in the correct medical term.

1. Removal and examination of the first lymph node to which cancer cells are likely to spread from a primary tumor is called a(n) ____________________.
2. A(n) ____________________ is a blood test for a substance produced by tumor cells found in elevated levels in patients with ovarian cancer.
3. A blood test for a substance made only by the prostate, elevated levels of which may indicate prostate cancer in its early stages, is called ____________________.
4. A type of protein present on some breast cancer cells to which estrogen attaches is called ____________________.
5. The removal of a sample of skin for laboratory analysis using a scalpel to slice the specimen from the site is called a(n) ____________________.
6. A(n) ____________________ is the removal of a sample of skin using a hollow instrument.
7. A procedure using an ultrasound imaging device on the tip of an endoscope for evaluation of bowel wall and adjacent structures is known as a(n) ____________________.
8. An x-ray examination of the breasts used to detect tumors is called ____________________.
9. A(n) ____________________ is a diagnostic test that uses ultrasound to visualize the prostate gland.
10. A(n) ____________________ is a visual examination of the tissues of the cervix and vagina using a lighted instrument.

TERM CONSTRUCTION

Exercise 15

Given their meanings, build a medical term from the appropriate combining form and suffix.

Use Combining Form for	Use Suffix for	Term
vagina	process of examining	1. ____________________
cancer	tumor or neoplasm	2. ____________________
thorax, chest	process of examining	3. ____________________
breast	process of recording	4. ____________________

Surgical Interventions

Term	Pronunciation	Meaning
General Surgical Intervention		
brachytherapy; *syn.* seed implantation	brak'ē-thār'ă-pē; sēd im'plan-tā'shŭn	procedure by which radioactive "seeds" are placed inside cancerous tissue and positioned to kill nearby cancer cells
cryosurgery	krī'ō-sŭr'jĕr-ē	the use of freezing temperatures to destroy tissue
debulking surgery	dē-bŭlk'ing sŭr'jĕr-ē	excision of a major part of a tumor that cannot be completely removed
palliative surgery	pal'ē-ă-tiv sŭr'jĕr-ē	surgery that is performed to relieve pain or other symptoms but not to cure the cancer or prolong a patient's life
radiofrequency ablation (RFA)	rā'dē-ō-frē'kwĕn-sē ab-lā'shŭn	procedure in which a surgical oncologist (cancer specialist) uses a small probe to deliver heat from radiofrequency energy to kill cancerous tissue; used primarily to treat liver, prostate, kidney, bone, and breast cancer
reconstructive surgery	rē'kon-strŭk'tiv sŭr'jĕr-ē	surgery performed to return function and appearance to a specific area of the body after removal of a tumor
Related to the Integumentary System		
Mohs surgery	mōz sŭr'jĕr-ē	surgical procedure that involves removing and examining a piece of tumor in the skin bit by bit until the entire lesion is removed
Related to the Musculoskeletal System		
amputation	amp'yū-tā'shŭn	surgical removal of an entire limb
limb salvage surgery	lim salvăj sŭr'jĕr-ē	surgical procedure in which only the cancerous section of bone is removed but nearby muscles, tendons, and other structures are left intact
Related to the Nervous System		
craniectomy	krā'nē-ek'tŏ-mē	excision of part of the cranium to access the brain
stereotactic radiosurgery	ster'ē-ō-tak'tik rā'dē-ō-sŭr'jĕr-ē	radiation therapy technique for treating brain tumors by aiming high-dose radiation beams directly at the tumors
Related to the Special Senses		
enucleation	ē-nū'klē-ā'shŭn	removal of an eyeball
iridectomy	ir'i-dek'tŏ-mē	excision of part of the iris (for very small melanomas)
Related to the Endocrine System		
parathyroidectomy	par'ă-thī-royd-ek'tŏ-mē	excision of all or some of the parathyroid glands
thyroidectomy	thī'roy-dek'tŏ-mē	excision of the thyroid gland
transsphenoidal resection	tranz-sfē-noy'dăl rē-sek'shŭn	excision of a pituitary adenoma by making an incision through the sphenoid bone (the nose to the bottom of the skull) where the pituitary gland is located
Related to the Blood and Immune System		
bone marrow transplant (BMT)	bōn ma'rō trans'plant	transfer of bone marrow from one person to another

(continued)

Surgical Interventions *(continued)*

Term	Pronunciation	Meaning
peripheral stem cell transplant	pĕr-if'ĕr-ăl stem sel trans'plant	the collection and freezing of stem cells from the blood, which are then reintroduced into the patient after chemotherapy
Related to the Lymphatic System		
lymphadenectomy	lim-fad'ĕ-nek'tŏ-mē	excision of a lymph node
Related to the Respiratory System		
laryngectomy	lar'in-jek'tŏ-mē	excision of all or part of the larynx, usually to treat cancer of the larynx
lobectomy	lō-bek'tŏ-mē	excision of a lobe (of the lung)
pneumonectomy	nū'mō-nek'tŏ-mē	excision of the lung
wedge resection	wej rē-sek'shŭn	excision of part of a lobe of the lung (**Figure 16-21**)
Related to the Digestive System		
colectomy	kŏ-lek'tŏ-mē	excision of all or part of the colon
esophagectomy	ĕ-sof-ă-jek'tŏ-mē	excision of the diseased portion of the esophagus and all associated tissues that might contain cancer
gastrectomy; *syn.* Billroth I operation and Billroth II operation	gas-trek'tŏ-mē; bil'rōt op-ĕr-ā'shŭn	excision of part or all of the stomach
pancreaticoduodenectomy; *syn.* Whipple operation	pan'krē-at'ĭ-kō-dū-od'en-ek'tŏ-mē; wip'ĕl op-ĕr-ā'shŭn	excision of all or part of the pancreas together with the duodenum and usually the distal stomach
Related to the Urinary System		
cystectomy	sis-tek'tŏ-mē	surgical removal of part or all of the bladder
fulguration	ful'gŭr-ā'shŭn	destruction of tissue by means of high-frequency electric current; commonly used to remove tumors from inside the bladder

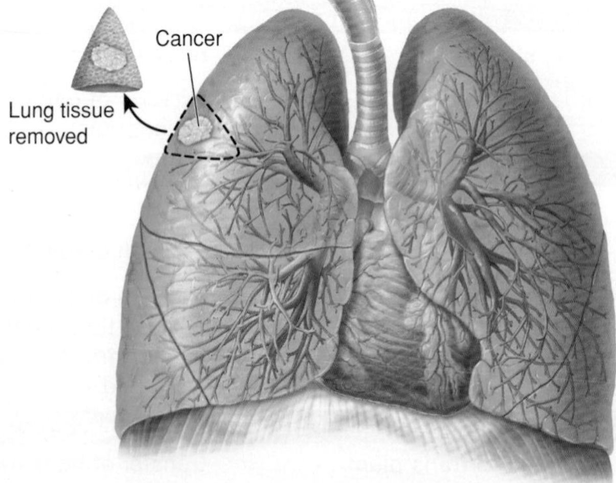

Figure 16-21 Wedge resection of the lung.

Surgical Interventions

Term	Pronunciation	Meaning
nephrectomy	ne-frek'tŏ-mē	excision of a kidney
transurethral resection of bladder tumor (TURB)	trans-yŭr-ē'thrăl rē-sek'shŭn uv blad'ĕr tū'mŏr	excision of a tumor from the bladder through the urethra using a resectoscope
Related to the Male Reproductive System		
prostatectomy; *syn.* transurethral resection of the prostate (TURP)	pros'tă-tek'tŏ-mē; trans-yŭr-ē'thrăl rē-sek'shŭn uv pros'tāt	removal of prostate tissue through the urethra using a resectoscope
Related to the Female Reproductive System		
loop electrosurgical excision procedure (LEEP)	lūp ĕ-lek'trō-sĭr'jik-ăl ek-sizh'ŭn prŏ-sē'jŭr	gynecologic procedure that uses a thin, low-voltage electrified wire loop to cut out cancerous tissue in the cervix
mastectomy	mas-tek'tŏ-mē	excision of a breast done to remove a malignant tumor
modified radical mastectomy	mod'i-fīd rad'i-kăl mas-tek'tŏ-mē	excision of a breast along with some of the underlying muscle and lymph nodes in the adjacent armpit (**Figure 16-22B**)
radical mastectomy	rad'i-kăl mas-tek'tŏ-mē	excision of the breast as well as the underlying muscles and lymph nodes in the adjacent armpit (**Figure 16-22C**)
simple mastectomy	simp'ĕl mas-tek'tŏ-mē	excision of a breast, leaving the underlying muscles and the lymph nodes intact (**Figure 16-22A**)
myomectomy	mī'ō-mek'tŏ-mē	excision of a myoma (benign neoplasm), specifically a uterine myoma

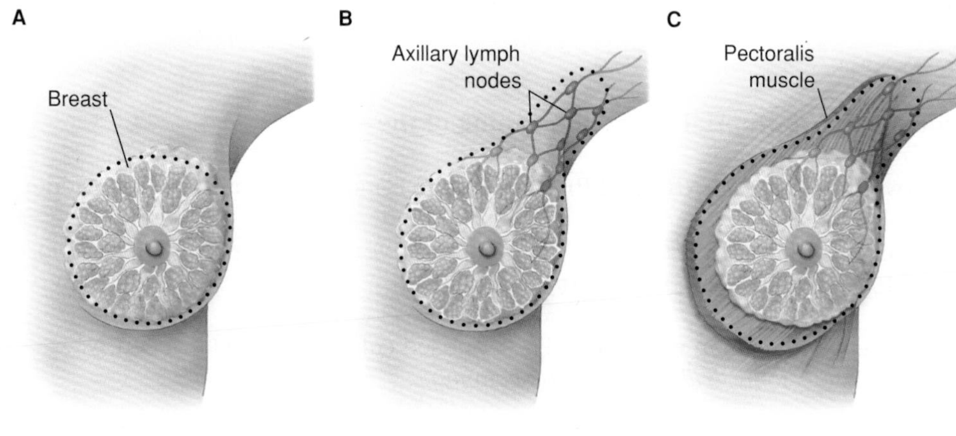

Figure 16-22 Types of mastectomies. **A.** Simple mastectomy. **B.** Modified radical mastectomy. **C.** Radical mastectomy.

Therapeutic Procedures

Term	Pronunciation	Meaning
external beam radiation	eks-tĕr'năl bēm rā'dē-ā'shŭn	procedure by which a beam of high-energy radiation is applied externally directly to the tumor to minimize damage to other tissues
radiation therapy	rā'dē-ā'shŭn thār'ă-pē	the use of high-energy x-rays or other particles to kill cancer cells

Exercises: Surgical Interventions and Therapeutic Procedures

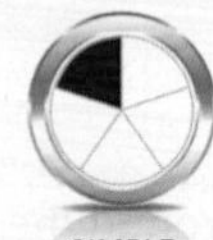
SIMPLE RECALL

Exercise 16

Write the correct medical term for the meaning given.

1. use of heat from radiofrequency energy to kill cancerous tissue ____________
2. use of high-energy x-rays or other particles to kill cancer cells ____________
3. excision of a breast done to remove a malignant tumor ____________
4. transfer of bone marrow from one person to another ____________
5. use of an electrified wire loop to cut out cancerous tissue in the cervix ____________
6. surgical removal of an entire limb ____________
7. destruction of tissue using high-frequency electric current to remove tumors from the bladder ____________
8. process of removing and examining a piece of tumor in the skin bit by bit until the entire lesion is removed ____________
9. excision of a major part of a tumor that cannot be completely removed ____________
10. collection and freezing of stem cells from the blood and then reintroducing them into the patient after chemotherapy ____________

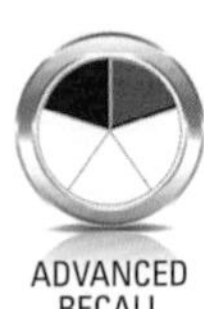
ADVANCED RECALL

Exercise 17

Circle the term that is most appropriate for the meaning of the sentence.

1. The patient underwent a (*TURP, TURBT, LEEP*) procedure to remove a tumor from her bladder.
2. Although her cancer could not be cured, Mrs. Johnson underwent (*reconstructive, debulking, palliative*) surgery to relieve her pain and symptoms.
3. The patient is a 51-year-old woman with recently diagnosed colon cancer who recently underwent a subtotal (*colectomy, iridectomy, myomectomy*).
4. The patient had a (*Billroth, Whipple, Mohs*) operation to stop the spread of cancer to various digestive organs and lymph nodes.
5. Mr. McDowell has had no bone pain since his (*thyroidectomy, limb salvage surgery, craniectomy*) for metastatic cancer of the femur.
6. Mrs. Elias was scheduled for a (*thyroidectomy, parathyroidectomy, transsphenoidal resection*) for removal of a pituitary adenoma.
7. The surgeon performed a (*pneumonectomy, wedge resection, lobectomy*) to remove the small tumor located in the lobe of the patient's lung.

8. Because of the malignant nature of Mrs. Harmon's cancer, the surgeon removed the breast as well as the underlying muscles and lymph nodes in the adjacent armpit; this procedure is known as a (*simple, modified radical, radical*) mastectomy.

9. The patient underwent (*wedge resection, transsphenoidal resection, stereotactic radiosurgery*) to treat his brain tumor.

10. Mr. O'Malley had small pellets of radioactive material applied directly to a cancer lesion during a procedure called (*radiation therapy, reconstructive surgery, brachytherapy*).

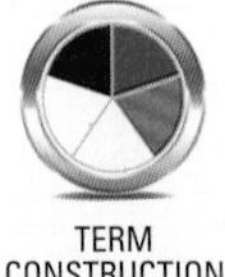
TERM CONSTRUCTION

Exercise 18

Using the given suffix, build a medical term for the meaning given.

Suffix	Meaning of Medical Term	Medical Term
-ectomy	excision of all or part of the esophagus	1. ______
-ectomy	excision of the thyroid gland	2. ______
-ectomy	excision of all or part of the stomach	3. ______
-ectomy	excision of a breast	4. ______
-ectomy	excision of one or both kidneys	5. ______
-ectomy	excision of a lymph node	6. ______
-ectomy	excision of a myoma	7. ______
-ectomy	excision of a lobe (of the lung)	8. ______

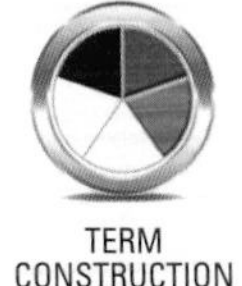
TERM CONSTRUCTION

Exercise 19

Break the given medical term into its word parts, and define each part. Then define the medical term.

For example:

laparotomy	*word parts:*	lapar/o, -tomy
	meanings:	abdomen, incision
	term meaning:	incision into the abdomen
1. pneumonectomy	*word parts:*	______
	meanings:	______
	term meaning:	______
2. colectomy	*word parts:*	______
	meanings:	______
	term meaning:	______

3. cystectomy *word parts:* ______________________

meanings: ______________________

term meaning: ______________________

4. thyroidectomy *word parts:* ______________________

meanings: ______________________

term meaning: ______________________

5. laryngectomy *word parts:* ______________________

meanings: ______________________

term meaning: ______________________

6. iridectomy *word parts:* ______________________

meanings: ______________________

term meaning: ______________________

7. craniectomy *word parts:* ______________________

meanings: ______________________

term meaning: ______________________

8. gastrectomy *word parts:* ______________________

meanings: ______________________

term meaning: ______________________

Medications and Drug Therapies

Term	Pronunciation	Meaning
aromatase inhibitors	ă-rō′mă-tās in-hib′i-tŏrz	group of drugs designed to reduce estrogen levels in a woman's body and stop the growth of cancer cells that depend on estrogen to live and grow
chemoprevention	kē′mō-prē-ven′shŭn	the use of drugs or other agents to inhibit or prevent disease
chemotherapy	kē′mō-thār′ă-pē	regimen of therapy that uses chemicals to treat cancer (**Figure 16-23**)
adjuvant chemotherapy	ad′jū-vănt kē′mō-thār′ă-pē	chemotherapy given in addition to surgery to destroy remaining residual tumor or to reduce the risk of recurrence

Medications and Drug Therapies

Term	Pronunciation	Meaning
interstitial chemotherapy	in′tĕr-stish′ăl kē′mō-thār′ă-pē	placement of chemotherapy drugs directly into a tumor
intrathecal chemotherapy	in′tră-thē′kăl kē′mō-thār′ă-pē	delivery of chemotherapy drugs into the subarachnoid space by lumbar puncture
palliative chemotherapy	pal′ē-ă-tiv kē′mō-thār′ă-pē	chemotherapy that is given to relieve pain or other symptoms of cancer but not to cure it
epidermal growth factor receptor (EGFR) inhibitor therapy	ep′i-dĕr′măl grōth fak′tŏr rĕ-sep′tŏr in-hib′i-tŏr thār′ă-pē	drugs that interfere with the growth of individual cancer cells
hormonal therapy	hōr-mōn′ăl thār′ă-pē	use of hormones to stop a tumor from growing, to relieve symptoms caused by a tumor, or to replace the hormone that is needed by the body to function properly after a body part is removed due to cancer
immunotherapy; *syn.* biologic therapy	im′yū-nō-thār′ă-pē; bī′ŏ-loj′ik thār′ă-pē	method of boosting the body's natural defenses to fight cancer by using materials made either by the body or in a laboratory to bolster, target, or restore immune system function

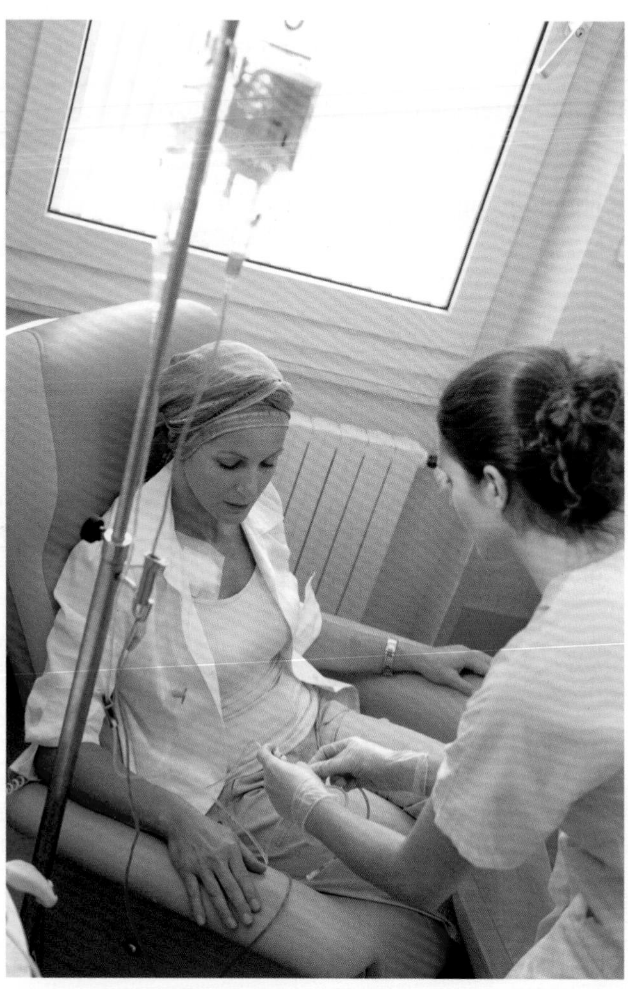

Figure 16-23 Patient with cancer undergoing chemotherapy.

Exercise: Medications and Drug Therapies

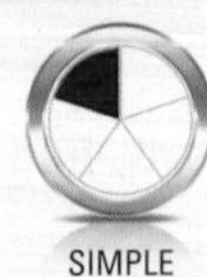
SIMPLE RECALL

Exercise 20

Write the correct medication or drug therapy term for the meaning given.

1. chemotherapy given in addition to surgery ____________
2. use of hormones to stop a tumor from growing or relieve symptoms caused by a tumor ____________
3. delivery of chemotherapy drugs into the subarachnoid space by lumbar puncture ____________
4. group of drugs designed to reduce estrogen levels in a woman's body and stop the growth of cancer cells ____________
5. method of boosting the body's natural defenses to fight cancer ____________
6. chemotherapy given to relieve pain only ____________
7. regimen of therapy that uses chemicals to kill cancer cells ____________
8. the use of drugs or other agents to inhibit or prevent disease ____________
9. use of drugs that interfere with the growth of individual cancer cells ____________
10. placement of chemotherapy drugs directly into a tumor ____________

Specialties and Specialists

Term	Pronunciation	Meaning
gynecologic oncology	gī′nĕ-kŏ-loj′ik ong-kol′ŏ-jē	medical specialty concerned with the diagnosis and treatment of cancers of the female reproductive system
gynecologic oncologist	gī′nĕ-kŏ-loj′ik ong-kol′ŏ-jist	physician who specializes in the care and treatment of women with gynecologic cancers
medical oncology	med′i-kăl ong-kol′ŏ-jē	medical specialty concerned with the use of medical and chemotherapeutic treatments of cancer
medical oncologist	med′i-kăl ong-kol′ŏ-jist	physician who specializes in treating cancer with chemotherapy
oncology	ong-kol′ŏ-jē	medical specialty concerned with the physical, chemical, and biologic properties and features of cancers
oncologist	ong-kol′ŏ-jist	physician who specializes in the science of oncology

Specialties and Specialists

Term	Pronunciation	Meaning
pediatric oncology	pē-dē-at′rik ong-kol′ŏ-jē	medical specialty concerned with the diagnosis and treatment of childhood cancers and blood diseases
pediatric oncologist	pē-dē-at′rik ong-kol′ŏ-jist	physician who specializes in the treatment of childhood cancers and blood diseases
radiation oncology	rā′dē-ā′shŭn ong-kol′ŏ-jē	radiologic specialty concerned with radiation treatment as the main mode of treatment for cancer
radiation oncologist; *syn.* radiotherapist	rā′dē-ā′shŭn ong-kol′ŏ-jist; rā′dē-ō-ther′ă-pist	physician who specializes in treating cancer with high-energy x-rays to destroy cancerous cells
surgical oncology	sŭr′ji-kăl ong-kol′ŏ-jē	surgical specialty concerned with the surgical aspects of cancer
surgical oncologist	sŭr′ji-kăl ong-kol′ŏ-jist	physician who specializes in the surgical aspects of cancer, including biopsy and tumor staging and resection

■ Exercise: Specialties and Specialists

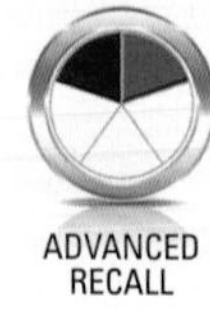
ADVANCED RECALL

Exercise 21

Match each type of medical specialty or specialist with its description.

medical oncology	surgical oncology	radiation oncology
pediatric oncology	gynecologic oncology	surgical oncologist
radiation oncologist	medical oncologist	pediatric oncologist
gynecologic oncologist		

1. medical specialty concerned with the diagnosis and treatment of cancers of the female reproductive system __________
2. radiologic specialty concerned with radiation treatment as the main mode of treatment for cancer __________
3. surgical specialty concerned with the surgical management of malignant tumors __________
4. medical specialty concerned with the diagnosis and treatment of childhood cancers and blood diseases __________
5. physician who specializes in the care and treatment of women with gynecologic cancers __________
6. physician who specializes in treating cancer with chemotherapy __________
7. medical specialty concerned with the use of medical and chemotherapeutic treatments of cancer __________

8. physician who specializes in the treatment of childhood cancers and blood diseases ____________

9. physician who specializes in treating cancer with high-energy x-rays to destroy cancer cells ____________

10. physician who specializes in the surgical aspects of cancer, including biopsy and tumor staging and resection ____________

Abbreviations

Abbreviation	Meaning
AFP	alpha fetoprotein
BCC	basal cell carcinoma
BMT	bone marrow transplant
CA	cancer, carcinoma
DCIS	ductal carcinoma in situ
DRE	digital rectal examination
EGFR	epidermal growth factor receptor
ERCP	endoscopic retrograde cholangiopancreatography
EUS	endoscopic ultrasound
FNA	fine-needle aspiration
GCT	germ cell tumor
GIST	gastrointestinal stromal tumor
hCG	human chorionic gonadotropin
HIDA	hepatobiliary iminodiacetic acid
LEEP	loop electrosurgical excision procedure
LP	lumbar puncture
MEN	multiple endocrine neoplasia
MRCP	magnetic resonance cholangiopancreatography
NHL	non-Hodgkin lymphoma
PSA	prostate-specific antigen
RFA	radiofrequency ablation
SCC	squamous cell carcinoma
SPECT	single photon emission computed tomography
TNM staging	tumor node metastasis
TRUS	transrectal ultrasound
TURB	transurethral resection of bladder tumor
TURP	transurethral resection of prostate
UV	ultraviolet

Exercises: Abbreviations

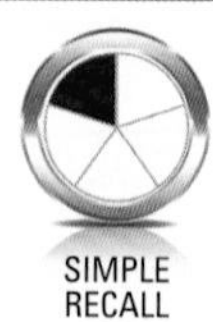
SIMPLE RECALL

Exercise 22

Write the meaning of each abbreviation used in these sentences.

1. A **GIST** is one of the most common tumors found in the gastrointestinal tract.

   ____

2. One form of breast cancer is called **DCIS.**

   ____

3. A patient who has prostate cancer may undergo treatment with a **TURP.**

   ____

4. A **HIDA** scan is a type of imaging study called a nuclear medicine scan that tracks the flow of bile from the liver.

   ____

5. A **BMT** is used to treat patients whose bone marrow has been destroyed by chemotherapy.

   ____

6. In an **RFA** procedure, the physician applies heat from radiofrequency energy directly onto the tumor to kill cancerous tissue.

   ____

7. A **TRUS** is ultrasound imaging of the prostate done through the rectum.

   ____

8. **EGFR**s are drugs that interfere with the growth of individual cancer cells.

   ____

9. A procedure using MRI and injectable dye to examine problems in the bile ducts, gallbladder, and pancreas is called **MRCP.**

   ____

10. An **EUS** is a procedure using an ultrasound imaging device on the tip of an endoscope for evaluation of the bowel wall and adjacent structures.

    ____

11. **SPECT** is a type of nuclear imaging test that shows how blood flows to tissues and organs.

    ____

12. The substance produced by tumor cells in the body found in elevated levels in patients with ovarian cancer is **AFP.**

    ____

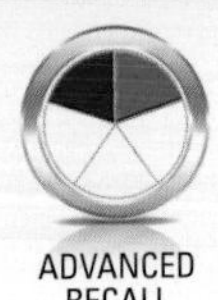

Exercise 23

Match each abbreviation with the appropriate description.

CA	TURB	FNA	BCC
PSA	LP	LEEP	MEN
ERCP	SCC	NHL	hCG

1. procedure to remove cerebrospinal fluid from the spinal cord ____________
2. procedure that uses a needle to aspirate material for examination ____________
3. general term for a group of diseases characterized by an abnormal uncontrolled growth of cells ____________
4. surgical treatment for bladder cancer ____________
5. procedure using x-ray and injectable dye to examine disorders in the bile ducts, gallbladder, and pancreas ____________
6. use of a low-voltage wire loop to remove cancerous tissue ____________
7. blood test for prostate cancer ____________
8. the most common form of skin cancer ____________
9. elevated levels may indicate cancer in the testis, ovary, liver, stomach, pancreas, or lung ____________
10. a group of disorders characterized by functioning tumors in more than one endocrine gland ____________
11. lymphoma other than Hodgkin disease ____________
12. a cancer that begins in the squamous cells ____________

WRAPPING UP

- Oncology is the study of cancer.
- Cancer can affect any of the body's organ system.
- In this chapter, you learned medical terminology including word parts, prefixes, suffixes, adjectives, conditions, tests, procedures, medications, specialties, and abbreviations related to oncology.

Chapter Review

Understanding Term Structure

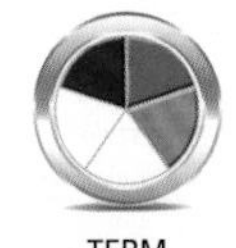
TERM CONSTRUCTION

Exercise 24

Break the given medical term into its word parts, and define each part. Then define the medical term. (Note: You may need to use word parts from other chapters.)

For example:

laparotomy	*word parts:*	lapar/o, -tomy
	meanings:	abdomen, incision
	term meaning:	incision into the abdomen

1. rhabdomyosarcoma *word parts:* ____________________

meanings: ____________________

term meaning: ____________________

2. myoma *word parts:* ____________________

meanings: ____________________

term meaning: ____________________

3. nephroma *word parts:* ____________________

meanings: ____________________

term meaning: ____________________

4. bronchoscopy *word parts:* ____________________

meanings: ____________________

term meaning: ____________________

5. meningioma *word parts:* ____________________

meanings: ____________________

term meaning: ____________________

6. endoscopy *word parts:* ____________________

meanings: ____________________

term meaning: ____________________

7. osteosarcoma *word parts:* ______________________________

meanings: ______________________________

term meaning: ______________________________

8. neuroma *word parts:* ______________________________

meanings: ______________________________

term meaning: ______________________________

9. iridectomy *word parts:* ______________________________

meanings: ______________________________

term meaning: ______________________________

10. laparoscopy *word parts:* ______________________________

meanings: ______________________________

term meaning: ______________________________

Comprehension Exercises

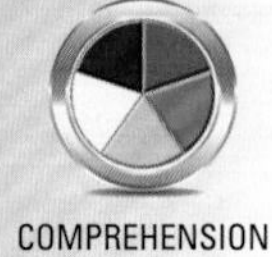

COMPREHENSION

Exercise 25

Fill in the blank with the correct term.

1. The common sites for gastrointestinal tract cancer are the colon and rectum; together, these are referred to as ______________________________ cancer.
2. A technique used to destroy cancer cells using extreme cold is ______________________________.
3. During a(n) ______________________________, a physician is able to view both the urethra and the bladder using a lighted scope.
4. When a tumor is nonmalignant, it is said to be ______________________________.
5. Too much exposure to the sun can result in a(n) ______________________________, the most dangerous type of skin cancer.
6. A(n) ______________________________ is another name for a pancreaticoduodenectomy.
7. To remove a tumor in the bladder, a surgeon may perform at the tumor site ______________________________, which is the use of high-frequency electric current to destroy tissue.
8. A(n) ______________________________ involves use of a scalpel to remove skin for examination.

9. A radiologist analyzes the images in a(n) ______________________________ for signs of early breast cancer.

10. A(n) ______________________________ is a fast-growing malignant tumor of the bone-forming cells (osteoblasts) of the body.

Exercise 26

COMPREHENSION

Write a short answer for each question.

1. What is the difference between a simple mastectomy and radical mastectomy?

____

2. What is the difference between Hodgkin lymphoma and non-Hodgkin lymphoma?

____

3. What is the name of the procedure used to surgically reduce the size of a tumor that cannot be completely removed by removing as much of it as possible? ______________________________

____

4. What is the purpose of palliative surgery? ______________________________

____

5. Which type of brain cancer starts from small, star-shaped cells? ______________________________

____

6. What is the difference between a chondroma and a chondrosarcoma? ______________________________

____

7. What is the function of oncogenes? ______________________________

____

8. How is external beam radiation delivered to treat a tumor? ______________________________

____

9. How do aromatase inhibitors stop the growth of cancer cells? ______________________________

____

10. Are sarcomas benign or malignant? ______________________________

____

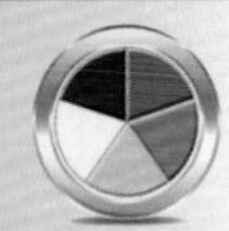

Exercise 27

COMPREHENSION **Circle the letter of the best answer to the following questions.**

1. Which of the following is mismatched?

A. bladder cancer—cystectomy
B. lymphoma—lymphadenectomy
C. melanoma—mastectomy
D. pancreatic cancer—Whipple operation

2. Benign is another word for

A. harmful.
B. nonmalignant.
C. invasive.
D. brightly colored.

3. What is another name for the Billroth operations I and II?

A. colectomy
B. Mohs surgery
C. endoscopy
D. gastrectomy

4. A retinoblastoma is a cancerous tumor involving the

A. cornea.
B. iris.
C. retina.
D. sclera.

5. A procedure used to remove the prostate as a cancer treatment is called

A. LEEP.
B. TURB.
C. TURP.
D. EGFR.

6. A tumor of the kidney is referred to as a

A. nephroma.
B. melanoma.
C. myoma.
D. leukemia.

7. A Wilms tumor is a type of cancer that affects

A. the elderly
B. children
C. fetuses
D. young men

8. Which type of surgery returns the function and appearance of an area of the body after a tumor has been removed?

A. palliative surgery
B. reconstructive surgery
C. debulking surgery
D. cryosurgery

9. Chemotherapy given in addition to surgery is called

A. adjuvant.
B. chemoprevention.
C. interstitial.
D. intrathecal.

10. The specialist who treats cancers only in women is called a(n)

A. pediatric oncologist.
B. oncologist.
C. gynecologic oncologist.
D. radiation oncologist.

Application and Analysis

CASE STUDIES

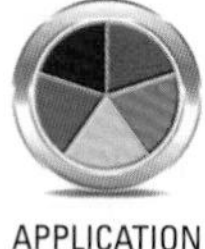

Exercise 28

APPLICATION

Read the case studies, and circle the correct letter for each of the questions.

CASE 16-1

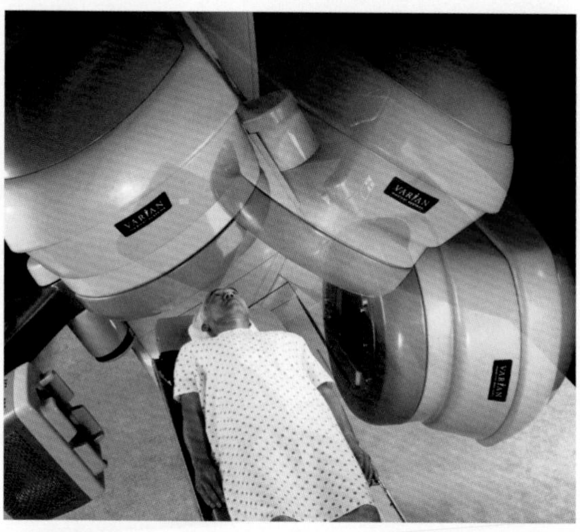

Figure 16-24 Patient undergoing radiation therapy.

Ms. Kumar has come in for her regularly scheduled clinic visit. She was previously diagnosed with metastatic left breast cancer and underwent a left mastectomy. She then received a five-year course of aromatase inhibitor therapy. She had recurrence of the cancer along with a suspicious left intramammary lymph node and the presence of multiple bony metastases. She recently underwent a course of palliative radiation therapy (**Figure 16-24**) for bony metastasis. She will be rescheduled for follow-up. In addition, a PET scan has been ordered for the patient, which will be completed next week.

1. What kind of imaging study is the patient about to undergo?

A. aromatase inhibitor therapy
B. PET
C. palliative radiation therapy
D. none of the above

2. What treatment did the patient receive for her bony metastases?

A. therapy that uses chemicals to treat cancer
B. placement of chemotherapy drugs directly into a tumor
C. the use of high-energy x-rays or other particles to kill cancer
D. drugs designed to reduce estrogen levels in a woman's body

3. How long did the patient take aromatase inhibitors?

A. five years
B. two years
C. one week
D. one year

4. What kind of radiation therapy did the patient receive?

A. reconstructive
B. systemic
C. adjuvant
D. palliative

5. What surgical treatment did the patient receive for her breast cancer?

A. lumpectomy
B. colectomy
C. mastectomy
D. adenectomy

CASE 16-2

Mr. Able came into the clinic for a regularly scheduled follow-up visit for squamous cell cancer of the base of the tongue. He is five years postop with no recurrence found. He speaks covering his tracheostomy and is easily understood. His tracheostomy site was found to be clean, dry, and intact. His neck was edematous and firm. The temporomandibular joint (TMJ) was tender to palpation. His oropharynx was not examined due to patient's inability to open his mouth. His abdomen has a left J feeding tube. He seems to be doing very well. An x-ray of his jaw was ordered to evaluate his TMJ symptoms.

6. Where is the TMJ located?

A. in the chest
B. in the face
C. in the neck
D. in the abdomen

7. How long has the patient been cancer-free?

A. two years
B. four years
C. five years
D. patient is not cancer-free

8. A tracheostomy is defined as a(n)

A. excision of part of the trachea.
B. creation of an artificial opening in the trachea.
C. incision into the trachea.
D. excision of the entire trachea.

9. The return of cancer is called

A. recurrence.
B. remission.
C. metastasis.
D. postoperative.

10. What does the term *edematous* mean?

A. hydrated
B. stiff
C. red
D. swollen

MEDICAL RECORD ANALYSIS

MEDICAL RECORD 16-1

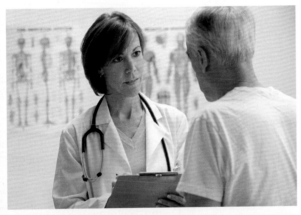

A physician's assistant works closely with the physician and can perform various medical tasks.

You are a physician's assistant working in a surgical oncology clinic. Mr. Lowe is a patient who is being seen for a carcinoma of the nose with subsequent evaluation of that lesion. You are reviewing the record of his visit to assist in his postoperative care.

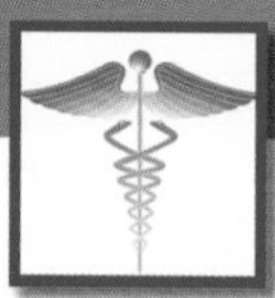

Medical Record

CLINIC NOTE

SUBJECTIVE: The patient is a 50-year-old male with a 10-year history of a nasal lesion. He initially described it as being a possible infection of his hair follicle that progressed. The patient never did seek medical attention for this and over the course of these years he has noticed that his nose has slowly started to disappear. He has recently been using a self-made nasal prosthesis made out of silicone. The patient does have a history of sun exposure as a child but no significant occupational exposure. He also has no history of smoking. He was seen by an outside physician and had a biopsy of his lesion performed, which was consistent with basal cell carcinoma.

OBJECTIVE: Temperature 99.6, pulse 96, respirations 16. He is alert and oriented, in no apparent distress. What remains of the nose shows only some septal cartilage and nasal bones with skin covering; otherwise he has no ala of nose and no lower or upper lateral cartilages. He does have an ulcerative lesion along the nasolabial fold on the left side. There is surrounding skin and mucosal ulceration and some friable tissue that bleeds with any extensive manipulation.

Anterior rhinoscopy demonstrates no obvious masses.

ASSESSMENT: Basal cell carcinoma of the nose.

PLAN: At this time, the patient is a candidate for a total rhinectomy as well as possible skin graft, possible lip resection, possible primary lip repair, possible nasolabial flap. We would like to have the patient admitted to the hospital postoperatively. The patient was informed about the risks and benefits of the procedure, which include but are not limited to bleeding, infection, pain, nasal obturator stenosis, cosmetic defect, recurrence, need for additional surgery, psychosocial impact, lip and oral incompetence, and numbness. Informed consent was obtained today.

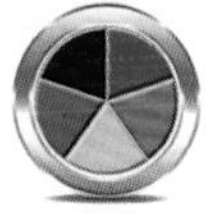

APPLICATION

Exercise 29

Write the appropriate medical terms used in this medical record on the blanks after their meanings. Note that not all the terms appear in the chapter, but you should be able to identify these terms based on word parts that are included in this chapter.

1. narrowing of a canal or orifice ____________________
2. the formation of an ulcer ____________________
3. process of examining the nose ____________________
4. malignant cancer of epithelial tissue ____________________
5. surgical removal of the nose ____________________

MEDICAL RECORD 16-2

Ms. Collins was admitted to the hospital last week for definitive surgical treatment of her left breast cancer. You, as an oncology nurse, are reviewing her record in anticipation of talking to the patient about future chemotherapy.

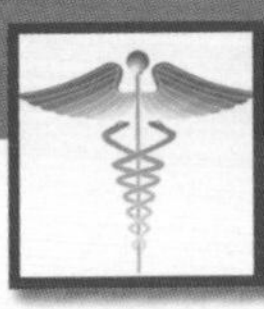

Medical Record

OPERATIVE REPORT

PREOPERATIVE DIAGNOSIS: Recurrent infiltrative poorly differentiated ductal carcinoma of the breast.

POSTOPERATIVE DIAGNOSIS: Recurrent infiltrative poorly differentiated ductal carcinoma of the breast.

OPERATION: Left simple mastectomy.

INDICATIONS FOR PROCEDURE: The patient is a 46-year-old female with history of left breast carcinoma diagnosed at an outside hospital. She then underwent excisional biopsy with chemotherapy and radiation therapy. The patient was referred for evaluation of continuously enlarging left breast mass; biopsy performed revealed recurrent infiltrative poorly differentiated ductal carcinoma with features of metastatic carcinoma. It was recommended that the patient undergo a left simple mastectomy. The patient agreed to the procedure and signed the consent form.

DESCRIPTION OF PROCEDURE: The patient was taken to the operating room and placed in supine position on the operating table. The left breast and arm were prepped and draped in the standard sterile surgical fashion. An elliptic incision was made to encompass the entire left breast. This incision extended from the sternum in the direction to the axilla up to the lateral margin of the left breast. The knife was used to cut down the dermis and then Bovie electrocautery was used to take this incision down to the breast tissue. Meticulous hemostasis was achieved throughout. Flaps were raised medially to the sternum, laterally to the pectoralis major lateral border, inferiorly to the mammary crease, and superior to the clavicle. The dissection was carried down to the level of the pectoralis fascia. At that time, the pectoralis minor was dissected from the overlying breast tissue, and this proceeded in a medial to lateral dissection. The dissection continued laterally, freeing up the edge of the pectoralis minor muscle.

After meticulous hemostasis was achieved, a #10 J-P drain was placed. The skin was closed in two layers, one with interrupted 4-0 Maxon sutures for the dermis, and the second with 4-0 Vicryl in a subcuticular fashion. Dry dressings were applied. The patient was revived from anesthesia, extubated, and transferred to the recovery room in stable condition.

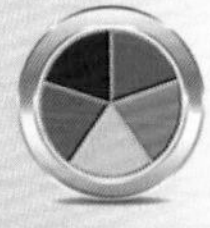

APPLICATION

Exercise 30

Read the medical report, and circle the correct letter for each of the questions.

1. What type of biopsy did the patient undergo during an earlier procedure?

   A. incisional
   B. excisional
   C. fine-needle aspiration
   D. punch biopsy

2. What was used to access the breast tissue during the operation?

   A. J-P drains
   B. Bovie electrocautery
   C. Flaps
   D. A knife

3. What type of mastectomy did the patient undergo?

   A. radical
   B. simple
   C. suprapubic
   D. modified radical

4. What kind of carcinoma was found in the patient's left breast?

   A. benign
   B. simple
   C. ductal
   D. lymph-dependent

5. What type of sutures was used to close the uppermost layer of skin?
   A. Maxon
   B. catgut
   C. Vicryl
   D. both Maxon and Vicryl

6. What type of surgery might the patient have in the future to improve the appearance of her chest?
   A. debulking surgery
   B. reconstructive surgery
   C. chemotherapy
   D. brachysurgery

Bonus Question

7. What is the main difference in the type of breast cancer that this patient has and ductal carcinoma in situ (DCIS), defined earlier in the chapter? ______________________________

____

Pronunciation and Spelling

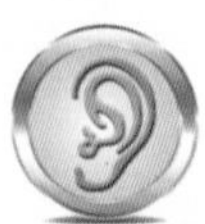
AUDITORY

Exercise 31

Review the Chapter 16 terms in the Dictionary/Audio Glossary in the Student Resources on thePoint, and practice pronouncing each term, referring to the pronunciation guide as needed.

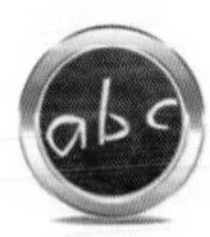

SPELLING

Exercise 32

Circle the correct spelling of each term.

1.	cranectomy	craniectomy	crenectomy
2.	fulguration	fulgeration	fuljuration
3.	rabdomyoma	rhabdomioma	rhabdomyoma
4.	thiroidectomy	thyroidectomy	thyrodectomy
5.	condrosarcoma	chondrosarcoma	chondrasacoma
6.	criosurgery	cyrosurjery	cryosurgery
7.	gleoma	glioma	glyoma
8.	leiomyosarcoma	liomyosarcoma	leomiosarcoma
9.	mamography	mammographe	mammography
10.	feochromocytoma	pheochromocytoma	pheocrhomcitoma
11.	brakytherapy	brachytherapy	brachytherape
12.	cholescintigraphy	colescintriphy	cholesintrigraphy
13.	lipomma	lipoma	lypoma
14.	nefrectome	nephrectomy	nephrictomy
15.	pallitive	palliative	pallative

Media Connection

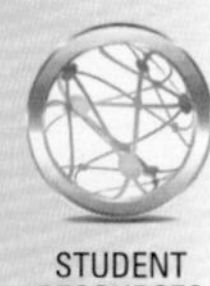
STUDENT RESOURCES

Exercise 33

Complete each of the following activities available with the Student Resources on thePoint. Check off each activity as you complete it, and record your score for the Chapter Quiz in the space provided.

Chapter Exercises

____ Flash Cards

____ Concentration

____ Abbreviation Match-Up

____ Roboterms

____ Word Anatomy

____ Fill the Gap

____ Break It Down

____ True/False Body Building

____ Quiz Show

____ Complete the Case

____ Medical Record Review

____ Look and Label

____ Image Matching

____ Spelling Bee

____ **Chapter Quiz** *Score:*________%

Additional Resources

____ Dictionary/Audio Glossary

____ Health Professions Careers: Physician's Assistant

____ Health Professions Careers: Oncology Nurse

Glossary of Prefixes, Suffixes, and Combining Forms

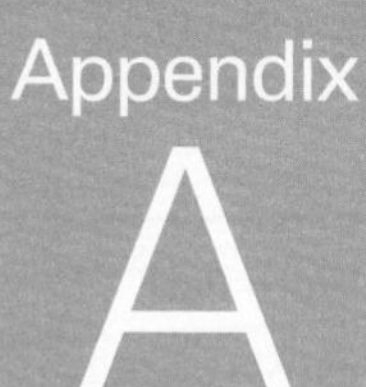

Word Part	Meaning
a-	without, not
ab-	away from
abdomin/o	abdomen
ablat/o	to take away
-ac	pertaining to
acr/o	extremity, tip
ad-	to, toward
aden/o	gland
adenoid/o	adenoid
adip/o	fat
adren/o	adrenal glands
adrenal/o	adrenal glands
-al	pertaining to
albumin/o	albumin
-algia	pain
aliment/o	nourishment, nutrition
alveol/o	alveolus
amni/o	amnion
amnion/o	amnion
an-	without, not
an/o	anus
andr/o	male
andro-	masculine, male
angi/o	vessel, vascular
ankyl/o	stiff
ante-	before
antero-	front
anti-	against
anxi/o	fear, worry
aort/o	aorta
appendic/o	appendix
-ar	pertaining to
-arche	beginning
arteri/o	artery
arthr/o	joint
articul/o	joint
-ary	pertaining to
-ase	enzyme
aspir/o	to breathe in or suck in
-asthenia	weakness
atel/o	incomplete
ather/o	fatty, fatty deposit
atri/o	atrium
ausculat/o	listening
auto-	self, same
bacteri/o	bacteria
balan/o	glans penis
basi-	base
baso-	base
bi-	two, twice
bi/o	life
bil/o	bile
bin-	two, twice
bio-	life
blast/o	immature cell
blephar/o	eyelid
brachi/o	arm
brady-	slow
bronch/o	bronchus (windpipe)
bronchi/o	bronchus (windpipe)
bucc/o	cheek
burs/o	bursa
calc/i	calcium
cancer/o	cancer
capn/i	carbon dioxide
capn/o	carbon dioxide
carcin/o	cancer
cardi/o	heart

(continued)

Word Part	Meaning
carp/o	carpal (wrist) bone
cec/o	cecum
-cele	herniation, protrusion
-centesis	puncture to remove fluid (aspirate)
cephal/o	head
cerebell/o	cerebellum (little brain)
cerebr/o	brain, cerebrum
cervic/o	neck, cervix (neck of uterus)
cheil/o	lip
chem/o	chemical, drug
chlor/o	green
chol/e	bile
cholecyst/o	gallbladder
chondr/o	cartilage
chondro-	cartilage
chori/o	chorion (membrane)
choroido-	the choroid
chrom/o	color
chromat/o	color
-cide	substance that kills
circum-	around
-clasia	to break
-clast	to break
clavic/o	clavicle
clavicul/o	clavicle
col/o	colon (section of large intestine)
colon/o	colon (section of large intestine)
colp/o	vagina
conjunctiv/o	conjunctiva
contra-	against
cor/e	pupil (of the eye)
cor/o	pupil (of the eye)
corne/o	cornea
coron/o	encircling, crown
cortic/o	cortex
cortic/o	outer portion of an organ, cortex
cost/o	rib
crani/o	cranium, skull
crin/o	to secrete
cry/o	cold

Word Part	Meaning
crypt-	hidden
cutane/o	skin
cyan/o	blue
cyst/o	fluid-filled sac (urinary bladder)
cyt/o	cell
-cyte	cell
dacry/o	tears, lacrimal (tear) duct
de-	away from, cessation, without
dent/o	tooth
derm/o	skin
dermat/o	skin
di-	two
diaphragmat/o	diaphragm
dipl/o	double, two
dips/o	thirst
dis-	separate
disc/o	disc or disk
diverticul/o	diverticulum (pouch opening from a tubular organ)
duoden/o	duodenum
dur/o	hard, dura mater
dys-	painful, difficult, abnormal
ect-	outer, outside
ecto-	outer, outside
electr/o	electric, electricity
em-	in
embry/o	embryo, immature form
embryon/o	embryo, immature form
-emia	blood (condition of)
en-	in, within
encephal/o	brain
end-	in, within
endo-	in, within
endocrin/o	endocrine
enter/o	small intestine
enur/o	to urinate in
epi-	on, upon, following
epididym/o	epididymis
epiglott/o	epiglottis
episi/o	vulva (external genitalia; wrapper)
erythr/o	red

Word Part	Meaning
-esis	condition of
esophag/o	esophagus
esthesi/o	sensation, perception
eu-	true, good, normal
ex-	out of, away from
exo-	out of, away from
fasci/o	fascia, band
femor/o	femur
fet/o	fetus
fibr/o	fiber
fibul/o	fibula
fund/o	fundus (part farthest from opening or exit)
galact/o	milk
gangli/o	ganglion
ganglion/o	ganglion
gastr/o	stomach
-gen	origin, production
-genesis	originating, producing
-genic	originating, producing
gestat/o	from conception to birth
glomerul/o	glomerulus
gluc/o	glucose, sugar
gluco-	glucose (sugar)
glucos/o	glucose, sugar
glyc/o	glucose, sugar
glycos/o	glucose, sugar
granul/o	granules
gravid/o	pregnancy
gyn/o	woman
gynec/o	woman
hallucin/o	to wander in one's mind
hem/o	blood
hemat/o	blood
hemi-	half
hepat/o	liver
herni/o	hernia (protrusion)
hetero-	other, different
hidr/o	sweat
hist/o	tissue
homeo-	same, alike

Word Part	Meaning
homo-	same, alike
hormon/o	hormone
humer/o	humerus
hydr/o	water, fluid
hyper-	above normal, excessive
hypn/o	sleep, hypnosis
hypo-	below normal, deficient
hyster/o	uterus (womb)
-ia	condition of
-iasis	condition of
-ic	pertaining to
ictero-	jaundice (yellow)
ile/o	ileum
ili/o	ilium
im-	not
immun/o	immune, safe
in-	not
infra-	below, beneath
inter-	between, among
intra-	within, inside
ir/o	iris
irid/o	iris
ischi/o	ischium
-ism	condition of
iso-	equal, alike
jejun/o	jejunum
kal/i	potassium
kary/o	nucleus
kerat/o	cornea, hard
kerat/o	hard, cornea
kinesi/o	movement
kinet/o	movement
kyph/o	humpback
labi/o	lip
lacrim/o	tears, lacrimal (tear) duct
lact/o	milk
lamin/o	lamina (plate)
lapar/o	abdomen
laryng/o	larynx
latero-	side

(continued)

Word Part	Meaning
lei/o	smooth
leio-	smooth
leuk/o	white
lingu/o	tongue
lip/o	fat
-lith	stone, calculus
lith/o	stone, calculus
lob/o	lobe
-logy	study of
lord/o	curved, bent
lumb/o	lumbar region, lower back
lymph/o	lymph
-lysis	destruction, breakdown, separation
macro-	large, long
mal-	bad, poor
-malacia	softening
mamm/o	breast, mammary gland
mandibul/o	mandible (lower jaw bone)
mast/o	breast, mammary gland
maxill/o	maxilla (upper jaw bone)
meat/o	meatus (opening)
medi/o	middle
mediastin/o	mediastinum (middle septum)
mega-	large, oversize
megalo-	large, oversize
-megaly	enlargement
melan/o	black, dark
men/o	menstruation
menisc/o	meniscus
menstru/o	menstruation
ment/o	mind, mental
meta-	change, beyond
metr/o	uterus
metri/o	uterus
-metry	measurement of
micro-	small
mono-	one
morph/o	form, shape
muc/o	mucus
multi-	many

Word Part	Meaning
muscul/o	muscle
my/o	muscle
myc/o	fungus
myel/o	bone marrow, spinal cord
myos/o	muscle
mys/o	muscle
narc/o	stupor, numbness, sleep
nas/o	nose
nat/o	birth
natr/i	sodium
necr/o	death
neo-	new
nephr/o	kidney
neur/o	nerve, nerve tissue
neutr/o	neutral
noct/i	night
non-	not
normo-	normal, usual
nucle/o	nucleus
nulli-	none
numer/o	number
ocul/o	eye
odont/o	tooth
olig/o	scanty, few
-oma	tumor or neoplasm
omphal/o	umbilicus, navel
onc/o	tumor
onych/o	nail
oophor/o	ovary
ophthalm/o	eye
opt/o	vision, eye
or/o	mouth
orch/o	testis, testicle
orchi/o	testis, testicle
orchid/o	testis, testicle
oste/o	bone
ovari/o	ovary
ox/a	oxygen
ox/o	oxygen
pachy/o	thick

Word Part	Meaning
palat/o	palate
pan-	all, entire
pancreat/o	pancreas
para-	beside
parathyroid/o	parathyroid glands
-partum	childbirth, labor
patell/o	patella (knee cap)
path/o	disease
-pathy	disease
pector/o	chest
ped/o	foot
pelv/i	pelvis, pelvic cavity
pelv/o	pelvis
peps/o	digestion
per-	through
peri-	around, surrounding
perine/o	perineum (area between the anus and vulva)
-pexy	surgical fixation
phag/o	eat, swallow
phalang/o	phalanges (bones of digits)
pharyng/o	pharynx (throat)
phas/o	speech
phleb/o	vein
phon/o	sound, voice
-phonia	condition of the voice
phot/o	light
phren/o	diaphragm
phren/o	mind
plas/o	growth, formation
-plasia	formation, growth
-plasty	surgical repair, reconstruction
pleur/o	rib, side, pleura (lung)
pneum/o	lung, air
pneumat/o	lung, air
pneumon/o	lung, air
pod/o	foot
poli/o	gray matter
poly-	many, much
polyp/o	polyp
post-	after, behind

Word Part	Meaning
postero-	back
pre-	before
presby/o	related to aging
pro-	before, promoting
proct/o	rectum, anus
prostat/o	prostate
proximo-	near point of origin
pseudo-	false
psych/o	mind, mental
pub/o	pubis
pulmon/o	lung
pupill/o	pupil (of the eye)
py/o	pus
pyel/o	renal pelvis
pylor/o	pylorus
quad-	four
quadri-	four
rachi/o	spine
radi/o	x-rays, radiation
radi/o	radius
radicul/o	nerve root
re-	again, backward
rect/o	rectum
ren/o	kidney
retin/o	retina
retro-	backward, behind
rhabd/o	striated muscle
rhin/o	nose
rhytid/o	wrinkle
-rrhage	flowing forth
-rrhagia	flowing forth
-rrhaphy	suture
-rrhea	flow, discharge
sacr/o	sacrum
salping/o	salpinx, uterine tube, fallopian tube
sarc/o	muscle, flesh
scapul/o	scapula (shoulder blade)
-schisis	to split
schiz/o	split
scler/o	hard, sclera

(continued)

Word Part	Meaning
scoli/o	crooked, twisted
-scopy	viewing, examining, or observing with an instrument
seb/o	sebum (an oily secretion)
semi-	half, partly
sept/o	septum, thin wall
sial/o	saliva
sigmoid/o	sigmoid colon
sinus/o	sinus, hollow space
soci/o	social, society
somn/i	sleep
somn/o	sleep
son/o	sound, sound waves
sperm/o	sperm, spermatozoon
spermat/o	sperm, spermatozoon
sphygm/o	pulse
spin/o	spine
spir/o	breathe
spondyl/o	vertebra
squam/o	scale-like structure
-stenosis	stricture, narrowing
stern/o	sternum (breastbone)
steth/o	chest
stomat/o	mouth
-stomy	surgical opening
sub-	below, beneath
super-	above
supra-	above
sym-	together, with
syn-	together, with
synovi/o	synovial joint or fluid
tachy-	rapid, fast
tars/o	tarsal bones
tel-	end
ten/o	tendon
tend/o	tendon
tendin/o	tendon
test/o	testis, testicle
testicul/o	testis, testicle

Word Part	Meaning
thalam/o	thalamus
thorac/o	thorax, chest
thromb/o	blood clot
thym/i	mind, soul, emotion
thym/o	thymus gland
thym/o	mind, soul, emotion
thyr/o	thyroid gland
thyroid/o	thyroid gland
toc/o	labor, birth
-tomy	incision
ton/o	tension, pressure, tone
tonsill/o	tonsil
trache/o	trachea
trans-	across, through
tri-	three
trich/o	hair
-tripsy	crushing
troph/o	nourishment
-trophy	development, nourishment
uln/o	ulna
ultra-	excess, beyond
uni-	one
ur/o	urine, urinary system/tract
ure-	urea, urine
ureter/o	ureter
urethr/o	urethra
-uria	urine, urination
urin/o	urine, urinary system/tract
uter/o	uterus
vagin/o	vagina
valv/o	valve
valvul/o	valve
varic/o	swollen or twisted vein
vas/o	duct, vessel, vas deferens
vas/o	blood vessel
vascul/o	blood vessel
ven/i	veins
ven/o	veins
ventricul/o	ventricle, normal cavity
ventro-	belly

Word Part	Meaning
vertebr/o	vertebra
vesic/o	fluid-filled sac (urinary bladder)
vesicul/o	fluid-filled sac (seminal vesicle)
viscer/o	internal organs
vulv/o	vulva (external genitalia; wrapper)
xanth/o	yellow
xer/o	dry
-y	condition of

Appendix B Word Part Lookup by Meaning

Meaning	Word Part
abdomen	abdomin/o
abdomen	lapar/o
above	super-
above	supra-
above normal, excessive	hyper-
across, through	trans-
adenoid	adenoid/o
adrenal glands	adren/o
adrenal glands	adrenal/o
after, behind	post-
again, backward	re-
against	anti-
against	contra-
albumin	albumin/o
all, entire	pan-
alveolus	alveol/o
amnion	amni/o
amnion	amnion/o
anus	an/o
aorta	aort/o
appendix	appendic/o
arm	brachi/o
around	circum-
around, surrounding	peri-
artery	arteri/o
atrium	atri/o
away from	ab-
away from, cessation, without	de-
back	postero-
backward, behind	retro-
bacteria	bacteri/o
bad, poor	mal-
base	basi-
base	baso-

Meaning	Word Part
before	ante-
before	pre-
before, promoting	pro-
beginning	-arche
belly	ventro-
below normal, deficient	hypo-
below, beneath	infra-
below, beneath	sub-
beside	para-
between, among	inter-
bile	bil/o
bile	chol/e
birth	nat/o
black, dark	melan/o
blood	hem/o
blood	hemat/o
blood (condition of)	-emia
blood clot	thromb/o
blood vessel	vas/o
blood vessel	vascul/o
blue	cyan/o
bone	oste/o
bone marrow, spinal cord	myel/o
brain	encephal/o
brain, cerebrum	cerebr/o
breast, mammary gland	mamm/o
breast, mammary gland	mast/o
breathe	spir/o
bronchus (windpipe)	bronch/o
bronchus (windpipe)	bronchi/o
bursa	burs/o
calcium	calc/i
cancer	cancer/o
cancer	carcin/o

Meaning	Word Part
carbon dioxide	capn/i
carbon dioxide	capn/o
carpal (wrist) bone	carp/o
cartilage	chondr/o
cartilage	chondro-
cecum	cec/o
cell	-cyte
cell	cyt/o
cerebellum (little brain)	cerebell/o
change, beyond	meta-
cheek	bucc/o
chemical, drug	chem/o
chest	pector/o
chest	steth/o
childbirth, labor	-partum
chorion (membrane)	chori/o
choroid	choroido-
clavicle	clavic/o
clavicle	clavicul/o
cold	cry/o
colon (section of large intestine)	col/o
colon (section of large intestine)	colon/o
color	chrom/o
color	chromat/o
condition of	-esis
condition of	-ia
condition of	-iasis
condition of	-ism
condition of	-y
condition of the voice	-phonia
conjunctiva	conjunctiv/o
cornea	corne/o
cornea, hard	kerat/o
cortex	cortic/o
cranium, skull	crani/o
crooked, twisted	scoli/o
crushing	-tripsy
curved, bent	lord/o
death	necr/o
destruction, breakdown, separation	-lysis

Meaning	Word Part
development, nourishment	-trophy
diaphragm	diaphragmat/o
diaphragm	phren/o
digestion	peps/o
disc or disk	disc/o
disease	-pathy
disease	path/o
diverticulum (pouch opening from a tubular organ)	diverticul/o
double, two	dipl/o
dry	xer/o
duct, vessel, vas deferens	vas/o
duodenum	duoden/o
eat, swallow	phag/o
electric, electricity	electr/o
embryo, immature form	embry/o
embryo, immature form	embryon/o
encircling, crown	coron/o
end	tel-
endocrine	endocrin/o
enlargement	-megaly
enzyme	-ase
epididymis	epididym/o
epiglottis	epiglott/o
equal, alike	iso-
esophagus	esophag/o
excess, beyond	ultra-
extremity, tip	acr/o
eye	ocul/o
eye	ophthalm/o
eyelid	blephar/o
false	pseudo-
fascia, band	fasci/o
fat	adip/o
fat	lip/o
fatty, fatty deposit	ather/o
fear, worry	anxi/o
femur	femor/o
fetus	fet/o
fiber	fibr/o
fibula	fibul/o

(continued)

Meaning	Word Part
flow, discharge	-rrhea
flowing forth	-rrhage
flowing forth	-rrhagia
fluid-filled sac (seminal vesicle)	vesicul/o
fluid-filled sac (urinary bladder)	cyst/o
fluid-filled sac (urinary bladder)	vesic/o
foot	ped/o
foot	pod/o
form, shape	morph/o
formation, growth	-plasia
four	quad-
four	quadri-
from conception to birth	gestat/o
front	antero-
fundus (part farthest from opening or exit)	fund/o
fungus	myc/o
gallbladder	cholecyst/o
ganglion	gangli/o
ganglion	ganglion/o
gland	aden/o
glans penis	balan/o
glomerulus	glomerul/o
glucose, sugar	gluco-
glucose, sugar	gluc/o
glucose, sugar	glucos/o
glucose, sugar	glyc/o
glucose, sugar	glycos/o
granules	granul/o
gray matter	poli/o
green	chlor/o
growth, formation	plas/o
hair	trich/o
half	hemi-
half, partly	semi-
hard, cornea	kerat/o
hard, dura mater	dur/o
hard, sclera	scler/o
head	cephal/o
heart	cardi/o
hernia (protrusion)	herni/o

Meaning	Word Part
herniation, protrusion	-cele
hidden	crypt-
hormone	hormon/o
humerus	humer/o
humpback	kyph/o
ileum	ile/o
ilium	ili/o
immature cell	blast/o
immune, safe	immun/o
in	em-
in, within	en-
in, within	end-
in, within	endo-
incision	-tomy
incomplete	atel/o
internal organs	viscer/o
iris	ir/o
iris	irid/o
ischium	ischi/o
jaundice (yellow)	ictero-
jejunum	jejun/o
joint	arthr/o
joint	articul/o
kidney	nephr/o
kidney	ren/o
labor, birth	toc/o
lamina (plate)	lamin/o
large, long	macro-
large, oversize	mega-
large, oversize	megalo-
larynx	laryng/o
life	bi/o
life	bio-
light	phot/o
lip	cheil/o
lip	labi/o
listening	ausculat/o
liver	hepat/o
lobe	lob/o
lumbar region, lower back	lumb/o

Meaning	Word Part
lung	pulmon/o
lung, air	pneum/o
lung, air	pneumat/o
lung, air	pneumon/o
lymph	lymph/o
male	andr/o
mandible (lower jaw bone)	mandibul/o
many	multi-
many, much	poly-
masculine, male	andro-
maxilla (upper jaw bone)	maxill/o
measurement of	-metry
meatus (opening)	meat/o
mediastinum (middle septum)	mediastin/o
meniscus	menisc/o
menstruation	men/o
menstruation	menstru/o
middle	medi/o
milk	galact/o
milk	lact/o
mind	phren/o
mind, mental	ment/o
mind, mental	psych/o
mind, soul, emotion	thym/i
mind, soul, emotion	thym/o
mouth	or/o
mouth	stomat/o
movement	kinesi/o
movement	kinet/o
mucus	muc/o
muscle	muscul/o
muscle	my/o
muscle	myos/o
muscle	mys/o
muscle, flesh	sarc/o
nail	onych/o
near point of origin	proximo-
neck, cervix (neck of uterus)	cervic/o
nerve root	radicul/o
nerve, nerve tissue	neur/o

Meaning	Word Part
neutral	neutr/o
new	neo-
night	noct/i
none	nulli-
normal cavity, ventricle	ventricul/o
normal, usual	normo-
nose	nas/o
nose	rhin/o
not	im-
not	in-
not	non-
nourishment	troph/o
nourishment, nutrition	aliment/o
nucleus	kary/o
nucleus	nucle/o
number	numer/o
on, upon, following	epi-
one	mono-
one	uni-
origin, production	-gen
originating, producing	-genesis
originating, producing	-genic
other, different	hetero-
out of, away from	ex-
out of, away from	exo-
outer portion of an organ, cortex	cortic/o
outer, outside	ect-
outer, outside	ecto-
ovary	oophor/o
ovary	ovari/o
oxygen	ox/a
oxygen	ox/o
pain	-algia
painful, difficult, abnormal	dys-
palate	palat/o
pancreas	pancreat/o
parathyroid glands	parathyroid/o
patella (knee cap)	patell/o
pelvis	pelv/o
pelvis, pelvic cavity	pelv/i

(continued)

Meaning	Word Part
perineum (area between the anus and vulva)	perine/o
pertaining to	-ac
pertaining to	-al
pertaining to	-ar
pertaining to	-ary
pertaining to	-ic
phalanges (bones of digits)	phalang/o
pharynx (throat)	pharyng/o
polyp	polyp/o
potassium	kal/i
pregnancy	gravid/o
prostate	prostat/o
pubis	pub/o
pulse	sphygm/o
puncture to remove fluid (aspirate)	-centesis
pupil (of the eye)	cor/e
pupil (of the eye)	cor/o
pupil (of the eye)	pupill/o
pus	py/o
pylorus	pylor/o
radius	radi/o
rapid, fast	tachy-
rectum	rect/o
rectum, anus	proct/o
red	erythr/o
related to aging	presby/o
renal pelvis	pyel/o
retina	retin/o
rib	cost/o
rib, side, pleura (lung)	pleur/o
sacrum	sacr/o
saliva	sial/o
salpinx, uterine tube, fallopian tube	salping/o
same, alike	homeo-
same, alike	homo-
scale-like structure	squam/o
scanty, few	olig/o
scapula (shoulder blade)	scapul/o
sclera, hard	scler/o
sebum (an oily secretion)	seb/o

Meaning	Word Part
self, same	auto-
sensation, perception	esthesi/o
separate	dis-
septum, thin wall	sept/o
side	latero-
sigmoid colon	sigmoid/o
sinus, hollow space	sinus/o
skin	cutane/o
skin	derm/o
skin	dermat/o
sleep	somn/i
sleep	somn/o
sleep, hypnosis	hypn/o
slow	brady-
small	micro-
small intestine	enter/o
smooth	lei/o
smooth	leio-
social, society	soci/o
sodium	natr/i
softening	-malacia
sound, sound waves	son/o
sound, voice	phon/o
speech	phas/o
sperm, spermatozoon	sperm/o
sperm, spermatozoon	spermat/o
spine	rachi/o
spine	spin/o
split	schiz/o
sternum (breast bone)	stern/o
stiff	ankyl/o
stomach	gastr/o
stone, calculus	-lith
stone, calculus	lith/o
striated muscle	rhabd/o
stricture, narrowing	-stenosis
study of	-logy
stupor, numbness, sleep	narc/o
substance that kills	-cide
surgical fixation	-pexy

Meaning	Word Part
surgical opening	-stomy
surgical repair, reconstruction	-plasty
suture	-rrhaphy
sweat	hidr/o
swollen or twisted vein	varic/o
synovial joint or fluid	synovi/o
tarsal bones	tars/o
tears, lacrimal (tear) duct	dacry/o
tears, lacrimal (tear) duct	lacrim/o
tendon	ten/o
tendon	tend/o
tendon	tendin/o
tension, pressure, tone	ton/o
testis, testicle	orch/o
testis, testicle	orchi/o
testis, testicle	orchid/o
testis, testicle	test/o
testis, testicle	testicul/o
thalamus	thalam/o
thick	pachy/o
thirst	dips/o
thorax, chest	thorac/o
three	tri-
through	per-
thymus gland	thym/o
thyroid gland	thyr/o
thyroid gland	thyroid/o
tissue	hist/o
to break	-clasia
to break	-clast
to breathe in or suck in	aspir/o
to secrete	crin/o
to split	-schisis
to take away	ablat/o
to urinate in	enur/o
to wander in one's mind	hallucin/o
to, toward	ad-
together, with	sym-
together, with	syn-
tongue	lingu/o

Meaning	Word Part
tonsil	tonsill/o
tooth	dent/o
tooth	odont/o
trachea	trache/o
true, good, normal	eu-
tumor	onc/o
tumor or neoplasm	-oma
two	di-
two, twice	bi-
two, twice	bin-
ulna	uln/o
umbilicus, navel	omphal/o
urea, urine	ure-
ureter	ureter/o
urethra	urethr/o
urine, urinary system/tract	ur/o
urine, urinary system/tract	urin/o
urine, urination	-uria
uterus	metr/o
uterus	metri/o
uterus	uter/o
uterus (womb)	hyster/o
vagina	colp/o
vagina	vagin/o
valve	valv/o
valve	valvul/o
vein	phleb/o
veins	ven/i
veins	ven/o
ventricle	ventricul/o
vertebra	spondyl/o
vertebra	vertebr/o
vessel, vascular	angi/o
viewing, examining, or observing with an instrument	-scopy
vision, eye	opt/o
vulva (external genitalia; wrapper)	episi/o
vulva (external genitalia; wrapper)	vulv/o
water, fluid	hydr/o
weakness	-asthenia
white	leuk/o

(continued)

Meaning	Word Part
within, inside	intra-
without, not	a-
without, not	an-
woman	gyn/o

Meaning	Word Part
woman	gynec/o
wrinkle	rhytid/o
x-rays, radiation	radi/o
yellow	xanth/o

Laboratory Tests and Values

Appendix C

ROUTINE URINALYSIS

Test	Normal Value	Clinical Significance
General Characteristics and Measurements		
Color	Pale yellow to amber	Color change can be due to concentration or dilution, drugs, metabolic or inflammatory disorders
Odor	Slightly aromatic	Foul odor typical of urinary tract infection, fruity odor in uncontrolled diabetes mellitus
Appearance (clarity or turbidity)	Clear to slightly hazy	Cloudy urine occurs with infection or after refrigeration; may indicate presence of bacteria, cells, mucus, or crystals
Specific gravity	1.003–1.030	Decreased in diabetes insipidus, acute renal failure, water intoxication; increased in liver disorders, heart failure, dehydration
pH	4.5–8.0	Acid urine accompanies acidosis, fever, high protein diet; alkaline urine in urinary tract infection, metabolic alkalosis, vegetarian diet
Chemical Determinations		
Glucose	Negative	Glucose present in uncontrolled diabetes mellitus, steroid excess
Ketones	Negative	Present in diabetes mellitus and in starvation
Protein	Negative	Present in kidney disorders, such as glomerulonephritis, acute kidney failure
Bilirubin	Negative	Breakdown product of hemoglobin; present in liver disease or in bile blockage
Urobilinogen	0.2–1.0 Ehrlich units/dL	Breakdown product of bilirubin; increased in hemolytic anemias and in liver disease; remains negative in bile obstruction
Blood (occult)	Negative	Detects small amounts of blood cells, hemoglobin, or myoglobin; present in severe trauma, metabolic disorders, bladder infections
Nitrite	Negative	Product of bacterial breakdown of urine; positive result suggests urinary tract infection and needs to be followed up with a culture of the urine
Microscopic		
Red blood cells	0–3 per high-power field	Increased because of bleeding within the urinary tract from trauma, tumors, inflammation, or damage within the kidney
White blood cells	0–4 per high-power field	Increased by kidney or bladder infection
Renal epithelial cells	Occasional	Increased number indicates damage to kidney tubules
Casts	None	Hyaline casts normal; large number of abnormal casts indicates inflammation or a systemic disorder
Crystals	Present	Most are normal; may be acid or alkaline
Bacteria	Few	Increased in urinary tract infection or contamination from infected genitalia
Others		Any yeasts, parasites, mucus, spermatozoa, or other microscopic findings would be reported here

COMPLETE BLOOD COUNT (CBC)

Test	Normal Value[a]	Clinical Significance
Red blood cell (RBC) count	Men: 4.2–5.4 million/mL Women: 3.6–5.0 million/mL	Decreased in anemia; increased in dehydration, polycythemia
Hemoglobin (Hb)	Men: 13.5–17.5 g/dL Women: 12–16 g/dL	Decreased in anemia, hemorrhage, and hemolytic reactions; increased in dehydration, heart and lung disease
Hematocrit (Hct) or packed cell volume (PCV)	Women: 37–47%	Decreased in anemia; increased in polycythemia, dehydration
Red blood cell (RBC) indices (examples)	Men: 40–50%	These values, calculated from the RBC count, Hb, and Hct, give information valuable in the diagnosis and classification of anemia
Mean corpuscular volume (MCV)	87–103 mL/red cell	Measures the average size or volume of each RBC: small size (microcytic) in iron-deficiency anemia; large size (macrocytic) typical of pernicious anemia
Mean corpuscular hemoglobin (MCH)	26–34 pg/red cell	Measures the weight of hemoglobin per RBC; useful in differentiating types of anemia in a severely anemic patient
Mean corpuscular hemoglobin concentration (MCHC)	31–37 g/dL	Defines the volume of hemoglobin per RBC; used to determine the color or concentration of hemoglobin per RBC
White blood cell (WBC) count	5,000–10,000/mL	Increased in leukemia and in response to infection, inflammation, and dehydration; decreased in bone marrow suppression
Platelets	150,000–350,000/mL	Increased in many malignant disorders; decreased in disseminated intravascular coagulation (DIC) or toxic drug effects; spontaneous bleeding may occur at platelet counts less than 20,000 mL
Differential (peripheral blood smear)	40–74%	A stained slide of the blood is needed to perform the differential. The percentages of the different WBCs are estimated, and the slide is microscopically checked for abnormal characteristics in WBCs, RBCs, and platelets
WBCs		
Segmented neutrophils (SEGs, POLYs)	0–3%	Increased in bacterial infections; low numbers leave person very susceptible to infection
Immature neutrophils (band cells or BANDs)	20–40%	Increased when neutrophil count increases
Lymphocytes (LYMPHs)	2–6%	Increased in viral infections; low numbers leave person dangerously susceptible to infection
Monocytes (MONOs)	1–4%	Increased in specific infections
Eosinophils (EOs)	0.5–1%	Increased in allergic disorders
Basophils (BASOs)	0–1%	Increased in allergic disorders

[a]Values vary depending on instrumentation and type of test.

BLOOD CHEMISTRY TESTS

Test	Normal Value	Clinical Significance
Basic Panel: An Overview of Electrolytes, Waste Product Management, and Metabolism		
Blood urea nitrogen (BUN)	7–18 mg/dL	Increased in renal disease and dehydration; decreased in liver damage and malnutrition
Carbon dioxide (CO_2) (includes bicarbonate)	23–30 mmol/L	Useful to evaluate acid–base balance by measuring total carbon dioxide in the blood: increased in vomiting and pulmonary disease; decreased in diabetic acidosis, acute renal failure, and hyperventilation
Chloride (Cl)	98–106 mEq/L	Increased in dehydration, hyperventilation, and congestive heart failure; decreased in vomiting, diarrhea, and fever
Creatinine	0.6–1.2 mg/dL	Produced at a constant rate and excreted by the kidneys; increased in kidney disease
Glucose	Fasting: 70–110 mg/dL Random: 85–125 mg/dL	Increased in diabetes and severe illness; decreased in insulin overdose or hypoglycemia
Potassium (K)	3.5–5 mEq/L	Increased in renal failure, extensive cell damage, and acidosis; decreased in vomiting, diarrhea, and excess administration of diuretics or IV fluids
Sodium (Na)	101–111 mEq/L or 135–148 mEq/L (depending on test)	Increased in dehydration and diabetes insipidus; decreased in overload of IV fluids, burns, diarrhea, or vomiting
Additional Blood Chemistry Tests		
Alanine aminotransferase (ALT)	10–40 U/L	Used to diagnose and monitor treatment of liver disease and to monitor the effects of drugs on the liver; increased in myocardial infarction
Albumin	3.8–5.0 g/dL	Albumin holds water in blood; increased levels are seen with dehydration; decreased levels in liver disease and kidney disease
Albumin-globulin ratio (A/G ratio)	Greater than 1	Low A/G ratio signifies a tendency for edema because globulin is less effective than albumin at holding water in the blood
Alkaline phosphatase (ALP)	20–70 U/L (varies by method)	Enzyme of bone metabolism; increased in liver disease and metastatic bone disease; decreased in zinc deficiency and hypothyroidism
Amylase	21–160 U/L	Used to diagnose and monitor treatment of acute pancreatitis and to detect inflammation of the salivary glands
Aspartate aminotransferase (AST)	0–41 U/L (varies)	Enzyme present in tissues with high metabolic activity; increased in myocardial infarction and liver disease; low levels are normally found in the blood
Bilirubin, total	0.2–1.0 mg/dL	Breakdown product of hemoglobin from red blood cells; increased when excessive red blood cells are being destroyed or in liver disease; lower than normal levels are usually not a health concern
Calcium (Ca)	8.8–10.0 mg/dL	Increased in excess parathyroid hormone production and in cancer; decreased in alkalosis, elevated phosphate in renal failure, and excess IV fluids
Cholesterol	120–220 mg/dL desirable range	Screening test used to evaluate risk of heart disease; levels of 200 mg/dL or greater indicate increased risk of heart disease and warrant further investigation; sudden decreases in cholesterol levels *may* increase the risk of cancer, depression, and anxiety and preterm birth in pregnant women

(continued)

Test	Normal Value	Clinical Significance
Creatine kinase (CK)	Men: 38–174 U/L Women: 96–140 U/L	Increased enzyme level indicates myocardial infarction or damage to skeletal muscle. When elevated, specific fractions (isoenzymes) are tested for; decreased levels may be found with septicemia
Gamma-glutamyl transferase (GGT)	Men: 6–26 U/L Women: 4–18 U/L	Used to diagnose liver disease and to test for chronic alcoholism
Globulins	2.3–3.5 g/dL	Proteins active in immunity; help albumin keep water in blood
High-density lipoproteins (HDLs)	Men: 30–70 mg/dL Women: 30–85 mg/dL	Used to evaluate the risk of heart disease
Iron, serum (Fe)	Men: 75–175 mg/dL Women: 65–165 m/dL	Increased in hemolytic conditions; decreased in iron deficiency and anemia
Lactic dehydrogenase (LDH or LD)	95–200 U/L (normal ranges vary greatly)	Enzyme released in many kinds of tissue damage, including myocardial infarction, pulmonary infarction, and liver disease
Lipase	4–24 U/L (varies with test)	Enzyme used to diagnose pancreatitis
Low-density lipoproteins (LDLs)	80–140 mg/dL	Used to evaluate the risk of heart disease
Magnesium (Mg)	1.3–2.1 mEq/L	Vital in neuromuscular function; increased levels may occur with Addison disease, dehydration, and chronic renal failure; decreased levels may occur in malnutrition, alcoholism, pancreatitis, diarrhea
Phosphorus (P) (inorganic)	2.7–4.5 mg/dL	Increased in response to calcium; main reservoir is in bone; elevated in kidney disease; decreased in excess parathyroid hormone
Protein, total	6–8 g/dL	Increased in dehydration, multiple myeloma; decreased in kidney disease, liver disease, poor nutrition, severe burns, excessive bleeding
Serum glutamic oxaloacetic transaminase (SGOT)		SGOT is former name for AST; see aspartate aminotransferase (AST)
Serum glutamic pyruvic transaminase (SGPT)		SGPT is former name for ALT; see alanine aminotransferase (ALT)
Thyroid-stimulating hormone (TSH)	0.5–6 mU/L	Produced by pituitary to promote thyroid gland function; increased when thyroid gland is not functioning; decreased in hyperthyroidism, pituitary gland damage, excessive thyroid hormone medication
Thyroxin (T4)	5–12.5 mg/dL (varies)	Screening test of thyroid function; increased in hyperthyroidism; decreased in myxedema and hypothyroidism
Triglycerides	Men: 40–160 mg/dL Women: 35–135 mg/dL	An indication of ability to metabolize fats; increased triglycerides and cholesterol indicate high risk of atherosclerosis; decreased in low fat diet, hyperthyroidism, and malnutrition
Triiodothyronine (T3)	120–195 mg/dL	Elevated in specific types of hyperthyroidism; decreased in hypothyroidism with high TSH
Uric acid	Men: 3.5–7.2 mg/dL Women: 2.6–6.0 mg/dL	Produced by breakdown of ingested purines in food and nucleic acids; elevated in kidney disease, gout, and leukemia; decreased in kidney disease, chronic alcohol use, and lead poisoning

Adapted from Cohen, BJ. *Memmler's The Human Body in Health and Disease.* 11th ed. Baltimore, MD: Lippincott Williams & Wilkins, 2009. Updated using www.labtestsonline.org by the American Association for Clinical Chemistry.

Abbreviations

Appendix D

Abbreviation	Meaning
APR	abdominoperineal resection
AB	abortion
Ab	antibody
ABG	arterial blood gas
ACB	aortocoronary bypass
ACS	acute coronary syndrome
ACTH	adrenocorticotropic hormone
ADH	antidiuretic hormone
ADHD	attention deficit hyperactivity disorder
ADL	activities of daily living
AFB	acid-fast bacilli
AFP	alpha fetoprotein
Ag	antigen
AIDS	acquired immunodeficiency syndrome
ALS	amyotrophic lateral sclerosis
ANA	antinuclear antibody test
AP	anteroposterior (from front to back)
ARDS	acute respiratory distress syndrome
ARF	acute renal failure
ASHD	arteriosclerotic heart disease
AV	arteriovenous, atrioventricular
b.i.d.	twice a day (Latin, *bis in die*)
BAL	bronchoalveolar lavage
BCC	basal cell carcinoma
BE	barium enema
BM	bowel movement
BMA	bone marrow aspiration
BMT	bone marrow transplant
BOOP	bronchiolitis obliterans with organizing pneumonia
BP	blood pressure
BPH	benign prostatic hyperplasia; benign prostatic hypertrophy
BT	blood transfusion

Abbreviation	Meaning
BUN	blood urea nitrogen
Bx	biopsy
C	Celsius, centigrade (temperature)
C-section	cesarean section
C&S	culture and sensitivity
C1 to C7	cervical vertebrae 1 to 7
CA	cancer, carcinoma
CABG	coronary artery bypass graft
CAD	coronary artery disease
CAM	complementary and alternative medicine
cath	catheter; catheterize; catheterization
CBC	complete blood count
cc	cubic centimeter
CF	cystic fibrosis
CHF	congestive heart failure
CK	creatine kinase
cm	centimeter
CMG	cystometrogram
CNS	central nervous system
COPD	chronic obstructive pulmonary disease
CP	cerebral palsy
CPAP	continuous positive airway pressure
CPR	cardiopulmonary resuscitation
CRF	chronic renal failure
CSF	cerebrospinal fluid
CT	computed tomography (type of x-ray)
CTS	carpal tunnel syndrome
CVA	cerebrovascular accident
CVS	chorionic villus sampling
CXR	chest x-ray
D&C	dilatation and curettage; dilation and curettage
DC	doctor of chiropractic medicine

(continued)

Abbreviation	Meaning
DCIS	ductal carcinoma in situ
DCT	distal convoluted tubule
DDS	doctor of dental surgery
DOB	date of birth
DRE	digital rectal examination
DS	Doppler sonography
DTR	deep tendon reflex
DVT	deep vein thrombosis, deep venous thrombosis
Dx	diagnosis
EBV	Epstein–Barr virus
ECG or EKG	electrocardiography
ED	erectile dysfunction
ED&C	electrodesiccation and curettage
EDC	estimated date of confinement
EDD	estimated date of delivery
EEG	electroencephalogram
EGD	esophagogastroduodenoscopy
EGFR	epidermal growth factor receptor
EMG	electromyogram
ENT	ears, nose, throat
EPO	erythropoietin
ER, ED	emergency room, emergency department
ERCP	endoscopic retrograde cholangiopancreatography
ESR	erythrocyte sedimentation rate
ESRD	end-stage renal disease
ESWL	extracorporeal shock wave lithotripsy
EUS	endoscopic ultrasound
F	Fahrenheit (temperature)
Fe	iron
FNA	fine-needle aspiration
FS	frozen section
FSH	follicle-stimulating hormone
Fx, fx	fracture
g, gm	gram
GBS	group B streptococcus
GCT	germ cell tumor
GERD	gastroesophageal reflux disease
GI	gastrointestinal

Abbreviation	Meaning
GIST	gastrointestinal stromal tumor
GTT	glucose tolerance test
GU	genitourinary
GXT	graded exercise test
GYN	gynecology; gynecologist
H&P	history and physical (examination)
hCG	human chorionic gonadotropin
HCT, Hct, ht	hematocrit
HGB, Hb, Hgb	hemoglobin
HIDA	hepatobiliary iminodiacetic acid
HIV	human immunodeficiency virus
HM	Holter monitor
HPV	human papillomavirus
HRT	hormone replacement therapy
HSG	hysterosalpingogram
Ht	height
HTN	hypertension
Hx	history
I&D	incision and drainage
IBS	irritable bowel syndrome
ICU	intensive care unit
ILD	interstitial lung disease
INH	isoniazid; isonicotinic acid hydrazide
IOL	intraocular lens
IOP	intraocular pressure
ITP	idiopathic thrombocytopenic purpura
IVF	in vitro fertilization
IVP	intravenous pyelogram; intravenous pyelography
IVU	intravenous urogram; intravenous urography
kg	kilogram
KUB	kidneys, ureters, and bladder (x-ray)
L	liter
L1 to L5	lumbar vertebrae 1 to 5
lab	laboratory
LASIK	laser-assisted in situ keratomileusis
LEEP	loop electrosurgical excision procedure
LES	lower esophageal sphincter
LH	luteinizing hormone

Abbreviation	Meaning
LMP	last menstrual period
LP	lumbar puncture
m	meter
mg	milligram
MD	doctor of medicine, muscular dystrophy
MEN	multiple endocrine neoplasia
MG	myasthenia gravis
mg	milligram
MI	myocardial infarction
mL	milliliter
mm	millimeter
MRA	magnetic resonance angiography
MRCP	magnetic resonance cholangiopancreatography
MRI	magnetic resonance imaging
MS	multiple sclerosis
MUGA	multiple uptake gated acquisition
NG	nasogastric
NHL	non-Hodgkin lymphoma
NICU	neonatal intensive care unit
noc	night
noct.	night (Latin, *nocte*)
NPO, npo	nothing by mouth (don't eat or drink) (Latin, *non per os*)
NSAID	nonsteroidal antiinflammatory drug
OA	osteoarthritis
OB	obstetrics; obstetrician
OB/GYN	obstetrics/gynecology
OCD	obsessive-compulsive disorder
OD	doctor of optometry; right eye (oculus dexter)
ORIF	open reduction, internal fixation
OS	left eye (oculus sinister)
OU	each eye or both eyes (oculus uterque)
oz	ounce
P	pulse rate
p.c.	after meals (Latin, *post cibum*)
p.r.n.	as needed (Latin, *pro re nata*)
PA	physician's assistant
PAD	peripheral arterial disease
PCT	proximal convoluted tubule

Abbreviation	Meaning
Peds	pediatrics
PET	positron emission tomography
PFTs	pulmonary function tests
PID	pelvic inflammatory disease
PLT	platelet or platelet count
POC	products of conception
postop, post-op	postoperative (after surgery)
PPD	purified protein derivative, purified protein derivative of tuberculin
preop, pre-op	preoperative (before surgery)
PRK	photorefractive keratectomy
PSA	prostate-specific antigen
pt	patient
PT	physical therapy, physical therapist, prothrombin time
PTCA	percutaneous transluminal coronary angioplasty
PTH	parathyroid hormone
PTSD	posttraumatic stress disorder
PUD	peptic ulcer disease
PVC	premature ventricular contraction
Px	prognosis
q.i.d.	four times a day (Latin, *quarter in die*)
R	respiratory rate
RA	rheumatoid arthritis
RAD	reactive airway disease
RAIU	radioactive iodine uptake
RBC	red blood cell; red blood cell count
RF	rheumatoid factor, respiratory failure
RFA	radiofrequency ablation
RHD	rheumatic heart disease
ROM	range of motion
Rx	prescription
SAB	spontaneous abortion
SCC	squamous cell carcinoma
SG	specific gravity
SLE	systemic lupus erythematosus
SOB	shortness of breath
SPECT	single photon emission computed tomography

(continued)

Abbreviation	Meaning
STAT, stat	immediately
STD	sexually transmitted disease
STI	sexually transmitted infection
SUI	stress urinary incontinence
Sx	symptom
T	temperature
T1 to T12	thoracic vertebrae 1 to 12
T_3	triiodothyronine
T_4	thyroxine
TAB	therapeutic abortion
TAH	total abdominal hysterectomy
TB	tuberculosis
TEE	transesophageal echocardiography
TIA	transient ischemic attack
TIP	transurethral incision of the prostate
TNM staging	tumor node metastasis
TPN	total parenteral nutrition
Tr	treatment
TRUS	transrectal ultrasound
TSH	thyroid-stimulating hormone

Abbreviation	Meaning
TUIP	transurethral incision of the prostate
TURB	transurethral resection of bladder tumor
TURP	transurethral resection of the prostate
Tx, Tr	treatment
UA	urinalysis
UGI	upper gastrointestinal
URI	upper respiratory infection
UTI	urinary tract infection
UV	ultraviolet
V/Q	ventilation-perfusion (scan)
VA	visual acuity
VATS	video-assisted thoracoscopic surgery
VCUG	voiding cystourethrogram; voiding cystourethrography
VD	venereal disease
VF	visual field
VS	vital signs
vWD	von Willebrand disease
WBC	white blood cell; white blood cell count
Wt	weight

DANGEROUS ABBREVIATIONS, ACRONYMS, AND SYMBOLS

The Joint Commission (www.jointcommission.org) originally issued a list of dangerous abbreviations, acronyms, and symbols that should not be used in health care. In 2010, this list was integrated into the Information Management standards. Organizations that wish to be accredited by the Joint Commission must develop and implement a list of abbreviations not to be used.

Official "Do Not Use" List

Do Not Use	Potential Problem	Use Instead
U (unit)	Mistaken for 0 (zero), 4 (four), or cc	Write "unit"
IU (international unit)	Mistaken for IV (intravenous) or 10 (ten)	Write "international unit"
Q.D., QD, q.d., qd (daily)	Mistaken for each other	Write "daily"
Q.O.D., QOD, q.o.d, qod (every other day)	Period after the Q mistaken for "I" and the "O" mistaken for "I"	Write "every other day"
Trailing zero (X.0 mg)[a]	Decimal point is missed	Write "X mg"
Lack of leading zero (.X mg)	Dosage error	Write "0.X mg"
MS	Can mean morphine sulfate or magnesium sulfate	Write "morphine sulfate." Write "magnesium sulfate"
MSO_4 and $MgSO_4$	Confused for one another	Write "morphine sulfate." Write "magnesium sulfate"

[a]Exception: A trailing zero may be used only where required to demonstrate the level of precision of the value being reported, such as for laboratory results, imaging studies that report size of lesions, or catheter/tube sizes. It may not be used in medication orders or other medication-related documentation.

An abbreviation on the "do not use" list should not be used in any of its forms—upper or lower case, with or without periods (e.g., Q.D., QD, or qd). Any of those variations may be confusing and could be misinterpreted.

In addition, the Joint Commission has identified the following error-prone abbreviations for possible future inclusion on the official "do not use" list.

Additional Abbreviations, Acronyms, and Symbols

Do Not Use	Potential Problem	Use Instead
> (greater than)	Mistaken for 7 (seven) or the letter "L;" confused for one another	Write "greater than"
< (less than)	Mistaken for 7 (seven) or the letter "L;" confused for one another	Write "less than"
Abbreviations for drug names	Misinterpreted due to similar abbreviations for multiple drugs	Write drug names in full
Apothecary units	Unfamiliar to many practitioners; confused with metric units	Use metric units
@	Mistaken for 2 (two)	Write "at"
cc (for cubic centimeter)	Mistaken for U (units) when poorly written	Write "mL" or "ml" or "milliliters" ("mL" is preferred)
µg (for microgram)	Mistaken for mg (milligrams), resulting in 1,000-fold overdose	Write "mcg" or "micrograms"

Appendix E Complementary and Alternative Medicine Terms

Term	Meaning
acupressure	A treatment involving the application of pressure to those areas of the body used in acupuncture.
acupuncture	A traditional Chinese therapeutic technique involving puncturing the skin with fine needles to influence the flow of *qi* (vital energy).
African medicine	Traditional African therapeutic techniques based on naturopathic medicine, designed to treat the physical, mental, and spiritual causes of disease.
Alexander technique	A system of educational therapy involving the use of minimal effort for maximum movement to improve posture and alleviate pain.
allopathy	A term used to describe conventional Western medicine in contrast to alternative or complementary medicine.
Alpha Calm Therapy	A therapeutic technique involving guided imagery and hypnosis.
alternative medicine	A general term for therapeutic practices that fall outside the realm of evidence-based, mainstream medicine and are intended as replacements for conventional medical treatments. Alternative medical therapies fall into five main groups: complete medical systems (such as homeopathy and Chinese medicine), mind–body interventions (such as visualization and yoga), manipulative and body-based methods (such as chiropractic and massage), biologically based therapies (such as herbalism and macrobiotics), and energy therapies (such as qi gong and vibrational medicine).
Ama-Deus	A South American Indian system of healing.
apitherapy	Treatment of illness involving the administration of honeybee stings.
applied kinesiology	The use of muscle testing to identify illness. Applied kinesiology is based on the theory that weakness in certain muscles is associated with imbalances in the body.
aromatherapy	A form of treatment involving the use of concentrated oils from plants with healing properties.
art therapy	A therapy involving the use of artistic expression to promote emotional well-being.
Ayurveda (ī′yŭr-ved′dă)	A form of natural medicine, traditional in India, that provides an integrated approach to preventing and treating illness through lifestyle intervention and natural therapy. It involves *nadis* (canals) that carry *prana* (energy) throughout the body, *chakras* (centers of consciousness) that connect body and soul, and *marmas* (points on the body beneath which vital structures connect).
Bach flower therapy	A system of diagnosis and treatment, developed by British physician Edward Bach, that involves the use of flower essences.
biofeedback	A method of treatment that uses monitors to help patients recognize physiologic information of which they are normally unaware. Using this method, patients can learn to consciously control involuntary bodily processes such as blood pressure, temperature, gastrointestinal functioning, and brain wave activity.
bodywork	A group of therapeutic techniques that involve exercising or manipulating the body to produce healing.
Bowen technique	A form of bodywork developed by Australian Tom Bowen, in which certain body areas are lightly touched to stimulate energy flow.
chelation therapy	The administration of *chelating agents* (drugs that bind and remove certain materials from the body) to treat or prevent illness.

Term	Meaning
Chinese medicine	An ancient health care system, traditional in China, based on the concept that disease results from disruption of *qi* (vital energy) and imbalance of *yin* (negative energy) and *yang* (positive energy). Chinese medicine encompasses several therapies, including herbal and nutritional therapy, restorative physical exercises, meditation, acupuncture, and massage.
chiropractic	A diagnostic and therapeutic system based on the concept that disease results from nervous system malfunction. Treatment involves manipulation and adjustment of body structures, particularly the spinal column, to relieve local and distant physical ailments.
complementary medicine	A general term for therapeutic techniques intended to accompany and support mainstream, evidence-based medical treatments.
craniosacral therapy	A diagnostic and therapeutic system in which the bones of the skull are manipulated to remove impediments to cerebrospinal fluid flow, with the goals of stress relief, pain alleviation, and overall health improvement.
crystal therapy	A treatment that uses stones and crystals, which serve as conduits for healing energy, to restore function.
cupping	A treatment that consists of attaching a cup to the skin and evacuating the air within to increase local blood flow.
curanderismo	A Mexican-American traditional form of medicine encompassing acupuncture and homeopathy. From the Spanish *curar* (to treat or cure).
Feldenkrais method	A form of bodywork, developed by Israeli physicist Moshe Feldenkrais, that includes private instruction (*Functional Integration*), and group instruction (*Awareness through Movement*).
Gerson therapy	A dietary therapy by German physician Max Gerson, which involves sodium restriction, potassium supplementation, fat restriction, periodic protein restriction, and coffee enemas.
guided imagery	A technique in which patients imagine or visualize certain scenarios to improve health or promote healing.
herbal medicine	The practice of creating or prescribing plant-derived remedies for medical conditions.
holistic medicine	A general term for therapies, such as yoga, that emphasize the unity of body, mind, and spirit.
homeopathy	A therapeutic system based on the concept that a disease may be treated with minute doses of drugs that cause the same symptoms in healthy people as the disease itself. Substances are *potentized* (diluted) to prepare *remedies* (pharmacologic therapies) for patients. Homeopathic medicine is practiced in a holistic fashion, incorporating the elements of body, mind, and spirit.
hydrotherapy	The internal and external use of water for the treatment of disease.
hypnosis	The induction of trance to treat a wide variety of conditions such as substance addiction, pain, and phobias.
Kneipping	A system of natural healing developed by Dominican priest Sebastian Kneipp, based on the principles of hydrotherapy and herbalism.
Korean medicine	A form of medicine, traditional in Korea, which encompasses acupuncture and moxibustion.
macrobiotics	A vegetarian dietary therapy promoting health and longevity.
magnet therapy	A therapy in which magnetic fields are applied to the body using magnetic field-generating machines, mattresses, or blankets.
massage therapy	A therapeutic system involving muscle manipulation to reduce tension and pain, promote relaxation, or diminish symptoms of muscular or neurologic diseases.
meridian therapy	A therapeutic method that involves rhythmic breathing, visualization, and moving one's hands along *meridians,* lines along the body that are said to represent channels through which *qi* (vital energy) flows.
moxibustion	A traditional Chinese medical therapy that involves burning *moxa* (mugwort, or *Artemisia vulgaris*) and placing it at certain points on the body to stimulate *qi* (vital energy).

(continued)

Term	Meaning
myofascial release	Type of soft tissue treatment aimed at relaxing contracted muscles and improving blood and lymph flow by using a hands-on technique of gentle, sustained pressure and stretching to eliminate pain and restore normal function.
naturopathy	A therapeutic system involving the use of heat, water, light, air, and massage for treatment of disease. The discipline is composed of various alternative medical therapies, including homeopathy, herbal medicine, acupuncture, hydrotherapy, and manipulative therapy.
orthomolecular medicine	A therapeutic modality and preventative medicine strategy involving the use of natural substances found in food, such as vitamins, amino acids, and minerals, to treat and prevent disease. Supplementation with relatively large doses of vitamins (*megavitamin therapy*) is sometimes used.
qi gong	A component of Chinese medicine that uses physical movement, breathing regulation, and meditation to achieve optimum health. From the Mandarin *qi* (breath), and *gong* (work or technique).
reflexology	The practice of stimulating certain points on the body, most commonly on the feet, to improve health.
Reiki (rā'kē)	A therapy based on the theory that spiritual energy is channeled through a Reiki practitioner, healing the patient's body and spirit. From the Japanese *rei* (spirit or soul) and *ki* (energy or life force).
Rolfing	A form of myofascial massage, developed by American chemist Ida P. Rolf, that involves deep soft tissue manipulation to release stored tension and manually realign body structures.
shiatsu	A massage technique that originated in Japan, in which the thumbs, palms, fingers, and elbows are used to place pressure at certain points on the body.
spinal decompression therapy	Type of traction used to relieve back pain by gently stretching the spine. The stretching relieves pressure on the vertebral discs and spinal nerves, which promotes fluid movement and healing.
tai chi	An ancient Chinese martial art involving a combination of intentional, leveraged movement and focused breathing to improve health and longevity.
Trager	A form of bodywork, developed by Milton Trager, MD, which combines physical movement with meditation.
vibrational medicine	A general term for therapeutic modalities based on the concept that disease originates in subtle energy systems, which are affected by environmental, nutritional, spiritual, and emotional factors. Examples of vibrational medicine therapies include acupuncture, aromatherapy, homeopathy, crystal healing, and orthomolecular medicine.
yoga	A system of exercises for the improvement of physical and spiritual health, derived from Hindu tradition.

Rules for Forming Plurals

Appendix E

Some medical terms also add an -s (or -es) to make a plural, but many do not. They have special endings related to their origins in Greek or Latin. The following table shows some of the special plural endings common in medical terms.

Singular Ending	Example	Plural Ending	Example
a	vertebra	ae	vertebrae
en	lumen	ina	lumina
ex, ix, yx	index	ices	indices
is	testis	es	testes
on	spermatozoon	a	spermatozoa
um	diverticulum	a	diverticula
us	nucleus	i	nuclei
x, nx	phalanx	ges, nges	phalanges

Appendix G

Health-Related Websites

■ GENERAL

eMedicine.com
http://www.emedicine.com

Institute for Safe Medication Practices
http://www.ismp.org/

Joint Commission
http://www.jointcommission.org/

Lab Tests Online (public resource on clinical laboratory testing)
http://www.labtestsonline.org/

Mayo Clinic
http://www.mayoclinic.com

Medline Plus
http://medlineplus.gov/

Medline Plus–Drugs, Supplements, and Herbals Information
http://www.nlm.nih.gov/medlineplus/druginformation.html

OR-Live
http://www.or-live.com/archives.cfm

Radiology Info (resource explaining radiologic procedures and therapies)
http://www.radiologyinfo.org/

Rx List (drug information)
http://www.rxlist.com

Science-Based Medicine
https://www.sciencebasedmedicine.org

U.S. Department of Health and Human Services (HHS)
http://www.hhs.gov/

U.S. Food and Drug Administration
http://www.fda.org

United States Pharmacopeia (sets standards to ensure the quality of medicines)
http://www.usp.org

University of Cambridge The Naked Scientists
http://www.thenakedscientists.com/HTML/

BLOOD

AIDS information
http://www.aidsinfonyc.org

Aplastic Anemia and MDS (myelodysplastic syndromes)
http://www.aamds.org/aplastic/

Blood Information
http://www.bloodbook.com/index.html

Blood Transfusion and Surgery
http://www.yoursurgery.com/proceduredetails.cfm?br=7&proc=7

TheBody.com (AIDS and HIV information)
http://www.thebody.com/index.html

National Hemophilia Foundation (all bleeding disorders)
http://www.hemophilia.org/home.htm

CARDIOVASCULAR SYSTEM

American Heart Association
http://www.americanheart.org/

American College of Cardiology
http://www.acc.org

Angioplasty.org
http://www.angioplasty.org

Cardiothoracic Surgery Network
http://www.ctsnet.org/

Cardiothoracic Surgery Network Video Gallery
http://www.ctsnet.org/section/videogallery/

ECG Library
http://www.ecglibrary.com

The Franklin Institute Online (heart basics)
http://www.fi.edu/learn/heart/index.html

Heart Anatomy
http://www-medlib.med.utah.edu/WebPath/CVHTML/CVIDX.html#1

TheHeart.org
http://www.theheart.org

Heart Surgery Forum
http://www.hsforum.com/stories/storyReader$3387

Karolinska Institute
http://www.mic.ki.se/diseases/C14.html

Medical University of South Carolina (cardiovascular perfusion)
http://www.musc.edu/perfusion/interven.htm

Medtronic
http://www.medtronic.com/physician/cardiology.html

National Heart, Lung and Blood Institute
http://www.NHLBI.nih.gov/

PBS NOVA Cut to the Heart
http://www.pbs.org/wgbh/nova/heart/

St. Jude Medical Heart Library
http://www.heartlibrary.com/

University of California, San Diego, Medical Center
http://www.health.ucsd.edu/labref

COMPLEMENTARY AND ALTERNATIVE MEDICINE

The Alternative Medicine Homepage
http://www.pitt.edu/~cbw/altm.html

American Botanical Council
http://www.herbalgram.org

American Herbalists Guild
http://www.americanherbalistsguild.com

American Herbal Pharmacopoeia
http://www.herbal-ahp.org

American Herbal Products Association
http://www.ahpa.org

The American Holistic Medical Association
http://www.holisticmedicine.org

Ayurvedic Foundation
http://www.ayur.com

Health Action Network Society
http://www.hans.org

HealthWorld Online
http://www.healthy.net

The Herb Society of America
http://www.herbsociety.org

Homeopathy Home
http://www.homeopathyhome.com

The International Association for the Study of Traditional Asian Medicine
http://www.iastam.org/home.htm

National Center for Complementary and Alternative Medicine (National Institutes of Health)
http://nccam.nih.gov

Naturopathic Medicine Network
http://www.pandamedicine.com

Reuters Health News
http://www.reutershealth.com

DIGESTIVE SYSTEM

American College of Gastroenterology–Patient Information Link
http://www.acg.gi.org

American Society of Colon and Rectal Surgeons–Patient Education Link
http://www.fascrs.org

Colon Cancer Alliance
http://www.ccalliance.org/

Crohn's and Colitis Foundation of America
http://www.ccfa.org/

***H. pylori* and Ulcers**
http://www.cdc.gov/ulcer/

United Ostomy Association
http://www.uoa.org/

ENDOCRINE SYSTEM

American Diabetes Association
http://www.diabetes.org

Little People of America, Inc. (dwarfism information and support site)
http://www.lpaonline.org/

National Adrenal Diseases Foundation
http://www.medhelp.org/nadf/

Pituitary Network Association
http://www.pituitary.com/

INTEGUMENTARY SYSTEM

Site sponsored by the American Academy of Dermatology
http://www.skincarephysicians.com/

Indiana University, Department of Dermatology Homepage
http://www.iupui.edu/~derm/home.html

Johns Hopkins University, Dermatology Image Atlas
http://dermatlas.med.jhmi.edu/derm/

Lupus Foundation of America
http://www.lupus.org/newsite/index.html

National Institute of Arthritis and Musculoskeletal and Skin Diseases (health information related to musculoskeletal and integumentary systems)
http://www.niams.nih.gov/hi/index.htm

The National Organization for Albinism and Hypopigmentation (NOAH)
http://www.albinism.org/

Skin Cancer Foundation
http://www.skincancer.org/

University of Iowa, Department of Dermatology Homepage
http://tray.dermatology.uiowa.edu/home.html

University of Iowa, Dermatologic Image Database
http://tray.dermatology.uiowa.edu/DermImag.htm

University of Texas South Western Medical Center at Dallas, Department of Dermatology, glossary of common skin diseases and therapies
http://www.swmed.edu/home_pages/derma/glossary.htm

LYMPHATIC SYSTEM

Leukemia and Lymphoma Society
http://www.leukemia-lymphoma.org/hm_lls

Lymphoma Research Foundation
http://www.lymphoma.org/

National Heart, Lung and Blood Institute
http://www.NHLBI.nih.gov/

MALE AND FEMALE REPRODUCTIVE SYSTEMS AND OBSTETRICS

American College of Obstetrics and Gynecology–Patient Education
http://www.acog.org/

American Society of Plastic and Reconstructive Surgeons (breast augmentation)
http://www.plasticsurgery.org

American Society of Reproductive Medicine
http://www.asrm.com

American Urological Association–Patient Information
http://www.auanet.org/

Centers for Disease Control and Prevention (sexually transmitted diseases)
http://www.cdc.gov/

MENTAL HEALTH

American Psychiatric Association
http://www.psych.org

Autism Society of America
http://www.autism-society.org/

National Association of Anorexia Nervosa and Associated Disorders
http://www.anad.org/

National Attention Deficit Association
http://www.add.org/

National Depressive and Manic Depressive Association
http://ndmda.org/

National Institute of Mental Health
http://www.nimh.nih.gov

Schizophrenia
http://www.schizophrenia.com/

■ MUSCULOSKELETAL SYSTEM

American Academy of Orthopaedic Surgeons
http://www.aaos.org/

The American Orthopaedic Society for Sports Medicine
http://www.sportsmed.org/sml/index.asp

Arthritis Foundation
http://www.arthritis.org/

Medical News Today
http://www.medicalnewstoday.com/sections/bones/

Muscular Dystrophy Association
http://www.mdausa.org/

National Institute of Arthritis and Musculoskeletal and Skin Diseases
http://www.niams.nih.gov/hi/index.htm

National Institutes of Health (osteoporosis and related bone diseases)
http://www.osteo.org

National Osteoporosis Foundation
http://www.nof.org/

Orthopaedics.com
http://www.orthopaedics.com/

Scoliosis Research Society
http://www.srs.org/

Southern California Orthopaedic Institute
http://www.scoi.com/

University of Washington Orthopaedics and Sports Medicine
http://www.orthop.washington.edu/

Wayne State School of Medicine
http://www.med.wayne.edu/diagRadiology/RSNA2003/Overview.htm

Wheeless' Textbook of Orthopaedics presented by Duke Orthopaedics
http://www.wheelessonline.com/

■ NERVOUS SYSTEM

Alzheimer Association
http://www.alz.org/

American Epilepsy Society
http://www.aesnet.org/

American Sleep Apnea Association
http://sleepapnea.org/

American Stroke Association
http://www.strokeassociation.org/presenter.jhtml?identifier=1200037

Epilepsy Foundation
http://www.efa.org/index.cfm

Huntington's Disease Society of America
http://www.hdsa.org/

Hydrocephalus
http://www.patientcenters.com/hydrocephalus/news/whatishydro.html

Hydrocephalus Association
http://www.hydroassoc.org/

Myasthenia Gravis Foundation of America, Inc.
http://www.myasthenia.org/

National Multiple Sclerosis Society
http://www.nmss.org/

National Stroke Association
http://www.stroke.org/

Parkinson's Disease Foundation
http://www.pdf.org/index.cfm

Spina Bifida Association
http://www.sbaa.org/

Spine-Health
http://www.spine-health.com/dir/dir01.html#surgery

Whole Brain Atlas from Harvard Medical School
http://www.med.harvard.edu/AANLIB/home.html

ONCOLOGY (CANCER)

OncoLink
http://www.oncolink.com/

Susan G. Komen Breast Cancer Foundation
http://www.komen.org/

Testicular Cancer Resource Center
http://tcrc.acor.org/index.html

RESPIRATORY SYSTEM

American Academy of Allergy, Asthma and Immunology
http://www.aaaai.org/

American Association for Respiratory Care (professional site for respiratory care including career description, patient education link)
http://www.aarc.org/

American Lung Association
http://www.lungusa.org/

American Sleep Apnea Association
http://sleepapnea.org/

The Auscultation Assistant
http://www.wilkes.med.ucla.edu/lungintro.htm

Cystic Fibrosis Foundation
www.cff.org

It's Time to Focus on Lung Cancer site
http://www.lungcancer.org/

The National Emphysema Foundation
http://www.emphysemafoundation.org/

National Heart, Lung and Blood Institute
http://www.NHLBI.nih.gov/

The R.A.L.E. Repository
http://www.rale.ca/

SPECIAL SENSES

American Academy of Ophthalmology
http://www.aao.org

American Optometric Association—Link to Eye Conditions
http://www.aoanet.org/

American Society of Cataract and Refractive Surgery
http://www.ascrs.org/

American Speech-Language-Hearing Association
http://www.asha.org/

Eye Care America
http://www.eyecareamerica.org/

LASIK Institute
http://www.lasikinstitute.org/

Medem Medical Library–Eye Health
http://www.medem.com/medlb/sub_detaillb.cfm?parent_id=30&act=disp

National Eye Institute
http://www.nei.nih.gov/

National Institute on Deafness and Other Communication Disorders
http://www.nidcd.nih.gov/

URINARY SYSTEM

American Urological Association–Patient Information
http://www.auanet.org/

American Urologic Association Foundation
http://www.auafoundation.org/

Bladder Health Council
http://www.incontinence.org/

Lab Tests Online–Public resource on clinical laboratory testing
http://www.labtestsonline.org/

National Kidney Foundation
http://www.kidney.org/

United Ostomy Association (urostomy [urinary diversion] information)
http://www.uoa.org

Key English-to-Spanish Health Care Phrases

Appendix H

INTRODUCTORY PHRASES

English	Spanish	Spanish Pronunciation
please[a]	por favor	por fah-vor
thank you	gracias	*grah*-see-ahs
good morning	buenos días	*bway*-nos *dee*-ahs
good afternoon	buenas tárdes	*bway*-nas *tar*-days
good evening	buenas noches	*bway*-nas *noh*-chays
my name is	mi nombre es	me *nohm*-bray ays
yes/no	si/no	see/no
What is your name?	¿Cómo se llama?	¿Koh-moh say *yah*-mah?
How old are you?	¿Cuántos años tienes?	¿*Kwan*-tohs ahn-yos tee-*ayn*-ays?
Do you understand me?	¿Me entiende?	¿Me ayn-tee-*ayn*-day?
Speak slower.	Habla más despacio.	*Ah*-blah mahs days-*pah*-see-oh
Say it once again.	Repítalo, por favor.	Ray-*pee*-tah-loh, por fah-vor.
physician	médico	*may*-dee-koh
hospital	hospital	*oh*-spee-tahl
midwife	comadre	koh-*mah*-dray
native healer	curandero	ku-ran-*day*-roh

[a]You should begin or end any request with the word PLEASE (POR FAVOR).

GENERAL

English	Spanish	Spanish Pronunciation
zero	cero	say-roh
one	uno	oo-noh
two	dos	dohs
three	tres	trays
four	cuatro	*kwah*-troh
five	cinco	*sin*-koh
six	seis	says
seven	siete	see-*ay*-tay

(continued)

English	Spanish	Spanish Pronunciation
eight	ocho	oh-choh
nine	nueve	new-*ay*-vay
ten	diez	*dee*-ays
hundred	ciento, cien	see-*en*-toh, see-*en*
Monday	lunes	*loo*-nays
Tuesday	martes	*mar*-tays
Wednesday	miércoles	mee-*er*-cohl-ays
Thursday	jueves	*hway*-vays
Friday	viernes	vee-*ayr*-nays
Saturday	sábado	*sah*-bah-doh
Sunday	domingo	doh-*ming*-oh
right	derecho	day-*ray*-choh
left	izqierdo	ees-kee-*ayr*-doh
early in the morning	temprano por la mañana	tehm-*prah*-noh por lah mah-*nyah*-na
in the daytime	en el dìa	ayn el *dee*-ah
at noon	a mediodía	ah meh-dee-oh-*dee*-ah
at bedtime	al acostarse	al ah-kos-*tar*-say
at night	por la noche	por la *noh*-chay
today	hoy	oy
tomorrow	mañana	mah-*nyah*-nah
yesterday	ayer	ai-*yer*
week	semana	say-*may*-nah
month	mes	mace

■ PARTS OF THE BODY

English	Spanish	Spanish Pronunciation
the head	la cabeza	la kah-*bay*-sah
the eye	el ojo	el *o*-hoh
the ears	los oídos	lohs o-*ee*-dohs
the nose	la nariz	la nah-*reez*
the mouth	la boca	lah *boh*-kah
the tongue	la lengua	la *len*-gwah
the neck	el cuello	el koo-*eh*-yoh
the throat	la garganta	lah gar-*gan*-tah
the skin	la piel	la pee-el
the bones	los huesos	lohs oo-*ay*-sos

English	Spanish	Spanish Pronunciation
the muscles	los músculos	lohs *moos*-koo-lohs
the nerves	los nervios	lohs *nayhr*-vee-ohs
the shoulder blades	las paletillas	lahs pah-lay-*tee*-yahs
the arm	el brazo	el *brah*-soh
the elbow	el codo	el *koh*-doh
the wrist	la muñeca	lah moon-*yeh*-kah
the hand	la mano	lah *mah*-noh
the chest	el pecho	el *pay*-choh
the lungs	los pulmones	lohs puhl-*moh*-nays
the heart	el corazón	el koh-rah-*son*
the ribs	las costillas	lahs kohs-*tee*-yahs
the side	el flanco	el *flahn*-koh
the back	la espalda	lay ays-*pahl*-dah
the abdomen	el abdomen	el ahb-*doh*-men
the stomach	el estómago	el ays-*toh*-mah-goh
the leg	la pierna	lah pee-ehr-nah
the thigh	el muslo	el *moos*-loh
the ankle	el tobillo	el toh-*bee*-yoh
the foot	el pie	el *pee*-ay
urine	urino	u-*re*-noh

■ DISEASES

English	Spanish	Spanish Pronunciation
allergy	alergia	ah-*layr*-hee-ah
anemia	anemia	ah-*nay*-mee-ah
cancer	cancer	kahn-sayr
chickenpox	varicela	vah-ree-*say*-lah
diabetes	diabetes	dee-ah-bay-tees
diphtheria	difteria	deef-*tay*-ree-ah
German measles	rubéola	roo-*bay*-oh-lah
gonorrhea	gonorrea	gon-noh-*ree*-ah
heart disease	enfermedad del corazón	ayn-*fayr*-may-dahd del koh-rah-*son*
lead poisoning	envenenamiento con plomo	ayn-vay-nay-nah-mee-*ayn*-toh kohn *ploh*-moh
liver disease	enfermedad del hígado	ayn-*fayr*-may-dahd del *ee*-gah-doh
measles	sarampión	sah-rahm-pee-*ohn*
tuberculosis	tuberculosis	too-*bayr*-koo-lohs-sees

SIGNS AND SYMPTOMS

English	Spanish	Spanish Pronunciation
Do you have stomach cramps?	¿Tiene calambres en el estómago?	¿Tee-*ay*-nay kah-*lahm*-brays ayn el ays-*toh*-mah-goh?
chills?	escalofrios?	ays-kah-loh-*free*-ohs?
an attack of fever	un ataque de fiebre?	oon ah-*tah*-kay day fee-*ay*-bray?
hemorrhage?	hemoragia?	ay-moh-*rah*-hee-ah?
nosebleeds?	hemoragia por la nariz?	ay-moh-*rah*-hee-ah por-lah nah-*rees*?
unusual vaginal bleeding?	hemoragia vaginal fuera de los periodos?	ay-moh-*rah*-hee-ah *vah*-hee-nahl foo-*ay*-rah day lohs pay-ree-*oh*-dohs?
hoarseness?	ronquera?	rohn-*kay*-rah?
a sore throat?	le duele la garganta?	lay doo-*ay*-lay lah gahr-*gahn*-tah?
Does it hurt to swallow?	¿Le duele al tragar?	¿Lay doo-ay-lay ahl trah-gar?
Do you have any difficulty in breathing?	¿Tiene difficultad al respirar?	¿Tee-*ay*-nay dee-fee-kool-*tahd* ahl rays-*pee*-rahr?
Does it hurt you to breathe?	¿Le duele al respirar?	¿Lay doo-*ay*-lay ahl rays-*pee*-rahr?
How does your head feel?	¿Cómo siente la cabeza?	¿*Koh*-moh see-*ayn*-tay lah kah-*bay*-sah?
Is your memory good?	¿Es buena su memoria?	¿Ays *bway*-nah soo may-*moh*-ree-ah?
Do you have any pain the head?	¿Le duele la cabeza?	¿Lay doo-*ay*-lay lah kah-*bay*-sah?
Do you feel dizzy?	¿Tiene usted vértigo?	¿Tee-ay-nay ood-*stayd vehr*-tee-goh?
Are you tired?	¿Está usted cansado?	¿Ay-*stah* oo-*stayd* kahn-*sah*-doh?
Can you eat?	¿Puede comer?	¿*Pway*-day koh-*mer*?
Do you have a good appetite?	¿Tiene usted buen apetito?	¿Tee-*ay*-nay oo-*stayd* bwayn ah-pay-*tee*-toh?
How are your stools?	¿Cómo son sus heces fecales?	¿*Koh*-moh sohn soos *bay*-says fay-*kal*-ays?
Are they regular?	¿Son regulares?	¿Sohn ray-goo-*lah*-rays?
Are you constipated?	¿Está estreñido?	¿Ay-*stah* ays-trayn-*yee*-do?
Do you have diarrhea?	¿Tiene diarrea?	¿Tee-*ay*-nay dee-ah-*ray*-ah?
Do you have any difficulty urinating?	¿Tiene dificultad en orinar?	¿Tee-*ay*-nay dee-fee-kool-*tahd* ayn oh-ree-*nahr*?
Do you urinate involuntarily?	¿Orina sin querer?	¿Oh-*ree*-nah seen kay-rayr?
How long have you felt this way?	¿Desde cuándo se siente asi?	¿*Days*-day *kwan*-doh say see-*ayn*-tay ah-see?
What diseases have you had?	¿Qué enfermedades ha tenido?	¿Kay ayn-fer-may-*dah*-days hah tay-*nee*-doh?
Do you hear voices?	¿Tiene los voces?	¿Tee-*ay*-nay los *vo*-ses?

EXAMINATION

English	Spanish	Spanish Pronunciation
Remove your clothing.	Quítese su ropa.	*Key*-tay-say soo *roh*-pah.
Put on this gown.	Pongáse la bata.	Pohn-*gah*-say lah *bah*-tah.
We need a urine specimen.	Es necesário una muestra de su orina.	Ays nay-*say*-sar-ee-oh oo-nah moo-*ay*-strah day oh-*ree*-nah.
Be seated.	Siéntese.	See-*ayn*-tay-say.

English	Spanish	Spanish Pronunciation
Recline.	Acuestése.	Ah-*cways*-tay-say.
Sit up.	Siéntese.	See-*ayn*-tay-say.
Stand.	Parése.	*Pah*-ray-say.
Bend your knees.	Doble las rodíllas.	*Doh*-blay lahs roh-*dee*-yahs.
Relax your muscles.	Reláje los músculos.	Ray-*lah*-hay lohs *moos*-koo-lohs.
Try to...	Atente...	Ah-*tayn*-tay...
Try again.	Atente ótra vez.	Ah-*tayn*-tay *oh*-tra vays.
Do not move.	No se muéva.	Noh say moo-*ay*-vah.
Turn on (or to) your left side.	Voltese a su lado izquierdo.	Vohl-*tay*-say ah soo *lah*-doh is-key-*ayr*-doh.
Turn on (or to) your right side.	Voltése a su lado derécho.	Vohl-*tay*-say ah soo *lah*-doh day-*ray*-choh.
Take a deep breath.	Respíra profúndo.	Ray-*speer*-rah pro-*foon*-doh.
Hold your breath.	Deténga su respiración.	Day-*tayn*-gah soo ray-speer-ah-see-*ohn.*
Don't hold your breath.	No deténga su respiración.	Noh day-*tayn*-gah soo ray-speer-ah-see-*ohn.*
Cough.	Tosa.	*Toh*-sah.
Open your mouth.	Abra la boca.	*Ah*-brah lah *boh*-kah.
Show me...	Enséñeme...	Ayn-*sayn*-yay-may...
Here?	¿Aquí?	¿Ah-*kee*?
There?	¿Allí?	¿Ah-*yee*?
Which side?	¿En qué lado?	¿Ayn kay *lah*-doh?
Let me see your hand.	Enséñeme la mano.	Ayn-*sehn*-yay-may lah *mah*-noh.
Grasp my hand.	Apriete mi mano.	Ah-*pree*-ay-tay mee *mah*-noh.
Raise your arm.	Levante el brazo.	Lay-*vahn*-tay el *brah*-soh.
Raise it more.	Más alto.	Mahs *ahl*-toh.
Now the other.	Ahora el otro.	Ah-*oh*-rah el *oh*-troh.

■ TREATMENT

English	Spanish	Spanish Pronunciation
It is necessary.	Es necessario.	Ays neh-say-*sah*-ree-oh.
An operation is necessary.	Una operación es necesaria.	Oo-nah oh-peh-rah-see-*ohn* ays neh-say-*sah*-ree-ah.
a prescription	una receta	*oo*-na ray-say-tah
Use it regularly.	Tómelo con regularidad.	*Toh*-may-loh kohn ray-goo-*lah*-ree-dad.
Take one teaspoonful three times daily (in water).	Toma una cucharadita tres veces al dia, con agua.	*Toh*-may oo-na koo-chah-rah-*dee*-tah trays *vay*-says ahl *dee*-ah, kohn ah-gwah.
Gargle.	Haga gargaras.	*Ah*-gah gar-*gah*-rahs.
Use injection.	Use una inyección.	*Oo*-say *oo*-nah in-*yek*-see-ohn.
oral contraceptives	una pildora	*oo*-nah peel-*doh*-rah
a pill	una pastilla	*oo*-nah pahs-*tee*-yah
a powder	un polvo	oon *pohl*-voh
before meals	antes de las comidas	*ahn*-tays day lahs koh-*mee*-dahs
after meals	despues de las comidas	*days*-poo-ehs day lahs koh-mee-dahs

(continued)

English	Spanish	Spanish Pronunciation
every day	todos los día	*toh*-dohs lohs *dee*-ah
every hour	cada hora	*kah*-dah *oh*-rah
Breathe slowly–like this (in this manner).	Respire despacio–asi.	Rays-*pee*-ray days-*pah*-see-oh–ah-*see.*
Remain on a diet.	Estar a dieta.	Ays-*tar* a dee-*ay*-tah.

■ ADDITIONAL

English	Spanish	Spanish Pronunciation
Do you have pain?	¿Tiéne dolor?	¿Tee-*ay*-nay doh-*lohr*?
Where is the pain?	¿Adónde es el dolor?	¿Ah-*dohn*-day ays ayl doh-*lohr*?
Do you want medication for your pain?	¿Quiére medicación para su dolor?	¿Kee-*ay*-ray may-dee-kah-see-*ohn pah*-rah soo doh-*lohr*?
Are you comfortable?	¿Estás cómodo	¿Ay-*stahs koh*-moh-doh
Are you thirsty?	¿Tiéne sed?	¿Tee-*ay*-nay sayd?
You may not eat/drink.	No cóma/béba.	Noh *koh*-mah/bay-*bah.*
You can only drink water.	Solo puede tomar agua.	Soh-loh *pway*-day toh-mar *ah*-gwah.
Apply bandage to...	Ponga una vendaje a...	*Pohn*-gah *oo*-nah vehn-*dah*-hay ah...
Apply ointment.	Aplíquese unguento.	Ah-*plee*-kay-say oon-goo-*ayn*-toh.
Keep very quiet.	Estese muy quieto.	Ays-*tay*-say moo-ay key-*ay*-toh.
You must not speak.	No debe hablar.	No day-bay ah-blahr.
It will sting.	Va ardér.	Vah ahr-*dayr.*
You will feel pressure.	Vá a sentír presión.	Vah ah sayn-*teer* pray-see-*ohn.*
I am going to...	Voy a...	Voy ah...
Count (take) your pulse.	Tomár su púlso.	Toh-*marh* soo *pool*-soh.
Take your temperature.	Tomár su temperatúra.	Toh-*marh* soo taym-pay-rah-*too*-rah.
Take your blood pressure.	Tomar su presión.	Toh-*mahr* soo pray-see-*ohn.*
Give you pain medicine.	Dárle medicación para dolór.	*Dahr*-lay may-dee-kah-see-*ohn* pah-rah doh-*lohr.*
You should (try to)...	Trate de...	*Trah*-tay day...
Call for help/assistance.	Llamar para asisténcia.	Yah-*mahr* pah-rah ah-sees-*tayn*-see-ah.
Empty your bladder.	Orinar.	Oh-ree-*nahr.*
Do you still feel very weak?	¿Se siente muy débil todavía?	¿Say see-*ayn*-tay moo-ee *day*-beel toh-dah-*vee*-ah?
It is important to...	Es importánte que...	Ays eem-por-*tahn*-tay kay...
Walk (ambulate).	Caminar.	Kah-mee-*narh.*
Drink fluids.	Beber líquidos.	Bay-*bayr lee*-kee-dohs.

From Rosdahl CB (1995). *Textbook of Basic Nursing.* 6th ed. Philadelphia, PA: J.B. Lippincott.

Metric Measurements

Appendix I

Unit	Abbreviation	Metric Equivalent	U.S. Equivalent
		Units of Length	
Kilometer	km	1,000 meters	0.62 miles; 1.6 km/mile
Meter[a]	m	100 cm; 1,000 mm	39.4 inches; 1.1 yards
Centimeter	cm	1/100 m; 0.01 m	0.39 inches; 2.5 cm/inch
Millimeter	mm	1/1,000 m; 0.001 m	0.039 inch; 25 mm/inch
Micrometer	µm	1/1,000 mm; 0.001 mm	
		Units of Weight	
Kilogram	kg	1,000 g	2.2 lb
Gram[a]	g	1,000 mg	0.035 oz.; 28.5 g/oz
Milligram	mg	1/1,000 g; 0.001 g	
Microgram	mcm	1/1,000 mg; 0.001 mg	
		Units of Volume	
Liter[a]	L	1,000 mL	1.06 qt
Deciliter	dL	1/10 L; 0.1 L	
Milliliter	mL	1/1,000 L; 0.001 L	0.034 oz.; 29.4 mL/oz
Microliter	mcL	1/1,000 mL; 0.001 mL	

[a]Basic unit.

Answers to Exercises

Chapter 1

Exercise 1

1. bone
2. heart
3. brain, cerebrum
4. lung
5. skin

Exercise 2

1. crani
2. cardi
3. gastr
4. colo, colon
5. nephr, ren

Exercise 3

1. painful, difficult, abnormal
2. inside, within
3. around, surrounding
4. after, behind
5. many, much

Exercise 4

1. pre-
2. inter-
3. a-, an-
4. supra-, super-
5. sub-, infra-

Exercise 5

1. -tomy
2. -ium
3. -gram
4. -al
5. -logy
6. -algia
7. -itis
8. -ectomy
9. -ism
10. -oma

Exercise 6

1. neur/o
2. gastr/o
3. nephr/o, ren/o
4. cardi/o
5. crani/o
6. oste/o
7. pulmon/o
8. cerebr/o
9. dermat/o
10. col/o, colon/o

Exercise 7

1. intracranial
2. subpulmonary
3. cardiogram
4. ostealgia
5. gastrotomy

Exercise 8

1. glomeruli
2. varicoses
3. ova
4. larynges
5. ulcers

Exercise 9

Practice until your pronunciation matches that heard in the Audio Glossary in the Student Resources.

Exercise 10

1. arthr/o / -itis
   -joint / inflammation
   inflammation of joint
2. pulmon/o / -ary
   lung / pertaining to
   pertaining to the lung
3. colon/o / -itis
   colon / inflammation
   inflammation of colon
4. oste/o / -al
   bone / pertaining to
   pertaining to bone
5. cardi/o / -tomy
   heart / incision
   incision into the heart

Exercise 11

1. dermatitis
2. pericardial
3. neurology
4. osteoma
5. renal

Exercise 12

1. below, beneath
2. osteoma
3. colonoscopy
4. skin
5. stomach
6. between
7. heart
8. lungs or lung
9. without, not
10. lymphoma

Exercise 13

1. D
2. B
3. A
4. D
5. B
6. B
7. A
8. B
9. C
10. B

Exercise 14

1. carditis
2. phenomena
3. pericardial
4. gastrectomy
5. nuclei
6. osteoarthritis
7. cardiography
8. vertebrae
9. dermatitis
10. cardiopulmonary

Chapter 2

Exercise 1

1. uni-, mono-
2. bi-, di-
3. tri-
4. quad-, quadri-
5. multi-, poly-

Exercise 2

1. half
2. half
3. many, much
4. one
5. four

Exercise 3

1. against
2. not
3. away from, cessation, without
4. without, not
5. separate

Exercise 4

1. inter-
2. post-
3. per-, trans-
4. super-, supra-
5. en-, end-, endo-, intra-

Exercise 5

1. outer, outside
2. away from
3. before
4. below, beneath
5. together, with

Exercise 6

1. hetero-
2. normo-
3. mega-, megalo-, macro-
4. oligo-
5. homo-, homeo-, iso-
6. micro-

Exercise 7

1. dys-
2. eu-
3. hyper-
4. pan-
5. iso-
6. hypo-

Exercise 8

1. rapid, fast
2. new

3. slow
4. again, backward
5. false

Exercise 9

1. large, enlargement
2. abnormal condition
3. condition, disease, or disorder
4. state or condition
5. flow, discharge

Exercise 10

1. -algia
2. -itis
3. -rrhea
4. -emia
5. -oma
6. -pathy

Exercise 11

1. puncture to remove fluid
2. surgical removal
3. surgical opening
4. surgical repair, reconstruction

Exercise 12

1. -tomy
2. -rrhaphy
3. -stomy
4. -ectomy

Exercise 13

1. instrument for measuring
2. process of recording
3. pertaining to
4. process of examining, examination
5. record, recording
6. pertaining to
7. study of
8. pertaining to

Exercise 14

1. -logist
2. -oid
3. -ium
4. -ary
5. -genic
6. -scope

Exercise 15

1. intensive care unit
2. red blood cell
3. pulse rate
4. history and physical
5. activities of daily living
6. emergency department
7. liter
8. treatment
9. ears, nose, and throat
10. laboratory

Exercise 16

1. Sx
2. VS
3. Dx
4. Ht
5. STAT
6. p.r.n.
7. R
8. BP
9. Rx
10. noct.
11. PT
12. Hx

Exercise 17

1. im-
2. ad-
3. poly-
4. per-
5. intra-
6. exo-
7. hemi-
8. hetero-
9. hypo-
10. dys-

Exercise 18

1. -osis
2. -rrhaphy
3. -gram
4. -tomy
5. -emia
6. -pathy
7. -ar
8. -plasty
9. -graphy
10. -ium

Exercise 19

1. bisect
2. submandibular
3. cavitary
4. cardiotomy
5. psychology
6. endoscope
7. polyarthritis
8. thrombosis
9. panarthritis
10. semiconscious

Exercise 20

1. myositis
2. lobectomy
3. cardiopathy
4. intercostal
5. postnasal
6. microbiologist
7. lymphoma
8. dermatoid
9. cranioplasty
10. tenorrhaphy

Exercise 21

1. mononeural
2. hemiplegia
3. ectoderm
4. infrasonic
5. pericarditis
6. megalosplenia
7. heterogeneous
8. bradycardia
9. diarrhea
10. heterogenic
11. myalgia
12. cystorrhaphy
13. osteogenesis
14. edematous
15. gastrotomy

Exercise 22

Practice until your pronunciation matches that heard in the Audio Glossary in the Student Resources.

Chapter 3

Exercise 1

1. fiber
2. death
3. muscle
4. tumor
5. water, watery fluid
6. disease
7. nerve
8. blood
9. smooth
10. form, shape

Exercise 2

1. gluc/o
2. blast/o
3. viscer/o
4. hist/o
5. -pathy
6. -osis
7. oste/o
8. lip/o
9. -cyte
10. aden/o

Exercise 3

1. histology
2. exacerbation
3. somatic
4. lesion
5. chronic
6. idiopathic
7. acute
8. gene
9. necrosis
10. homeostasis

Exercise 4

1. group of organs with related functions; body system
2. localized physical changes in tissue characterized by redness, heat, pain, and swelling, in response to an injury
3. any virus, microorganism, or other substance that causes disease
4. lessening in severity of disease symptoms
5. pertaining to the internal organs
6. study of cells
7. study of the cause of disease
8. grouping of two or more tissues that are integrated to perform a specific function
9. sum of the normal chemical and physical changes occurring in tissue
10. excessive growth of tissue

Exercise 5

1. exacerbation
2. nucleus
3. systemic
4. tissue
5. idiopathic
6. cytoplasm
7. cytology
8. pathogen

Exercise 6

1. thorax, chest
2. neck
3. lumbar region, lower back
4. abdomen
5. pelvis

Exercise 7

1. abdominocentesis
2. thoracoplasty
3. pelvimeter

4. lumbar
5. cervicectomy
6. podalgia

Exercise 8
1. thorax
2. spinal cavity (vertebral canal)
3. umbilical region
4. abdomen
5. cranium

Exercise 9
1. limb
2. abdominal region above (superior to) the umbilical region
3. space within the chest occupied by the lungs, heart, and other organs
4. muscle between the abdominal and thoracic cavities
5. abdominal region to left or right of hypogastric region

Exercise 10
1. abdominal
2. hypochondriac
3. four
4. cranial
5. thoracic

Exercise 11
1. below
2. within
3. tail
4. back
5. front
6. on, following
7. side
8. head
9. around
10. back

Exercise 12
1. between the vertebrae
2. surrounding the heart
3. posterior to the cecum
4. pertaining to the middle of the carpal bone
5. pertaining to a high number

Exercise 13
1. distal
2. supine
3. superior
4. superficial
5. lateral
6. anterior
7. anteroposterior
8. ventral
9. cephalad
10. Fowler position

Exercise 14
1. lying face up
2. below or downward
3. vertical plane dividing the body into anterior and posterior halves
4. nearer the trunk or attachment point
5. toward the tail
6. horizontal plane dividing the body into upper (superior) and lower (inferior) halves
7. pertaining to both sides
8. body in standard reference position: standing erect, arms at the sides, palms facing forward
9. pertaining to the middle
10. pertaining to the back

Exercise 15
1. side
2. sagittal
3. deep
4. unilateral
5. posterior
6. distal
7. anterior or ventral
8. superior
9. decubitus
10. proximal

Exercise 16
1. black, dark
2. blue
3. yellow
4. green
5. white
6. red
7. color

Exercise 17
1. erythrocyte
2. xanthoderma
3. melanoma
4. chromaturia
5. leukocyte
6. blue discoloration of skin and other tissues

Exercise 18
1. surgical removal of lobe
2. after surgery
3. incision through the chest wall into the pleural (lung) space
4. above the clavicle (collar bone)
5. disease affecting a lymph node
6. organ enlargement
7. condition of bluish discoloration of the skin and other tissues

Exercise 19
1. cranial cavity
2. spinal cavity (vertebral canal)
3. thoracic cavity
4. diaphragm
5. abdominal cavity
6. pelvic cavity
7. abdominopelvic cavity

Exercise 20
1. right hypochondriac region
2. epigastric region
3. left hypochondriac region
4. right lumbar region
5. umbilical region
6. left lumbar region
7. right iliac region
8. hypogastric (suprapubic) region
9. left iliac region

Exercise 21
1. fibr/o / -osis
   fiber / abnormal condition
   abnormal condition of fibrous tissue
2. path/o / -genic
   disease / producing
   causing disease or abnormality
3. hem/o / -stasis
   blood / stopping
   stopping of bleeding
4. neur/o / -blast
   nerve / immature cell
   immature nerve cell
5. oste/o / necr/o / -osis
   bone / death / abnormal condition
   abnormal condition of death of bone tissue
6. cervic/o / brachi/o / -al
   neck / arm / pertaining to
   pertaining to the neck and arm
7. crani/o / cerebr/o / -al
   cranium, skull / brain, cerebrum
   pertaining to the skull and brain
8. super- / lateral
   above / side
   at the side and above
9. viscer/o / -megaly
   internal organs / enlargement
   enlargement of internal organs
10. hyper- / glyc/o / -emia
    above, excessive / glucose, sugar / blood (condition of)
    condition of above normal blood glucose

Exercise 22
1. hyperplasia
2. abnormal
3. study of form or shape
4. condition of lipids (fat) in the blood
5. remission
6. left lumbar
7. anteroposterior
8. Fowler or semirecumbent
9. blue
10. exacerbation

Exercise 23
1. the edge nearest the trunk (in direction of shoulder)
2. standing erect, arms at the sides, palms facing forward (anteriorly)
3. a group of organs with related functions
4. the cell nucleus
5. when it persists
6. study of the cause of a disease
7. a cavity is space (occupied by internal organs)
8. in the anatomic position, it is the posterior surface (back) of the hand
9. having a yellow discoloration of the skin
10. somatic condition

Exercise 24
1. B
2. A
3. D
4. C
5. A
6. B
7. D
8. C
9. D
10. B

Exercise 25
1. pulmonary
2. thoracotomy
3. lobectomy

4. lateral
5. proximally
6. distally

Exercise 26
1. bronchogenic
2. segmentectomy
3. lymphadenectomy
4. endotracheal
5. bronchoscopy
6. intercostal
7. subcutaneous

Exercise 27
Practice until your pronunciation matches that heard in the Audio Glossary in the Student Resources.

Exercise 28
1. chromosome
2. diaphragm
3. homeostasis
4. cephalad
5. cytoplasm
6. erythrocyte
7. decubitus
8. umbilical
9. pathogen
10. leukocyte
11. inflammation
12. cytology
13. metabolism
14. cyanosis
15. nuclei

Chapter 4

Exercise 1
1. epidermis
2. sudoriferous glands
3. skin, cutaneous membrane, or integument
4. sebaceous glands
5. subcutaneous layer or hypodermis
6. arrector pili muscles
7. dermis
8. epidermis
9. hair
10. sebum

Exercise 2
1. nail
2. hair follicle
3. sudoriferous glands
4. melanocytes
5. sebaceous glands
6. keratinocytes
7. keratin
8. adipocytes

Exercise 3
1. hair
2. wrinkle
3. nail
4. skin
5. fat
6. sebum (an oily secretion)
7. dry
8. skin
9. hard
10. red
11. sweat
12. cold

Exercise 4
1. xanth/o
2. seb/o
3. cyan/o
4. derm/o, dermat/o, cutane/o
5. electr/o
6. erythr/o
7. pachy/o
8. py/o
9. myc/o
10. melan/o
11. necr/o
12. hidr/o
13. kerat/o, scler/o

Exercise 5
1. softening
2. below, beneath
3. disease
4. inflammation
5. through
6. around, beside, near
7. instrument used to cut
8. eating
9. within
10. flowing, discharge
11. across, through
12. formation, growth
13. life

Exercise 6
1. inflammation of the skin
2. flow or discharge of pus
3. study of fungus
4. abnormal condition of sweating
5. excision or surgical removal of a nail

Exercise 7
1. xeroderma
2. dermatome
3. dermatologist
4. rhytidoplasty
5. necrosis
6. onychomalacia
7. melanocyte

Exercise 8
1. an- / hidr/o / -osis
   without, not / sweat / abnormal condition
   abnormal condition of not sweating
2. erythr/o / -derma
   red / skin condition
   condition of reddening of the skin
3. scler/o / -derma
   hard / skin
   condition of hardening of the skin
4. seb/o / -rrhea
   sebum / flow, discharge
   flow or discharge of oil or sebum
5. onych/o / -phagia
   nail / eating
   eating (one's) nails (nail biting)
6. rhytid/o / -ectomy
   wrinkle / excision, surgical removal
   surgical removal of wrinkles
7. trans- / derm/o / -al
   across, through / skin / pertaining to
   pertaining to across or through the skin
8. epi- / derm/o / -al
   on, following / skin / pertaining to
   pertaining to (the layer of skin) on top of the dermis
9. sub- / cutane/o / -ous
   below, beneath / skin / pertaining to
   pertaining to below or beneath the skin
10. myc/o / -osis
    fungus / abnormal condition
    abnormal condition of fungus
11. kerat/o / -genic
    hard / originating, producing
    producing hardness

Exercise 9
1. hyperplasia
2. atypical
3. purulent
4. indurated
5. integumentary
6. dysplasia
7. circumscribed
8. adipose

Exercise 10
1. erythematous
2. turgor
3. cyanosis
4. pallor
5. exfoliation
6. eschar
7. pruritic
8. diaphoresis

Exercise 11
1. full-thickness burn
2. papule
3. pustule
4. varicella
5. superficial burn; first-degree burn
6. cellulitis
7. herpes zoster; shingles
8. psoriasis
9. eczema
10. herpes simplex
11. keloid
12. jaundice
13. lesion
14. abrasion

Exercise 12
1. wheal
2. nevus
3. decubitus ulcer
4. nodule
5. scabies
6. cicatrix
7. rosacea
8. gangrene
9. contusion
10. tinea pedis

Exercise 13
1. vesicle
2. macule
3. verruca
4. pediculosis
5. tinea capitis
6. comedo

7. urticaria
8. paronychia
9. cyst
10. impetigo
11. burn
12. abscess

Exercise 14
1. tuberculosis skin test
2. scratch test
3. biopsy
4. culture and sensitivity
5. frozen section

Exercise 15
1. surgical repair of the skin
2. the use of heat, cold, electric current, or caustic chemicals to destroy tissue
3. skin grafting using skin from another species; xenograft
4. the act of cutting out

Exercise 16
1. incision and drainage
2. incision
3. irrigation
4. sutured
5. debrided
6. dermatoautoplasty

Exercise 17
1. rhytid/o wrinkle
2. derm/o skin
3. cry/o cold
4. electr/o electric, electricity
5. rhytid/o wrinkle
6. derm/o skin

Exercise 18
1. steroid
2. antiinfective
3. antifungal
4. pediculicide
5. antiinflammatory
6. liquid nitrogen
7. antipruritic
8. intralesional injection
9. scabicide

Exercise 19
1. medical aesthetician
2. dermatologist
3. dermatology

Exercise 20
1. purified protein derivative of tuberculin
2. culture and sensitivity
3. incision and drainage

Exercise 21
1. FS
2. bx
3. ED&C

Exercise 22
1. epidermis
2. dermis
3. subcutaneous layer (hypodermis)
4. sebaceous gland
5. arrector pili muscle
6. hair follicle
7. sudoriferous (sweat) gland

Exercise 23
1. hidr/o sweat
2. kerat/o hard
3. cry/o cold
4. dermat/o skin
5. scler/o hard
6. onych/o; myc/o nail; fungus
7. rhytid/o wrinkle
8. py/o pus
9. lip/o fat
10. seb/o sebum
11. dermat/o; myc/o skin; fungus
12. cutane/o skin

Exercise 24
1. an- / hidr/o / -osis
without, not / sweat / abnormal condition
abnormal condition of not sweating
2. erythr/o / cyan/o / -osis
red / blue / abnormal condition
abnormal condition characterized by red and blue coloring
3. trich/o / -pathy
hair / disease
disease of the hair
4. py/o / -derma
pus / skin condition'
condition of pus in the skin
5. para- / onych/o / -ia
beside / nail / pertaining to
pertaining to beside the nail (nail infection)
6. dermat/o / -logist
skin / one who specializes in
physician who specializes in the skin
7. trans- / derm/o / -al
across, through / skin / pertaining to
pertaining to across or through the skin
8. dermat/o / heter/o / -plasty
skin / other, different / surgical
repair, reconstruction surgical repair or reconstruction of the skin using skin from another species
9. pachy/o / -derma
thick / skin condition
condition of thick skin
10. onych/o / -malacia
nail / softening
softening of the nail
11. cyan/o / -osis
blue / abnormal condition
abnormal condition characterized by blue coloring
12. onych/o / -phagia
nail / to eat
to eat one's nails (nail biting)
13. intra- / derm/o / -al
within / skin / pertaining to
pertaining to within the skin
14. xer/o / -derma
dry / skin condition
condition of dry skin

Exercise 25
1. epidermis, dermis, and subcutaneous (hypodermis) layer (in any order)
2. arrector pili
3. comedo
4. sudoriferous
5. medical aesthetician
6. abscess
7. rhytidoplasty
8. adipocytes
9. indurated
10. vitiligo
11. Tinea
12. excoriation
13. furuncle
14. necrosis
15. tinea pedis
16. albinism
17. fissure

Exercise 26
1. B
2. C
3. B
4. C
5. D
6. D
7. A
8. C
9. B

Exercise 27
1. dermabrasion
2. circumscribed
3. debridement
4. carbuncle
5. tinea
6. impetigo
7. urticaria
8. paronychia
9. scratch
10. dermatome

Exercise 28
1. A
2. B
3. D
4. C
5. D
6. A
7. B
8. D

Exercise 29
1. C
2. D
3. A
4. the back of the foot

Exercise 30
1. B
2. A
3. C
4. pertaining to the nose and stomach

Exercise 31
Practice until your pronunciation matches that heard in the Audio Glossary in the Student Resources.

Exercise 32
1. anhidrosis
2. cicatrix
3. dermatomycosis
4. onychophagia

5. urticaria
6. psoriasis
7. gangrene
8. tinea
9. dysplasia
10. pruritic
11. keratogenic
12. xeroderma
13. jaundice
14. erythematous
15. arrector pili muscles

Chapter 5

Exercise 1

1. humerus
2. metacarpal bones
3. scapula
4. sternum
5. diaphysis
6. tendon
7. fascicle
8. calcaneus
9. axial skeleton
10. vertebrae

Exercise 2

1. moving away from the body's midline
2. band of strong connective tissue that connects bones or cartilage at a joint
3. the site where bones come together; joint
4. bending foot upward the tibia
5. the socket of the hip bone where the femur articulates
6. the skull
7. lower jawbone
8. a joint that moves freely; the joint cavity contains synovial fluid; diarthrosis
9. upper jawbone
10. dense connective tissue attached to bone in many joints
11. the growth area of a long bone
12. muscle tone; tonus

Exercise 3

1. patella
2. meniscus
3. unstriated
4. Fascia
5. fibula
6. ilium
7. lamina
8. clavicle
9. metaphysis
10. tibia
11. bursa
12. ischium, pubis
13. vertebrae
14. tarsal
15. flexion

Exercise 4

1. endosteum
2. compact bone
3. radius
4. carpal bones
5. spongy bone
6. sacrum
7. intervertebral disc
8. ulna
9. epiphyseal plate
10. osteocyte

Exercise 5

1. clavicle
2. humerus
3. cancellous
4. ligament
5. insertion
6. antagonist
7. striated, unstriated
8. synovial
9. eversion
10. suture
11. ligaments
12. sacrum

Exercise 6

1. cranium, skull
2. lumbar region, lower back
3. crooked, twisted
4. bone
5. sternum
6. maxilla
7. cartilage
8. carpals
9. tendon
10. vertebra
11. fascia, band
12. muscle
13. mandible
14. sacrum
15. femur

Exercise 7

1. cost/o
2. tars/o
3. lei/o
4. fibul/o
5. burs/o
6. arthr/o, articul/o
7. pelv/i, pelv/o
8. thorac/o
9. ischi/o
10. clavic/o, clavicul/o
11. lamin/o
12. cervic/o
13. menisc/o
14. phalang/o

Exercise 8

1. surgical repair, reconstruction
2. weakness
3. below, beneath
4. development, nourishment
5. excision, surgical removal
6. growth
7. suture
8. together, with
9. to split
10. to break

Exercise 9

1. inflammation of bone
2. condition of bent forward
3. muscle pain
4. inflammation of a bursa
5. inflammation of the maxilla
6. below the scapula
7. relating to the pelvis
8. inflammation of a tendon
9. between vertebrae
10. surgical repair of a joint

Exercise 10

1. myositis
2. cranioplasty
3. patellectomy
4. tenorrhaphy
5. arthralgia
6. intracranial
7. tarsectomy
8. meniscitis
9. discectomy
10. chondroplasty

Exercise 11

1. intercostal
2. femoral
3. intervertebral
4. ischiofemoral
5. synovial
6. pelvic
7. subscapular
8. carpal

Exercise 12

1. humeral
2. intercostal
3. substernal
4. suprapatellar
5. cranial
6. sacral
7. intervertebral
8. intracranial
9. lumbar
10. costovertebral
11. submandibular
12. lumbosacral

Exercise 13

1. scoliosis
2. tendonitis or tendinitis
3. fracture
4. chondromalacia
5. bursitis
6. osteoporosis
7. rickets
8. tenodynia
9. spondylarthritis
10. ankylosing spondylitis
11. kyphosis
12. arthralgia
13. arthritis
14. osteomalacia

Exercise 14

1. myasthenia
2. polymyositis
3. gout
4. strain, sprain
5. rheumatoid arthritis
6. fibromyalgia
7. bursolith
8. atrophy
9. carpal
10. dyskinesia
11. tenosynovitis

Exercise 15

1. arthritis
2. arthralgia
3. rachischisis
4. maxillitis
5. tenodynia
6. bursitis

7. myalgia
8. arthrochondritis
9. osteomalacia

Exercise 16

1. hyper- / -trophy
   above, excessive / development
   excessive development (of a part or organ)
2. scoli/o / -osis
   crooked, twisted / abnormal condition
   abnormal condition of crooked or twisted (spine)
3. crani/o / -schisis
   cranium, skull / split
   split skull
4. carp/o / -ptosis
   carpal bones / dropping
   dropping of the carpal bones
5. ankyl/o / -osis
   stiff / abnormal condition
   abnormal condition of stiffening (of a joint)
6. burs/o / -lith
   bursa / stone
   calculus (stone) in a bursa
7. a- / -trophy
   not, without / development
   without (absence of) development
8. oste/o / -itis
   bone / inflammation
   inflammation of bone
9. brady- / kines/o / -ia
   slow / movement / condition of
   condition of slow movement
10. poly- / myos/o / -itis
    many, much / muscle / inflammation
    inflammation of many muscles

Exercise 17

1. computed tomography
2. electromyogram
3. arthrography
4. nuclear medicine imaging
5. radiography
6. creatine kinase
7. uric acid
8. rheumatoid factor

Exercise 18

1. bone densitometry
2. range of motion testing
3. bone scan
4. arthroscopy
5. magnetic resonance imaging
6. erythrocyte sedimentation rate
7. synovial fluid analysis

Exercise 19

1. synovectomy
2. reduction
3. myorrhaphy
4. chondrectomy
5. arthroclasia
6. discectomy
7. traction
8. cranioplasty
9. spondylosyndesis
10. osteoclasis
11. patellectomy
12. osteoclast
13. chondroplasty
14. meniscectomy
15. maxillotomy
16. arthroplasty

Exercise 20

1. ostectomy
2. bursectomy
3. craniotomy
4. myoplasty
5. orthosis
6. open reduction, internal fixation
7. laminectomy
8. tenorrhaphy
9. arthrocentesis
10. prosthesis

Exercise 21

1. myoplasty
2. chondrectomy
3. arthrodesis
4. tenorrhaphy
5. craniotomy

Exercise 22

1. oste/o / -clasis
   bone / to break
   intentional fracture of bone (to correct deformity)
2. my/o / -rrhaphy
   muscle / suture
   suture of a muscle
3. arthr/o / -plasty
   joint / surgical repair, reconstruction
   surgical repair of a joint
4. phalang/o / -ectomy
   phalanges / excision, surgical removal
   excision of a phalanges
5. rachi/o / -tomy
   spine / incision
   incision into the spine
6. disc/o / -ectomy
   vertebral disc / excision, surgical removal
   excision of (part or all) of a vertebral disc
7. chondr/o / -plasty
   cartilage / surgical repair, reconstruction
   surgical repair of cartilage
8. arthr/o / -centesis
   joint / puncture to aspirate
   puncture to aspirate (fluid) from a joint
9. synov(i)/o / -ectomy
   synovial joint / excision, surgical or fluid removal
   excision of (part or all of) a synovial membrane
10. oste/o / -ectomy
    bone / excision, surgical removal
    excision of bone

Exercise 23

1. skeletal muscle relaxant
2. analgesic
3. corticosteroid
4. nonsteroidal antiinflammatory drug (NSAID)

Exercise 24

1. chiropractor
2. podiatrist
3. orthotist
4. osteopath
5. rheumatologist
6. orthopedist

Exercise 25

1. magnetic resonance imaging
2. myasthenia gravis
3. Second cervical vertebra
4. muscular dystrophy
5. range of motion
6. open reduction, internal fixation
7. electromyogram
8. carpal tunnel syndrome
9. rheumatoid arthritis
10. nonsteroidal antiinflammatory drug
11. erythrocyte sedimentation rate, rheumatoid factor, creatine kinase

Exercise 26

1. T4
2. Fx
3. CT
4. L3
5. MRI
6. OA

Exercise 27

1. vertebrae
2. carpal bones
3. phalanges
4. tarsal bones
5. cranium
6. mandible
7. clavicle
8. acromion
9. scapula
10. sternum
11. humerus
12. femur
13. patella

Exercise 28

1. tendons
2. biceps brachii
3. origins
4. insertion
5. humer/o
6. ten/o, tend/o, tendin/o

Exercise 29

1. ankyl/o / -osis
   stiff / abnormal condition
   abnormal condition of stiffening (of a joint)
2. carp/o / -ptosis
   carpal bones / dropping
   dropping of the carpal bones; wrist-drop

3. electr/o / my/o / -gram
electricity / muscle / record, recording
recording of a muscle's electrical activity
4. myo / -itis
muscle / inflammation
inflammation of muscle
5. kyph/o / -osis
humpback / abnormal condition
abnormal condition of humpback
6. intra- / crani / o/-al
within / skull / pertaining to
pertaining to within the skull
7. poly- / my/o / -itis
many, much / muscle / inflammation
inflammation of many muscles
8. supra- / patell/o / -ar
above / patella / pertaining to
pertaining to above the patella
9. ten/o / -dynia
tendon / pain
pain in a tendon
10. arthr/o / -centesis
joint / puncture to aspirate
puncture to aspirate (fluid) from a joint
11. chondr/o / -ectomy
cartilage / excision, surgical removal
surgical removal of cartilage
12. cost/o / vertebr/o / -al
rib / vertebra / pertaining to
pertaining to the ribs and vertebrae
13. sub- / mandibul/o / -ar
below, / mandible / pertaining to beneath, below
pertaining to below the mandible
14. oste/o / arthr/o / -itis
bone / joint / inflammation
inflammation of bone and joint
15. my/o / -rrhaphy
muscle / suture
suture of a muscle
16. oste/o / -malacia
bone / softening
softening of bones
17. arthr/o / -scopy
joint / process of examining, examination
process of examining (the interior of) a joint
18. my/o / -algia
muscle / pain
muscle pain
19. spondyl/o / arthr/o/ / -itis
vertebra / joint / inflammation
inflammation of a vertebral joint

Exercise 30

1. adduction
2. Orthotics
3. arthroplasty
4. podiatrist
5. prosthesis
6. Carpal tunnel syndrome
7. compact
8. exostosis
9. Fibromyalgia
10. Extension
11. bone scan
12. dystrophy
13. rheumatoid arthritis (RA)
14. range of motion (ROM)
15. hyperkinesia
16. Chiropractic
17. dorsiflexion
18. orthopedics

Exercise 31

1. A suture is an immovable joint, such as one that joins the skull bones together.
2. Ligaments attach bones to bones.
3. Metacarpal bones are found in the hand.
4. Osseous means it is composed of bone (or bony) tissue.
5. Osteopathy is school of medicine emphasizing manipulative measures in addition to techniques of conventional medicine.
6. A tenorrhaphy is done when a tendon is partly or completely separated (torn).
7. Rickets results from a vitamin D deficiency in childhood.
8. Arthrodesis surgically stiffens the joint.
9. Uric acid crystals are deposited in the joint.
10. An x-ray image (arthrogram) of a joint using a contrast dye is produced.
11. The insertion is the movable end of the muscle and it is the end of the muscle attached to bone that moves during muscle contraction.
12. The xiphoid process is the inferior portion of the sternum.
13. Cardiac muscle (striated, involuntary) muscle is the third type of muscle tissue.
14. Rachiotomy is another term for a laminotomy.

Exercise 32

1. C
2. D
3. A
4. D
5. A
6. D
7. B
8. A
9. B
10. D
11. A
12. A
13. C
14. A

Exercise 33

1. A
2. D
3. B
4. C
5. B
6. C
7. D
8. A
9. D
10. B
11. A

Exercise 34

1. paraspinal
2. sacral
3. myofascial
4. range of motion
5. the knees; "bilateral total knee replacement"

Exercise 35

1. arthralgia
2. myalgia
3. arthritis
4. range of motion
5. rheumatoid arthritis
6. inflammation in many joints

Exercise 36

Practice until your pronunciation matches that heard in the Audio Glossary in the Student Resources.

Exercise 37

1. laminotomy
2. osteoarthritis
3. rheumatology
4. tenodynia
5. osseous
6. clavicle
7. myorrhaphy
8. vertebrae
9. fibromyalgia
10. dorsiflexion
11. ankylosis
12. polymyositis
13. fascia
14. osteoporosis
15. intervertebral

Chapter 6

Exercise 1

1. pons
2. occipital lobe
3. cerebrum
4. central nervous system (CNS)
5. cerebellum
6. ventricle
7. temporal lobe
8. parietal lobe
9. frontal lobe
10. brainstem

Exercise 2

1. portion of the central nervous system contained in the vertebral canal that conducts nerve impulses to and from the brain and body
2. outer layer of the cerebrum; controls higher mental functions
3. whitish cordlike structure that transmits stimuli from the central nervous system to another area of the body or from the body to the central nervous system
4. groove or depression on the surface of the brain
5. thin inner layer of the meninges that attaches directly to the brain and spinal cord
6. part of the nervous system external to the brain and spinal cord that consists

of all other nerves throughout the body
7. part of the brainstem that contains reflex centers associated with eye and head movements
8. 12 pairs of nerves that emerge from the brain
9. part of the central nervous system contained within the cranium
10. three membranous coverings of the brain and spinal cord

Exercise 3
1. ganglion
2. spinal nerves
3. neuron
4. arachnoid mater
5. cerebrospinal fluid
6. gyrus
7. neuroglia
8. dura mater
9. diencephalon

Exercise 4
1. entire brain
2. glue, neuroglia
3. brain, cerebrum
4. nerve
5. hard, dura mater
6. meninges
7. cerebellum (little brain)
8. nerve root
9. sleep
10. mind, mental
11. ganglion
12. thalamus
13. cranium, skull
14. sensation, perception
15. speech
16. vertebra
17. bone marrow, spinal cord
18. spine
19. mind, mental
20. gray matter

Exercise 5
1. gli/o
2. ventricul/o
3. encephal/o
4. anxi/o
5. myel/o
6. cerebell/o
7. cortic/o
8. gangli/o
9. thalam/o
10. schiz/o
11. spin/o
12. thym/i, thym/o
13. cerebr/o
14. ment/o, phren/o, psych/o,
15. spondyl/o, vertebr/o
16. esthesi/o
17. dur/o
18. hallucin/o
19. narc/o

Exercise 6
1. one who specializes in
2. half
3. attraction for
4. excited state, obsession
5. abnormal fear, aversion to, sensitivity to
6. many, much
7. four
8. condition of
9. incision
10. above, excessive
11. partial or incomplete paralysis
12. below, deficient
13. paralysis
14. on, upon, following
15. relating to or caused by stroke or seizure

Exercise 7
1. inflammation of the brain
2. incision into the skull
3. x-ray study of the spinal cord (specifically, the subarachnoid space and its contents)
4. pertaining to glia or neuroglia
5. condition of difficulty speaking
6. pertaining to the spine
7. pertaining to the cerebellum
8. one who specializes in the mind
9. splitting of the mind
10. condition of loss of sensation
11. disease of the spinal nerve roots
12. disease involving many nerves

Exercise 8
1. myelitis
2. craniotomy
3. neuropathy
4. glioma
5. cranial
6. dysesthesia
7. meningitis
8. subdural
9. meningioma
10. encephalopathy

Exercise 9
1. pertaining to the meninges
2. pertaining to the cranium or skull
3. pertaining to on or outside the dura mater
4. pertaining to the cerebrum
5. pertaining to a lack of blood flow
6. pertaining to a nerve root
7. pertaining to the mind

Exercise 10
1. bipolar
2. dural
3. neural
4. glial
5. ictal
6. postictal
7. cerebellar
8. ischemic
9. subdural

Exercise 11
1. cerebr/o; cerebrum
2. radicul/o; nerve root
3. ment/o; mind
4. dur/o; dura mater
5. spin/o; spine
6. cerebell/o; cerebellum (little brain)

Exercise 12
1. concussion
2. stupor
3. coma
4. parkinsonism, Parkinson disease
5. disorientation
6. stroke
7. multiple sclerosis (MS)
8. cerebral aneurysm
9. cerebral embolism
10. amnesia
11. amyotrophic lateral sclerosis (ALS), Lou Gehrig disease
12. paraplegia

Exercise 13
1. obsessive-compulsive disorder (OCD)
2. anxiety
3. attention deficit hyperactivity disorder (ADHD)
4. posttraumatic stress disorder (PTSD)
5. paranoia
6. delusions
7. compulsion
8. depression
9. catatonia
10. agoraphobia
11. autism
12. delirium

Exercise 14
1. poly- / neur/o / -itis
   many, much / nerve / inflammation
   inflammation of many nerves
2. radicul/o / -pathy
   nerve roots / disease
   disease of the nerve roots
3. a- / phas/o / -ia
   without, not / speech / condition of
   condition of without speech
4. mening/o / myel/o / -cele
   meninges / spinal bone / herniation, marrow, cord protrusion
   herniation or protrusion of the meninges and spinal cord
5. encephal/o / -itis
   brain / inflammation of
   inflammation of the brain
6. hemi- / -paresis
   half / partial or incomplete paralysis
   partial paralysis of half of the body
7. neur/o / -algia
   nerve / pain
   pain in a nerve
8. schiz/o / -phrenia
   split / the mind
   splitting of the mind
9. sub- / dur/o / -al
   below, / hard, dura / pertaining to beneath matter
   pertaining to below the dura matter (deep to the dura mater)
10. poli/o / myel/o / -itis
    gray matter / bone marrow / inflammation of spinal cord
    inflammation of the gray matter of the spinal cord

Exercise 15
1. Glasgow coma scale (GCS)
2. evoked potential studies
3. Babinski sign
4. positron emission tomography
5. cerebral angiography

Exercise 16
1. lumbar puncture
2. polysomnography
3. magnetic resonance imaging (MRI)
4. deep tendon reflex (DTR)
5. electroencephalography (EEG)
6. myelogram

Exercise 17
1. neuroplasty
2. craniectomy
3. laminectomy
4. craniotomy
5. radicotomy
6. neurolysis
7. ganglionectomy
8. psychotherapy

Exercise 18
1. neuroplasty
2. ganglionectomy
3. rhizotomy or radicotomy
4. craniectomy

Exercise 19
1. anticonvulsant
2. antidepressant
3. antianxiety agent, anxiolytic
4. antiinflammatory
5. sedative
6. analgesic
7. neuroleptic
8. epidural injection

Exercise 20
1. drug that reduces anxiety
2. drug used treat mental illnesses
3. drug that provides loss of sensation
6. drug that promotes sleep

Exercise 21
1. psychologist
2. neurology
3. psychiatry
4. psychiatrist
5. EEG technician
6. psychology
7. neurologist

Exercise 22
1. cerebral palsy
2. transient ischemic attack
3. lumbar puncture
4. multiple sclerosis
5. cerebral spinal fluid
6. obsessive-compulsive disorder
7. magnetic resonance imaging
8. cerebrovascular accident

Exercise 23
1. EEG
2. CVA
3. ALS
4. PTSD
5. ADHD
6. PET
7. CNS
8. DTR

Exercise 24
1. frontal lobe
2. cerebral cortex
3. parietal lobe
4. occipital lobe
5. cerebellum
6. brain stem
7. temporal lobe

Exercise 25
1. pia mater
2. arachnoid mater
3. dura mater

Exercise 26

1. meningi/o / -cyte
   meninges / cell
   cell of the meninges
2. neur/o / -pathy
   nerve / disease
   disease of a nerve
3. crani/o / cerebr/o / -al
   cranium, skull / brain, / pertaining to cerebrum
   pertaining to the skull and brain
4. quadri- / -paresis
   four / partial or incomplete paralysis
   partial paralysis in four limbs
5. radicul/o / myel/o / -pathy
   nerve root / bone marrow, spinal cord / disease
   disease involving the spinal cord and the nerve roots
6. electr/o / encephal/o / -graphy
   electric, electricity / brain / writing, description
   electrical recording of brain activity
7. encephal/o / -scopy
   brain / process of examining, examination
   process of examining the brain
8. poli/o / dys- / -trophy
   gray matter / painful, / development, difficult, nourishment abnormal
   wasting of the gray matter of the nervous system
9. spondyl/o / -osis
   vertebra / abnormal condition
   abnormal condition of the vertebra`
10. ganglion/o / -ectomy
    ganglion / excision, surgical removal
    excision of a ganglion

Exercise 27
1. hallucinations
2. Lethargy
3. ataxia
4. Bell palsy
5. sleep apnea
6. Alzheimer disease
7. anesthesia
8. electroencephalography (EEG)
9. shingles
10. paranoia
11. Cerebral palsy (CP)
12. meningitis
13. Radiculopathy
14. migraine
15. cerebral thrombosis
16. cerebrum
17. gyri
18. brainstem
19. Syncope
20. epilepsy

Exercise 28
1. D
2. C
3. A
4. B
5. B
6. B
7. C
8. D
9. C
10. B
11. B
12. B
13. C
14. C

Exercise 29
1. C
2. C
3. D
4. A
5. D
6. C
7. D
8. B

Exercise 30
1. B
2. C
3. B
4. B
5. C

Exercise 31
1. aphasia
2. cerebrovascular accident
3. transient ischemic attack
4. electroencephalogram
5. seizure
6. Lamictal and Dilantin
7. carotid endarterectomy

Exercise 32
Practice until your pronunciation matches that heard in the Audio Glossary in the Student Resources.

Exercise 33
1. cerebrum
2. encephalopathy
3. temporal
4. delusion
5. Alzheimer
6. schizophrenia
7. radiculopathy
8. catatonia
9. cerebellum

10. myelopathy
11. anesthesia
12. neuropathy
13. parietal
14. hallucination
15. seizure

Chapter 7

Exercise 1

1. lens
2. vitreous humor
3. choroid
4. orbit
5. iris
6. conjunctiva
7. pupil
8. cornea
9. optic nerve
10. nasolacrimal ducts

Exercise 2

1. retina
2. sclera
3. lacrimal ducts
4. choroid
5. tarsal glands, meibomian glands
6. lens
7. conjunctiva
8. lacrimal glands
9. pupil
10. aqueous humor

Exercise 3

1. tarsal glands
2. retina
3. aqueous humor
4. optic nerve
5. cornea
6. vitreous humor
7. lacrimal glands
8. iris
9. sclera

Exercise 4

1. eye
2. tears or tear ducts
3. iris
4. pupil (of the eye)
5. tears or lacrimal (tear) ducts
6. cornea
7. eye
8. pupil (of the eye)
9. cornea
10. eyelid

Exercise 5

1. conjunctiv/o
2. scler/o
3. phot/o
4. blephar/o
5. ton/o
6. presby/o
7. dipl/o
8. opt/o
9. ir/o or irid/o
10. retin/o

Exercise 6

1. paralysis
2. vision
3. prolapse, drooping, sagging
4. two, twice
5. destruction, breakdown, separation
6. flow, discharge
7. surgical fixation
8. softening
9. surgical repair, reconstruction
10. process of examining, examination
11. dilation, stretching
12. abnormal fear, aversion to, sensitivity to

Exercise 7

1. ir/o
2. retin/o
3. pupill/o
4. conjunctiv/o
5. scler/o
6. corne/o

Exercise 8

1. conjunctivitis
2. diplopia
3. blepharoptosis
4. pupillometer
5. photophobia
6. retinopathy
7. iridoplegia
8. keratoplasty
9. sclerotomy
10. ophthalmologist

Exercise 9

1. instrument for examining the eye
   eye
   instrument for examining
2. measurement of vision
   vision, eye
   measurement of
3. involuntary movement of the eyelid
   eyelid
   involuntary movement
4. discharge of tears
   tears or lacrimal (tear) duct
   flow, discharge
5. vision loss that is age-related
   related to aging
   vision
6. surgical fixation of the retina
   retina
   surgical fixation
7. dilation of the pupil
   pupil
   dilation, stretching
8. inflammation of the iris
   iris
   inflammation
9. instrument for measuring pressure
   tension, pressure
   instrument for measuring
10. disease of the cornea
    cornea
    disease

Exercise 10

1. pertaining to the eye
2. pertaining to tears
3. pertaining to vision
4. within or inside the eye
5. pertaining to the iris
6. pertaining to the conjunctiva
7. pertaining to the eye
8. pertaining to the sclera
9. ability of the eye to adjust focus on near objects

Exercise 11

1. intraocular
2. binocular
3. blepharal
4. pupillary
5. retinal
6. optic
7. corneal
8. iridial

Exercise 12

1. ophthalmic
2. conjunctival
3. optic
4. intraocular
5. corneal
6. blepharal
7. binocular

Exercise 13

1. involuntary rhythmic movements of the eye
2. any disease of the retina
3. softening of the iris
4. inflammation of the eyelid
5. clouding of the lens of the eye, which causes poor vision
6. abnormal protrusion of one or both eyeballs
7. stone in the lacrimal sac or lacrimal ducts
8. excessive dryness of the conjunctiva and cornea, usually associated with vitamin A deficiency; dry eyes
9. group of diseases of the eye characterized by increased intraocular pressure that damages the optic nerve
10. any disease of the eyes

Exercise 14

1. astigmatism
2. Hyperopia
3. Color blindness
4. amblyopia
5. diplopia
6. presbyopia
7. nyctalopia
8. Myopia
9. macular degeneration
10. photophobia
11. ophthalmia

Exercise 15

1. diabetic retinopathy
2. ophthalmoplegia
3. dacryoadenitis
4. chalazion
5. dacryocystitis
6. hordeolum
7. pterygium
8. retinitis pigmentosa
9. strabismus
10. detached retina

Exercise 16

1. scler/o / -malacia
   hard, sclera / softening
   softening of the sclera
2. kerat/o / -itis
   cornea / inflammation
   inflammation of the cornea

3. irid/o / -plegia
   iris / paralysis
   paralysis of the iris
4. dacry/o / -rrhea
   tears or tear ducts / flow, discharge
   discharge of tears
5. blephar/o / -spasm
   eyelid / involuntary movement
   involuntary movement of the eyelid
6. scler/o / -itis
   hard, sclera / inflammation
   inflammation of the sclera
7. conjunctiv/o / -itis
   conjunctiva / inflammation
   inflammation of the conjunctiva
8. ophthalm/o / -algia
   eye / pain
   pain in the eye
9. blephar/o / -ptosis
   eyelid / prolapse, drooping, sagging
   sagging eyelid
10. kerat/o / -malacia
   cornea / softening
   softening of the cornea

Exercise 17
1. instrument used for measuring pressure within the eye
2. instrument used for examining the interior of the eye through the pupil
3. examination of the retina
4. instrument used for measuring the curvature of the cornea
5. measurement of the pupil

Exercise 18
1. visual field assessment
2. Snellen chart
3. pupillometry
4. fluorescein angiography
5. refraction
6. extraocular movement assessment

Exercise 19
1. fluorescein angiography
2. retinoscopy
3. Snellen chart
4. refraction
5. tonometer
6. visual acuity

Exercise 20
1. pupill/o / -meter
   pupil / instrument for measuring
   instrument for measuring the pupil
2. ton/o / -metry
   tension, pressure / measurement of
   measurement of pressure (within the eye)
3. ophthalm/o / -scopy
   eye / process of examining, examination
   examination of the eye
4. kerat/o / -meter
   cornea / instrument for measuring
   instrument for measuring (the curvature of) the cornea
5. retin/o / -scopy
   retina / process of examining, examination
   examination of the retina
6. ophthalm/o / -scope
   eye / instrument for examining
   instrument for examining (the interior of) the eye

Exercise 21
1. enucleation
2. cryoretinopexy
3. vitrectomy
4. photorefractive keratectomy (PRK)
5. cataract extraction
6. retinal photocoagulation
7. laser-assisted in situ keratomileusis (LASIK)

Exercise 22
1. Phacoemulsification
2. trabeculectomy
3. dacryocystotomy
4. scleral buckling
5. keratoplasty
6. blepharoplasty
7. intraocular lens (IOL) implant

Exercise 23
1. tomy
2. blepharo
3. ectomy
4. kerato
5. ectomy
6. irido

Exercise 24
1. mydriatic
2. corticosteroid
3. prostaglandin
4. miotic
5. hypotonic

Exercise 25
1. optometry
2. ophthalmology
3. optician
4. ophthalmologist
5. optometrist

Exercise 26
1. each eye; both eyes (oculus uterque)
2. extraocular movement
3. intraocular lens
4. left eye (oculus sinister)
5. visual field

Exercise 27
1. visual acuity
2. laser-assisted in situ keratomileusis
3. right eye (oculus dexter)
4. photorefractive keratectomy
5. intraocular pressure

Exercise 28
1. smallest auditory ossicle shaped like a stirrup
2. receptor for hearing located inside the cochlea; the organ of hearing
3. passage leading inward from the auricle to the tympanic membrane (eardrum)
4. middle auditory ossicle that is shaped like an anvil
5. external portion of the ear that directs sound waves
6. largest auditory ossicle that is shaped like a hammer or club
7. three small bones (malleus, incus, stapes) of the middle ear that transmit sound waves
8. waxy substance produced by glands of the external auditory canal; earwax
9. inner ear, which is made up of a series of semicircular ducts (canals), the vestibule, and the cochlea

Exercise 29
1. vestibule
2. semicircular canals
3. auditory ossicles
4. tympanic membrane
5. auditory tube
6. mastoid cells
7. auricle
8. cochlea
9. external auditory canal

Exercise 30
1. auditory ossicles
2. mastoid cells
3. labyrinth
4. cerumen
5. spiral organ or organ of Corti
6. semicircular ducts
7. vestibule
8. auditory tube or pharyngotympanic tube or eustachian tube
9. tympanic membrane

Exercise 31
1. hearing
2. pain
3. vestibule
4. ear
5. hearing, sound
6. hard, sclera
7. painful, difficult, abnormal
8. cochlea

Exercise 32
1. labyrinth/o
2. -ectomy
3. -stomy
4. scler/o
5. dys-
6. ot/o

Exercise 33
1. inflammation of the labyrinth or inner ear
2. surgical opening into the middle ear
3. inflammation of the mastoid cells (infection in the air cell system of the mastoid process)
4. flow or discharge from the ear
5. instrument for measuring hearing
6. incision into the tympanic membrane (eardrum)
7. excision of the stapes

Exercise 34
1. vestibulotomy
2. aural
3. acoustic
4. cochleitis
5. sclerosis
6. otalgia
7. myringitis

Exercise 35

1. pertaining to the ear
2. pertaining to hearing or sound
3. pertaining to the ear
4. pertaining to the tympanic membrane
5. pertaining to a vestibule
6. pertaining to hearing
7. pertaining to the cochlea

Exercise 36

1. aural
2. vestibular
3. tympanic
4. acoustic
5. labyrinthine
6. mastoid

Exercise 37

1. aural
2. labyrinthine
3. auditory
4. otic
5. mastoid
6. tympanic

Exercise 38

1. otomycosis
2. otosclerosis
3. tinnitus
4. cholesteatoma
5. cerumen impaction
6. presbycusis
7. vertigo
8. acoustic neuroma

Exercise 39

1. otitis media
2. sensorineural hearing loss
3. presbycusis
4. otitis externa
5. conductive hearing loss
6. dysacusis

Exercise 40

1. sensorineural hearing loss
2. Otitis externa
3. conductive hearing loss
4. Otopyorrhea
5. Ménière disease
6. tympanic membrane perforation
7. otitis media

Exercise 41

1. ot/o/-algia; otalgia
2. labyrinth/o/-itis; labyrinthitis
3. ot/o/-rrhea; otorrhea
4. mastoid/o/-it is; mastoiditis
5. myring/o/-itis; myringitis

Exercise 42

1. unit of measure of frequency or pitch of sound
2. record of hearing (presented in graph form)
3. use of an otoscope to examine the external auditory canal and tympanic membrane
4. measurement of middle ear function
5. unit for expressing the intensity of sound
6. record of middle ear function (presented in graph form)

Exercise 43

1. audiometer
2. audiometry
3. audiogram
4. tympanometer

Exercise 44

1. otoscope
2. tympanogram
3. audiometer
4. otoscopy
5. tympanometry
6. audiogram

Exercise 45

1. labyrinthectomy
2. mastoidotomy
3. stapedectomy
4. ear lavage
5. otoplasty

Exercise 46

1. cochlear implant
2. myringotomy or tympanostomy
3. myringotomy; tympanostomy tube placement
4. tympanoplasty
5. mastoidectomy

Exercise 47

1. mastoidotomy
2. stapedectomy
3. tympanostomy
4. tympanoplasty

Exercise 48

1. otic
2. antibiotic
3. ceruminolytic

Exercise 49

1. otology
2. audiologist
3. otorhinolaryngology
4. audiology
5. otologist
6. otorhinolaryngologist

Exercise 50

1. eyes, ears, nose, and throat
2. each ear, both ears (auris utraque)
3. hertz
4. otitis media
5. decibel
6. right ear (auris dexter)

Exercise 51

1. ears, nose, and throat
2. otitis externa
3. left ear (auris sinister)
4. electronystagmography
5. tympanic membrane

Exercise 52

1. cornea
2. iris
3. pupil
4. lens
5. anterior chamber
6. posterior chamber
7. sclera
8. choroid
9. retina
10. optic nerve

Exercise 53

1. auricle
2. tympanic membrane
3. external auditory canal
4. ossicles
5. semicircular ducts
6. cochlea
7. vestibule
8. auditory (pharyngotympanic) tube

Exercise 54

1. ophthalm/o / -ic
   eye / pertaining to
   pertaining to the eye
2. audi/o / -meter
   hearing / instrument for measuring
   instrument for measuring hearing
3. blephar/o / -itis
   eyelid / inflammation
   inflammation of the eyelid
4. tympan/o / -stomy
   tympanic membrane, eardrum / surgical opening
   surgical opening into the tympanic membrane (eardrum)
5. irid/o / -malacia
   iris / softening
   softening of the iris
6. labyrinth/o / -itis
   labyrinth, inner ear / inflammation
   inflammation of the labyrinth
7. retin/o / -pathy
   retina / disease
   disease of the retina
8. acous/o / -tic
   hearing, sound / pertaining to
   pertaining to hearing or sound
9. pupill/o / -meter
   pupil / instrument for measuring
   instrument for measuring the pupil
10. staped/o / -ectomy
    stapes / excision, surgical removal
    excision of the stapes
11. ton/o / -meter
    tension, pressure / instrument for measuring
    instrument for measuring pressure
12. vestibul/o / -ar
    vestibule / pertaining to
    pertaining to a vestibule
13. scler/o / -tomy
    hard, sclera / incision
    incision into the sclera
14. ot/o / -scopy
    ear / process of examining, examination
    examination of the ear

Exercise 55

1. discharge from the ear
   ear
   flow, discharge
2. examination of the eye
   eye
   process of examining, examination

3. measurement of vision
   vision
   measurement of
4. inflammation of the tympanic membrane
   tympanic membrane, eardrum
   inflammation
5. discharge of pus from the ear
   ear
   pus
   flow, discharge
6. discharge of tears
   tears
   flow, discharge
7. pertaining to the ear
   ear
   pertaining to
8. age-related vision loss
   related to aging
   vision
9. recording of hearing
   hearing
   record, recording
10. excision of (part of) the mastoid process of the temporal bone
    mastoid process
    excision, surgical removal
11. inflammation of the conjunctiva
    conjunctiva
    inflammation
12. measurement of middle ear (function)
    middle ear
    measurement of
13. surgical repair of the cornea
    cornea
    surgical repair, reconstruction
14. age-related hearing loss
    related to aging
    hearing

Exercise 56
1. otorhinolaryngologist
2. optometrist
3. audiologist
4. otologist
5. ophthalmologist

Exercise 57
1. cochlea
2. ossicles
3. retina
4. cerumen impaction
5. lacrimal glands
6. Ménière disease
7. otitis externa
8. Astigmatism
9. Presbycusis
10. mydriatic
11. hypotonic
12. Detached retina
13. laser-assisted in situ keratomileusis (LASIK)
14. xerophthalmia
15. fluorescein angiography
16. ear lavage
17. Snellen test
18. stapedectomy
19. Prostaglandins
20. Cryoretinopexy

Exercise 58
1. myopia
2. a spinning sensation; commonly used to mean dizziness
3. impaired vision
4. diplopia
5. photophobia
6. hyperopia is farsightedness, myopia is nearsightedness
7. to soften earwax
8. myringotomy

Exercise 59
1. C
2. A
3. D
4. C
5. D
6. A
7. B
8. A
9. C
10. D
11. B
12. B
13. D
14. D
15. A
16. B
17. D
18. B
19. B
20. A

Exercise 60
1. B
2. D
3. D
4. C
5. A
6. B
7. A
8. C
9. B
10. D

Exercise 61
1. C
2. A
3. B

Exercise 62
1. corneal
2. intraocular
3. microkeratome
4. keratography
5. speculum

Exercise 63
1. audiometry
2. otorrhea
3. otic
4. tympanoplasty
5. dysacusis
6. tympanic membrane perforation
7. tympanic
8. tinnitus
9. tympanostomies
10. conductive hearing loss
11. toward the front of the body and above or upward
12. a significant conductive hearing loss in the right ear

Exercise 64
Practice until your pronunciation matches that heard in the Audio Glossary in the Student Resources.

Exercise 65
1. tarsal
2. choroid
3. vitreous
4. corneal
5. ophthalmology
6. chalazion
7. diplopia
8. glaucoma
9. nystagmus
10. presbyopia
11. pterygium
12. strabismus
13. fluorescein
14. refraction
15. Snellen
16. pupillometry
17. acuity
18. cataract
19. mydriatic
20. optician

Chapter 8

Exercise 1
1. pituitary gland
2. adrenal glands, suprarenal glands
3. islets of Langerhans
4. thyroid gland
5. parathyroid glands
6. pineal gland, pineal body
7. hypothalamus
8. thymus gland
9. ovaries

Exercise 2
1. growth hormone
2. thyroxine
3. follicle-stimulating hormone
4. parathyroid hormone
5. prolactin
6. oxytocin
7. aldosterone
8. melatonin
9. insulin

Exercise 3
1. parathyroid hormone (PTH)
2. Thymosin
3. Adrenocorticotrophic hormone (ACTH)
4. luteinizing hormone (LH)
5. thyroid-stimulating hormone (TSH)
6. Thyroxine (T_4), triiodothyronine (T_3)
7. antidiuretic hormone (ADH)
8. testes
9. ovaries
10. cortisol

Exercise 4
1. glucose, sugar
2. cortex
3. thyroid gland
4. potassium
5. to secrete

6. thirst
7. glucose, sugar
8. sodium

Exercise 5
1. excision or surgical removal of an adrenal gland
2. deficiency of calcium
3. pertaining to a hormone
4. enlargement of the head, face, hands, and feet
5. incision into the thyroid gland
6. inflammation of the thymus gland
7. excision or surgical removal of a parathyroid gland
8. one who specializes in the endocrine system

Exercise 6
1. condition of a deficient thyroid gland
   below, deficient
   thyroid gland
   condition of
2. pertaining to the pancreas
   pancreas
   pertaining to
3. resembling a normal thyroid gland
   good, normal
   thyroid gland
   resembling
4. glucose or sugar in the urine
   glucose, sugar
   urine, urination
5. condition of excessive glucose in the blood
   above, excessive
   glucose, sugar
   blood
6. disease of an adrenal gland
   adrenal gland
   disease
7. condition of much (excessive) thirst
   many, much
   thirst
   condition of
8. abnormal condition of a gland
   gland
   abnormal condition

Exercise 7
1. cortical
2. exogenous
3. pancreatic
4. thymic
5. endogenous

Exercise 8
1. euthyroid
2. pancreatic
3. metabolism
4. thymic
5. exogenous

Exercise 9
1. thym/o; thymus gland
2. cortic/o; cortex
3. adren/o; adrenal glands
4. thyroid/o; thyroid gland
5. pancreat/o; pancreas
6. hormon/o; hormone

Exercise 10
1. polydipsia
2. Hashimoto thyroiditis, Hashimoto disease
3. exophthalmos
4. acidemia
5. thyrotoxicosis
6. hirsutism
7. ketosis
8. Type 1 diabetes mellitus
9. myxedema
10. polyuria
11. adenomegaly
12. hyperthyroidism
13. Type 2 diabetes mellitus

Exercise 11
1. gigantism
2. Addison disease
3. congenital hypothyroidism
4. acromegaly
5. hypothyroidism
6. Graves disease
7. diabetes insipidus
8. Diabetic ketoacidosis
9. Cushing syndrome
10. adrenalitis
11. Goiter
12. tetany

Exercise 12
1. hyponatremia
2. hyperkalemia
3. hypercalcemia
4. polyuria
5. glycosuria
6. hyperglycemia
7. calcipenia
8. polydipsia
9. hypocalcemia

Exercise 13
1. glucosuria, glycosuria
2. endocrinopathy
3. acromegaly
4. adrenomegaly
5. thyroiditis
6. adenitis
7. pancreatitis
8. calcipenia
9. adrenopathy
10. thyromegaly

Exercise 14
1. above, excess / parathyroid glands / condition of
2. below, deficient / parathyroid glands / condition of
3. above, excessive / calcium / blood (condition of)
4. below, deficient / calcium / blood (condition of)
5. above, excessive / glucose, sugar / blood (condition of)
6. below, deficient / glucose / blood (condition of)
7. above, excessive / sodium / blood (condition of)
8. below, deficient / sodium / blood (condition of)
9. above, excessive / potassium / blood (condition of)
10. below, deficient / potassium / blood (condition of)

Exercise 15
1. glucometer
2. thyroid function tests
3. glucose tolerance test (GTT)
4. radioactive iodine uptake test (RIU); ^{131}I uptake test
5. thyroid scan
6. thyroid-stimulating hormone level

Exercise 16
1. thyroxine level
2. glucose tolerance test
3. blood glucose
4. fasting blood glucose
5. electrolyte panel
6. glycosylated hemoglobin

Exercise 17
1. excision of the thyroid gland
2. excision of an adrenal gland
3. excision of the thymus gland
4. excision of the thyroid and parathyroid glands

Exercise 18
1. thyroid gland
2. adrenalectomy
3. incision
4. thyroid

Exercise 19
1. pancreat/o; pancreas
2. thyroid/o; thyroid gland
3. aden/o; gland
4. parathyroid/o; parathyroid gland
5. thym/o; thymus gland

Exercise 20
1. insulin therapy
2. antithyroid
3. hormone replacement therapy (HRT)
4. antidiabetic
5. continuous subcutaneous insulin infusion; insulin pump

Exercise 21
1. endocrinology
2. endocrinologist

Exercise 22
1. diabetes insipidus
2. thyroid-stimulating hormone
3. fasting blood glucose
4. antidiuretic hormone
5. parathyroid hormone
6. glucose tolerance test
7. radioactive iodine uptake
8. triiodothyronine
9. glycosylated hemoglobin alpha 1c

Exercise 23
1. ACTH
2. DM
3. FSH
4. T_4
5. DKA
6. CSII
7. DI
8. GH
9. LH

Exercise 24
1. pituitary gland
2. thyroid
3. adrenal gland
4. testis
5. pineal gland
6. parathyroid glands
7. thymus gland
8. pancreas
9. ovary

Exercise 25
1. pancreat/o / -ic
   pancreas / pertaining to
   pertaining to the pancreas
2. adrenal/o / -itis
   adrenal gland / inflammation
   inflammation of an adrenal gland
3. glucos/o / -uria
   glucose, sugar / urine, urination
   glucose in the urine
4. acr/o / -megaly
   extremity, tip / enlargement
   enlargement of the extremities
5. cortic/o / -al
   cortex / pertaining to
   pertaining to the cortex
6. calc/i / -penia
   calcium / deficiency
   deficiency of calcium
7. thyroid/o / -tomy
   thyroid gland / incision
   incision into the thyroid gland

Exercise 26
1. thym/o; thymus gland
2. thyr/o; thyroid gland
3. kal/i; potassium
4. adrenal/o; adrenal gland
5. natr/i; sodium
6. endocrin/o or crin/o; endocrine or to secrete
7. pancreat/o; pancreas
8. dips/o; thirst

Exercise 27
1. hyperthyroidism
2. glucose tolerance test (GTT)
3. adrenalectomy
4. antidiuretic hormone (ADH)
5. Islets of Langerhans
6. polyuria
7. euthyroid
8. congenital hypothyroidism
9. diabetes insipidus
10. endocrinologist

Exercise 28
1. A
2. D
3. B
4. D
5. A
6. B
7. B
8. B
9. C
10. B

Exercise 29
1. C
2. B
3. B
4. A
5. C
6. B
7. D
8. B

Exercise 30
1. endogenous
2. polyuria
3. blood glucose testing
4. pancreatitis
5. glycosuria

Exercise 31
1. C
2. B
3. A
4. C
5. B

Exercise 32
1. hyperthyroidism
2. thyromegaly or goiter
3. exophthalmos
4. thyroid scan
5. thyroidectomy
6. hemostasis
7. lying face up

Exercise 33
Practice until your pronunciation matches that heard in the Audio Glossary in the Student Resources.

Exercise 34
1. pituitary
2. pancreas
3. CORRECT
4. CORRECT
5. euthyroid
6. diabetes
7. exophthalmos
8. hirsutism
9. CORRECT
10. CORRECT
11. myxedema
12. CORRECT
13. CORRECT
14. glycosylated
15. CORRECT

Chapter 9

Exercise 1
1. leukocyte, white blood cell (WBC)
2. platelets, thrombocytes
3. blood
4. lymphocyte
5. plasma
6. spleen
7. granulocyte
8. agranulocyte
9. monocyte
10. eosinophil
11. basophil
12. erythrocyte, red blood cell (RBC)
13. hemoglobin
14. bone marrow
15. serum

Exercise 2
1. essential trace element necessary for hemoglobin to transport oxygen in red blood cells
2. soldier-like cell that protects the body and inactivates antigens
3. agent or substance that provokes an immune response
4. any virus, microorganism, or other substance that causes disease
5. protection against disease
6. hormone released by kidneys that stimulates red blood cell production in bone marrow
7. formation of blood cells and other formed elements
8. type of granulocyte that fights against bacterial infections; stains a neutral pink
9. any of the various plasma components involved in the clotting process
10. protein substance present in the red blood cells of most people capable of inducing intense antigenic reactions

Exercise 3
1. erythrocyte
2. Hemoglobin
3. formed elements
4. Histamine
5. antibodies
6. antigens
7. bone marrow
8. spleen
9. erythropoietin
10. leukocyte
11. macrophage
12. serum

Exercise 4
1. Rh factor
2. coagulation
3. antibody
4. fibrin
5. leukocyte
6. hemoglobin
7. pathogen
8. platelet
9. phagocytosis

Exercise 5
1. B
2. T
3. spleen
4. erythrocyte, red blood cell (RBC)
5. fibrin
6. granulocyte
7. macrocyte
8. Fibrinogen
9. macrophage

Exercise 6
1. blood
2. disease
3. blood clot
4. immune, safe
5. white
6. red
7. eat, swallow
8. granules
9. vein
10. color
11. neutral
12. formation, growth

Exercise 7
1. thromb/o
2. plas/o
3. lymph/o
4. neutr/o
5. hem/o, hemat/o
6. erythr/o
7. leuk/o
8. phag/o
9. cyt/o
10. nucle/o

Exercise 8
1. self, same
2. flowing forth
3. one
4. base
5. many, much
6. attraction for, liking
7. deficiency
8. destruction, breakdown, separation
9. production, formation
10. large, long
11. small
12. blood (condition of)
13. origin, production
14. abnormal condition

Exercise 9
1. study of veins
2. flowing forth of blood (bleeding)
3. blood clotting cell
4. red (blood) cell
5. attraction for neutral (stain)

Exercise 10
1. leukocyte
2. thrombolysis
3. mononucleosis
4. pancytopenia
5. polycythemia
6. erythropoiesis
7. phlebology

Exercise 11
1. hemorrhagic
2. systemic
3. Rejection
4. predisposition
5. Hemolytic
6. cytopathic
7. autoimmunity

Exercise 12
1. hemostasis
2. rejection
3. proliferative
4. inflammatory
5. virulent
6. hypersensitive
7. hemopoietic
8. systemic

Exercise 13
1. bleed
2. bleeding
3. platelets
4. transport
5. iron
6. produce
7. destruction
8. clotting
9. increase
10. low

Exercise 14
1. platelets
2. pernicious
3. Sjögren syndrome
4. lymph nodes
5. sickle cell anemia
6. autoimmune disease
7. coagulate
8. polycythemia
9. blood
10. autoimmune
11. joints

Exercise 15
1. deficiency in all types of (blood) cells
2. abnormal condition of (increase of white blood cells with) one nucleus
3. pertaining to without formation or growth (pertaining to aplasia, characterized by defective regeneration)
4. attraction for blood (tendency to bleed)
5. inflammation of a joint

Exercise 16
1. hemochromatosis
2. hemophilia
3. thrombocytopenia
4. thrombosis
5. hemorrhage

Exercise 17
1. Sjögren syndrome
2. EBV antibody test
3. cross-matching
4. prothrombin time
5. HGB
6. inflammation
7. differential white blood count
8. hematocrit
9. pathogen, antibiotic
10. ANA

Exercise 18
1. blood smear
2. red blood cell count
3. hemogram
4. platelet count
5. albumin
6. bilirubin
7. white blood cell count

Exercise 19
1. plasmapheresis
2. bone marrow transplant
3. splenectomy
4. blood transfusion
5. blood component therapy
6. autologous blood
7. homologous blood
8. apheresis

Exercise 20
1. splenectomy
2. vaccinations
3. phlebotomy
4. blood transfusions
5. aspiration
6. immunizations
7. immunosuppression

Exercise 21
1. anticoagulant
2. vaccine
3. antibiotic
4. antiserum, immune serum
5. hemostatic agent, procoagulant
6. immunosuppressant
7. antihistamine
8. thrombolytic agent

Exercise 22
1. allergology
2. rheumatologist
3. hematologist
4. hematology
5. immunology
6. allergist
7. immunologist
8. rheumatology

Exercise 23
1. prothrombin time, von Willebrand disease
2. bone marrow aspiration, bone marrow transplant
3. complete blood count
4. erythrocyte sedimentation rate
5. hemoglobin, hematocrit
6. red blood cells, white blood cells
7. idiopathic thrombocytopenic purpura, blood transfusions
8. antibody, antigens
9. culture and sensitivity

Exercise 24
1. Fe
2. PLT
3. ESR
4. EPO
5. ANA
6. EBV
7. SLE
8. RA

Exercise 25
1. neutrophil
2. eosinophil
3. basophil
4. lymphocyte
5. monocyte

Exercise 26
1. hem/o / stasis
   blood / stopped, standing still
   stopped bleeding
2. erythr/o / -cyte
   red / cell
   red (blood) cell

3. hemat/o / -poiesis
   blood / production, formation
   blood (cell) production or formation
4. thromb/o / cyt/o / -penia
   blood clot / cell / deficiency
   deficiency of blood clotting cells
5. path/o / -gen
   disease / origin, production
   disease-producing
6. cyt/o / path/o / -ic
   cell / disease / pertaining to
   pertaining to cell disease
7. a- / plas/o / -tic
   without / formation, growth / pertaining to
   pertaining to without formation or growth
8. chromat/o / -ic
   color / pertaining to
   pertaining to color
9. an- / -emia
   without / blood (condition of)
   condition of without blood cells
10. hem/o / chromat/o / -osis
    blood / color / abnormal condition
    abnormal condition of blood color
11. hem/o / -philia
    blood / attraction for
    attraction for blood
12. granul/o / -cyte
    granules / cell
    cell containing granules
13. lymph/o / cyt/o / -ic
    lymph / cell / pertaining to
    pertaining to a lymph cell
14. hem/o / -rrhage
    blood / flowing forth
    flowing forth of blood
15. mono- / nucle/o / -osis
    one / nucleus / abnormal condition
    abnormal condition of one nucleus

Exercise 27

1. antibodies
2. Antigens
3. vaccination or immunization
4. Hemorrhagic or blood loss
5. Thrombocytopenia
6. Inflammation
7. erythrocyte sedimentation rate
8. white

Exercise 28

1. to decrease rejection of the donor organ
2. erythrocytes, leukocytes, platelets, or red blood cells, white blood cells, thrombocytes
3. anticoagulant
4. erythrocyte sedimentation rate (ESR)
5. Antigens are agents or substances that produce an immune response; antibodies protect the body and inactivate antigens.
6. clotting or coagulation
7. leukocytes (macrophages)
8. mononuclear leukocytes
9. bone marrow
10. autologous blood transfusion
11. Rheumatoid arthritis is an autoimmune disease, and immunosuppressants reduce the normal immune response.
12. A vaccine is the preparation composed of a weakened or killed pathogen, and a vaccination is the administration of a vaccine.
13. "Systemic" is a term that means affecting the whole body, and this disease can affect the entire body.
14. culture and sensitivity (C&S)
15. in the bone marrow

Exercise 29

1. D
2. D
3. B
4. D
5. B
6. C
7. A
8. A
9. C
10. A
11. D
12. D

Exercise 30

1. B
2. D
3. C
4. A
5. D
6. A
7. C
8. B
9. D
10. B

Exercise 31

1. hemolytic
2. thrombocytopenia
3. NKA
4. as needed
5. anti- / bi/o / -tic
   opposing, / life / pertaining to against
   pertaining to against life

Exercise 32

1. B
2. C
3. D
4. A
5. A

Exercise 33

1. systemic lupus erythematosus
2. erythrocyte sedimentation rate
3. white blood count
4. Epstein–Barr virus test
5. antinuclear antibody test
6. hematuria

Exercise 34

Practice until your pronunciation matches that heard in the Audio Glossary in the Student Resources.

Exercise 35

1. erythrocyte
2. granulocyte
3. leukocyte
4. neutrophil
5. eosinophil
6. agranulocyte
7. erythropoietin
8. phagocytosis
9. hemoglobin
10. hemorrhagic
11. virulent
12. proliferation
13. immunosuppressant
14. thalassemia
15. thrombocytopenia

Chapter 10

Exercise 1

1. atrium
2. venule
3. myocardium
4. aortic valve
5. septum
6. arteriole
7. superior vena cava and inferior vena cava
8. heart
9. endocardium
10. pericardium

Exercise 2

1. clear fluid consisting of fluctuating amounts of white blood cells and a few red blood cells that accumulates in tissue and is removed by the lymphatic capillaries
2. vessel carrying blood away from the heart
3. vessel carrying blood to the heart
4. microscopic thin-walled lymph vessels that pick up lymph, proteins, and waste from body tissues
5. largest artery that carries oxygenated blood away from the heart
6. tubular structures that transport blood
7. vessels transporting lymph from body tissues to the venous system
8. the largest lymph vessels that transport lymph to the venous system
9. small bean-shaped masses of lymphatic tissue that filter bacteria and foreign material from the lymph
10. heart valve between the right atrium and right ventricle

Exercise 3

1. atria
2. outer
3. endocardium
4. bicuspid
5. aorta
6. artery
7. capillaries
8. vein
9. capillary

10. tricuspid
11. two
12. pericardium
13. arteriole
14. heart

Exercise 4
1. pulmonary valve
2. myocardium
3. lumen
4. lymph
5. septum
6. apex

Exercise 5
1. lymph nodes
2. ventricles
3. arteries
4. aortic valve
5. pericardium
6. lumen
7. capillary
8. ducts
9. lymph
10. inferior

Exercise 6
1. atrium
2. muscle
3. blood vessel
4. vessel, vascular
5. vein
6. electric, electricity
7. artery
8. heart
9. normal cavity, ventricle
10. lung
11. encircling, crown
12. vein
13. blood vessel
14. chest, thorax
15. valve

Exercise 7
1. scler/o
2. sphygm/o
3. varic/o
4. lymph/o
5. valv/o, valvul/o
6. aort/o
7. arteri/o
8. atri/o
9. cardi/o
10. steth/o, thorac/o

Exercise 8
1. stricture, narrowing
2. small
3. rapid, fast
4. across, through
5. within
6. between
7. in, within
8. instrument for recording
9. slow
10. on, following
11. around, surrounding
12. tissue, structure
13. pertaining to
14. three
15. away from, cessation, without
16. pertaining to destruction, breakdown, separation

Exercise 9
1. inflammation of a vein
2. study of the heart
3. heart muscle tissue
4. abnormal condition of blood clot
5. recording of a vein (x-ray image of veins)
6. surgical removal of fatty deposit
7. resembling lymph
8. imaging of the aorta

Exercise 10
1. angioplasty
2. thoracic
3. arteriole
4. venule
5. vascular
6. adenoid
7. lymphopathy
8. sonography

Exercise 11
1. above
2. paroxysmal
3. patent
4. narrowed
5. cyanotic
6. Systole
7. diastole

Exercise 12
1. constriction
2. cardiovascular
3. cyanotic
4. precordial
5. varicose
6. oxygenate
7. thoracic
8. ischemic
9. atrioventricular
10. deoxygenate

Exercise 13
1. sphygm/o; pulse
2. cardi/o; vascul/o; heart; blood vessel
3. varic/o; swollen or twisted vein
4. arteri/o; ven/o; artery; vein
5. thromb/o; blood clot

Exercise 14
1. weakening
2. hardening
3. high
4. low
5. narrowing
6. death
7. valve
8. lack of
9. irregular
10. regular
11. early
12. abnormal
13. edema
14. chest pain
15. cramping
16. outside

Exercise 15
1. backward
2. fluid
3. narrowed
4. filariae
5. myocardial infarction
6. angina pectoris
7. cardiac arrest
8. cyanotic
9. circulation
10. tachycardia
11. phlebitis
12. decrease
13. embolus
14. blood clot
15. varicose
16. coronary occlusion

Exercise 16
1. angiostenosis
2. palpitation
3. arrhythmia
4. lymphedema
5. occlusion
6. plaque
7. mitral valve stenosis
8. lymphadenitis
9. dysrhythmia
10. cardiomegaly

Exercise 17
1. bradycardia
2. pericarditis
3. endocardium
4. interventricular
5. pericardium
6. tachycardia
7. polyarteritis

Exercise 18
1. lymph/o / angi/o / -itis
   lymph / vessel, vascular / inflammation
   inflammation of a lymphatic vessel
2. lymph/o / aden/o / -pathy
   lymph / gland / disease
   disease of the lymph nodes
3. thromb/o / phleb/o / -itis
   blood clot / vein / inflammation
   inflammation of a vein (with formation of a) blood clot
4. cardi/o / my/o / -pathy
   heart / muscle / disease
   disease of the heart muscle
5. endo- / cardi/o / -itis
   in, within / heart / inflammation
   inflammation within the heart (inflammation of the endocardium)
6. cardi/o / valvul/o / -itis
   heart / valve / inflammation
   inflammation of the valves of the heart
7. my/o / cardi/o / -itis
   muscle / heart / inflammation
   inflammation of the heart muscle
8. tel- / angi/o / -ectasia
   end / vessel, vascular / dilation, stretching
   dilation of end (or terminal) vessels

Exercise 19
1. Holter monitor
2. arteriography
3. lymphangiography
4. angioscopy

5. auscultation
6. electrocardiography
7. SPECT
8. sonography
9. percussion
10. magnetic resonance angiography

Exercise 20

1. exercise stress test, graded exercise test (GXT), or stress electrocardiogram
2. echocardiography
3. transesophageal echocardiography
4. multiple uptake gated acquisition (MUGA) scan or single photon emission computed tomography (SPECT) scan
5. coronary angiography or cardiac catheterization
6. exercise
7. heart ventricles
8. radiofrequency waves
9. sphygmomanometer
10. auscultation; stethoscope

Exercise 21

1. electrolyte panel
2. cardiac enzyme tests
3. cardiac troponin
4. lipid panel
5. C-reactive protein

Exercise 22

1. sonography
2. venography
3. ventriculography
4. aortography
5. angiography

Exercise 23

1. adenectomy
2. percutaneous transluminal coronary angioplasty (PTCA)
3. embolectomy
4. valvuloplasty
5. atherectomy
6. lymphadenectomy
7. lymphadenotomy

Exercise 24

1. valve replacement
2. cardioversion
3. endarterectomy
4. cardiac pacemaker
5. PTCA
6. stent
7. CABG
8. aortocoronary bypass

Exercise 25

1. angioplasty
2. aneurysmectomy
3. pericardiocentesis
4. adenectomy
5. valvotomy

Exercise 26

1. valvul/o / -plasty
   valve / surgical repair, reconstruction
   surgical repair or reconstruction of a valve
2. angi/o / -plasty
   vessel, vascular / surgical repair, reconstruction
   surgical repair reconstruction of a vessel
3. ather/o / -ectomy
   fatty deposit / excision, surgical removal
   excision or surgical removal of fatty plaque
4. phleb/o / -ectomy
   vein / excision, surgical removal
   excision or surgical removal of vein
5. valv/o / -tomy
   valve / incision
   incision into a valve

Exercise 27

1. vasoconstrictor
2. anticoagulant
3. thrombolytic therapy
4. vasodilator
5. hemostatic agent
6. antiarrhythmic agent
7. nitroglycerin
8. hypolipidemic agent

Exercise 28

1. cardiology
2. lymphedema therapy
3. cardiologist
4. cardiac electrophysiology
5. lymphedema therapist
6. cardiac electrophysiologist

Exercise 29

1. congestive heart failure
2. aortocoronary bypass
3. single photon emission computed tomography
4. arteriosclerotic heart disease
5. deep vein thrombosis
6. premature ventricular contraction
7. blood pressure
8. acute coronary syndrome
9. hypertension
10. coronary artery bypass graft

Exercise 30

1. Holter monitor
2. percutaneous transluminal coronary angioplasty
3. magnetic resonance angiogram
4. atrioventricular
5. transesophageal echocardiogram
6. coronary artery disease
7. rheumatic heart disease
8. graded exercise test
9. myocardial infarction
10. peripheral arterial disease

Exercise 31

1. ECG
2. MRI
3. MRA
4. DS
5. MUGA

Exercise 32

1. superior vena cava
2. right atrium
3. endocardium
4. right ventricle
5. inferior vena cava
6. left atrium
7. epicardium
8. left ventricle
9. myocardium
10. apex

Exercise 33

1. cervical lymph nodes
2. axillary lymph nodes
3. mediastinal lymph nodes
4. inguinal lymph nodes

Exercise 34

1. angi/o / -stenosis
   vessel / stricture, narrowing
   narrowing of a blood vessel
2. phleb/o / -itis
   vein / inflammation
   inflammation of a vein
3. electr/o / cardi/o / -graphy
   electric, electricity / heart / recording writing, description
   recording of the electrical conduction of the heart
4. atri/o / ventricul/o / -ar
   atrium / ventricle / pertaining to
   pertaining to the atrium and ventricle
5. tachy- / cardi/o / -ia
   rapid, fast / heart / condition of
   condition of fast heart (rate)
6. inter- / ventricul/o / -ar
   between / ventricle / pertaining to
   pertaining to between the ventricles
7. thromb/o / -osis
   blood clot / abnormal condition
   abnormal condition of a blood clot
8. poly- / arteri/o / -itis
   many, much / artery / inflammation
   inflammation of many arteries
9. thromb/o / phleb/o / -itis
   blood clot / vein / inflammation
   inflammation of a vein (related to) a blood clot
10. cardi/o / my/o / -pathy
    heart / muscle / disease
    disease of the heart muscle
11. arteri/o / scler/o / -osis
    artery / hard / abnormal condition
    abnormal condition of hardening of the arteries
12. sphygm/o / -ic
    pulse / pertaining to
    pertaining to the pulse
13. ven/o / -graphy
    vein / recording, writing, description
    recording of a vein (image of vein after injection with a dye)
14. brady- / cardi/o / -ia
    slow / heart / condition of
    condition of slow heart (rate)

15. ather/o- / scler/o / -osis
fatty deposit / hard / abnormal condition
abnormal condition of hardening due to fatty deposits
16. my/o / cardi/o / -ium
muscle / heart / tissue, structure
heart muscle tissue
17. valvul/o / -tomy
valve / incision
incision into a valve
18. lymph/o / aden/o / -pathy
lymph / gland / disease
disease of a lymph gland
19. lymph/o / angi/o / -itis
lymph / vessel, vascular / inflammation
inflammation of a lymph vessel
20. thromb/o / -lytic
blood clot / pertaining to destruction, breakdown, separation
pertaining to destruction of a blood clot

Exercise 35
1. myocardium
2. septum
3. cardiologist
4. pulmonary
5. aorta
6. diastole
7. telangiectasia
8. varicose
9. flutter
10. fibrillation
11. Elephantiasis
12. intermittent claudication
13. ischemia
14. myocardial infarction
15. cardiac
16. deep vein thrombosis
17. premature ventricular contraction
18. murmurs
19. open
20. inflammation

Exercise 36
1. hemostatic agent
2. the wrist or neck
3. within a blood vessel
4. cholesterol, high-density lipoprotein (HDL), low-density lipoprotein (LDL), and triglycerides
5. hypotension is blood pressure that is below normal and hypertension is persistently elevated (high) blood pressure
6. stethoscope and sphygmomanometer
7. angina pectoris
8. pericardiocentesis
9. tapping on body parts
10. to view an image of the beating heart
11. defibrillation and drug therapy
12. bradycardia
13. to stop a fibrillation or during cardiac arrest
14. coronary artery bypass (aortocoronary bypass) and coronary artery bypass graft (CABG)
15. it is inflated at the site of stenosis, thereby enlarging the lumen

Exercise 37
1. A
2. B
3. A
4. B
5. D
6. A
7. A
8. B
9. A
10. B
11. D
12. B
13. D
14. C
15. A
16. D
17. C
18. C
19. B
20. D

Exercise 38
1. B
2. C
3. A
4. A
5. D
6. C
7. D
8. D
9. D
10. B
11. C

Exercise 39
1. cardiovascular
2. echocardiogram
3. graded exercise test
4. myocardial infarction
5. ventricular
6. cyanosis
7. arteriosclerosis
8. atherosclerosis

Exercise 40
1. B
2. D
3. A
4. C
5. A
6. redness

Exercise 41
Practice until your pronunciation matches that heard in the Audio Glossary in the Student Resources.

Exercise 42
1. aneurysm
2. lymphangiitis
3. valvoplasty
4. telangiectasia
5. Doppler
6. sphygmomanometer
7. vasoconstrictor
8. diastole
9. auscultation
10. elephantiasis
11. paroxysmal
12. ischemic
13. dysrhythmia
14. arrhythmia
15. claudication

Chapter 11

Exercise 1
1. lobes
2. expiration, exhalation
3. epiglottis
4. eupnea
5. larynx
6. pharynx, throat
7. inspiration, inhalation
8. diaphragm
9. nose
10. external respiration, breathing
11. nasal septum
12. bronchi
13. alveoli
14. visceral layer; visceral pleura
15. sputum; phlegm

Exercise 2
1. nose and pharynx
2. cilia, mucous membranes
3. trachea
4. larynx
5. epiglottis
6. bronchus
7. bronchioles
8. diaphragm
9. paranasal sinuses
10. carina
11. parietal layer
12. pleural cavity
13. respiration

Exercise 3
1. internal respiration
2. glottis
3. adenoid
4. mediastinum
5. lungs
6. pleura
7. patent
8. thorax

Exercise 4
1. carbon dioxide
2. trachea
3. epiglottis
4. thorax, chest
5. to breathe in or suck in
6. septum, thin wall
7. rib, side, pleura (lung)
8. mediastinum (middle septum)
9. bronchus (windpipe)
10. mucus
11. tonsil
12. listening
13. lung, air
14. lung
15. incomplete

Exercise 5
1. pect/o, pector/o, thorac/o
2. tonsill/o
3. phon/o

4. thorac/o
5. pharyng/o
6. laryng/o
7. pleur/o
8. spir/o
9. lob/o
10. bronch/o, bronchi/o
11. sinus/o
12. nas/o, rhin/o
13. diaphragmat/o, phren/o
14. ox/o, ox/a
15. capn/o, capn/i

Exercise 6
1. through
2. below, deficient
3. in
4. breathing
5. rapid, fast
6. flowing forth
7. all, entire
8. involuntary movement
9. paralysis
10. herniation, protrusion
11. excision, surgical removal
12. blood (condition of)
13. process of examining, examination
14. without, not
15. a writing, description

Exercise 7
1. -metry
2. -al, -ar, -ary, -ic
3. -rrhea
4. -phonia
5. -emia
6. -centesis
7. -ectasis
8. dys-
9. -stomy
10. per-
11. eu-
12. -plasty
13. -itis
14. -cele
15. -tomy

Exercise 8
1. excision or surgical removal of the adenoids
2. inflammation of the alveoli
3. instrument for examination of the bronchus
4. herniation or protrusion of the diaphragm
5. inflammation of the epiglottis
6. instrument for examining the larynx
7. pertaining to the lobes of the lung
8. pertaining to the nose
9. involuntary movement of the pharynx
10. inflammation of the pleura

Exercise 9
1. pneumonitis
2. septoplasty
3. tracheotomy
4. thoracostomy
5. tonsillitis
6. sinusitis
7. laryngitis
8. lobar
9. alveolar
10. pharyngitis

Exercise 10
1. pertaining to or suffering from apnea
2. pertaining to the trachea
3. pertaining to the diaphragm
4. pertaining to a low level of oxygen
5. pertaining to pleurisy
6. pertaining to respiration
7. pertaining to the tonsil
8. pertaining to within the trachea
9. pertaining to the mediastinum
10. pertaining to mucus or a mucous membrane

Exercise 11
1. thoracic
2. bronchial
3. pleural
4. alveolar
5. diaphragmatic
6. lobar
7. anoxic
8. pharyngeal
9. intercostal
10. pectoral

Exercise 12
1. pulmonary, lobar
2. thoracic
3. pharyngeal
4. mediastinal
5. lobar

Exercise 13
1. lob/o; lobe
2. phren/o; diaphragm
3. pleur/o; rib, side, pleura (lung)
4. nas/o; nose
5. pulmon/o; lung

Exercise 14
1. hypoxemia
2. tonsillitis
3. upper respiratory infection (URI)
4. bronchiectasis
5. bronchitis
6. pleural effusion
7. rhinitis
8. tracheorrhagia
9. epistaxis
10. lobar pneumonia
11. pharyngitis
12. pansinusitis
13. atelectasis
14. pneumonitis
15. rhonchi
16. dyspnea
17. rubs
18. wheeze
19. chronic obstructive pulmonary disease (COPD)

Exercise 15
1. pulmonary edema
2. bronchopneumonia
3. influenza
4. hemothorax
5. empyema
6. pertussis
7. pansinusitis
8. adult respiratory distress syndrome
9. pleuritis
10. tuberculosis
11. pulmonary embolism

Exercise 16
1. croup
2. asthma
3. hypoxia
4. pneumococcal pneumonia
5. rales
6. interstitial lung disease
7. pulmonary embolism
8. bronchiolitis obliterans with organizing pneumonia
9. emphysema
10. reactive airway disease
11. Cheyne–Stokes respiration

Exercise 17
1. pneumon/o / -ia
lung / condition of
condition of the lung
2. a- / -phonia
without, not / condition of the voice
condition of without a voice (loss of voice)
3. bronchi/o / -ectasis
bronchus / dilation, stretching
dilation of the bronchi
4. bronch/o / pneumon/o / -ia
bronchus / lung / condition
condition of the bronchus and lung
5. laryng/o / -spasm
larynx / involuntary movement
involuntary movement of the larynx
6. pleur/o / -itis
pleura / inflammation
inflammation of the pleura
7. a- / -pnea
without, not / breathing
not breathing
8. laryng/o / -itis
larynx / inflammation
inflammation of the larynx
9. pneumon/o / -itis
lung / inflammation
inflammation of the lung
10. sinus/o / -itis
sinus / inflammation
inflammation of the sinus(es)
11. trache/o / -itis
trachea / inflammation
inflammation of the trachea
12. diaphragmat/o / -cele
diaphragm / herniation, protrusion
herniation of the diaphragm
13. nas/o / pharyng/o / -itis
nose / pharynx / inflammation
inflammation of the nose and pharynx
14. -dys / -phonia
painful, difficult, / condition of the voice
condition of vocal difficulty (difficulty producing sound)

15. pharyng/o / -itis
pharynx / inflammation
inflammation of the pharynx

Exercise 18
1. Computed tomography
2. chest radiograph
3. V/Q scan
4. PPD test
5. Bronchoalveolar lavage
6. magnetic resonance imaging
7. VATS
8. spirometry

Exercise 19
1. pulse oximetry
2. arterial blood gases (ABGs)
3. percussion
4. acid-fast bacilli (AFB) smear
5. radiography
6. laryngoscopy
7. pulmonary function tests (PFTs)
8. polysomnography
9. auscultation
10. peak flow monitoring

Exercise 20
1. thoracoscopy
2. rhinoscopy
3. pharyngoscopy
4. bronchoscopy
5. laryngoscopy

Exercise 21
1. thoracotomy
2. adenoidectomy
3. tracheoplasty
4. hyperbaric medicine
5. mechanical ventilation
6. aspiration
7. continuous positive airway pressure (CPAP) therapy
8. tracheotomy
9. laryngotracheotomy
10. tracheostomy tube
11. bronchoplasty
12. endotracheal intubation
13. pneumonectomy
14. incentive spirometry

Exercise 22
1. tracheotomy
2. tonsillectomy
3. rhinoplasty
4. thoracentesis
5. CPR

Exercise 23
1. septoplasty
2. laryngectomy
3. thoracentesis
4. bronchoscopy
5. thoracotomy

Exercise 24
1. laryng/o / -scope
larynx / instrument for examination
instrument for examination of the larynx
2. rhin/o / -plasty
nose / surgical repair, reconstruction
surgical repair of the nose
3. laryng/o / -stomy
larynx / surgical opening
surgical opening in the larynx
4. pneumon/o / -ectomy
lung / excision, surgical removal
surgical removal of a lung
5. sinus/o / -tomy
sinus / incision
incision into the sinus
6. bronch/o / -plasty
bronchus / surgical repair, reconstruction
surgical repair of the bronchus
7. thorac/o / -centesis
thorax / puncture to aspirate
puncture to aspirate the thorax (pleural cavity)
8. trache/o / -tomy
trachea / incision
incision into the trachea
9. adenoid/o / -ectomy
adenoid / excision, surgical removal
excision of the adenoid
10. trache/o / -stomy
trachea / surgical opening
surgical opening of the trachea

Exercise 25
1. nebulizer
2. expectorant
3. corticosteroid
4. antitussive
5. antihistamine
6. bronchodilator
7. antibiotic
8. decongestant
9. antitubercular drug

Exercise 26
1. otorhinolaryngologist
2. pulmonologist
3. otorhinolaryngology
4. pulmonology

Exercise 27
1. reactive airway disease
2. computed tomography (scan)
3. upper respiratory infection
4. ventilation–perfusion (scan)
5. tuberculosis
6. cardiopulmonary resuscitation
7. magnetic resonance imaging
8. purified protein derivative
9. video-assisted thoracoscopic surgery
10. arterial blood gas
11. continuous positive airway pressure
12. bronchoalveolar lavage

Exercise 28
1. chronic obstructive pulmonary disease, interstitial lung disease
2. pulmonary function tests, cystic fibrosis
3. acute respiratory distress syndrome
4. acid-fast bacilli, bronchiolitis obliterans with organizing pneumonia
5. chest x-ray

Exercise 29
1. nasal cavity
2. nasal septum
3. nose
4. epiglottis
5. larynx
6. bronchi
7. bronchioles
8. paranasal sinuses
9. pharyngeal tonsil (adenoids)
10. tonsils
11. pharynx
12. glottis
13. trachea
14. mediastinum
15. lung
16. diaphragm

Exercise 30
1. frontal sinus
2. nasal cavity
3. nose
4. oral cavity
5. epiglottis
6. sphenoid sinus
7. nasopharynx
8. oropharynx
9. tonsils
10. laryngopharynx
11. larynx
12. esophagus

Exercise 31
1. laryng/o / -eal
larynx / pertaining to
pertaining to the larynx
2. rhin/o / -rrhea
nose / -flow, discharge
discharge from the nose
3. pulmon/o / -ary
lung / pertaining to
pertaining to the lung
4. phren/o / -spasm
diaphragm / involuntary movement
involuntary movement of the diaphragm
5. thorac/o / -tomy
thorax / surgical incision
surgical incision into the thorax
6. tachy- / -pnea
fast / breathing
fast breathing (rate)
7. thorac/o / -ic
thorax / pertaining to
pertaining to the thorax
8. bronch/o / -spasm
bronchus / involuntary movement
involuntary movement of the bronchus
9. pulmon/o / -logy
lung / study of
study of the lungs
10. bronch/o / -scopy
bronchus / process of examining, examination
process of examining the bronchus

Exercise 32
1. visceral layer
2. alveoli
3. epiglottis
4. tachypnea
5. Hemothorax
6. asthma
7. laryngospasm
8. upper respiratory
9. Stridor
10. pharynx

Exercise 33
1. larynx, trachea, bronchi, and lungs
2. glottis or vocal cords
3. the anatomic region formed by the sternum, the thoracic vertebrae, and the ribs, extending from the neck to the diaphragm
4. three lobes make up the right lung and two lobes make up the left lung
5. tracheostomy or tracheotomy
6. pulmonary fibrosis
7. to aspirate fluid from the chest cavity
8. a mask is used to pump constant pressurized air through the nasal passages to keep the airway open
9. flow and volume of air inspired and expired by the lungs
10. windpipe

Exercise 34
1. B
2. A
3. D
4. B
5. D
6. B
7. B
8. B
9. C
10. D

Exercise 35
1. B
2. D
3. A
4. C
5. C
6. B
7. A
8. C
9. B
10. A

Exercise 36
1. erythema
2. tuberculosis
3. rhonchi
4. auscultation
5. wheezing
6. bilateral
7. to rule out active tuberculosis

Exercise 37
1. bronchitis
2. sputum
3. dyspnea
4. pulmonary embolism
5. pulmonary
6. pulmonologist

Exercise 38
Practice until your pronunciation matches that heard in the Audio Glossary in the Student Resources.

Exercise 39
1. alveolar
2. pulmonary
3. CORRECT
4. diaphragm
5. pneumopleuritis
6. pleuralgia
7. CORRECT
8. CORRECT
9. tonsillar
10. dyspnea

Chapter 12

Exercise 1
1. jejunum
2. appendix; vermiform appendix
3. gallbladder
4. mouth; oral cavity
5. palate
6. pharynx
7. fundus
8. liver
9. ileum
10. anus
11. salivary glands
12. bile

Exercise 2
1. duodenum
2. pancreas
3. esophagus
4. sigmoid colon
5. pylorus
6. rectum
7. cecum
8. descending colon
9. uvula
10. rugae

Exercise 3
1. stomach
2. teeth
3. transverse
4. tongue
5. water
6. cardia
7. three
8. saliva
9. body
10. ascending

Exercise 4
1. duodenum
2. mouth
3. pancreas
4. small intestine
5. lip
6. saliva
7. liver
8. cheek
9. anus
10. digestion
11. pharynx
12. anus, rectum
13. pylorus
14. colon
15. sigmoid colon
16. tooth
17. abdomen

Exercise 5
1. jejun/o
2. appendic/o
3. phag/o
4. hemat/o, hem/o
5. gastr/o
6. esophag/o
7. bucc/o
8. rect/o
9. polyp/o
10. cholecyst/o
11. cec/o
12. lingu/o
13. ile/o
14. dent/o, odont/o
15. col/o, colon/o
16. lith/o
17. palat/o
18. bil/o, chol/e
19. herni/o
20. abdomin/o, lapar/o
21. aliment/o

Exercise 6
1. in, within
2. crushing
3. enzyme
4. around, surrounding
5. surgical opening
6. abnormal condition
7. one who specializes in
8. herniation, protrusion
9. origin, production
10. enlargement
11. backward, behind
12. prolapse, drooping, sagging
13. viewing or examining with an instrument
14. meal
15. after, behind
16. above, excessive
17. pain
18. softening
19. a writing, a description
20. vomiting
21. instrument for examination
22. puncture to aspirate
23. stricture, narrowing
24. record, recording
25. suture
26. pain
27. incision

Exercise 7
1. inflammation of the pancreas
2. instrument for examination of the sigmoid colon
3. pertaining to nourishment
4. surgical opening into the colon
5. surgical removal or excision of the gallbladder
6. inflammation of a diverticulum

Exercise 8
1. proctologist
2. hepatitis
3. buccal
4. lithotripsy

5. abdominocentesis
6. anoplasty
7. gastrectomy
8. colonoscopy

Exercise 9
1. esophagitis
2. appendectomy
3. gastroscopy
4. colostomy
5. cheilorrhaphy
6. laparotomy
7. cholecystogram
8. oral
9. alimentary
10. hepatitis
11. pancreatopathy

Exercise 10

1. gastr/o / enter/o / -logist

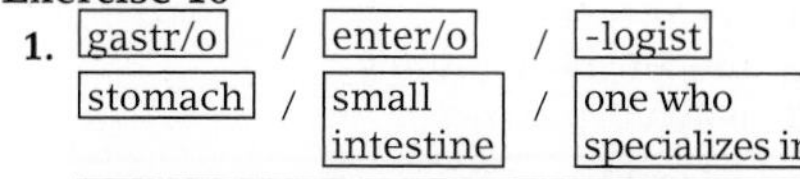

stomach / small intestine / one who specializes in

one who specializes in the treatment of the stomach and small intestine

2. dys- / peps/o / -ia

painful, / digestion / pertaining to difficult, abnormal

pertaining to painful digestion (heartburn)

3. hyper- / -emesis

above, excessive / -vomiting

condition of excessive vomiting

4. col/o / -ectomy

colon / surgical removal, excision

surgical removal of the colon

5. herni/o / -rrhaphy

hernia / suture

suture of a hernia

6. dys- / phag/o / -ia

painful, difficult, abnormal / eat, swallow / condition of

condition of painful swallowing

7. chol/e / lith/o / -iasis

gall, bile / stone, calculus / abnormal condition

abnormal condition of gallstones

8. hemat/o / -emesis

blood / -vomiting

vomiting blood

9. rect/o / -cele

rectum / -herniation, protrusion

herniation of the rectum

10. palat/o / -plasty

palate / surgical repair, reconstruction

surgical repair of the palate

11. ile/o / -stomy

ileum / surgical opening

surgical opening into the ileum

12. sub- / lingu/o / -al

below, beneath / tongue / pertaining to

pertaining to below or beneath the tongue

Exercise 11
1. eructation
2. occult
3. feces
4. peristalsis
5. mastication
6. halitosis
7. digestion
8. bolus
9. defecation
10. bloody stools

Exercise 12
1. deglutition
2. melena
3. inguinal
4. nausea
5. flatus
6. chyme
7. vomit
8. anorexia

Exercise 13
1. ascites
2. anorexia nervosa
3. volvulus
4. gastroesophageal reflux disease
5. Crohn disease
6. ileus
7. incontinence
8. pruritus ani
9. gastric ulcer
10. hiatal hernia

Exercise 14
1. diverticula
2. peritonitis
3. constipation
4. anorexia nervosa
5. dysentery
6. peptic ulcer disease
7. cirrhosis
8. irritable bowel syndrome
9. polyp
10. intussusception

Exercise 15
1. pancreatitis
2. gastralgia
3. polyposis
4. gastroenteritis
5. hepatomegaly
6. cholelithiasis
7. cholecystitis

Exercise 16
1. polyp/o; polyp
2. hepat/o; liver
3. diverticul/o; diverticulum
4. esophag/o; esophagus
5. cholecyst/o; gallbladder
6. stomat/o; mouth
7. hemat/o; blood
8. appendic/o; appendix
9. phag/o; eat, swallow
10. cheil/o; lip

Exercise 17
1. stool culture
2. barium swallow
3. endoscopy
4. paracentesis
5. hemoccult test

Exercise 18
1. proctoscopy
2. flexible sigmoidoscopy
3. colonoscopy
4. abdominal ultrasound
5. barium enema
6. cholecystogram
7. esophagogastroduodenoscopy

Exercise 19
1. abdomin/o; abdomen
2. cholecyst/o; gallbladder
3. lapar/o; abdomen
4. sigmoid/o; sigmoid colon
5. colon/o; colon
6. proct/o; rectum, anus

Exercise 20
1. surgical incision into the abdominal cavity
2. suturing of the tongue
3. removal of the stomach
4. process of feeding a patient through nasogastric intubation
5. surgical repair of the roof of the mouth
6. removal of a section of the stomach
7. a connection made surgically between two structures, such as adjacent parts of the intestine
8. crushing of gallstones
9. surgical removal of the appendix
10. surgical construction of an artificial opening between the ileum and the body exterior; done to bypass a damaged part of the ileum

Exercise 21
1. bariatric surgery
2. abdominoperineal resection
3. gavage
4. palatoplasty
5. anastomosis
6. cholecystectomy
7. gastric lavage
8. nasogastric intubation
9. TPN
10. gastric bypass

Exercise 22
1. colostomy; col/o / -stomy
2. pancreatography; pancreat/o / -graphy
3. periodontal; peri- / odont/o / -al
4. cheilorrhaphy; cheil/o / -rrhaphy
5. ileotomy; ile/o / -tomy
6. cholelithotripsy; cholecyst/o / lith/o / -tripsy
7. polypectomy; polyp/o / -ectomy
8. hemicolectomy; hemi- / colon/o / -ectomy
9. abdominoplasty; abdomin/o / -plasty

Exercise 23
1. surgical repair of the palate
palate
surgical repair
2. surgical construction of an artificial opening between the colon and the body exterior; done to bypass a damaged part of the colon
colon
surgical opening
3. suture of a hernia
hernia
suture

4. surgical construction of an artificial opening between the ileum and the body exterior; done to bypass a damaged part of the ileum
   ileum
   incision
5. surgical removal of the appendix
   appendix
   surgical removal, excision
6. suturing of the tongue
   tongue
   suturing

Exercise 24
1. antidiarrheal
2. laxative, cathartic
3. antacid
4. emetic
5. antiemetic

Exercise 25
1. medical specialty concerned with diagnosis and treatment of disorders of the gastrointestinal tract
2. physician who specializes in proctology
3. medical specialty concerned with diagnosis and treatment of disorders of the anus and rectum
4. physician who specializes in gastroenterology
5. branch of medicine concerned with the prevention and control of obesity and allied diseases

Exercise 26
1. gastrointestinal
2. barium enema
3. total parenteral nutrition
4. esophagogastroduodenoscopy
5. nasogastric
6. upper gastrointestinal
7. gastroesophageal reflux disease

Exercise 27
1. IBS
2. BM
3. PUD
4. APR
5. BE

Exercise 28
1. mouth
2. pharynx
3. liver
4. duodenum
5. gallbladder
6. ascending colon
7. cecum
8. appendix
9. salivary glands
10. esophagus
11. stomach
12. pancreas
13. transverse colon
14. descending colon
15. sigmoid colon
16. rectum
17. anus

Exercise 29
1. duodenum
2. jejunum
3. ascending colon
4. ileum
5. cecum
6. appendix
7. left colic (splenic) flexure
8. transverse colon
9. descending colon
10. sigmoid colon
11. rectum
12. anus

Exercise 30
1. surgical repair of the pylorus
   pylorus
   surgical repair
2. herniation of the esophagus
   esophagus
   herniation, protrusion
3. stomach pain
   stomach
   pain
4. softening of the mouth
   mouth
   softening
5. enlargement of the liver
   liver
   enlargement
6. process of examining through the abdominal wall into the stomach
   abdomen
   stomach
   technique of producing images
7. instrument used to examine the anus
   anus
   instrument to examine
8. eating (biting) the lip
   lip
   eat, swallow
9. surgical opening between the sigmoid colon and rectum
   sigmoid colon
   rectum
   surgical opening
10. inflammation of the small intestine and colon
   small intestine
   colon
   inflammation
11. narrowing of the rectum
   rectum
   stricture, narrowing
12. suturing of the lip
   lip
   suturing
13. teeth pain
   teeth
   pain
14. disease of the appendix
   appendix
   disease
15. incision into gallbladder to remove gall stones
   gall, bile
   stone, calculus
   incision
16. surgical opening into the jejunum
   jejunum
   surgical opening
17. surgical removal of the esophagus and stomach
   esophagus
   stomach
   surgical removal
18. drooping of the rectum
   rectum
   prolapse, drooping, sagging

Exercise 31
1. sial/o; saliva
2. aliment/o; nourishment, nutrition
3. pylor/o; pylorus
4. pharyng/o; pharynx
5. duoden/o; duodenum
6. gastr/o; enter/o; stomach; small intestine
7. hepat/o; liver
8. palat/o; palate
9. bucc/o; pharyng/o cheek; pharynx
10. dent/o; tooth
11. cec/o; cecum
12. proct/o; rectum, anus
13. polyp/o; polyp

Exercise 32
1. abdominocentesis
2. proctologist
3. occult blood test; hemoccult test
4. gastroesophageal reflux disease (GERD)
5. hyperemesis
6. pancreatolithectomy
7. gastroenterostomy

Exercise 33
1. B
2. A
3. C
4. A
5. C
6. B
7. A
8. C
9. C
10. A
11. D
12. A
13. C
14. C
15. D

Exercise 34
1. C
2. B
3. B
4. C
5. B
6. C

Exercise 35
1. gastrointestinal
2. diarrhea
3. constipation
4. bowel movement
5. nausea
6. anal
7. peptic ulcer
8. a deep furrow, cleft, slit or tear in the anus

Exercise 36
1. C
2. A
3. A
4. C

5. to decrease the reflux of acid from the stomach to the esophagus

Exercise 37

Practice until your pronunciation matches that heard in the Audio Glossary in the Student Resources.

Exercise 38

1. rugae
2. cecum
3. tongue
4. regurgitation
5. ileus
6. feces
7. occult
8. pylorus
9. uvula
10. gavage
11. nausea
12. mastication
13. polyposis
14. palate
15. incontinence

Chapter 13

Exercise 1

1. opening that carries urine from the urethra to the outside of the body
2. one of two narrow tubes that carry urine from the kidneys to the bladder
3. one of two bean-shaped organs that remove wastes from the blood and help maintain fluid and electrolyte balance in the body
4. microscopic functional unit of the kidney that forms urine
5. a reservoir in each kidney that collects urine

Exercise 2

1. glomerulus
2. renal cortex
3. glomerular capsule
4. urethra
5. urinary bladder
6. trigone of bladder
7. urine

Exercise 3

1. meat/o
2. olig/o
3. ur/o, urin/o
4. nephr/o, ren/o
5. hydr/o
6. pyel/o
7. noct/i
8. lith/o
9. enur/o

Exercise 4

1. -stomy
2. -lith
3. -cele
4. -scopy
5. -ptosis
6. -emia
7. -iasis, esis
8. -stenosis

Exercise 5

1. nephr/o
2. py/o
3. urethr/o
4. son/o
5. vesic/o
6. ureter/o
7. hydr/o

Exercise 6

1. hematuria
2. ureterostenosis
3. lithotripsy
4. uremia
5. glomerulitis
6. ureterolith
7. sonogram
8. cystoscopy

Exercise 7

1. pyuria
2. hematuria
3. albuminuria
4. glycosuria or glucosuria
5. oliguria
6. bacteriuria
7. polyuria
8. dysuria

Exercise 8

1. nephr/o / -megaly
   kidney / enlargement
   enlargement of the kidney
2. cyst/o / scope
   fluid-filled sac / instrument for (urinary bladder) examination
   instrument for examining the bladder
3. noct/i / -uria
   night / urine, urination
   urination at night
4. ureter/o / -stomy
   ureter / surgical opening
   creation of a surgical opening into a ureter
5. ren/o / -gram
   kidney / recording
   recording of kidney (function)
6. nephr/o / -lysis
   kidney / destruction, breakdown, separation
   separation of the kidney (freeing of the kidney from inflammatory adhesions)
7. vesicul/o/ / -ar
   fluid-filled sac (urinary bladder) / pertaining to
   pertaining to the urinary bladder
8. nephr/o / -rrhaphy
   kidney / suture
   suturing of the kidney

Exercise 9

1. to pass urine
2. pertaining to the kidney
3. pertaining to the urinary bladder
4. to urinate
5. pertaining to the urethra
6. pertaining to urine

Exercise 10

1. micturition
2. vesical
3. meatal
4. genitourinary
5. nephric
6. urinate
7. ureteral

Exercise 11

1. urin/o / -ary
   urine, urinary system/tract / pertaining to
   pertaining to urine or the urinary system/tract
2. ren/o / -al
   kidney / pertaining to
   pertaining to the kidney
3. cyst/o / -ic
   fluid-filled sac (urinary bladder) / pertaining to
   pertaining to the urinary bladder
4. urethr/o / -al
   urethra / pertaining to
   pertaining to the urethra
5. ureter/o / -al
   ureter / pertaining to
   pertaining to the ureter

Exercise 12

1. stricture
2. enuresis
3. renal calculus, nephrolith
4. nephrolithiasis
5. renal failure
6. urethral stenosis
7. urinary tract infection
8. uremia
9. hypospadias
10. anuria
11. hydronephrosis
12. polyuria

Exercise 13

1. stress urinary incontinence
2. diuresis
3. hydroureter
4. nocturia
5. urinary suppression
6. polycystic kidney disease
7. urinary retention
8. nephroptosis
9. hematuria
10. urge incontinence
11. epispadias
12. urethral stenosis
13. renal hypertension
14. nocturnal enuresis
15. end-stage renal disease

Exercise 14

1. ureter/o / -lith
2. protein/o / -uria
3. albumin/o / -uria
4. ur/o / -emia
5. urethr/o / -itis
6. glycos/o / -uria
7. ureter/o / -itis
8. pyel/o / nephr/o / -itis
9. nephr/o / lith/o / -iasis
10. glomerul/o / nephr/o / -itis

Exercise 15
1. ureterolith
2. pyuria
3. cystitis
4. nephroptosis
5. cystocele
6. dysuria
7. polyuria
8. pyelitis
9. oliguria
10. ureterocele
11. nephritis
12. cystolith
13. bacteriuria
14. nephromegaly
15. ureterostenosis

Exercise 16
1. creatinine clearance test
2. cystoscope
3. kidneys, ureters, and bladder (KUB) x-ray
4. renogram
5. urinalysis (UA)
6. specific gravity (SG)
7. urethroscopy
8. intravenous pyelography (IVP), intravenous urography (IVU)
9. nephrogram
10. blood urea nitrogen (BUN)

Exercise 17
1. cystometrogram
2. retrograde pyelogram
3. urodynamics
4. nephrosonography
5. voiding cystourethrogram
6. nephrotomogram
7. urinometer
8. urinalysis

Exercise 18
1. nephroscopy
2. cystogram
3. nephrography
4. urethroscope
5. cystoscopy
6. renogram
7. cystography
8. nephroscope

Exercise 19
1. procedure of inserting a tube through the urethra into the bladder to drain it of urine
2. incision into the bladder to remove a stone
3. surgical fixation of a floating kidney
4. creating a surgical opening into the bladder
5. incision into the renal pelvis to remove a stone
6. excision of a ureter
7. repair of the urethra
8. surgical removal of the bladder
9. breaking up of renal or ureteral calculi by focused ultrasound energy

Exercise 20
1. hemodialysis
2. kidney transplant or renal transplant
3. Nephrolithotomy
4. Ureterostomy
5. peritoneal dialysis
6. Cystoplasty
7. vesicourethral suspension
8. nephrotomy

Exercise 21
1. lith/o / -tomy
   stone, calculus / incision
   incision (to remove a) stone or calculus
2. cyst/o / -rrhaphy
   fluid-filled sac (urinary bladder) / suture
   suturing the urinary bladder
3. ureter/o / -tomy
   ureter / incision
   incision into the bladder
4. nephr/o / -ectomy
   kidney / excision, surgical removal
   excision or surgical removal of the kidney
5. pyel/o / -plasty
   renal pelvis / surgical repair, reconstruction
   repair of the renal pelvis
6. meat/o / -tomy
   meatus / incision
   incision into a meatus
7. lith/o / -tripsy
   stone, calculus / crushing
   crushing of a stone or calculus
8. nephr/o / -lysis
   kidney / destruction, breakdown, separation
   separation of the kidney (from adhesions)
9. urethr/o / -tomy
   urethra / incision
   incision into a urethra

Exercise 22
1. urinary analgesic
2. antibiotic
3. diuretic
4. antibacterial

Exercise 23
1. nephrologist
2. urology
3. urologist
4. nephrology

Exercise 24
1. urinary tract infection
2. intravenous pyelogram, intravenous pyelography
3. end-stage renal disease
4. specific gravity
5. catheter, catheterize, catheterization
6. voiding cystourethrogram, voiding cystourethrography
7. blood urea nitrogen
8. acute renal failure
9. genitourinary
10. intravenous urogram, intravenous urography

Exercise 25
1. kidneys, ureters, and bladder (x-ray)
2. extracorporeal shock wave lithotripsy
3. chronic renal failure
4. urinalysis
5. stress urinary incontinence

Exercise 26
1. inferior vena cava
2. abdominal aorta
3. bladder
4. urethra
5. kidneys
6. ureters

Exercise 27
1. renal artery
2. renal vein
3. renal pelvis
4. ureter
5. calyx
6. renal cortex
7. renal medulla

Exercise 28
1. cyst/o; fluid-filled sac (urinary bladder)
2. meat/o; meatus
3. urethr/o; urethra
4. hemat/o; blood
5. cyst/o; fluid-filled sac (urinary bladder)
6. ren/o; kidney
7. ureter/o; ureter
8. py/o; pus
9. pyel/o; renal pelvis
10. urethr/o; urethra
11. glycos/o; glucose, sugar
12. nephr/o; kidney
13. vesic/o; bladder
14. noct/i; night
15. ur/o; urine, urinary system/tract
16. cyst/o; fluid-filled sac (urinary bladder)
17. nephr/o; kidney
18. urethr/o; urethra
19. olig/o; scanty, few
20. ureter/o; ureter

Exercise 29
1. ureter/o / -lith
   ureter / stone, calculus
   stone or calculus in the ureter
2. glycos/o / -uria
   glucose, sugar / urine, urination
   glucose or sugar in the urine
3. nephr/o / -ptosis
   kidney / prolapse, drooping, sagging
   drooping of the kidney
4. ureter/o / -stenosis
   ureter / stricture, narrowing
   narrowing of the ureter
5. nephr/o / -tomy
   kidney / incision
   incision into the kidney
6. ur/o / -emia
   urine, urinary system/tract / blood (condition of)
   condition of urine in the blood

7. pyel/o / -itis
renal pelvis / inflammation
inflammation of the renal pelvis
8. glomerul/o / nephr/o / -itis
glomerulus / kidney / inflammation
inflammation of the glomeruli of the kidney

Exercise 30
1. specific gravity
2. KUB
3. hydroureter
4. catheterization
5. proteinuria
6. hemodialysis
7. stress urinary incontinence (SUI)
8. renal hypertension
9. vesicourethral suspension
10. nephroptosis
11. cystometrogram
12. urinalysis
13. urinary retention
14. nocturnal enuresis
15. hypospadias

Exercise 31
1. the amount of urea in the blood
2. a kidney
3. urine sample
4. the kidney stone may obstruct the flow of urine
5. to release wastes (urine) from the body
6. to surgically crush the stone in the bladder
7. the kidney
8. a nephrologist
9. urinary analgesic
10. urine
11. bladder and urethra
12. catheterization
13. urology
14. make an incision to remove a stone from an organ
15. the kidney
16. a ureter
17. cystogram
18. urinometer
19. an antibacterial and an antibiotic
20. the kidney

Exercise 32
1. D
2. B
3. D
4. A
5. B
6. A
7. B
8. D
9. C
10. A
11. C
12. A
13. C
14. A
15. D

Exercise 33
1. B
2. A
3. C
4. D
5. C

Exercise 34
1. oliguria
2. nocturnal enuresis
3. pyelonephritis
4. hydronephrosis
5. urinalysis
6. catheterization
7. SG
8. urinary retention
9. hydroureter
10. KUB
11. a stone in the urinary tract

Exercise 35
1. C
2. B
3. D
4. A
5. C
6. B
7. B
8. pertaining to through the vagina

Exercise 36
Practice until your pronunciation matches that heard in the Audio Glossary in the Student Resources.

Exercise 37
1. glomerulus
2. meatus
3. cystic
4. CORRECT
5. CORRECT
6. nephromegaly
7. CORRECT
8. cystocele
9. diuresis
10. CORRECT
11. hydroureter
12. CORRECT
13. CORRECT
14. urinalysis
15. cystoscopy

Chapter 14

Exercise 1
1. prepuce, foreskin
2. scrotum
3. seminal vesicles
4. sperm, spermatozoon
5. vas deferens, ductus deferens
6. bulbourethral glands
7. penis
8. seminiferous tubules

Exercise 2
1. testosterone
2. glans penis
3. epididymis
4. semen
5. prostate gland
6. testis

Exercise 3
1. prostate
2. sperm, spermatozoon
3. male
4. fluid-filled sac (seminal vesicle)
5. testis, testicle
6. glans penis
7. epididymis
8. sperm, spermatozoon
9. duct, vessel, vas deferens
10. testis, testicle

Exercise 4
1. crypt-
2. -lysis
3. -ism
4. -cele
5. -tomy
6. an-
7. -pexy
8. -plasty
9. –stomy
10. -genesis

Exercise 5
1. orchi/o, testicul/o
2. balan/o
3. vesicul/o
4. vas/o
5. prostat/o

Exercise 6
1. vasectomy
2. andropathy
3. prostatolith
4. vesiculitis
5. spermatogenesis
6. balanorrhea
7. orchiopexy

Exercise 7
1. prostatic
2. testicular
3. condom
4. ejaculation
5. epididymal
6. spermatic
7. balanic

Exercise 8
1. spermicide
2. testicular
3. balanic
4. prostatic
5. puberty
6. epididymal
7. condom

Exercise 9
1. testicul/o testis; testicle
2. prostat/o; prostate
3. balan/o; glans penis
4. epididym/o; epididymis
5. sperm/o; sperm, spermatozoon

Exercise 10
1. inflammation of the prostate
2. abnormal persistent and painful erection of the penis
3. absence of sperm; inability to produce sperm
4. abnormal discharge from the glans penis
5. inflammation of the epididymis
6. narrowing of the penis foreskin opening that prevents it from being retracted over the glans penis
7. a wart-like lesion on the genitals

Exercise 11
1. chlamydia
2. Genital herpes
3. varicocele
4. Gonorrhea
5. acquired immunodeficiency syndrome
6. hydrocele
7. Benign prostatic hypertrophy
8. erectile dysfunction

Exercise 12
1. human papillomavirus (HPV)
2. benign prostatic hyperplasia (BPH), benign prostatic hypertrophy (BPH)
3. human immunodeficiency virus (HIV)
4. sexually transmitted disease (STD) or venereal disease (VD) or sexually transmitted infection (STI)
5. spermatocele
6. testicular torsion
7. syphilis
8. Peyronie disease

Exercise 13
1. spermat/o / -cele
2. prostat/o / -itis
3. balan/o / -rrhea
4. a- / sperm/o / -ia
5. orchid/o / -itis
   orch/o/ -itis
   test/o/ -itis
6. balan/o / -itis
7. crypt/o / orchid/o / -ism
8. epididym/o / -itis

Exercise 14
1. andr/o / -pathy
   male / disease
   disease found in males
2. prostat/o / -lith
   prostate / stone
   stone in the prostate
3. balan/o / -itis
   glans penis / inflammation
   inflammation of the glans penis
4. olig/o / sperm/o / -ia
   few, scanty / sperm, spermatozoon / condition of
   deficiency of sperm
5. an- / orch/o / -ism
   without, not / testis, testicle / condition of
   condition of being without a testis
6. prostat/o / -rrhea
   prostate / discharge
   discharge from the prostate
7. crypt- / orchid/o / -ism
   hidden / testis, testicle / condition of
   condition of hidden testes

Exercise 15
1. transrectal ultrasound
2. digital rectal examination
3. prostatic-specific antigen

Exercise 16
1. surgical reconnecting of the vasa deferentia in a male with a vasectomy to restore fertility; vasectomy reversal operation
2. operation to remove the prepuce (foreskin) from the penis
3. removal of one or both testes
4. incision into the prostate to remove a stone
5. removal of the prostate through the urethra using a resectoscope; used to treat benign prostatic hyperplasia
6. device that is surgically placed in the penis to produce an erection; used to treat erectile dysfunction (ED)

Exercise 17
1. orchioplasty
2. epididymectomy
3. prostatolithotomy
4. orchiectomy
5. vasectomy
6. prostatectomy

Exercise 18
1. epididymectomy
2. orchioplasty
3. vesiculectomy
4. orchidotomy
5. vasectomy

Exercise 19
1. orchi/o / -tomy
   testis, testicle / incision
   incision into a testis
2. balan/o / -plasty
   glans penis / surgical repair, reconstruction
   surgical repair of the glans penis
3. prostat/o / -ectomy
   prostate / excision, surgical removal
   excision (removal) of the prostate
4. orchi/o / -pexy
   testis, testicle / surgical fixation
   surgical fixation (treatment) of a testis
5. vas/o / -ectomy
   duct, vessel / excision, surgical removal
   surgical excision of the vas deferens

Exercise 20
1. impotence agent
2. antiretroviral
3. vasodilator
4. antiviral

Exercise 21
1. urology
2. urologist

Exercise 22
1. benign prostatic hyperplasia, benign prostatic hypertrophy
2. transurethral incision of the prostate
3. erectile dysfunction
4. human immunodeficiency virus
5. prostatic-specific antigen
6. sexually transmitted infection
7. transrectal ultrasound
8. transurethral incision of the prostate

Exercise 23
1. transurethral resection of the prostate
2. sexually transmitted disease
3. digital rectal examination
4. human papillomavirus
5. acquired immunodeficiency syndrome
6. benign prostatic hyperplasia or benign prostatic hypertrophy

Exercise 24
1. prostate gland
2. vas deferens
3. penis
4. glans penis
5. prepuce (foreskin)
6. epididymis
7. seminal vesicle
8. testis
9. scrotum

Exercise 25
1. testicul/o; testis, testicle
2. prostat/o; prostate
3. balan/o; glans penis
4. orch/o; testis, testicle
5. epididym/o; epididymis
6. sperm/o; sperm, spermatozoon
7. vesicul/o; fluid-filled sac (seminal vesicle)
8. andr/o; male

Exercise 26
1. excision of the vas deferens
   duct, vessel, vas deferens
   excision
2. discharge from the prostate
   prostate
   discharge
3. inflammation of the glans penis
   glans penis
   inflammation
4. pertaining to the epididymis
   epididymis
   pertaining to
5. surgical fixation of the testes (surgical treatment of an undescended testicle)
   testis, testicle
   surgical fixation
6. stone in the prostate
   prostate
   stone
7. repair of a testis
   testis, testicle
   surgical repair, reconstruction
8. excision of the seminal vesicle
   fluid-filled sac (seminal vesicle)
   excision, surgical removal

Exercise 27
1. through sexual contact
2. to reverse a vasectomy and regain the ability to reproduce
3. testosterone
4. secretions from the testes, seminal glands, prostate gland, and bulbourethral glands
5. spermatocele
6. human papillomavirus (HPV) infection
7. prostate gland
8. prepuce or foreskin

9. cryptorchidism
10. vasectomy
11. in the erectile tissues inside the penis

Exercise 28
1. B
2. D
3. B
4. C
5. A
6. C
7. A
8. D
9. C
10. B
11. D
12. C
13. B
14. A
15. A
16. D
17. B
18. B

Exercise 29
1. D
2. B
3. C
4. B
5. D
6. A

Exercise 30
1. digital rectal examination
2. dysuria
3. hydrocele
4. orchiopexy
5. transrectal ultrasound

Exercise 31
1. D
2. B
3. A
4. D
5. D
6. transrectal ultrasound and needle biopsy

Exercise 32
1. orchialgia
2. balanorrhea
3. spermicide
4. condyloma
5. urethritis

Exercise 33
1. D
2. A
3. B
4. C
5. B
6. an accumulation of an excessive amount of watery fluid in cells, tissues, or serous cavities (exact answer will vary depending on dictionary used)

Exercise 34
Practice until your pronunciation matches that heard in the Audio Glossary in the Student Resources.

Exercise 35
1. scrotum
2. spermatozoon
3. semen
4. prostate gland
5. coitus
6. epididymis
7. balanorrhea
8. aspermia
9. phimosis
10. hydrocele
11. prostatitis
12. varicocele
13. chlamydia
14. condyloma
15. syphilis

Chapter 15

Exercise 1
1. placenta
2. lactiferous ducts
3. endometrium
4. breasts or mammary glands
5. genitalia
6. ovum
7. amnion
8. umbilical cord
9. nipple
10. fundus
11. areola
12. corpus luteum
13. vesicular ovarian follicles, graafian follicles
14. greater vestibular glands, Bartholin glands
15. zygote

Exercise 2
1. outer layer of the uterus that covers the body of the uterus and part of the cervix
2. fluid that encases the fetus and provides a cushion for the fetus as the mother moves
3. tubular, lower portion of the uterus that opens into the vagina
4. hormone secreted by the fertilized ovum soon after conception
5. female gamete or sex cell; when fertilized by a sperm, it develops into an ovum and is capable of developing into a new individual
6. outermost membrane surrounding the fetus
7. tubular structures that carry the oocyte from the ovary to the uterus
8. period of development from fertilization until birth
9. subdivisions of the lobes of the mammary gland that make breast milk
10. hormone that stimulates breast growth and milk secretion
11. pear-shaped organ located in the middle of the pelvis that supports a growing embryo and fetus and is the site of menstruation
12. part of the labia that covers and protects the female external genital organs
13. the developing organism from conception until the end of the eighth week of gestation

Exercise 3
1. corpus luteum
2. labia
3. Fimbriae
4. mons pubis
5. ovulation
6. introitus
7. labia minora
8. ovaries
9. vagina
10. zygote

Exercise 4
1. vulva
2. fetus
3. cervical os
4. lactation
5. effacement
6. gamete
7. lochia
8. vagina
9. lobules of mammary gland
10. ovaries

Exercise 5
1. endometrium
2. clitoris
3. labia
4. perineum
5. mammary glands
6. genitalia
7. adnexa
8. myometrium

Exercise 6
1. fundus
2. pelvis, pelvic cavity
3. cervix, neck (neck of uterus)
4. breast, mammary gland
5. from conception to birth
6. pubis
7. salpinx, uterine tube, fallopian tube
8. vagina
9. pregnancy
10. scanty, few
11. uterus
12. milk
13. birth
14. chorion
15. perineum

Exercise 7
1. vagin/o, colp/o
2. gyn/o, gynec/o
3. my/o
4. salping/o
5. mamm/o, mast/o
6. cephal/o
7. gravid/o
8. perine/o
9. hydr/o
10. toc/o
11. men/o, menstru/o
12. cervic/o
13. galact/o, lact/o
14. vulv/o, episi/o
15. pub/o

Exercise 8
1. above
2. surgical repair, reconstruction
3. incision

4. none
5. herniation, protrusion
6. measurement of
7. flow, discharge
8. condition of
9. new
10. beginning
11. suture
12. puncture to aspirate
13. before
14. in, within
15. childbirth, labor

Exercise 9
1. flowing forth (of blood) from the uterus
2. study of woman
3. excision or surgical removal of the uterus
4. record (image) of the breast
5. incision into the vulva
6. suture of the vagina
7. excision or surgical removal of (one or both) ovaries
8. inflammation of the cervix
9. surgical repair or reconstruction of the vagina
10. excision or surgical removal of (one or both) salpinges (uterine tubes)

Exercise 10
1. gynecologist
2. hysteroscopy
3. colporrhaphy
4. omphalocele
5. vaginitis
6. mammography
7. amniotomy
8. fetal
9. embryology
10. mastectomy

Exercise 11
1. suprapubic
2. intrauterine
3. menarche
4. estimated date of confinement
5. stillbirth
6. para
7. prenatal
8. meconium
9. primigravida

Exercise 12
1. chorionic
2. nullipara
3. transabdominal
4. neonate
5. congenital
6. cystic
7. gestational
8. gravida

Exercise 13
1. in vitro
2. ovarian
3. uterine
4. postpartum
5. neonatal
6. perineal
7. menses
8. date of birth
9. last menstrual period
10. nulligravida

Exercise 14
1. fet/o; fetus
2. vagin/o; vagina
3. pelv/i; pelvis
4. metri/o; uterus
5. abdomin/o, pelv/i; abdomen, pelvis
6. embry/o; embryo
7. abdomin/o; abdomen
8. ovari/o; ovary

Exercise 15
1. sexually transmitted disease (STD)
2. oligohydramnios
3. gastroschisis
4. cervical dysplasia
5. Turner syndrome
6. ectopic pregnancy
7. menopause
8. atrial septal defect
9. cleft lip
10. nuchal cord
11. abortion, spontaneous abortion
12. toxoplasmosis
13. rupture of membranes
14. patent ductus arteriosus
15. abruptio placenta
16. tetralogy of Fallot
17. bacterial vaginosis
18. pelvic inflammatory disease (PID)
19. atresia
20. breech pregnancy

Exercise 16
1. metrorrhagia
2. dyspareunia
3. infertility
4. polycystic ovary syndrome
5. ventricular septal defect
6. Braxton Hicks
7. gestational diabetes
8. eclampsia
9. postpartum depression
10. atrophic vaginitis
11. spina bifida
12. uterine prolapse
13. cleft palate
14. placenta previa
15. prolapsed cord
16. congenital
17. jaundice of newborn
18. incomplete abortion
19. adenomyosis

Exercise 17

1. a- / men/o / -rrhea
   without, not / menstruation / flow, discharge
   without (absence of) menstrual flow

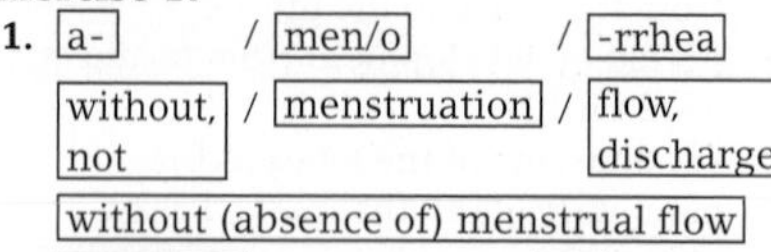

2. salping/o / itis
   salpinx, uterine tube, fallopian tube / inflammation
   inflammation of the salpinx
3. mast/o / -itis
   breast / inflammation
   inflammation of the breast
4. endo- / metri/o / -osis
   in, within / uterus / abnormal condition
   abnormal condition within the uterus (endometrium)
5. vulv/o / -dynia
   vulva / pain
   pain in the vulva
6. micro- / cephal/o / -y
   small / head / condition of
   condition of abnormally small head
7. my/o / -oma
   muscle (uterus) / tumor
   tumor of the uterus
8. omphal/o / -cele
   umbilicus, navel / herniation, protrusion
   herniation of the umbilical cord
9. mast/o / -dynia
   breast / pain
   pain in the breast
10. -dys / men/o / -rrhea
    painful, difficult / menstruation / flow, discharge
    painful or difficult menstrual flow

Exercise 18
1. fetoscope
2. transvaginal ultrasound
3. hysterosalpingography
4. Apgar
5. TORCH panel
6. quad marker screen
7. Papanicolaou test

Exercise 19
1. pelvic ultrasound
2. colposcopy
3. pregnancy test
4. mammography
5. chorionic villus sampling (CVS)
6. amniocentesis
7. TORCH panel

Exercise 20
1. puncture to aspirate (fluid) from the amnion (amniotic sac)
2. instrument for examination of the vagina
3. process of recording the uterus and salpinges (uterine tubes); radiography of the uterus and uterine tubes
4. process of recording the breast; radiography of the breasts
5. instrument for examining (listening to) the fetus
6. process of examining the vagina; examination of the vagina and cervix by means of an endoscope

Exercise 21
1. dilatation and curettage
2. myomectomy
3. pessary
4. total abdominal hysterectomy
5. cerclage
6. vaginal hysterectomy
7. induction of labor
8. in vitro fertilization (IVP)
9. loop electrosurgical excision procedure (LEEP) or loop excision
10. amniotomy or artificial rupture of membranes

Exercise 22

1. tubal ligation
2. cryosurgery
3. salpingo-oophorectomy
4. salpingectomy
5. therapeutic abortion
6. cesarean section

Exercise 23

1. mammoplasty
2. amniotomy
3. mastopexy
4. hysteroplasty or uteroplasty
5. episiotomy

Exercise 24

1. salping/o / oophor/o / -ectomy
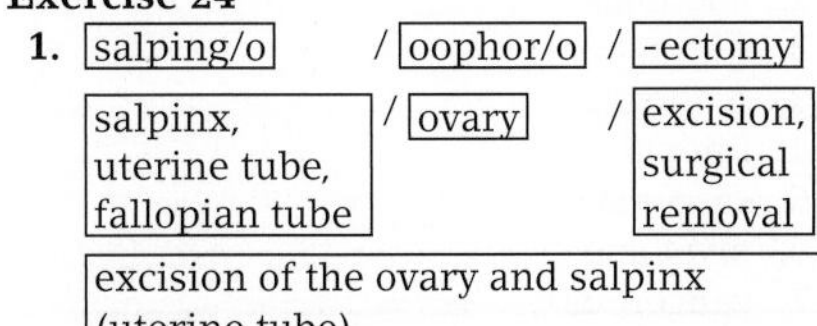
salpinx, uterine tube, fallopian tube / ovary / excision, surgical removal
excision of the ovary and salpinx (uterine tube)
2. colp/o / -rrhaphy
vagina / suture
suture of the vagina
3. uter/o / -tomy
uterus / incision
incision of the uterus
4. mamm/o / -plasty
breast, mammary gland / surgical repair, reconstruction
surgical repair of the breast
5. hyster/o / -ectomy
uterus / excision, surgical removal
excision of the uterus
6. episi/o / -tomy
vulva / incision
incision of the vulva
7. salping/o / -ectomy
salpinx, uterine tube, fallopian tube / excision, surgical removal
excision of a salpinx (uterine tube)
8. oophor/o / -ectomy
ovary / excision, surgical removal
excision of an ovary
9. mast/o / -pexy
breast, mammary gland / surgical fixation
surgical fixation of the breast (plastic surgery to elevation and reshape a drooping breast)
10. vulv/o / -ectomy
vulva / excision, surgical removal
excision of all or part of the vulva

Exercise 25

1. oxytocin
2. abortifacient
3. contraceptive
4. ovulation induction
5. tocolytic
6. hormone replacement therapy (HRT)

Exercise 26

1. midwife
2. neonatal intensive care unit
3. reproductive endocrinology
4. neonatology
5. obstetrics
6. pediatrics
7. neonatologist
8. midwifery
9. reproductive endocrinologist
10. gynecology
11. obstetrician
12. pediatrician
13. gynecologist

Exercise 27

1. total abdominal hysterectomy
2. spontaneous abortion
3. abortion
4. pelvic inflammatory disease
5. sexually transmitted disease

Exercise 28

1. neonatal intensive care unit
2. obstetrician
3. hormone replacement therapy
4. total abdominal hysterectomy
5. therapeutic abortion
6. estimated date of delivery
7. last menstrual period
8. in vitro fertilization
9. dilatation and curettage or dilation and curettage
10. loop electrosurgical excision procedure

Exercise 29

1. D&C
2. CVS
3. HSG
4. GYN
5. DOB
6. hCG

Exercise 30

1. peritoneal cavity
2. ovary
3. uterine tube
4. uterus
5. clitoris
6. labium minus
7. labium majus
8. vagina
9. cervix

Exercise 31

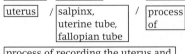

1. hyster/o / salping/o / -graphy
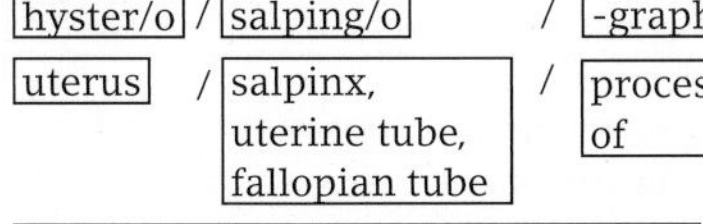
uterus / salpinx, uterine tube, fallopian tube / process of
process of recording the uterus and salpinges; radiography of the uterus and uterine tubes
2. episi/o / -tomy
vulva / incision
incision of the vulva
3. colp/o / -rrhaphy
vagina / suture
suturing the vagina
4. endo- / cervic/o / -al
in, within / cervix / pertaining to
pertaining to within the cervix
5. pelv/i / -metry
pelvis / measurement of
measurement of the pelvis
6. oophor/o / -ectomy
ovary / excision, surgical removal
excision of an ovary
7. mamm/o / -graphy
breast, mammary gland / process of recording
process of recording the breast; radiography of the breast
8. metr/o / -rrhagia
uterus / flowing forth
flowing forth (of blood) from the uterus between periods
9. olig/o / men/o / -rrhea
scanty, few / menstruation / flow, discharge
scanty discharge (of blood) during menstruation
10. mamm/o / -plasty
breast / surgical repair, reconstruction
surgical repair of the breast
11. salping/o / -ectomy
salpinx, uterine tube, fallopian tube / excision, surgical removal
surgical removal of a salpinx (uterine tube)
12. colp/o / -scopy
vagina / process of examining, examination
process of examining the vagina (and cervix)
13. vagin/o / -itis
vagina / inflammation
inflammation of the vagina
14. cervic/o / -itis
cervix / inflammation
inflammation of the cervix

Exercise 32

1. ectopic
2. nulligravida
3. Infertility
4. In vitro fertilization
5. Cesarean section
6. nuchal cord

Exercise 33

1. salpingo-oophorectomy
2. embryo
3. uterine tube (salpinx or fallopian tube)
4. Nulligravida refers to a woman who has had no pregnancies; primigravida refers to a woman who has had a single pregnancy; gravida refers to a woman who is pregnant.
5. perimetrium (outer layer); myometrium (muscular middle layer); endometrium (inner layer)
6. Gynecology deals with the functions and diseases of the female genital tract as well as endocrinology and reproductive health. Obstetrics deals with childbirth and the care of the mother.

7. anywhere other than the lining of the uterus
8. Rupture of membranes is a spontaneous rupture of the amniotic sac. An amniotomy is an artificial (purposeful) tearing of the amniotic sac to induce labor.
9. to test for various problems in the fetus, such as genetic defects, fetal infections, or fetal lung immaturity

Exercise 34
1. D
2. A
3. B
4. A
5. C
6. B
7. B
8. D

Exercise 35
1. C
2. B
3. A
4. C
5. A
6. B
7. A
8. C
9. A
10. D

Exercise 36
1. sexually transmitted disease
2. endocervical curettage
3. colposcopy
4. stenosis
5. patient has been pregnant 3 times
6. Papanicolaou test

Exercise 37
1. Prenatal
2. cervix
3. episiotomy
4. neonatologist
5. Apgar score
6. to enlarge the vagina and assist childbirth

Exercise 38

Practice until your pronunciation matches that heard in the Audio Glossary in the Student Resources.

Exercise 39
1. hysterectomy
2. suprapubic
3. cervicitis
4. cystic
5. laparotomy
6. mastectomy
7. endometrial
8. ovulation
9. perimetrium
10. mammography
11. placenta
12. clitoris
13. areola
14. colposcopy
15. zygote

Chapter 16

Exercise 1
1. disease
2. cancer
3. tumor
4. cancer
5. cold
6. black, dark
7. white
8. muscle, flesh
9. x-rays, radiation
10. abdomen

Exercise 2
1. cyt/o
2. kary/o
3. chem/o
4. cancer/o, carcin/o
5. rhabd/o
6. squam/o
7. plas/o
8. bi/o
9. ablat/o
10. sarc/o

Exercise 3
1. change, beyond
2. viewing, examining, or observing with an instrument
3. tumor
4. origin, production
5. within
6. bad, poor
7. smooth
8. new
9. painful, difficult, abnormal
10. originating, producing
11. beside
12. across, through

Exercise 4
1. tumor of the bone
2. tumor of cartilage
3. tumor of smooth muscle
4. cancerous tumor
5. condition of white blood cells (type of cancer)
6. tumor of the muscle
7. pertaining to a duct

Exercise 5
1. cytology
2. squamous
3. leiomyoma
4. melanoma
5. adenoma
6. lymphoma
7. myeloma
8. nephroma
9. angioma
10. neuroma

Exercise 6
1. benign
2. malignant
3. myelomas
4. melanoma
5. glandular tissue
6. oncogenic
7. recurrence
8. neuroma
9. malignant
10. lipoma
11. malignant neoplasm

Exercise 7
1. carcinoma
2. benign
3. lesion
4. dysplasia
5. tumor
6. cancer
7. in situ
8. invasion
9. metastasis

Exercise 8
1. adenoma
2. fibroma
3. pathogenic
4. lipoma
5. sarcoma
6. myeloma
7. cancerous
8. fibrosarcoma

Exercise 9
1. lymphoma
2. bronchogenic carcinoma
3. leiomyoma
4. chondroma
5. osteosarcoma
6. liposarcoma
7. lymphangioma
8. Wilms tumor
9. melanoma
10. glioma
11. osteofibroma
12. giant cell tumor
13. rhabdomyoma
14. mesothelioma
15. germ cell tumor (GCT)

Exercise 10
1. Leukemia
2. GIST
3. Wilms
4. Hodgkin
5. pheochromocytoma
6. bone
7. chondrosarcoma
8. giant cell tumor
9. retinoblastoma
10. meningioma

Exercise 11
1. medulloblastoma
2. ductal carcinoma in situ
3. oat cell carcinoma
4. squamous cell carcinoma
5. basal cell carcinoma
6. neuroblastoma
7. Kaposi sarcoma

Exercise 12
1. nephroma
2. lymphoma
3. leukemia
4. glioma
5. adenoma
6. leiomyoma
7. leiomyosarcoma
8. astrocytoma
9. carcinoma
10. rhabdomyosarcoma

Exercise 13

1. radionuclide scan
2. Endoscopic retrograde cholangiopancreatography
3. cholescintigraphy
4. fine-needle aspiration
5. lumbar puncture
6. Pap test
7. tumor marker
8. thoracoscopy
9. single photon emission computed tomography scan
10. hCG

Exercise 14

1. sentinel lymph node biopsy
2. alpha-fetoprotein (AFP) test
3. prostate-specific antigen (PSA) test
4. estrogen receptors
5. shave biopsy
6. punch biopsy
7. endoscopic ultrasound
8. mammography
9. transrectal ultrasound
10. colposcopy

Exercise 15

1. colposcopy
2. carcinoma
3. thoracoscopy
4. mammography

Exercise 16

1. radiofrequency ablation
2. radiation therapy
3. mastectomy
4. bone marrow transplant (BMT)
5. loop electrosurgical excision procedure (LEEP)
6. amputation
7. fulguration
8. Mohs surgery
9. debulking surgery
10. peripheral stem cell transplant

Exercise 17

1. TURBT
2. palliative
3. colectomy
4. Whipple
5. limb salvage surgery
6. transsphenoidal resection
7. wedge resection
8. radical
9. stereotactic radiosurgery
10. brachytherapy

Exercise 18

1. esophagectomy
2. thyroidectomy
3. gastrectomy
4. mastectomy
5. nephrectomy
6. lymphadenectomy
7. myomectomy
8. lobectomy

Exercise 19

1. pneumon/o / -ectomy
   lung / excision, surgical removal
   excision of the lung
2. col/o/ / -ectomy
   colon / excision, surgical removal
   excision of (all or part of) the colon
3. cyst/o / -ectomy
   bladder / excision, surgical removal
   excision of the (urinary) bladder
4. thyroid/o / -ectomy
   thyroid gland / excision, surgical removal
   excision of the thyroid gland
5. laryng/o / -ectomy
   larynx / excision, surgical removal
   excision of (all or part of) the larynx
6. irid/o / -ectomy
   iris / excision, surgical removal
   excision of (part of) the iris
7. crani/o / -ectomy
   skull, cranium / excision, surgical removal
   excision of (part of) the cranium
8. gastr/o / -ectomy
   stomach / excision, surgical removal
   excision of (all or part of) the stomach

Exercise 20

1. adjuvant chemotherapy
2. hormonal therapy
3. intrathecal chemotherapy
4. aromatase inhibitors
5. immunotherapy, biologic therapy
6. palliative chemotherapy
7. chemotherapy
8. chemoprevention
9. epidermal growth factor receptor (EGFR) inhibitor therapy
10. interstitial chemotherapy

Exercise 21

1. gynecologic oncology
2. radiation oncology
3. surgical oncology
4. pediatric oncology
5. gynecologic oncologist
6. medical oncologist
7. medical oncology
8. pediatric oncologist
9. radiation oncologist
10. surgical oncologist

Exercise 22

1. gastrointestinal stromal tumor
2. ductal carcinoma in situ
3. transurethral resection of prostate
4. hepatobiliary iminodiacetic acid
5. bone marrow transplant
6. radiofrequency ablation
7. transrectal ultrasound
8. epidermal growth factor receptors
9. magnetic resonance cholangiopancreatography
10. endoscopic ultrasound
11. single photon emission computed tomography
12. alpha fetoprotein

Exercise 23

1. LP
2. FNA
3. CA
4. TURB
5. ERCP
6. LEEP
7. PSA
8. BCC
9. hCG
10. MEN
11. NHL
12. SCC

Exercise 24

1. rhabd/o / my/o / sarc/o/-oma
   striated / muscle / muscle, flesh
   (malignant) tumor of striated muscle
2. my/o / -oma
   muscle / tumor
   (benign) tumor of muscle
3. nephr/o / -oma
   kidney / tumor
   tumor of the kidney
4. bronch/o / -scopy
   bronchus / viewing, examining, or observing with an instrument
   examining the bronchial tree through a bronchoscope
5. meningi/o / -oma
   meninges / tumor
   (benign) tumor of the meninges
6. endo- / -scopy
   in, within / viewing, examining, or observing with an instrument
   examining the interior using an endoscope
7. oste/o / sarc/o / -oma
   bone / muscle, flesh / tumor
   (malignant) tumor of bone arising from osteoblasts
8. neur/o / -oma
   nerve / tumor
   tumor of a nerve
9. irid/o / -ectomy
   iris / excision, surgical removal
   excision or surgical removal of the iris
10. lapar/o / -scopy
    abdomen / viewing, examining, or observing with an instrument
    examining the abdomen with a laparascope

Exercise 25

1. colorectal
2. cryotherapy
3. cystoscopy
4. benign
5. melanoma
6. Whipple operation
7. fulguration
8. shave biopsy
9. mammogram
10. osteosarcoma

Exercise 26

1. A simple mastectomy is the removal of a breast in which the underlying muscles and the lymph nodes are left intact. A radical mastectomy is the removal of the breast as well as the underlying muscles and lymph nodes in the adjacent armpit.
2. Hodgkin lymphoma is indicated by the presence of Reed-Sternberg cells. Non-Hodgkin lymphoma is a type of lymphoma other than the Hodgkin type.
3. debulking
4. to relieve pain and other symptoms but not to cure cancer
5. astrocytoma
6. A chondroma is benign and a chondrosarcoma is malignant.
7. Oncogenes are genes that cause normal cells to grow out of control and become cancer cells.
8. A beam of high-energy radiation is applied externally directly to the tumor while minimizing damage to other tissues.
9. They reduce estrogen levels in a woman's body and stop the growth of cancer cells that depend on estrogen to live and grow.
10. malignant

Exercise 27

1. C
2. B
3. D
4. C
5. C
6. A
7. B
8. B
9. A
10. C

Exercise 28

1. B
2. C
3. A
4. D
5. C
6. B
7. C
8. B
9. A
10. D

Exercise 29

1. stenosis
2. ulceration
3. rhinoscopy
4. carcinoma
5. rhinectomy

Exercise 30

1. B
2. B
3. B
4. C
5. C
6. B
7. Ductal carcinoma in situ (DCIS) is breast cancer that is confined to the ducts and has not spread into the tissue of the breast. This patient's cancer has become invasive so has obviously spread into the tissues of the breast.

Exercise 31

Practice until your pronunciation matches that heard in the Audio Glossary in the Student Resources.

Exercise 32

1. craniectomy
2. fulguration
3. rhabdomyoma
4. thyroidectomy
5. chondrosarcoma
6. cryosurgery
7. glioma
8. leiomyosarcoma
9. mammography
10. pheochromocytoma
11. brachytherapy
12. cholescintigraphy
13. lipoma
14. nephrectomy
15. palliative

FIGURE CREDITS

Figure 2-3. Copyright © Jochen Sand/Digital Vision/GettyImages.

Figure 3-1. Nath JL. *Using Medical Terminology: A Practical Approach.* Baltimore: Lippincott Williams & Wilkins, 2005.

Figure 3-2. Modified from Nath JL. *Using Medical Terminology: A Practical Approach.* Baltimore: Lippincott Williams & Wilkins, 2005.

Figure 3-3. Anatomical Chart Company.

Figure 3-4. Nath JL. *Using Medical Terminology: A Practical Approach.* Baltimore: Lippincott Williams & Wilkins, 2005.

Figure 3-5. Nath JL. *Using Medical Terminology: A Practical Approach.* Baltimore: Lippincott Williams & Wilkins, 2005.

Figure 3-6. Nath JL. *Using Medical Terminology: A Practical Approach.* Baltimore: Lippincott Williams & Wilkins, 2005.

Figure 3-7. Anatomical Chart Company.
Figure Labeling 1. Modified from Nath JL. *Using Medical Terminology: A Practical Approach.* Baltimore: Lippincott Williams & Wilkins, 2005.
Figure Labeling 2. Anatomical Chart Company.
Photo of nurse practitioner with patient. Copyright © Martin Barraud/OJO Images/GettyImages

Figure 4-1. Anatomical Chart Company.

Figure 4-2. Image provided by Stedman's, Dr. Barankin Collection.

Figure 4-3. Ills: Anatomical Chart Company. Photos: From Riordan CL, McDonough M, Davidson JM, et al. Noncontact laser Doppler imaging in burn depth analysis of the extremities. *J Burn Care Rehabil.* 2003;24:177–186.

Figure 4-4. From Fleisher GR, Ludwig W, Baskin MN. *Atlas of Pediatric Emergency Medicine.* Philadelphia, PA: Lippincott Williams & Wilkins; 2003: Fig. 11–37.

Figure 4-5. From Weber J, Kelley J. *Health Assessment in Nursing.* 2nd ed. Philadelphia, PA: Lippincott Williams & Wilkins; 2003.

Figure 4-6. From Bickley LS. *Bates' Guide to Physical Examination and History Taking.* 8th ed. Philadelphia, PA: Lippincott Williams & Wilkins; 2003.

Figure 4-7. From Goodheart HP. *Goodheart's Photoguide of Common Skin Disorders.* 2nd ed. Philadelphia, PA: Lippincott Williams & Wilkins; 2003.

Figure 4-8. From Weber J, Kelley J. *Health Assessment in Nursing.* 2nd ed. Philadelphia, PA: Lippincott Williams & Wilkins; 2003.

Figure 4-9. From Smeltzer SC, Bare BG. *Textbook of Medical-Surgical Nursing.* 9th ed. Philadelphia, PA: Lippincott Williams & Wilkins; 2000.

Figure 4-10. From Fleisher GR, Ludwig S, Henretig FM. *Textbook of Pediatric Emergency Medicine.* 5th ed. Philadelphia, PA: Lippincott Williams & Wilkins; 2005.

Figure 4-11. From Tasman W, Jaeger E. *The Wills Eye Hospital Atlas of Clinical Ophthalmology.* 2nd ed. Lippincott Williams & Wilkins; 2001.

Figure 4-12. From Goodheart HP. *Goodheart's Photoguide of Common Skin Disorders.* 2nd ed. Philadelphia, PA: Lippincott Williams & Wilkins; 2003.

Figure 4-13. From Willis MC. *Medical Terminology: A Programmed Learning Approach to the Language of Health Care.* 2nd ed. Baltimore, MA: Lippincott Williams & Wilkins; 2007.

Figure 4-14. From Bickley LS. *Bates' Guide to Physical Examination and History Taking.* 8th ed. Philadelphia, PA: Lippincott Williams & Wilkins; 2003.

Figure 4-15. From Hall JC. *Sauer's Manual of Skin Diseases.* 9th ed. Philadelphia, PA: Lippincott Williams & Wilkins; 2006.

Figure 4-16. Ill: Anatomical Chart Company. Photo: Image provided by Stedman's, Dr. Barankin Collection.

Figure 4-17. From Berg D, Worzala K. *Atlas of Adult Physical Diagnosis.* Philadelphia, PA: Lippincott Williams & Wilkins; 2006.

Figure 4-18. From Neville B, et al. *Color Atlas of Clinical Oral Pathology.* Philadelphia, PA: Lea & Febiger; 1991. Used with permission.

Figure 4-19. Image provided by Stedman's, Dr. Barankin Collection.

Figure 4-20. From Berg D, Worzala K. *Atlas of Adult Physical Diagnosis.* Philadelphia, PA: Lippincott Williams & Wilkins; 2006.

Figure 4-21. From Goodheart HP. *Goodheart's Photoguide of Common Skin Disorders.* 2nd ed. Philadelphia, PA: Lippincott Williams & Wilkins; 2003.

Figure 4-23. From F. Malzieu/Photo Researchers, Inc.

Figure 4-25. Image provided by Stedman's, Dr. Barankin Collection.

Figure 4-26. From Goodheart HP. *Goodheart's Photoguide of Common Skin Disorders.* 2nd ed. Philadelphia, PA: Lippincott Williams & Wilkins; 2003.

Figure 5-1. From Nath JL. *Using Medical Terminology: A Practical Approach.* Baltimore, MD: Lippincott Williams & Wilkins; 2005.

Figure 5-2. From Cohen BJ. *Medical Terminology: An Illustrated Guide.* 5th ed. Baltimore, MD: Lippincott Williams & Wilkins; 2007.

Figure 5-3. From Nath JL. *Using Medical Terminology: A Practical Approach.* Baltimore, MD: Lippincott Williams & Wilkins; 2005.

Figure 5-4. From Tank PW, Gest TR. *Lippincott Williams & Wilkins Atlas of Anatomy.* Baltimore, MD: Lippincott Williams & Wilkins; 2008.

Figure 5-6. From *Stedman's Medical Dictionary.* 28th ed. Baltimore, MD: Lippincott Williams & Wilkins; 2006.

Figure 5-8. From Premkumar K. *The Massage Connection, Anatomy and Physiology.* 2nd ed. Baltimore, MD: Lippincott Williams and Wilkins; 2004.

Figure 5-9. From Nath JL. *Using Medical Terminology: A Practical Approach.* Baltimore, MD: Lippincott Williams & Wilkins; 2005.

Figure 5-10. From Braun MB, Simonson SJ. *Introduction to Massage Therapy.* 2nd ed. Baltimore, MD: Lippincott Williams & Wilkins; 2007.

Figure 5-12. From *Granger, Neuromuscular Therapy Manual.* Baltimore, MD: Lippincott Williams & Wilkins; 2010, and Anatomical Chart Company.

Figure 5-13. From Nath JL. *Using Medical Terminology: A Practical Approach.* Baltimore, MD: Lippincott Williams & Wilkins; 2005.

Figure 5-14. From Yochum TR, Rowe LJ. *Yochum and Rowe's Essentials of Skeletal Radiology.* 3rd ed. Philadelphia, PA: Lippincott Williams & Wilkins; 2004.

Figure 5-15. **B.** From Nath JL. *Using Medical Terminology: A Practical Approach.* Baltimore, MD: Lippincott Williams & Wilkins; 2005.

Figure 5-16. Image from Rubin E, Farber JL. *Pathology.* 3rd ed. Philadelphia, PA: Lippincott Williams & Wilkins; 1999.

Figure 5-17. **A.** Copyright © Photodisc/Jim Wehtje/GettyImages. **B.** From Strickland JW, Graham TJ. *Master Techniques in Orthopaedic Surgery: The Hand.* 2nd ed. Philadelphia, PA: Lippincott Williams & Wilkins; 2005.

Figure 5-18. **A.** From Cohen BJ. *Medical Terminology.* 4th ed. Philadelphia, PA: Lippincott Williams & Wilkins; 2003. **B.** From Koval KJ, Zuckerman JD. *Atlas of Orthopaedic Surgery: A Multimedial Reference.* Philadelphia, PA: Lippincott Williams & Wilkins; 2004.

Figure 5-19. From Daffner RH. *Clinical Radiology The Essentials.* 3rd ed. Philadelphia, PA: Lippincott Williams & Wilkins; 2007.

Figure 5-20. From *Rockwood and Wilkins' Fractures in Children.* Lippincott Williams & Wilkins; 2014.

Figure 5-21. From Deep Light Productions/Photo Researchers, Inc.

Figure 5-22. From Cohen BJ. *Medical Terminology.* 4th ed. Philadelphia, PA: Lippincott Williams & Wilkins; 2003.

Figure 5-25. From Koval KJ, Zuckerman JD. *Atlas of Orthopaedic Surgery: A Multimedia Reference.* Philadelphia, PA: Lippincott Williams & Wilkins; 2004.

Figure 5-26. From Strickland JW, Graham TJ. *Master Techniques in Orthopaedic Surgery: The Hand.* 2nd ed. Philadelphia, PA: Lippincott Williams & Wilkins; 2005.

Figure 5-27. Photo courtesy of Drive Medical Design & Manufacturing, Port Washington, NY.

Figure 5-28. Photos courtesy of U.S. Orthotics, Tampa, FL.

Figure 5-29. Anatomical Chart Company.

Figure 5-30. From Jackson DW. *Master Techniques in Orthopaedic Surgery: Reconstructive Knee Surgery.* Philadelphia, PA: Lippincott Williams & Wilkins; 2007.

Figure 6-1. Modified from Bear MF, Connors BW, Parasido MA. *Neuroscience: Exploring the Brain.* 3rd ed. Philadelphia, PA: Lippincott Williams & Wilkins; 2006.

Figure 6-2. Modified from Bear MF, Connors BW, Parasido MA. *Neuroscience: Exploring the Brain.* 3rd ed. Philadelphia, PA: Lippincott Williams & Wilkins; 2006.

Figure 6-3. Anatomical Chart Company.

Figure 6-5. Copyright © Hulton Archive/Stringer/GettyImages.

Figure 6-7. Modified from Anatomical Chart Company.

Figure 6-10. Modified from Anatomical Chart Company.

Figure 6-12. From O'Doherty N. *Atlas of the Newborn.* Philadelphia, PA: JB Lippincott; 1979:254, with permission.

Figure 6-14. From Daffner RH. *Clinical Radiology: The Essentials.* 3rd ed. Philadelphia, PA: Lippincott Williams & Wilkins; 2007.

Figure 6-15. From Bickley LS, Szilagyi P. *Bates' Guide to Physical Examination and History Taking.* 8th ed. Philadelphia, PA: Lippincott Williams & Wilkins; 2003.

Figure 6-18. Simon Fraser/RVI, Newcastle upon Tyne/Photo Researchers, Inc.

Figure 6-19. Normal: From Snell MD. *Clinical Anatomy.* 7th ed. Lippincott Williams & Wilkins; 2003. Multiple sclerosis: Ronald L. *Eisenberg, an Atlas of Differential Diagnosis.* 4th ed. Philadelphia, PA: Lippincott Williams & Wilkins; 2003.

Figure 6-20. From Willis MC. *Medical Terminology: A Programmed Learning Approach to the Language of Health Care.* 2nd ed. Baltimore, MD: Lippincott Williams & Wilkins; 2007.

Figure 6-22. From Fleisher GR, Ludwig S, Baskin MN. *Atlas of Pediatric Emergency Medicine.* Philadelphia, PA: Lippincott Williams & Wilkins; 2004.

Figure 7-1. Modified from Anatomical Chart Company.

Figure 7-2. Modified from Tank PW, Gest TR. *Lippincott Williams & Wilkins Atlas of Anatomy.* Baltimore, MD: Lippincott Williams & Wilkins; 2008.

Figure 7-3. From Tasman W, Jaeger E. *The Wills Eye Hospital Atlas of Clinical Ophthalmology.* 2nd ed. Lippincott Williams & Wilkins; 2001.

Figure 7-4. From Rubin E, Farber JL. *Pathology.* 4th ed. Philadelphia, PA: Lippincott Williams & Wilkins; 2005.

Figure 7-5. From Tasman W, Jaeger E. *The Wills Eye Hospital Atlas of Clinical Ophthalmology.* 2nd ed. Lippincott Williams & Wilkins; 2001.

Figure 7-6. Anatomical Chart Company.

Figure 7-7. From Nath JL. *Using Medical Terminology: A Practical Approach.* Baltimore, MD: Lippincott Williams & Wilkins; 2005.

Figure 7-9. Image provided by Stedman's.

Figure 7-10. **A.** From Bickley LS, Szilagyi P. *Bates' Guide to Physical Examination and History Taking.* 8th ed. Philadelphia, PA: Lippincott Williams & Wilkins; 2003. **B.** McConnell TH. *The Nature of Disease Pathology for the Health Professions.* Philadelphia, PA: Lippincott Williams & Wilkins; 2007. **C, D.** From Tasman W, Jaeger E. *The Wills Eye Hospital Atlas of Clinical Ophthalmology.* 2nd ed. Lippincott Williams & Wilkins; 2001.

Figure 7-11. Bill Bachmann/Photo Researchers, Inc.

Figure 7-12. LifeART image copyright © 2015 Lippincott Williams & Wilkins. All rights reserved.

Figure 7-13. **A.** Anatomical Chart Company.

Figure 7-14. Anatomical Chart Company.

Figure 7-15. Anatomical Chart Company.

Figure 7-17. From Moore KL, Dalley AF II. *Clinical Oriented Anatomy.* 4th ed. Baltimore, MD: Lippincott Williams & Wilkins; 1999.

Figure 7-18. © Barbara Sauder/iStockphoto.

Figure 7-19. **A.** From Moore KL, Dalley AF II. *Clinical Oriented Anatomy.* 4th ed. Baltimore, MD: Lippincott Williams & Wilkins; 1999. **B.** From Taylor C, Lillis C, LeMone P. *Fundamentals of Nursing: The Art and Science of Nursing Care.* 4th ed. Philadelphia, PA: Lippincott Williams & Wilkins; 2001.

Figure 7-21. Anatomical Chart Company.

Figure 7-22. Courtesy of Larry E. Humes, PhD.

Figure 8-1. From Westheimer R, Lopater S. *Human Sexuality: A Psychosocial Perspective.* Baltimore, MD: Lippincott Williams & Wilkins; 2002.

Figure 8-2. Anatomical Chart Company.

Figure 8-6. From McConnell TH. *The Nature of Disease Pathology for the Health Professions.* Philadelphia, PA: Lippincott Williams & Wilkins; 2007.

Figure 8-8. From Rubin E. *Essential Pathology.* 3rd ed. Philadelphia, PA: Lippincott Williams & Wilkins; 2000.

Figure 8-9. From Goodheart HP. *Photoguide of Common Skin Disorders.* 2nd ed. Philadelphia, PA: Lippincott Williams & Wilkins; 2003.

Figure 8-13. From Klossner NJ, Hatfield N. *Introductory Maternity and Pediatric Nursing.* Philadelphia, PA: Lippincott Williams & Wilkins; 2005.

Figure 8-14. From Smeltzer SC, Bare BG. *Textbook of Medical-Surgical Nursing.* 12th ed. Philadelphia, PA: Lippincott Williams & Wilkins; 2010. Courtesy of Medtronic Diabetes.

Figure 8-15. Southern Illinois University/Photo Researchers, Inc.

Figure 8-16. Olivier Voisin/Photo Researchers, Inc.

Figure 8-17. Spencer Grant/Photo Researchers, Inc.

Figure 8-18. From Eisenberg RL. *An Atlas of Differential Diagnosis.* 4th ed. Philadelphia, PA: Lippincott Williams & Wilkins; 2003.

Figure 9-1. From Cohen BJ. *Medical Terminology.* 5th ed. Philadelphia, PA: Lippincott Williams & Wilkins; 2007.

Figure 9-2. From Willis MC. *Medical Terminology: A Programmed Learning to the Language of Health Care.* 2nd ed. Baltimore, MD: Lippincott Williams & Wilkins; 2007.

Figure 9-3. From Cohen BJ. *Medical Terminology.* 5th ed. Philadelphia, PA: Lippincott Williams & Wilkins; 2007.

Figure 9-4. From Nath JL. *Using Medical Terminology.* 2nd ed. Philadelphia, PA: Lippincott Williams & Wilkins; 2013.

Figure 9-5. From Cohen BJ. *Medical Terminology.* 5th ed. Philadelphia, PA: Lippincott Williams & Wilkins; 2007.

Figure 9-6. From Nath JL. *Using Medical Terminology.* 2nd ed. Philadelphia, PA: Lippincott Williams & Wilkins; 2013.

Figure 9-7. From Cohen BJ. *Medical Terminology.* 5th ed. Philadelphia, PA: Lippincott Williams & Wilkins; 2007.

Figure 9-8. From Cohen BJ. *Memmler's The Human Body in Health and Disease.* 11th ed. Baltimore, MD: Lippincott Williams & Wilkins; 2008.

Figure 9-11. From Cohen BJ. *Medical Terminology.* 5th ed. Philadelphia, PA: Lippincott Williams & Wilkins; 2007.

Figure 9-12. From Cohen BJ. *Medical Terminology.* 5th ed. Philadelphia, PA: Lippincott Williams & Wilkins; 2007.

Figure 9-17. From Springhouse. *Lippincott's Visual Encyclopedia of Clinical Skills.* Philadelphia, PA: Wolters Kluwer Health; 2009.

Figure 9-18. **A.** Russ Curtis/Photo Researchers, Inc. **B.** Aaron Haupt/Photo Researchers, Inc.

Figure 9-19. Dr P. Marazzi/Photo Researchers, Inc.

Figure 9-20. Anatomical Chart Company.

Figure 10-2. From McArdle WD, Katch KI, Katch VL. *Exercise Physiology.* 7th ed. Baltimore, MD: Lippincott Williams & Wilkins; 2009.

Figure 10-3. Anatomical Chart Company.

Figure 10-4. From Premkumar K. *The Massage Connection Anatomy and Physiology.* Baltimore, MD: Lippincott Williams & Wilkins; 2004.

Figure 10-10. From Nath JL. *Using Medical Terminology: A Practical Approach.* Baltimore, MD: Lippincott Williams & Wilkins; 2005.

Figure 10-11. From Brant WE, Helms CA. *Fundamentals of Diagnostic Radiology.* 3rd ed. Philadelphia, PA: Lippincott Williams & Wilkins; 2007.

Figure 10-12. Anatomical Chart Company.

Figure 10-15. Anatomical Chart Company.

Figure 10-19. From Willis MC. *Medical Terminology: A Programmed Learning Approach to the Language of Health Care.* 2nd ed. Baltimore, MD: Lippincott, Williams & Wilkins; 2007.

Figure 10-20. From Bickley LS. *Bates' Guide to Physical Examination and History Taking.* 8th ed. Philadelphia, PA: Lippincott Williams & Wilkins; 2003.

Figure 10-22. From Cohen BJ. *Medical Terminology.* 5th ed. Philadelphia, PA. Lippincott Williams & Wilkins; 2007.

Figure 10-24. From Willis MC. *Medical Terminology: A Programmed Learning Approach to the Language of Health Care.* 2nd ed. Baltimore, MD: Lippincott Williams & Wilkins; 2007.

Figure 10-25. Copyright © Comstock Images/GettyImages.

Figure 10-26. From Smeltzer SC, Bare BG, Hinkle J, et al. *Brunner and Suddarth's Textbook of Medical Surgical Nursing.* 12th ed. Philadelphia, PA: Lippincott Williams & Wilkins; 2009.

Figure 10-27. From Smeltzer SC, Bare BG, Hinkle J, et al. *Brunner and Suddarth's Textbook of Medical Surgical Nursing.* 12th ed. Philadelphia, PA: Lippincott Williams & Wilkins; 2009.

Figure 10-28. LifeART image copyright © 2011 Lippincott Williams & Wilkins. All rights reserved.

Figure 10-29. LifeART image copyright © 2011 Lippincott Williams & Wilkins. All rights reserved.

Figure 10-31. Anatomical Chart Company.

Figure 11-1. Anatomical Chart Company.

Figure 11-2. From Nath JL. *Using Medical Terminology: A Practical Approach.* Baltimore, MD: Lippincott Williams & Wilkins; 2005.

Figure 11-5. Anatomical Chart Company.

Figure 11-6. Anatomical Chart Company.

Figure 11-7. Anatomical Chart Company.

Figure 11-8. Anatomical Chart Company.

Figure 11-9. From Yochum TR, Rowe LJ. *Yochum and Rowe's Essentials of Skeletal Radiology.* 3rd ed. Philadelphia, PA: Lippincott Williams & Wilkins; 2004.

Figure 11-10. From **A.** Brant WE, Helms CA. *Fundamentals of Diagnostic Radiology.* 3rd ed. Philadelphia, PA: Lippincott Williams & Wilkins; 2007. **B.** Fleisher GR, et al. *Textbook of Pediatric Emergency Medicine.* 5th ed. Philadelphia, PA: Lippincott Williams & Wilkins; 2005.

Figure 11-11. From Smeltzer SC, Bare BG, Hinkle J, et al. *Brunner and Suddarth's Textbook of Medical Surgical Nursing.* 12th ed. Philadelphia, PA: Lippincott Williams & Wilkins; 2009.

Figure 11-12. Anatomical Chart Company.

Figure 11-15. **A.** From Southern Illinois University/Photo Researchers, Inc. **B.** From Crapo JD, Glassroth J, Karlinsky JB, et al. *Baum's Textbook of Pulmonary Diseases.* 7th ed. Philadelphia, PA: Lippincott Williams & Wilkins; 2004.

Figure 11-16. Copyright © Lifesize/Monica Rodriguez/GettyImages.

Figure 11-17. From Willis MC. *Medical Terminology: The Language of Health Care.* 2nd ed. Baltimore, MD: Lippincott Williams & Wilkins; 2005.

Figure 11-18. From Cohen BJ. *Medical Terminology.* 5th ed. Philadelphia, PA: Lippincott Williams & Wilkins; 2007.

Figure 11-20. Photo courtesy of Respironics, Inc. Murrysville, PA (from Willis Programmed, 2e).

Figure 11-22. From Smeltzer SC, Bare BG, Hinkle J, et al. *Brunner and Suddarth's Textbook of Medical Surgical Nursing.* 12th ed. Philadelphia, PA: Lippincott Williams & Wilkins; 2009.

Figure 11-23. **A.** Courtesy of Tyco Health care/Nelicor Puritan Bennett, Pleasanton, CA. **B.** Smeltzer SC, Bare BG, Hinkle J, et al. *Brunner and Suddarth's Textbook of Medical Surgical Nursing.* 12th ed. Philadelphia, PA: Lippincott Williams & Wilkins; 2009.

Figure 11-24. From Moore KL, Agur AM, Dalley AF. *Essential Clinical Anatomy.* 4th ed. Baltimore, MD: Lippincott Williams & Wilkins; 2010.

Figure 11-25. From Pillitteri A. *Maternal & Child Health Nursing: Care of the Childbearing & Childrearing Family.* 6th ed. Philadelphia, PA: Lippincott Williams & Wilkins; 2010.

Figure 11-26. From Stern EJ, Swensen SJ, Kanne JP. *High Resolution CT of the Chest: Comprehensive Atlas.* 3rd ed. Philadelphia, PA: Lippincott Williams & Wilkins; 2010.

Figure 12-1. From Nath JL. *Using Medical Terminology: A Practical Approach.* Baltimore, MD: Lippincott Williams & Wilkins; 2005.

Figure 12-3. From Nath JL. *Using Medical Terminology: A Practical Approach.* Baltimore, MD: Lippincott Williams & Wilkins; 2005.

Figure 12-4. From Nath JL. *Using Medical Terminology: A Practical Approach.* Baltimore, MD: Lippincott Williams & Wilkins; 2005.

Figure 12-5. Modified from Anatomical Chart Company.

Figure 12-6. Anatomical Chart Company.

Figure 12-7. From Willis MC. *Medical Terminology: A Programmed Learning Approach to the Language of Health Care.* 2nd ed. Baltimore, MD: Lippincott Williams & Wilkins; 2007.

Figure 12-8. From Rubin R, Strayer DS, Rubin E. *Rubin's Pathology: Clinicopathologic Foundations of Medicine.* 5th ed. Baltimore, MD: Lippincott Williams & Wilkins; 2008.

Figure 12-9. From Willis MC. *Medical Terminology: A Programmed Learning Approach to the Language of Health Care.* 2nd ed. Baltimore, MD: Lippincott Williams & Wilkins; 2007.

Figure 12-13. Modified from LifeART image copyright © 2011 Lippincott Williams & Wilkins. All rights reserved.

Figure 12-14. From Mulholland MW, Maier RV, et al. *Greenfield's Surgery Scientific Principles and Practice.* 4th ed. Philadelphia, PA: Lippincott Williams & Wilkins; 2006.

Figure 12-15. From Cohen BJ. *Medical Terminology.* 5th ed. Philadelphia, PA: Lippincott Williams & Wilkins; 2007.

Figure 12-16. MIXA/Punchstock.

Figure 12-17. From Snell RS. *Clinical Anatomy by Regions.* 8th ed. Philadelphia, PA: Lippincott Williams & Wilkins; 2008.

Figure 12-18. From Cohen BJ. *Medical Terminology.* 5th ed. Philadelphia, PA: Lippincott Williams & Wilkins; 2007.

Figure 12-19. **A.** Kronenberger J, Durham LS, Woodson D. *Lippincott Williams & Wilkins' Comprehensive Medical Assisting.* 3rd ed. Baltimore, MD: Lippincott Williams & Wilkins; 2008. **B.** Smeltzer SC, Bare BG, Hinkle J, et al. *Brunner and Suddarth's Textbook of Medical Surgical Nursing.* 12th ed. Philadelphia, PA: Lippincott Williams & Wilkins; 2009.

Figure 12-21. From Smeltzer SC, Bare BG, Hinkle J, et al. *Brunner and Suddarth's Textbook of Medical Surgical Nursing.* 12th ed. Philadelphia, PA: Lippincott Williams & Wilkins; 2009.

Figure 12-22. From Smeltzer SC, Bare BG, Hinkle J, et al. *Brunner and Suddarth's Textbook of Medical Surgical Nursing.* 12th ed. Philadelphia, PA: Lippincott Williams & Wilkins; 2009.

Figure 12-23. From Willis MC. *Medical Terminology: A Programmed Learning Approach to the Language of Health Care.* 2nd ed. Baltimore, MD: Lippincott Williams & Wilkins; 2007.

Figure 13-6. From Nath JL. *Using Medical Terminology: A Practical Approach.* Baltimore, MD: Lippincott Williams & Wilkins; 2005.

Figure 13-7. Anatomical Chart Company.

Figure 13-8. From McConnell TH. *The Nature of Disease Pathology for the Health Professions.* Philadelphia, PA: Lippincott Williams & Wilkins; 2007.

Figure 13-9. From Mulholland MW, Maier RV, Doherty GM, et al. *Greenfield's Surgery Scientific Principles and Practice.* 4th ed. Philadelphia, PA: Lippincott Williams & Wilkins; 2006.

Figure 13-14. From Nath JL. *Using Medical Terminology: A Practical Approach.* Baltimore, MD: Lippincott Williams & Wilkins; 2005.

Figure 13-16. From Premkumar K. *The Massage Connection Anatomy and Physiology.* Baltimore, MD: Lippincott Williams & Wilkins; 2004.

Figure 13-17. From McClatchey KD, ed. *Clinical Laboratory Medicine.* 2nd ed. Philadelphia, PA: Lippincott Williams & Wilkins; 2002.

Figure 14-1. Modified from Anatomical Chart Company.

Figure 14-2. Anatomical Chart Company.

Figure 14-10. From Goodheart HP. *Goodheart's Photoguide of Common Skin Disorders.* 2nd ed. Philadelphia, PA: Lippincott Williams & Wilkins; 2003.

Figure 14-11. Image from Rubin E, Farber JL. *Pathology.* 3rd ed. Philadelphia, PA: Lippincott Williams & Wilkins; 1999.

Figure 14-12. From Nath JL. *Using Medical Terminology: A Practical Approach.* Baltimore, MD: Lippincott Williams & Wilkins; 2005.

Figure 14-15. From Nath JL. *Using Medical Terminology: A Practical Approach.* Baltimore, MD: Lippincott Williams & Wilkins; 2005.

Figure 14-16. © 2010 Intuitive Surgical, Inc.

Figure 15-6. Reprinted with permission from Pillitteri A. *Maternal and Child Health Nursing.* 4th ed. Philadelphia, PA: Lippincott Williams & Wilkins; 2003.

Figure 15-10. Anatomical Chart Company.

Figure 15-11. From Pillitteri A. *Maternal and Child Nursing.* 4th ed. Philadelphia, PA: Lippincott, Williams & Wilkins; 2003.

Figure 15-13. Anatomical Chart Company.

Figure 15-15. From Nettina SM. *Lippincott Manual of Nursing Practice.* 9th ed. Philadelphia, PA: Wolters Kluwer Health; 2010.

Figure 15-18. Anatomical Chart Company.

Figure 15-19. Deep Light Productions/Photo Researchers, Inc.

Figure 15-20. Sonograms: From Willis MC. *Medical Terminology: A Programmed Learning Approach to the Language of Health Care.* 2nd ed. Baltimore, MD: Lippincott Williams & Wilkins; 2007.

Figure 15-24. From Klossner NJ, Hatfield N. *Introductory Maternity and Pediatric Nursing.* Philadelphia, PA: Lippincott Williams & Wilkins; 2005.

Figure 16-1. From McConnell TH. *The Nature of Disease Pathology for the Health Professions.* Philadelphia, PA: Lippincott Williams & Wilkins; 2007.

Figure 16-5. Neuroma figure: CNRI/Photo Researchers, Inc. All other figs: From Cagle PT. *Color Atlas and Text of Pulmonary Pathology.* Philadelphia, PA: Lippincott Williams & Wilkins; 2005.

Figure 16-12. From Rubin R, Strayer DS, Rubin E. *Rubin's Pathology: Clinicopathologic Foundations of Medicine.* 5th ed. Baltimore, MD: Lippincott Williams & Wilkins; 2008.

Figure 16-13. Anatomical Chart Company.

Figure 16-14. From Rubin R, Strayer DS, Rubin E. *Rubin's Pathology: Clinicopathologic Foundations of Medicine.* 5th ed. Baltimore, MD: Lippincott Williams & Wilkins; 2008.

Figure 16-15. Anatomical Chart Company.

Figure 16-16. John Bavosi/Photo Researchers, Inc.

Figure 16-21. Modified from Anatomical Chart Company.

Figure 16-23. Véronique Burger/Photo Researchers, Inc.

Figure 16-24. From Varian Medical Systems, Palo Alto, CA, with permission.

STEDMAN'S Anatomy Atlas

Skeletal Anatomy, Anterior View 768
Skeletal Anatomy, Posterior View 769
The Skull, Anterior and Posterior Views 770
Muscular System, Anterior View 771
Muscular System, Posterior View 772
Spinal and Cranial Nerves 773
Cerebral Hemispheres 774
Anatomy of the Heart, Anterior View 775
Arterial System, Anterior View 776
Venous System, Anterior View 777
Respiratory System, Anterior View 778
Lymphatic System, Anterior View 779
Digestive System, Anterior View 780
Urinary System, Anterior View 781
Male and Female Urogenital Systems, Midsagittal View 782

Skeletal Anatomy, Anterior View

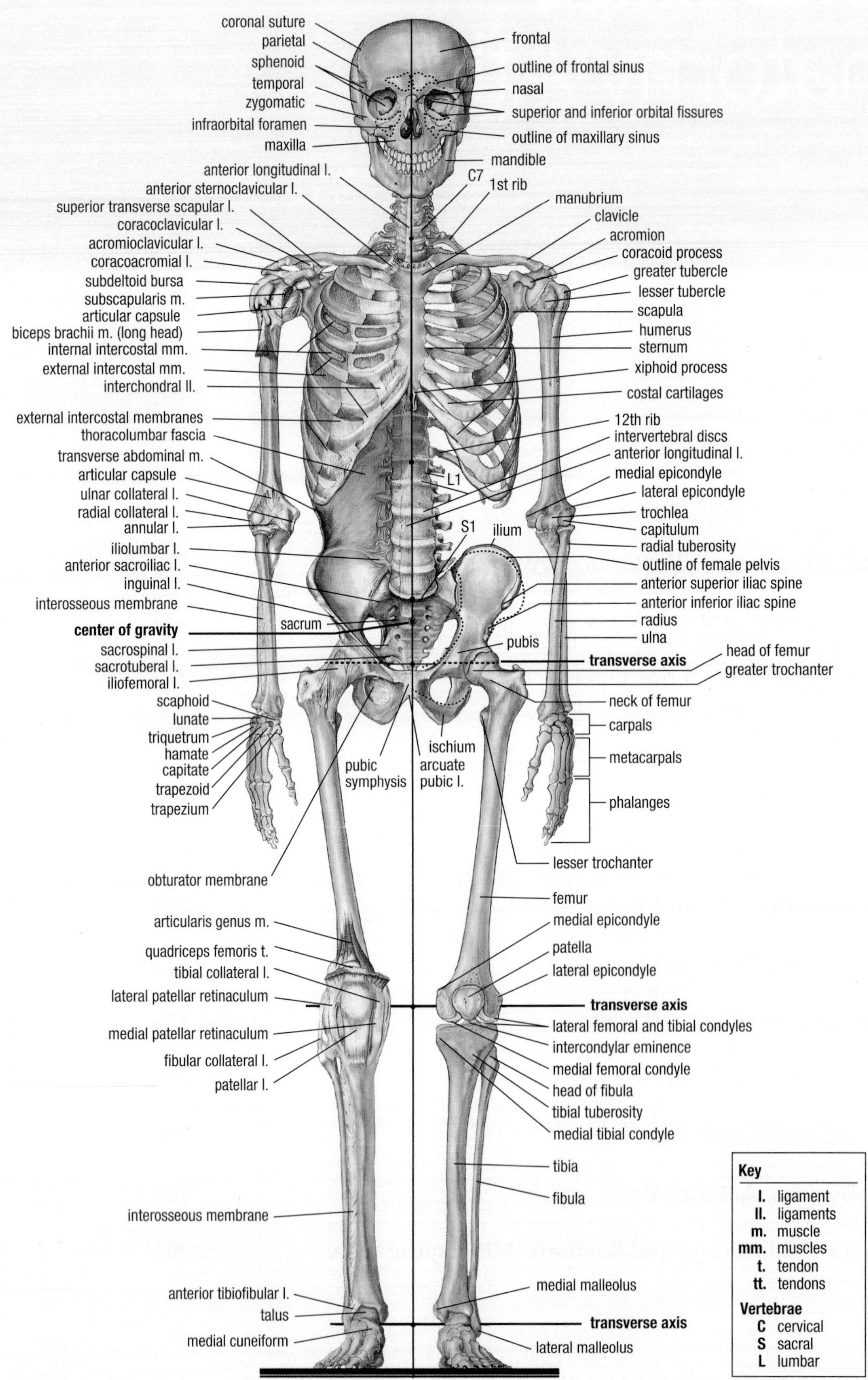
coronal suture
parietal
sphenoid
temporal
zygomatic
infraorbital foramen
maxilla
anterior longitudinal l.
anterior sternoclavicular l.
superior transverse scapular l.
coracoclavicular l.
acromioclavicular l.
coracoacromial l.
subdeltoid bursa
subscapularis m.
articular capsule
biceps brachii m. (long head)
internal intercostal mm.
external intercostal mm.
interchondral ll.
external intercostal membranes
thoracolumbar fascia
transverse abdominal m.
articular capsule
ulnar collateral l.
radial collateral l.
annular l.
iliolumbar l.
anterior sacroiliac l.
inguinal l.
interosseous membrane
center of gravity
sacrospinal l.
sacrotuberal l.
iliofemoral l.
scaphoid
lunate
triquetrum
hamate
capitate
trapezoid
trapezium
obturator membrane
articularis genus m.
quadriceps femoris t.
tibial collateral l.
lateral patellar retinaculum
medial patellar retinaculum
fibular collateral l.
patellar l.
interosseous membrane
anterior tibiofibular l.
talus
medial cuneiform
frontal
outline of frontal sinus
nasal
superior and inferior orbital fissures
outline of maxillary sinus
mandible
C7
1st rib
manubrium
clavicle
acromion
coracoid process
greater tubercle
lesser tubercle
scapula
humerus
sternum
xiphoid process
costal cartilages
12th rib
intervertebral discs
anterior longitudinal l.
medial epicondyle
lateral epicondyle
trochlea
capitulum
radial tuberosity
outline of female pelvis
anterior superior iliac spine
anterior inferior iliac spine
radius
ulna
L1
S1
ilium
sacrum
pubis
transverse axis
head of femur
greater trochanter
neck of femur
carpals
metacarpals
phalanges
ischium
arcuate pubic l.
pubic symphysis
lesser trochanter
femur
medial epicondyle
patella
lateral epicondyle
transverse axis
lateral femoral and tibial condyles
intercondylar eminence
medial femoral condyle
head of fibula
tibial tuberosity
medial tibial condyle
tibia
fibula
medial malleolus
transverse axis
lateral malleolus
Key
l. ligament
ll. ligaments
m. muscle
mm. muscles
t. tendon
tt. tendons
Vertebrae
C cervical
S sacral
L lumbar

Skeletal Anatomy, Posterior View

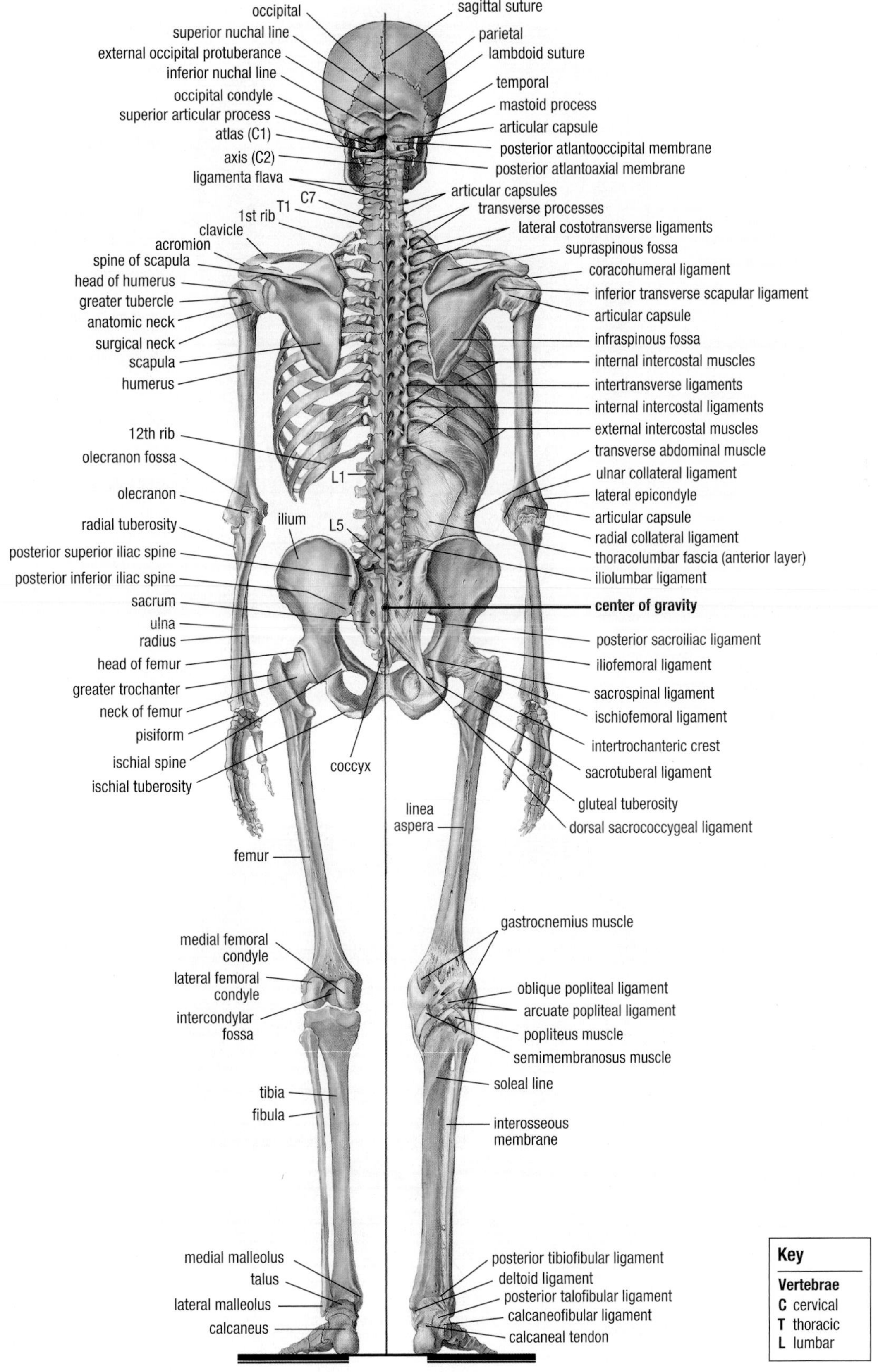
occipital
superior nuchal line
external occipital protuberance
inferior nuchal line
occipital condyle
superior articular process
atlas (C1)
axis (C2)
ligamenta flava
C7
T1
1st rib
clavicle
acromion
spine of scapula
head of humerus
greater tubercle
anatomic neck
surgical neck
scapula
humerus
12th rib
olecranon fossa
olecranon
radial tuberosity
posterior superior iliac spine
posterior inferior iliac spine
sacrum
ulna
radius
head of femur
greater trochanter
neck of femur
pisiform
ischial spine
ischial tuberosity
L1
ilium
L5
coccyx
linea aspera
femur
medial femoral condyle
lateral femoral condyle
intercondylar fossa
tibia
fibula
medial malleolus
talus
lateral malleolus
calcaneus
sagittal suture
parietal
lambdoid suture
temporal
mastoid process
articular capsule
posterior atlantooccipital membrane
posterior atlantoaxial membrane
articular capsules
transverse processes
lateral costotransverse ligaments
supraspinous fossa
coracohumeral ligament
inferior transverse scapular ligament
articular capsule
infraspinous fossa
internal intercostal muscles
intertransverse ligaments
internal intercostal ligaments
external intercostal muscles
transverse abdominal muscle
ulnar collateral ligament
lateral epicondyle
articular capsule
radial collateral ligament
thoracolumbar fascia (anterior layer)
iliolumbar ligament
center of gravity
posterior sacroiliac ligament
iliofemoral ligament
sacrospinal ligament
ischiofemoral ligament
intertrochanteric crest
sacrotuberal ligament
gluteal tuberosity
dorsal sacrococcygeal ligament
gastrocnemius muscle
oblique popliteal ligament
arcuate popliteal ligament
popliteus muscle
semimembranosus muscle
soleal line
interosseous membrane
posterior tibiofibular ligament
deltoid ligament
posterior talofibular ligament
calcaneofibular ligament
calcaneal tendon

Key

Vertebrae
C cervical
T thoracic
L lumbar

The Skull, Anterior and Posterior Views

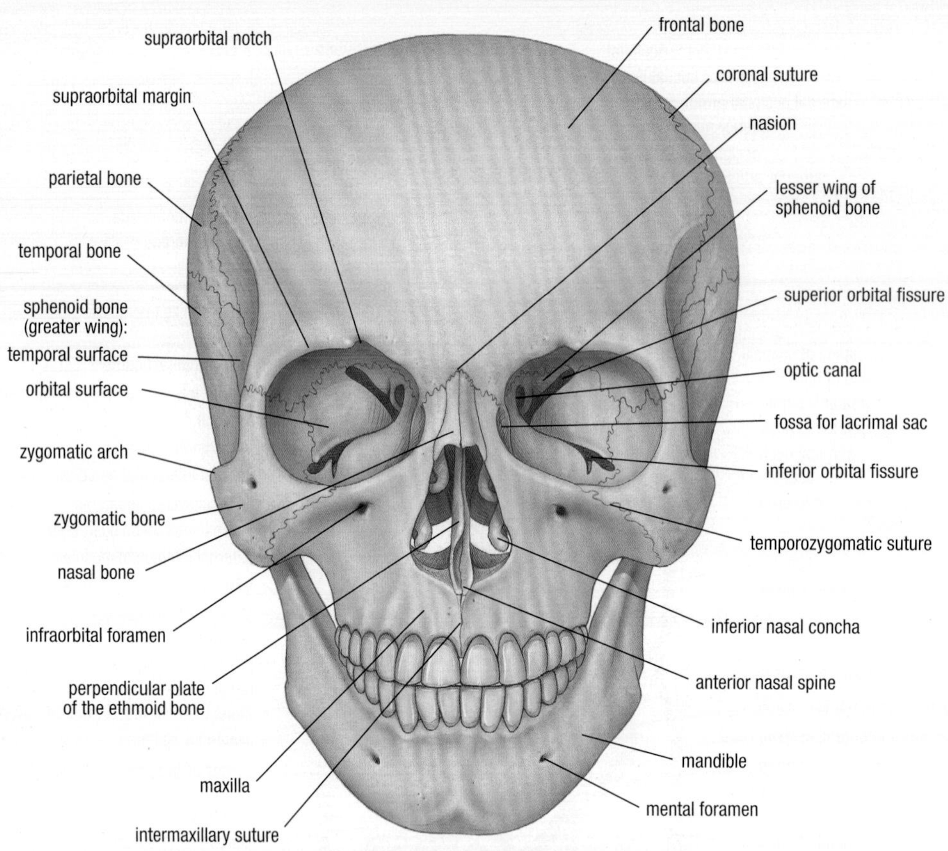

frontal bone
supraorbital notch
coronal suture
supraorbital margin
nasion
parietal bone
lesser wing of sphenoid bone
temporal bone
sphenoid bone (greater wing):
temporal surface
orbital surface
superior orbital fissure
optic canal
fossa for lacrimal sac
zygomatic arch
inferior orbital fissure
zygomatic bone
temporozygomatic suture
nasal bone
infraorbital foramen
inferior nasal concha
perpendicular plate of the ethmoid bone
anterior nasal spine
mandible
maxilla
mental foramen
intermaxillary suture

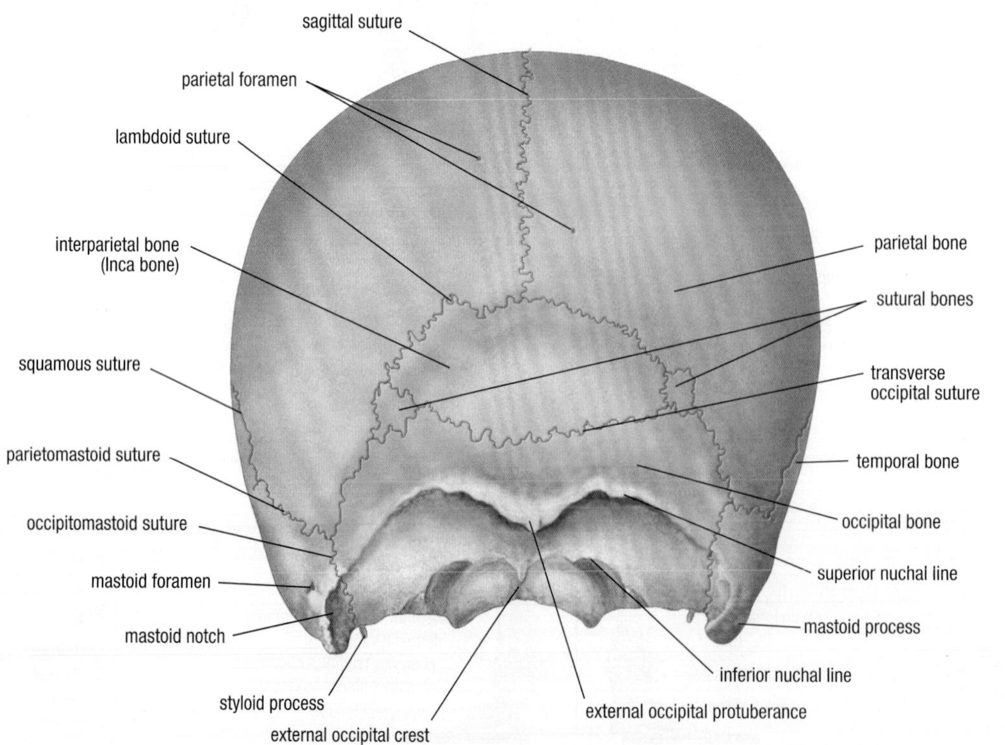

sagittal suture
parietal foramen
lambdoid suture
interparietal bone (Inca bone)
parietal bone
sutural bones
squamous suture
transverse occipital suture
parietomastoid suture
temporal bone
occipitomastoid suture
occipital bone
superior nuchal line
mastoid foramen
mastoid notch
mastoid process
inferior nuchal line
styloid process
external occipital protuberance
external occipital crest

Muscular System, Anterior View

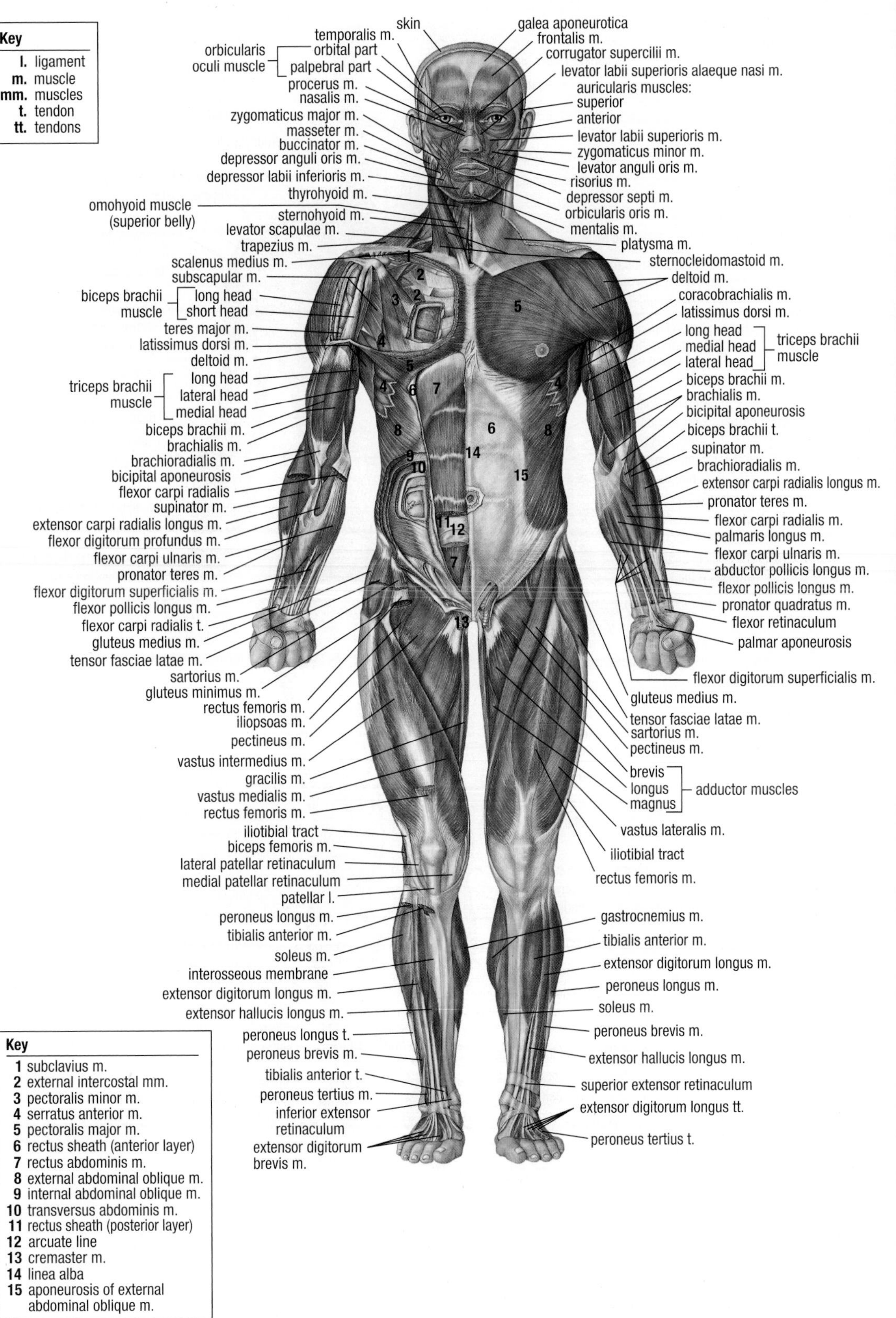
Key
l. ligament
m. muscle
mm. muscles
t. tendon
tt. tendons
skin
temporalis m.
orbicularis oculi muscle
orbital part
palpebral part
procerus m.
nasalis m.
zygomaticus major m.
masseter m.
buccinator m.
depressor anguli oris m.
depressor labii inferioris m.
thyrohyoid m.
omohyoid muscle (superior belly)
sternohyoid m.
levator scapulae m.
trapezius m.
scalenus medius m.
subscapular m.
biceps brachii muscle
long head
short head
teres major m.
latissimus dorsi m.
deltoid m.
triceps brachii muscle
long head
lateral head
medial head
biceps brachii m.
brachialis m.
brachioradialis m.
bicipital aponeurosis
flexor carpi radialis
supinator m.
extensor carpi radialis longus m.
flexor digitorum profundus m.
flexor carpi ulnaris m.
pronator teres m.
flexor digitorum superficialis m.
flexor pollicis longus m.
flexor carpi radialis t.
gluteus medius m.
tensor fasciae latae m.
sartorius m.
gluteus minimus m.
rectus femoris m.
iliopsoas m.
pectineus m.
vastus intermedius m.
gracilis m.
vastus medialis m.
rectus femoris m.
iliotibial tract
biceps femoris m.
lateral patellar retinaculum
medial patellar retinaculum
patellar l.
peroneus longus m.
tibialis anterior m.
soleus m.
interosseous membrane
extensor digitorum longus m.
extensor hallucis longus m.
peroneus longus t.
peroneus brevis m.
tibialis anterior t.
peroneus tertius m.
inferior extensor retinaculum
extensor digitorum brevis m.
galea aponeurotica
frontalis m.
corrugator supercilii m.
levator labii superioris alaeque nasi m.
auricularis muscles:
superior
anterior
levator labii superioris m.
zygomaticus minor m.
levator anguli oris m.
risorius m.
depressor septi m.
orbicularis oris m.
mentalis m.
platysma m.
sternocleidomastoid m.
deltoid m.
coracobrachialis m.
latissimus dorsi m.
long head
medial head
lateral head
triceps brachii muscle
biceps brachii m.
brachialis m.
bicipital aponeurosis
biceps brachii t.
supinator m.
brachioradialis m.
extensor carpi radialis longus m.
pronator teres m.
flexor carpi radialis m.
palmaris longus m.
flexor carpi ulnaris m.
abductor pollicis longus m.
flexor pollicis longus m.
pronator quadratus m.
flexor retinaculum
palmar aponeurosis
flexor digitorum superficialis m.
gluteus medius m.
tensor fasciae latae m.
sartorius m.
pectineus m.
brevis
longus
magnus
adductor muscles
vastus lateralis m.
iliotibial tract
rectus femoris m.
gastrocnemius m.
tibialis anterior m.
extensor digitorum longus m.
peroneus longus m.
soleus m.
peroneus brevis m.
extensor hallucis longus m.
superior extensor retinaculum
extensor digitorum longus tt.
peroneus tertius t.
Key
1 subclavius m.
2 external intercostal mm.
3 pectoralis minor m.
4 serratus anterior m.
5 pectoralis major m.
6 rectus sheath (anterior layer)
7 rectus abdominis m.
8 external abdominal oblique m.
9 internal abdominal oblique m.
10 transversus abdominis m.
11 rectus sheath (posterior layer)
12 arcuate line
13 cremaster m.
14 linea alba
15 aponeurosis of external abdominal oblique m.

Muscular System, Posterior View

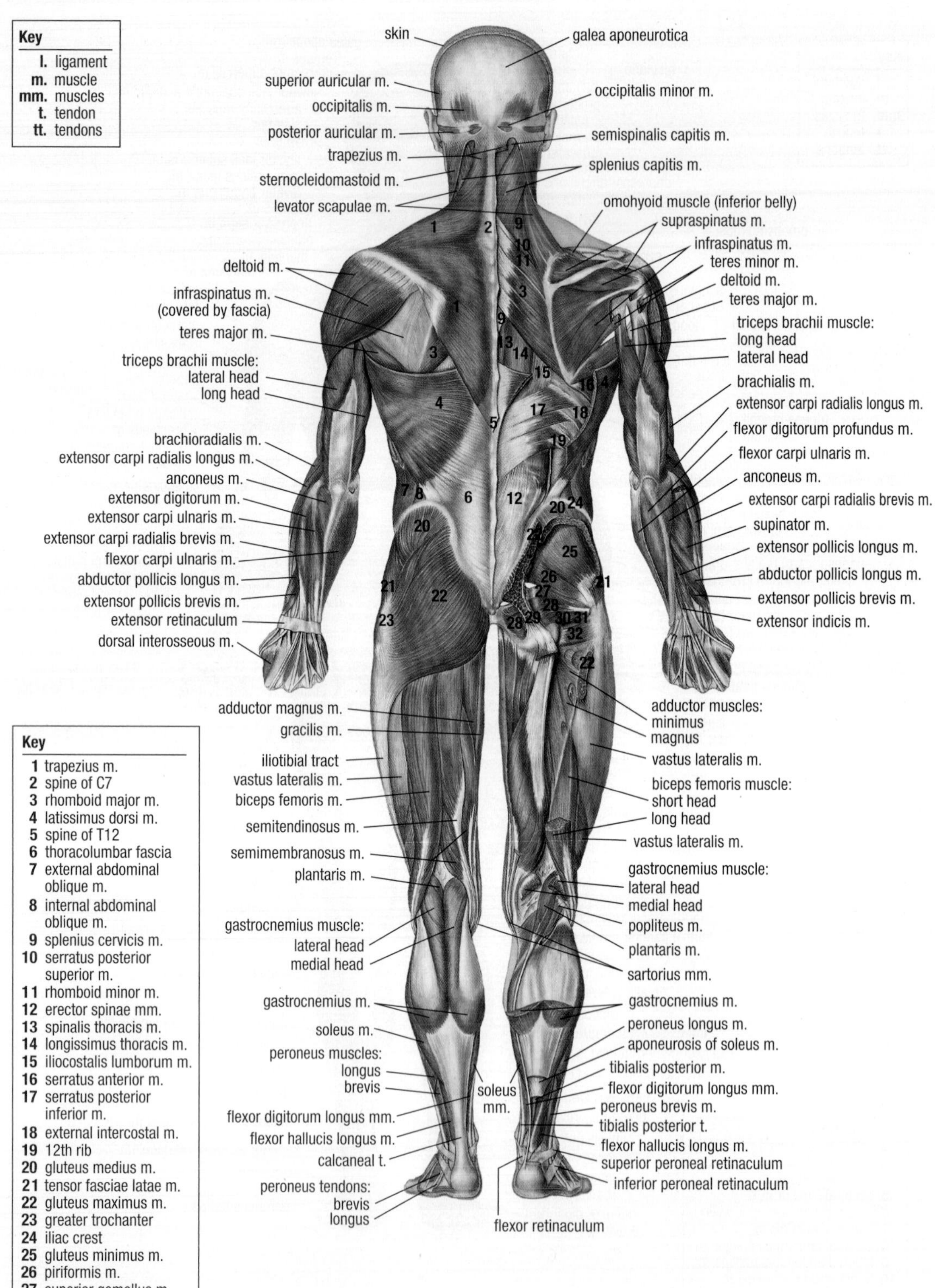

Key

- **l.** ligament
- **m.** muscle
- **mm.** muscles
- **t.** tendon
- **tt.** tendons

Key

1. trapezius m.
2. spine of C7
3. rhomboid major m.
4. latissimus dorsi m.
5. spine of T12
6. thoracolumbar fascia
7. external abdominal oblique m.
8. internal abdominal oblique m.
9. splenius cervicis m.
10. serratus posterior superior m.
11. rhomboid minor m.
12. erector spinae mm.
13. spinalis thoracis m.
14. longissimus thoracis m.
15. iliocostalis lumborum m.
16. serratus anterior m.
17. serratus posterior inferior m.
18. external intercostal m.
19. 12th rib
20. gluteus medius m.
21. tensor fasciae latae m.
22. gluteus maximus m.
23. greater trochanter
24. iliac crest
25. gluteus minimus m.
26. piriformis m.
27. superior gemellus m.
28. obturator internus m.
29. sacrotuberal l.
30. inferior gemellus m.
31. obturator externus m.
32. quadratus femoris m.

Spinal and Cranial Nerves

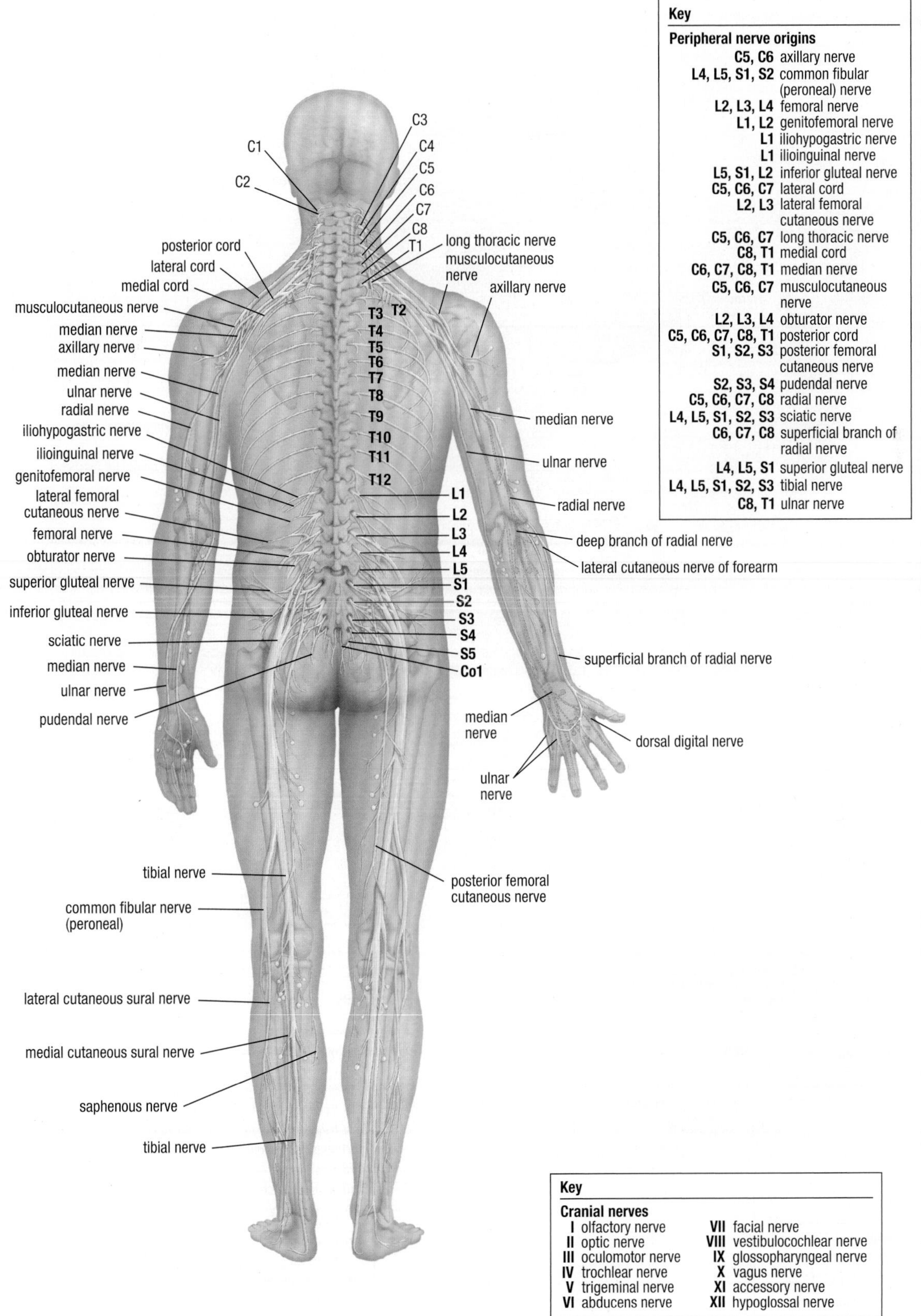

Key

Peripheral nerve origins

C5, C6	axillary nerve
L4, L5, S1, S2	common fibular (peroneal) nerve
L2, L3, L4	femoral nerve
L1, L2	genitofemoral nerve
L1	iliohypogastric nerve
L1	ilioinguinal nerve
L5, S1, L2	inferior gluteal nerve
C5, C6, C7	lateral cord
L2, L3	lateral femoral cutaneous nerve
C5, C6, C7	long thoracic nerve
C8, T1	medial cord
C6, C7, C8, T1	median nerve
C5, C6, C7	musculocutaneous nerve
L2, L3, L4	obturator nerve
C5, C6, C7, C8, T1	posterior cord
S1, S2, S3	posterior femoral cutaneous nerve
S2, S3, S4	pudendal nerve
C5, C6, C7, C8	radial nerve
L4, L5, S1, S2, S3	sciatic nerve
C6, C7, C8	superficial branch of radial nerve
L4, L5, S1	superior gluteal nerve
L4, L5, S1, S2, S3	tibial nerve
C8, T1	ulnar nerve

Key

Cranial nerves

I	olfactory nerve	**VII**	facial nerve
II	optic nerve	**VIII**	vestibulocochlear nerve
III	oculomotor nerve	**IX**	glossopharyngeal nerve
IV	trochlear nerve	**X**	vagus nerve
V	trigeminal nerve	**XI**	accessory nerve
VI	abducens nerve	**XII**	hypoglossal nerve

Cerebral Hemispheres

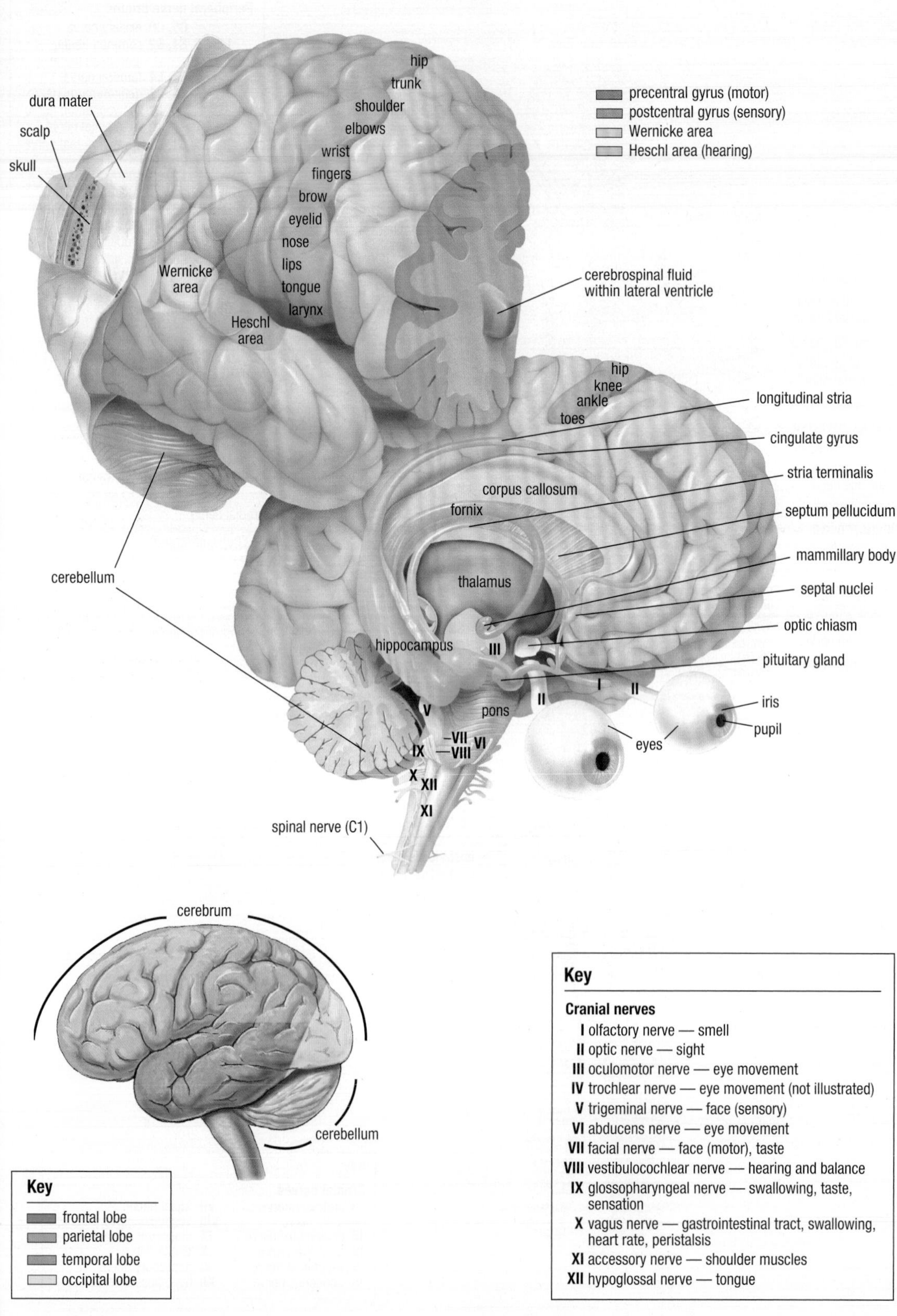

Key

- frontal lobe
- parietal lobe
- temporal lobe
- occipital lobe

Key

Cranial nerves

I olfactory nerve — smell
II optic nerve — sight
III oculomotor nerve — eye movement
IV trochlear nerve — eye movement (not illustrated)
V trigeminal nerve — face (sensory)
VI abducens nerve — eye movement
VII facial nerve — face (motor), taste
VIII vestibulocochlear nerve — hearing and balance
IX glossopharyngeal nerve — swallowing, taste, sensation
X vagus nerve — gastrointestinal tract, swallowing, heart rate, peristalsis
XI accessory nerve — shoulder muscles
XII hypoglossal nerve — tongue

Anatomy of the Heart, Anterior View

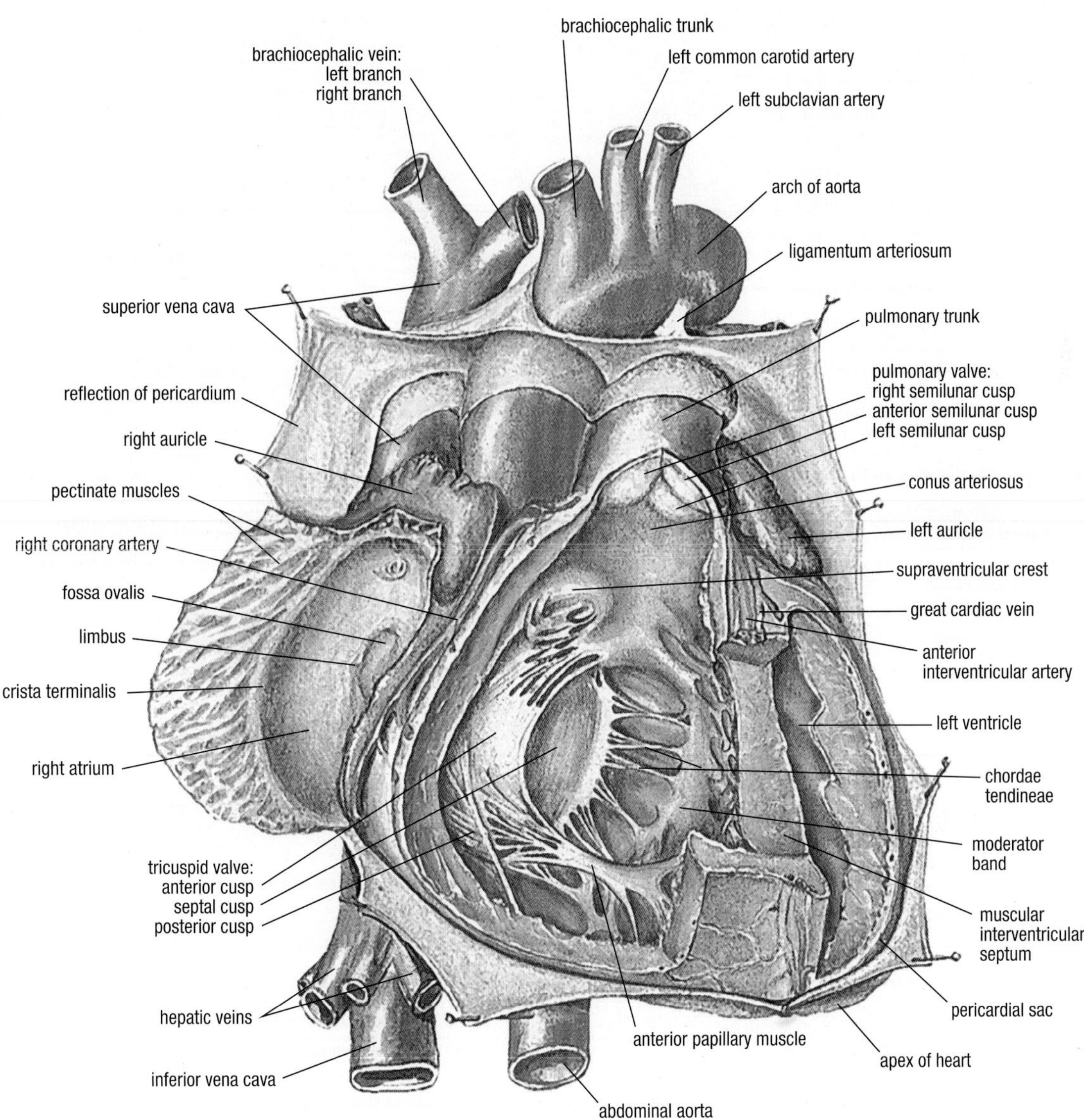
brachiocephalic trunk
brachiocephalic vein:
left branch
right branch
left common carotid artery
left subclavian artery
arch of aorta
ligamentum arteriosum
superior vena cava
pulmonary trunk
reflection of pericardium
pulmonary valve:
right semilunar cusp
anterior semilunar cusp
left semilunar cusp
right auricle
conus arteriosus
pectinate muscles
left auricle
right coronary artery
supraventricular crest
fossa ovalis
great cardiac vein
limbus
anterior
interventricular artery
crista terminalis
left ventricle
right atrium
chordae
tendineae
moderator
band
tricuspid valve:
anterior cusp
septal cusp
posterior cusp
muscular
interventricular
septum
pericardial sac
hepatic veins
anterior papillary muscle
apex of heart
inferior vena cava
abdominal aorta

Arterial System, Anterior View

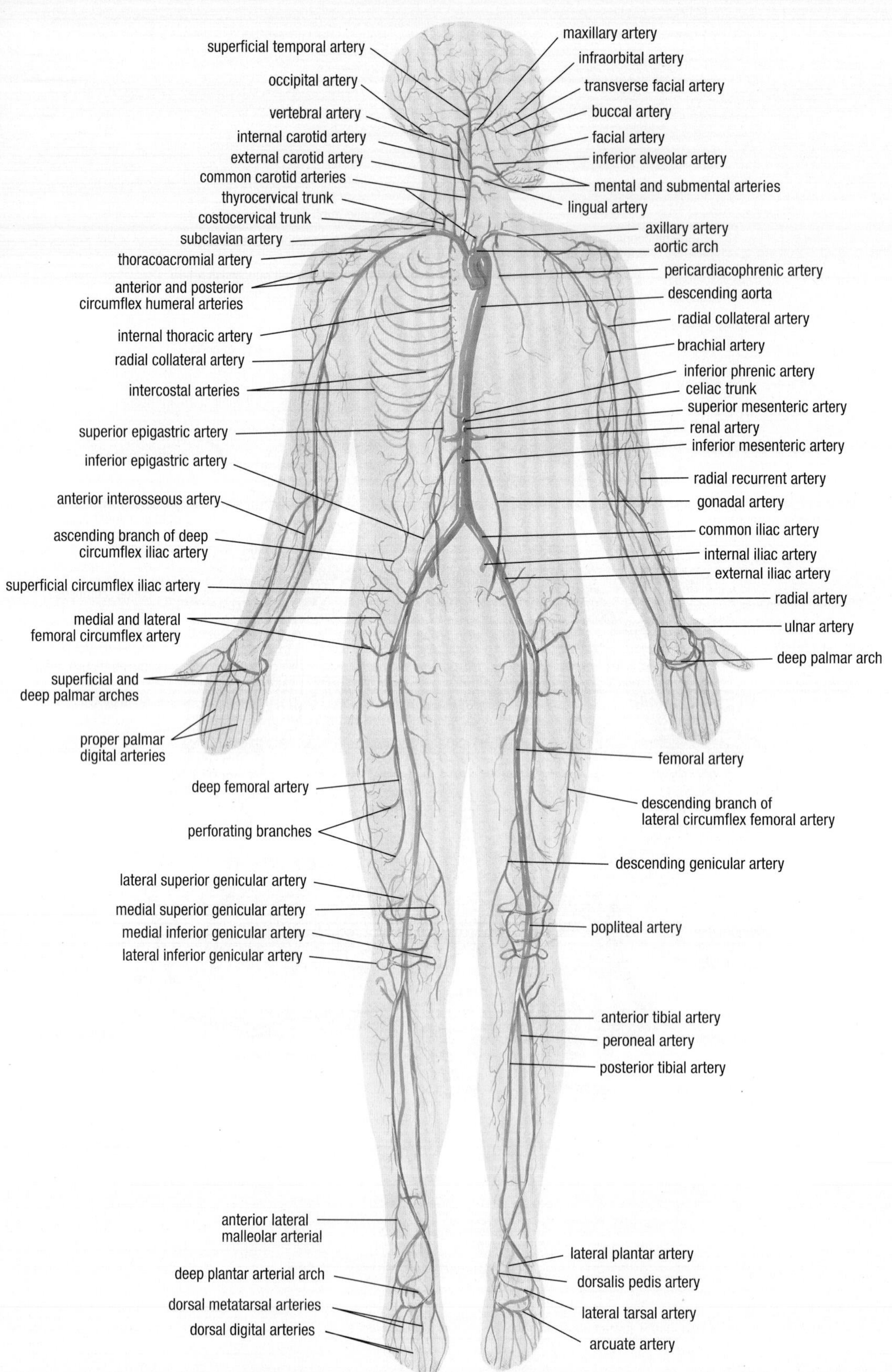
superficial temporal artery
occipital artery
vertebral artery
internal carotid artery
external carotid artery
common carotid arteries
thyrocervical trunk
costocervical trunk
subclavian artery
thoracoacromial artery
anterior and posterior circumflex humeral arteries
internal thoracic artery
radial collateral artery
intercostal arteries
superior epigastric artery
inferior epigastric artery
anterior interosseous artery
ascending branch of deep circumflex iliac artery
superficial circumflex iliac artery
medial and lateral femoral circumflex artery
superficial and deep palmar arches
proper palmar digital arteries
deep femoral artery
perforating branches
lateral superior genicular artery
medial superior genicular artery
medial inferior genicular artery
lateral inferior genicular artery
anterior lateral malleolar arterial
deep plantar arterial arch
dorsal metatarsal arteries
dorsal digital arteries
maxillary artery
infraorbital artery
transverse facial artery
buccal artery
facial artery
inferior alveolar artery
mental and submental arteries
lingual artery
axillary artery
aortic arch
pericardiacophrenic artery
descending aorta
radial collateral artery
brachial artery
inferior phrenic artery
celiac trunk
superior mesenteric artery
renal artery
inferior mesenteric artery
radial recurrent artery
gonadal artery
common iliac artery
internal iliac artery
external iliac artery
radial artery
ulnar artery
deep palmar arch
femoral artery
descending branch of lateral circumflex femoral artery
descending genicular artery
popliteal artery
anterior tibial artery
peroneal artery
posterior tibial artery
lateral plantar artery
dorsalis pedis artery
lateral tarsal artery
arcuate artery

Imagery © Anatomical Chart Company

Venous System, Anterior View

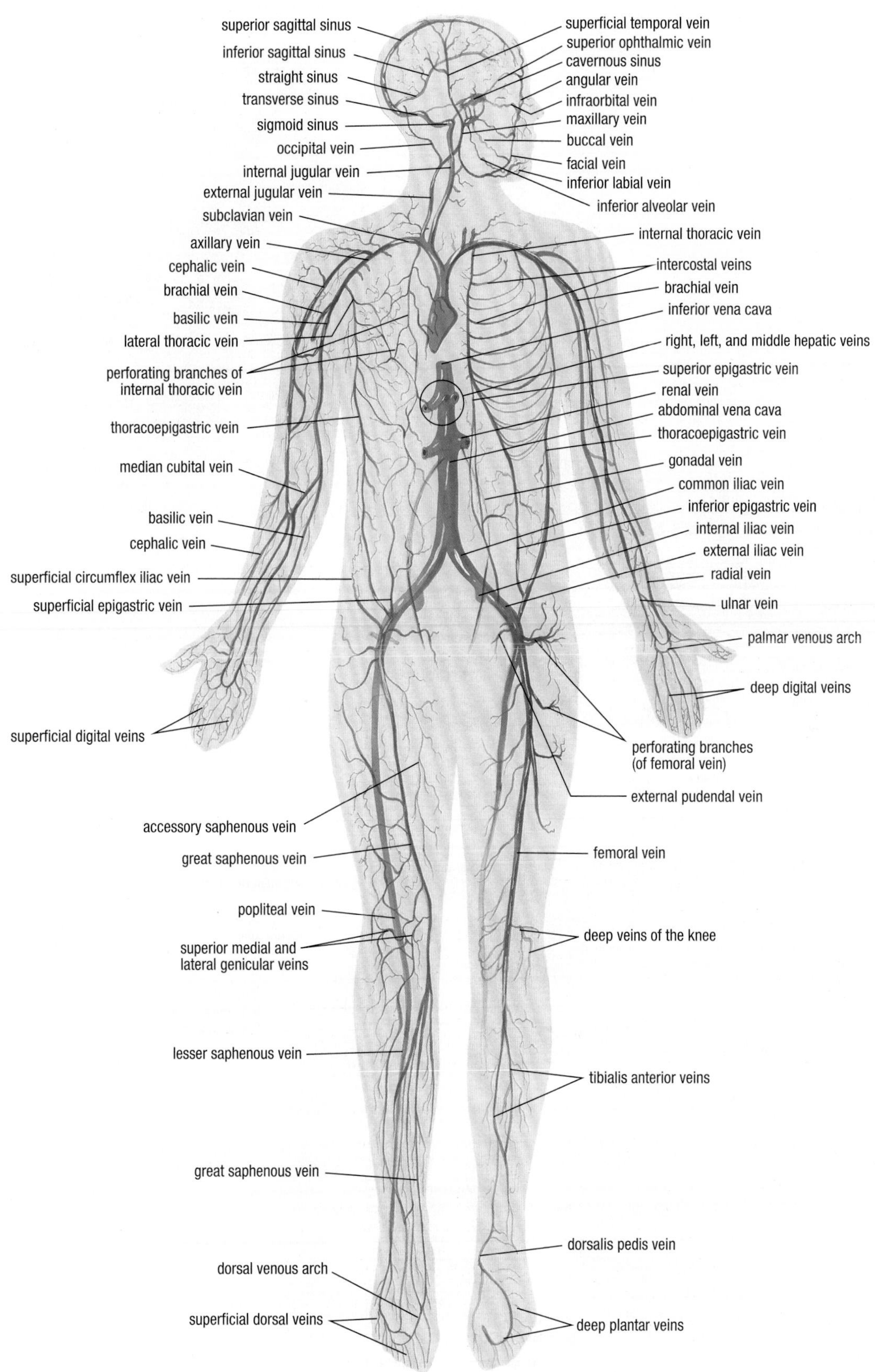
superior sagittal sinus
inferior sagittal sinus
straight sinus
transverse sinus
sigmoid sinus
occipital vein
internal jugular vein
external jugular vein
subclavian vein
axillary vein
cephalic vein
brachial vein
basilic vein
lateral thoracic vein
perforating branches of internal thoracic vein
thoracoepigastric vein
median cubital vein
basilic vein
cephalic vein
superficial circumflex iliac vein
superficial epigastric vein
superficial digital veins
accessory saphenous vein
great saphenous vein
popliteal vein
superior medial and lateral genicular veins
lesser saphenous vein
great saphenous vein
dorsal venous arch
superficial dorsal veins
superficial temporal vein
superior ophthalmic vein
cavernous sinus
angular vein
infraorbital vein
maxillary vein
buccal vein
facial vein
inferior labial vein
inferior alveolar vein
internal thoracic vein
intercostal veins
brachial vein
inferior vena cava
right, left, and middle hepatic veins
superior epigastric vein
renal vein
abdominal vena cava
thoracoepigastric vein
gonadal vein
common iliac vein
inferior epigastric vein
internal iliac vein
external iliac vein
radial vein
ulnar vein
palmar venous arch
deep digital veins
perforating branches (of femoral vein)
external pudendal vein
femoral vein
deep veins of the knee
tibialis anterior veins
dorsalis pedis vein
deep plantar veins

Respiratory System, Anterior View

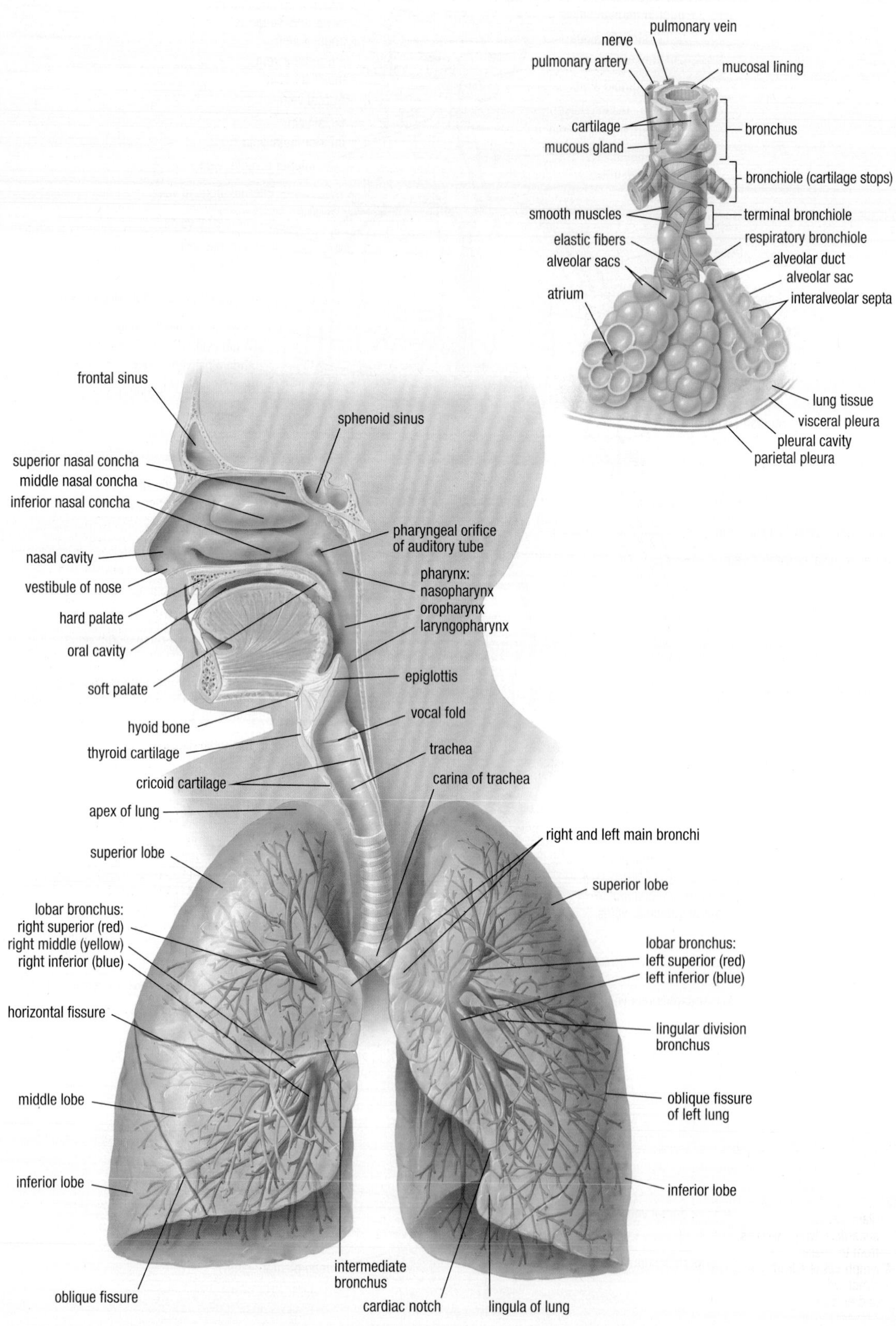
pulmonary vein
nerve
pulmonary artery
mucosal lining
cartilage
mucous gland
bronchus
bronchiole (cartilage stops)
smooth muscles
terminal bronchiole
elastic fibers
respiratory bronchiole
alveolar sacs
alveolar duct
alveolar sac
atrium
interalveolar septa
lung tissue
visceral pleura
pleural cavity
parietal pleura
frontal sinus
sphenoid sinus
superior nasal concha
middle nasal concha
inferior nasal concha
pharyngeal orifice of auditory tube
nasal cavity
vestibule of nose
pharynx:
nasopharynx
oropharynx
laryngopharynx
hard palate
oral cavity
soft palate
epiglottis
hyoid bone
vocal fold
thyroid cartilage
trachea
cricoid cartilage
carina of trachea
apex of lung
right and left main bronchi
superior lobe
superior lobe
lobar bronchus:
right superior (red)
right middle (yellow)
right inferior (blue)
lobar bronchus:
left superior (red)
left inferior (blue)
horizontal fissure
lingular division bronchus
middle lobe
oblique fissure of left lung
inferior lobe
inferior lobe
intermediate bronchus
oblique fissure
cardiac notch
lingula of lung

Lymphatic System, Anterior View

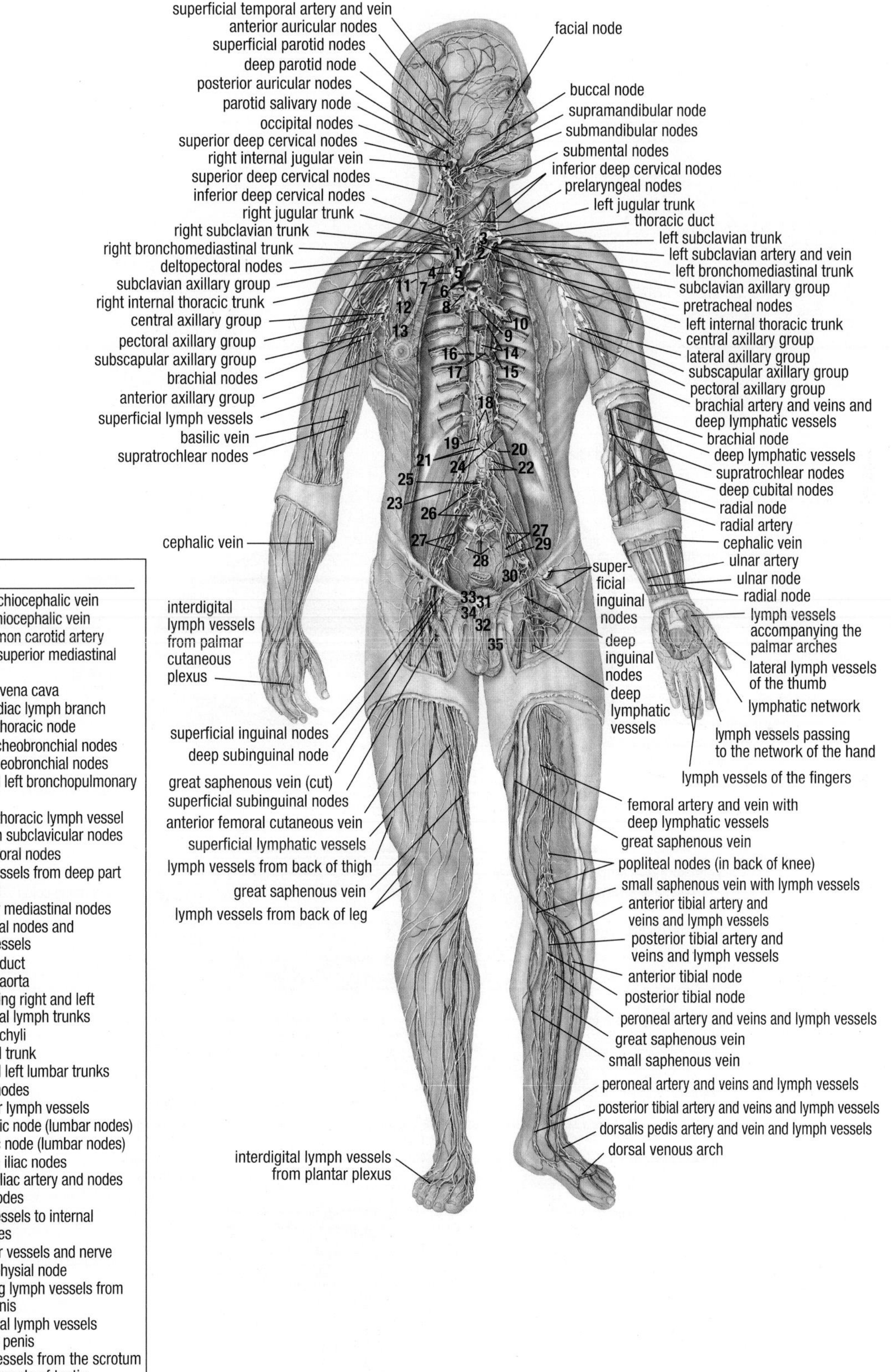

Key

1 right brachiocephalic vein
2 left brachiocephalic vein
3 left common carotid artery
4 anterior superior mediastinal nodes
5 superior vena cava
6 right cardiac lymph branch
7 internal thoracic node
8 right tracheobronchial nodes
9 left tracheobronchial nodes
10 right and left bronchopulmonary nodes
11 internal thoracic lymph vessel ending in subclavicular nodes
12 interpectoral nodes
13 lymph vessels from deep part of breast
14 posterior mediastinal nodes
15 intercostal nodes and lymph vessels
16 thoracic duct
17 thoracic aorta
18 descending right and left intercostal lymph trunks
19 cisterna chyli
20 intestinal trunk
21 right and left lumbar trunks
22 lumbar nodes
23 testicular lymph vessels
24 retroaortic node (lumbar nodes)
25 preaortic node (lumbar nodes)
26 common iliac nodes
27 internal iliac artery and nodes
28 sacral nodes
29 lymph vessels to internal iliac nodes
30 obturator vessels and nerve
31 presymphysial node
32 collecting lymph vessels from glans penis
33 superficial lymph vessels from the penis
34 lymph vessels from the scrotum
35 lymph vessels of testis and epididymis

Digestive System, Anterior View

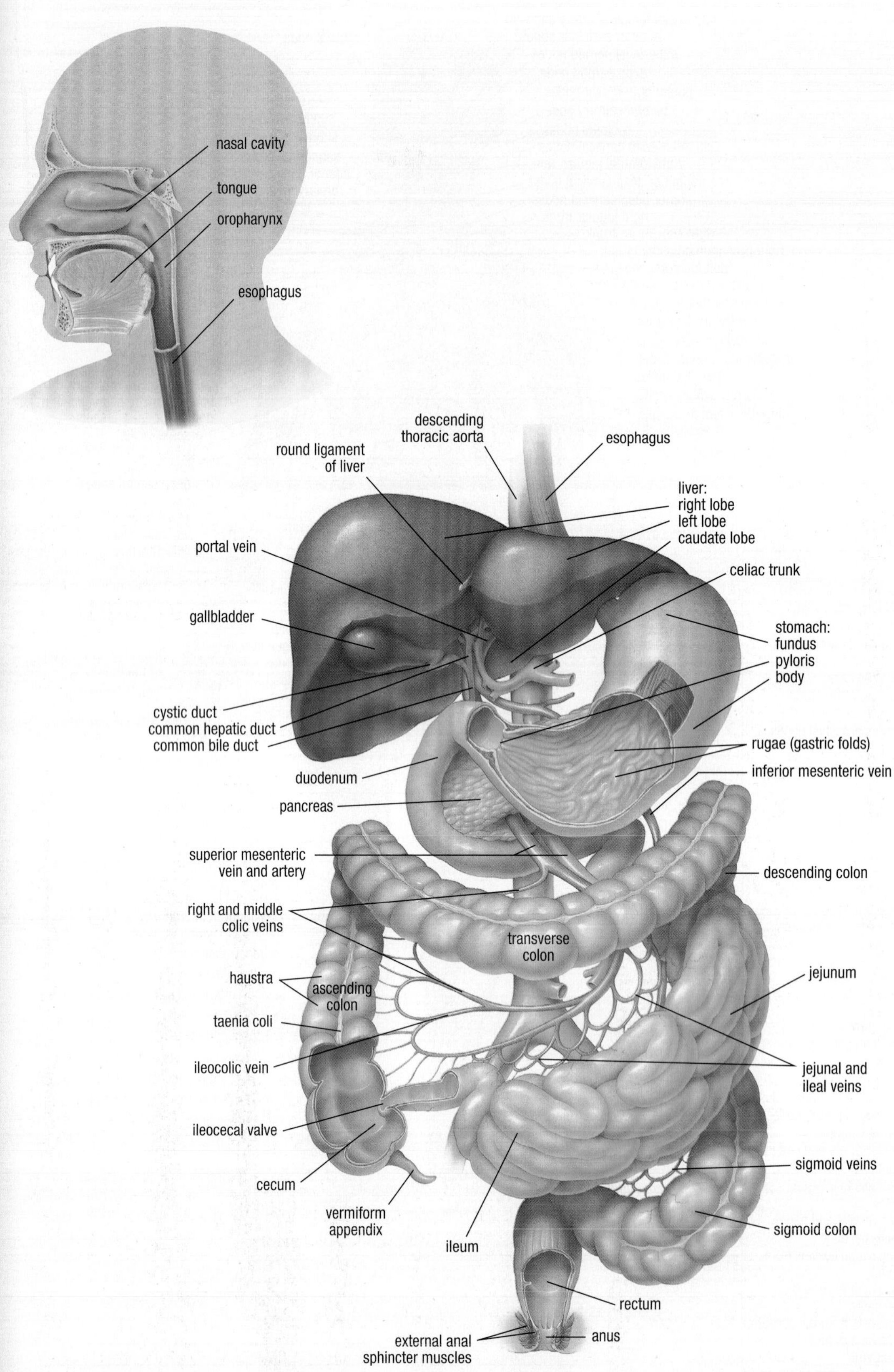

Urinary System, Anterior View

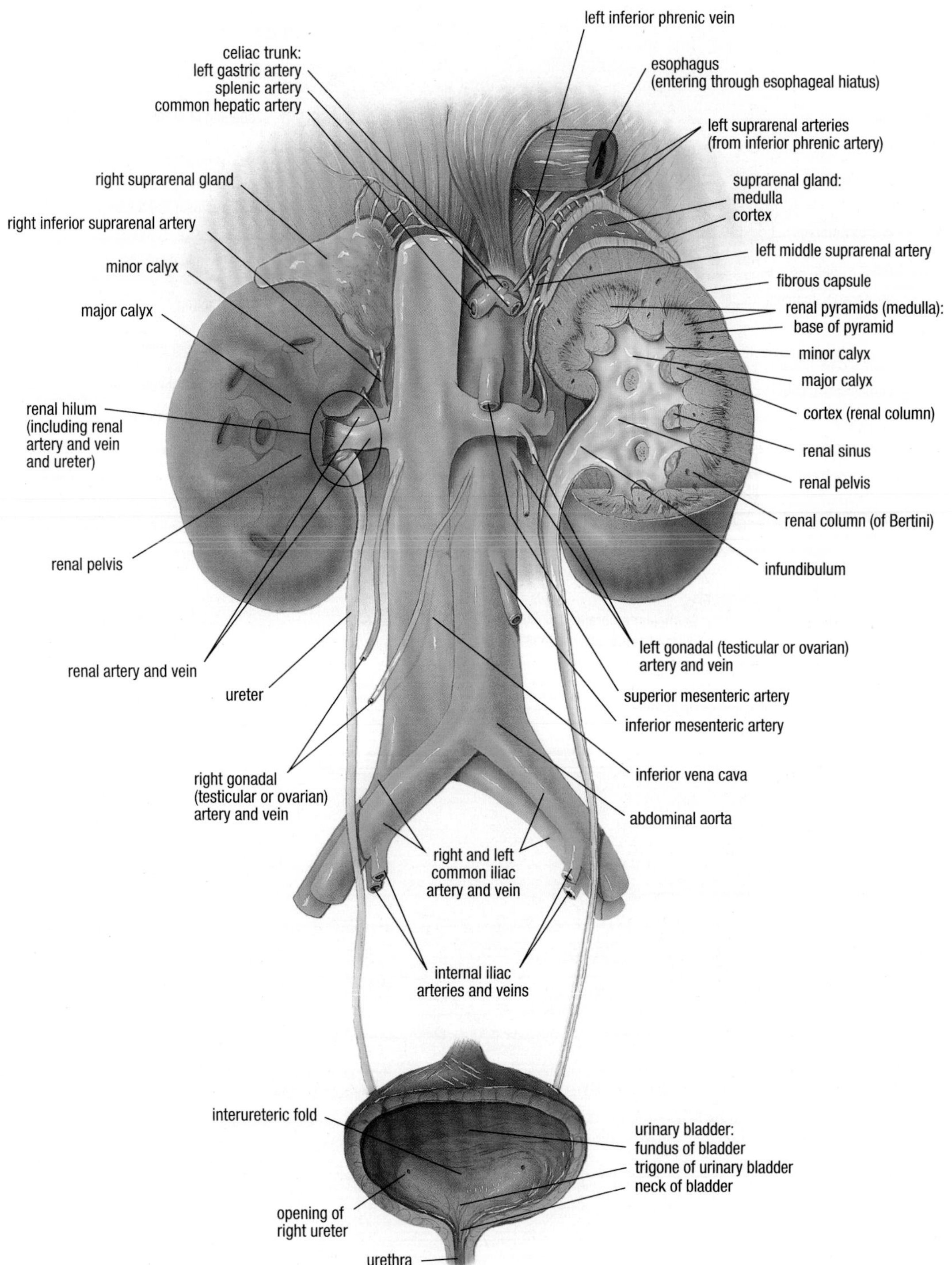
left inferior phrenic vein
celiac trunk:
left gastric artery
splenic artery
common hepatic artery
esophagus
(entering through esophageal hiatus)
left suprarenal arteries
(from inferior phrenic artery)
right suprarenal gland
suprarenal gland:
medulla
cortex
right inferior suprarenal artery
left middle suprarenal artery
minor calyx
fibrous capsule
major calyx
renal pyramids (medulla):
base of pyramid
minor calyx
major calyx
renal hilum
(including renal
artery and vein
and ureter)
cortex (renal column)
renal sinus
renal pelvis
renal column (of Bertini)
renal pelvis
infundibulum
left gonadal (testicular or ovarian)
artery and vein
renal artery and vein
ureter
superior mesenteric artery
inferior mesenteric artery
right gonadal
(testicular or ovarian)
artery and vein
inferior vena cava
abdominal aorta
right and left
common iliac
artery and vein
internal iliac
arteries and veins
interureteric fold
urinary bladder:
fundus of bladder
trigone of urinary bladder
neck of bladder
opening of
right ureter
urethra

Male and Female Urogenital Systems, Midsagittal View

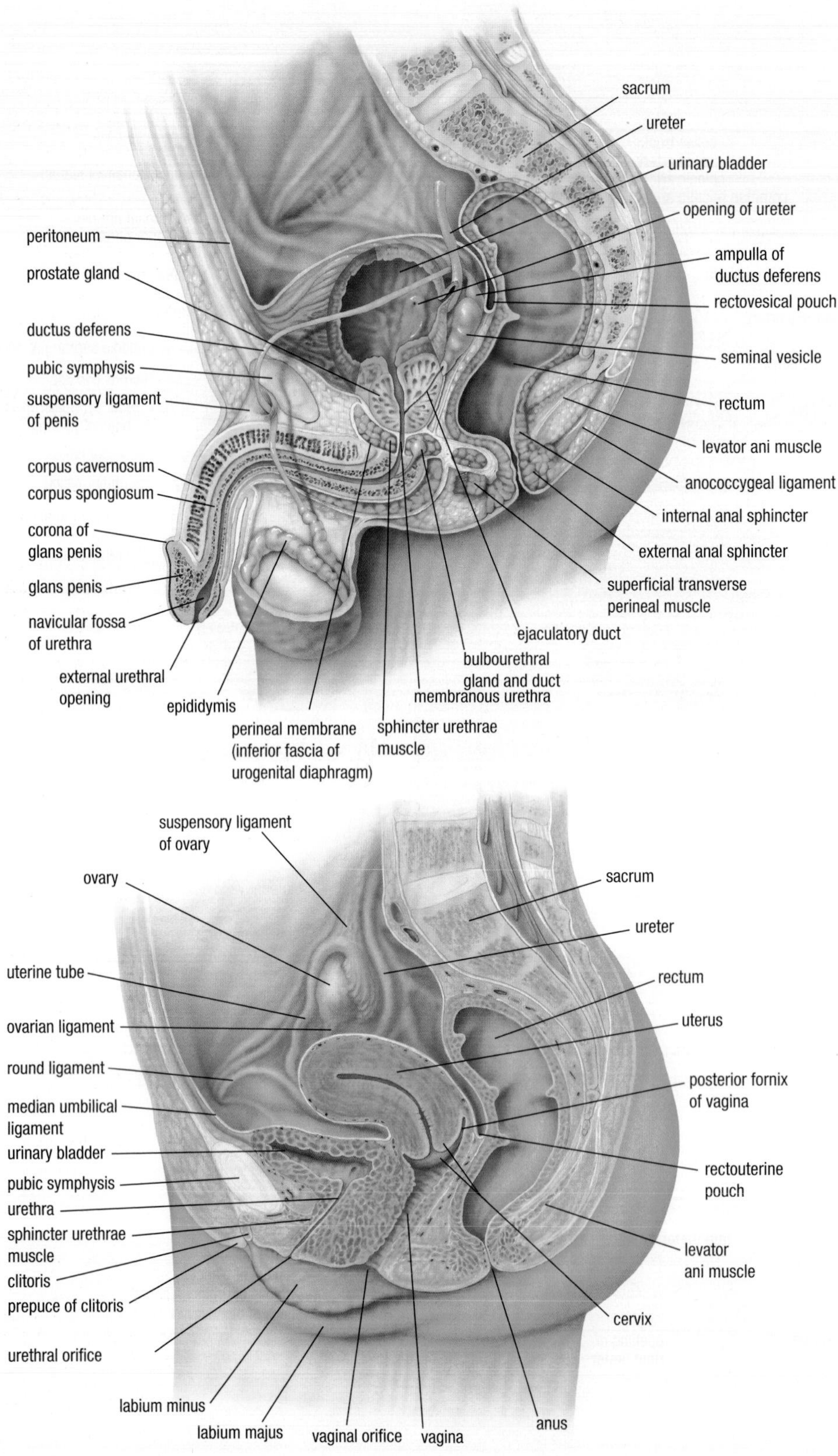
sacrum
ureter
urinary bladder
opening of ureter
ampulla of
ductus deferens
rectovesical pouch
seminal vesicle
rectum
levator ani muscle
anococcygeal ligament
internal anal sphincter
external anal sphincter
superficial transverse
perineal muscle
ejaculatory duct
bulbourethral
gland and duct
membranous urethra
sphincter urethrae
muscle
perineal membrane
(inferior fascia of
urogenital diaphragm)
epididymis
external urethral
opening
navicular fossa
of urethra
glans penis
corona of
glans penis
corpus spongiosum
corpus cavernosum
suspensory ligament
of penis
pubic symphysis
ductus deferens
prostate gland
peritoneum
suspensory ligament
of ovary
ovary
uterine tube
ovarian ligament
round ligament
median umbilical
ligament
urinary bladder
pubic symphysis
urethra
sphincter urethrae
muscle
clitoris
prepuce of clitoris
urethral orifice
labium minus
labium majus
vaginal orifice
vagina
anus
cervix
levator
ani muscle
rectouterine
pouch
posterior fornix
of vagina
uterus
rectum
ureter
sacrum

■ INDEX

Note: Page numbers followed by f refer to figures.

A

A-, 6, 23, 75, 417
-a, 10, 709
Ab-, 24
AB (abortion), 604, 622
Ab (antibody), 314, 336
Abbreviations, 31–33, 701–705. *See also* specific abbreviations
  dangerous, 704–705
  for diagnosis and treatment, 32
  Joint Commission "Do Not Use" list of, 32, 705
  other, 33
  for practice areas and specialists, 32
  for prescriptions, 32
  for units of measurement, 32
ABCD signs of melanoma, 648, 648f
Abdomen, 48
Abdominal aortic aneurysm, infrarenal, 368f
Abdominal cavity, 49, 49f
Abdominal divisions, 47–50
  combining forms for, 47
  terms for, 48–49, 50f
Abdominal ultrasound, 484, 484f
Abdomin/o, 47
Abdominocentesis, 484
Abdominopelvic, 598
Abdominopelvic cavity, 49f
Abdominopelvic regions, 49, 50, 50f
  epigastric, 49, 50f
  four quadrants of, 49, 50f
  hypogastric (suprapubic), 49, 50f
  left hypochondriac, 49, 50f
  left iliac, 49, 50f
  left lumbar, 49, 50f
  right hypochondriac, 49, 50f
  right iliac, 49, 50f
  right lumbar, 49, 50f
  umbilical, 49, 50f
Abdominoperineal (A&P) resection, 487
Abdominoplasty, 29, 487
Abduct, 24
Abduction, 114, 115, 116f
ABG (arterial blood gas), 434, 447
Ablat/o, 638
Abortifacient, 619
Abortion (AB), 604, 622
  incomplete, 604
  spontaneous, 604, 622
  therapeutic, 616, 622
Abrasion, 82
Abruptio placentae, 604
Abscess, 82
-ac, 6, 7, 29
ACB (aortocoronary bypass), 383, 389
Accessory pancreatic duct, 273f
Accommodation, 218
Acetabulum, 111, 112f
Acidemia, 283
Acid-fast bacilli (AFB) smear, 434, 434f, 447
Acidosis, 283
Acne, 82
-acousis, 240
Acous/o, 240
Acoustic, 242
Acoustic neuroma, 244
Acquired immunodeficiency syndrome (AIDS), 560, 570
Acr/o, 47, 279
Acromegaly, 283, 283f
Acromion, 111, 112f
Acronyms, 32, 704–705
ACS (acute coronary syndrome), 367, 389
ACTH (adrenocorticotropic hormone), 275, 275f, 296
Activities of daily living (ADL), 33
-acusis, 240
Acute, 44
Acute coronary syndrome (ACS), 367, 389
Acute renal failure (ARF), 535
Acute respiratory distress syndrome (ARDS), 424, 447
Ad-, 24
AD (auris dexter), 253
Addison disease, 283, 284f
Adduct, 24
Adduction, 114, 115, 116f
Adductor longus, 117f
Adductor magnus, 117f
Adenectomy, 293, 385
Adenitis, 283
Aden/o, 42, 279, 361
Adenocarcinoma, 644
Adenoidectomy, 440
Adenoid/o, 416
Adenoids, 411
Adenoma, 645
Adenomegaly, 283
Adenomyosis, 602
ADH (antidiuretic hormone), 276, 296
ADHD (attention deficit hyperactivity disorder), 182, 194
Adip/o, 75
Adipocytes, 73, 73f
Adipose, 80
Adipose tissue, 73f
Adjuvant chemotherapy, 666
ADL (activities of daily living), 33
Adnexa, 587
Adrenal glands, 272, 273f,
Adrenalectomy, 293
Adrenaline, 276, 277f
Adrenalitis, 284
Adrenal/o, 279
Adrenalopathy, 284
Adren/o, 279
Adrenocorticotropic hormone (ACTH), 275, 275f, 296
Adrenomegaly, 284
-ae, 10, 709
AFB (acid-fast bacilli), 434, 434f, 447
Afebrile, 23
Afferent arteriole, 510
AFP (alpha-fetoprotein), 610, 622, 670
A/G ratio (albumin-globulin ratio), 715
Ag (antigen), 314, 336
Agonist, 116, 117f
Agoraphobia, 183
Agranulocyte, 313
AIDS (acquired immunodeficiency syndrome), 560, 570
Airway, 413
-al, 7, 29, 171, 279, 362, 418
Alanine aminotransferase (ALT), 715
Albinism, 27, 82, 82f
Albumin, 327, 715
Albumin-globulin ratio (A/G ratio), 715
Albumin/o, 512
Albuminuria, 518
Aldosterone, 276
-algia, 7, 27, 123, 240, 418, 469
Alkalemia, 284
Alkaline phosphatase (ALP), 715
Allergist, 335
Allergology, 335
ALP (alkaline phosphatase), 715
Alpha cell, 273f
Alpha-fetoprotein (AFP), 610, 622, 670
Alpha fetoprotein (AFP) test, 655
ALS (amyotrophic lateral sclerosis), 176, 177f, 194
ALT (alanine aminotransferase), 715
Alveolar, 422
Alveoli, 413
Alveol/o, 416
Alzheimer disease, 176, 177f
Amblyopia, 220
Amenorrhea, 602
Amnesia, 176
Amni/o, 594
Amniocentesis, 28, 611
Amnion, 588
Amnionic, 598
Amnionic fluid, 588
Amnion/o, 594
Amniotic, 598
Amniotomy, 616
Amputation, 661
Amylase, 715

Amyotrophic lateral sclerosis (ALS), 176, 177f, 194
An-, 6, 23, 75, 417, 554
ANA (antinuclear antibody) test, 329, 336
Anaerobic, 23
Analgesic, 146, 192
Analysis. *See also specific topics*
of medical terms, 14–15
of synovial fluid, 136
Anarchism, 557
Anastomosis, 487
Anatomic position, 54, 54f
Andro-, 554
Andr/o, 553
Andropathy, 557
Anemia, 323
aplastic, 323
hemorrhagic, 324
iron deficiency, 323
pernicious, 324, 324f
sickle cell, 324
Anesthetic, 192
Aneurysm, 367
cerebral, 178
infrarenal abdominal aortic, 368f
Aneurysmectomy, 382
Angina pectoris, 367
Angi/o, 361
Angiography
cerebral, 187
coronary, 378, 378f
fluorescein, 227
lymphangiography, 380
magnetic resonance, 378, 389
Angioplasty, 382
coronary, 384, 384f
percutaneous transluminal coronary, 384, 384f, 390
Angioscopy, 378
Angiostenosis, 367
Ankyl/o, 121
Ankylosing spondylitis, 128
Ankylosis, 128
Anorexia, 475
Anorexia nervosa, 477
Anoxic, 422
Answers to exercises, 727–762
Antacid, 492
Antagonist, 116, 117f
Ante-, 594
Anterior, 53, 54f
Anterior root, 165
Anterior/posterior repair, 614
Antero-, 52
Anteroposterior (AP), 33, 53, 54f
Anti-, 23
Antianxiety agent, 192
Antiarrhythmic agent, 388
Antibacterial, 23, 534
Antibiotic, 252, 334, 445, 534
Antibody (Ab), 314, 336
Anticoagulant, 334, 388
Anticonvulsant, 192
Antidepressant, 192
Antidiabetic, 294
Antidiarrheal, 492
Antidiuretic hormone (ADH), 276, 296
Antiemetic, 492
Antifungal, 94
Antigen (Ag), 314, 336
Antihistamine, 334, 445
Anti-infective, 94
Anti-inflammatory, 94, 192
Antinuclear antibody (ANA) test, 329, 336
Antipruritic, 94
Antiretroviral, 569
Antiserum, 334
Antithyroid, 294
Antitubercular drug, 445
Antitussive, 445
Antiviral, 569
Anuria, 518
Anus, 465
Anxiety, 182
Anxi/o, 170
Anxiolytic, 192
Aorta, 356
Aortic stenosis, 367
Aortic valve, 355
Aort/o, 361
Aortocoronary bypass (ACB), 383, 389
Aortography, 378
AP (anteroposterior), 33, 53, 54f
Apex, 353
Apgar score, 611
Aphasia, 178
versus aphagia, 184
Apheresis, 331, 331f
Aphonia, 424
Aplastic anemia, 323
Apnea, 424
Apneic, 422
Appearance, of urine, 697
Appendectomy, 28, 487
Appendicular skeleton, 110, 111, 112f
Appendix, 464
APR (abdominoperineal resection), 493
Aqueous humor, 210f, 211
-ar, 29, 171, 362, 418
Arachnoid mater, 167, 167f
-arche, 595
ARDS (acute respiratory distress syndrome), 424, 447
Areola, 585
ARF (acute renal failure), 535
Aromatase inhibitors, 666
Arrector pili muscles, 73, 73f
Arrhythmia, 371
Arterial blood gases (ABGs), 434, 447
Arterial stent, 385f
Arterial system (anterior view), 776f
Arteries, 356f
Arteri/o, 361
Arteriography, 378
Arteriole, 356
Arteriosclerosis, 367
Arteriosclerotic heart disease (ASHD), 367, 389
Arteriovenous (AV), 365, 389
Artery, 356
Arthralgia, 128
Arthritis, 9, 128, 129f
knee, 129f
Arthr/o, 121
Arthrocentesis, 140, 141f
Arthrochondritis, 128
Arthroclasia, 140
Arthrodesis, 140
Arthrography, 136
Arthroplasty, 140
Arthroscopy, 136, 137f
Articular, 29
Articulations, 114
Articul/o, 121
Artificial rupture of membranes, 616
-ary, 7, 29, 362, 418
AS (auris sinister), 253
Ascending colon, 464
Ascites, 477, 478f
ASD (atrial septal defect), 605
-ase, 469
ASHD (arteriosclerotic heart disease), 367, 389
Aspartate aminotransferase (AST), 699
Aspermia, 557
Aspiration, 440
Aspir/o, 416
AST (aspartate aminotransferase), 699
-asthenia, 123, 595
Asthma, 424
Astigmatism, 220
Astrocytoma, 650
Ataxia, 178
Atelectasis, 424
atel/o, 416
Atherectomy, 382
Ather/o, 361
Atherosclerosis, 367
Athlete's foot. *See* Tinea pedis
Atomizer, 445
Atresia, 605
Atrial septal defect (ASD), 605
Atri/o, 361
Atrioventricular (AV), 365, 389
Atrium, 353
Atrophic vaginitis, 602
Atrophy, 128
Attention deficit hyperactivity disorder (ADHD), 182, 194
Atypical, 80
AU (auris utraque), 253
Audi/o, 240
Audiogram, 247, 263f
Audiologist, 252
Audiology, 252
Audiometer, 247
Audiometry, 247, 247f
Auditory, 242
Auditory canal, external, 236, 237f
Auditory ossicles, 236, 237, 237f, 238f
Auditory tube, 236, 237, 237f
Aural, 243
Aur/i, 240
Auricle, 237, 237f
Auris dexter (AD), 253
Auris sinister (AS), 253
Auris utraque (AU), 253

Aur/o, 240
Ausculat/o, 417
Auscultation, 379, 435, 435f
Autism, 183
Auto-, 318
Autograft, 91
Autoimmune disease, 284, 324
Autoimmunity, 321
Autologous blood, 331
AV (arteriovenous), 365, 389
Axial skeleton, 111, 112f

B

B cell, 313
B lymphocyte, 313
Babinski sign, 187, 187f
Bacteria, in urine, 697
Bacterial endocarditis, 369f
Bacterial pneumonia, 427
Bacterial vaginosis, 602
Bacteri/o, 512
bacteriuria, 518
BAL (bronchoalveolar lavage), 435, 447
Balanic, 556
Balanitis, 557
Balan/o, 553
Balanoplasty, 565
Balanorrhea, 558
Band cells, 698
BANDs (immature neutrophils), 698
Bariatric surgery, 488
Bariatrics, 493
Barium enema (BE), 478f, 484, 493
Barium swallow, 484
Bartholin glands, 588
Basal cell carcinoma (BCC), 647, 648f, 670
Basal ganglia, 165
Basi-, 318
Baso-, 318
Basophils (BASOs), 313, 698
BASOs (basophils), 313, 698
BCC (basal cell carcinoma), 647, 648f, 670
BE (barium enema), 478f, 484, 493
Becker, muscular dystrophy, 131
Bedsore, 83
Bell palsy, 178, 178f
Benign, 642
Benign prostatic hyperplasia (BPH), 558, 558f, 570
Beta cells, 273f
Bi-, 22, 23, 171, 214
Biceps brachii, 117f, 118f
Biceps femoris, 117f
b.i.d. (twice a day), 32
Bilateral, 22, 23, 53, 54f
Bile, 465
Bile duct, common, 273f
Bilirubin, 327
  total, blood, 699
  urine, 697
Billroth operation (I& II), 662
Bin-, 214
Binocular, 218
Bio-, 75
Bi/o, 638
Biologic therapy, 667
Biopsy (bx), 90, 95, 656
Bipolar, 175
Bipolar disorder, 183
Birth canal, 587
Blackhead, 82
Bladder cancer, 652
Blast/o, 42
Blepharal, 218
Blepharitis, 220
Blephar/o, 213
Blepharoplasty, 231
Blepharoptosis, 220, 221f
Blepharospasm, 220
Blood, 311
  autologous, 331
  component therapy, 331
  homologous, 331
  occult, in urine, 697
Blood and immune system, 310–336
  anatomy and physiology of, 311–315
    functions of, 311
    structures in, 310, 310f
    terms for, 311–315
  cancer terms for, 650–651, 657–658, 661–662
  medical terms in, 321–336
    abbreviations, 336
    adjectives and other related terms, 321–322
    medications and drug therapies, 334
    specialties and specialists, 335
    surgical interventions and therapeutic procedures, 331, 332f
    symptoms and medical conditions, 323–325, 323f–325f
    tests and procedures, 327–329, 328f–329f
  word parts for, 318–319
    combining forms, 318–319
    prefixes, 319
    suffixes, 318
Blood chemistry tests, 699–700
Blood component therapy, 331
Blood glucose, 291, 291f
Blood loss anemia, 324
Blood pressure (BP), 33, 389
  monitoring, 379
Blood smear, 327
Blood sugar, 291, 291f
Blood transfusion (BT), 331, 336
Blood urea nitrogen (BUN), 525, 535, 699
Blood vessels, 356
BM (bowel movement), 475, 493
BMA (bone marrow aspiration), 331, 332f, 336, 657
BMT (bone marrow transplant), 331, 336, 661, 670
Body, 463
  areas of, 47–50
    combining forms for, 47
    terms for, 48–49, 49f
  as a whole, 44, 45f
Body cavities, 47–49
  combining forms for, 47
  terms for, 48–49, 49f
Body directions, positions, and planes, 51–58
  terms for, 53–58
    directional, 53, 54f
    planes, 54, 55f
    positional, 54, 54f
  word parts for, 51–52
Body planes, 55–56, 56f
Body structures, in health and disease, 42–44
  terms in, 44, 45f
  word parts for, 42
Body systems, 44, 45f, 61–62. *See also specific systems*
Boil, 84
Bolus, 475
Bone densitometry, 136
Bone marrow, 110, 311
Bone marrow aspiration (BMA), 331, 332f, 336, 657
Bone marrow biopsy, 658
Bone marrow transplant (BMT), 331, 336, 661, 670
Bone scan, 136, 137f, 657
Bones, 110–114. *See also specific bones*
  cancellous, 110, 111f
  compact, 110, 111f
  densitometry, 136
  scan, 136, 137f
  spongy, 110, 111f
BOOP (bronchiolitis obliterans with organizing pneumonia), 425, 447
Bowel movement (BM), 475, 493
Bowman capsule, 510
BP (blood pressure), 33, 379, 389
BPH (benign prostatic hyperplasia; benign prostatic hypertrophy), 558, 558f, 570
Brachialis, 117f
Brachi/o, 47
Brachioradialis, 117f
Brachytherapy, 661
Brady-, 27, 362
Bradycardia, 27, 371
Bradykinesia, 128
Brain, 164f, 165, 166f
Brainstem, 165, 166f
Braxton Hicks contractions, 604
Breasts, 585
Breathing
  external respiration, 414
  process, 414, 414f
Breech pregnancy, 604
Bronchi, 413
Bronchial, 422
Bronchiectasis, 424
Bronchi/o, 417
Bronchioles, 413
Bronchiolitis obliterans with organizing pneumonia (BOOP), 425, 447
Bronchitis, 425
Bronch/o, 417
Bronchoalveolar lavage (BAL), 435, 447
Bronchodilator, 445
Bronchogenic carcinoma, 651
Bronchoplasty, 440

Bronchopneumonia, 427
Bronchoscopy, 435
Bruise, 83
BT (blood transfusion), 331, 336
Building terms, 16
Bulbourethral glands, 550
BUN (blood urea nitrogen), 525, 535, 699
Bunion, 128
Burn
  full-thickness burn, 82, 83f
  partial-thickness burn, 82, 83f
  superficial burn, 82, 83f
Bursa(ae), 114, 115f
Bursectomy, 140
Bursitis, 128
Burs/o, 121
Bursolith, 128
Bx (biopsy), 90, 95, 656

C

C (Celsius/centigrade), 32
CABG (coronary artery bypass graft), 383–384, 389
CA (cancer), 642
Ca (calcium), blood, 699
CAD (coronary artery disease), 368, 389
Calcaneal tendon, 117f
Calcaneus, 111, 112f
Calc/i, 279
Calcipenia, 284
Calcium (Ca), blood, 699
Calyx, 509
CAM (complementary and alternative medicine), 32, 706–708, 712
Cancellous bones, 110, 111f
Cancer (CA), 642
Cancer/o, 638
Cancerous, 642
Capillary, 356
Capn/I, 417
Capn/o, 417
Carbon dioxide (CO_2), blood, 699
Carbuncle, 82
Carcin/o, 638
Carcinogen, 642
Carcinogenic, 29
Carcinoma (CA), 645
Cardi, 4
Cardia, 463
Cardiac, 6–7, 29
Cardiac arrest, 367
Cardiac catheterization, 378
Cardiac cycle, 353
Cardiac electrophysiologist, 388
Cardiac electrophysiology, 388
Cardiac muscle, 116, 118f
Cardiac pacemaker, 383
Cardiac tamponade, 367
Cardi/o, 8, 16, 361
Cardiologist, 388
Cardiology, 8, 388
Cardiomegaly, 28, 367
Cardiomyopathy, 368
Cardiopathy, 368
Cardiopulmonary resuscitation (CPR), 440, 447
Cardiovalvulitis, 368
Cardiovascular, 365
Cardiovascular and lymphatic systems, 352–391
  anatomy and physiology of, 352–354
    functions of cardiovascular system in, 352, 353f
    functions of lymphatic system in, 352, 353f
    structures of cardiovascular system in, 352, 353f
    structures of lymphatic system in, 352
    terms for, 353–358
  medical terms in, 353–358
    abbreviations, 389–390
    adjectives and other related terms, 365–366
    medications and drug therapies, 388
    specialties and specialists, 388
  surgical interventions and therapeutic procedures, 382–385
    test and procedures, 377–380, 378f, 380f
  word parts for, 361–362
    combining forms, 361–362
    prefixes, 362
    suffixes, 362
Cardioversion, 383
Carditis, 9, 16
Carina, 413
Carpal, 126
Carpal bones, 111, 112f
Carpal tunnel syndrome (CTS), 128
Carpectomy, 140
Carp/o, 121
Carpoptosis, 128
Cartilage, 114
Case reports, 102–103
Casts, urine, 697
Cataract, 220, 221f, 223f
Cataract extraction, 231
Catatonia, 183
Cathartic, 492
Catheterization (cath), 529
Cauda equina, 165
Caudad, 53, 54f
Caudal, 51
Cauterization, 91
Cavities, body, 47–49
  combining forms for, 47
  terms for, 48–49, 49f
CBC (complete blood count), 328, 336, 698
cc (cubic centimeter), 32
Cecum, 464
-cele, 418, 469, 512, 554, 595
Cell, 44, 45f
  chromosome, 44, 45f
  cytoplasm, 44
  gene, 44
  nucleus, 44, 45f
Cellulitis, 82, 83f
-centesis, 28, 123, 418, 469, 595
Centigrade (C), 32
Centimeter (cm), 32, 725
Central nervous system (CNS), 164f, 165, 194
Cephalad, 53, 54f
Cephal/o, 51, 594
Cerclage, 616
Cerebellar, 175
Cerebell/o, 170
Cerebellum, 165, 166f
Cerebr, 4
Cerebral, 175
Cerebral aneurysm, 178
Cerebral angiography, 187
Cerebral cortex, 166, 166f
Cerebral embolism, 178, 178f
Cerebral hemispheres, 774f
Cerebral palsy (CP), 178, 194
Cerebral thrombosis, 178, 178f
Cerebr/o, 8, 170
Cerebrospinal fluid (CSF), 167, 194
Cerebrovascular accident (CVA), 179, 179f, 194
Cerebrum, 166, 166f
Cerumen, 237, 237f
Cerumen impaction, 244
Ceruminolytic, 252
Cervical conization, 658
Cervical dysplasia, 602
Cervical os, 587
Cervical vertebrae, 113, 113f
Cervicitis, 602
Cervic/o, 47, 122, 593
Cervix, 587
Cesarean section (C-section), 616, 622
CF (cystic fibrosis), 425, 447
Chalazion, 220, 221f
Chem/o, 638
Chemoprevention, 666
Chemotherapy, 666
Chest, 102, 413
Chest radiograph (CXR), 434, 447
Cheyne-Stokes respiration, 425
CHF (congestive heart failure), 368, 389
Chicken pox. *See* Varicella
Chime, 475
Chiropractic, 146
Chiropractor, 146
Chlamydia, 560
Chloride (Cl), blood, 699
Chlor/o, 57
Chloroma, 58
Cholecystectomy, 488
Cholecystitis, 477
Cholecystogram, 484
Cholelithiasis, 477, 478f
Cholelithotripsy, 488
Cholescintigraphy, 658
Cholesteatoma, 244, 245f
Cholesterol, blood, 699
Chondrectomy, 140
Chondro-, 639
Chondr/o, 121
Chondroma, 649f
Chondromalacia, 129
Chondroplasty, 140
Chondrosarcoma, 649
Chori/o, 594
Chorion, 588
Chorionic, 598

Chorionic villus sampling (CVS), 612, 622
Choroid, 210f, 211
Choroido-, 214
Chromat/o, 318
Chromaturia, 58
Chrom/o, 57, 318
Chromosome, 44, 45f
Chronic, 44
Chronic obstructive pulmonary disease (COPD), 425, 447
Chronic renal failure (CRF), 535
Cicatrix, 82
-cide, 76
Cilia, 412
Circum-, 52
Circumcision, 565, 565f
Circumduction, 114, 116f
Circumscribed, 80
Cirrhosis, 477
CK (creatine kinase), 136, 700
Cl (chloride), blood, 699
Clarity, of urine, 697
-clasia, 123
-clasis, 123
-clast, 123
Claustrophobia, 183
Clavicle, 111, 112f
Clavic/o, 121
Clavicul/o, 121
Cleft lip, 605, 605f
Cleft palate, 605, 605f
Clitoris, 588
Clonus, 179
Closed fractures, 130f
Clotting disorder, 325
Clotting factors, 314
cm (centimeter), 32, 725
CMG (cystometrogram), 526, 535
CNS (central nervous system), 164f, 165, 194
CO_2 (carbon dioxide), blood, 699
Coagulation, 314
Coarctation of the aorta, 368
Coccyx, 113, 113f
Cochlea, 238
Cochlear, 243
Cochlear implant, 249, 250f
Cochle/o, 240
Coitus, 556
Cold sores, 84
Colectomy, 662
Collecting duct, 510
Colo, 4
Col/o, 8, 468
Colon, 4, 464
Colon cancer, 652
Colon/o, 8, 468
Colonoscopy, 484
Color
  combining forms for, 57
  terms for, 58
  of urine, 697
Color blindness, 220
Colostomy, 29, 488
Colostomy sites, 488f
Colp/o, 593
Colporrhaphy, 614
Colposcope, 612
Colposcopy, 612, 612f, 658
Coma, 179
Combining forms, 683–689
Combining vowels, 8
Comedo, 82
Comminuted fracture, 130f
Common bile duct, 273f
Compact bones, 110, 111f
Complementary and alternative medicine (CAM), 32, 706–708, 712
Complete blood count (CBC), 328, 336, 698
Compound fractures, 130f
Compulsion, 183
Computed tomography (CT), 33, 138, 138f, 434, 447. *See also* Single photon emission computed tomography (SPECT)
Conception, 588
Condom, 556
Conductive hearing loss, 244
Condyloma, 560
Cone biopsy, 658
Congenital, 598
Congenital hypothyroidism, 284
Congestive heart failure (CHF), 368, 389
Conjunctiva, 210, 210f
Conjunctival, 218
Conjunctivitis, 221
Conjunctiv/o, 213
Consent forms, 58
Constipation, 477
Constriction, 365
Continuous positive airway pressure (CPAP) therapy, 440, 440f, 447
Continuous subcutaneous insulin infusion (CSII), 294, 294f, 296
Contra-, 23
Contraception, 23
Contraceptive, 619
Contusion, 83
COPD (chronic obstructive pulmonary disease), 425, 447
Cord
  nuchal, 604, 604f
  prolapsed, 605
  spinal, 164f, 165, 167
  umbilical, 589f, 590
  vocal, 411, 412f
Cor/e, 213
Cornea, 210f, 211
Corneal, 218
Corne/o, 213
Cor/o, 213
Coronal plane, 54, 55f
Coronary angiography, 378, 378f
Coronary artery bypass graft (CABG), 383–384, 389
Coronary artery disease (CAD), 368, 389
Coronary circulation, 353
Coronary occlusion, 368
Coron/o, 361
Corpus luteum, 586
Cortical, 282
Cortic/o, 170, 279
Corticosteroid, 146, 233, 445
Cortisol, 276
Costectomy, 140
Cost/o, 122, 417
Costovertebral, 126
CP (cerebral palsy), 178, 194
CPAP (continuous positive airway pressure), 440, 440f, 447
CPR (cardiopulmonary resuscitation), 440, 447
Crackles, 428
Crani, 4
Cranial, 7, 29, 126, 175
Cranial cavity, 49, 49f
Cranial nerves, 164f, 165, 168, 773f
Craniectomy, 190, 191f
craniectomy, 661
Crani/o, 8, 122, 170
Craniopathy, 28
Cranioplasty, 140, 190, 191f
Cranioschisis, 129
Craniotomy, 3, 140, 190, 191f
Cranium, 48, 111, 112f
C-reactive protein (CRP), 377
Creatine kinase (CK), 136, 700
Creatinine, blood, 699
Creatinine clearance test, 525
CRF (chronic renal failure), 535
Crin/o, 279
Crohn disease, 477
Crossed eyes, 224
Crossmatching, 328
Croup, 425
CRP (C-reactive protein), 377
Cry/o, 75, 213, 638
Cryoretinopexy, 231
Cryosurgery, 91, 91f, 614, 661
Crypt-, 554
Cryptorchidism, 558, 558f
Crystals, urine, 697
C&S (culture and sensitivity), 90, 95, 328, 336
C-section (cesarean section), 616, 622
CSF (cerebrospinal fluid), 167, 194
CSII (continuous subcutaneous insulin infusion), 294, 294f, 296
CT (computed tomography), 33, 138, 138f, 147, 434, 447
CT intravenous pyelogram, 526f
CTS (carpal tunnel syndrome), 128, 147
Cubic centimeter (cc), 32
Culture and sensitivity (C&S), 90, 95, 328, 336
Curvature of spine, 129, 129f
Cushing syndrome, 284, 284f
Cutane/o, 75
Cutaneous membrane, 72
CVA (cerebrovascular accident), 179, 179f, 194
CVS (chorionic villus sampling), 612, 622
CXR (chest x-ray), 434, 447
Cyan/o, 57, 75
Cyanosis, 58, 80
Cyanotic, 365

Cyst, 83, 83f
Cystectomy, 529, 662
Cystic, 516, 598
Cystic fibrosis (CF), 425, 447
Cystitis, 518
Cyst/oa, 512
Cystocele, 518
Cystogram, 30, 526, 526f
Cystography, 526
Cystolith, 518
Cystolithotomy, 529
Cystometrogram (CMG), 526, 535
Cystoplasty, 529
Cystorrhaphy, 29, 529
Cystoscope, 526
Cystoscopy, 526, 526f
Cystostomy, 529
-cyte, 42, 319
Cyt/o, 42, 318, 638
Cytology, 44
Cytopathic, 321
Cytoplasm, 44

D

Dacry/o, 213
Dacryoadenitis, 221
Dacryocystitis, 221
Dacryocystotomy, 231
Dacryolith, 221
Dacryorrhea, 221
Date of birth (DOB), 598, 622
dB (decibel), 247, 253
D&C (dilatation and curettage; dilation and curettage), 614, 614f, 622
DC (doctor of chiropractic medicine), 32
DCIS (ductal carcinoma in situ), 652, 653f, 670
DCT (distal convoluted tubule), 510, 535
DDS (doctor of dental surgery), 32
De-, 23, 171, 362
Deaminase, 23
Debridement, 91
Debulking surgery, 661
Decibel (dB), 247, 253
Deciliter (dL), 725
Decongestant, 445
Decubitus, 54
Decubitus ulcer, 83, 104, 104f
Deep, 53, 54f
Deep tendon reflex (DTR), 187, 194
Deep vein thrombosis (DVT), 371, 389
Defecation, 475
Defibrillation, 383
Deglutition, 475
Delirium, 183
Deltoid, 117f
Delusion, 183
Dementia, 183
Dentist, 30
Dent/o, 468
Deoxygenate, 365
Depression, 183
-derma, 76
Dermabrasion, 91
Dermat, 4
Dermat/o, 8, 75
Dermatoautoplasty, 91
Dermatoheteroplasty, 91
Dermatologist, 30, 94
Dermatology, 8, 30, 94
Dermatome, 83, 91, 91f, 92
Dermatoplasty, 91
Dermis, 72, 73f
Derm/o, 75
Descending colon, 464
Detached retina, 221, 221f
Detrusor muscle, 510
Di-, 22, 23
DI (diabetes insipidus), 284, 296
Diabetes insipidus (DI), 284, 296
Diabetes mellitus (DM), 284, 285, 296
Diabetic ketoacidosis (DKA), 285, 296
Diabetic retinopathy, 221, 223f
Diagnosis (Dx), 32
Diagnostic test reports, 59
Diaphoresis, 80
Diaphragm, 48, 413
Diaphragmatic, 422
Diaphragmat/o, 417
Diaphragmatocele, 425
Diaphysis, 110, 111f
Diarrhea, 28, 477
Diarthric, 22, 23
Diarthrosis, 114, 115f
Diastole, 365
Diencephalon, 167
Differential count, 328
Differential (peripheral blood smear) count, 698
Differential white blood count, 328
Differentiation, 642
Digestion, 475
Digestive system, 44, 45f
  anatomy and physiology, 462–465
    functions of, 462
    organs and structures in, 462, 463f
    terms for accessory digestive organs in, 465, 465f
    terms for primary digestive structures and organs in, 462–465, 463f–465f
  anterior view, 780f
  cancer terms for, 652, 658, 662
  medical terms in, 475
    abbreviations, 493–494
    adjectives and other related, 475–476, 476f
    medications and drug therapies, 492
    specialties and specialists, 493
    surgical interventions and therapeutic procedures, 487–489, 488f–489f
    symptoms and medical conditions, 477–481, 478f–481f
    tests and procedures, 484–486, 484f–485f
  word parts for, 467
    combining forms, 468
    prefixes, 468
    suffixes, 469
Digital rectal examination (DRE), 564, 564f, 570, 658, 670
Dilatation and curettage (D&C), 614, 614f, 622
Dipl/o, 213
Diplopia, 221
Dips/o, 279
Dipstick urinalysis, 525
Direction, in prefixes, 24–25
Directional terms, 53, 54f
Dis-, 23
Disarticulate, 23
Discectomy, 140, 141f
Disc/o, 122
Disk (disc)
  herniated, 131, 131f
  normal, 131f
Disorientation, 179
Distal, 53, 54f
Distal convoluted tubule (DCT), 510, 535
Diuresis, 519
Diuretic, 534
Diverticulitis, 14, 477
Diverticul/o, 468
Diverticulum, 14, 477
Divisions of abdomen, 47–50
  combining forms for, 47
  terms for, 48–49, 50f
DKA (diabetic ketoacidosis), 285, 296
DM (diabetes mellitus), 284, 285, 296
DOB (date of birth), 598, 622
Doctor of chiropractic medicine (DC), 32
Doctor of dental surgery (DDS), 32
Doctor of medicine (MD), 32, 148
Doctor of optometry (OD), 32
Doppler sonography (DS), 379, 389
Dorsal, 51, 53, 54f
Dorsal recumbent, 54
Dorsal root, 165
Dorsiflexion, 114, 116f
Down syndrome, 606
DRE (digital rectal examination), 564, 564f, 570, 658, 670
DS (Doppler sonography), 379, 389
DTR (deep tendon reflex), 187, 194
Duchenne, muscular dystrophy, 131
Ductal carcinoma in situ (DCIS), 652, 653f, 670
Ductless glands, 272, 273f
Ductus deferens, 552
Duoden/o, 468
Duodenum, 464
Dura mater, 167, 167f
Dural, 175
Dur/o, 170
DVT (deep vein thrombosis), 371, 389
Dx (diagnosis), 32
-dynia, 469
Dys-, 6, 26, 240, 417, 512, 594, 639
Dysacousia, 244
Dysacusis, 244
Dysentery, 477
Dyskinesia, 129
Dysmenorrhea, 602
Dyspareunia, 602
Dyspepsia, 26, 477
Dysphagia, 477
Dysphonia, 425

Dysplasia, 80, 642
Dyspnea, 425
Dysrhythmia, 371
Dystocia, 604
Dystrophy, 129
Dysuria, 519

E

Ear, 236–253
- anatomy and physiology of, 236–238
  - functions of, 236
  - structures in, 236, 237f
  - terms for, 237–238, 237f, 238f
- medical terms in, 242–253
  - abbreviations, 253
  - adjectives and other related terms, 242–243
  - medical conditions, 244–245
  - medications and drug therapies, 252
  - specialties and specialists, 252
  - surgical interventions and therapeutic procedures, 249–250, 249f–250f
  - tests and procedures, 247–248
- word parts for, 240–241
  - combining forms, 240
  - prefixes, 240
  - suffixes, 240

Ear lavage, 249
Ears, nose, and throat (ENT), 32, 253
EBV (Epstein-Barr virus), 329, 336
ECG (electrocardiography), 379, 389
Echocardiography, 379, 379f
Eclampsia, 604
Ect-, 24
-ectasia, 214, 362, 418
-ectasis, 214
Ecto-, 24, 594
Ectoderm, 24
-ectomy, 7, 28, 76, 123, 240, 418
Ectopic pregnancy, 604
Eczema, 84, 84f
ED (emergency department), 32
ED (erectile dysfunction), 558, 570
ED&C (electrodesiccation and curettage), 91
EDC (estimated date of confinement), 599, 622
EDD (estimated date of delivery), 599, 622
Edema, 371
Edematous, 29
EEG (electroencephalography), 187, 187f, 194
EENT (eyes, ears, nose, and throat), 253
Effacement, 588
Efferent arteriole, 510
EGD (esophagogastroduodenoscopy), 484, 493
EGFR (epidermal growth factor receptor), 670
Ejaculation, 550, 556
Electr/o, 75, 361
Electrocardiogram, 379
Electrocardiography (ECG/EKG), 379, 389
Electrodesiccation and curettage (ED&C), 91
Electroencephalography (EEG), 187, 187f, 194
Electroencephalography (EEG) technician, 193
Electrolyte panel, 291, 377
Electromyogram (EMG), 138, 139f, 148
Electronystagmography (ENG), 248, 253
Elephantiasis, 371
em-, 417
Embolectomy, 383
Embolus, 368
Embry/o, 588, 594
Embryonic, 598
Embryon/o, 594
Emergency department (ED), 32
Emergency room (ER), 32
-emesis, 469
Emetic, 492
EMG (electromyogram), 138, 139f, 148
-emia, 27, 279, 319, 418, 512
Emphysema, 425, 426f
Empyema, 425
En-, 24
-en, 10, 709
Encephalitis, 180
Encephal/o, 170
End-, 24
Endarterectomy, 384
Endemic, 24
Endo-, 24, 362, 468, 594
Endocarditis, 369, 369f
Endocardium, 24, 353
Endocrine, 272
Endocrine glands, 272, 273f
Endocrine system, 271–297
- anatomy and physiology of, 272–277
  - functions of, 272
  - structures in, 272
  - terms for, 272–277
    - glands and organs, 272–274, 273f–274f
    - hormones, 275–276, 275f, 277f
- cancer terms for, 650, 661
- medical terms in, 282–296
  - abbreviations, 296
  - adjectives and other related terms, 282
  - medical conditions, 283–287
  - medications and drug therapies, 294
  - specialties and specialists, 295
  - surgical interventions and therapeutic procedures, 293
  - tests and procedures, 291–292
- word parts for, 279–280
  - combining forms, 279
  - prefixes, 279
  - suffixes, 279–280

Endocrin/o, 279
Endocrinologist, 295
Endocrinology, 295
Endocrinopathy, 285
Endogenous, 282
Endometrial, 598
Endometrial biopsy, 658
Endometriosis, 602, 602f
Endometritis, 602
Endometrium, 587
Endoscopic colon polypectomy, 489f
Endoscopic retrograde cholangiopancreatography (ERCP), 658, 670
Endoscopic ultrasound (EUS), 658, 670
Endoscopy, 30, 435, 484
Endosteum, 110, 111f
Endotracheal, 422
Endotracheal intubation, 440, 441f
End-stage renal disease (ESRD), 519, 535
ENG (electronystagmography), 248, 253
English-to-Spanish healthcare phrases, 719–724
- diseases, 721
- examination, 722–723
- general, 719–720, 724
- introductory phrases, 719
- parts of body, 720–721
- signs and symptoms, 722
- treatment, 723–724

ENT (ears, nose, and throat), 32, 253
Enter/o, 468
Enucleation, 231, 661
Enuresis, 519
Enur/o, 512
EOM (extraocular movement), 227, 235
EOs (eosinophils), 698
Eosinophils (EOs), 698
Epi-, 52, 75, 171, 362
Epicardium, 353
Epidermal growth factor receptor (EGFR) inhibitor therapy, 667
Epidermis, 72, 73f, 73
Epididymal, 556
Epididymectomy, 565
Epididymis, 551
Epididymitis, 558
Epididym/o, 553
Epidural, 175
Epidural injection, 192
Epigastric region, 49, 50f
Epiglottis, 412, 417
Epiglott/o, 417
Epilepsy, 180
Epinephrine, 276, 277f
Epiphysial plate, 110, 111f
Epiphysis, 110, 111f
Episi/o, 593
Episiotomy, 616
Epispadias, 519, 519f
Epistaxis, 425
EPO (erythropoietin), 336
Eponyms, 3
Epstein-Barr virus (EBV), 336
Epstein-Barr virus (EBV) antibody test, 329
ER (emergency room), 32
ERCP (endoscopic retrograde cholangiopancreatography), 658, 670
Erectile dysfunction (ED), 558, 570
Eructation, 475
Erythematous, 80

Erythr/o, 57, 75, 318
Erythrocyte, 312
Erythrocyte sedimentation rate (ESR), 136, 148, 328, 336
Erythrocytes, 58
Erythropoietin (EPO), 336
-es, 10, 709
Eschar, 80
-esis, 512
Esophagectomy, 662
Esophag/o, 468
Esophagogastroduodenoscopy (EGD), 484, 493
Esophagus, 463
ESR (erythrocyte sedimentation rate), 136, 148, 328, 336
ESRD (end-stage renal disease), 519, 535
Esthesi/o, 170
Estimated date of confinement (EDC), 599, 622
Estimated date of delivery (EDD), 599, 622
Estrogen, 276Estrogen receptor test, 655
ESWL (extracorporeal shock wave lithotripsy), 529, 529f, 535
Etiology, 44
Eu-, 26, 171, 279, 417
Eupeptic, 26
Euphoria, 183
Eupnea, 413
EUS (endoscopic ultrasound), 658, 670
Eustachian tube, 237
Euthyroid, 282
Eversion, 114, 116f
Evoked potential studies, 188
Ewing sarcoma, 649
Ewing tumor, 649
Ex-, 24
-ex, 10, 709
Exacerbation, 44
Excessive sleep disorder, 181
Excision, 91
Excoriation, 84
Exercise stress test, 380, 380f
Exfoliation, 80
Exhalation, 413, 414f
Exhale, 24
Exo-, 24
Exoenzyme, 24
Exogenous, 282
Exophthalmos, 222, 285, 285f
Exophthalmus, 222
Exostosis, 130
Expectorant, 445
Expiration, 413, 414f
Extension, 114, 116f
Extensor digitorum longus, 117f
External auditory canal, 237, 237f
External auditory meatus, 237, 237f
External beam radiation, 663
External oblique, 117f
External respiration, 414
External urethral orifice, 510
Extracorporeal shock wave lithotripsy (ESWL), 529, 529f, 535
Extraocular movement (EOM), 227, 235
Extremity, 48
Eye, 210–235
  anatomy and physiology of, 210–211
    functions of, 210
    inner layer, 210f, 211
    middle layer, 210f, 211
    outer layer, 210f, 211
    structures in, 210, 210f
    terms for, 210–211, 210f, 211f
  documentation involving, 227
  medical terms in, 218–235
    abbreviations, 235
    adjectives and other related terms, 218–219
    medical conditions, 220–224
    medications and drug therapies, 233
    specialties and specialists, 234
    surgical interventions and therapeutic procedures, 231–232, 232f
    tests and procedures, 227–228, 228f, 229f
  word parts for, 213–214
    combining forms, 213–214
    prefixes, 214
    suffixes, 214
Eyelids, 210
Eyes, ears, nose, and throat (EENT), 253

F

F (Fahrenheit), 32
Fahrenheit (F), 32
Fallopian tubes, 586
False labor, 604
Fascia, 116
Fascicle, 117, 118f
Fasci/o, 122
FAST, 179
Fasting blood glucose (FBG), 291, 296
FBG (fasting blood glucose), 291, 296
Fe (iron), serum, 312, 336, 700
Fecal Occult Blood Test, 475
Feces, 475
Female reproductive system, 584f. *See also* Reproductive system, female
Femoral, 126
Femor/o, 122
Femur, 111, 112f
Fertilization, 588
Fetal, 599
Fetal ultrasound, 612
Fet/o, 594
Fetoscope, 612
Fetus, 588
Fibrillation, 371, 372f
Fibrin, 314
Fibrinogen, 314
Fibr/o, 42
Fibroma, 645
Fibromyalgia, 130
Fibromyoma, 603
Fibrosarcoma, 645
Fibula, 111, 112f
Fibul/o, 122
Filariae, 371
Fimbriae, 586
Fine-needle aspiration (FNA), 656, 656f, 670
First-degree burn. *See* Superficial burn
Fissure, 84, 84f
Flatus, 475
Flexible sigmoidoscopy, 484
Flexion, 114, 116f
Flu, 425
Fluorescein angiography, 227
Flutter, 371, 372f
FNA (fine-needle aspiration), 656, 656f, 670
Follicle-stimulating hormone (FSH), 275, 275f, 296
Follow-up note, 59
Foreskin, 551
Formed elements, 311
Fowler position, 54
Fracture (fx), 130, 130f, 148
  closed, 130f
  compound, 130f
  greenstick, 130f
  open, 130f
  simple, 130f
  spiral, 130f
  transverse, 130f
Frontal lobe, 166, 166f
Frontal plane, 54, 55f
Frontalis, 117f
Frozen section (FS), 90, 95
FS (frozen section), 90, 95
FSH (follicle-stimulating hormone), 275, 275f, 296
Fulguration, 662
Full-thickness burn, 82, 83f
Fund/o, 594
Fundus, 210f, 211, 463, 587
Furuncle, 84
Fx (fracture), 130, 130f, 148

G

g (gram), 32, 725
Galact/o, 594
Gallbladder, 465
Gamete, 551, 588
Gamma-glutamyl transferase (GGT), 700
Gangli/o, 170
Ganglion, 168
Ganglionectomy, 190
Ganglion/o, 170
Gangrene, 84
Gastr, 4, 4f
Gastrectomy, 488, 662
Gastric bypass surgery, 488
Gastric lavage, 489
Gastric resection, 489
Gastric ulcer, 4f, 479
Gastritis, 3, 4f, 27
Gastr/o, 8, 468
Gastrocnemius, 117f
Gastroenteritis, 479
Gastroenterologist, 493
Gastroenterology, 493

Gastroesophageal reflux disease (GERD), 493
Gastrointestinal (GI), 493
Gastrointestinal stromal tumor (GIST), 652, 670
Gastrointestinal tract, 4f
Gastroschisis, 606
Gastroscope, 30
Gastroscopy, 30
Gastrotomy, 3, 4f, 29
Gavage, 489
GBS (group B streptococcus), 610, 622
GCS (Glasgow coma scale), 188, 188f
GCT (germ cell tumor), 652, 670
-gen, 319, 469, 639
Gene, 44
-genesis, 29, 554
-genic, 29, 76, 639
Genital herpes, 560
Genital wart, 561
Genitalia, 586
Genitourinary (GU), 516, 535
GERD (gastroesophageal reflux disease), 493
Germ cell tumor (GCT), 652, 670
-ges, 10, 709
Gestational, 588, 599
Gestational diabetes, 604
Gestat/o, 594
GGT (gamma-glutamyl transferase), 700
GH (growth hormone), 275, 275f, 296
GI (gastrointestinal), 493
Giant cell tumor, 649
Gigantism, 285, 286f
GIST (gastrointestinal stromal tumor), 652, 670
Glands, 272
Glans penis, 551
Glasgow coma scale (GCS), 188, 188f
Glaucoma, 222, 223f
Glia, 168
Glial, 175
Glial cells, 168
Gli/o, 170
Glioma, 650
Globulins, blood, 700
Glomerular capsule, 510
Glomerul/o, 512
Glomerulonephritis, 519
Glomerulus, 509
Glossary, of combining forms, prefixes, and suffixes, 683–689
Glossorrhaphy, 489
Glottis, 412
Glucagon, 276
Gluco-, 512
Gluc/o, 42, 279
Glucometer, 291, 291f
Glucose
  blood, 699
  urine, 697
Glucose tolerance test (GTT), 291, 296
Glucos/o, 279
Glucosuria, 285, 519
Gluteus maximus, 117f
Gluteus medius, 117f
Glyc/o, 42, 279, 512
Glycos/o, 279, 512
Glycosuria, 285, 519
Glycosylated hemoglobin, 291
Glycosylated hemoglobin alpha 1c (HbA_{1c}), 291, 296
gm (gram), 32
Goiter, 285, 286f
Gonad, 551
Gonorrhea, 560
Gout, 130
Graafian follicles, 586
Gracilis, 117f
Graded exercise test (GXT), 380, 380f, 389
Graft, 384
-gram, 7, 30, 171, 362, 469
Gram (g), 32, 725
Gram (gm), 32
Granul/o, 318
Granulocyte, 313
-graph, 362
-graphy, 30, 362, 418, 469
Graves disease, 285
gravida, 599
gravid/o, 594
greater vestibular glands, 588
Greenstick fractures, 130f
Group B streptococcus (GBS), 610, 622
Growth hormone (GH), 275, 275f, 296
GTT (glucose tolerance test), 291, 296
GU (genitourinary), 516, 535
GXT (graded exercise test), 380, 380f, 389
GYN (gynecologist), 32, 620, 622
GYN (gynecology), 32, 620, 622
Gynec/o, 593
Gynecologic oncologist, 668
Gynecologic oncology, 668
Gynecologist (GYN), 32, 620, 622
Gynecology (GYN), 32, 620, 622
Gyn/o, 593
Gyrus, 166

H

Haematologist, 335
Haemophilia, 325
Haemorrhoids, 479
Hair, 73, 73f
Hair follicle, 73, 73f
Halitosis, 475
Hallucination, 183
Hallucin/o, 170
Hashimoto disease, 285
Hashimoto thyroiditis, 285
Hb (hemoglobin), 312, 328, 336, 698
HbA_{1c} (glycosylated hemoglobin alpha 1c), 291, 296
hCG (human chorionic gonadotropin), 588, 622, 656, 670
HCT (hematocrit), 328, 329f, 336, 698
Hct (hematocrit), 328, 329f, 336, 698
HDLs (high-density lipoproteins), 700
Head, eyes, ears, nose, and throat (HEENT), 227
Health care provider patient care notes, 59
Health-related websites, 710–718
Heart, 353, 775f
HEENT (Head, eyes, ears, nose, and throat), 227
Height (Ht), 33
Hemat/o, 42, 318, 468, 512
Hematochezia, 475
Hematocrit (HCT, Hct, ht), 328, 329f, 336, 698
Hematology, 335
Hematopoiesis, 311
Hematopoietic, 321
Hematuria, 519
Hemi-, 22, 171
Hemiparesis, 180, 180f
Hemiplegia, 22
Hem/o, 42, 318, 468
Hemoccult test, 484
Hemochromatosis, 325
Hemodialysis, 530, 530f
Hemoglobin (HGB, Hgb, Hb), 312, 328, 336, 698
Hemogram, 328
Hemolytic, 321
Hemopoiesis, 311
Hemopoietic, 321
Hemorrhagic, 322
Hemorrhagic anemia, 324
Hemostasis, 322
Hemostatic agent, 334, 388
Hemothorax, 425
Hepatic flexure, 464
Hepat/o, 468
Hepatobiliary iminodiacetic acid (HIDA) scan, 658, 670
Hepatomegaly, 479
Herniated nucleus pulposus, 131, 131f
Herni/o, 468
Herniorrhaphy, 489
Herpes simplex, 84
Herpes zoster, 84, 85f, 180, 180f
Hertz (Hz), 248, 253
Hetero-, 26
Heterogeneous, 26
HGB (hemoglobin), 312, 328, 336, 698
Hgb (hemoglobin), 312, 328, 336, 698
Hiatal hernia, 480, 480f
HIDA (hepatobiliary iminodiacetic acid), 658, 670
Hidr/o, 75, 76
High-density lipoproteins (HDLs), blood, 700
Hindbrain, 165, 166f
Hip bone, 111, 112f
  ilium, 112
  ischium, 112
  pubis, 112
Hirsutism, 286, 287f
Histamine, 314
Hist/o, 42
Histology, 44
History (hx), 32
History and physical (H&P) examination, 32, 58

HIV (human immunodeficiency virus), 560, 570
Hives. *See* Urticaria
HM (Holter monitor), 380, 389
Hodgkin disease, 650
Holter monitor (HM), 380, 389
Homeo-, 26
Homeometric, 26
Homeostasis, 44
Homo-, 26
Homogeneous, 26
Homologous blood, 331
Hordeolum, 222
Hormonal therapy, 667
Hormone replacement therapy (HRT), 294, 619, 622
Hormones, 272
Hormon/o, 279
Hospital records, 58–59
H&P (history and physical examination), 32, 58
HPV (human papillomavirus), 560, 570
HRT (hormone replacement therapy), 294, 619, 622
HSG (hysterosalpingogram), 612, 622
Ht (height), 33
ht (hematocrit), 328, 329f, 336, 698
HTN (hypertension), 26, 369, 389
Human chorionic gonadotropin (hCG), 588, 622, 656, 670
Human immunodeficiency virus (HIV), 560, 570
Human papillomavirus (HPV), 560, 570
Humeral, 126
Humer/o, 122
Humerus, 112, 112f, 118f
Hx (history), 32
Hydr/o, 42, 76, 512, 594
Hydrocele, 558
Hydrocephalus, 180, 181f
Hydronephrosis, 519, 520f
Hydroureter, 519
Hymen, 588
Hyoid, 112, 112f
Hyper-, 26, 171, 279, 468
Hyperbaric medicine, 441
Hypercalcemia, 286
Hyperkalemia, 286
Hyperkinesia, 131
Hypernatremia, 286
Hyperopia, 222, 222f
Hyperparathyroidism, 286
Hyperplasia, 44, 80
Hypersensitive, 322
Hypertension (HTN), 26, 369, 389
Hypertensive, 25f
Hyperthyroidism, 286
Hypertrophy, 131
Hypn/o, 170
Hypnotic, 192
Hypo-, 26, 171, 279, 417
Hypocalcemia, 286
Hypochondriac region, 49, 50f
Hypodermis, 72
Hypogastric, 5
Hypogastric (suprapubic) region, 49, 50f
Hypoglycemia, 26, 286
Hypokalemia, 286
Hypolipidemic agent, 388
Hyponatremia, 286
Hypoparathyroidism, 286
Hypospadias, 519, 519f
Hypotension, 369
Hypotensive, 25f
Hypothalamus, 272, 273f
Hypothyroidism, 287
Hypotonic, 233
Hypoxemia, 27
Hypoxia, 425
Hypoxic, 422
Hysterectomy, 615
Hyster/o, 593
Hysterosalpingography (HSG), 612, 622
Hysterotomy, 615, 615f
Hz (Hertz), 248, 253

I

-i, 10, 709
^{131}I uptake test, 291, 292f, 296
-ia, 7, 10, 27, 171, 595
-iasis, 469, 512
-iatrist, 171
IBS (irritable bowel syndrome), 480, 493
-ic, 7, 29, 279, 362, 418
-ices, 10, 709
-icle, 362
Ictal, 175
-ictal, 171
Ictero-, 214
ICU (intensive care unit), 32
I&D (incision and drainage), 91, 95
Idiopathic, 44
Idiopathic thrombocytopenic purpura (ITP), 325, 336
-ies, 10
ILD (interstitial lung disease), 426, 426f, 447
Ile/o, 468
Ileostomy, 489
ileum, 464
Ileus, 480
Iliac region, 49, 50f
Ili/o, 122
Iliofemoral, 126
Ilium, hip bone, 112
Im-, 23
Immature neutrophils (BANDs), 698
Immediately (STAT), 33
Immune serum, 334
Immunity, 314
Immunization, 331
Immun/o, 318
Immunologist, 335
Immunology, 335
Immunosuppressant, 334
Immunosuppression, 331
Immunotherapy, 667
Impetigo, 84, 85f
Impotence agent, 569
Impotent, 23
In-, 23, 417
In situ, 642
In vitro, 599
In vitro fertilization (IVF), 616, 622
-ina, 10, 709
Incentive spirometry, 441, 441f
Incision, 91
Incision and drainage (I&D), 91, 95
Incoherence, 180
Incompetent, 23
Incomplete abortion, 604
Incontinence, 480
Incus, 237
Induction of labor, 616
Indurated, 80
Inferior, 51, 53, 54f
Inferior vena cava, 357
Infertility, 604
Inflammation, 44
Inflammatory, 322
Influenza, 425
Infra-, 6, 24, 52
Infraspinatus, 117f
Infrasplenic, 24
Inguinal, 475
INH (isoniazid; isonicotinic acid hydrazide), 447
Inhalation, 414, 414f
Insertion of muscles, 117, 118f
Inspiration, 414, 414f
Insulin, 276
Insulin pump, 294
Insulin therapy, 294
Integument, 72
Integumentary, 80
Integumentary system, 72–95
  anatomy and physiology of, 72–73
    functions of, 72
    organs and structures in, 72, 73f
    terms for, 72–73, 73f
  medical terms in, 80–95
    abbreviations, 95
    adjectives and other related terms, 80
    medical conditions, 82–88, 82f–87f
    medications and drug therapies, 94
    surgical interventions and therapeutic procedures, 91–92, 91f–92f
    tests and procedures, 90
  word parts for, 75–76
    combining forms, 75
    prefixes, 75
    suffixes, 76
Intensive care unit (ICU), 32
Inter-, 6, 24, 52, 123, 362
Intercostals, 24, 126, 422
Intermittent claudication, 369
Internal respiration, 414
Interstitial chemotherapy, 667
Interstitial lung disease (ILD), 426, 426f, 447
Intervertebral, 126
Intervertebral disc, 114
Intra-, 6, 24, 52, 75, 123, 362, 639
Intra-articular, 24
Intracranial, 126
Intraductal carcinoma, 652
Intralesional injection, 94

Intraocular, 218
Intraocular lens (IOL) implant, 231, 235
Intraocular melanoma, 650
Intraocular pressure (IOP), 235
Intrathecal chemotherapy, 667
Intrauterine, 599
Intravenous pyelography (IVP), 526, 526f, 535
Intravenous urography (IVU), 526, 535
Introitus, 588
Intussusception, 480, 480f
Invasion, 642
Inversion, 114, 116f
IOL (intraocular lens), 231, 235
-ion, 10
IOP (intraocular pressure), 235
Iridal, 219
Iridectomy, 231, 661
Iridial, 219
Irid/o, 213
Iridomalacia, 222
Iridoplegia, 222
Iridotomy, 231
Iris, 210f, 211
Iritis, 222
Ir/o, 213
Iron (Fe), 312, 336, 700
Iron deficiency anemia, 323
Irrigation, 91
Irritable bowel syndrome (IBS), 480, 493
-is, 10, 709
Ischemia, 369
Ischemic, 175, 365
Ischi/o, 122
Ischiofemoral, 126
Ischium, hip bone, 112
Islets of Langerhans, 272, 273f
-ism, 7, 27, 279, 554, 595
Iso-, 26
Isomorphous, 26
Isoniazid (INH), 447
-ist, 30
ITP (idiopathic thrombocytopenic purpura), 325, 336
-itis, 7, 27, 76, 123, 418
-ium, 7, 10, 30, 362
IVF (in vitro fertilization), 616, 622
IVP (intravenous pyelogram; intravenous pyelography), 526, 526f, 535
IVU (intravenous urogram; intravenous urography), 526, 535
-ix, 10, 709

J

Jaundice, 84
Jaundice of newborn, 606
Jejun/o, 468
Jejunum, 464
Joint Commission "Do Not Use" List, 705
Joint movements, 114
Joints, 110, 114

K

K (potassium), blood, 699
Kal/i, 279
Kaposi sarcoma, 3, 648f
Kardia, 195
Kary/o, 638
Keloid, 84, 85f
Keratin, 73
Keratinocytes, 73
Keratitis, 222
Kerat/o, 75, 213
Keratomalacia, 222
Keratometer, 227
Keratoplasty, 231
Ketones, urine, 697
Ketosis, 287
Kg (kilogram), 32
kg (kilogram), 32
Kidney, 509
Kidney transplant, 530
Kidneys, ureters, and bladder (KUB) x-ray, 526, 535
Kilogram (kg), 32, 725
Kilometer (km), 725
Kinesi/o, 122
Kinet/o, 122
Knee
  arthritis, 129f
  arthroscopic examination of, 137f
Knee brace, 143f
Knee joint, 115f
KUB (kidneys, ureters, and bladder) x-ray, 526, 535
Kyph/o, 122
Kyphosis, 129, 129f

L

L (liter), 32. 725
lab (laboratory), 33
Labia, 588
Labia majora, 588
Labi/o, 468
Laboratory (lab), 33
Laboratory reports, 59
Laboratory tests, 697–700. *See also specific systems and tests*
Labyrinth, 236, 238
Labyrinthectomy, 249
Labyrinthine, 243
Labyrinthitis, 244
Labyrinth/o, 240
Lacrimal, 219
Lacrimal ducts, 210, 210f, 211f
Lacrimal glands, 210, 211f
Lacrim/o, 213
Lactation, 588
Lactic dehydrogenase (LDH/LD), 700
Lactiferous ducts, 585
Lactiferous sinuses, 585
Lact/o, 594
Lamina, 112, 112f
Laminectomy, 140, 190
Lamin/o, 122
Laminotomy, 140
Lapar/o, 468, 638
Laparoscopy, 484, 486f
Laparotomy, 489, 615
Large intestine, 464, 464f
Laryngeal, 422
Laryngectomy, 441, 662
Laryngitis, 426
Laryng/o, 417
Laryngoscopy, 435
Laryngospasm, 426
Laryngotracheotomy, 441
Larynx, 412
Laser-assisted in situ keratomileusis (LASIK), 231, 235
LASIK (laser-assisted in situ keratomileusis), 231, 235
Last menstrual period (LMP), 599, 622
Lateral, 53, 54f
Lateral recumbent, 54
Lateral rotation, 116f
Latero-, 52
Latissimus dorsi, 117f
Laxative, 492
LDH (lactic dehydrogenase), 700
LDLs (low-density lipoproteins), blood, 700
LEEP (loop electrosurgical excision procedure), 615, 622, 663, 670
Left colic flexure, 464
Left hypochondriac region, 49, 50f
Left iliac region, 49, 50f
Left lower quadrant (LLQ), 49, 50f
Left lumbar region, 49, 50f
Left splenic flexure, 464
Left upper quadrant (LUQ), 49, 50f
Leio-, 639
Lei/o, 42, 122
Leiomyoma, 603, 649
Leiomyosarcoma, 649
Lens, 210f, 211
-lepsis, 171
-lepsy, 171
LES (lower esophageal sphincter), 463, 493
Lesion, 44, 84, 642
Lethargy, 180
Leukemia, 650
Leuk/o, 57, 318, 638
Leukocytes (white blood cells), 58, 312, 697
LH (luteinizing hormone), 275, 275f, 296
Ligament, 114
Limb salvage surgery, 661
Lingu/o, 468
Lipase, blood, 700
Lipid panel, 377
Lipid profile, 377
Lip/o, 42, 75
Lipoma, 645
Liposarcoma, 645, 649
Liquid nitrogen, 94
Liter (L), 32, 725
-lith, 554
-lith stone, 513
lith/o, 468, 512
Lithotomy, 530, 604
Lithotripsy, 531
Liver, 465
L1–L5, 148
LLQ (left lower quadrant), 49, 50f

LMP (last menstrual period), 599, 622
Lobar, 422
Lobar pneumonia, 427
Lobectomy, 441, 662
Lobes, 413
Lobes of mammary gland, 585
Lob/o, 417
lobules of mammary gland, 585
lochia, 588
-logist, 30, 76, 171, 469
-logy, 7, 30, 76, 469
Loop electrosurgical excision procedure (LEEP), 615, 622, 663, 670
Loop excision, 615
Lord/o, 122
Lordosis, 129, 129f
Lou Gehrig disease, 176, 177f
Low-density lipoproteins (LDLs), blood, 700
Lower esophageal sphincter (LES), 463, 493
LP (lumbar puncture), 188, 188f, 194, 658, 670
Lumbar, 127
Lumbar puncture (LP), 188, 188f, 194, 658, 670
Lumbar region, 49, 50f
Lumbar vertebrae, 113, 113f
Lumb/o, 47, 122
Lumbocostal, 127
Lumbosacral, 127
Lumen, 356
Lungs, 413
LUQ (left upper quadrant), 49, 50f
Luteinizing hormone (LH), 275, 275f, 296
Lymph, 312, 358
Lymph capillaries, 358
Lymph ducts, 358
Lymph glands, 358
Lymph node, 312, 358
Lymphadenectomy, 385, 662
Lymphadenitis, 371
Lymphadenopathy, 371
Lymphadenotomy, 385
Lymphangiitis, 371
Lymphangiography, 380
Lymphangioma, 650
Lymphatic system, 311, 357f, 779f
Lymphatic vessels, 358
Lymphedema, 371
Lymphedema therapist, 388
Lymphedema therapy, 388
Lymph/o, 318, 361
Lymphocytes (LYMPHs), 313, 698
Lymphoid, 30
Lymphoma, 651
LYMPHs (lymphocytes), 313, 698
-lysis, 214, 319, 554
-lysis destruction, 513
-lytic, 362

M

m (meter), 32, 725
Macro-, 26, 318
Macrocyte, 312
Macrophage, 313
Macrosomia, 26
Macular degeneration, 222, 223f
Macular rash, 102
Macule, 84
Magnesium (Mg), blood, 700
Magnetic resonance angiography (MRA), 378, 389
Magnetic resonance cholangiopancreatography (MRCP), 658, 670
Magnetic resonance imaging (MRI), 33, 138, 139f, 148, 189, 189f, 194, 378, 389, 434, 447
Main pancreatic duct, 273f
Mal-, 639
-malacia, 76, 214, 469
Male urethra, 552
Malignant, 642
Malignant neoplasm, 645
Malleus, 237
Mammary glands, 585
Mamm/o, 594
Mammography, 612, 658, 659f
Mammoplasty, 615
Mandible, 112, 112f
Mandibul/o, 122
Mania, 183
-mania, 171
Mantoux test, 90
Masseter, 117f
Mastectomy, 663
Mastication, 475
Mastitis, 602
Mast/o, 594
Mastodynia, 602
Mastoid, 243
Mastoid cells, 237
Mastoidectomy, 249
Mastoiditis, 244
Mastoid/o, 240
Mastoidotomy, 249
mastopexy, 615
Maxilla, 112, 112f
Maxillitis, 131
Maxill/o, 122
Maxillotomy, 140
MCHC (mean corpuscular hemoglobin concentration), 698
MCV (mean corpuscular volume), 698
MD (doctor of medicine), 32, 148
MD (muscular dystrophy), 131, 148
Mean corpuscular hemoglobin (MCH), 698
Mean corpuscular hemoglobin concentration (MCHC), 698
Mean corpuscular volume (MCV), 698
Meaning, word part lookup by, 690–696
Meatal, 516
Meato-, 240
Meat/o, 512
Meatotomy, 531
Mechanical ventilation system, 441, 441f
Meconium, 599
Medial, 53, 54f
Medial rotation, 116f
Mediastinal, 422
Mediastin/o, 417
Mediastinum, 413
Medical aesthetician, 94
Medical oncologist, 668
Medical oncology, 668
Medical records, 58–59
Medical terms, 2–16
  analysis of, 14–15
  building of, 16
  for complementary and alternative medicine, 706–708
  derivation of, 3
  parts of, 3–10
    combining vowels added to roots, 8
    prefixes, 5–6
    putting parts together in, 9
    suffixes, 6–7
    word roots, 3–4, 4f
  plural endings in, 10, 709
  pronunciations for, 12–13
  spelling of, 11, 11f
  use of, 2, 2f
Medi/o, 51
Medulla oblongata, 165
Medullary cavity, 110, 111f
Medulloblastoma, 650
Mega-, 26
Megadose, 26
Megalo-, 26
Megalosplenia, 26
-megaly, 28, 279, 469
Meibomian cyst, 220, 221f
Meibomian glands, 211
Melan/o, 57, 75, 638
Melanocytes, 73
Melanoma, 58, 645, 648
Melatonin, 276
Melena, 475
MEN (multiple endocrine neoplasia), 650, 670
Menarche, 599
Ménière disease, 244
Ménière syndrome, 244
Meningeal, 175
Meninges, 167, 167f
Meningi/o, 170
Meningioma, 650
Meningitis, 180
Mening/o, 170
Meningomyelocele, 180, 181f
Meniscectomy, 140
Meniscitis, 131
Menisc/o, 122
Meniscus, 114
Men/o, 593
Menopause, 602
Menorrhagia, 602
Menses, 599
Menstrual cycle, 586
Menstruation, 599
Menstru/o, 593
Mental, 175
Ment/o, 170
Mesencephalon, 165

Mesothelioma, 651
Meta-, 639
Metabolism, 44, 282
Metacarpal bones, 112, 112f
Metaphysis, 110, 111f
Metastasis, 642
Metastatic ovarian cancer, 643f
Metatarsal bones, 112, 112f
-meter, 30, 214
Meter (m), 32, 725
Metric measurement, 725
Metri/o, 593
Metr/o, 593
Metrorrhagia, 602
-metry, 214, 418, 595
mg (milligram), 32, 725
MG (myasthenia gravis), 131, 148
Mg (magnesium), blood, 700
Micro-, 26, 318, 594
Microcardia, 26
Microcephaly, 606
Microgram (mcm), 725
Microliter (mcL), 725
Micrometer (μm), 725
Microscope, 30
Micturate, 516
Micturition, 516
Midbrain, 165
Midwife, 620
Midwifery, 620
Migraine, 181
Milligram (mg), 32, 725
Milliliter (mL), 32, 725
Millimeter (mm), 32, 725
MI (myocardial infarction), 369, 369f, 389
Miotic, 233
Mitral valve, 355
Mitral valve prolapse, 369
Mitral valve replacement, 385f
Mitral valve stenosis, 369
mL (milliliter), 32, 725
mm (millimeter), 32, 725
Modified radical mastectomy, 663
Mohs surgery, 661
Mole, 84
Mono-, 22, 318
Monocytes (MONOs), 313, 698
Mononeural, 22
Mononucleosis, 325
Mononucleosis spot test, 329
MONOs (monocytes), 313, 698
Mons pubis, 588
Morph/o, 42
Mouth, 462
MRA (magnetic resonance angiography), 378, 389
MRCP (magnetic resonance cholangiopancreatography), 658, 670
MRI (magnetic resonance imaging), 33, 138, 139f, 148, 189, 189f, 194, 378, 389, 434, 447
MS (multiple sclerosis), 181, 194
Muc/o, 417
Mucous, 422
MUGA (multiple uptake gated acquisition), 378, 389
Multi-, 22, 594
Multicellular, 22
Multiple endocrine neoplasia (MEN), 650, 670
Multiple sclerosis (MS), 181, 194
Multiple uptake gated acquisition (MUGA), 378, 389
Murmur, 369
Muscles, 110, 115
  insertion of, 117, 118f
  origin of, 117
  skeletal, 117, 118f
  smooth, 117, 118f
  tonicity, 117
Muscular dystrophy (MD), 131, 148
Muscular system
  anterior view, 771f
  posterior view, 772f
Muscul/o, 122
Musculoskeletal system, 109–149
  anatomy and physiology of, 110–118
    functions of, 110
    structures in, 110
    terms for, 110–118
      bone structure, 110, 111f
      joints and joint movements, 114–115, 115f, 116f
      muscles, 115–117, 117f–118f
      skeleton and bones, 111–114, 111f–113f
  cancer terms for, 649, 657, 661
  medical terms in, 126–148
    abbreviations, 147–148
    adjectives and other related terms, 126–127
    medical conditions, 128–132, 129f–133f
    medications and drug therapies, 146
    specialties and specialists, 146–147
    surgical interventions and therapeutic procedures, 140–142, 141f–143f
    tests and procedures, 136, 137f–139f, 138
  word parts for, 121–123
    combining forms, 121–122
    prefixes, 123
    suffixes, 123
Myalgia, 27, 131
Myasthenia gravis (MG), 131, 148
Myc/o, 75
Mydriatic, 233
Myel/o, 122, 170
Myelogram, 189
Myeloma, 646
My/o, 42, 122, 361, 593
Myocardial, 9
Myocardial infarction (MI), 369, 369f, 389
Myocarditis, 369
Myocardium, 30, 353
Myoma, 603
Myomectomy, 615, 663
Myometrium, 587
Myopia, 222, 222f
Myoplasty, 140
Myorrhaphy, 140
Myositis, 132
Myos/o, 42
Myringitis, 244
Myring/o, 240, 241
Myringotomy, 249, 250f
Mys/o, 122
Myxedema, 287

N

Na (sodium), blood, 699
Nail, 73
Narc/o, 170
Narcolepsy, 181
Nasal, 422
Nasal cavity, 411, 412f
Nasal septum, 411
Nas/o, 417
Nasogastric (NG) intubation, 489, 493
Nasolacrimal ducts, 211, 211f
Nasopharyngitis, 426
Nasopharyngoscopy, 435
Nat/o, 594
Natr/i, 279
Nausea, 475
Nebulizer, 445
Necr/o, 42, 75
Necrosis, 44
Neo-, 27, 594, 639
Neonatal, 599
Neonatal intensive care unit (NICU), 620, 622
Neonate, 27, 599
Neonatologist, 620
Neonatology, 620
Neoplasm, 646
Nephr, 4
Nephrectomy, 531, 663
Nephric, 516
Nephritis, 519
Nephr/o, 8, 512
Nephrogram, 527
Nephrography, 527
Nephrolith, 519
Nephrolithiasis, 519
Nephrolithotomy, 531
Nephrologist, 534
Nephrology, 9, 534
Nephrolysis, 531
Nephroma, 652
Nephromegaly, 519
Nephron, 509
Nephron loop, 510
Nephropexy, 531
Nephroptosis, 519
Nephroscope, 527
Nephroscopy, 527
Nephrosonography, 527
Nephrotomogram, 527
Nephrotomy, 531
Nerve, 168
Nerve roots, 165
Nervous system, 164, 164f

Nervous system and mental health, 163–196
  anatomy and physiology of, 164–168
    functions of, 165
    structures in, 164–165, 164f
    terms related to, 165–168, 166f, 167f
  medical terms in, 175–195
    abbreviations, 194–195
    adjectives and other related terms, 175
    diagnostic procedures, 187–189
    medical conditions, 176–184
    medications and drug therapies, 192
    specialties and specialists, 193
    surgical interventions and therapeutic procedures, 190–191, 191f
  word parts for, 170–171
    combining forms, 170
    prefixes, 171
    suffixes, 171
Neural, 175
Neuralgia, 181
Neuritis, 181
Neur/o, 8, 42, 170
Neuroblastoma, 650
Neuroglia, 168
Neuroleptic, 192
Neurologist, 193
Neurology, 193
Neurolysis, 191
Neuroma, 646
Neuron, 168
Neuropathy, 181
Neuroplasty, 191
Neurosis, 183
Neurotransmitters, 165
Neutr/o, 318
Neutrophils, 313
  immature, 698
  segmented, 698
Nevus, 84
Newborn, 599
NG (nasogastric), 489, 493
-nges, 709
NHL (non-Hodgkin lymphoma), 651, 670
NICU (neonatal intensive care unit), 620, 622
Night blindness, 222
Nipple, 586
Nitrite, urine, 697
Nitroglycerin, 388
noct. (night), 32
Noct/I, 512
Nocturia, 520
Nocturnal enuresis, 520
Nodule, 84, 85f
Noise-induced hearing loss, 247
Non-, 23
Non-Hodgkin lymphoma (NHL), 651, 670
Noninfectious, 23
Non-small cell carcinoma, 651
Nonsteroidal anti-inflammatory drug (NSAID), 146, 148
Noradrenaline, 276, 277f
Norepinephrine, 276, 277f
Normo-, 26
Normotensive, 25f, 26
Nose, 411
Note
  follow-up, 59
  health care provider patient care, 58–59
Nothing by mouth (NPO), 33
NPO (nothing by mouth), 33
NSAID (nonsteroidal anti-inflammatory drug), 146, 148
Nuchal cord, 604, 604f
Nucle/o, 42, 318
Nucleus, 44, 45f
Nulli-, 594
Nulligravida, 599
Nullipara, 599
Number, in prefixes, 22
-nx, 709
Nyctalopia, 222
Nystagmus, 222

O

OA (osteoarthritis), 9, 132, 148
Oat cell carcinoma, 651, 651f
OB (obstetrics; obstetrician), 32, 620, 622
Obliques, 117f
Obsessive-compulsive disorder (OCD), 183, 194
Obstetric ultrasound, 612
Obstetrician (OB), 32, 620, 622
Obstetrics (OB), 32, 620, 622
Occipital lobe, 166, 166f
Occipitalis, 117f
Occlusion, 369
Occult blood, 475
Occult blood test, 484
OCD (obsessive-compulsive disorder), 183, 194
Ocular, 219
Ocul/o, 213
Oculus dexter (OD), 235
Oculus sinister (OS), 235
Oculus uterque (OU), 235
OD (doctor of optometry), 32
OD (oculus dexter), 235
Odont/o, 468
Odor, of urine, 697
OE (otitis externa), 244, 253
-oid, 30, 280, 362
Oil glands, 72
-ole, 362
Olig/o, 512, 594
Oligohydramnios, 605
Oliguria, 520
OM (otitis media), 244, 245f, 253
-oma, 7, 28, 42, 639
Omphal/o, 594
Omphalocele, 606
-on, 10, 709
Onc/o, 638
Oncogenes, 642
Oncogenic, 642
Oncologist, 668
Oncology, 668
Oncology and cancer terms, 637–672
  medical terms in, 642–646
    abbreviations, 670
    diagnostic procedures, 656–658
    laboratory tests, 655–656
    medications and drug therapies, 666–667
    specialties and specialists, 668–669
    surgical interventions, 661–663
    therapeutic procedures, 663
  word parts for, 638–639
    combining forms, 638
    prefixes, 639
    suffixes, 639
Onych/o, 75
Oocyte, 586
Oophorectomy, 615
Oophor/o, 593
Open fractures, 130f
Open reduction, internal fixation (ORIF), 140, 148
Ophthalmalgia, 222
Ophthalmia, 224
Ophthalmic, 219
Ophthalm/o, 213, 214
Ophthalmologist, 234
Ophthalmology, 234
Ophthalmopathy, 224
Ophthalmoplegia, 224
Ophthalmoscope, 227, 228f
Ophthalmoscopy, 227, 228f
-opia, 214
-opsia, 214
Optic, 219
Optic nerve (CN I), 210f, 211
Optician, 234
Opt/o, 214
Optometrist, 234
Optometry, 234
Oral cavity, 462
Orbicularis oculi, 117f
Orbicularis oris, 117f
Orbit, 210
Orchidectomy, 565
Orchid/o, 553
Orchidopexy, 565
Orchiectomy, 565
Orchi/o, 553
Orchiopexy, 565
Orchioplasty, 565
Orchiotomy, 565
Orchitis, 558
Orch/o, 553
Orchotomy, 565
Organ, 44
Organ of Corti, 238
Organ system, 44
ORIF (open reduction, internal fixation), 140, 148
Origin of muscles, 117
Or/o, 468
Orthopaedics, 147
Orthopaedist, 147

Orthopedics, 147
Orthopedist, 147
Orthopnea, 426
Orthosis, 142, 143f
Orthotics, 147
Orthotist, 147
OS (oculus sinister), 235
-osis, 28, 42, 123, 280, 319
Osseous, 127
Ost, 4
Ostectomy, 140
Osteitis, 132
Oste/o, 8, 42, 122
Osteoarthritis (OA), 9, 132, 148
Osteoblast, 110, 111f
Osteochondritis, 132
Osteoclasis, 141
Osteoclast, 110, 111f, 141, 143
Osteocyte, 110, 111f
Osteofibroma, 649
Osteogenesis, 29
Osteoma, 28
Osteomalacia, 132
Osteomyelitis, 132
Osteonecrosis, 132
Osteopath, 147
Osteopathy, 147
Osteoporosis, 28, 132, 132f
Osteosarcoma, 649, 649f
Otalgia, 244
Otic, 243, 252
Otitis externa (OE), 244, 253
Otitis media (OM), 244, 245f, 253
Ot/o, 240
Otologist, 252
Otology, 252
Otomycosis, 244
Otoplasty, 249
Otopyorrhea, 244
Otorhinolaryngologist, 252, 446
Otorhinolaryngology, 252, 446
Otorrhea, 244
Otosclerosis, 244
Otoscope, 248, 248f
Otoscopy, 248
OU (oculus uterque), 235
Ounce (oz), 32
-ous, 7, 29
Ovarian, 599
Ovaries, 272, 273f, 586
Ovari/o, 593
Ovulation, 590
Ovulation induction, 619
Ovum, 586
Ox/a, 417
Ox/o, 417
OXT (oxytocin), 276, 619
Oxygenate, 365
Oxytocin (OXT), 276, 619
oz (ounce), 32

P

P (pulse rate), 33
PA (physician's assistant), 32
Pachy/o, 75
Packed cell volume (PCV), 311, 698
PAD (peripheral arterial disease), 370, 389
Palate, 462
Palat/o, 468
Palatoplasty, 489
Palliative chemotherapy, 667
Palliative surgery, 661
Pallor, 80
Palpitation, 371
Pan-, 26, 417
Pancreas, 465
Pancreatectomy, 293
Pancreatic, 282
Pancreatic duct, 273f
Pancreaticoduodenectomy, 662
Pancreatitis, 287, 480
Pancreat/o, 279, 468
Pancytopenia, 325
Panic disorder, 183
Panlobar, 26
Pansinusitis, 427
Papanicolaou (Pap) test, 610, 656
Papule, 84, 85f
Para, 599, 639
Para-, 75, 171
Paracentesis, 484
Paranasal sinuses, 411, 412f
Paranoia, 183
Paraplegia, 181
Parathyroid glands, 272, 273f
Parathyroid hormone (PTH), 276, 296
Parathyroidectomy, 293, 661
Parathyroid/o, 279
-paresis, 171
Paresthesia, 181
Parietal layer, 413
Parietal lobe, 166, 166f
Parkinson disease, 181
Parkinsonism, 181
Paronychia, 84, 85f
Paroxysmal, 365
Partial-thickness burn, 82, 83f
-partum, 595
Patella, 112, 112f
Patellectomy, 141
Patell/o, 122
Patent, 365, 414
Patent ductus arteriosus (PDA), 606
Path/o, 42, 318, 638
Pathogen, 44, 314
-pathy, 28, 42, 76, 554
Patient (pt), 32
Patient care notes, health care provider, 58–59
p.c. (after meals), 32
PCT (proximal convoluted tubule), 510, 535
PCV (packed cell volume), 311, 698
PDA (patent ductus arteriosus), 606
Peak flow monitoring, 437
Pectoral, 422
Pectoralis major, 117f
Pector/o, 417
Pediatric oncologist, 669
Pediatric oncology, 669
Pediatrician, 620
Pediatrics (peds), 32, 620
Pediculicide, 94
Pediculosis, 86
Ped/o, 47
Peds (pediatrics), 32, 620
Pelv/i, 47, 122, 593
Pelvic, 127, 599
Pelvic bone, 111, 112f
Pelvic cavity, 49, 49f
Pelvic inflammatory disease (PID), 603, 622
Pelvic ultrasound, 612
Pelvimetry, 612
Pelvis, 48
Pelv/o, 122
-penia, 280, 319
Penile implant, 565
Penis, 551
Peps/o, 468
Peptic ulcer, 481
Peptic ulcer disease (PUD), 481, 493
Per-, 24, 75, 417
Percussion, 380, 437
Percutaneous, 24
Percutaneous transluminal coronary angioplasty (PTCA), 384, 384f, 390
Peri-, 6, 24, 52, 362, 468
Pericardiocentesis, 384
Pericarditis, 24, 370, 370f
Pericardium, 8, 355
Perimetrium, 587
Perineal, 599
Perine/o, 593
Perineum, 588
Periosteum, 110, 111f
Peripheral arterial disease (PAD), 370, 389
Peripheral nervous system (PNS), 164, 164f, 165, 168
Peripheral stem cell transplant, 662
Peristalsis, 476
Peritoneal dialysis, 531, 531f
Peritonitis, 481
Peritubular capillaries, 510
Pernicious anemia, 324, 324f
Peroneus longus, 117f
Pertussis, 426
Pessary, 615
PET (positron emission tomography), 189, 189f, 194
-pexy, 214, 554, 595
Peyronie disease, 559, 559f
PFTs (pulmonary function tests), 437, 447
pH, of urine, 697
Phacoemulsification, 231
-phagia, 76
Phag/o, 318, 468
Phagocytosis, 314, 315f
Phalangectomy, 141
Phalanges, 112, 112f
Phalang/o, 122
Pharyngeal, 422
Pharyngeal tonsil, 411
Pharyngitis, 427

Pharyng/o, 417, 468
Pharyngoscopy, 437
Pharyngotympanic tube, 237
Pharynx, 411, 412f, 463
Phas/o, 170
Pheochromocytoma, 650, 650f
-phile, 171
-philia, 171, 319
Phimosis, 559, 559f
Phlebectomy, 385
Phlebitis, 371
Phleb/o, 318, 361
Phlebotomy, 331, 332f
Phobia, 183
-phobia, 171, 214
-phonia, 418
Phon/o, 417
Phosphorus (P), inorganic, blood, 700
Phot/o, 214
Photophobia, 224
Photorefractive keratectomy (PRK), 231, 235
-phrenia, 171
Phrenic, 422
Phren/o, 170, 417
Physical therapist (PT), 32
Physical therapy (PT), 32
Physician's assistant (PA), 32
-physis, 123
Pia mater, 167, 167f
PID (pelvic inflammatory disease), 603, 622
Pineal body, 273f, 274
Pineal gland, 273f, 274
Pinna, 237, 237f
Pitting edema, 371, 373f
Pituitary adenoma, 650
Pituitary gland, 166f, 273f, 274
Placenta, 590
Placenta previa, 605, 605f
Plane, 51, 54, 55f
Planes, body, 54, 55f
Plantar flexion, 114, 116f
Plaque, 370
-plasia, 42, 76, 595
Plasma, 311
Plasmapheresis, 331
Plas/o, 318, 638
-plasty, 29, 76, 123, 214, 418, 554, 595
Platelet count (PLT), 328, 336, 698
Platelets (PLT), 313, 336
-plegia, 171, 214, 418
Pleura, 413
Pleural, 422
Pleural cavity, 413
Pleural effusion, 427
Pleuritic, 422
Pleuritis, 427
Pleur/o, 417
Pleuroscopy, 658
PLT (platelet count), 328, 336, 698
PLT (platelets), 313, 336
Plural endings, 10–11, 709
-pnea, 418
Pneumat/o, 417
Pneum/o, 417
Pneumococcal pneumonia, 427
Pneumonectomy, 442, 662
Pneumonia, 27, 427
Pneumonitis, 427
Pneumon/o, 417
Pneumothorax, 427, 427f
PNS (peripheral nervous system), 164, 164f, 165, 168
Podiatrist, 147
Podiatry, 147
Pod/o, 47
-poiesis, 319
Poli/o, 170
Poliomyelitis, 182, 182f
Poly-, 6, 22, 171, 279, 318, 512, 594
Polyarteritis, 22, 370
Polycystic kidney disease, 520, 520f
Polycystic ovary syndrome, 603, 603f
Polycythemia, 325
Polydipsia, 287
Polymyositis, 132
Polyneuritis. *See* Polyneuropathy
Polyneuropathy, 182
Polyp, 481
Polypectomy, 489
Polyp/o, 468
Polyposis, 481
Polysomnography, 189, 437
Polyuria, 287, 521
Pons, 165
Pore, 73f
-porosis, 123
Portable nebulizer, 445f
Position, in prefixes, 24–25
Positron emission tomography (PET), 189, 189f, 194
Post-, 6, 24, 468, 594
Posterior, 53, 54f
Posterior root, 165
Postero-, 52
Postictal, 175
Postmortem, 24
Postop (postoperative), 33
Post-op (postoperative), 33
Postoperative (postop, post-op), 33
Postpartum, 599
Postpartum depression, 605
Postprandial, 282, 476
Postsurgical, 5
Posttraumatic stress disorder (PTSD), 183, 194
Potassium (K), blood, 699
PPD (purified protein derivative), 90, 95, 434, 447
-prandial, 469
Pre-, 6, 24, 594
Precancerous, 24
Precordial, 365
Predisposition, 322
Preeclampsia, 605
Prefixes, 5–6, 22–27. *See also specific prefixes and systems*
  direction in, 24–25
  glossary of, 683–689
  negation in, 23–24
  other, 27
  position in, 24–25
  relative characteristics in, 25–27, 25f
  with same meaning, 23
  time in, 24–25
Pregnancy, 588
Pregnancy test, 610
Premature ventricular contraction (PVC), 371, 372f
Prenatal, 599
Preop (preoperative), 33
Pre-op (preoperative), 33
Preoperative (preop, pre-op), 33
Prepuce, 551
Presbycusis, 245
Presby/o, 214
Presbyopia, 224
Prescription (Rx), 32
Priapism, 559
Primigravida, 599
PRK (photorefractive keratectomy), 231, 235
p.r.n. (as needed), 32
Pro-, 318
Procoagulant, 334
Proct/o, 468
Proctologist, 493
Proctology, 493
Proctoscopy, 484
Progesterone, 276
Prognosis (Px), 32
Prolactin, 275, 275f, 590
Prolapsed cord, 605
Proliferative, 322
Pronation, 114, 115, 116f
Prone, 54
Pronunciation key, 12–13
Prostaglandin, 233
Prostate biopsy, 658
Prostate gland, 551
Prostatectomy, 565, 663
Prostate-specific antigen (PSA) test, 564, 570, 656, 670
Prostatic, 556
Prostatic calculus, 559
Prostatitis, 559
Prostat/o, 553
Prostatolith, 559
Prostatolithotomy, 565
Prostatorrhea, 559
Prosthesis, 142
Protein
  total, blood, 700
  urine, 697
Proteinuria, 521
Prothrombin time (PT), 328, 336
Proximal, 53, 54f
Proximal convoluted tubule (PCT), 510, 535
Proximo-, 52
Pruritic, 80
Pruritus ani, 481
PSA (prostate-specific antigen), 564, 570, 656, 670
Pseudo-, 27
Pseudomalignancy, 27
Psoriasis, 86, 86f

Psychiatrist, 193
Psychiatry, 193
Psych/o, 170
Psychologist, 193
Psychology, 193
Psychosis, 183
Psychotherapy, 191
Psychotropic, 192
PTCA (percutaneous transluminal coronary angioplasty), 384, 384f, 390
Pterygium, 224, 224f
PTH (parathyroid hormone), 276, 296
-ptosis, 214, 469, 513
pt (patient), 32
PT (physical therapist), 32
PT (physical therapy), 32
PT (prothrombin time), 328, 336
PTSD (posttraumatic stress disorder), 183, 194
Puberty, 556
Pubis, hip bone, 112
Pub/o, 122, 594
PUD (peptic ulcer disease), 481, 493
Pulmon, 4
Pulmonary, 29, 422
Pulmonary edema, 427
Pulmonary embolism, 428, 428f, 429
Pulmonary fibrosis, 426
Pulmonary function tests (PFTs), 437, 447
Pulmonary valve, 355
Pulmon/o, 8, 361, 417
Pulmonologist, 446
Pulmonology, 446
Pulse, 380
Pulse oximetry, 437, 437f
Pulse rate (P), 33
Punch biopsy, 657, 657f
Pupil, 210f, 211
Pupillary, 219
Pupill/o, 214
Pupillometer, 228
Pupillometry, 228
Purified protein derivative (PPD) test, 90, 95, 434, 447
Purulent, 80
Pustule, 86, 86f
PVC (premature ventricular contraction), 371, 372f
Px (prognosis), 32
Pyelitis, 521
Pyel/o, 512
Pyelolithotomy, 531
Pyelonephritis, 521
Pyeloplasty, 531
Pyloric sphincter, 463
Pylor/o, 468
Pylorus, 463
Py/o, 75, 512
Pyuria, 521

Q

q.i.d. (four times a day), 32
Quad-, 22
Quad marker screen, 610
Quadri-, 22, 171
Quadruplets, 22

R

R (respiratory rate), 33
RA (rheumatoid arthritis), 132, 133f, 148, 325, 336
Rachi/o, 122
Rachiotomy, 140
Rachischisis, 132
RAD (reactive airway disease), 428, 447
Radiation oncologist, 669
Radiation oncology, 669
Radiation therapy, 663
Radical mastectomy, 663
Radicotomy, 191
Radicular, 175
Radicul/o, 170
Radiculopathy, 182
Radi/o, 122, 638
Radioactive iodine uptake test (RIU), 291, 292f, 296
Radiofrequency ablation (RFA), 661, 670
Radiographer, 30f
Radiography, 30, 138, 434
Radiologist, 30f
Radionuclide scan, 657
Radiotherapist, 669
Radius, 112f, 113
Rales, 428
Range of motion (ROM) testing, 138, 148
Raynaud disease, 370, 370f
Raynaud syndrome. *See* Raynaud disease
RBC (red blood cell, red blood cell count), 33, 58, 312, 326, 328, 336, 697
Re-, 27
Reactivate, 27
Reactive airway disease (RAD), 428, 447
Read, write, speak, listen, 13
Reconstructive surgery, 661
Records, medical, 58–59
Rect/o, 468
Rectum, 465
Rectus abdominis, 117f
Rectus femoris, 117f
Recurrence, 643
Red blood cell count (RBC), 328, 336
Red blood cell (RBC) indices, 698
Red blood cells (RBCs), 33, 58, 312, 336, 697
Reduction, 141
Reed–Sternberg cells, 650, 650f
Refraction, 228, 229f
Regional enteritis, 477
Regurgitate, 476
Rejection, 322
Relative characteristics, in prefixes, 25–26, 25f
Remission, 44, 643
Ren, 4
Renal artery, 509
Renal calculus, 519
Renal corpuscle, 509
Renal cortex, 509
Renal epithelial cells, urine, 697
Renal failure, 519, 521
Renal hypertension, 521
Renal medulla, 509
Renal pelvis, 509
Renal transplant, 530
Renal vein, 509
Ren/o, 8, 512
Renogram, 527
Reports, 58–59
Reproductive endocrinologist, 620
Reproductive endocrinology, 620
Reproductive system, female, 583–624
  anatomy and physiology of, 584–585
    functions of, 584
    organs and structures in, 584, 584f
    terms for, 585–590, 586f
  cancer terms for, 652, 658, 663
  medical terms in, 598–599
    abbreviations, 622
    adjectives and other related terms, 598–599
    medical conditions, 602–606
    medications and drug therapies, 619
    specialties and specialists, 620
    surgical interventions and therapeutic procedures, 614–616, 314f–316f
    tests and procedures, 610–612, 611f
  word parts for, 593–595
    combining forms, 594
    prefixes, 594
    suffixes, 595
Reproductive system, male, 550–571
  anatomy and physiology of, 550
    functions of, 550
    structures in, 550
    terms for, 550–552
  cancer terms for, 658, 663
  medical terms in, 556
    medical conditions, 557–560
    abbreviations, 570
    adjectives and other related terms, 556–557
    medications and drug therapies, 569
    specialties and specialists, 569
    surgical interventions and therapeutic procedures, 565–566, 565f, 567f
    symptoms and medical conditions, 602
    tests and procedures, 564–565
  word parts for, 553–554
    combining forms, 553
    prefixes, 553
    suffixes, 554
Respiration, 414
Respiratory, 422
Respiratory failure (RF), 428, 447
Respiratory rate (R), 33

Respiratory system, 409–448
anatomy and physiology of, 410–414
functions of, 411
structures in, 410, 410f
terms for, 411–414
lower respiratory tract, 411, 411f
respiration, 413, 414f
upper respiratory tract, 411, 411f
anterior view, 778f
cancer terms for, 651, 658, 662
medical terms in, 422–448
abbreviations, 447
adjectives and other related terms, 422–424
medications and drug therapies, 445, 446f
specialties and specialists, 446
surgical interventions and therapeutic procedures, 440–442, 440f–442f
symptoms and medical conditions, 424–429, 425f–429f
tests and procedures, 434–438, 435f–436f
word parts for, 416–418
combining forms, 416–417
prefixes, 417
suffixes, 418
Respiratory tract, 412f
Retina, 210f, 211
Retinal, 219
Retinal photocoagulation, 232
Retinal tear, 221f, 224
Retinitis pigmentosa, 224
Retin/o, 214
Retinoblastoma, 650
Retinopathy, 224
Retinoscopy, 228
Retro-, 52, 468
Retrograde pyelogram, 527
RF (respiratory failure), 428, 447
RF (rheumatoid factor), 136, 148
RFA (radiofrequency ablation), 661, 670
Rh factor, 312
Rhabd/o, 122, 638
Rhabdomyoma, 649
Rhabdomyosarcoma, 649
RHD (rheumatic heart disease) 370, 370f, 390
Rheumatic heart disease (RHD) 370, 370f, 390
Rheumatoid arthritis (RA), 132, 133f, 148, 325, 336
Rheumatoid factor (RF), 136, 148
Rheumatoid factor test, 329
Rheumatologist, 147, 335
Rheumatology, 147, 335
Rhinitis, 428
Rhin/o, 417
Rhinoplasty, 442
Rhinoscopy, 437
Rhizotomy, 191
Rhomboideus, 117f
Rhonchi, 428
Rhytidectomy, 91
Rhytid/o, 75
Rhytidoplasty, 91, 92f
Ribs, 112f, 113
Rickets, 132
Right colic flexure, 464
Right hypochondriac region, 49, 50f
Right iliac region, 49, 50f
Right lower quadrant (RLQ), 49, 50f
Right lumbar region, 49, 50f
Right upper quadrant (RUQ), 49, 50f
RIU (radioactive iodine uptake test), 291, 292f, 296
RLQ (right lower quadrant), 49, 50f
ROM (range of motion), 138, 148
Roots
combining vowels added to roots, 8
word, 3–4, 4f
Rosacea, 86
Rotation, 114, 116f
-rrhage, 319, 595
-rrhagia, 418, 595
-rrhaphy, 29, 123, 469, 595
-rrhea, 28, 76, 214, 418, 554, 595
Rubs, 428
Rugae, 463
Rupture of membranes, 605
RUQ (right upper quadrant), 49, 50f
Rx (prescription), 32

S

SAB (spontaneous abortion), 604, 622
Sacral, 127
Sacr/o, 122
Sacrovertebral, 127
Sacrum, 113, 113f
Sagittal plane, 54, 55f
Saliva, 462
Salivary glands, 462
Salpingectomy, 615
Salpinges, 586
Salpingitis, 603
Salping/o, 593
Salping-ooophorectomy, 615
Sarc/o, 42, 638
Sarcoma, 646
Sartorius, 117f
Scabicide, 94
Scabies, 86, 86f
Scapula, 112f, 113
Scapul/o, 122
Scar, 82
SCC (squamous cell carcinoma), 649, 649f, 670
-schisis, 123
Schiz/o, 170
Schizophrenia, 183
Scintigraphy, 380
Sclera, 210f, 211
Scleral, 219
Scleral buckling, 232, 232f
Scleritis, 224
Scler/o, 75, 214, 240, 361
Scleromalacia, 224
Sclerotomy, 232
Scoli/o, 122
Scoliosis, 129, 129f
-scope, 30, 469
-scopy, 30, 214, 418, 469, 513, 595, 639
Scratch test, 90
Scrotum, 551
Sebaceous, 80
Sebaceous glands, 73, 73f
Seb/o, 75
Sebum, 73
Second-degree burn. *See* Partial-thickness burn
Sedative, 192
*See*d implantation, 661
Segmented neutrophils (SEGs, POLYs), 698
Seizure, 182
Semen, 551
Semi-, 22
Semicircular canals, 238
Semicircular ducts, 238
Semimembranosus, 117f
Seminal glands, 551
Seminal vesicles, 551
Seminiferous tubules, 552
Semirecumbent, 22, 54
Semitendinosus, 117f
Sensorineural hearing loss, 245
Sentinel lymph node biopsy, 657
Septicaemia, 325
Sept/o, 417
Septoplasty, 442
Septum, 353
Serratus anterior, 117f
Serum, 311
Serum glutamic oxaloacetic transaminase (SGOT), 700
Serum glutamic pyruvic transaminase (SGPT), 700
Sexually transmitted disease (STD), 560, 570, 603, 622
Sexually transmitted infection (STI), 570
SG (specific gravity), 525, 535, 697
SGOT (serum glutamic oxaloacetic transaminase), 700
SGPT (serum glutamic pyruvic transaminase), 700
Shave biopsy, 657
Shingles, 84, 85f, 180, 180f
Shortness of breath (SOB), 447
sial/o, 468
Sickle cell anemia, 324
Sigmoid colon, 464
Sigmoid/o, 468
Simple fractures, 130f
Simple mastectomy, 663
Single photon emission computed tomography (SPECT) scan, 379, 390, 657, 670
Sinus rhythm, 371, 372f
Sinusitis, 428
Sinus/o, 417
Sinusotomy, 442
-sis, 319
Sjögren syndrome, 325
Skeletal muscle relaxant, 146
Skeletal muscles, 117, 117f, 118f

Skeleton. *See also specific bones*
anterior view, 112f, 768f
appendicular, 110
axial, 110
posterior view, 769f
thorax, 111
Skin. *See* Integumentary system
Skin layer, 72
Skull
anterior view, 770f
posterior view, 770f
Sleep apnea, 182
SLE (systemic lupus erythematosus), 325, 336
Small cell carcinoma, 651
Small intestine, 464, 464f
Smooth muscles, 117, 118f
Snellen chart, 228, 229f
SOB (shortness of breath), 447
Soci/o, 170
Sodium (Na), blood, 699
Soft palate, 462
Somatic, 44
Somn/i, 170
Somn/o, 170
Son/o, 361, 512
Sonography, 379
Spanish healthcare phrases, 719–724
diseases, 721
examination, 722–723
general, 719–720, 724
introductory phrases, 719
parts of body, 720–721
signs and symptoms, 722
treatment, 723–724
-spasm, 214, 418
Spastic colon, 480
Specialty reports, 59
Specific gravity (SG), 524, 535, 697
SPECT (single photon emission computed tomography), 379, 390, 657, 670
Spelling, 11, 11f
Sperm, 552
Spermatic, 556
Spermatic cord, 552
Spermat/o, 553
Spermatocele, 559, 559f
Spermatozoon, 552
Spermicide, 556
Sperm/o, 553
Sphygmic, 366
Sphygm/o, 361
Sphygmomanometer, 380
Spina bifida, 606, 606f
Spinal cavity, 49, 49f
Spinal cord, 164f, 165, 167
Spinal nerves, 164f, 165, 168, 773f
Spine, curvature of, 129, 129f
Spin/o, 170
Spiral fractures, 130f
Spiral organ, 238
Spir/o, 417
Spirometry, 437
Spleen, 312
Splenectomy, 331
Spondylarthritis, 132
Spondyl/o, 122, 170
Spondylosyndesis, 141, 141f
Spongy bones, 110, 111f
Spontaneous abortion (SAB), 604, 622
Sprain, 132
Sputum, 414
Squam/o, 638
Squamous cell carcinoma (SCC), 649, 649f, 670
Stapedectomy, 249
Staped/o, 240
Stapes, 237
-stasis, 42
STAT (immediately), 33
STD (sexually transmitted disease), 560, 570, 603, 622
-stenosis, 362, 370, 469, 513
Stenotic, 366
Stent, 385
Stereotactic biopsy, 657
Stereotactic radiosurgery, 661
Sterilization, 616
Stern/o, 122
Sternoclavicular, 127
Sternocleidomastoid, 117f
Sternoid, 127
Sternum, 112f, 113
Steroid, 94
Steth/o, 361
Stethoscope, 380
STI (sexually transmitted infection), 570
Stillbirth, 599
Stomach, 44, 45f, 463, 464f
Stomat/o, 468
-stomy, 29, 240, 418, 469, 513, 554
Stool culture, 484
Strabismus, 224
Strain, 132
Stress, 379
Stress electrocardiogram, 380
Stress marks, 12
Stress urinary incontinence (SUI), 521, 535
Stricture, 521
Stridor, 428
Stroke, 179, 179f
Stupor, 182
Sty, 222
Sub-, 6, 24, 52, 75, 123
Subcostal, 127
Subcutaneous, 24
Subcutaneous layer, 72, 73f
Subdural, 175
Subdural hematoma, 182, 182f
Submandibular, 127
Submaxillary, 127
Subscapular, 127
Substernal, 127
Sudoriferous, 80
Sudoriferous glands, 73, 73f
Suffixes, 6–7, 22, 22f, 27–30. *See also specific suffixes*
in conditions/diseases, 27–28
different suffixes with same root, 30f
glossary of, 683–689
other, 29–30
in surgery, 28–29
SUI (stress urinary incontinence), 521, 535
Sulcus, 166
Super-, 6, 24, 52
Superficial, 53, 54f
Superficial burn, 82, 83f
Superinfection, 24
Superior, 51, 53, 54f
Superior vena cava, 357
Supination, 114, 115, 116f
Supine, 54
Supra-, 6, 24, 52, 123, 594
Suprapatellar, 127
Suprapubic, 599
Suprapubic region, 49, 50f
Suprarenal, 24
Suprarenal glands, 272, 273f
Suprascapular, 127
Supraventricular, 366
Surgical oncologist, 669
surgical oncology, 669
Suture, 91, 92f, 114
Sweat glands, 72
Sx (symptom), 32
Sym-, 24, 123
Symbols, 704–705
Joint Commission "Do Not Use" List, 705
Symphysis, 24, 114
Symptom (Sx), 32
Syn-, 24, 123
Syncopal episode, 182
Syncope, 182
Synovectomy, 142
Synovial, 127
Synovial fluid, 114
Synovial fluid analysis, 136
Synovial joint, 114, 115f
Synovi/o, 122
Syphilis, 560
Syphilitic chancres, 561f
Systemic, 44, 322
Systemic lupus erythematosus (SLE), 325, 336
Systole, 366

T

T (temperature), 33
T_3 (triiodothyronine), 276, 296, 700
T_4 (thyroxine), 276, 296, 700
T cell, 313
T lymphocyte, 313
TAB (therapeutic abortion), 616, 622
Tachy-, 27, 362, 417
Tachycardia, 27, 371, 372f
Tachypnea, 428
TAH (total abdominal hysterectomy), 615, 622
Tarsal bones, 112f, 113
Tarsal glands, 211
Tarsectomy, 142
Tars/o, 122
TB (tuberculosis), 429, 447
Teeth, 462

TEE (transesophageal echocardiography), 379, 390
Tel-, 362
Telangiectasia, 371
Temperature (T), 33
Temporal lobe, 166, 166f
Temporalis, 117f
Tendinitis, 132
Tendin/o, 122
Tend/o, 122
Tendon, 114
Tendonitis, 132
Ten/o, 122
Tenodynia, 132
Tenorrhaphy, 142, 142f
Tenosynovitis, 132
Tensor fasciae latae, 117f
Teres major, 117f
Teres minor, 117f
Term analysis, 14–15
Terms, medical. *See* Medical terms; *specific systems; specific terms*
Testes, 273f, 274
Testicles, 273f, 274, 552
Testicular torsion, 559
Testicul/o, 553
Testis, 552
Testitis, 558
Test/o, 553
Testosterone, 276, 552
Tetany, 287
Tetralogy of Fallot, 606
Thalam/o, 170
Thalassemia, 324
Therapeutic abortion (TAB), 616, 622
Thermometer, 30
Third-degree burn. *See* Full-thickness burn
Thoracentesis, 442
Thoracic, 366, 422
Thoracic cavity, 49, 49f
Thoracic vertebrae, 113, 113f, 148
Thorac/o, 47, 122, 361, 417
Thoracoscopy, 437, 658
Thoracotomy, 442
Thorax, 48, 111, 413
Throat, 411, 463
Thromb/o, 318, 361
Thrombocyte, 313
Thrombocytopenia, 325
Thrombolytic agent, 334
Thrombolytic therapy, 388
Thrombophlebitis, 371
Thrombosis, 325
Thrombotic, 366
Thrombus, 370
Thymectomy, 293
Thym/i, 170
Thymic, 282
Thym/o, 170, 279
Thymosin, 276
Thymus gland, 273f, 274
Thyr/o, 279
Thyroid function tests, 291
Thyroid gland, 274, 274f
Thyroid scan, 291, 292f
Thyroidectomy, 293, 661
Thyroiditis, 287
Thyroid/o, 279
Thyroidotomy, 293
Thyroid-stimulating hormone (TSH), 275, 275f, 291, 296, 700
Thyromegaly, 287
Thyroparathyroidectomy, 293
Thyrotoxicosis, 287
Thyroxine (T_4), 276, 296, 700
Thyroxine level, blood test, 291
TIA (transient ischemic attack), 182, 194
Tibia, 112f, 113
Tibialis anterior, 117f
Tic, 182
Time, in prefixes, 24–25
Tinea, 86, 86f
Tinea capitis, 87
Tinea pedis, 87
Tinnitus, 245
Tiny muscles, 72
TIP (transurethral incision of the prostate), 566, 570
Tissue, 44, 45f
TM (tympanic membrane), 237, 237f, 253
TNM staging (tumor node metastasis), 643, 644f, 670Toc/o, 594
Tocolytic, 619
-tome, 76
-tomy, 7, 29, 171, 418, 469, 554, 595
Tongue, 462
Tonic–clonic seizure, 182
Ton/o, 122, 214
Tonometer, 228
Tonometry, 228
Tonsillar, 422
Tonsillectomy, 442
Tonsillitis, 429
Tonsill/o, 417
Tonsils, 411, 412f
TORCH panel, 610, 611f
Total abdominal hysterectomy (TAH), 615, 622
Total parenteral nutrition (TPN), 489, 493
Tourette syndrome, 182
Toxoplasmosis, 605
TPN (total parenteral nutrition), 489, 493
Tr (treatment), 32
Trabecular bones, 110, 111f
Trabeculectomy, 232
Trachea, 412, 412f
Tracheal, 422
Tracheitis, 429
Trache/o, 417
Tracheoplasty, 442
Tracheorrhagia, 429
Tracheostomy, 442, 442f
Tracheostomy tube, 442
Traction, 142, 142f
Trans-, 24, 75, 362, 639
Transabdominal, 599
Transection, 24
Transesophageal echocardiography (TEE), 379, 390
Transient ischemic attack (TIA), 182, 194
Transitional cell carcinoma, 652
Translucent plate, 73
Transrectal ultrasound (TRUS), 570, 658, 670
Transsphenoidal resection, 661
Transurethral incision of the prostate (TUIP/TIP), 566, 570
Transurethral resection of bladder tumor (TURB), 663, 670
Transurethral resection of prostate (TURP), 566, 570, 663, 670
Transvaginal, 599
Transvaginal ultrasound, 612
Transverse colon, 464
Transverse fractures, 130f
Transverse plane, 54, 55f
Trapezius, 117f
Treatment (Tr), 32
Treatment (Tx), 32
Tri-, 22, 362
Triceps brachii, 117f
Trich/o, 75
Tricuspid valve, 355
Triglycerides, blood, 700
Trigone of bladder, 510
Triiodothyronine (T_3), 276, 296, 700
Trimester, 22
-Tripsy, 469, 513
-trophia, 214
Troph/o, 42
-trophy, 123
TRUS (transrectal ultrasound), 570, 658, 670
TSH (thyroid-stimulating hormone), 275, 275f,, 291, 296, 700
T1–T12 (thoracic vertebrae 1–12), 148
Tubal ligation, 616
Tube placement, 250
Tubectomy, 615
Tuberculosis (TB), 429, 429f, 447
Tuberculosis skin test, 90
TUIP (transurethral incision of the prostate), 566, 570
Tumor, 646
Tumor marker test, 656
Tumor staging, 643
TURB (transurethral resection of bladder tumor), 663, 670
Turgor, 80
Turner syndrome, 606
TURP (transurethral resection of prostate), 566, 570, 663, 670
Tx (treatment), 32
Tympanic, 243
Tympanic membrane (TM), 237, 237f, 253
Tympanic membrane perforation, 245
Tympan/o, 240, 241
Tympanogram, 248
Tympanometer, 248
Tympanometry, 248
Tympanoplasty, 250

Tympanostomy, 249, 250, 250f
Type 1 diabetes mellitus, 285
Type 2 diabetes mellitus, 285

U

UA (urinalysis), 525, 535, 697
UGI (upper gastrointestinal), 484, 493
Ulcerative colitis, 481
-ule, 362
Ulna, 112f, 113
Uln/o, 122
Ultra-, 26
Ultrasonography, 26, 379
Ultraviolet (UV), 670
-um, 10, 709
Umbilical cord, 590
Umbilical region, 49, 50f
Uni-, 22
Unilateral, 22, 53, 54f
Upper gastrointestinal series (UGI), 484, 493
Upper respiratory infection (URI), 429, 447
Ure-, 512
Uremia, 521
Ureter, 510
Ureteral, 516
Ureterectomy, 531
Ureteritis, 521
Ureter/o, 512
Ureterocele, 521
Ureterolith, 521
Ureterostenosis, 521
Ureterostomy, 531
Ureterotomy, 531
Urethra, 510
Urethral, 516
Urethral stenosis, 521
Urethritis, 521
urethr/o, 512
Urethroplasty, 531
Urethroscope, 527
Urethroscopy, 527
Urethrotomy, 531
Urge incontinence, 521
URI (upper respiratory infection), 429, 447
-uria, 280, 513
Uric acid, 700
Uric acid test, 136
Urinalysis (UA), 525, 535, 697
Urinary, 516
Urinary analgesic, 534
Urinary bladder, 510
Urinary retention, 521
Urinary suppression, 521
Urinary system, 508, 508f, 518f
  anatomy and physiology of, 508–510
    functions of, 508
    organs and structures in, 509f
    terms in, 509, 509f
  anterior view, 781f
  cancer terms for, 652, 662–663
  medical terms in, 516–536
    abbreviations, 535
    adjectives and other related terms, 516
    medications and drug therapies, 534
    specialties and specialists, 534
    surgical interventions and therapeutic procedures, 529–531, 529f–531f
    symptoms and medical conditions, 518–521, 519f–520f
    tests and procedures, 525–527
  word parts for, 512–513
  combining forms, 512
    prefixes, 512
    suffixes, 512–513
Urinary tract infection (UTI), 521, 535
Urinate, 516
Urine, 510
Urin/o, 512
Urinometer, 525
Ur/o, 512
Urobilinogen, urine, 697
Urodynamics, 527
Urogenital system (male and female, midsagittal view), 782f
Urologist, 534, 569
Urology, 534, 569
Urothelial carcinoma, 652
Urticaria, 87
-us, 10, 709
Uterine, 599
Uterine fibroid, 603, 603f
Uterine prolapse, 603
Uterine tubes, 586
Uter/o, 594
Uterotomy, 615
Uterus, 587
UTI (urinary tract infection), 521, 535
UV (ultraviolet), 670
Uvula, 462

V

VA (visual acuity), 228, 235
Vaccination, 331
Vaccine, 334
Vagina, 587
Vaginal hysterectomy, 615
Vaginal orifice, 588
Vagin/o, 594
Valve replacement, 385
Valv/o, 361
Valvotomy, 385
Valvul/o, 361
Valvuloplasty, 385
Varicella, 87
Varic/o, 361
Varicocele, 559
Varicose, 366
Varicose vein, 371, 373f
Vas, 4
Vas deferens, 552
Vascul/o, 361
Vasectomy, 566
Vas/o, 361, 553
Vasoconstrictor, 388
Vasodilator, 388, 569
Vasopressin, 276
Vasovasostomy, 566
Vastus lateralis, 117f
Vastus medialis, 117f
VATS (video-assisted thoracoscopic surgery), 437, 438f, 447
VCUG (voiding cystourethrogram), 527, 535
VD (venereal disease), 560, 570
Veins, 357, 357f
Venereal disease (VD), 560, 570
Ven/i, 361
Venipuncture, 331
Ven/o, 361
Venography, 379
Venotomy, 331
Venous system (anterior view), 777f
Ventilation–perfusion (V/Q) scan, 434, 435f, 447
Ventral, 53, 54f
Ventral root, 165
Ventricle, 167, 353
Ventricular septal defect (VSD), 606
Ventricul/o, 170, 361
Ventriculography, 379
Ventro-, 52
Venule, 357
Vermiform appendix, 464
Verruca, 87
Vertebra, 113, 113f
  cervical vertebrae, 113, 113f
  coccyx, 113, 113f
  lumbar vertebrae, 113, 113f
  sacrum, 113, 113f
  thoracic vertebrae, 113, 113f
Vertebr/o, 122, 170
Vertex, 605
Vertigo, 245
Vesical, 516
Vesicle, 87, 87f
Vesic/o, 512
Vesicourethral suspension, 531
Vesicular ovarian follicles, 586
Vesiculectomy, 566
Vesicul/o, 512, 553
Vestibular, 243
Vestibule, 238, 588
Vestibul/o, 240
Vestibulocochlear nerve (CN VIII), 238
VF (visual field), 228, 235
Video-assisted thoracoscopic surgery (VATS), 437, 438f, 447
Virulent, 322
Visceral, 44
Visceral layer, 413
Viscer/o, 42
Visual acuity (VA) testing, 228, 235
Visual field (VF) testing, 228, 235
Vital signs (VS), 33
Vitiligo, 87, 87f
Vitrectomy, 232
Vitreous humor, 210f, 211
Voiding cystourethrogram (VCUG), 527, 535
Volvulus, 481
Vomit, 476

von Willebrand disease (vWD), 325, 336
Vowels, combining, 8
V/Q (ventilation–perfusion), 434, 435f, 447
VS (vital signs), 33
VSD (ventricular septal defect), 606
Vulva, 587
Vulvectomy, 615
Vulv/o, 594
Vulvodynia, 603

W

WBC (white blood cell) count, 328, 329f, 336, 698
WBCs (white blood cells), 33, 58, 311f, 313, 313f, 336, 697
Websites, health-related, 710–718
  blood, 711
  cardiovascular system, 711–712
  complementary and alternative medicine, 712
  digestive system, 713
  endocrine system, 713
  general, 710
  integumentary system, 713–714
  lymphatic system, 714
  mental health, 714–715
  musculoskeletal system, 715
  nervous system, 715–716
  oncology, 716
  reproductive systems and obstetrics, 714
  respiratory system, 716–717
  special senses, 717
  urinary system, 717–718
Wedge resection, 662
Weight (Wt), 33
Wheal, 87, 87f
Wheeze, 429
Whipple operation, 662
White blood cell (WBC), 33, 58, 311f, 313, 313f, 336, 697White blood cell (WBC) count, 328, 329f, 336, 698
Whooping cough, 427
Wilms tumor, 652, 652f
Windpipe, 412, 412f
Womb, 587
Word parts, 3–10, 22, 22f. *See also specific word parts*
  for body directions, positions, and planes, 51–52
  combining vowels added to roots, 8
  lookup by meaning of, 690–696
  prefixes in, 5–6 (*See also* Prefixes)
  putting parts together in, 9
  suffixes in, 6–7 (*See also* Suffixes)
  word roots, 3–4, 4f
Word roots, 3–4, 4f
Word structure, 1–16
  medical terms in, 2–16
    analysis of, 14–15
    building of, 16
    derivation of, 3
    parts of, 3–10 (*See also* Word parts)
    plural endings in, 10
    pronunciations for, 12–13
    spelling of, 11, 11f
    use of, 2
  plural endings in, 709
Wrist-drop, 128
Wt (weight), 33

X

-x, 10, 709
Xanth/o, 57, 75
Xanthoderma, 58, 87
Xenograft, 91
Xer/o, 75
Xerophthalmia, 224
Xiphoid process, 113

Y

-y, 10, 319
-yx, 709

Z

Zygomaticus, 117f
zygote, 590